Diseases of
the Colon

Gastroenterology and Hepatology

Executive Editor

J. Thomas LaMont, M.D.

Chief, Division of Gastroenterology
Beth Israel Hospital
Boston, Massachusetts
and
Charlotte F. and Irving W. Rabb Professor of Medicine
Harvard Medical School
Boston, Massachusetts

Diseases of the Colon

edited by

Steven D. Wexner
Cleveland Clinic Florida
Weston, Florida, U.S.A.

Neil Stollman
University of California–San Francisco
San Francisco, California, U.S.A.

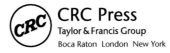

CRC Press
Taylor & Francis Group
Boca Raton London New York

CRC Press is an imprint of the
Taylor & Francis Group, an **informa** business

CRC Press
Taylor & Francis Group
6000 Broken Sound Parkway NW, Suite 300
Boca Raton, FL 33487-2742

First issued in paperback 2019

© 2010 by Taylor & Francis Group, LLC
CRC Press is an imprint of Taylor & Francis Group, an Informa business

No claim to original U.S. Government works

ISBN-13: 978-0-8247-2999-8 (hbk)
ISBN-13: 978-0-367-39034-1 (pbk)

A CIP record for this book is available from the British Library.

Library of Congress Cataloging-in-Publication Data available on application

**Visit the Taylor & Francis Web site at
http://www.taylorandfrancis.com**

**and the CRC Press Web site at
http://www.crcpress.com**

This book is dedicated to two groups of people.

First, to my family: my loving wife, Nicolette, and my children, Wesley, Marisa, Trevor, and Gabriella. Their love motivates me to succeed in projects such as this one. As always, it is valuable time away from them that allows my academic activities to flourish. I thank them and I love them very much for their support, understanding, and encouragement.

Second, to two of Cleveland Clinic Florida's major philanthropic supporters: Mr. Nick Caporella and Dr. Daniel Dosoretz. Their vision, philanthropy, and altruism has allowed me to pursue my quest for continued growth and development in my specialty. Many other friends, supporters, and grateful patients have followed the lead of these two gentlemen and recognized the need for generous gifts to Cleveland Clinic Florida to allow me to continue to research and to publish. The culmination of those efforts is reflected in, in part, the production of this book.

Steven D. Wexner, M.D.

I am fortunate to have received guidance from many mentors throughout my career, for which I am grateful, but none has been as kind, supportive, and ultimately formative than Arvey Rogers, M.D., who has fostered my curiosity, my intellect, my skills, and, above all, my compassion. I remain deeply appreciative and thankful. Equally, I wish to thank my wonderful family, Lisa, Benjamin, and Natalie, who has indulged my efforts with support and tolerated my absences with grace.

Neil Stollman, M.D.

Preface

Some specialties, such as psychiatry, are mainly solitary endeavors where a physician and a patient may work together. Other specialties, such as primary care, function as a central hub, surrounded by various specialists who can consult as needed. In contrast, diseases of the colon require an in-depth collaboration between gastroenterologists and colorectal surgeons.

In considering this endeavor at its inception, we noted that there were numerous books on general gastroenterology, usually authored, naturally, by gastroenterologists; likewise, numerous texts on colonic surgery have been authored by surgeons. We sought to closely integrate these two allied specialties. Granted, some gastroenterology textbooks include chapters written by surgeons and vice versa. However, these books did not seem to be fusions between the disciplines. Therefore, we designed a book that would require intimate cooperation in writing each chapter, which certainly mirrors the interdisciplinary relationships practiced every day by our two specialties. This methodology ensures that the reader will acquire a significant fund of knowledge from the allied specialty. Surgeons will learn how gastroenterologists approach a problem and vice versa. Their insights will be invaluable and will improve the efficiency of their approach to these disorders.

To fulfill this goal, we have provided a current compendium of most major colonic disorders, and in almost all cases, have required that the chapter be coauthored by at least one surgeon and one gastroenterologist. In doing so, this unique mixture hopefully highlights the often-differing emphasis that our two skill sets bring to the care of our patients. Our aim was to provide a useful, definitive, and concise reference source for internists, gastroenterologists, and general and colorectal surgeons, as well as residents and fellows in these disciplines. From this publication the reader will learn all facets of both the medical and surgical management of the entire gamut of disorders of the colon.

We have been extremely fortunate in having many of the world's experts in their respective areas agree to participate, and we are grateful to them. In fact, a number of our authors have commented to us that being "forced" to approach their topic with a (often new) coauthor from the sister discipline was quite enlightening, and brought them new insights into their respective topics. We know our readers will share these insights and find that having both viewpoints simultaneously presented will provide a well-balanced and ultimately useful guide to the care of these patients. These presentations will allow the readers to appropriately adjust their practice to the interdisciplinary levels discussed in these chapters.

In addition to the number of experts, the editors are very indebted to Ms. Elektra McDermott, who has shepherded this project ably, tirelessly, and wisely from inception to completion. Equally, we thank Sandra Beberman at Informa Healthcare, who saw the value in this collaborative effort early on and has championed it throughout.

This work will be a useful tool for our fellow practitioners, who strive daily to provide exceptional care to their patients with colonic disorders, and to the patients who we humbly and gratefully serve.

Steven D. Wexner
Neil Stollman

Contents

Part III.   DIAGNOSTICS, IMAGING AND THERAPEUTIC TECHNIQUES FOR COLONIC EVALUATION AND INTERVENTION

Part VII. NEOPLASTIC DISORDERS OF THE COLON

Part VIII. INFLAMMATORY (NONINFECTIOUS) BOWEL DISORDERS

Contributors

Joseph Ahn Department of Medicine, Hepatology Division, Rush University Medical Center, Chicago, Illinois, U.S.A.

Shmuel Avital Department of Surgery, Tel-Aviv Sourasky Medical Center and the Sackler Faculty of Medicine, Tel-Aviv University, Tel-Aviv, Israel

Kamran Ayub Division of Gastroenterology, Department of Internal Medicine, University of Washington, Seattle, Washington, U.S.A.

David E. Beck Department of Colon and Rectal Surgery, Ochsner Clinic Foundation, New Orleans, Louisiana, U.S.A.

Mitchell Bernstein Division of Colon and Rectal Surgery, College of Physicians and Surgeons, Columbia University, and Anorectal Physiology Laboratory and The Continence Center, St. Luke's/ Roosevelt Hospital Center, New York, New York, U.S.A.

Scott J. Boley Department of Surgery, Albert Einstein College of Medicine, Montefiore Medical Center, Bronx, New York, U.S.A.

Lawrence J. Brandt Division of Gastroenterology, Departments of Medicine and Surgery, Albert Einstein College of Medicine, Montefiore Medical Center, Bronx, New York, U.S.A.

Elizabeth Broussard Department of Medicine, University of Washington School of Medicine, Harborview Medical Center, Seattle, Washington, U.S.A.

Adriane Budavari Department of Medicine, Mayo Clinic Scottsdale, Scottsdale, Arizona, U.S.A.

Eileen Bulger Department of Surgery, University of Washington School of Medicine, Seattle, Washington, U.S.A.

John P. Cello Department of Medicine and Surgery, University of California–San Francisco, San Francisco, California, U.S.A.

Raúl Cutait Department of Surgery, Syrian-Lebanese Hospital, São Paulo, Brazil

Julio Studart de Moraes Department of Gastroenterology, Policlínica Geral do Rio de Janeiro, Rio de Janeiro, Brazil

John K. DiBaise Division of Gastroenterology and Hepatology, Mayo Clinic Scottsdale, Scottsdale, Arizona, U.S.A.

Kelli Bullard Dunn Division of Surgical Oncology, Roswell Park Cancer Institute, and the State University of New York at Buffalo, Buffalo, New York, U.S.A.

Eli D. Ehrenpreis Section of Gastroenterology, Department of Medicine, University of Chicago Hospitals, University of Chicago Medical Center, Chicago, Illinois, U.S.A.

Rami Eliakim Division of Gastroenterology, Department of Medicine, Rappaport School of Medicine, Rambam Medical Center and Technion–Israel Institute of Technology, Haifa, Israel

Anton Emmanuel Departments of Gastroenterology and Neurogastroenterology, University College Hospital, London, U.K.

Jeffrey M. Fox Department of Internal Medicine and Gastroenterology, The Pernaneate Medical Group, Inc., San Rafael, California, U.S.A.

Laura Gladstone Division of Colon and Rectal Surgery, Swedish Medical Center, Seattle, Washington, U.S.A.

Steven A. Guarisco Department of Gastroenterology, Ochsner Clinic Foundation, New Orleans, Louisiana, U.S.A.

Heinz Hammer Department of Gastroenterology, University Clinic Medical School Graz, Graz, Austria

Arthur Harris Division of Gastroenterology and Hepatology, Weill Medical College at Cornell University, New York, New York, U.S.A.

Steve Heymen UNC Center for Functional GI and Motility Disorders, University of North Carolina at Chapel Hill, Chapel Hill, North Carolina, U.S.A.

Roger Hurst Department of Surgery, University of Chicago Medical Center, Chicago, Ilinois, U.S.A.

J. Marcio N. Jorge Division of Colorectal Surgery, Department of Gastroenterology, University of São Paulo, São Paulo, Brazil

Orit Kaidar-Person Department of Colorectal Surgery, Cleveland Clinic Florida, Weston, Florida, U.S.A.

Richard E. Karulf Division of Colon and Rectal Surgery, Department of Surgery, University of Minnesota, Minneapolis, Minnesota, U.S.A.

Jeffry A. Katz Case Western Reserve University School of Medicine, University Hospitals of Cleveland, Cleveland, Ohio, U.S.A.

Han Kuijpers Department of General Surgery, Ziekenhuis Gelderse Vallei Hospital, Ede, The Netherlands

Jorge Andres Larach Department of Colorectal Surgery, Cleveland Clinic Florida, Weston, Florida, U.S.A.

Jimmy S. Levine Minnesota Gastroenterology, Minneapolis, Minnesota, U.S.A.

Nancy Lewis Division of Medical Sciences, Fox Chase Cancer Center, Philadelphia, Pennsylvania, U.S.A.

Warren Lichliter Department of Colon and Rectal Surgery, Baylor University Medical Center, Dallas, Texas, U.S.A.

Chad J. Long Department of Medicine, University of Chicago Hospitals, University of Chicago Medical Center, Chicago, Illinois, U.S.A.

Martin Luchtefeld Ferguson Clinic, MMPC, Grand Rapids, and Michigan State University, East Lansing, Michigan, U.S.A.

Robert D. Madoff Division of Colon and Rectal Surgery, Department of Surgery, University of Minnesota, Minneapolis, Minnesota, U.S.A.

Uma Mahadevan Department of Gastroenterology, University of California–San Francisco, San Francisco, California, U.S.A.

Jorge Marcet Department of Surgery, University of South Florida, Tampa, Florida, U.S.A.

Michael Meyers Department of Surgery, University of North Carolina, Chapel Hill, North Carolina, U.S.A.

David E. Milkes Department of Veterans Affairs, Palo Alto Health Care System, Stanford University School of Medicine, Stanford, California, U.S.A.

Peter J. Molloy Division of Gastroenterology, Department of Medicine, Western Pennsylvania Hospital, Clinical Campus of Temple University School of Medicine, Pittsburgh, Pennsylvania, U.S.A.

Hélio Moreira, Jr. Colorectal Service, Department of Surgery, Medical School of the Federal University of Goiás, Goiânia, Goiás, Brazil

Omar S. Nehme Division of Gastroenterology, Indiana University School of Medicine, Indianapolis, Indiana, U.S.A.

Juan J. Nogueras Department of Colorectal Surgery, Cleveland Clinic Florida, Weston, Florida, U.S.A.

H. Juergen Nord Department of Medicine, University of South Florida, Tampa, Florida, U.S.A.

Kevin W. Olden Division of Gastroenterology, Mayo Clinic Scottsdale, Scottsdale, Arizona, U.S.A.

Gregory D. Olds Henry Ford Hospital, Detroit, Michigan, U.S.A.

Lucia Oliveira Department of Anorectal Physiology, Policlínica Geral do Rio de Janeiro, Rio de Janeiro, Brazil

Derek Patel Division of Gastroenterology, Department of Medicine, University of California–San Diego, San Diego, California, U.S.A.

Johann Pfeifer Department of General Surgery, University Clinic Medical School Graz, Graz, Austria

Owais Rahim Division of Gastroenterology, Department of Medicine, Western Pennsylvania Hospital, Clinical Campus of Temple University School of Medicine, Pittsburgh, Pennsylvania, U.S.A.

Jeffrey B. Raskin Division of Gastroenterology, Miami Miller School of Medicine, University of Miami/Jackson Memorial Medical Center, Miami, Florida, U.S.A.

Thomas E. Read Division of Colon and Rectal Surgery, Department of Surgery, Western Pennsylvania Hospital, Clinical Campus of Temple University School of Medicine, Pittsburgh, Pennsylvania, U.S.A.

Harry L. Reynolds Case Western Reserve University School of Medicine, University Hospitals of Cleveland, Cleveland, Ohio, U.S.A.

Joffre Marcondes Rezende Gastroenterology Service, Department of Internal Medicine, Medical School of the Federal University of Goiás, Goiânia, Goiás, Brazil

Raul Rosenthal Bariatric Institute, Cleveland Clinic Florida, Weston, Florida, U.S.A.

Mara R. Salum Department of Surgery, Syrian-Lebanese Hospital, São Paulo, Brazil

Dana R. Sands Department of Colorectal Surgery, Cleveland Clinic Florida, Weston, Florida, U.S.A.

Laurence R. Sands Division of Colon and Rectal Surgery, University of Miami School of Medicine, Miami, Florida, U.S.A.

William Schecter Department of Clinical Surgery, University of California–San Francisco, and Department of Surgery, San Francisco General Hospital, San Francisco, California, U.S.A.

Lawrence R. Schiller Department of Gastroenterology, Baylor University Medical Center, Dallas, Texas, U.S.A.

Roanne R. E. Selinger Division of Gastroenterology, Department of Internal Medicine, University of Washington, Seattle, Washington, U.S.A.

Elin Sigurdson Division of Medical Sciences, Fox Chase Cancer Center, Philadelphia, Pennsylvania, U.S.A.

Roy M. Soetikno Department of Veterans Affairs, Palo Alto Health Care System, Stanford University School of Medicine, Stanford, California, U.S.A.

Neil Stollman Division of Gastroenterology, University of California–San Francisco, San Francisco, and East Bay Endosurgery, Oakland, California, U.S.A.

Christina M. Surawicz Department of Medicine, University of Washington School of Medicine, Harborview Medical Center, Seattle, Washington, U.S.A.

Alex Teixeira Department of Gastroenterology, Brockton Hospital, Brockton, Massachusetts, U.S.A.

Jonathan P. Terdiman Department of Medicine, University of California–San Francisco, San Francisco, California, U.S.A.

Ruedi F. Thoeni Department of Radiology, University of California–San Francisco, San Francisco, California, U.S.A.

Jon S. Thompson Department of Surgery, University of Nebraska Medical Center, Omaha, Nebraska, U.S.A.

Raymond Thornton Department of Radiology, University of California–San Francisco, San Francisco, California, U.S.A.

Hagit Tulchinsky Colon and Rectal Surgery, Department of Surgery, Rabin Medical Center, Beilinson Campus, Petah Tikva, and Sakler School of Medicine, Tel Aviv University, Tel Aviv, Israel

Madhulika G. Varma Department of Surgery, University of California–San Francisco, San Francisco, California, U.S.A.

David Weinberg Gastroenterology Section, Divisions of Medical and Population Sciences, Fox Chase Cancer Center, Philadelphia, Pennsylvania, U.S.A.

Samir M. Yebara Department of Colorectal Surgery, Cleveland Clinic Florida, Weston, Florida, U.S.A.

Tonia Young-Fadok Division of Colon and Rectal Surgery, Mayo Clinic Scottsdale, Scottsdale, Arizona, U.S.A.

Oded Zmora Colon and Rectal Surgery, Department of Surgery and Transplantation, Sheba Medical Center, Tel Hashomer, and Sakler School of Medicine, Tel Aviv University, Tel Aviv, Israel

1 ▌ Colonic Development, Embryology, Structure, and Function

J. Marcio N. Jorge
*Division of Colorectal Surgery, Department of Gastroenterology, University of São Paulo,
São Paulo, Brazil*

INTRODUCTION

Galen (1) (129–200 A.D.) was the first to describe the anatomy of the anal sphincter and its role in continence and defecation. In 1543, the anatomist Andreas Vesalius (2) published the first illustrations with an in-depth description of the anatomy of the anorectum and pelvic floor. However, the anatomy of this region is so intrinsically related to its physiology that many aspects are appreciated only in the living. Therefore, it is a region in which the colorectal surgeon has advantages over the anatomist with experience relative to in vivo dissection as well as physiological and endoscopic examinations. Recent advances in both anorectal physiology and surgical techniques have renewed the interest in more detailed studies of anatomy (3–9). Recently a novel virtual reality model has been designed to teach anorectal pelvic floor anatomy, pathology, and surgery (10). This virtual reality technology was proposed to improve visualization of three-dimensional structures over conventional media on the premise that it supports stereoscopic vision, viewer-centered perspective, large angles of view, and interactivity.

EMBRYOLOGY

The colon is a capacious tube described in humans to be somewhere between the short, straight type with a rudimentary cecum, such as that of the carnivores, and a long sacculated colon with a capacious cecum, such as that of the herbivores. The primitive gut tube develops from the endodermal roof of the yolk sac. At the beginning of the third week of development, it can be divided into three regions: the foregut in the head fold, the hindgut with its ventral allantoic outgrowth in the smaller tail fold, and, between these two portions, the midgut, which, at this stage, opens ventrally into the yolk sac (Fig. 1). After the stages of "physiologic herniation," "return to the abdomen," and "fixation," the midgut progresses below the major pancreatic papilla to form the small intestine, the ascending colon, and the proximal two-thirds of the transverse colon. This segment is supplied by the midgut (superior mesenteric) artery, with corresponding venous and lymphatic drainage. The sympathetic innervation of the midgut and, likewise, the hindgut originates from T8 to L2, via splanchnic nerves and the autonomic abdominopelvic plexuses. The parasympathetic outflow to the midgut is derived from the 10th cranial nerve (vagus) with preganglionic cell bodies in the brain stem.

The distal colon (distal third of the transverse colon), the rectum, and the anal canal above the dentate line are all derived from the hindgut. Therefore, this segment is supplied by the hindgut [inferior mesenteric artery (IMA)] artery, with corresponding venous and lymphatic drainage. Its parasympathetic outflow comes from S2, S3, and S4 via splanchnic nerves.

The dentate line marks the fusion between endodermal and ectodermal tubes, where the terminal portion of the hindgut or cloaca fuses with the proctodeum, an ingrowth from the anal pit. The cloaca originates at the portion of the rectum below the pubococcygeal line, whereas the hindgut originates above it. Before the fifth week of development, the intestinal and urogenital tracts terminate in conjunction with the cloaca. At the sixth week, the urorectal septum migrates caudally and the two tracts are separated. The cloacal part of the anal canal, which has both endodermal and ectodermal elements, forms the anal transitional zone

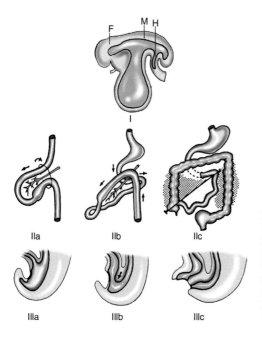

Figure 1 Embryology of the colon, rectum, and anus I- The primitive tube, at the third week of development, can be divided into three regions: the foregut (**F**) in the head fold, the hindgut (**H**) with its ventral allantoic outgrowth in the tail fold, and the midgut (**M**) between these two portions; IIa-IIc- stages of development of the midgut: physiologic herniation (a), return to the abdomen (b), and fixation 9c); IIIa-IIIc- The urogenital septum migrates caudally, at the sixth week, and separates the urogenital and intestinal tracts.

after breakdown of the anal membrane. During the tenth week, the anal tubercles, a pair of ectodermal swellings around the proctodeal pit, fuse dorsally to form a horseshoe-shaped structure and anteriorly to create the perineal body. The cloacal sphincter is separated by the perineal body into urogenital and anal portions [external anal sphincter (EAS)]. The internal anal sphincter (IAS) is formed later (6th to 12th week) from enlarging fibers of the circular layer of the rectum (11,12). The sphincters apparently migrate during their development; the external sphincter grows cephalad and the internal sphincter moves caudally. Concomitantly, the longitudinal muscle descends into the intersphincteric plane (11).

COLON

The colon (from the Greek *koluein*, "to retard") is a capacious tube, averaging approximately 150 cm, which roughly surrounds the loops of the small bowel as an arch. Its diameter gradually decreases from 7.5 cm at the cecum to 2.5 cm at the sigmoid, but it can be substantially augmented by distension. Anatomic differences between the small and large intestines include position, caliber, degree of fixation, and, in the colon, the presence of three distinct characteristics: the teniae coli, the haustra, and the appendices epiploicae (Fig. 2). The three taeniae coli—anterior (tenia libera), posteromedial (tenia mesocolica), and posterolateral (tenia omentalis)—represent bands of the outer longitudinal coat of muscle that traverse the colon from the base of the appendix to the rectosigmoid junction, where they merge. The muscular longitudinal layer is actually a complete coat around the colon, although it is considerably thicker at the teniae (13). The haustra or haustral sacculations are outpouchings of bowel wall between the teniae; they are caused by the relative shortness of the teniae—about one-sixth shorter than the length of bowel wall (14). The haustra are separated by the plicae semilunares or crescentic folds of the bowel wall, which give the colon its characteristic radiographic appearance when filled with air or barium. The appendices epiploicae are small appendages of fat that protrude from the serosal aspect of the colon.

Cecum and Ascending Colon

The ileum terminates in the posteromedial aspect of the cecum, and the angulation between these two structures is maintained by the superior and inferior ileocecal ligaments. Viewed from the cecal lumen, the ileocecal junction is represented by a narrow, transversely situated slit-like opening—the ileocecal valve (valve de Bauhin). A circular sphincter, the ileocecal sphincter, originates from a slight thickening of the muscular layer of the terminal ileum.

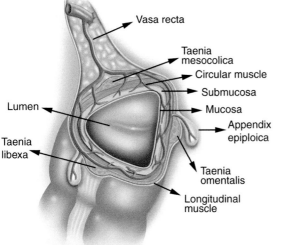

Figure 2 Structure of the colon.

A competent ileocecal valve is related, in colonic obstruction, to the critical closed-loop type of colonic obstruction, but ileocecal competence is not always demonstrated on barium enema studies. Therefore, instead of preventing reflux of the colonic contents into the ileum, more likely, the ileocecal valve acts by regulating ileal emptying, as the ileocecal sphincter seems to relax in response to the entrance of food in the stomach (15). Similar to the gastroesophageal junction, extrasphincteric factors apparently play a role in prevention of reflux from the colon to the ileum. Kumar and Phillips (16) found that the competence of the ileocecal junction, detected in 93% of human autopsy specimens, was not impaired by the removal of a strip of mucosa or a circular muscle; however, division of the superior and inferior ileocecal ligaments rendered the junction incompetent in all specimens.

The vermiform appendix arises from the posteromedial aspect of the cecum about 3.0 cm below the ileocecal junction. The confluence of the three teniae is a useful guide to locate the base of the appendix. The appendix, due to its great mobility, may occupy, possibly at different times in the same individual, a variety of positions: retrocecal (65%), pelvic (31%), subcecal (2.3%), preileal (1.0%), and postileal (0.4%) (17).

The cecum is entirely invested with the peritoneum; however, its mobility is usually limited by a small mesocecum. In about 5% of individuals, the peritoneal covering is absent posteriorly; it then rests directly on the iliacus and psoas major muscles (18). Conversely, an abnormally mobile cecum-ascending colon, due to an anomaly of fixation, can be found in 10% to 22% of cases (14). In this case, a long mesentery is present, and the cecum may assume abnormal positions and originate a volvulus.

The ascending colon, extending from the level of the ileocecal junction to the right colic or hepatic flexure, is approximately 15 cm long. The ascending colon is covered with the peritoneum anteriorly and on both sides, and fragile adhesions between the right abdominal wall and its anterior aspect, known as Jackson's membrane, may exist (19). Similar to the descending colon, on its posterior surface, the ascending colon is devoid of the peritoneum, as it is replaced by an areolar tissue (Toldt fascia), which resulted from an embryological process of fusion or coalescence of the mesentery to the parietal posterior peritoneum (20). In the lateral peritoneal reflection, this process is represented by the white line of Toldt, which is more evident at the descending-sigmoid junction. This line serves as a guide to start mobilization of the ascending, descending, or sigmoid colon.

Transverse Colon

The transverse colon is relatively fixed at each flexure; in between flexures, it is completely invested with the peritoneum and suspended by a transverse mesocolon, which provides variable mobility; the nadir of the transverse colon may reach the hypogastrium. The greater omentum is fused on the anterosuperior aspect of the transverse colon, and intercoloepiploic dissection is necessary to mobilize the colon or to enter the lesser sac of the peritoneum. The left colic flexure (splenic flexure) is situated beneath the lower angle of the spleen and firmly attached to the diaphragm by the phrenocolic ligament, which also forms a shelf to support the spleen. Because of the risk of hemorrhage, mobilization of the splenic flexure should be approached with great care and preceded by dissection upward along the descending colon and from the midtransverse colon toward the splenic flexure. This flexure, when compared to the hepatic flexure, is more acute, higher, and more deeply situated.

Descending and Sigmoid Colon

Similar to the ascending colon, the descending colon is covered by the peritoneum only on its anterior and lateral aspects; however, the descending colon is narrower and more dorsally situated than is the ascending colon. The sigmoid colon, extending from the lower end of the descending colon at the pelvic brim to the proximal limit of the rectum, varies dramatically in length (15 to 50 cm, mean 38 cm) and configuration. More commonly, the sigmoid colon is a mobile, omega-shaped loop, completely invested by the peritoneum.

Both the anatomy and function of the rectosigmoid junction have been a matters of substantial controversy, and both surgeons and anatomists diverge in opinion. Some authors considered it as a clearly defined segment as it is the narrowest part of the large intestine; in fact, it is usually well characterized endoscopically, as a narrow and sharply angulated segment. However, this segment is also considered, at least externally, a "no-man's land" region, which, to most surgeons, comprises the last 5 to 8 cm of the sigmoid and the uppermost 5 cm of the rectum (18,21). O'Beirne (22) has postulated that because the rectum is usually emptied and contracted, the sigmoid plays a role in continence as the fecal reservoir. Subsequently, a thickening of the circular muscle layer between the rectum and sigmoid was described as a rectosigmoid sphincter (23) or pylorus sigmoidorectalis (24).

Stoss (6), in a recent study of 39 human cadavers, found the rectosigmoid junction situated at 6 to 7 cm below the sacral promontory, and it was macroscopically identified as the point where the tenia libera and the tenia omentalis fuse to form a single anterior tenia, and also where both haustra and mesocolon terminate. Under microdissection, this segment was characterized by conspicuous strands of longitudinal muscle fibers with curved interconnecting fibers between the longitudinal and circular muscle layers, allowing synergistic interplay between these two layers. This author concluded that although the rectosigmoid does not comply with the definition of an anatomical sphincter, it might be regarded as a functional sphincter, because mechanisms of active dilating occlusion and passive "kinking" occlusion do exist.

RECTUM

The rectum is 12 to 15 cm long; however both proximal and distal limits of the rectum are debatable. The rectosigmoid junction is considered at the level of S3 by anatomists and at the sacral promontory by surgeons. Likewise, the distal limit is regarded as the muscular anorectal ring by surgeons and as the dentate line by anatomists.

The rectum is characterized by three lateral curves, which correspond, on the intraluminal aspect, to the folds or valves of Houston (Figs. 3A and B) (25,26).There are usually three folds: two on the left side (at 7–8 cm and at 12–13 cm) and one on the right side (at 9–11 cm). The middle valve is the most consistent one (Kohlrausch's plica) and corresponds to the level of the anterior peritoneal reflection. The rectal valves do not contain all the rectal wall layers, representing an excellent location for rectal biopsy because they are an easy target, with minimal risk of perforation (19). The valves of Houston must be negotiated during rectosigmoidoscopy and they disappear after straightening of the rectum, which is attributed to the 5 cm length gained during rectal mobilization.

The upper third of the rectum is invested by the peritoneum on both its anterior and lateral aspects; the middle rectum is only anteriorly covered by the peritoneum, as the posterior peritoneal reflection is usually 12 to 15 cm from the anal verge; and finally, the lower third of the rectum is entirely extraperitoneal, as the anterior peritoneal reflection occurs at 9 to 7 cm from the anal verge, in men, and a little lower, 7.5 to 5 cm from the anal verge, in women.

(A) **(B)**

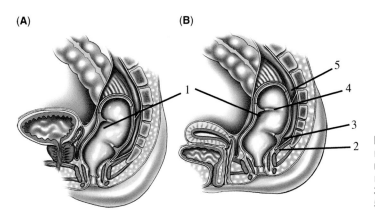

Figure 3 Sagittal diagram of the rectum and rectosigmoid junction in males (**A**) and females (**B**): 1-middle rectal valve, 2- levator ani muscles, 3-mesorectum, 4-presacral fascia, 5-rectosacral Waldeyer's fascia.

The rectum is, therefore, entirely extraperitoneal on its posterior aspect. According to anatomists, the rectum is characterized by the absence of a mesorectum. However, the areolar tissue on the posterior aspect of the rectum, containing terminal branches of the IMA and enclosed by the fascia propria, is often referred to by surgeons as the mesorectum. A more distinct mesorectum, however, may be noted in patients with procidentia. The mesorectum may be a metastatic site from a rectal cancer and can be removed without clinical sequelae, because no functionally significant nerves pass through it (27).

Anatomical Relationships of the Rectum
Ureter
In resections of the right and left colon, identification of the ureters is mandatory, because injury of its abdominal or pelvic portions may occur. On either side, the ureter, on its inferomedial course, rests upon the psoas muscle and is crossed obliquely by the spermatic vessels, anteriorly, and the genitofemoral nerve, posteriorly. The right ureter lies lateral to the inferior vena cava and in addition, is, anteriorly crossed by the right colic and ileocolic arteries and by the root of the mesentery and the terminal ileum. On its pelvic portion, the ureter crosses the pelvic brim, in front of, or a little lateral to, the bifurcation of the common iliac artery and descends abruptly between the peritoneum and the internal iliac artery. In the female, as the ureter traverses the posterior layer of the broad ligament and the parametrium, it passes laterally to the uterus and the upper part of the vagina; at this point, it is enveloped by the vesical and vaginal venous plexuses and crossed above and lateromedially by the uterine artery. The mesosigmoid is attached to the pelvic walls in an inverted V shape, composing a recess, the intersigmoid fossa. The left ureter lies immediately underneath this fossa, and is crossed on its anterior surface by the spermatic, left colic, and sigmoid vessels.

Fascial Attachments of the Rectum and the Presacral Space

The fascia propria of the rectum is then an extension of the pelvic fascia, which encloses the rectum, and fat, nerves, and blood and lymphatic vessels, present mainly in the lateral and posterior extraperitoneal portion of the rectum.

The lateral ligaments or lateral stalks of the rectum, distal condensations of the fascia propria of the rectum, form a roughly triangular structure with a base on the lateral pelvic wall and an apex attached on the lateral aspect of the rectum. As pointed out by Church et al. (3), these ligaments have been the subject of "anatomical confusion and misconception." They comprise essentially connective tissue and nerves; the middle rectal artery does not traverse the lateral stalks of the rectum, but sends minor branches through them, unilaterally or bilaterally, in about 25% of cases (28). Consequently, division of the lateral stalks during rectal mobilization carries a 1:4 chance of bleeding. However, from a practical point of view, the stalks rarely require ligation; electrocautery is sufficient in the vast majority of cases. Furthermore, ligation of the stalks implies leaving behind lateral mesorectal tissue. Such remnants may preclude obtaining adequate lateral (29) or mesorectal (27,30) margins during cancer surgery.

The presacral fascia is a thickened part of the parietal endopelvic fascia, which covers the concavity of the sacrum and coccyx, nerves, the middle sacral artery, and presacral veins. Intraoperative rupture of the presacral fascia may cause troublesome hemorrhage, related to the underlying presacral veins, in 4.6% to 7% of cases after surgery for rectal neoplasms (31–33). These veins are avalvular and communicate, via basivertebral veins, with the internal vertebral venous system. This system can attain, in the lithotomy position, hydrostatic pressures of 17 to 23 cm H_2O, about two to three times the normal pressure of the inferior vena cava (31). In addition, the adventitia of the basivertebral veins adheres firmly, by structures "in anchor," to the sacral periosteum at the level of the ostia of the sacral foramina, found mainly at the level of S3–S4 (31). Consequently, despite its venous nature, presacral hemorrhage can be fatal, due to the high hydrostatic pressure, and difficult to control, due to retraction of the vascular stump into the sacral foramen.

Both the rectosacral and the visceral pelvic fascia are important anatomical landmarks during rectal mobilization. The rectosacral fascia is an anteroinferior-directed thick fascial reflection from the presacral fascia, at the S4 level, to the fascia propria of the rectum, just above the anorectal ring. The rectosacral fascia is classically, but improperly, known as the fascia of Waldeyer; William Waldeyer, in fact, described the entire pelvic fascia but did not emphasize, specifically, the rectosacral fascia (34). Anteriorly, the extraperitoneal rectum is separated from the prostate and the seminal vesicles or vagina by a fascial investment, first reported in 1836 by Denonvilliers as the prostatoperitoneal membrane. The so-called visceral pelvic fascia or Denonvilliers' fascia has become important as colorectal surgeons become ever more concerned with pelvic surgical anatomy in order to improve not only the oncological but also the functional outcome after rectal excision (35).

Innervation of the Rectum

The sympathetic and parasympathetic components of the autonomic innervation of the large intestine closely follow the blood supply. The sympathetic supply arises from L1, L2, and L3. Preganglionic fibers, via lumbar sympathetic nerve synapse in the preaortic plexus, and the postganglionic fibers follow the branches of the IMA and superior rectal artery to the upper rectum and left colon. The lower rectum is innervated by the presacral nerves, which are formed by fusion of the aortic plexus and lumbar splanchnic nerves. Just below the sacral promontory, the presacral nerves form the hypogastric plexus (or superior hypogastric plexus). (Fig. 4A). Two main hypogastric nerves, on either side of the rectum, carry sympathetic innervation from the hypogastric plexus to the pelvic plexus. The pelvic plexus lies on the lateral side of the pelvis at the level of the lower third of the rectum, adjacent to the lateral stalks.

(A)   **(B)**

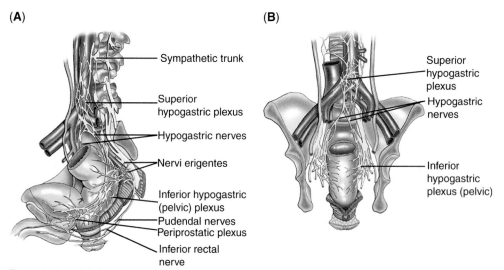

Figure 4   Lateral (**A**) and frontal (**B**) view of the parasympathetic and sympathetic nerve supply to the rectum and sphincters.

The parasympathetic supply derives from S2, S3, and S4. These fibers emerge through the sacral foramen and are called the nervi erigenti (Fig. 4B). They pass laterally, forward, and upward to join the sympathetic hypogastric nerves at the pelvic plexus. From the pelvic plexus, combined postganglionic parasympathetic and sympathetic fibers are distributed to the upper rectum and left colon, via inferior mesenteric plexus, and directly, to the lower rectum and upper anal canal. The periprostatic plexus, a subdivision of the pelvic plexus situated on the Denonvilliers' fascia, supplies the prostate, seminal vesicles, corpora cavernosa, vas deferens, urethra, ejaculatory ducts, and bulbourethral glands. Erection of the penis is mediated by both parasympathetic (arteriolar vasodilatation) and sympathetic (inhibition of vasoconstriction) inflow, whereas ejaculation is primarily mediated by parasympathetic activity.

Urinary and sexual dysfunction is commonly seen after a variety of pelvic surgical procedures, including low anterior resection and abdominoperineal resection. All pelvic nerves lie in the plane between the peritoneum and the endopelvic fascia and are endangered during rectal dissection. Injury to the autonomic nerves may occur in several points: During flush ligation of the IMA, close to the aorta, the sympathetic preaortic nerves may be injured. Lesions of both superior hypogastric plexus and hypogastric nerves may occur during dissection at the sacral promontory or in the presacral region; in this case, sympathetic denervation with intact nervi erigentes results in retrograde ejaculation and bladder dysfunction. The nervi erigentes are located in the posterolateral aspect of the pelvis, and, at the point of fusion with the sympathetic nerves, they are closely related to the middle hemorrhoidal artery. An isolated injury of these nerves may completely abolish erectile function (36). The pelvic plexus may be damaged either by excessive traction on the rectum, particularly laterally, or during division of the lateral stalks, when it is done closer to the pelvic lateral wall. Finally, dissection close to the seminal vesicles and prostate may damage the periprostatic plexus (mixed parasympathetic and sympathetic injury), resulting in erectile impotence and flaccid neurogenic bladder; sexual function may be preserved by dissection below the Denonvilliers' fascia.

Permanent bladder paresis occurs in 7% to 59% of patients after abdominoperineal resection of the rectum (37). The incidence of impotence after low anterior resection and abdominoperineal resection is about 15% and 45%, respectively (38). The overall incidence of sexual dysfunction after proctectomy may reach up to 100% for malignant disease (39,40); however, these rates are much lower, 0% to 6% (36,41), for benign conditions such as inflammatory bowel disease. This occurs because dissections performed for benign disease are closer to the bowel wall and avoid injuring the nerves (42). Sexual complications after rectal surgery predominate in males; conversely, they are probably underdiagnosed in females (43). Some discomfort during intercourse is reported in 30% (44) and dyspareunia in 10% (45), after proctocolectomy and ileostomy. Some authors believe that the sexual function in women is primarily mediated by impulses carried by the pudendal nerves, which are covered by dense endopelvic fascia and therefore more protected from operative injury, compared to the more easily damaged nervi erigentes (36).

Anal Canal

Although representing a relatively small segment of the digestive tract, the anal canal has a peculiar anatomy and a complex physiology, which accounts for both its vital role in continence and its susceptibility to a variety of diseases. There are two distinct definitions for the anal canal. The "surgical" or "functional" anal canal extends for approximately 4 cm from the anal verge to the anorectal ring. The "anatomical" or "embryological" anal canal is shorter (2 cm), extending from the anal verge to the dentate line—the level that corresponds to the proctodeal membrane (Fig. 5) (46).

Lining of the Anal Canal

The lining of the anal canal consists of an upper mucosal and a lower cutaneous segment. The dentate (pectinate) line represents the "saw-toothed" junction of the ectoderm and the endoderm, and therefore, represents an important landmark between two distinct origins of venous and lymphatic drainage, nerve supply, and epithelial lining. Above the dentate line, the intestine has sympathetic and parasympathetic innervation and the venous and lymphatic drainage and the arterial supply are to and from the hypogastric vessels. Distally to the dentate line, the anal

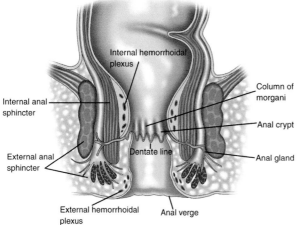

Internal hemorrhoidal plexus

Internal anal sphincter

External anal sphincter

Dentate line

External hemorrhoidal plexus

Anal verge

Column of morgani

Anal crypt

Anal gland

Figure 5   The anal canal.

canal has somatic nerve supply, and its vascularization is related to the inferior hemorrhoidal system. The upper anal canal contains a rich profusion of both free and organized sensory nerve endings, especially in the vicinity of the anal valves (47). Anal sensation is carried in the inferior rectal branch of the pudendal nerve and is thought to play a role in anal continence.

The pectinate or dentate line corresponds to a line of anal valves, which represent remnants of the proctodeal membrane. Above each valve, there is a little pocket known as an anal sinus or crypt. A variable number of glands, 4 to 12, more concentrated in the posterior quadrants, are connected to the anal crypts. More than one gland may open into the same crypt, while half the crypts have no communication. The anal gland ducts, in an outward and downward route, enter the submucosa, two-thirds of these enter the IAS, and half of these terminate into the intersphincteric plane (48). Obstruction of these ducts, presumably by accumulation of foreign material in the crypts, may cause perianal abscesses and fistulas (49).

Above the dentate line, 8 to 14 longitudinal folds, known as the rectal columns (columns of Morgagni), have their bases connected in pairs to each valve at the dentate line. At the lower end of the columns are the anal papillae. The mucosa in the area of the columns consists of several layers of cuboidal cells and acquires a deep purple color due to the underlying internal hemorrhoidal plexus. This 0.5 to 1 cm strip of mucosa above the dentate line is known as the anal transition or cloacogenic zone, and it is the source of some anal tumors. Above this area, the epithelium changes to a single layer of cuboidal columnar cells.

The anal verge (white line of Hilton) marks the lowermost edge of the anal canal, and it is usually the level of reference for measurements taken during colonoscopy. Others prefer to evert the anus and consider the dentate line as a landmark because it is more precise (50); the difference between the two is nearly 1 cm. Distally to the anal verge, the lining becomes thicker and pigmented and acquires hair follicles, glands, including large apocrine glands, and other features of normal skin. For this reason, perianal hidradenitis suppurativae, inflammation of the apocrine glands, may be excised with preservation of the anal canal.

Based on a recent histologic review of cadaver dissections, it was found that the mean distance of aganglionic bowel from the dentate line was 6.6 mm (range, 0–21 mm) in Meissner's plexus and 5.1 mm (range, 0–15 mm) in Auerbach's plexus. Therefore, the normal aganglionic segment in adults is 2 cm or less from the dentate line, and, rectal biopsy needs to be performed above this point (51).

Muscles of the Anorectal Region

Based on phylogenetic studies, it was found that two muscle groups derive from the cloaca: "sphincter" and "lateral compressor" groups (Fig. 6) (52). The sphincteric group is present in almost all animals. In higher mammals, this group is divided into ventral (urogenital) and dorsal (anal) groups; in primates, the latter forms, the EAS. The lateral compressor or pelvicaudal group is subdivided, in reptiles and mammals, in lateral and medial compartments. The homologue of the lateral compartment is, apparently, the ischiococcygeus, and,

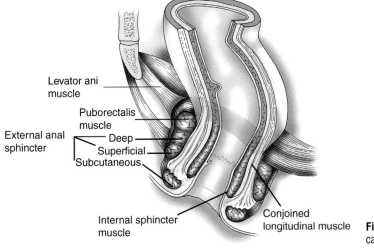

Levator ani
muscle

Puborectalis
muscle

External anal
sphincter

Deep

Superficial

Subcutaneous

Internal sphincter
muscle

Conjoined
longitudinal muscle

Figure 6 Muscles of the anal canal.

of the medial pelvicaudal compartment, the pubo- and ileococcygeus. In addition, most primates possess a variable-sized group of muscle fibers close to the inner border of the medial pelvicaudal muscle, which attach the rectum to the pubis; these fibers are more distinct and known in man as the puborectalis (PR) muscle.

Internal Anal Sphincter

The IAS represents the distal, 2.5 to 4 cm long, condensation of the inner circular muscle layer of the rectum (Fig. 6). The lower rounded edge of the IAS can be palpated on physical examination, about 1.2 cm distal to the dentate line; the groove between it and the EAS, the intersphincteric sulcus, can be visualized or easily palpated. The different echogenic patterns of the anal sphincters facilitate their visualization during endosonography. The IAS is a 2 to 3 mm thick circular band and shows a uniform hypoechogenicity. The PR and the EAS, despite their mixed linear echogenicity, the PR and EAS are both predominantly hyperechogenic, and the distinction is made by their position and shape, and topography (9,53).

As a smooth muscle in a state of continuous maximum contraction, the IAS represents, due to both intrinsic myogenic and extrinsic autonomic neurogenic properties, a natural barrier to the involuntary loss of stool. The IAS is supplied by sympathetic (L5) and parasympathetic (S2, S3, and S4) nerves following the same route as the nerves to the rectum. A gradual increase in pressures is noted from proximal to distal in the anal canal; the highest resting pressures are usually recorded 1 to 2 cm cephalad to the anal verge. This high-pressure zone or functional anal canal length, which corresponds anatomically to the condensation of the smooth muscle fibers of the IAS, is shorter in women (2–3 cm) as compared to men (2.5–3.5 cm) (48,54). Interestingly, although parity may contribute to this difference, nulliparous women still have significantly shorter functional anal canals than men (54).

The anal canal is also relatively asymmetric on its radial profile; the normal values for the radial asymmetry index are 10% or lesser (54–56). This functional asymmetry is found for both resting- and squeeze-pressure profiles; it follows the inherent anatomic asymmetry in the arrangement of the sphincter muscles. In the upper third of the anal canal, higher pressures are found posteriorly, due to the activity of the PR along with the deep portion of the EAS, whereas in the lower third, pressures are higher anteriorly, due to the posteriorly directed superficial loop of the EAS.

Conjoined Longitudinal Muscle

Whereas the inner circular layer of the rectum gives rise to the IAS, the outer longitudinal layer, at the level of the anorectal ring, mixes with some fibers of the levator ani muscle to form the conjoined longitudinal muscle (Fig. 6). This muscle descends between the IAS and EAS, and ultimately some of its fibers, referred to as the corrugator cutis ani muscle, traverse the lowermost part of the EAS to insert into the perianal skin.

There is still a great deal of controversy and speculation about the anatomy of the conjoined longitudinal muscle. Other sources for the striated component of the conjoined longitudinal muscle include the PR and deep EAS (57), the pubococcygeus and top loop of the EAS (58), and lower fibers of the PR (59). On its descending course, the conjoined longitudinal muscle may give rise to medial extensions that cross the IAS to contribute the smooth muscle of submucosa (sustentator tunicae mucosae, musculus submucosae ani) (60).

Possible functions of the conjoined longitudinal muscle include its role in attaching the anorectum to the pelvis and action as a skeleton supporting and binding the rest of the internal and external sphincter complex together (61). Shafik (58) ascribes its main role during defecation, causing shortening and widening of the anal canal and eversion of the anal orifice, and proposes the term "evertor ani muscle." Haas and Fox (62) consider that the meshwork composed by the conjoined longitudinal muscle may minimize functional deterioration of the sphincters after its surgical division, and act as a support against hemorrhoidal and rectal prolapses. Finally, the conjoined longitudinal muscle and its extensions to the intersphincteric plane divide the adjacent tissues into subspaces and may play a role in the containment of sepsis (8).

External Anal Sphincter

The EAS is the elliptical cylinder of striated muscle that envelops the entire length of the inner tube of smooth muscle, but it ends slightly more distal to the terminus of the IAS. The EAS was initially described by including three divisions: subcutaneous, superficial, and deep (57). Subsequently, Goligher et al. (63) described the EAS as a simple continuous sheet of muscle, which forms, along with the PR and levator ani, one funnel-shaped sheet of skeletal muscle; the deepest part of the EAS is intimately related to the PR muscle, which is actually considered a component of both the levator ani and EAS muscle complexes. Others considered the EAS as being composed by a deep compartment (deep sphincter and PR) and a superficial compartment (subcutaneous and superficial sphincter) (10,64). The EAS is innervated on each side by the inferior rectal branch (S2 and S3) of the pudendal nerve and the perineal branch of S4. Despite the fact that the PR and EAS have somewhat different innervations, these muscles seem to act as an indivisible unit (7). After unilateral transection of a pudendal nerve, the EAS function is still preserved due to the crossover of the fibers at the spinal cord level.

Oh and Kark (64) also noted differences in the arrangement of the EAS according to gender and site around the anal canal. In the male, the upper half of the EAS is enveloped anteriorly by the conjoined longitudinal muscle, while the lower half is crossed by it. In the female, the entire EAS is grossly encapsulated by a mixture of fibers derived from both longitudinal and IAS muscles. Based on an embryological study, it was found that the EAS also seems to be subdivided into two parts, superficial and deep, however without any connection with the PR (7). Shafik (4) proposed the three U-shaped loop system concept, in which each loop is a separate sphincter with distinct attachments, muscle bundle directions, and innervations and each loop complements the others to help maintain continence. However, clinical experience has not supported Shafik's tripartite scheme; the EAS is more likely a one-muscle unit, not divided into layers or laminae, attached by the anococcygeal ligament posteriorly to the coccyx and anteriorly to the perineal body. Based on dissection studies, the EAS does not seem to be a complete circle in certain planes, neither in the male nor in the female. Whereas generally the whole EAS complex is thicker in the male than in the female, the anterior part of the EAS is thick in the female and thinner and more elongated in the male. These gender differences of the ventral part of the EAS, already present in fetuses, may account for difficulties in interpretation of endoanal ultrasound, and consequently, overreporting of obstetric injuries (65).

Levator Ani

The levator ani muscle is the major component of the pelvic floor. Also known as the pelvic diaphragm, the levator ani muscle is a pair of broad, symmetrical sheets composed of three striated muscles: iliococcygeus, pubococcygeus, and PR (Figs. 7A and B). A variable fourth component, the ischiococcygeus or coccygeus, is, in humans, rudimentary and represented by a few muscle fibers on the surface of the sacrospinous ligament (66). Ileococcygeus fibers arise from the ischial spine and posterior part of the obturator fascia and course inferiorly and medially to insert into the lateral aspects of S3 and S4, the coccyx, and the anococcygeal raphe. The pubococcygeus arises from the posterior aspect of the pubis and the anterior part of the obturator fascia, runs dorsally alongside the anorectal junction to decussate with fibers

(A)

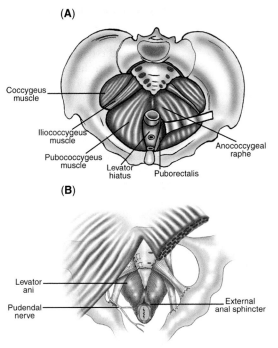

Coccygeus muscle

Iliococcygeus muscle

Pubococcygeus muscle

Levator hiatus

Puborectalis

Anococcygeal raphe

(B)

Levator ani

Pudendal nerve

External anal sphincter

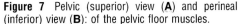

Figure 7 Pelvic (superior) view (**A**) and perineal (inferior) view (**B**): of the pelvic floor muscles.

of the opposite side at the anococcygeal raphe and to insert into the anterior surface of the fourth sacral and first coccygeal segments.

The levator hiatus consists of an elliptical space situated between the two pubococcygeus muscles where the lower rectum, urethra, and the dorsal vein of either the penis in men or the vagina in women pass through it. The hiatal ligament, originating from the pelvic fascia, maintains the intrahiatal viscera together and prevents their constriction during levator ani contraction; a dilator function has been attributed to the anococcygeal raphe, due to its criss-cross arrangement (11).

The PR muscle is a U-shaped strong loop of striated muscle, which slings the anorectum junction to the back of the pubis. The anorectal angle, the result of the anatomic configuration of the U-shaped sling of PR muscle around the anorectal junction, is thought to maintain gross fecal continence. Different theories have been postulated to explain the importance of the PR and the anorectal angle in the maintenance of fecal continence. Parks et al. (67) considered that increasing intra-abdominal pressure forces the anterior rectal wall down into the upper anal canal, occluding it by a type of flap valve mechanism creating an effective seal. Subsequently it was demonstrated that the flap mechanism does not occur; instead a continued sphincteric occlusion-like activity attributed to the PR was noted (68,69).

The PR is the most medial portion of the levator muscle and is situated immediately cephalad to the deep component of the external sphincter. The anorectal ring, the upper end of the sphincter, more precisely, the PR and the upper border of the IAS, is an easily recognized boundary of the anal canal on physical examination,. Despite lacking embryological significance, the anorectal ring is of clinical relevance because division of this structure, as during surgery for abscesses and fistula, will inevitably result in fecal incontinence. Because the junction between the two muscles is indistinct, and they have similar innervation (pudendal nerve), the PR has been regarded, by some authors, as a part of the EAS and not of the levator ani complex (11,64). Anatomical and phylogenetic studies suggest that the PR is either a part of the levator ani (13) or of the EAS (50,59). Based on microscopic examinations in human embryos, Levi et al. (7) observed that the PR has a common primordium with the ileo- and pubococcygeus muscles; the PR is, in different stages of development, never connected with the EAS. Additionally, neurophysiologic studies have implied that the innervation of these muscles may not be the same, because stimulation of sacral nerves resulted in electromyographic activity in the ipsilateral PR muscle, but not in the EAS (70). This is, therefore, a controversial issue, and as a consequence of all this evidence, the PR has been considered as belonging in both muscle groups, the EAS and the levator ani (71).

Skeletal Muscle Responses

The levator ani is supplied by sacral roots (S2, S3, and S4) on its pelvic surface and by the perineal branch of the pudendal nerve on its inferior surface. The PR receives additional innervation from the inferior rectal nerves. Garavoglia et al. (72) suggested three types of striated muscular function in the mechanism of continence: lateral compression (pubococcygeus), sphincteric (deep EAS), and angulation (PR). The EAS along with the pelvic floor muscles, unlike other skeletal muscles, which are usually inactive at rest, maintains continuous unconscious resting electrical tone by a reflex arc at the cauda equine level. During maximal squeeze efforts, intra-anal pressures usually reach two or three times their baseline resting tone; however, due to muscular fatigue, maximal voluntary contraction of the EAS can be sustained for only 40 to 60 seconds. Histological studies have shown that EAS, PR, and levator ani muscles have a predominance of type I fibers, which is characteristic of skeletal muscles of tonic contractile activity (72). In response to conditions of threatened continence, such as increased intra-abdominal pressures and rectal distension, the EAS and PR muscles reflexly or voluntarily contract further to prevent fecal leakage. The automatic continence mechanism is then formed by the resting tone, maintained by the IAS, and magnified by reflex EAS contraction. This extra pressure gradient is essential to minimize voluntary attention to the sphincter.

Perianal and Pararectal Spaces

Potential spaces of clinical significance in the anorectal region include ischiorectal, perianal, intersphincteric, submucous, superficial postanal, deep postanal, supralevator, and retrorectal spaces. The ischiorectal fossa is subdivided by a thin horizontal fascia into two spaces: the ischiorectal and perianal spaces. The ischiorectal space comprises the upper two-thirds of the ischiorectal fossa. It is a pyramid-shaped space situated, on both sides, between the anal canal and lower part of the rectum, medially, and the sidewall of the pelvis, laterally. On the superolateral wall, the pudendal nerve and the internal pudendal vessels run in the pudendal canal (Alcock's canal). The ischiorectal fossa contains fat and the inferior rectal vessels and nerves. The perianal space surrounds the lower part of the anal canal. The external hemorrhoidal plexus lies in the perianal space and communicates with the internal hemorrhoidal plexus at the dentate line. This space is the typical site of anal hematomas, perianal abscesses, and anal fistula tracts. The perianal space also encloses the subcutaneous part of the EAS, the lowest part of the IAS, and fibers of the longitudinal muscle. These fibers function as a septa, dividing the space into a compact arrangement, which may account for the severe pain caused by a perianal hematoma or abscess (19).

The intersphincteric space is a potential space between the IAS and the EAS. Its importance lies in the genesis of perianal abscesses, because most of the anal glands end in this space. The submucous space is situated between the IAS and the mucocutaneous lining of the anal canal. This space contains the internal hemorrhoidal plexus and the muscularis submucosae ani. Above, it is continuous with the submucous layer of the rectum, and inferiorly, it ends at the level of the dentate line. The superficial postanal space is interposed between the anococcygeal ligament and the skin. The deep postanal space, also known as the retrosphincteric space of Courtney, is situated between the anococcygeal ligament and the anococcygeal raphe (73). Both postanal spaces communicate posteriorly with the ischiorectal fossa and are potential sites of horseshoe abscesses.

The supralevator spaces are situated between the peritoneum superiorly and the levator ani inferiorly. Medially, these bilateral spaces are related to the rectum and, laterally, to the obturator fascia. Supralevator abscesses may occur as a result of upward extension of cryptoglandular source or from a pelvic origin. The retrorectal space is located between the fascia propria of the rectum anteriorly and the presacral fascia posteriorly. Laterally are the lateral rectal ligaments, inferiorly is the rectosacral ligament and, above, it is continuous with the retroperitoneum. The retrorectal space is a site for embryological remnants and the rare presacral tumors.

Arterial Supply

The superior and inferior mesenteric arteries nourish the entire large intestine, and the limit between the two territories is the junction between the proximal two-thirds and the distal third

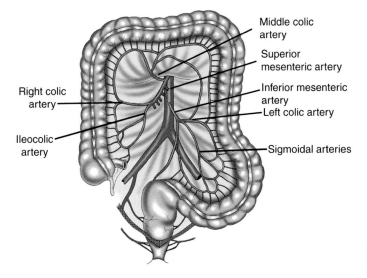

Figure 8 The arterial supply of the large intestine.

of the transverse colon (Fig. 8). The superior mesenteric artery originates from the aorta behind the superior border of the pancreas at L1 and supplies the cecum, appendix, ascending colon, and most of the transverse colon. After passing behind the neck of the pancreas and antero-medial to the uncinate process, the superior mesenteric artery crosses the third part of the duodenum and continues downward and to the right along the base of the mesentery. From its left side arises a series of 12 to 20 jejunal and ileal branches. From its right side, the colic branches arise as the middle, right, and ileocolic arteries.

The superior and inferior rectal (or hemorrhoidal) arteries represent the major blood supply to the anorectum (Fig. 9). The contribution of the middle rectal artery (middle hemorrhoidal artery) varies inversely with the magnitude of the superior rectal artery, which may explain its variable and controversial anatomy. Some authors report absence of the middle rectal artery in 40% to 88% (74,75), whereas others identified it in 94% to 100% of specimens (28,76). The middle rectal artery is more prone to be injured during low anterior resection, when anterolateral dissection of the rectum, close to the pelvic floor, is performed from the prostate and seminal vesicles or from the upper part of the vagina (19). Although scarce in extramural anastomoses, the anorectum has a profuse intramural anastomotic network, which probably accounts for the fact that division of both superior rectal and middle rectal artery does not result in necrosis of the rectum. This tenet is fundamental to ileoanal reservoir surgery.

The paired inferior rectal artery is a branch of the internal pudendal artery, which is a branch of the internal iliac artery. The inferior rectal artery arises within the pudendal canal and is, on its course, entirely extrapelvic; it traverses the obturator fascia, the ischiorectal fossa, and the

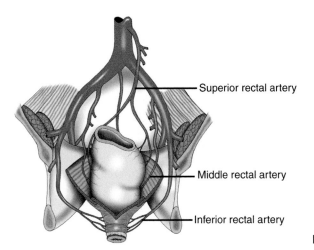

Figure 9 The arterial supply of the anorectum.

EAS to reach the submucosa of the anal canal and ultimately ascend in this plane. The inferior rectal artery needs to be ligated during the perineal stage of the abdominoperineal resection. Klosterhalfen et al. (5), based on postmortem angiographic, manual, and histologic preparations, found two topographic variants of the inferior rectal artery. In the so-called type I, the most common (85%), the posterior commissure is less perfused than the other sections of the anal canal. In addition, the blood supply may be jeopardized by contusion of the vessels passing vertically through the muscle fibers of the IAS during increased sphincter tone. These authors then postulated that, in a pathogenetic model of the primary anal fissure, the resulting decrease in blood supply would lead to a relevant ischemia at the posterior commissure.

Venous Drainage

Blood from the rectum along with the left colon, via the inferior mesenteric vein, reaches the intrahepatic capillary bed through the portal vein. The anorectum also drains, via middle and inferior rectal veins, to the internal iliac vein and then to the inferior vena cava. Although it is still a controversial subject, the presence of anastomoses among these three venous systems may explain the lack of correlation between hemorrhoids and portal hypertension (77).

The paired inferior and middle rectal veins and the single superior rectal vein originate from three anorectal arteriovenous plexuses. The external rectal plexus, situated subcutaneously around the anal canal below the dentate line, constitutes, when dilated, the external hemorrhoids. The internal rectal plexus, which originates the internal hemorrhoids, is situated submucosally around the upper anal canal, above the dentate line. The perirectal or perimuscular rectal plexus drains to the middle and inferior rectal veins.

Lymphatic Drainage

The lymphatic drainage of the large intestine, similar to the venous drainage, basically follows its arterial supply. The lymph nodes in the rectum are particularly numerous and situated between the peritoneum and the bowel wall, equivalent to the epicolic group in the colon, are known as "nodules of Gerota." Lymph from the upper two-thirds of the rectum drains exclusively upward, via superior rectal vessels, to the inferior mesenteric nodes and then to the para-aortic nodes. Lymphatic drainage from the lower third of the rectum occurs not only cephalad, along the superior rectal and inferior mesentery arteries, but also laterally, along the middle rectal vessels to the internal iliac nodes. Studies using lymphoscintigraphy fail to demonstrate communications between inferior mesenteric and internal iliac lymphatics (78). In the anal canal, the dentate line is the landmark for two different systems of lymphatic drainage: above, to the inferior mesenteric and internal iliac nodes; and below, along the inferior rectal lymphatics to the superficial inguinal nodes, or less frequently, along the inferior rectal artery. Block and Enquist (79) have demonstrated that in the female, after injection of dye 5 cm above the anal verge, lymphatic drainage may also spread to the posterior vaginal wall, uterus, cervix, broad ligament, fallopian tubes, ovaries, and cul-de-sac. After injection of dye at 10 cm above the anal verge, spread occurred only to the broad ligament and cul-de-sac, and at the 15 cm level, no spread to the genitals was seen.

Physiology

Anorectal physiology is complex and mechanisms responsible for both fecal continence and defecation are diverse and interrelated. The high incidence of functional intestinal disorders, and, more recently, the technological progress in functional testing have led to a great deal of research in this area. To evaluate the different aspects of anorectal function, methods such as colonic transit times, anorectal manometry, defecography, electromyography, and pudendal nerve latency have gained widespread popularity (80). These methods allow better understanding of normal and disordered anorectal function. Thus, potentially disabling and highly prevalent disorders such as fecal incontinence and chronic idiopathic constipation can be stratified in several causative diagnoses with distinctive therapeutic approaches (81–83).

Factors Maintaining Fecal Continence

Continence is maintained by the interaction of multiple mechanisms, including stool consistency and delivery of colonic contents to the rectum, rectal capacity and compliance, anorectal sensation, the function of the anal sphincter mechanism, and the pelvic floor muscles and nerves.

Colon: Contractile Activity, Myoelectric Activity, and Movements

Colonic motility studies are of limited use due to the relative inaccessibility of the proximal colon. Three types of colonic motor patterns were classically described in humans, based on colonic manometric findings by Adler et al. (84). Type I contractions are monophasic waves of low amplitude (5–10 cm H_2O) and short duration (5–10 seconds) of a mean frequency of 10/min. Type II contractions represent about 90% of all normal manometric recording activity and correspond to combined contraction/relaxation haustral movements. These contractions occur in bursts of 2/min and they are of longer duration (25–30 seconds) and of higher amplitude (15–30 cm H_2O). Type III contractions are of low amplitude (less than 10 cm H_2O); they over-impose type I or II contractions and represent a change in basal pressure. Waves of larger amplitude and longer duration (so-called type IV waves) have been described, mainly in patients with ulcerative colitis and diarrhea. Subsequently, two other phenomena were recognized: giant motor contractions and migrating motor complex (85). Giant motor contractions are high-amplitude, rapidly propagated contraction waves, usually seen on walking and following meals, and frequently accompanied by an urge to defecate. The migrating motor complex is a periodic motor activity represented by rhythmic bursts of activity, usually with aboral migration. This activity has been described only in canines; in the human this activity has been found only in the stomach and small bowel (86).

Two types of activity have been detected in colonic electromyographic recordings, rhythmic slow waves and spike bursts (12). Slow waves originate in the circular muscle of the colon; they represent the basal electrical activity. They are events of low frequency, varying from 11 cycles/min in the proximal colon to 6 cycles/min in the sigmoid. In the rectum, the slow wave frequency is about 20 cycles/min, and this distal gradient is thought to inhibit the aboral flow. Spike bursts are associated with short- and long-type contractions, which last 3 to 4 seconds and about 10 to 11 seconds, respectively. Long spike burst activity increases for two hours after each meal and is significantly reduced during sleep. However, to date, colonic myoelectrical activity has not been accurately correlated with colonic organized movements.

The simplest and most easily interpreted colonic transit evaluation requires ingestion of radio-opaque markers and quantification of these markers on abdominal radiographs. The mean values for normal total colonic transit time are about 32 and 41 hours for men and women, respectively. The mean segmental transit times are 12, 14, and 11 hours for right colon, left colon, and rectosigmoid, respectively (87,88). Colonic transit times are related to three types of movements: segmentation, mass, and retrograde movements (85).

Segmentations, also known as haustrations, mixing, or nonpropulsive movements, are large circular constrictions of about 30 seconds' duration occurring at 60-second intervals. The combined contractions of the circular layer and the taeniae coli lead to an outward bulging of the unstimulated segment of the intestine into the haustra, and the fecal bolus is "slowly dug into and rolled over." This movement entails retrograde and anterograde movements of contents within a segment and allows gradual exposure of the fecal bolus to the surface of the large intestine to presumably enhance colonic absorption.

Mass or propulsive movements are responsible for propelling large amounts of feces over long segments of the colon. From a constrictive ring at a distended or irritated point in the colon, a 20 cm or longer segment contracts as a unit and forces the fecal bolus distally within this segment. During a mass movement, the haustrations completely disappear. This type of movement occurs only a few times a day, and is more often seen in the transverse, descending, and sigmoid colons. In fact, these segments may empty together into the rectum to elicit defecation. Finally, retrograde movements may occur, particularly in the transverse ascending segment and are thought to retard distal progression of the fecal bolus.

Colonic Absorption, Stool Volume, and Consistency

The colon absorbs water, sodium, and chloride and secretes potassium and bicarbonate. In healthy individuals, colonic absorption of water reduces the 1000 to 1500 mL of fluid that enters the colon each day to about 100 to 150 mL (89). Continence mechanisms are designed to handle the daily elimination of formed stool. Liquid stool emptied rapidly into the rectum results in great stress on the sphincters and even in normal subjects, phasic flows of liquid stool may occasionally produce urgency and incontinence.

Rectosigmoid Junction
Despite the fact that the rectum is a highly capacious and compliant, during defecation, a two-step pattern of emptying is usually noted; first the sigmoid empties into the rectum and then the rectum evacuates. These facts have suggested an active role of the sigmoid in fecal continence, either as a reservoir or as a functional sphincter (6).

Rectal Capacity and Compliance
Rectal contents must be accommodated if defecation is to be delayed. This deferral of the call to stool is possible through the mechanism of rectal compliance. The nondiseased rectum has elastic properties, which allow it to maintain a low intraluminal pressure while being filled, in order to preserve continence. Contrasted with the high capacity and compliance characteristics of the normal rectum, significantly decreased compliance has been demonstrated in incontinent patients.

Whether poor rectal compliance is a cause or a consequence of fecal incontinence is controversial. The fact that no difference has been found in rectal compliance between patients with idiopathic and those with traumatic incontinence, suggests that decreased rectal compliance is rather a consequence of an incompetent anal sphincter (90). However, it is also plausible that if rectal compliance deteriorates, smaller volumes of feces will result in higher intraluminal pressures, causing urgency and incontinence. This mechanism was observed primarily in patients with ulcerative colitis and radiation proctitis (91,92). Sphincter-saving operations can be associated with incontinence, and the loss of the rectal reservoir is thought to be the main factor; the formation of neorectal pouches, whether ileal or colonic, improves compliance (93,94).

Motility of the Rectum and Anal Canal
The rectum has low resting pressure, about 5 mmHg, with infrequent small-amplitude contractions, at a frequency of about 5 to 10 cycles/min. High-amplitude contractions, up to 100 cm H_2O, of low frequency have been demonstrated, some of which appear to propagate (95). The anal canal typically shows overlapping of resting tone with small oscillations of pressure and with frequency of about 15 cycles/min and amplitude of 10 cm H_2O. Pressure in the anal canal is approximately 10 to 14 times higher than in the rectal canal and slow waves are occasionally observed in the anal canal, with a higher frequency distally. This gradient is thought to play a role in anal continence, by propelling the contents back into the rectum, thereby keeping the anal canal empty.

Rectal Sensation
Rectal sensation involves various complex mechanisms. The rectum itself does not have receptors; proprioceptors are more likely situated in the levators, PR, and anal sphincters. Autonomous smooth muscle and voluntary skeletal muscles are triggered by distinct mechanisms with different thresholds. Diseases such as altered mental conditions (encephalopathy, dementia, and stroke) and sensory neuropathy (diabetes) may selectively reduce conscious sensation and awareness of rectal fullness. Although these patients may not recognize or respond to threats to continence, the autonomic pathways, which mediate the rectoanal inhibitory reflex, may be intact. A fecal bolus in the rectum results in reflex relaxation of the IAS. In these patients, that relaxation occurs before a sensation of rectal distension, which results in both fecal impaction and subsequent overflow incontinence. High conscious rectal sensory thresholds have been observed in patients with fecal incontinence and in 28% of cases, it is most likely the primary cause (96). Although incontinence has been divided into two major groups, sphincter motor dysfunction and sensory deficiency, these disturbances are probably interactive.

Rectoanal Inhibitory Reflex and Anal Sensation
The rectoanal inhibitory reflex, characterized by transient EAS contraction and pronounced IAS reflex relaxation in response to rectal distension, was first described by Gowers in 1877 (Fig. 10) (97). This reflex enables rectal contents to come into contact with the highly sensitive epithelial lining of the upper anal canal. By providing accurate distinction between flatus and feces, this "sampling" mechanism is thought to have a role in the fine adjustment of anal

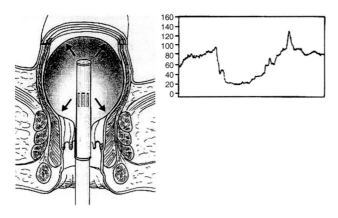

Figure 10 Manometric tracing shows relaxation of the internal anal sphincter during inflation of the balloon.

continence (47). Both reduced anal sensation and defective sampling mechanisms are probably important factors in the pathogenesis of fecal incontinence. When both are abnormal, the patient may be completely unaware of impending incontinence.

Internal Anal Sphincter

The IAS is a smooth muscle in a state of continuous maximum contraction. This tone, which provides a natural barrier to the involuntary loss of stool, is due to both intrinsic myogenic and extrinsic autonomic neurogenic properties. In the composition of the resting tone of the anal canal, the IAS is responsible for 50% to 85%, the EAS accounts for 25% to 30%, and the remaining 15% is attributed to expansion of the anal cushions (98,99).

Although the IAS relaxes in response to rectal distension, it gradually reacquires its tone as the rectum accommodates to the distension. Pronounced impairment of the IAS function without compensatory increase in the activity of the EAS results in fecal incontinence (100).

Skeletal Muscle Responses

The EAS, along with the pelvic floor muscles, maintains continuous unconscious resting electrical tone by unlike other skeletal muscles, that are usually inactive at rest, the EAS along with the pelvic floor muscles maintains continuous unconscious resting electrical tone level, unlike other skeletal muscles, that are usually inactive at rest. Histological studies have shown that the EAS, PR, and levator ani muscles have a predominance of type I fibers, which is characteristic of skeletal muscles of tonic contractile activity (101). In response to conditions of threatened continence, such as increased intra-abdominal pressures and rectal distension, the EAS and PR muscles reflexly or voluntarily contract further to prevent fecal leakage. Due to muscular fatigue, maximal voluntary contraction of the EAS can be sustained for only 40 to 60 seconds. The automatic continence mechanism is then formed by the resting tone, maintained by the IAS, and magnified by reflex EAS contraction. This extra pressure gradient is essential to minimize voluntary attention to the sphincters and, therefore, optimize continence.

PR Muscle and the Anorectal Angle

The anorectal angle represents the result of the anatomic configuration of the U-shaped sling of the PR muscle around the anorectal junction. Whereas the anal sphincters are responsible for closure of the anal canal to retain gas and liquid stool, the PR muscle and the anorectal angle are designed to maintain gross fecal continence. Different theories have been postulated to explain the importance of the PR muscle and the anorectal angle in the maintenance of fecal continence. Parks et al. (67) considered that increasing intra-abdominal pressure forces the anterior rectal wall down into the upper anal canal, occluding it by a type of flap valve mechanism, thus creating an effective seal. Subsequently, it was demonstrated that the flap mechanism in fact does not occur; instead, a continued sphincteric occlusion-like activity attributed to the PR was noted (68).

Sequence of Defecation

Defecation is a complex and incompletely understood phenomenon, related to several integrated mechanisms, all under influence of the central nervous system. Defecation is triggered by filling of the rectum from the sigmoid colon. At a conscious level, rectal distension is interpreted via stretch receptors located in the pelvic floor muscles as a desire to defecate. Rectal distension also initiates the rectoanal inhibitory reflex. The IAS relaxation, by opening the upper anal canal, exposes the rectal contents to the highly sensitive anal mucosa; differentiation between flatus and stool can then be made. This "sampling" mechanism determines the urgency of defecation. Meanwhile, the simultaneous EAS reflex contraction maintains continence. If defecation is to be deferred, conscious contraction of the EAS assisted by the mechanism of rectal compliance yields time for recuperation of the IAS function.

If the call to stool is answered, either the sitting or squatting positions are assumed, and the anorectal angle is then "opened." Increase in both intrarectal and intra-abdominal pressures results in reflex relaxation in the EAS, IAS and PR muscles; at this point, defecation may occur without straining.

Nevertheless, some degree of straining is usually necessary to initiate rectal evacuation. Straining will ensure further relaxation of the anal sphincter muscles and the anorectal angle becomes even more obtuse. Consequently, pelvic floor descending and funneling occurs, and the rectal contents are expelled by direct transmission of the increased abdominal pressure through the relaxed pelvic floor.

REFERENCES

1. Galen (129–200 A.D.) De Sedis Musculis, as quoted by Levy E. Anorectal Musculature. Am J Surg 1936; 32:141–198.
2. Vesalii Bruxellensis Andreae. De humani corporis fabrica de Recti Intestini Musculis. 1st ed. 1543:228.
3. Church JM, Raudkivi PJ, Hill GL. The surgical anatomy of the rectum—a review with particular relevance to the hazards of rectal mobilisation. Int J Colorect Dis 1987; 2:158–166.
4. Shafik A. A concept of the anatomy of the anal sphincter mechanism and the physiology of defecation. Dis Colon Rectum 1987; 30:970–982.
5. Klosterhalfen B, Vogel P, Rixen H, Mitterman C. Topography of the inferior rectal artery. A possible cause of chronic, primary anal fissure. Dis Colon Rectum 1989; 32:43–52.
6. Stoss F. Investigations of the muscular architecture of the rectosigmoid junction in humans. Dis Colon Rectum 1990; 33:378–383.
7. Levi AC, Borghi F, Garavoglia M. Development of the anal canal muscles. Dis Colon Rectum 1991; 34:262–266.
8. Lunniss PJ, Phillips RKS. Anatomy and function of the anal longitudinal muscle. Br J Surg 1992; 79:882–884.
9. Tjandra JJ, Milsom Jw, Stolfi VM,et al. Endoluminal ultrasound defines anatomy of the anal canal and pelvic floor. Dis Colon Rectum 1992; 35:465–470.
10. Dobson HD, Pearl RK, Orsay CP, et al. Virtual reality: new method of teaching anorectal and pelvic floor anatomy. Dis Colon Rectum 2003; 46:349–352.
11. Shafik A. A new concept of the anatomy of the anal sphincter mechanism and the physiology of defecation II. Anatomy of the levator ani muscle with special reference to puborectalis. Invest Urol 1975; 13:175–182.
12. Pemberton JH. Anatomy and physiology of the anus and the rectum. In: Zuidema GD, ed. Shackelford's Surgery of the Alimentary Tract. Philadelphia: WB Saunders, 1991:242–273.
13. Paramore RH. The Hunterian lectures on the evolution of the pelvic floor in non-mammalian vertebrates and pronograde mammals. Lancet 1910; 1:1393–1399, 1459–1467.
14. Romolo JL. Congenital lesions: intussusception and volvulus. In: Zuidema GD, ed. Shackelford's Surgery of the Alimentary Tract. Philadelphia: WB Saunders, 1991:45–51.
15. Guyton AC. Textbook of Medical Physiology. Philadelphia: WB Saunders, 1986:754–769.
16. Kumar D, Phillips SF. The contribution of external ligamentous attachments to function of the ileocecal junction. Dis Colon Rectum 1987; 30:410–416.
17. Wakeley CPG.The position of the vermiform appendix as ascertained by an analysis of 10,000 cases. J Anat 1983; 67:277–283.
18. Goligher J. Surgery of the anus, rectum and colon. London: BaillièreTindall, 1984:1–47.
19. Nivatvongs S, Gordon PH. Surgical anatomy. In: Gordon PH, Nivatvongs S, eds. Principle and Practice of Surgery for the Colon, Rectum and Anus. St Louis: Quality Medical Publishing Inc, 1992:3–37.
20. Skandalakis JE, Gray SW, Ricketts R. The colon and rectum. In: Skandalakis JE, Gray SW, eds. Embryology for Surgeons. The Embryological Basis for the Treatment of Congenital Anomalies. Baltimore: Williams & Wilkins, 1994:242–281.
21. Ewing MR. The significance of the level of the peritoneal reflection in the surgery of rectal cancer. Br J Surg 1952; 39:495–500.

22. O'Beirne J. New views of the process of defecation and their application to the pathology and treatment of diseases of the stomach, bowels and other organs. Dublin: Hodges and Smith, 1833.
23. Mayo WJ. A study of the rectosigmoid. Surg Gynecol Obstet 1917; 25:616–621.
24. Cantlie J. The sigmoid flexure in health and disease. J Trop Med Hyg 1915; 18:1–7.
25. Houston J. Observation on the mucous membrane of the rectum. Dublin Hospital Reports Commun Med Surg 1830; 5:158–165.
26. Abramson DJ. The valves of Houston in adults. Am J Surg 1978; 136:334–336.
27. Heald RJ, Husband EM, Ryall RD. The mesorectum in rectal cancer surgery—the clue to pelvic recurrence? Br J Surg 1982; 69:613–616.
28. Boxall TA, Smart PJG, Griffiths JD. The blood-supply of the distal segment of the rectum in anterior resection. Brit J Surg 1963(50):399–404.
29. Cawthorn SJ, Parums DV, Gibbs NM, et al. Extent of mesorectal spread and involvement of lateral resection margin as prognostic factors after surgery for rectal cancer. Lancet 1990; 335:1055–1059.
30. Quirke P, Durdey P, Dixon MF, Williams NS. Local recurrence of rectal adenocarcinoma due to inadequate surgical resection. Histopathological study of lateral tumour spread and surgical excision. Lancet 1986; 1:996–998.
31. Quinyao W, Weijin S, Youren Z, Wenqing Z, Zhengrui H. New concepts in severe presacral hemorrhage during proctectomy. Arch Surg 1985; 120:1013–1020.
32. Zama N, Fazio VW, Jagelman DG, Lavery IC, Weakley FL, Church JM. Efficacy of pelvic packing in maintaining hemostasis after rectal excision for cancer. Dis Colon Rectum 1988; 31:923–928.
33. Jorge, JMN, Habr-Gama A, Souza Jr AS, Kiss DR, Nahas P, Pinotti HW. Rectal surgery complicated by massive presacral hemorrhage. Arq Bras Cir Dig 1990; 5:92–95.
34. Crapp AR, Cuthbertson AM. William Waldeyer and the rectosacral fascia. Surg Gynecol Obstet 1974; 138:252–256.
35. Lindsey I, Guy RJ, Warren BF, McC Mortensen NJ. Anatomy of Denonvilliers' fascia and pelvic nerves, impotence, and implications for the colorectal surgeon. Br J Surg 2000; 87:1288–1299.
36. Bauer JJ, Gerlent IM, Salky B, Kreel I. Sexual dysfunction following proctectomy for benign disease of the colon and rectum. Ann Surg 1983; 197:363–367.
37. Gerstenberg TC, Nielsen ML, Clausen S, Blaabjerg J, Lindenberg J. Bladder function after abdominoperineal resection of the rectum for anorectal cancer. Am J Surg 1980; 91:81–86.
38. Orkin BA. Rectal carcinoma: treatment. In: Beck DE, Wexner SD. Fundamentals of Anorectal Surgery. New York: McGraw-Hill, Inc. 1992:260–369.
39. Danzi M, Ferulano GP, Abate S, Califano G. Male sexual function after abdominoperineal resection for rectal cancer. Dis Colon Rectum 1983; 26:665–658.
40. Balslev I, Harling H. Sexual dysfunction following operation for carcinoma of the rectum. Dis Colon Rectum 1983; 26:785–788.
41. Walsh PC, Schlegel PN. Radical pelvic surgery with preservation of sexual function. Ann Surg 1988; 208:391–400.
42. Lee ECG, Dowling BL. Perimuscular excision of the rectum for Crohn's disease and ulcerative colitis. A conservative technique. Br J Surg 1972; 59:29–32.
43. Metcalf AM, Dozois RR, Kelly KA. Sexual function in women after proctocolectomy. Ann Surg 1986; 204:624–627.
44. Burnham WR, Lennard-Jones JE, Brooke BN. Sexual problems among married ileostomists. Gut 1977; 18:673–677.
45. Petter O, Gruner N, Reidar N, et al. Marital status and sexual adjustment after colectomy. Scand J Gastrol 1977; 12:193–197.
46. Nobles VP. The development of the human anal canal. J Anat 1984; 138:575.
47. Duthie HL, Gairns FW. Sensory nerve endings and sensation in the anal region in man. Br J Surg 1960; 47:585–595.
48. Lilius HG. Investigation of human fetal anal ducts and intramuscular glands and a clinical study of 150 patients. Acta Chir Scand (suppl) 1968; 383:1–88.
49. Parks AG. Pathogenesis and treatment of fistula-in-ano. Br Med J 1961; 1:463–469.
50. Ewing MR. The white line of Hilton. Proc R Soc Med 1954; 47:525–530.
51. Ricciardi R, Counihan TC, Banner BF, Sweeney WB. What is the normal aganglionic segment of anorectum in adults?. Dis Colon Rectum 1999; 42:380–382.
52. Wendell-Smith CP. Studies on the morphology of the pelvic floor. Ph.D. Thesis, University of London, 1967.
53. Cuesta MA, Meijer S, Derksen EJ, Boutkan H, Meuwissen SGM. Anal sphincter imaging in fecal incontinence using endosonography. Dis Colon Rectum 1992; 35:59–63.
54. Jorge JMN, Habr-Gama A. The value of sphincteric asymmetry index analysis in anal incontinence. Dis Colon Rectum 1997; 40:A14–A15.
55. Taylor BM, Beart RW, Phillips SF. Longitudinal and radial variations of pressure in the human anal sphincter. Gastroenterology 1984; 86:693–697.
56. Braun JC, Treutner KH, Dreuw B, Klimaszewski M, Schlumpelick V. Vectormanometry for differential diagnosis of fecal incontinence. Dis Colon Rectum 1994; 37:989–996.

57. Milligan ETC, Morgan CN. Surgical anatomy of the anal canal: with special reference to anorectal fistulae. Lancet 1934; 2:1150–1156.
58. Shafik A. A new concept of the anatomy of the anal sphincter mechanism and the physiology of defecation III. The longitudinal anal muscle: anatomy and role in sphincter mechanism. Invest Urol 1976; 13:271–277.
59. Lawson JON. Pelvic anatomy II. Anal canal and associated sphincters. Ann R Coll Surg Engl 1974; 54:288–300.
60. Roux C. Contribution to the knowledge of the anal muscles in man. Arch Mikr Anat 1881; 19:721–723.
61. Courtney H. Anatomy of the pelvic diaphragm and anorectal musculature as related to sphincter preservation in anorectal surgery. Am J Surg 1950; 79:155–173.
62. Haas PA, Fox TA. The importance of the perianal connective tissue in the surgical anatomy and function of the anus. Dis Colon Rectum 1977; 20:303–313.
63. Goligher JC, Leacock AG, Brossy JJ. The surgical anatomy of the anal canal. Br J Surg 1955; 43:51–61.
64. Oh C, Kark AE. Anatomy of the external anal sphincter. Br J Surg 1972; 59:717–723.
65. Fritsch H, Brenner E, Lienemann A, Ludwikowski B. Anal sphincter complex: reinterpreted morphology and its clinical relevance. Dis Colon rectum 2002; 45:188–194.
66. Williamson RCN, Mortensen NJMcC. Anatomy of the large intestine. In: Kirsner JB, Shorter RG, eds. Diseases of the Colon, Rectum and Anal Canal. Rochester, Minnesota: Williams & Wilkins, 1987:1–22.
67. Parks AG, Porter NH, Hardcastle J. The syndrome of the descending perineum. Proc R Soc Med 1966; 59:477–482.
68. Bartolo DCC, Roe AM, Locke-Edmunds JC, Virjee J, Mortensen NJMcC. Flap-valve theory of anorectal continence. Br J Surg 1986; 73:1012–1014.
69. Bannister JJ, Gibbons C, Read NW. Preservation of faecal continence during rises in intra-abdominal pressure: is there a role for the flap valve? Gut 1987; 28:1242–1245.
70. Percy JP, Swash M, Neill ME, Parks AG. Electrophysiological study of motor nerve supply of pelvic floor. Lancet 1981; 1:16–17.
71. Russell KP. Anatomy of the pelvic floor, rectum and anal canal. In: Smith LE, eds. Practical Guide to Anorectal Testing. New York: Ygaku-Shoin Medical Publishers, Inc, 1991:744–747.
72. Garavoglia M, Borghi F, Levi AC. Arrangement of the anal striated musculature. Dis Colon Rectum 1993; 36:10–15.
73. Courtney H. Posterior subsphincteric space. Its relation to posterior horseshoe fistula. Surg Gynecol Obstet 1949; 89:222–226.
74. Ayoub SF. Arterial supply of the human rectum. Acta Anat 1978; 100:317–327.
75. Didio LJA, Diaz-Franco C, Schemainda R, Bezerra AJC. Morphology of the middle rectal arteries: a study of 30 cadaveric dissections. Surg Radiol Anat 1986; 8:229–236.
76. Michels NA, Siddharth P, Kornblith PL, Park WW. The variant blood supply to the small and large intestines: its importance in regional resections. A new anatomic study based on four hundred dissections with a complete review of the literature. J Int Col Surg 1963; 39:127–170.
77. Bernstein WC. What are hemorrhoids and what is their relationship to the portal venous system? Dis Colon Rectum 1983; 26:829–834.
78. Miscusi G, Masoni L, Dell'Anna A, Montori A. Normal lymphatic drainage of the rectum and the canal anal revealed by lymphoscintigraphy. Coloproctology 1987; 9:171–174.
79. Block IR, Enquist IF. Studies pertaining to local spread of carcinoma of the rectum in females. Surg Gynecol Obstet 1961; 112:41–46.
80. Jorge JMN, Wexner SD. A practical guide to basic anorectal physiology. Contemp Surg 1993; 43:214.
81. Wexner SD, Jorge JMN. Colorectal physiological tests: use or abuse of technology? Eur J Surg 1994; 160:167–174.
82. Jorge JMN, Wexner SD. Etiology and management of fecal incontinence. Dis Colon Rectum 1993; 36:77–97.
83. Wexner SD, Daniel N, Jagelman DG. Colectomy for constipation: physiologic investigation is the key to success. Dis Colon Rectum 1991; 34:851–856.
84. Adler HF, Atkinson AJ, Ivy AC. Supplementary and synergistic action of stimulating drugs on motility of human colon. Surg Gynecol Obstet 1942; 74:809–813.
85. Kumar D, Wingate DL. Colorectal motility. In: Henry MM, Swash M, eds. Coloproctology and the Pelvic Floor. Oxford: Butterworth-Heinemann Ltd, 1992:72–85.
86. Sarna SK, Condon R, Cowles V. Colonic migrating and non-migrating motor complexes in dogs. Am J Physiol 1984; 246:G355–360.
87. Arhan P, Devroede G, Jehannin B, et al. Segmental colonic transit time. Dis Colon Rectum 1981; 24:625–629.
88. Jorge JMN, Habr-Gama A. Tempo de trânsito colônico total e segmentar: análise crítica dos métodos e estudo em indivíduos normais com marcadores radiopacos. Rev Bras Colo Proct 1991(11):55–60.
89. Phillips SF, Giller J. The contribution of the colon to the electrolyte and water absorption in man. J Lab Clin Med 1973; 81:733–746.
90. Rasmussen O, Christiensen B, Sorensen M, Tetzchner T, Christiansen J. Rectal compliance in the assessment of patients with fecal incontinence. Dis Colon Rectum 1990; 33:650–653.

91. Denis Ph, Colin R, Galmiche JP, et al. Elastic properties of the rectal wall in normal adults and in patients with ulcerative colitis. Gastroenterology 1979; 77:45–48.
92. Varma JS, Smith AN, Busuttil A. Correlation of clinical and manometric abnormalities of rectal function following chronic radiation injury. Br J Surg 1985; 72:875–878.
93. Parks AG, Nicholls RJ. Proctocolectomy without ileostomy for ulcerative colitis. Br Med J 1978; 2:85–88.
94. Wexner SD, James K, Jagelman DG. The double stapled ileal reservoir and ileoanal anastomosis: a prospective review of sphincter function and clinical outcome. Dis Colon Rectum 1991; 34:487–494.
95. Scharli AF, Kiesewetter WB. Defecation and continence: some new concepts. Dis Colon Rectum 1970; 13:81–107.
96. Buser WD, Miner PB Jr. Delayed rectal sensation with fecal incontinence. Dis Colon Rectum 1991; 34:744–747.
97. Gowers WR. The automatic action of the sphincter ani. Proc R Soc Lond 1877; 26:77–84.
98. Frenckner B, Euler CHRV. Influence of pudendal block on the function of the anal sphincters. Gut 1975; 16:482–489.
99. Lestar B, Penninckx F, Kerremans R. The composition of anal basal pressure. An in vivo and in vitro study in man. Int J Colorect Dis 1989; 4:118–122.
100. Sun WM, Read NW, Donnelly TC. Impaired internal anal sphincter in a subgroup of patients with idiopathic fecal incontinence. Gastroenterology 1989; 97:130–135.
101. Swash M. Histopathology of pelvic floor muscles in pelvic floor disorders. In: Henry MM, Swash M, eds. Coloproctology and the Pelvic Floor. London: Butterworth-Heinemann Ltd, 1992:173–183.

Part II | DISORDERS OF FUNCTION

2 | Colonic and Rectal Obstruction

Jorge Marcet
Department of Surgery, University of South Florida, Tampa, Florida, U.S.A.

H. Juergen Nord
Department of Medicine, University of South Florida, Tampa, Florida, U.S.A.

Orit Kaidar-Person
Department of Colorectal Surgery, Cleveland Clinic Florida, Weston, Florida, U.S.A.

INTRODUCTION

Obstruction of the large intestine is a serious medical problem requiring urgent attention and intervention. A variety of conditions can result in bowel obstruction, most commonly colorectal cancer, volvulus, and diverticular disease. The onset of obstruction may be gradual, as seen in patients with sigmoid cancer, or acute, as in those with sigmoid volvulus. Symptoms of obstruction include abdominal pain and distension and obstipation. Recent advances in medical care have changed the therapeutic approach to patients with obstruction, including more frequent use of one-stage surgical procedures and nonoperative methods for palliation. An understanding of the etiology of large bowel obstruction and the methodology for appropriate intervention is necessary to assure optimal outcome.

ETIOLOGY

In adults, the most common cause of colon obstruction is colonic adenocarcinoma (1). One study, which included 300 patients treated by emergent surgery for large bowel obstruction, found that colorectal cancer, volvulus, and diverticular disease accounted for 53%, 17%, and 12% of cases of colonic obstruction, respectively (Table 1) (2). In another series of 4583 patients with colorectal cancer, 16% presented with obstructive symptoms, and approximately half required emergency decompression (3). The splenic flexure was the most common location, accounting for 49% of the obstructing lesions. Left and right colonic obstructive lesions were equally distributed, each accounting for 23%. Only 6% of the obstructing tumors were located in the rectum. Obstruction from colon cancer tends to have an insidious onset as the neoplasm gradually envelops the bowel lumen. Most patients recount a history of symptoms of several months' duration.

Volvulus results from torsion of a portion of the intestine, along its long axis. This rotation results in a closed loop of intestine and an obstruction proximal to the volvulus. As a result, intestinal ischemia may occur from torsion of the mesentery. The volvulus occurs at sites where the colon is freely mobile and not fixed to the retroperitoneum, such as the sigmoid colon, cecum, and ascending colon and, rarely, the transverse colon.

Diverticular disease can cause colonic obstruction during an episode of diverticulitis from circumferential inflammation of the intestine or extrinsic compression from an abscess. Repeated episodes of diverticulitis or chronic diverticulitis cause fibrosis, which can lead to stricture and obstruction. Less common causes of mechanical bowel obstruction include hernia, inflammatory bowel disease, fecal impaction, ischemic stricture, radiation stricture, rectal or colonic intussusception, and presence of foreign body. Pseudo-obstruction, or Ogilvie's syndrome, is a nonobstructive form of colonic ileus that mimics the signs and symptoms of mechanical obstruction.

Table 1 Causes of Colon Obstruction Requiring Surgery

Cause	Percent
Colorectal cancer	53
Volvulus	17
Diverticular disease	12
Extrinsic obstruction from metastatic disease	6
Other	12
Stricture	
Hernia	
Fecal impaction	
Pseudo-obstruction	
Adhesions	

Source: From Ref. 2.

PATHOPHYSIOLOGY

Large bowel obstruction can result in alterations in the intestinal blood flow and in the intestinal flora. The duration and degree of obstruction, as well as the competency of the ileocecal valve, determine the local and systemic pathophysiologic consequences. A closed loop obstruction occurs when the ileocecal valve is competent. Obstruction causes accumulation of intestinal contents and swallowed air in the intestinal lumen. As intraluminal pressure increases, the capillary pressure is exceeded and blood flow to the colonic mucosa decreases (4). Impairment of water and electrolyte absorption and enhanced electrolyte secretion may result in transudation of fluids from the intravascular space into the intestinal lumen (5).

Experimental animal studies on colonic obstruction have shown that blood flow proximal to the obstruction actually increases (6). In one study using a pig model, blood flow in the cecum decreased while the flow in the left colon increased, suggesting a possible explanation of why perforation from large bowel obstruction usually occurs in the cecum (7). Another explanation for why the cecum is most likely to perforate in the obstructed colon is because it has the greatest diameter than that of other colonic segments. This follows the Law of Laplace in which tension on the wall of a vessel is proportional to the pressure times the radius.

Bacterial overgrowth, from loss of normal intestinal motility, plays an important role in the pathophysiology of intestinal obstruction. Bacterial translocation through the intestinal wall is more likely to occur in the obstructed bowel (8). In one study, patients with bowel obstruction were significantly more likely to have gut bacteria cultured in the mesenteric lymph nodes, and this resulted in a statistically significant increase in postoperative infections (9).

CLINICAL PRESENTATION

The clinical presentation will vary depending on the etiology of obstruction, the degree of obstruction, and the duration of symptoms. With partial obstruction, patients may complain of abdominal bloating and change in bowel habits, including a decrease in stool frequency, a decrease in the caliber of stools, alternating diarrhea and constipation, a decreased appetite, and intermittent abdominal distension. Symptoms of partial bowel obstruction often precede complete obstruction for weeks or months. With complete obstruction, patients have abdominal distension and pain, and cessation of bowel movements. These patients are of particular concern due to the risk of bowel perforation if the obstruction is not relieved in a timely manner.

Patients with a late presentation of colonic obstruction may have significant weight loss due to decreased food intake. When the ileocecal valve is compromised, nausea and vomiting may occur, resulting in dehydration and electrolyte abnormalities. Peritonitis may result from perforation secondary to colonic overdistension, ischemic necrosis, diverticulitis, or cancer. Pain may arise from intestinal distension by air, intestinal ischemia, infection, or a deeply invasive cancer.

Acute colonic obstruction most often occurs from a colonic volvulus. Patients may recount a history of similar symptoms that spontaneously resolved or required nonoperative intervention with resolution of symptoms.

EVALUATION
Clinical History

Patients are queried regarding the duration of symptoms, prior episodes of similar events, presence of blood in the stool, bloating, decrease in appetite, weight loss, vomiting, and pain. A history is obtained regarding prior abdominal surgery, intestinal diseases, and bowel habits. The patient's age also plays a role. While colorectal cancer increases significantly after the age of 50, most patients with malignant obstruction are in their sixth and seventh decades of life. A family history of colorectal polyps and cancer is also important to note.

Physical Exam

A general physical assessment is performed with emphasis on the vital signs and state of hydration. The abdomen is examined for distention, guarding, peritoneal signs, tympani on palpation, hernia, the presence of a mass, and ascites. Digital rectal examination evaluates for fecal impaction, a rectal mass, pain, anal or rectal stenosis, and gross or occult blood in the stool. Rigid proctosigmoidoscopy or flexible sigmoidoscopy is carefully undertaken, introducing minimal air into the rectum.

Diagnostic Studies

Initial laboratory assessment includes a complete blood count. The white blood cell count may be elevated due to dehydration or as a result of infection. Anemia, especially microcytic, in a patient with colonic obstruction alludes to a likely malignant etiology. Blood chemistry is analyzed for electrolyte abnormalities that may occur as a result of vomiting. An elevated blood urea nitrogen and creatinine may result from dehydration.

Abdominal X Rays

Plain abdominal radiography is a simple and noninvasive procedure with high diagnostic value. Radiographs may show colonic distention and help distinguish large bowel from small bowel obstruction. The classic radiological signs of proximal colon dilation and absence of air in the distal colon or rectum are pathognomonic for a mechanical colon obstruction. However, it has been demonstrated that the presence or absence of air in the rectum is not an important radiological sign in determining colon obstruction (10). If the ileocecal valve is compromised, the small intestine may also become distended. Small intestinal distension without large intestinal distension is indicative of a small bowel obstruction. In a review by Chapman et al. (11), the sensitivity of plain radiographs was 84% and the specificity was 72%, in the diagnosis of large bowel obstruction. Even when mechanical obstruction was correctly diagnosed, the site of obstruction was incorrectly identified in 35% of patients.

Sigmoid volvulus may appear on plain abdominal radiographs as a markedly distended ahaustral loop of bowel with a bent inner-tube appearance (bird's beak sign). In regard to cecal volvulus, the cecum may be displaced into another part of the abdomen, often toward the midline and the upper abdomen. A ''coffee bean'' shape has been described as a radiographic sign (12). In a review of 58 cases of colonic volvulus, Friedman et al. found that plain radiographs alone allowed diagnosis in 43% of patients (13).

Contrast Enema

If proctosigmoidoscopy fails to identify the cause of obstruction, a water-soluble contrast enema examination is indicated to confirm the diagnosis of mechanical large bowel obstruction. Barium is not used due to the risk of intraperitoneal extravasation. Furthermore, it may prevent the subsequent need for endoscopy if the barium cannot be fully evacuated. It is important to avoid colonic overdistension due to the risk of perforation.

The procedure is performed under fluoroscopic guidance using a tilt table, while instilling the water-soluble contrast by means of gravity. Prior bowel preparation is not required, therefore this test can be performed on an urgent basis. The contrast agent may abruptly stop at the site of a complete obstruction. Occasionally, a small amount of contrast is able to pass a partially obstructing lesion. In such cases, it is not necessary to continue the examination to fill the remainder of the colon. The purpose of the study is only to determine the site, degree, and type of obstruction. This study is not intended to provide accurate mucosal detail.

Water-soluble contrast enema examination of the colon was associated with a sensitivity and specificity of 96% and 98%, respectively (11).

Contrast enema can also distinguish distal colonic obstruction from pseudo-obstruction—a differentiation that may often be challenging. The high-osmolarity contrast medium is an excellent aid in cleansing the colon in preparation for endoscopic decompression in cases of pseudo-obstruction. A contrast enema can, at least temporarily, resolve a volvulus especially in the sigmoid colon.

Computed Tomography

Computed tomography (CT) may be useful when the etiology of the obstruction cannot be determined by the above-mentioned studies (14). This study may show bowel wall thickening and mesenteric fat stranding, characteristic of the radiographic changes noted in diverticulitis or diverticular abscess. When extrinsic compression of the colon wall is suspected, CT may identify a mass resulting from pelvic or intraperitoneal malignancy. If the etiology of large bowel obstruction is from suspected or known colorectal cancer, then CT of the abdomen and pelvis with intravenous contrast, and in cases of partial obstruction with oral contrast, is undertaken to preoperative disease staging.

Endoscopy

Colonoscopy is capable of localizing the obstruction and also has diagnostic and potentially therapeutic capabilities. The disadvantage inherent to endoscopic procedures in patients with large bowel obstruction is that the colon cannot be adequately prepped, because laxatives and colonic purges are contraindicated. A meticulous technique in which minimal air is introduced is paramount due to the risk of perforation in an already dilated proximal colon. Colonoscopy can unwind a sigmoid volvulus, but is less successful in realigning a cecal volvulus. Colonic strictures can be biopsied via colonoscopy, stented as a temporizing measure prior to surgery, or therapeutically dilated. In pseudo-obstruction, colonoscopy not only confirms the diagnosis but also deflates the colon, thus reducing the risk of perforation. Endoscopic placement of a long decompression tube to at least proximal to the splenic flexure will usually effectively treat this condition. In one study of 24 patients with suspected Ogilvie's syndrome, colonoscopy identified four patients (17%) with mechanical bowel obstruction (15).

Colonoscopic examination in the patient with large bowel obstruction is preferably performed after prepping the patient with a tap-water enema. Laxatives should never be given to a patient with suspected large bowel obstruction because increased colonic distension may occur, thereby increasing the risk of perforation. Colonoscopy is contraindicated in patients with peritoneal signs because the condition may worsen.

Caution should be taken with air insufflation because the bowel is already distended and additional air increases the risk of perforation. One modification of the usual technique is to shut off the air in the insufflation pump of the light source and, instead, infuse water manually or with a pump. The water sufficiently distends the bowel lumen, is transparent for proper mucosal visualization, and does not lead to overdistention with air or trapping of air proximal to the obstruction that cannot be aspirated. A similar technique is used for colonoscopy in the management of pseudo-obstruction.

Endoscopy can be performed at the bedside with minimal or no sedation. In most cases, it is not necessary to reach the cecum. The goal of endoscopy in these circumstances is to diagnose the cause of the obstruction and to intervene therapeutically, if necessary. For malignant obstruction, the location of the tumor is noted and a determination is made by the endoscopic appearance as to whether the tumor is intrinsic or extrinsic; biopsies are performed for tissue confirmation.

TREATMENT
Initial Management

The initial treatment of a suspected or known large bowel obstruction is to withhold all oral intake and stabilize the patient. Intravenous hydration is initiated and dehydration is corrected. Patients with vomiting, abdominal distension, or complete obstruction should have nasogastric tube decompression. However, in the absence of concomitant small bowel distension, a nasogastric tube is ineffective in decompressing a distended colon. Anemia, which is often seen in patients with colorectal cancer, is corrected by transfusion of packed red blood

Table 2   Treatment Options in Colon and Rectal Obstruction

Multistage resections
Two-stage resections (Hartmann's procedure)
Subtotal colectomy (one-stage resection)
Segmental resection with on-table lavage
Colostomy
Cecostomy
Debulking by endoscopic snare and electrocoagulation
Recanalization with neodymium-doped; yttrium aluminum garnet laser or argon plasma coagulator
Endoluminal stenting

cells, if necessary. Electrolyte abnormalities are corrected and rehydration is monitored by the urine output. Patients with heart disease may require central venous pressure monitoring and even Swan–Ganz catheterization for optimal surveillance of the cardiac function during intravenous fluid resuscitation. With suspected infection such as with diverticulitis, empiric broad-spectrum antibiotic therapy is instituted (Table 2).

Urgent Surgery

Patients with perforation or peritonitis are prepared for urgent surgery. Initial resuscitation with fluids, nasogastric tube decompression, and correction of electrolyte, coagulation, and hematologic abnormalities is expeditiously performed. Potential ostomy sites are marked on both sides of the abdomen and the patient is placed in the low lithotomy position, allowing for access to the abdomen and rectum. Broad-spectrum antibiotics for coverage of aerobic and anaerobic bacteria are started. Rapid sequence induction anesthesia is preferred to prevent aspiration of gastric contents, because the stomach may not have been adequately preoperatively decompressed. The abdomen is explored through a midline incision and specific care is taken to avoid rupture of a critically dilated colon. Initial assessment of the peritoneal cavity is undertaken to rule out perforation or ischemic bowel. Peritoneal fluid cultures are taken if the fluid is purulent or grossly contaminated.

The surgical treatment will depend on the etiology of the obstruction. The quickest procedure to facilitate resolution of the obstruction should be considered. The options for surgical treatment include proximal colostomy alone, resection of the obstructing lesion with proximal colostomy, or resection and reanastomosis with or without proximal diversion. In cases of abdominal gross contamination, resection of the obstructing lesion with proximal colostomy (Hartmann's procedure) is performed. A proximal diverting colostomy without resection may be considered in an unstable patient, in a patient with carcinomatosis, or when the surgeon is less experienced in the management of major colon resections. With the exception of carcinomatosis, the cause of obstruction can be investigated once the patient has recovered. If further surgery is contemplated to remove the source of obstruction, this is planned at least six weeks after the initial colostomy. Resection of the obstructing lesion, takedown of the colostomy, and primary anastomosis are done at the second surgery. In reality, this approach is rarely indicated.

For more than a century, unprepared bowel and the presence of feces in the lumen during bowel surgery were considered to be associated with higher rates of anastomotic leakage, anastomotic dehiscence, and septic complications. Mechanical bowel preparation was considered as an essential part of the preoperative preparation. However, reports from emergency trauma surgeries suggested that primary colonic anastomosis could be safely performed without prior bowel preparation. Currently, numerous prospective randomized trials and several meta-analyses have documented that there is no conclusive evidence that mechanical bowel preparation is associated with reduced rates of anastomotic leakage and septic complications after elective colorectal surgery; on the contrary, there is evidence that mechanical bowel preparation may be associated with an increased rate of anastomotic leakage and septic complications (16–19).The surgeon must remember that these trials have included only patients undergoing elective surgery. The bacterial flora in the emergency setting may be very different and therefore may not translate to the obstructed bowel. Moreover at the time of this writing, bowel preparation is routinely utilized in North America (20).

In cases of emergency surgery due to acute colonic obstruction, a single-stage procedure such as resection with a primary anastomosis is not the common practice. Different techniques such as intraoperative decompression and on-table bowel lavage have been used to allow bowel cleansing and decompression prior to primary anastomosis. However, a few studies demonstrated that resection and primary anastomosis could be performed with acceptable morbidity and mortality in cases of emergency large bowel conditions (such as malignant bowel obstruction) with ileocolic, ileorectal, or colocolonic anastomoses without the need for preoperative or intraoperative mechanical bowel preparation (21–23).

Intraoperative Decompression

Decompression of the large bowel, especially when massively distended, will facilitate subsequent intra-abdominal dissection and may reduce the risk of intraoperative rupture. This maneuver can be accomplished with a large-bore intravenous needle (12 or 14 gauge) or a rubber catheter. Prior to needle or catheter placement, a purse string suture is placed around the site of insertion and laparotomy sponges are placed around the operating field to protect against fecal spillage. The colonic gas is aspirated first because the liquid contents will often obstruct the catheter. The purse string suture is tied after removing the catheter, thus closing the hole in the colon. The insertion site is usually chosen within an area to be resected or converted to a stoma. Alternatively, the appendix can be removed and its base aperture can be used to facilitate this method.

Intraoperative Colonic Lavage

Contraindications to primary anastomosis include hemodynamic instability, markedly dilated bowel, ischemia, and intraperitoneal contamination. If there are no contraindications for a primary anastomosis, an intraoperative colonic lavage should be considered. Although the efficacy of intraoperative colonic lavage is still in dispute (22), several studies have suggested that this intervention is associated with a reduced rate of anastomotic dehiscence (24,25). On-table lavage is carefully undertaken in order to prevent contamination of the operative field. After resection of the obstructing lesion, the transected end of the proximal colon is brought over the side of the patient and allowed to empty into a large sterile bag. Alternatively, a large-bore tube, such as respirator tubing, can be secured in the colonic lumen and allowed to drain over the side of the table into a collection bag. The proximal colon is irrigated antegrade via a 12 or 14 French catheter placed through the appendiceal orifice. Warm saline is used for irrigation until the effluent is clear. Advantages of intraoperative colonic lavage in cases of acute colonic obstruction include the possibility of performing a single-stage procedure with primary anastomosis without the need for a stoma. Disadvantages of this procedure include prolonged operative time, the use of a large amount of solution to achieve proper irrigation, and a higher possibility for spillage and contamination. These data predate the ever-expanding pool of literature advocating the elimination of any bowel preparation.

Resection of the obstructing lesion and proximal colon with ileocolic or ileorectal anastomosis or a one-stage surgical procedure should be considered if the patient is stable and there are no contraindications to anastomosis. One prospective, nonrandomized study compared subtotal colectomy and intraoperative colonic lavage with primary anastomosis. The complication rate was significantly higher in the intraoperative lavage group (42% vs. 14%). The mean operating time was also significantly higher in the lavage group. Although early postoperative diarrhea was seen in approximately one-third of patients in the subtotal colectomy group, disabling diarrhea persisted in only two (6%) patients (22).

A cecostomy is sometimes indicated in the management of patients with colonic obstruction. The cecostomy functions to vent the colon, thus preventing overdistension by air. The cecostomy does not function in the same capacity as a colostomy in that it is not a reliable outlet for stool. A tube cecostomy is performed similar to an open gastrostomy tube insertion. A purse string suture of nonabsorbable material is placed around the cecostomy tube insertion site. Additional nonabsorbable sutures anchor the cecum to the abdominal wall. The tube is kept patent by daily irrigations. When decompression is no longer required, the tube is removed and the wound should close spontaneously. For long-term decompression, a sutured cecostomy helps avoid the problem of tube displacement or clogging. The serosal surface of the cecum is sutured to the peritoneum through a small right lower quadrant incision. Once the peritoneal cavity has been walled off, the cecum is opened and sutured to the skin (26). A sutured cecostomy requires that a colostomy appliance be worn. Another disadvantage to this procedure is that surgery is required for subsequent closure of the cecostomy. The treatment of cecal volvulus and colonic pseudo-obstruction is discussed in the following sections under the management of these conditions.

Endoluminal Decompression

In patients not requiring urgent surgery, diagnostic colonoscopy is performed and endoluminal treatments are considered. Endoluminal decompression may be performed by endoscopic tumor debulking, laser recanalization, or endoluminal stenting. Large exophytic tumors are debulked most efficiently using a large monopolar polypectomy snare. The neodymium-doped yttrium aluminum garnet laser is primarily used for coagulation of the intraluminal and exophytic portions of the tumor, which cannot be removed by snare resection. Coagulation of the entire cancer surface is done from the proximal to the distal end. Tumor necrosis and sloughing occurs over the next several days. Treatments can be repeated weekly until adequate recanalization occurs. The procedure is repeated at monthly intervals thereafter, or as necessary to maintain lumen patency or to stop bleeding. The laser is set to deliver one- to two-second pulses at 70 to 80 W. The tip of the laser-emitting fiber is held 5 to 10 mm from the tissue during the treatment. All persons in the treatment room, including the patient, wear protective goggles to shield the eyes from scattered laser light. One must be aware that coaxial gas (CO_2) insufflation has the potential for further colonic distention. Frequent aspiration is required during the procedure. The procedure is usually well tolerated and side effects such as rectal bleeding and drainage from sloughing of the necrotic tissues are minimal (27). Laser treatment only affects the intraluminal growth of the tumor, but fails to control the extraluminal growth. Yttrium aluminum garnet laser therapy, applied as the sole modality, is effective for short-term palliation of incurable colorectal cancer; however, in most patients, it is not adequate for long-term palliation (28).

Argon plasma coagulation is another coagulation alternative for ablation of any residual tumor after snare resection. All of these methods apply primarily for lesions in the rectosigmoid region. More proximal lesions are more difficult to manage and carry an increased risk for perforation. Complications include bleeding, perforation, and stricture formation especially in lesions involving two-thirds or more of the bowel circumference. Bacteremia occurs with laser therapy and patients in high-risk groups require antibiotic prophylaxis for subacute bacterial endocarditis.

Self-expandable metallic stents may serve as a bridging modality to definitive surgery and as a feasible nonsurgical palliation for patients with obstructing colorectal tumors. Patients presenting with obstructing colorectal cancer often have high operative mortality. Risk factors related to obstruction, such as electrolyte imbalance and dehydration, can be controlled by proper resuscitation and preparation of the patient. The use of self-expandable metallic stents in patients with high operative risk will allow bowel decompression and preparation prior to surgery, allow for a one-stage procedure without the need for stoma, and decrease morbidity and mortality from emergency surgery (29,30). Colonic stent placement is also an excellent alternative to a diverting stoma for patients with inoperable obstructing colorectal cancer. Colonic stents can offer the patients a cost-effective treatment option, and a better quality of life, without a permanent stoma (31,32). Nevertheless, a considerable number of patients will still require surgical palliation due to stent failure and stent-related complications (32). Self-expandable metallic stents may also be used as a temporary treatment of obstructions secondary to a plethora of benign colorectal diseases including ischemic stenosis, postoperative strictures, stenosis subsequent to diverticulitis, and fistulas (33).

Self-expandable metallic stents can be placed endoscopically, by interventional radiologists, with fluoroscopic guidance, or by a combined technique (34,35). Although all methods have comparable risks, the advantages of the endoscopic procedures include the possibility of obtaining a histologic specimen during the procedure, better fixation of the sigmoid provided by the scope than a guide wire alone, and easier access to more proximal parts of the colon (34). The combined endoscopic and radiographic procedure may have optimal results. Marking the proximal and distal ends of the tumor with luminal injection of radio-opaque contrast medium may help identify the tumor and determine its length. Currently, several types of stents are available, varying in shape, size, and coating. The major differences are the diameter, the length of the expanded stents, and the diameter of the delivery system. There are no prospective trials comparing the success rate of different stent types, although studies suggest that the use of fully coated stents is associated with a higher rate of stent migration (36). It is imperative to determine the degree of obstruction and to delineate the length of the stricture prior to stent application. The site of the lesion, degree of obstruction, length of the stricture, presence of a fistula proximal to obstruction, and operator preference will determined the technique, stent size and type, and number of stents inserted during the procedure. In the presence of a fistula, the use of a coated stent allows eliminating the retrograde stasis and sealing the opening of the fistula, thus serving two purposes in treating the fistula (33).

The stent should extend at least 1 to 2 cm beyond the lesion, and because the longest available Wallstent (Boston Scientific Europe, Hertfordshire, U.K.) is 10 cm long, lesions shorter than 7 cm usually have better rates of success when managed by expandable metallic stents. Longer lesions are suitable for stenting as well. Aviv et al. (37) report that out of 16 patients who were treated for malignant colonic obstruction using stenting, three patients had lesions longer than 7 cm and two or more stents were applied during the procedure, with no significant increase in the complication rate.

Complete obstruction represents a contraindication for colonic stenting because a minimal lumen diameter is required for guide wire placement; other contraindications include perforation, peritonitis, and hemodynamic instability. Rectal stenting of low rectal lesions, less than 4 cm from the anus, may cause incontinence and be considered as a contraindication for stent application (35).

Limitations of this procedure include the fact that these stents were primarily designed for the esophagus where insertion along a straight axis is usually easier. Appropriate guide wire placement beyond the tumor may be difficult due to intestinal looping and prosthesis insertion may likewise be challenging, if not impossible, if tumor stenosis is markedly angulated. Complications include stent malposition, migration, tumor ingrowth, stool impaction, and necrosis with the risk of perforation, peritonitis and abscess formation (35). Tumor ingrowth can be palliated with laser recanalization. Necrosis can result from pressure of the proximal or distal edges of the stent on normal mucosa, especially in cases of angulation.

In a systematic review evaluating the efficacy and safety of self-expandable metallic stents in the treatment of patients with malignant colonic obstruction, 54 studies were evaluated, with a total of 1198 patients. Stenting was performed as a definitive palliative procedure in 66% of the patients and as a bridge to surgery in 34% of the patients. Primary colorectal cancer was the reason for obstruction in 84% of the patients. The rectosigmoid area was the most frequent location for stent application (86%). Technical success in placement of the stent was achieved at the first attempt in 93% of the patients. The cumulative complication rates for perforation, migration, and recurrent obstruction were 3.76%, 11.81%, and 7.34%, respectively. The authors concluded that palliative colorectal stenting should be considered as the treatment of choice in patients with obstruction due to advanced colorectal cancer, when considering palliative treatment. Colonic stenting as a bridge to surgery appears to be a relatively safe option compared to emergency surgery, although there are no prospective randomized trials comparing both treatment modalities (30).

TREATMENT OF SPECIFIC CAUSES OF COLORECTAL OBSTRUCTION
Colorectal Cancer

Colorectal cancer is the most common cause of large bowel obstruction in the United States (2). Obstructive symptoms are a presenting complaint in 8% to 29% of cases (38). Patients requiring urgent management of obstructing colon cancer tend to have more advanced disease and a poorer prognosis than those undergoing elective resection.

The goal of colorectal cancer treatment is curative resection, preferably accomplished by a single-stage procedure. While cure for cancer is the ideal end point, this goal is not always realistic because patients often present with advanced disease. In these patients, palliative procedures with minimal morbidity should be considered to alleviate symptoms. The avoidance of a colostomy is also an important goal for these patients.

While surgery is the treatment of choice for most patients with obstructing colorectal cancer, endoluminal surgery or endoscopic relief of the obstruction may be indicated in select patients. Wide surgical resection, combined with chemotherapy and radiation therapy, as indicated, offers the best chance of cure in the majority of patients. Endoscopic treatments are reserved for patients in whom surgery is medically contraindicated, in those who refuse surgery, and in patients with a short life expectancy. As well, patients with partially or completely obstructing colonic lesions in whom recanalization of the lumen may allow temporary relief of obstruction, allowing time for more thorough preoperative evaluation and bowel preparation, may benefit from endoscopic treatment.

Surgery

Currently, the surgical approach most often favored is resection of the obstructing lesion with end colostomy or with primary anastomosis. Historically, management of malignant colonic obstruction was treated with multistage procedures, an approach less commonly employed today. The procedures were undertaken in three stages, including a transverse colostomy to relieve obstruction, followed by resection and reanastomosis, and completed by closure of the colostomy. The majority of patients underwent tumor resection at a second operation during the same hospitalization (39). Although postulated to reduce complications, several studies have shown that multistage procedures result in higher complication rates (40,41). The additional morbidity of the staged procedures is related to the formation and closure of the ostomy.

Proximal diversion without resection may be considered in the unstable patient without peritonitis. Additionally, if the surgeon is relatively inexperienced in the oncologic management of colorectal cancer, proximal diversion should be the procedure of choice.

All of the surgical procedures discussed may be amenable to laparoscopy. Moreover, the surgeon must clearly have advanced laparoscopic skills before contemplating operation of the obstructed bowel.

Resection with End Stoma

Resection with creation of a colostomy (Hartmann's procedure) is most commonly used for perforating lesions. This procedure has the advantage of removing the contaminating source from the peritoneal cavity and is also used in patients with obstructing lesions, to avoid the potential consequences of anastomotic failure. Other situations in which an anastomosis may be contraindicated include patients with active colitis, immunocompromised patients, or those with poor nutritional status. The perioperative morbidity for a Hartmann's procedure is low and thus the procedure is frequently used in the management of obstructing left colonic lesions. The main drawback is that a laparotomy is required in order to close the colostomy, considerably adding to the associated risks. Mortality as high as 7% and morbidity rates ranging from 20% to 30% have been reported for subsequent colostomy closure. Furthermore, 25% to 50% of patients do not have intestinal continuity restored due to poor operative risk or patient unwillingness (38,42).

One-Stage Surgical Procedures

Because proximal fecal loading has been postulated to impair anastomotic healing, surgeons have avoided one-stage procedures for obstructing large bowel lesions. However, because bacterial colonization of the small intestine is minimal, especially if the competency of the ileocecal valve is maintained, obstructing cancers of the right and transverse colon can be safely managed by resection and primary ileocolic anastomosis. Morbidity rates are similar to those for primary anastomosis in nonobstructed patients (3,43). Moreover, as stated above, numerous recent prospective randomized trials have shown that bowel preparation may be unnecessary in the elective setting.

For left-sided obstruction, several techniques are available in order to accomplish the ultimate goal of resection and primary anastomosis. These include on-table lavage of the proximal colon, subtotal colectomy, and preoperative decompression by endoluminal techniques.

Intraoperative lavage of the proximal colon was introduced as a means of decontaminating the unprepped bowel prior to anastomosis after resection of obstructing left colon cancer. Numerous reports have demonstrated the technical feasibility of intraoperative lavage, but results are variable, with anastomotic leak rates ranging from 5% to 10% and wound infection rates as high as 30% (44–47).Contraindications to segmental resection and intraoperative lavage include serosal tears or devitalized areas of the proximal bowel or when synchronous lesions are suspected in the proximal bowel.

Subtotal colectomy and primary anastomosis is considered by many surgeons as the optimal treatment for malignant left-sided colonic obstruction (48–50). Advantages to this approach include the avoidance of a bowel preparation, removal of the disease process, and avoidance of a colostomy with a single-stage operation. Morbidity and mortality are comparable to those in patients undergoing elective colonic resection. Diarrhea is common in the early postoperative period (51), but spontaneously resolves in the majority of patients (22).

Endoluminal Therapy
When obstruction is incomplete, endoluminal techniques can be employed for temporary relief. This allows for evaluation of the bowel proximal to the obstructing lesion and preoperative bowel preparation. These techniques are used to relieve the obstruction in preparation for surgery or can be used solely for palliation.

Laser
A number of studies have described the efficacy of laser therapy in palliation for colorectal malignancy (52–54). Laser photoablation provides palliation that compares favorably with radiation therapy, electrocoagulation, or cryotherapy with minimal morbidity in patients with advanced malignancy, or those in whom surgery is contraindicated. In one large series, recanalization of operable tumors was feasible in 97% of patients with lower gastrointestinal malignancies. Similarly, subjective improvement of symptoms occurred in 97% of patients, with a low procedure-related morbidity (3%) and mortality (0.5%) (55).

The cost of palliative surgery was found to be twice as high as palliative laser therapy in one study, which included patients with obstructing colorectal cancer (56). One major reason for this cost inequity is that laser treatments are usually outpatient procedures, whereas operated patients require hospitalization. Furthermore, fewer side effects and lower complication rates occurred in patients undergoing laser treatment versus surgical palliation. Palliative outcomes were comparable in patients treated by laser therapy, colostomy, or surgical resection.

Endoluminal Stents
Endoscopically placed intraluminal stents have been used successfully for temporary colonic decompression before an elective single-stage surgery. The most commonly used stent consists of a self-expanding metal mesh. In one prospective analysis of 72 patients with left-sided malignant obstruction, those treated by stent placement followed by elective surgery had a reduced need for colostomies (15% vs. 59% in the control group), a shorter hospitalization, and fewer severe complications than patients treated by emergent surgery (29).

To date, no comparative studies have evaluated the use of coagulation versus laser, or stents in the palliation of colorectal neoplasia. Most series are small, single-institution experiences without a control group of other treatment modalities. All newer palliation techniques should be measured against traditional treatments with palliative surgery, chemotherapy, and radiotherapy.

Radiation
External beam radiation for partly obstructing rectal cancers often resolves symptoms of obstruction, bleeding, and pain. While this is a frequently employed preoperative modality in patients with locally advanced rectal cancer, its use for obstructing colonic tumors is contraindicated due to the intolerability of the small bowel to radiation.

Diverticular Disease

Patients with partial colonic obstruction of suspected diverticular origin should have a trial of nonoperative management with bowel rest, intravenous hydration, and broad-spectrum antibiotics. If a diverticular abscess is discovered on CT scan, percutaneous drainage is undertaken. If there are no peritoneal signs or active infection, colonoscopy is attempted to exclude a malignancy. Upon patient improvement, a semielective resection is undertaken during the same hospitalization, after a gentle prep. In patients with acute diverticulitis or abscess, surgery is delayed for several weeks to allow the inflammation to subside. Those patients presenting with an acute obstruction are treated emergently as described in the section on Urgent Surgery.

Volvulus
Sigmoid Volvulus
In patients without peritoneal signs, nonoperative means of detorsing the bowel are initially attempted. Rigid proctosigmoidoscopy should be attempted initially as this may be expeditiously

undertaken at the patient's beside or in the emergency room setting. The endoscopist should be prepared for a rush of gas and liquid stool as the volvulus is reduced. A rectal tube is left in place to allow for continued colonic decompression.

Flexible sigmoidoscopy or colonoscopy is performed when the volvulus is beyond the reach of the proctosigmoidoscope. The added length with the fiberoptic scope allows the potential benefit of evaluating the sigmoid mucosa for evidence of ischemia (57). Clogging of the colonoscope channel by stool may limit decompression of the bowel; therefore a rectal tube should be left in place. This maneuver can be accomplished by back loading a very long suture through the biopsy channel of the colonoscope and tying it to the end of the rectal tube. Once the colonoscope is beyond the point of the volvulus, the suture is pulled until the tube is advanced to the desired point. Alternatively, the tube is advanced alongside the colonoscope ("piggybacked") and released once above the torsion of the volvulus. Any soft, large-bore tube can be used for this purpose. The tube is then attached to a urinary drainage bag to limit soiling.

Recurrence rates of 50% or greater have been reported after endoscopic decompression of sigmoid volvulus (57,58). Therefore, for patients who are acceptable surgical risks, definitive surgery should be performed during the same hospitalization. The most common surgical approach is sigmoid resection, perhaps laparoscopically. When megacolon is present, recurrence after sigmoid resection alone is high; therefore subtotal colectomy with ileorectostomy is recommended (59). An alternative procedure that has been successfully employed, which avoids bowel resection, is mesosigmoplasty (60). This technique involves a radial incision in the peritoneum of the sigmoid from the root of the mesentery to the apex near the bowel. The peritoneal incision is then closed in a transverse fashion, thus broadening the mesenteric attachment. However, the standard of care remains resection, generally with an anastomosis.

Cecal Volvulus

Cecal volvulus is treated similar to sigmoid volvulus, with an initial attempt at early endoscopic decompression followed by elective surgery for patients who are good surgical candidates. Surgical options include cecopexy, with or without cecostomy, and resection with or without anastomosis. Early surgical intervention is important to avoid loss of bowel viability.

A cecopexy is done by elevating a flap of parietal peritoneum in the right paracolic gutter and suturing it to the antimesenteric tinea of the right colon. The addition of cecostomy aids in fixing the colon in two planes and allows for decompression of the cecum. Anderson and Lee (61) reported that cecostomy and cecopexy was superior to cecopexy alone in a group of 49 patients undergoing treatment for cecal volvulus. Cecostomy and cecopexy has been associated with a lower mortality rate than resection and primary anastomosis, but with similar recurrence rates (62).

Colonic Pseudo-Obstruction

Colonic pseudo-obstruction is a functional disorder of the large intestine manifested by increasing colonic distension, which develops over one to seven days, usually following spinal or pelvic surgery, abdominal trauma, and other medical illnesses associated with narcotic use. Most patients will go to the intensive care unit and are critically ill with significant comorbidities. They present with abdominal distension, tympany, and various degrees of abdominal pain. Bowel sounds are usually present; peritoneal signs suggest peritonitis or colonic perforation.

Abdominal films show significant colonic distention, usually more in the right and transverse colon than in the left. Small bowel distension and air fluid levels are rare and are more indicative of true obstruction. The colon dilation is often out of proportion to the physical exam. A cecal dilation of 12 to 13 cm or more raises the concern of impending perforation and active intervention is warranted.

When intervention is necessary, a water-soluble enema is preferentially performed, serving two purposes. First, it definitively rules out a mechanical obstruction and, second, the high osmolarity often facilitates some colonic evacuation, rendering the colon more optimal for subsequent endoscopic decompression. In the absence of peritoneal signs, there is no risk involved with a carefully performed enema.

Conservative therapy includes correction of electrolyte abnormalities (including magnesium), cessation of all narcotics that could impair motility, insertion of a rectal tube, and positioning the patient on the right side allowing gas to rise toward the splenic flexure. Nasogastric suction is ineffective in the absence of small bowel distension and will not decompress the colon. Ambulation, whenever possible, is helpful.

Failure of these simple conservative measures warrants medical treatment with neostigmine. Neostigmine is an anticholinesterase agent that increases cholinergic activity. A 2-mg dose of intravenous neostigmine is safe and leads to rapid colon decompression in more than 90% of patients (63). Patients should be placed on a bedpan because rapid and significant passage of gas and stool occurs within a few minutes after administration. Patients should be monitored for bradycardia, hypotension, and bronchospasm during administration. Atropine should be kept available to reverse its effects, if necessary; some patients may require repeat dosing.

While neostigmine is the treatment of choice for acute colonic pseudo-obstruction, colonoscopic decompression should be considered for those patients who fail neostigmine or have a contraindication. As mentioned above (see section Endoscopic Therapy), the air insufflation pump at the light source is turned off and water is infused either manually or with a pump, through the operating channel of the endoscope. Water allows good visualization of the lumen direction and avoids colonic overdistension, especially of the more proximal portions, which can easily occur with standard air insufflation. Colonoscopic gas aspiration alone is ineffective in the long term because it leads to rapid redistention over time. Endoscopic placement of a colonic decompression tube over a previously placed guide wire is most effective. Fluoroscopic monitoring facilitates the procedure, but can be accomplished without X-ray if guide wire and tube length are carefully measured from maximal site of insertion to anus (measurement on colonoscope insertion shaft). A retrospective review of our experience suggests that it is unnecessary to place the decompression tube tip into the cecum or around the hepatic flexure. Decompression was effective in all cases where the tube was placed at last proximal to the splenic flexure (64). Endoscopic decompression is effective in more than 90% of patients and safe in experienced hands (65).

Surgery is indicated in patients in whom conservative measures fail and colonoscopy is unsuccessful. In these circumstances, a tube cecostomy is performed through a limited incision in the right lower quadrant. In patients with repeated episodes of pseudo-obstruction despite colonoscopic decompression, a cecostomy may be an alternative to repeated colonoscopies. A sutured cecostomy, constructed similar to a colostomy, is preferred over a tube cecostomy because the catheter is prone to obstruction, which may result in intraperitoneal contamination. This procedure has the disadvantage of requiring long-term care to manage the stoma. Bowel resection may be required if intestinal viability is suspected. Patients with a perforated bowel should have resection with ileostomy and mucus fistula and thorough cleansing of the peritoneal cavity.

REFERENCES

1. Buechter KJ, Boutsany C, Caillouette R, et al. Surgical management of the acutely obstructed colon: a review of 127 cases. Am J Surg 1988; 156:163–168.
2. Greenlee HB, Pienkos EJ, Vanderbilt PC. Acute large bowel obstruction. Arch Surg 1974; 108: 470–476.
3. Phillips RK, Hittinger R, Fry JS, et al. Malignant large bowel obstruction. Br J Surg 1985; 72:296–302.
4. Gatch WD, Culbertson CG. Circulatory disturbances caused by intestinal obstruction. Ann Surg 1935; 102:619.
5. Boley SJ, Agrawal GP, Warren AR, et al. Pathophysiologic effects of bowel distension on intestinal blood flow. Am J Surg 1969; 117:228–234.
6. Papanicolaou G, Ahn YK, Nikas DJ, Fielding P. Effect of large-bowel obstruction on colonic blood flow: an experimental study. Dis Colon Rectum 1989; 32:673–679.
7. Coxon JE, Dickson C, Taylor I. Changes in intestinal blood flow during the development of chronic large bowel obstruction. Br J Surg 1984; 71:795–798.
8. Sykes PA, Boulter KH, Schofield PF. The microflora of the obstructed bowel. Br J Surg 1976; 63:721–725.
9. Sagar PM, MacFie J, Sedman P, et al. Intestinal obstruction promotes gut translocation of bacteria. Dis Colon Rectum 1995; 38:640–644.
10. Wittenburg J. The diagnosis of colonic obstruction on plain abdominal radiographs: start with the cecum, leave the rectum to last. AJR 1993; 161:443–333.
11. Chapman A, Mc Namara M, Porter G. The acute contrast enema in suspected large bowel obstruction: value and technique. Clin Radiol 1992; 46:273–278.

12. Goosenberg EB, Greenfield SM, Kasama RK. Cecal volvulus update. Contemp Gastroenterol 1991; 4:11.
13. Friedman J, Odland M, Bubrick M. Experience with colonic volvulus. Dis Colon Rectum 1989; 32: 409–416.
14. Frager D. Intestinal obstruction: role of CT. Gastroenterol Clin North Am 2002; 31(3):777–779.
15. Gosche J, Sharpe J, Larson G. Colonic decompression for pseudo-obstruction of the colon. Am Surg 1989; 55:111–115.
16. Guenaga KF, Matos D, Castro AA, et al. Mechanical bowel preparation for elective colorectal surgery. Cochrane Database Syst Rev 2005; 25(1):CD001544.
17. Bucher P, Mermillod B, Gervaz P, et al. Mechanical bowel preparation for elective colorectal surgery: a meta-analysis. Arch Surg 2004; 139(12):1359–1364.
18. Slim K, Vicaut E, Panis Y, et al. Meta-analysis of randomized clinical trials of colorectal surgery with or without mechanical bowel preparation. Br J Surg 2004; 91(9):1125–1130.
19. Wille-Jorensen P, Guenaga KF, Matos D, et al. Pre-operative mechanical bowel cleansing or not? An updated meta-analysis. Colorectal Dis 2005; 7(4):304–310.
20. Zmora O, Wexner SD, Hajjar L, et al. Trends in preparation for colorectal surgery: survey of the members of the American society of colon and rectal surgeons. Am Surg 2003; 69(2):150–154.
21. Mealy K, Salman A, Arthur G. Definitive one-stage emergency large bowel surgery. Br J Surg 1988; 75(12):1216–1219.
22. Torralba JA, Robles R, Parrilla P, et al. Subtotal colectomy vs. intraoperative colonic irrigation in the management of obstructed left colon carcinoma. Dis Colon Rectum 1998; 41(1):18–22.
23. Dorudi S, Wilson NM, Heddle RM. Primary restorative colectomy in malignant left-sided large bowel obstruction. Ann R Coll Surg Engl 1990; 72:393–395.
24. Radcliffe AG, Dudley HAF. Intraoperative antegrade irrigation of the large intestine. Surg Gynecol Obstet 1983; 156:721–723.
25. Murray JJ, Schoetz DJ, Coller JA. Intraoperative colonic lavage and primary anastomosis in non-elective colon resection. Dis Colon Rectum 1991; 34:527–531.
26. Corman ML. Colon and Rectal Surgery. 3rd ed. Philadelphia: Lippincott-Raven Publishers, 1998.
27. Krasner N. Laser therapy in the management of benign malignant tumors in the colon rectum. Int J Colorect Dis 1989; 4:2–5.
28. Van Cutsem E, Boonem A, Geboes K, et al. Risk factors which determine long term outcome of neodymium-YAG laser palliation of colorectal cancer. Int J Colorect Dis 1989; 4:9–11.
29. Martinez-Santos C, Lobato RF, Frajedas JM, et al. Self expandable stent before elective surgery versus emergent surgery for the treatment of malignant colorectal obstructions: comparison of primary anastomosis and morbidity rates. Dis Colon Rectum 2002; 45:401–406.
30. Sebastian S, Johnston S, Geoghegan T, et al. Pooled analysis of the efficacy and safety of self-expanding metal stenting in malignant colorectal obstruction. Am J Gastroenterol 2004; 99(10):2051–2057.
31. Xinopoulos D, Dimitroulopoulos D, Theodosopoulos T, et al. Stenting or stoma creation for patients with inoperable malignant colonic obstructions? Results of a study and cost-effectiveness analysis. Surg Endosc 2004; 18(3):421–426.
32. Hunerbein M, Krause M, Moesta KT, et al. Palliation of malignant rectal obstruction with self-expanding metal stents. Surgery 2005; 137(1):42–47.
33. Paul L, Pinto I, Gomez H, et al. Metallic stents in the treatment of benign diseases of the colon: preliminary experience in 10 cases. Radiology 2002; 223(3):715–722.
34. Baron TH. Indications and results of endoscopic rectal stenting. J Gastrointest Surg 2004; 8(3):266–269.
35. Keymling M. Colorectal stenting. Endoscopy 2003; 35(3):234–238.
36. Choo IW, Do YS, Suh SW, et al. Malignant colorectal obstruction: treatment with a flexible covered stent. Radiology 1998; 206(2):415–421.
37. Aviv RI, Shyamalan G, Watkinson A, et al. Radiological palliation of malignant colonic obstruction. Clin Radiol 2002; 57(5):347–351.
38. Deans GT, Krukowski ZH, Irwin ST. Malignant obstruction of the left colon. Br J Surg 1994; 81:1270–1276.
39. Gutman M, Kaplan O, Skornick Y, et al. Proximal colostomy: still an effective measure in obstructing carcinoma of the large bowel. J Surg Oncol 1989; 41:210.
40. Sjodahl R, Franzen T, Nystrom P. Primary versus staged resection for acute obstructing colorectal carcinoma. Br J Surg 1992; 79:685–688.
41. Kronberg O. Acute obstruction from tumor in the left colon without spread: a randomized trial of emergency colostomy versus resection. Int J Colorectal Dis 1995; 10:1.
42. Isbister WH, Prasad J. The management of left-sided large bowel obstruction. Aust NZ J Surg 1996; 66:602.
43. Koruth NM, Hunter DC, Krukowski ZH, et al. Immediate resection in emergency large bowel surgery: a 7-year audit. Br J Surg 1985; 72:703.
44. Dudley HAF, Radcliffe AG, McGeehan D. Intraoperative irrigation of the colon to permit primary anastomosis. Br J Surg 1980; 67:80.
45. Foster ME, Johnson CD, Billings PJ, et al. Intraoperative antegrade lavage and anastomotic healing in acute colonic obstruction. Dis Colon Rectum 1986; 29:255.
46. Thomson WHF, Carter SC. On-table lavage to achieve safe restorative rectal and emergency left colonic resection without covering colostomy. Br J Surg 1986; 73:61.

47. Pollack AV, Playforth MJ, Evans M. Perioperative lavage of the obstructed left colon to allow safe primary anastomosis. Dis Colon Rectum 1987; 30:171.
48. Stephenson BM, Shandall AA, Farouk R, Griffith G. Malignant left-sided large bowel obstruction managed by subtotal/total colectomy. Br J Surg 1990; 77:1098–1102.
49. Tan SG, Nambiar R, Rauff A, et al. Primary resection and anastomosis in obstructed descending colon due to cancer. Arch Surg 1991; 126:748.
50. Arnaud JP, Bergamaschi R. Emergency subtotal/total colectomy with anastomosis for acutely obstructed carcinoma of the left colon. Dis Colon Rectum 1994; 37:685.
51. Ross S, Krukowski ZH, Munro A, Russell IT. Single-stage treatment for malignant left-sided colonic obstruction: a prospective randomized clinical trail comparing subtotal colectomy with segmental resection following intraoperative irrigation. Br J Surg 1995; 82:1622–1627.
52. Brown SG, Barr H, Matthewson K, et al. Endoscopic treatment of inoperable colorectal cancers with the ND-YAG laser. Br J Surg 1986; 73:949–952.
53. Brunetaud JM, Maunoury V, Ducrotte P, et al. Palliative treatment of rectosigmoid carcinoma by laser endoscopic ablation. Gastroenterol 1987; 92:663–668.
54. Mathews-Vligen EMH, Tytgat GNJ. Laser photocoagulation in the palliation of colorectal malignancies. Cancer 1986; 57:2212–2216.
55. Spinelli P, Mancini A, Dal Fante M. Endoscopic treatment of gastrointestinal tumors: indications and results of laser photocoagulation and photodynamic therapy. Semin Surg Onc 1995; 11:307–318.
56. Tache W, Paech S, Kruis W, et al. Comparison between endoscopic laser and different surgical treatments for palliation of advanced rectal cancer. Dis Colon Rectum 1993; 36:377–382.
57. Procaccino J, Labow SB. Transcolonic decompression of sigmoid volvulus. Dis Colon Rectum 1989; 32:349.
58. Ballantyne GH. Review of sigmoid volvulus: history and results of treatment. Dis Colon Rectum 1982; 25:494.
59. Morrissey TB, Deitch EA. Recurrence of sigmoid volvulus after surgical intervention. Am Surg 1994; 60:329.
60. Bagarani M, Conde AS, Longo R, et al. Sigmoid volvulus in West Africa: a prospective study on surgical treatments. Dis Colon Rectum 1993; 36:186.
61. Anderson J, Lee D. Acute cecal volvulus. Br J Surg 1981; 68:117.
62. Anderson JR, Welch GH. Acute volvulus of the right colon: an analysis of 69 patients. World J Surg 1986; 10:336.
63. Ponek RJ, Saunders MD, Kimmey MB. Neostigmine for the treatment of acute colonic pseudo-obstruction: a randomized double-blinded controlled trial. N Engl J Med 1999; 341:137–141.
64. Sherman FS, Nord HJ, Robinson BE. Acute colonic pseudo-obstruction: treatment by endoscopic decompression and proximal tube placement. Gastrointest Endosc 1997; 45:AB118.
65. Brothers TE, Strodel WE, Eckhauser FE. Endoscopy in colonic volvulus. Ann Surg 1987; 206:1.

3 | Incontinence

Lucia Oliveira
Department of Anorectal Physiology, Policlínica Geral do Rio de Janeiro, Rio de Janeiro, Brazil

Julio Studart de Moraes
Department of Gastroenterology, Policlínica Geral do Rio de Janeiro, Rio de Janeiro, Brazil

INTRODUCTION

Fecal incontinence is a disabling and distressing condition that can severely affect quality of life. This "silent affliction" is commonly diagnosed in elderly patients who reside in nursing homes. Because many individuals deny this condition to their general practitioners, the exact incidence of fecal incontinence remains unknown. However, the reported incidence in the literature varies from 0.1% to 5% of the general population (1–3). The prevalence of fecal incontinence is also difficult to estimate; one survey shows fecal incontinence appears to be more common than previously appreciated at 13.7% (4) among individuals seen by primary care physicians, compared to 7.8% as previously reported by Drossman et al. (5) in 1993. Additionally, they noted a progressive increase in the prevalence of fecal incontinence with increasing age and a predilection for males. However, due to obstetrical trauma in women under 45 years of age, fecal incontinence is eight times more frequent than in the age-equivalent male population (6). In a recent survey that included 15,904 adults aged 40 years or older and excluding residents of nursing homes 1.4% reported major fecal incontinence and 0.7% major fecal incontinence with bowel symptoms with impaired quality of life (7).

Fecal incontinence has a very prominent socioeconomic impact due to the necessity of a number of stoma appliances and products used by affected patients. The economic impact of fecal incontinence is tremendous with a cost of more than four million spent annually in the United States for diapers and other incontinence supplies (8,9). Furthermore, an estimated long-term cost of $17,166 per patient has been reported to treat fecal incontinence secondary to obstetric injury alone (10).

One of the main interests of modern society is to help maintain dignity and quality of life. Therefore, every effort should be made to achieve this aim and to help affected individual's return to an acceptable level of social and professional lifestyle.

While evaluating the patient's history, an effort should be made to adequately investigate the history of fecal and urinary incontinence, as many patients presenting with both conditions initially deny these problems to their physicians. Any involuntary loss of sphincter control can be objectively construed as fecal incontinence; this condition can also be defined as the loss of anal sphincter control or the inability to defer the call to stool to a socially acceptable time and place, resulting in an unwanted release of gas, liquid, or solid stool.

The mechanism of continence is complex and is dependent on a number of factors such as sphincter function, stool consistency, delivery of colonic contents, rectal capacity and compliance, anorectal sensation, and pelvic floor anatomy (11). Stool or gas passes into the rectum, which then distends, initiating the relaxation of the internal sphincter via the rectoanal inhibitory reflex. The rectal contents then enter the anal canal, whereby sampling in the sensitive anoderm occurs. If passage of rectal contents is unwanted, afferent stimulation via the pudendal nerves augment the tonic activity in the puborectalis that decreases the anorectal angle and stimulates the external sphincter mechanism, tightening and lengthening the anal canal. Any disruption of this process may lead to fecal incontinence. The presence of liquid feces alone can induce incontinent episodes even in healthy individuals.

CLINICAL EVALUATION

A careful history and physical examination is important in the evaluation of fecal incontinence and can help steer appropriate investigation and therapy for individuals (Table 1).

Table 1 Physical Examination

Abdominal examination	Palpation
Masses	Pinprick touch
Neurologic examination	Resting tone
Perineal sensation	Squeeze tone
Anal reflex	Puborectalis motion
Mental status	Muscular deficits
Perianal examination	Soft tissue scarring
Inspection	Rectal content
Excoriation	Rectal mass
Signs of infection	Evidence of internal prolapse
Perineal soiling	Rectocele
Scars	Endoscopy
Mucosal ectropion	Neoplasm
Prolapsing hemorrhoids	Solitary rectal ulcer
Rectal prolapse	Hemorrhoids
Patulous anus	Fistula
Loss of perineal body	IBD
Muscular deficit	
Perineal descent with valsalva	
Fistula	

Abbreviation: IBD, inflammatory bowel disease.

It is important to distinguish fecal incontinence of sufficient severity as to require surgical treatment from that of urgency and soiling, conditions that do not usually require surgery and are associated with minor anorectal conditions. This latter condition is known as pseudoincontinence and can be related to hemorrhoids, anal fissures, dermatologic anal conditions, or a variety of other benign or malignant anal disorders.

Fecal impaction can simulate fecal incontinence as liquid stool leaks, which then soils the patient's underwear. In children, these types of incontinent episodes are interpreted by the caregivers or parent as fecal incontinence. In fact, the presence of a fecal mass and the continuous stimulation of the internal anal sphincter relaxation produce a hypotonic anus that is unable to control liquid stool (Fig. 1). The most important factor to help maintain fecal continence is the sphincteric mechanism represented by the external and internal anal sphincters and the puborectalis muscle. Therefore, any traumatic, congenital, or iatrogenic injury to the sphincters can produce fecal incontinence. Obstetrical trauma and previous surgical procedures are the most common causes of disruption of the sphincter mechanism leading to fecal incontinence.

Disruption of the anal canal musculature produces fecal incontinence due to loss of the anal canal high-pressure zone, alterations in normal sampling mechanisms, or both. The etiology of fecal incontinence is outlined in Table 2. The degree of fecal incontinence is related to the type (solid, liquid, or gas), frequency, and duration of the incontinence. It is important to determine whether incontinence occurs during sleep, at rest, or during strenuous or moderate activity, as well as the impact of this condition on the patient's social and professional activities. In addition, a dietary and medication history should be noted, as well as any coexistent bladder and/or sexual disturbances. A medical history and review of systems

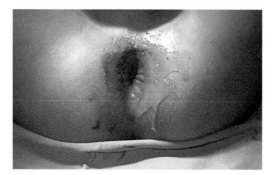

Figure 1 (*See color insert*) Young patient with rectal fecaloma producing hypotonic anus and soiling.

Table 2 Classification of Etiology of Anal Incontinence

Pseudoincontinence
Perineal soiling
   Rectal mucosal prolapse
   Hemorrhoidal prolapse
   Incomplete defecation
   Poor hygiene
   Fistula in ano
   Dermatologic condition
   Anorectal sexually transmitted disease
   Anorectal neoplasm
Overflow incontinence
Impaction
Encopresis
Antimotility drugs
Incontinence with normal pelvic floor
Diarrheal states
   Inflammatory bowel disease
   Short gut
   Laxative abuse
   Infection
     Parasites
     Bacteria
     Toxins
   Intermittent partial small bowel obstruction
Incontinence with abnormal pelvic floor function
Sphincter injury
   Obstetric
   Traumatic
   Iatrogenic
   Neoplastic
   Inflammatory
   Rectal prolapse
Congenital abnormalities
   Spina bifida
   Imperforate anus
   Myelomeningocele

Urgency
   Non-compliance rectum
   Irradiation
   Inflammatory bowel disease
   Absent rectal reservoir
   Irritable bowel syndrome

Psychotropic drugs
Rectal neoplasms

Systemic disease processes
   CNS/spinal cord
   Neoplasm
   Injury
   Dementia/stroke
   Multiple sclerosis
   Scleroderma
   Neuropathies (diabetic)

Pelvic floor denervation
   Pudendal nerve neuropathy
   Perineal descent syndrome
Traumatic
   Aging
   Neoplastic infiltration

Abbreviation: CNS, central nervous system.

may reveal systemic disorders predisposing to incontinence such as diabetes, alcoholism, and neurologic or connective tissue diseases. In the elderly, especially in institutional settings, fecal impaction, laxative overuse, hyperosmotic enteral feeding, and diarrheal states are common causes of fecal incontinence.

A number of fecal incontinence scales and scores have been proposed to objectively quantify the severity of this problem (Table 3) (12–24). However, when analyzing each scale, it is virtually impossible to make comparisons of the results among these various classifications. In addition, most of these classifications do not incorporate the frequency of incontinent episodes that can profoundly compromise the patient's quality of life.

Recently, an incontinence quality of life scale was proposed and then validated by the American Society of Colon and Rectal Surgeons (ASCRS) (25). This scale has helped to elucidate that quality of life issues are a crucial aspect in the treatment of fecal incontinence. For example, restoration of at least half of the baseline continence of an active, hard-working 45-year-old female can profoundly improve her quality of life. Conversely, an 87-year-old female who lives a sedentary life would not appreciate the same improvement in her quality of life.

Jorge and Wexner (26) introduced the Cleveland Clinic Florida Incontinence Scoring System (CCFISS) for fecal incontinence, modified from existing scoring systems (Table 4). They introduced a stratification relative to the frequency of incontinent episodes to gas, liquid, or solid stool, as well as any alteration in the patient's lifestyle; a perfect continence was graded as zero, whereas complete incontinence was scored as 20. This scoring system is simple, easy to apply, and can objectively evaluate patients with fecal incontinence. For these reasons, it has become the most commonly used scoring system. In fact, this scoring system was submitted to independent validation by Rothbarth et al., in 2001 (27), who demonstrated a correlation

Table 3 Different Classification or Scoring Systems for Fecal Incontinence in the Literature

Author	Scoring system
Kelly (12)	Points: 0–2 = poor; 2–4 = fair; 5–6 = good 0 = 50% accidents, always soiling, absent sphincters 1 = occasional accidents, occasional soiling, weak sphincters
Parks (13)	1 = normal 2 = difficult control of flatus and diarrhea 3 = no control of diarrhea 4 = no control of solid stool
Lane (14)	True incontinence = loss of feces without knowledge or control Partial incontinence = passage of flatus or mucus under same conditions Overflow incontinence = result of rectal distension without sphincter relaxation
Rudd (15)	1 = continence 2 = minor leak 3 = acceptable leak 4 = unsatisfactory major leak 5 = total failure
Holschneider (16)	Continence (resting tone at manometry > 16 mmHg) Partial continence (rt 9–15) Incontinence (rt < A8)
Keighley and Fielding (17)	Minor = fecal leakage once a month or less, to diarrhea Moderate = incontinence once a week to solid stool Severe = incontinence in most days, perineal pad
Corman (18)	Excellent = continent all time Good = continent but may require enemas Fair = incontinent for liquid stool Poor = incontinent for solid stool
Hiltunen (19)	Continent, partially continent, totally incontinent
Broden (20)	1 = none 2 = medium 3 = severe incontinence
Womack (21)	A = continence B = incontinence for liquid stool C = incontinence to flatus and diarrhea D = totally incontinent
Rainey (22)	A = continence B = incontinence to liquid stool C = incontinence to solid stool
Miller (23)	Grade I: incontinence less frequent than once a month Grade II: between once a month and once a week Grade III: more than once a week Score: flatus 1–3, fluid 4–6, solid 7–9
Pescatori (24)	Incontinence for A = flatus/mucus; B = diarrhea; C = solid stool 1 = occasionally 2 = weekly 3 = daily Score: from 0 (continence) to 6 (severe total incontinence)

between the CCFISS scores and the patient's quality of life: a CCFISS score above 9 was associated with a significant decrease in the patient's quality of life. The quality of life of the majority of patients with scores higher than 9 who were incontinent to solid stool more than once per week and required daily use of pads was significantly adversely affected.

Table 4 Cleveland Clinic Florida Fecal Incontinence Scoring System

Type of incontinence	Never	Rarely	Sometimes	Usually	Always
Solid	0	1	2	3	4
Liquid	0	1	2	3	4
Gas	0	1	2	3	4
Wears pad	0	1	2	3	4
Lifestyle alteration	0	1	2	3	4

Note: never, 0 (never); rarely, < 1/month; sometimes, < 1/week > 1/month; usually, < 1/day > 1/week; always, > 1/day; 0 = perfect continence; 20 = complete incontinence.
Source: From Ref. 26.

Based on these initial scoring systems, specifically on the CCFISS, a fecal incontinence severity index was proposed by Rockwood et al. in 1999 (28). Based on the type and frequency of incontinence, these authors assessed the scores of both surgeons and their patients related to incontinence to gas, mucus, liquid, and solid stool. Furthermore, they demonstrated that surgeon and patient ratings were similar, with only minor differences associated with accidental incontinence of solid stool.

As with other conditions, the impact of fecal incontinence on quality of life is receiving more attention. In fact, a definition of quality of life is a difficult aspect of patient assessment and is generally related to physical, psychological, and social well-being. In addition, quality of life should be subjectively assessed from the patient's point of view. Therefore, given the wide array of issues involved, conducting quality of life studies can be difficult. In 2002, Rockwood et al. (25) published a Fecal Incontinence Quality of Life (FIQL) scale, representing one of the first attempts in the development of a psychometric evaluation of quality of life tool designed to assess the impact of treatment for fecal incontinence. For this purpose, they utilized a correlation with the Short Form 36 Quality of Life Scale (SF-36) (29), which is a validated questionnaire commonly used to establish the validity of new condition-specific measures. Based on the SF-36, the FIQL scale contains 29 items comprising four scales or domains: (i) Lifestyle (10 items), (ii) coping/behavior (9 items), (iii) depression/self-perception (7 items), and (iv) embarrassment (3 items) (Table 5). A panel of experts was consulted to identify the quality of life–related domains adversely affected by fecal incontinence both in patients with fecal incontinence and in a control group. It was thereby demonstrated that these scales were both reliable and valid, each demonstrating stability over time and acceptable internal reliability.

The importance of using a scoring system is the possibility of objectively assessing the severity of fecal incontinence. Severity scores are also important in establishing the comparability of patients in order to effectively evaluate alternative methods of treatment. For this purpose, a Severity Index for Fecal Incontinence was created, demonstrating significant correlations with three of the four quality of life scales of incontinent patients (28).

Isolated sphincter dysfunction must be differentiated from metabolic or neurologic disorders that may clinically manifest as fecal incontinence. In most patients with sphincter injury, clinical evaluation by an experienced surgeon is adequate for preoperative evaluation and planning. Direct inspection of the perineum with adequate illumination is essential. Spreading the buttocks may reveal the presence of dermatitis, a patulous anus, loss of the perineal body, or a muscular deficit in the anorectal ring (Fig. 2). The presence of perineal soiling, scars from previous surgery or trauma, mucosal ectropion, prolapsing hemorrhoids, or complete rectal prolapse should be noted. A single glance at the perianal skin and undergarments may help to assess the degree and type of incontinence. Sensory alterations in the perianal area can be examined by a gentle touch and pinprick. The patient should be asked to strain in order to evaluate the presence of perineal descent, rectocele, or cystocele. In females, vaginal digital examination is important to examine the rectovaginal septum and the anterior sphincter bulk. Digital examination during resting and squeezing phases should also be performed. The external anal sphincter and the more proximal puborectalis muscle should each be examined. Digital examination may also exclude the presence of fecal impaction. Anoscopy and proctosigmoidoscopy may reveal the presence of inflammatory or neoplastic conditions or other disorders such as solitary rectal ulcer, colitis cystica profunda, or rectoanal intussusception. Finally, the ability of a patient to retain a 100-mL enema is a useful clinical guide in patients in whom fecal incontinence is suspected. If a patient is able to retain the enema for 10 minutes while ambulating, extensive evaluation may not be warranted.

Pelvic floor morphology and the presence of complex reflex mechanisms have made isolated evaluation of the components of the continence mechanism very difficult. However, an exponential growth in the knowledge of pelvic floor physiology has recently allowed the development and refinement of several investigative tools that allow a better diagnostic approach of these components.

INVESTIGATIONAL METHODS
Anal Manometry

Anal manometry is an objective method of studying the sphincter mechanism. This test is usually performed using a computerized perfusion system (Fig. 3). Measuring the pressures

Table 5 Fecal Incontinence Quality of Life Scale Composition

Scale 1: Lifestyle
I cannot do many of things I want to do.
I am afraid to go out.
It is important to plan my schedule (daily activities) around my bowel pattern.
I cut down on how much I eat before I go out.
It is difficult for me to get out and do things like going to a movie or to church.
I avoid traveling by plane or train.
I avoid travelling.
I avoid visiting friends.
I avoid going out to eat.
I avoid staying overnight away from home.
Scale 2: Coping/Behavior
I have sex less often than I would like to.
The possibility of bowel accidents is always on my mind.
I feel I have no control over my bowels.
Whenever I go someplace new, I specifically locate where the bathrooms are.
I worry about not being able to get to the toilet in time.
I worry about bowel accidents.
I try to prevent bowel accidents by staying very near a bathroom.
I can't hold my bowel movement long enough to get to the bathroom.
Whenever I am away from home, I try to stay near a restroom as much as possible.
Scale 3: Depression/Self Perception
In general, would you say your health is.
I am afraid to have sex.
I feel different from other people.
I enjoy life less.
I feel like I am not a healthy person.
I feel depressed.
During the past month, have you felt so sad, discouraged, hopeless, or had so many problems that you wondered
    if anything was worthwhile?
Scale 4: Embarrassment
I leak stool without even knowing it.
I worry about others smelling stool on me.
I feel ashamed.
Q1: In general, would you say your health is:
1 Excellent
2 Very Good
3 Fair
4 Poor
Q2: For each of the items, please indicate how much of the time the issue is a concern for you due to accidental bowel leakage.
    (If it is a concern for you for reasons other than accidental bowel leakage then check the box under Not Apply, N/A).

Due to accidental bowel leakage:	Most of the time	Some of the time	A little of the time	None of the time	N/A
a. I am afraid to go out.					
b. I avoid visiting friends.					
c. I avoid staying overnight away from home.					
d. It is difficult for me to get out and do things like going to a movie or to church.					
e. I cut down on how much I eat before I go out.					
f. Whenever I am away from home, I try stay near a restroom as much as possible.					
g. It is important to plan my schedule (daily activities) around my bowel pattern.					
h. I avoid traveling.					
i. I worry about not being able to get to the toilet in time.					
j. I feel I have no control over my bowels.					
k. I can't hold my bowel movement long enough to get to the bathroom.					
l. I leak stool without even knowing it.					

(*Continued*)

Table 5 Fecal Incontinence Quality of Life Scale Composition (*Continued*)

m. I try to prevent bowel accidents by
   staying very near a bathroom.
Q3: Due to accidental bowel leakage, indicate the extent to which you AGREE or DISAGREE with each of the following items.
   (If it is a concern for you for reasons other than accidental bowel leakage then check the box under Not Apply, N/A.)

Due to accidental bowel leakage:	Strongly agree	Some-what agree	Somewhat disagree	Strongly disagree
a. I feel ashamed.	1	2	3	4
b. I can not do many of the things I want to do.	1	2	3	4
c. I worry about bowel accidents.	1	2	3	4
d. I feel depressed.	1	2	3	4
e. I worry about others smelling stool on me.	1	2	3	4
f. I feel like I am not a healthy person.	1	2	3	4
g. I enjoy life less.	1	2	3	4
h. I have sex less often than I would like to.	1	2	3	4
i. I feel different from other people.	1	2	3	4
j. The possibility of bowel accidents is always on my mind.	1	2	3	4
k. I am afraid to have sex.	1	2	3	4
l. I avoid traveling by plane or train.	1	2	3	4
m. I avoid going out to eat.	1	2	3	4
n. Whenever I go someplace new, I specically locate where the bathrooms are.	1	2	3	4

Q4: During the past month, have you felt so sad, discouraged, hopeless, or had so many problems that you wondered if anything was worthwhile?
1 Extremely so—to the point that I have just about given up
2 Very much so
3 Quite a bit
4 Some—enough to bother me
5 A little bit
6 Not at all

in the rectum and anal canal at rest and during squeezing provides useful information regarding the internal and external anal sphincters. Manometry can also assess the presence of the rectoanal inhibitory reflex, rectal capacity, and compliance. In addition, the strength of the external anal sphincter can be evaluated through a sustained squeeze for a 40-second duration. The capacity of the external anal sphincter muscle to sustain the contraction, or the "fatigue index," is an important tool in assessing the sphincter status (Fig. 4). It is hypothesized that surgical resection of the rectum, inflammation, radiation, or neoplastic infiltration may decrease rectal compliance and therefore allow for a more rapid rise in rectal pressure with rectal filling. When rectal pressure becomes greater than anal sphincter pressure, incontinence results. Moreover, a small decrease in rectal capacity may contribute to incontinence. This situation may also occur after low colorectal or coloanal anastomosis.

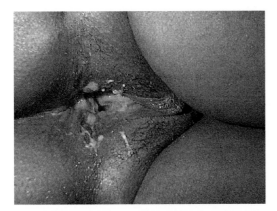

Figure 2 (*See color insert*) Patulous anus.

(A)   **(B)**

(C)   **(D)**

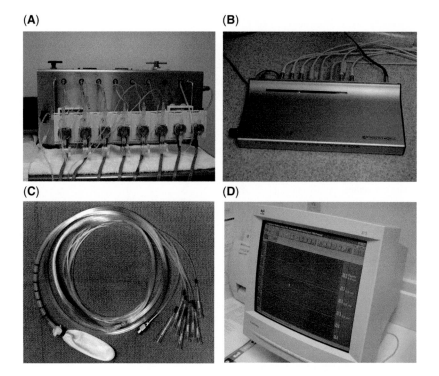

Figure 3 Manometry equipment: (**A**) perfusion system, (**B**) polygraph, (**C**) water-perfused catheter, and (**D**) monitor.

There are a number of methods for performing anal manometry, as well as various types of cathethers including air-filled balloons, fluid-filled balloons, or microtransducers (30). However, the most widely used method is the water-perfused system. The latest sophisticated manometric units provide a three-dimensional analysis of the anal sphincter mechanism. These systems utilize vector analysis and can demonstrate an assymetry index of the sphincter muscle (Fig. 5).

Although sphincter tone can be qualitatively perceived by digital examination, objective measurement requires anal manometry, which has proven to be both reliable and reproducible.

Direct traumatic injury is characterized by a low maximum voluntary contraction pressure, possibly a low resting pressure, a decrease in the length of the high-pressure zone, and impaired anal sensation. Patients with isolated external sphincter injury will have near-normal resting tone and reduced maximal contraction pressure. Isolated division of the internal sphincter muscle will result in decreased resting pressure with maintenance of normal maximal voluntary contraction pressures, as well as a decrease in anal canal sensation. Therefore, measurement of anal pressures can allow for therapeutic decisions based on

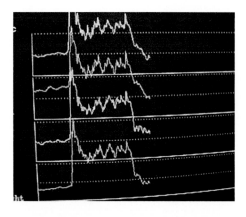

Figure 4 Fatigue index.

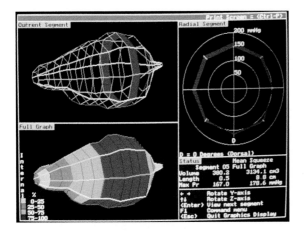

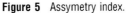

Figure 5 Assymetry index.

objective parameters. In addition, they provide a baseline for comparison following treatment. Nonetheless, it is important to note that the etiology of fecal incontinence cannot be determined by anal manometry alone. When combined with a clinical history and other complementary physiological tests, manometry can help to distinguish between fecal incontinence attributable to sphincter injury, neural lesion or neuropathy, or both. Normal manometric parameters are listed in Table 6.

Anal Ultrasonography

Anal ultrasonography is a painless and simple method of evaluating sphincter morphology and has been increasingly utilized in the assessment of incontinent patients, in many cases, replacing anal electromyography (EMG). Anal ultrasonography was introduced by Law and Bartram in 1989 (31) and allows for excellent assessment of both the external and the internal anal sphincter anatomy (Fig. 6). In addition, the puborectalis muscle can be visualized (Fig. 7). Anal ultrasonography utilizes an ultrasound scanner, an endoprobe, and a 7 or 10 MHz transducer that allows for a 360°evaluation of the anal canal circumference. The internal anal sphincter is described as a hypoechoic image, whereas the external anal sphincter and the puborectalis are seen as hyperechoic or mixed images. This procedure is well tolerated by patients, because it is relatively painless, is quick, and does not require bowel preparation or sedation.

When compared to EMG, ultrasonography is better tolerated by patients and more valuable in the evaluation of fecal incontinence. This is mainly due to the fact that it provides information relative to the integrity of the internal anal sphincter and its ability to detect occult sphincter defects in patients who would otherwise be erroneously labeled as having idiopathic fecal incontinence. Similarly, isolated anterior defects resulting from obstetrical trauma can be well demonstrated by anal ultrasonography (Fig. 8) (32,33). In addition, anal ultrasonography can be utilized for follow-up after surgical treatment of fecal incontinence (Fig. 9).

Electromyography

EMG entails recording of electrical activity generated by muscle fibers during voluntary contraction, during simulated defecation, while eliciting various reflexes, and at rest. The

Table 6 Normal Manometric Values

Resting pressure	40–70 mmHg
Squeeze pressure	100–180 mmHg
HPZ length	2–3 cm in females
	2.5–3.5 cm in males
Rectoanal inhibitory reflex	Present
Sensory threshold	10–30 cc
Rectal capacity	100–250 cc
Compliance	3–15 ccH$_2$0/mmHg

Abbreviation: HPZ, high pressure zone.

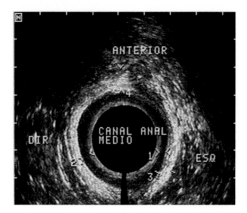

Figure 6 Normal ultrasound.

recordings of the external anal sphincter and puborectalis muscle activity are important in assessing patients with fecal incontinence. The EMG unit can record electrical muscular activity using cutaneous surface or anal plug, concentric needle, single-fiber, or monopolar wire electrodes. The latter method, although the most uncomfortable, has the ability to measure amplitude, duration, and number of phases of motor unit action potentials. In addition, information regarding innervation and functional status of individual motor units within the muscle can be obtained.

Sphincter damage may be seen as polyphasia, denervation, reinnervation, increased complexity of motor unit potentials during concentric needle examination, or increased fiber density during single-fiber examination. EMG potentials that are multiphasic and have an increased amplitude and duration are consistent with injury, denervation, and subsequent partial reinnervation of the puborectalis and external anal sphincter muscle fibers from adjacent intact neuromuscular units. If significant denervation has occurred, neurogenic pelvic floor dysfunction may result (Fig. 10) (34). Single-fiber EMG allows the investigator to measure "muscle fiber density." An increased fiber density indicates a damaged neuromuscular unit that has undergone partial reinnervation. Although single-fiber study is more quantitative than concentric needle examination, it is much more prolonged and painful.

EMG has been less utilized for the evaluation of patients with fecal incontinence since the introduction of anal ultrasonography. This is due to the fact that anal ultrasonography is more tolerable and provides adequate imaging of the internal and external sphincter complex, even when the defect is deep within the anal canal (35).

Currently, EMG is complementary to rather than exclusive of anal ultrasonography (36,37). Anal ultrasound provides information relative to sphincter anatomy (structure), whereas EMG assesses physiology (function) of the external anal sphincter.

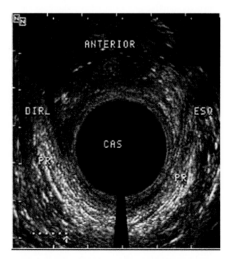

Figure 7 Puborectalis muscle at ultrasound.

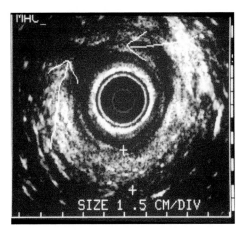

Figure 8 Anterior defect on ultrasound.

Pudendal Nerve Terminal Motor Latency Assessment

The external sphincter muscle and the puborectalis are both innervated by the pudendal nerve. Pudendal nerve terminal motor latency measures the length of time required for a fixed electrical stimulus to travel along the pudendal nerve between the ipsilateral ischial spine and the anal verge. Therefore, damage to this important nerve is one of the multiple mechanisms involved in fecal incontinence. The latency of the pudendal nerve may be increased in patients with abnormal perineal descent, rectal prolapse and neurogenic fecal incontinence (normal: 2.1 ± 0.2 msec). This technique is simple in which a digital exam is performed, and a special St. Mark's stimulator electrode is mounted on the examiner's index finger and positioned on the ischial spine (Fig. 11). The stimulating electrode is slowly moved as the optimal waveform is sought. The measurement of pudendal latency plays an important role in the evaluation of patients with fecal incontinence, particularly for those in whom a surgical procedure is being planned. It has already been demonstrated by multiple authors that pudendal neurophathy is associated with a poor outcome after sphincter repair (38–40). Specifically, it has been demonstrated that pudendal neuropathy is a predictor of poor outcome especially when there is bilateral nerve damage (41).

Other Imaging Methods

Other tests that may be helpful in the evaluation of fecal incontinence include cinedefecography and magnetic resonance imaging (MRI). The former is a radiographic method of evaluating the dynamics of defecation. It has not been routinely indicated for the evaluation of incontinent patients; however, in select patients, it may provide information relative to the presence of associated factors such as intussusception and increased perineal descent (Fig. 12).

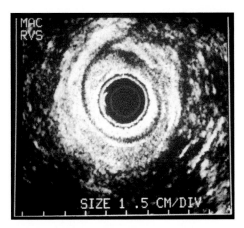

Figure 9 Postsphincteroplasty.

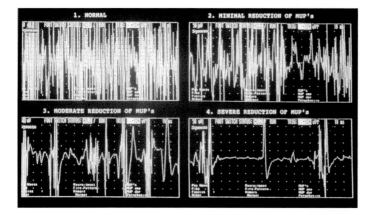

Figure 10 Electromyography.

Although cross-sectional imaging using MRI can delineate the anal sphincters, it cannot provide specific details unless a special endocoil is used. Initial reports in which radiologists had little experience with this method favored anal ultrasonography for the assessment of the anal sphincters. However, Rociu et al. (42), in a retrospective study comparing MRI and anal ultrasound in 22 patients who underwent both tests before surgery, demonstrated that there were no statistical differences between the two methods regarding the quality of images. Interestingly, external sphincter muscle atrophy was only detected by MRI, which was subsequently confirmed at the time of surgery in 100% of cases. Although anal ultrasound is a less expensive method, both tests are adequate for the evaluation of anal sphincter defects. This conclusion has been confirmed by Malouf et al. (43) in a series of 52 incontinent patients who underwent both diagnostic methods.

CONSERVATIVE TREATMENT

Various medical and surgical therapies exist for the treatment of fecal incontinence. None, however, is ideal. Understanding the complex mechanism of anal continence is the important initial step for adequate treatment of these patients. Various illnesses may cause changes in stool consistency or intestinal transit time that, even in the presence of a normal pelvic floor and sphincteric function, may account for fecal incontinence. Management of these patients should be directed toward correction of identifiable underlying causes. A thorough investigation of diarrheal disorders should be conducted. Patients with identifiable causes for diarrhea or rapid transit time should be medically managed, as indicated. Specific therapy in combination with constipating agents, dietary manipulation, or both will achieve satisfactory results in many patients. Some patients with loose stools may benefit from dietary restrictions such as lactose or gluten. In patients with known abnormal bile salt metabolism, the addition of cholestyramine may improve diarrhea and secondary incontinence. Patient education, bowel training, and laxatives should be employed to minimize straining. Underlying pathologic conditions such as colonic neoplasia and functional pelvic outlet obstruction should be excluded.

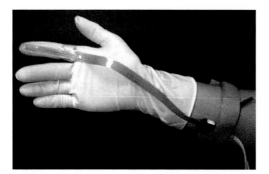

Figure 11 Pudendal nerve terminal motor latency study glove with St. Mark's stimulator.

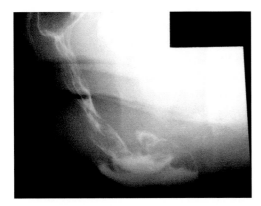

Figure 12 Defecography with internal invagination.

Fecal impaction can account for pseudoincontinence in individuals with otherwise normal pelvic floor function. Overflow incontinence caused by fecal impaction should be excluded by physical examination in all incontinent patients. These patients should be instructed to increase water and fiber intake. However, fiber can also cause or exacerbate fecal impaction. Therapies consisting of enemas, laxatives, and occasional disimpaction in combination with a good bowel regimen, patient education, and biofeedback (in selected cases) are successful in the majority of individuals. In addition, medications that can contribute to fecal impaction should be eliminated. Finally, manual extraction with or without fragmentation of the fecal bolus may be a necessary first-line measure, followed by repeated water enemas.

Patients with idiopathic diarrhea can be managed with antidiarrheal agents such as diphenoxylate and atropine or loperamide hydrochloride (44,45). Scars such as a keyhole deformity due to previous anorectal procedures can cause significant soiling. Nonoperative therapy including instruction in personal hygiene with careful cleaning of the everted anus should be undertaken. Bulk-forming or antimotility agents may help to produce formed stool and minimize leakage, once a semisolid stool is obtained. A piece of cotton gauze placed between the buttocks and over the deformity may help prevent skin irritation. Surgical correction may be necessary for patients with severe deformities.

Perineal strengthening exercises are simple to perform and can improve fecal incontinence in some patients. These patients are instructed to contract the perineal muscle and hold the contraction to a count of 10, repeating the maneuver at several intervals during each day.

An alternative for conservative treatment of anal incontinence is daily cleansing using colonic irrigation. Patients are instructed to fill their rectum with 500 to 1000 cc of water while seated on a toilet. This safe and inexpensive procedure prevents incontinent episodes by maintaining an empty bowel. However, this procedure is time consuming and does not provide a definite treatment for incontinence.

Perianal Electrical Stimulation

Perianal electrical stimulation has been reported to improve fecal incontinence (46). This procedure is usually indicated for treating a variety of conditions related to fecal incontinence. The rationale of this method is to decrease the susceptibility of the anal sphincters to fatigue and therefore to increase the squeeze pressures. A prospective study with 15 patients who underwent transanal electrostimulation after six months' follow-up demonstrated an improvement in sphincter function, as observed by anal manometry and clinical evaluation (47).

A recent search of the Cochrane Incontinence Group trials register reported only one eligible trial of electrical stimulation that included 40 participants (48). Findings of this trial suggested that electrical stimulation with anal biofeedback and exercise provides more short-term benefits than vaginal biofeedback and exercises for women with obstetric-related fecal incontinence. However, this data is insufficient and larger trials are required.

Recently, a method of electrical stimulation was developed in Brazil for the treatment of fecal incontinence (Viotti, São Paulo, Brazil). Two electrodes are positioned in the perianal area, and electrical stimulus varying from 4 to 36 mA are applied at intervals during 15-minute sessions (Fig. 13). The duration and frequency of the stimulus can be individually adjusted.

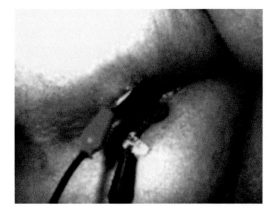

Figure 13 (*See color insert*) Electrical stimulation.

Currently, centers are randomizing nonsurgical candidates to either electrical stimulation or bio-feedback therapy. All patients are submitted to physiological evaluation to exclude sphincteric defects amenable to surgical treatment. The initial favorable experience with 10 patients has been promising. However, a long-term prospective randomized trial will be necessary to prove any definitive benefits of using electrical stimulation therapy for the treatment of fecal incontinence.

Radiofrequency

The development of the SECCA® device (Curon Medical, Minneapolis, Minnesota, U.S.A.) has made it possible to deliver temperature-controlled radiofrequency energy to the anorectal junction to treat fecal incontinence. The procedure is performed on an outpatient basis either in the endoscopy suite or in an ambulatory surgery center. Exclusion criteria include inflammatory bowel disease, chronic diarrhea, irritable bowel syndrome, pregnancy, and congenital or traumatic abnormalities of the external sphincter. The initial report in the literature was a small series that included 10 female patients with varying degrees of fecal incontinence (49). The most common complication was bleeding in four patients, which was conservatively treated. All parameters in a fecal incontinence–related quality of life scale were improved, and at six months, the majority of patients had eliminated the use of protective pads. Subsequently, the results of an extensive two-year study were published (50). The apparent durability of this procedure has initiated a multicenter study to evaluate the safety and efficacy of the SECCA® procedure. In this trial, 50 patients from five different centers were enrolled (51). The procedure was performed on an outpatient basis using local anesthesia. Of the 43 females and 7 males, a 70% resolution of incontinent symptoms was achieved. As previously demonstrated, all parameters in the FIQL scale were improved and only minor complications were reported.

Carbon Beads

The ACYST™ (Advanced UroScience Inc., St. Paul, Minnesota, U.S.A.) procedure utilizes microcarbon-coated beads that are injected into the anal canal and lower rectum in an outpatient setting. The long-term bulking effect in the tissue results from the combination of scar tissue and carbon-coated beads (52). However, this procedure has not yet been approved by the U.S. Food and Drug Administration (FDA) and is therefore still considered an investigational medical device. As with the SECCA® procedure, exclusion criteria include inflammatory bowel disease, chronic diarrhea, irritable bowel syndrome, pregnancy, and congenital or traumatic abnormalities of the external sphincter.

Anal Incontinence Plug

An anal plug was initially used for the control of colostomy output following abdominoperineal resection. This technique raised the idea for the development of an anal continence plug to be used in selected patients with fecal incontinence. Currently, available expandable plugs function in the capacity of an anal tampon. However, the estimated monthly cost per patient is approximately $500, and patients rarely tolerate their long-term use.

The Procon™ Incontinence Device was initially introduced by the AnaTech, LLC, Houston, Texas, U.S.A. as a 510K Class II FDA-approved device. This device is a small, flexible biochemically inert catheter with a distal motion sensor electrode (Fig. 14), which was designed to be placed in the rectal vault and held in place by a small balloon. A signaling device (beeper) worn on the patient's waist signifies when stool reaches the rectum, thereby preventing seepage and allowing adequate time to reach a bathroom, deflate the balloon, and evacuate. The possibility of warning patients of an imminent bowel movement has distinguished this device from other anal plugs. A single report in the literature was published in 2002, wherein the authors describe their initial experience with seven incontinent patients (53). The majority were females with a mean age of 72.7 years. The type of incontinence was idiopathic in four patients, two patients had a sphincter defect, and one had incontinence due to a neurogenic cause. The device was used for 14 consecutive days, wherein patients were asked to complete a quality of life diary and daily log of bowel activity prior to and after the completion of 14 days during which the patients wore the device. A statistically significant improvement in quality of life and a reduction in the incontinence score were noted, and the authors concluded that the Procon™ incontinence device is a promising device for select patients. However, adequate selection of suitable candidates is very important for this procedure; exclusion criteria are pediatric cases and patients with dementia or neurologic diseases.

At the time of this writing, the Procon2™ device is marketed by Incontinence Control Devices, Inc., Houston, TX, U.S.A. and after undergoing physical revision, another clinical trial is underway in order to reassess its safety and effectiveness.

Biofeedback

Among the nonoperative treatment modalities available for patients with incontinence, biofeedback therapy is the most widely used. However, a recent review of the Cochrane Incontinence Group on 23 articles related to biofeedback for fecal incontinence demonstrated that, in fact, there were only five eligible prospective randomized trials that included a total of 109 patients (54). These trials were small and employed a limited range of outcome measures. Furthermore, follow-up information was not consistently reported, and only two trials provided data in a form suitable for statistical analyses. Therefore, the limited number of identified trials coupled with their methodological weaknesses does not allow reliable objective assessment of the actual role of sphincter exercises and biofeedback therapy in the nonoperative management of fecal incontinence. Nonetheless, as stated above, biofeedback therapy is one of the most widely used nonsurgical methods for the treatment of fecal incontinence with reported success rates ranging from 50% to 90% (Table 7) (55–90).

Biofeedback is a behavioral therapy that is safe, noninvasive, and cost-effective. This therapy requires a quiet and comfortable environment and a well-motivated patient who can focus on an image, word, or phrase to remove distractions. Physiologic activity is monitored, and unconscious physiologic information is provided by audio or visual stimuli to allow the patient to gain control over these functions. Biofeedback is an interesting option

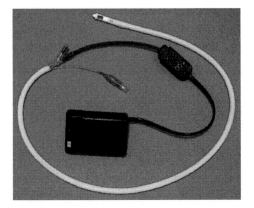

Figure 14 Procon™ incontinence device.

Table 7 Results of Biofeedback for Fecal Incontinence

Author	Year	Patients (*N*)	Mean age (years)	Mean follow-up (months)	Control group	BF system	Clinical improvement (%)
Haskell and Rovner (55)	1967	54	–	–	No	EMG	61
Engel et al. (56)	1974	6	41	0.6–60	No	Balloon	86
Cerulli et al. (57)	1979	50	47	0.4–108	No	Balloon	73
Goldenberg et al. (58)	1980	12	0.12–78	0.3–24	No	Balloon	83
Wald (59)	1981	17	48	15	No	Balloon	71
MacLeod (60)	1983	50	55	12	No	EMG	72
Wald (61)	1983	15	8	23	Yes	Balloon	47
Latimer et al. (62)	1984	26	30	6	Yes	NR	88
Wald and Tunugunta (63)	1984	11	52	0.7–24	Yes	Balloon	73
Whitehead et al. (64)	1985	18	73	6	Yes	Balloon	77
Buser and Miner (65)	1986	13	–	0.16–30	No	Balloon	92
Whitehead et al. (66)	1986	33	9	12	Yes	Balloon	64
MacLeod (67)	1987	113	56	0.6–60	No	EMG	63
Berti Riboli et al. (68)	1988	20	61	–	No	Balloon	84
Loening-Baucke (69)	1990	8	63	12	Yes	Balloon	38
Miner et al. (70)	1990	25	–	24	Yes	Balloon	76
Chiarioni et al. (71)	1993	14	49	14	Yes	Balloon	85
Salomon et al. (72)	1993	20	54	–	No	Water	60
Jensen and Lowry (73)	1993	43	55	–	No	NR	93
Souza et al. (74)	1994	28	–	–	Yes	NR	57
Arhan et al. (75)	1994	47	11	–	No	Balloon	50
Keck et al. (76)	1994	15	39	–	No	Balloon	73
Enck et al. (77)	1994	18	57	60	Yes	EMG	Yes
Ferrara et al. (78)	1995	32	55	–	Yes	EMG	Yes
Sangwan et al. (79)	1995	28	53	21	No	Balloon	75
Guillemot et al. (80)	1995	16	62	30	Yes	Balloon	25
van Tets et al. (81)	1996	12	48	3	No	EMG	0
Rao et al. (82)	1996	19	50	12	No	NR	53
Ko et al. (83)	1997	25	63	Not done	No	NR	87.5
Gilliland et al. (84)	1997	141	72 (10–100)	–	No	EMG	77.5
Karlboym et al. (85)	1997	28	46 (22–72)	14	No	EMG	43
Rieger et al. (86)	1997	19	63 (16–78)	6	No	EMG	23
Patankar et al. (87)	1997	25	66	Not done	No	NR	70
Patankar et al. (88)	1997	72	70	Not done	No	NR	83.3
Glia et al. (89)	1998	26	61	21 (12–46)	No	NR	53.7
Pager et al. (90)	2002	83	–	42	No	NR	75

Abbreviations: EMG, electromyography; NR, not reported; BF, biofeedback.

for the nonsurgical treatment of fecal incontinence, especially in patients who have failed to gain satisfactory function after an anatomically successful sphincter repair (91). The principle of biofeedback therapy is to exercise the sphincter muscles by training the mind to control somatic function in order to improve sphincter strength. This technique of retraining pelvic floor muscles was introduced by Arnold Kegel for the treatment of fecal incontinence (92,93). Using a perineometer, Kegel developed a variety of pelvic floor exercises, which today bear his name.

There are two methods for biofeedback training: one is in response to rectal distention using manometric techniques and the other is unrelated to rectal distention, using EMG. In the former method, the patients should have normal rectal sensation in order to recognize smaller distention volumes and increase the strength of external anal sphincter contraction in response to distention. The latter method, unrelated to rectal distention, is performed using an intra-anal plug connected to an EMG machine. Patients are instructed to contract and relax the sphincter anal muscles while the muscle activity is recorded and displayed on the computer screen. Patients are taught to contract and relax the sphincters in the initial learning process that requires 15 to 30 minutes. The aim of this method is to increase external sphincter strength. Treatment is supervised by a biofeedback therapist who evaluates patients during a six- to eight-week period. Both methods are effective, although some patients may respond better to one system than to the other.

Results are defined as "good" if patients achieve at least a 75% decrease in the frequency of incontinent episodes or if complete continence is restored. Conditions that may be predisposed to a poor biofeedback response include severe sphincteric lesions, low anterior resection, a keyhole deformity, obesity, or irritable bowel syndrome.

The exact mechanism by which biofeedback improves anal continence remains obscure, and further studies are necessary to elucidate this issue. Several investigators have attempted to study biofeedback mechanism for the treatment of fecal incontinence, but the results are contradictory. For example, some authors have reported an increase in sphincter pressures in patients with a successful outcome, whereas others (61,69,94) reported no noticeable difference in any of these pressures.

The reported success rates in the literature vary between 50% and 90% (54). Despite this overall enthusiasm, it was demonstrated that initial good results at six months can deteriorate after two years, and it may therefore be useful to reinforce this treatment after six months. A high level of motivation and intelligence are factors associated with the best results. Similarly, an understanding of biological muscle response to what the psychotherapist is asking the patient to do is crucial. The most optimal results of this therapy are usually obtained in patients with muscle weakness after anorectal surgery. Conversely, in patients with neurological involvement such as diabetic neuropathy, multiple sclerosis, or myelomeningocele, suboptimal results can be expected as rectal sensation is largely impaired or completely absent in 70% of patients. This observation was confirmed by van Tets et al. (81) who studied 12 patients with neurogenic incontinence who underwent biofeedback therapy. After a 12-week training period, none of the patients experienced an improvement in fecal incontinence.

Although it can be time consuming, biofeedback is completely free of any morbidity, causes minimal discomfort to the patient, and is a good option for incontinent patients with altered sphincter function.

In a long-term study of patients who were treated by biofeedback several years before, Enck et al. (77) reported that an improvement in continence was observed in 19 patients not only during treatment but also for several years thereafter. Another long-term study of clinical results of biofeedback therapy demonstrated that continence was improved at 6 and 30 months (80). One recent study evaluated the long-term outcomes of biofeedback in 83 patients and demonstrated that for many patients, an improvement continued subsequent to program completion (90).

Our personal experience includes 120 patients selected for biofeedback therapy, 66 of whom completed the entire biofeedback training program (95). These included 56 females and 10 males of a median age of 66 (10–82) years, who underwent a median of three (1–8) biofeedback sessions. The overall success of biofeedback was 84%. At a median follow-up period of 12.5 (1–43) months, the median prebiofeedback CCFSS was 11.8, and the median postbiofeedback score decreased to 5 ($p < 0.0001$). An increase in squeeze pressures was also noted after biofeedback therapy ($p = 0.0016$). One parameter that positively influenced outcome was the absence of muscle fatigue (61% of good outcome), whereas the presence of a severe sphincter defect determined poor outcome; there were no complications associated with this therapy.

Biofeedback therapy is a virtually harmless and inexpensive treatment that can improve fecal incontinence in approximately 75% of selected patients and is our preferred method of nonsurgical treatment for fecal incontinence.

Macroplasty

Augmentation of the anal sphincter muscle bulk has been performed in four uncontrolled studies using autologous fat injection, Teflon paste, or collagen injections (96–99). The satisfactory results obtained in these small trials stimulated the development of a new silicone substance to be injected for the same purpose. Recently, an injectable silicone biomaterial for fecal incontinence was proposed, and the results from a small series of six patients were published (100). These patients initially underwent anorectal physiologic testing during which poor internal sphincter function was detected. The trans-sphincteric injection of silicone-based biomaterial was performed under local anesthesia, with an improvement in five of the six patients. This method is a promising new tool for the treatment of fecal incontinence related to internal sphincter defects, and, certainly, new and larger series in the literature will demonstrate the potential benefits of this treatment modality.

Our initial experience with this new modality includes three female patients with a moderate degree of incontinence. The injections were positioned at three points around the anal circumference at 3, 7, and 11 hours, and all patients tolerated the procedure well (Fig. 15). At a follow-up of four months, all patients demonstrated an improvement in the number of incontinent episodes. The injected silicone was well positioned, as demonstrated by anal ultrasonography (Fig. 16).

Topical or Oral Drugs

The use of topical and oral medications such as phenylephrine (101) and amitriptyline (102) has been proposed in the treatment of fecal incontinence. The use of topical phenylephrine is a feasible method of increase resting anal tone as demonstrated with different concentrations by Cheetham in 2001 (101). Oral amitriptyline is effective in the reduction of incontinent episodes and improved symptoms in 89% of a small series of 18 patients (102). The successful results were reportedly due to the decrease in the amplitude and frequency of rectal motor complexes, as well as an increase in colonic transit times, resulting in firmer stool that are passed less frequently.

Selection of the treatment modality to be employed depends on a number of aspects such as the severity of symptoms, bioavailability, and patient cooperation. Moreover, the concomitant use of various methods can improve results. For patients where conservative options have failed or were insufficient due to the presence of neuromuscular damage, a number of surgical procedures are available.

SURGICAL TREATMENT

The determination of patients who will benefit from a surgical procedure is important, especially among females. A 29% incidence of sphincter injury after vaginal delivery was reported in the literature and could be detected by anal ultrasonography (103). These anterior isolated sphincter defects can be managed by overlapping sphincteroplasty with successful outcomes of 69% to 97% (104–107). Long-term function after anterior sphincteroplasty, however, is still in question, and recent studies have demonstrated that only less than 50% of patients remain continent after five years (108). Surgical techniques for patients with failed anterior sphincteroplasty include implantation of an artificial anal sphincter, performing a

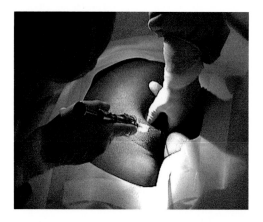

Figure 15 Macroplasty.

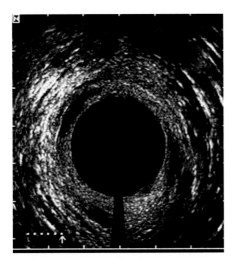

Figure 16 Ultrasound following macroplasty.

stimulated graciloplasty, or implantation of a sacral nerve stimulator (11,109). These three techniques are complex surgical procedures and are associated with a very high morbidity; hence, they should be used prudently in a very select group of patients. Table 8 demonstrates the various surgical procedures for fecal incontinence.

Preoperative Patient Preparation

Due to the risk of infection and an associated breakdown of the repair, intraoperative and postoperative broad-spectrum antibiotics are recommended for all patient procedures (110,111).

Despite the recent controversies regarding the use of mechanical bowel preparation for colorectal surgery, it is our policy to prepare all patients with a full oral bowel preparation (112). All patients are operated under general anesthesia. However, sphincter repairs can also be performed under spinal anesthesia.

For anterior sphincteroplasty, postanal repair, gluteus maximus transposition, and total pelvic floor repair, patients are usually placed in the prone jackknife position. For more

Table 8 Surgical Treatment of Fecal Incontinence

Anorectal muscle repair
  Perineorrhaphy
  Direct aposition
  Overlapping sphincteroplasty
  Internal sphincter repair
  Postanal repair
  Total pelvic floor repair
  Levatoroplasty
Neosphincter procedures
  Static anal encirclement
    Free muscle transplantation
    Sartorius, palmaris, longus
    Gluteus maximus transposition
    Gracilis transposition
    Thiersch operation
  Dynamic anal encirclement
    Stimulated gracilis neosphincter
    Artificial bowel sphincter
Intestinal diversion
    Colostomy
    Ileostomy
Other
    Continent colonic conduit
    Sacral nerve stimulation

complex procedures such as the gracilis muscle transposition and implantation of an artificial sphincter, the Lloyd–Davies or lithotomy positions are recommended.

Obstetric Damage

Various reports in the literature associating fecal incontinence with obstetrical trauma have brought the risk of sphincter injury to the attention of colorectal surgeons and obstetricians (113,114). Recognition of this etiologic factor of fecal incontinence in the female population has important implications; first, many incontinent patients do not seek medical attention due to embarrassment (115) and, second, the social and psychological impact is tremendous. Medicolegal issues have been increasingly reported (116), and the treatment of postpartum fecal incontinence has a very high cumulative cost (10).

Obsteric injury to the sphincters may be noted at the time of delivery or may be detected in the postpartum period. The reported incidence of sphincter injuries at the time of delivery ranges between 0.5% and 3% of vaginal deliveries (117,118). However, the use of anal ultrasonography has altered this view by identifying occult sphincter defects. A recent meta-analysis by Oberwalder et al. (119) reported the incidence of postpartum anal sphincter defects diagnosed by anal ultrasonography and associated incidences of fecal incontinence. A 27% incidence of anal sphincter defects in primiparous women and an 8.5% incidence of new sphincter defects in multiparous women were found. In addition, this analysis demonstrated that 29.7 % of anal sphincter defects were symptomatic, whereas no defects could be demonstrated in 3.4% of women with postpartum fecal incontinence. Utilizing a Bayesian calculation, the probability of postpartum fecal incontinence due to a sphincter defect was 76.8% to 82.8%, much higher than commonly estimated with at least two-thirds of occult defects being asymptomatic in the postpartum period.

A systematic review of national practice survey among colorectal surgeons and obstetricians conducted in the United Kingdom discussed the numerous aspects of obstetric damage and brought attention to the need for basic guidelines in the management and prevention of sphincter trauma (120). They reported a wide variation in the experience of repairing acute anal sphincter injury. The group with the largest experience were consultant obstetricians (46.5% undertaking ≥ 5 repairs/year), while only 10% of responding colorectal surgeons had similar levels of experience. Furthermore, there was extensive disparity in the definition of obstetric anal sphincter injury. While observational studies suggest that a new "overlap" repair using polydioxanone sutures (PDS) with antibiotic cover gives better functional results, there was a wide variation in practice with 337 (50%) consultants, 82 (55%) trainees, and 80 (89%) coloproctologists already using the "overlap" method for repair of the external sphincter. In addition, although over 50% of colorectal surgeons undertake long-term follow-up of their patients, less than 10% of obstetricians do the same. Finally, while over 70% of coloproctologists would recommend an elective cesarean section in a subsequent pregnancy, only 22% of obstetric consultants would adopt that policy.

One of the important issues involving obstetric injury to the anal sphincters is the inconsistent classification of perineal tears in the literature. Therefore, in 1999, a standardized classification was proposed by Sultan (121) (Table 9). For women who had a primary repair

Table 9 Classification of Perineal Tears

First degree
  Laceration of the vaginal epithelium or perineal skin only
Second degree
  Involvement of the vaginal epithelium, perineal skin, perineal muscles, and
  fascia but not the anal sphincter
Third degree
  Disruption of the vaginal epithelium, perineal skin, perineal body, and
    anal sphincter muscles. This should be subdivided into:
    Partial tear of the external sphincter involving less than 50% thickness
    Complete tear of the external sphincter
    Internal sphincter torn as well
Fourth degree
  A third-degree tear with disruption of the anal epithelium

Source: Frome Ref. 121.

at the time of delivery, information regarding the possibility of future sequelae is warranted. Furthermore, these patients should be assessed at 6 to 12 weeks postpartum by anorectal physiology and ultrasonography. A secondary repair should be offered for all symptomatic women who sustain a sphincter defect. In those cases, if the repair is successful, the patient should be advised to deliver any subsequent pregnancies by cesarian section.

Direct apposition of obstetric sphincter lacerations is usually performed at the time of injury, and satisfactory results can be achieved in a tension-free repair. However, hematoma formation, wound infection, faulty technique, or an unrecognized second sphincter injury can produce a poor outcome requiring a secondary repair (122–124).

In patients with severe traumatic lesions with gross contamination of the perianal region and associated pelvic injury, it is advisable to delay definitive sphincter repair. These patients are best managed with local debridement and a diverting colostomy. Secondary repair is performed only after all contaminated perineal wounds have healed and the inflammation has completely resolved. Despite numerous questions regarding obstetrical sphincter damage, which remain unanswered, there are some evidence-based data already established: (i) Forceps delivery and nulliparity are risk factors for recognized anal sphincter injury at the time of vaginal delivery (125,126). (ii) The performance of a midline episiotomy is associated with an increased risk of anal sphincter tear compared with delivery without an episiotomy (127), whereas mediolateral episiotomy seems to protect nulliparous women from sphincter damage (128). (iii) Forceps delivery is associated with a stronger risk factor for third-degree perineal tears than vacuum extraction, therefore the latter should be used for the prevention of fecal incontinence whenever possible (129). (iv) There is no difference in outcomes after primary repair of third-degree obstetric tear when an approximation or an overlapping technique is used.

Factors that Influence Surgical Results (Table 10)
Suture Material
Currently, there are no prospective randomized trials assessing the best suture material for sphincter repair. Although most texts describe the use of chromic catgut, monofilament suture materials such as PDS or polypropylene (Prolene) are thought to be superior to catgut due to a longer half-life. However, there is strong evidence that synthetic materials such as vicryl or polyglycolic acid (dexon) are preferable to catgut for perineal repairs (130).

Stool Softeners
Many surgeons adopt the use of stool softeners and oral fiber to avoid the passage of a hard fecal bolus that may theoretically disrupt the repair. Because there are no randomized trials comparing the use of stool softeners after sphincter repair, there are no formal contraindications for that practice. However, the use of bowel confinement has been shown to confer no benefit in terms of septic complications or functional outcomes (131).

Diversion
Diversion of the colon through a colostomy or ileostomy has not demonstrated any supported data in the management of acute sphincter trauma. A small randomized trial of 27 patients showed no conclusive evidence that diversion confers any benefit for those patients undergoing a secondary repair. In addition, it may be associated with higher morbidity and longer hospitalization times (132).

Table 10 Optimal Conditions for Sphincter Repair

Preoperative
   Absence of irritable bowel syndrome
   No previous repair
   Scar present
   Bilateral intact pudendal nerves
   Normal rectal sensation
   Asthenic patient
   Young patient
Intraoperative
   Overlapping scar
   Increased resting and squeeze pressure
   Increased high-pressure zone

Age

The exact reason for deterioration of continence over time remains unknown. However, a number of reports have shown that age, gender, and parity all affect anorectal function. Increasing age leads to perineal descent at rest and slowed pudendal nerve conduction in anorectal sensory function. There is a high correlation between age and the degree of sclerosis of the internal anal sphincter, leading to decreased resting pressures (133). In addition, muscle atrophy occurs with aging (134). Nonetheless, advanced age should not preclude an otherwise potentially useful sphincter repair.

Obesity

Regardless of which operation is utilized for fecal incontinence in obese patients, the outcomes are less successful, and preoperative counseling is required to avoid unexpected and disappointing results (135,136).

Neuropathy

While some authors are still reluctant to associate neuropathy with poor outcomes after sphincter repair, one multivariate analysis showed that bilateral neuropathy was the only factor predictive of failure following sphincteroplasty (40). In the same study, bilaterally normal pudendal nerves were predictive of success. In fact, many prior publications have related pudendal neuropathy with poor outcomes after sphincter repair (Table 11) (38–41,137–139). Although patients should not be denied a sphincter repair based on a prolonged pudendal nerve study, this evaluation is important in the patient's preoperative counseling and advisory discussion.

Irritable Bowel Syndrome

Any alteration in bowel habits leading to diarrheal states or an exacerbation of an underlying irritable bowel syndrome can cause symptomatic recurrence after sphincter repair (140). Therefore, preoperative patient selection is mandatory.

Hormonal Influence

The existence of estrogen receptors throughout the female genitourinary tract and in the pelvic floor musculature, particularly in the external anal sphincter, has been documented (141). Based on this knowledge, a beneficial effect of hormone replacement therapy in postmenopausal women with fecal incontinence has been suggested. Although there is no randomized trial to support this evidence, hormone replacement therapy may be an indication for postmenopausal women with fecal incontinence, provided that there is no contraindication for its use.

REPEAT SPHINCTER REPAIR

In some situations, a persistent defect is noted on anal ultrasound after primary sphincteroplasty. If the patient is symptomatic and the persistent defect seems to be the cause of these symptoms, a repeat repair is recommended. In a small series of 26 patients who underwent repeat sphincter repair, both the continence score and the ability to defer defecation were improved in 65% of patients undergoing a second or third repair (142).

Table 11 Influence of Pudendal Neuropathy on Outcome

Author	Year	Cases (no.)	Success without neuropathy (%)	Success with neuropathy (%)	p
Laurberg et al. (138)	1988	19	80	11	<0.05
Wexner et al. (38)	1991	16	92	50	NS
Simmang et al. (137)	1994	14	100	67	NS
Londono-Schimmer et al. (40)	1994	94	55	30	<0.001
Sitzler and Thomson (139)	1996	31	67	63	NS
Sangwan et al. (39)	1996	15	100	14	<0.005
Gilliland et al.	1997	76	63	16	<0.01

Abbreviation: NS, not significant.

In another retrospective study of 151 patients who underwent a sphincter repair, 36 patients had at least one previous repair. In that group, the outcome was successful in 61% of patients. Therefore, repeat sphincter repair should be considered in all cases (143).

SURGICAL PROCEDURES
Perineorrhaphy

Plication of the perineal body in conjunction with a vaginal colporrhaphy is performed by some surgeons. Development of the rectovaginal septum by sharp dissection is followed by an excision of excess vaginal mucosa and approximation of the transverse perineal musculature to reconstruct or reinforce the perineal body. Failure to recognize and repair concomitant injury of the anal sphincter mechanism is usually accompanied by continued fecal incontinence. Overlapping sphincteroplasty is clearly the operation of choice in incontinent patients with a functional, yet, anatomically disrupted sphincter muscle.

Direct Apposition

Initial direct surgical methods created to restore continence after sphincter injury involved identification, mobilization of external anal sphincter, excision of all scar tissue, and direct apposition of the muscles ends (Fig. 17). The results were disappointing, and there is now clear evidence that this type of repair is associated with poor outcomes as up to 59% of patients have some degree of persistent incontinence.

Overlapping Sphincteroplasty

Initial attempts to repair severe sphincter muscle injury carried a 40% failure rate possibly due to the inability of applying direct end-to-end sutures to maintain muscle integrity (144). Therefore, overlapping sphincter repair was introduced to minimize the risk of disruption and is currently the most commonly used surgical procedure for the treatment of anal sphincter defects (Fig. 18). After sterile preparation of the perianal area, a circumanal and bilateral nerve block is achieved using a mixture of 0.25% marcaine and 0.5% xylocaine with 1:200.000 units of epinephrine for adequate hemostasis and elevation of tissue planes, and to minimize post-operative pain. An anterior 120° to 160° curvilinear incision approximately 0.5 cm caudal and parallel to the outer edge of the anal verge is performed, allowing dissection and mobilization of the sphincter muscles and scar. The anterior dissection should be performed with the surgeon's contralateral index finger in the vagina. This maneuver is useful to gauge tissue thickness and to avoid inadvertent vaginal wall injury. Lateral dissection, where muscle anatomy is usually intact, can help the surgeon to identify the proper plane for dissection.

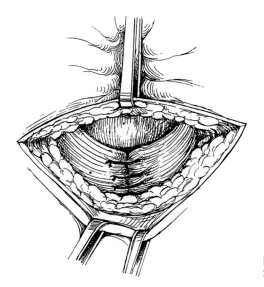

Figure 17 Direct sphincter repair. *Source*: From W. B. Saunders, London, U.K.

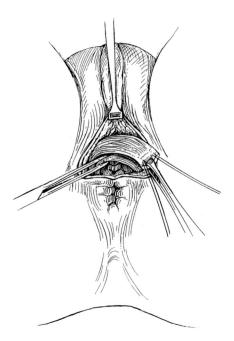

Figure 18 Overlapping sphincteroplasty. *Source*: From W. B. Saunders, London, U.K.

Care must be taken to preserve the pudendal nerve bundles that enter the muscles in the bilateral posterolateral positions. The intersphincteric space is then mobilized from lateral to medial to the area of the midline scar, and the external and internal anal sphincters are separated. After completion of the flap dissection, the scar tissue is divided through the midline. It is important to preserve all scar tissue in order to better anchor the sutures. A prospective trial comparing three types of repair (muscle to muscle, muscle to scar, and scar over scar) has highlighted the importance of scar preservation during sphincteroplasty (145).

The repair starts with apposition of the levator muscles using interrupted 2–0 polydioxane sutures. In addition, the internal anal sphincter can be also plicated using the same technique. These sutures should be placed far enough laterally to achieve a snug repair that can be best assessed using the index finger in the anal canal. Although it was demonstrated that this technique may improve continence by increasing the length of the high-pressure zone, it is an optional repair (104). Finally, the divided external sphincter overlap is performed with interrupted mattress type 2–0 polydioxane sutures, using the scar tissues for adequate suture fixation.

The anterior and lateral aspects of the wound are then closed with interrupted absorbable 2–0 polyglactin sutures in a V–Y fashion, leaving the central portion open for drainage. Wound packing is avoided, and patients are instructed to take daily sitz baths after the first postoperative day. On the third postoperative day, a regular diet and psyllium supplements are started, parenteral antibiotics are discontinued, and the bladder catheter is removed; the wound is generally completely closed within four to six weeks. Various series have demonstrated a 70% to 80% success rate after overlapping sphincteroplasty (Table 12) (38,39,41,104,135,137–139,146–153).

Although the long-term results of sphincter repair are less acceptable than in the initial years, this procedure is a good option for the treatment of fecal incontinence secondary to isolated or combined anterior sphincter defects (154). It has the advantages of a low incidence of perineal infection and restores normal anatomy and function.

Internal Sphincter Repair

Plication of the internal anal sphincter is performed in conjunction with overlapping sphincteroplasty in order to increase the high-pressure zone. However, because this is a thin and delicate muscle, this procedure does not appear to offer a clear benefit, because restoration of continence is achieved in 75% of patients with or without repairing the internal anal sphincter (155,156). In fact, a slight improvement in fecal continence was only demonstrated by Leroi et al. (157) in a small series of five patients who underwent isolated internal sphincter repair.

Table 12 Sphincteroplasty Series

Author	Year	Patients (N)	Age mean (range)	Women (%)	Obstetric (%)	Colostomy (%)	Good/excellent results (%)
Fang et al. (146)	1984	79	(17–68)	78	88	0	89
Laurberg et al. (138)	1988	19	(23–64)	100	100	–	47
Yoshioka et al. (147)	1989	27	34 (17–81)	52	70	37	74
Wexner et al. (38)	1991	16	54 (34–74)	100	90	0	76
Fleshman et al. (148)	1991	28	38 (22–75)	100	100	0	75
Engel et al. (149)	1994	55	32 (26–52)	100	100	24	76
Engel et al. (150)	1994	28	41 (22–66)	89	53	36	75
Simmang et al. (137)	1994	14	66 (51–81)	100	79	0	93
Londono-Schimmer et al. (40)	1994	128	43 (16–77)	78	64	15	50
Oliveira et al. (104)	1996	55	48 (27–72)	100	84	0	71
Felt-Bersma et al. (151)	1996	18	47 (29–72)	61	39	0	72
Nikiteas et al. (135)	1996	42	43	76	26	14	67
Sitzler et al. (139)	1997	31	42	87	64	80	74
Roche et al. (152)	1997	150	(60–90)	92	70		
Ternent et al. (153)	1997	16	44	100	100		62
Gilliland et al. (41)	1997	77	47 (25–80)	–	69	–	55

Postanal Repair

The technique of postanal repair was first introduced by Parks in 1975 (158) to restore the anorectal angle in incontinent patients with intact but poorly functioning sphincters and a flat anorectal angle. In this operation, a posterior levatorplasty was thought to improve continence by making the anorectal angle more acute and by lengthening the anal canal (Fig. 19). This procedure is particularly suited for idiopathic neurogenic incontinence and persistent incontinence following rectal prolapse repair. In addition, it can be employed in patients with poor resting pressures without a demonstrable sphincter defect, who have failed conservative measures and biofeedback therapy.

Unlike anterior sphincteroplasty, the U-shaped incision is performed posteriorly, approximately 5 cm caudal to the anal verge, which allows dissection of the sphincter muscles to Waldeyer's fascia where the levator complex is located; the Waldeyer's fascia is identified and divided by sharp dissection. The supralevator space is entered, the perirectal fat is pushed away, and the levator ani muscles are identified laterally. Plication of the ileococcygeous,

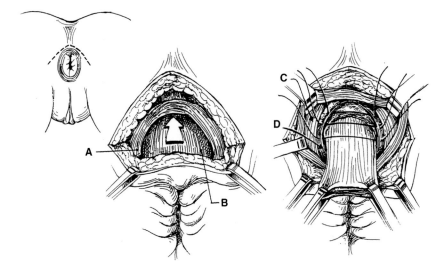

Figure 19 Postanal repair: (**A**) external anal sphincter; (**B**) internal anal sphincter; (**C**) puborectalis muscle; (**D**) levator ani muscle. *Source*: From W. B. Saunders, London, U.K.

pubococcygeous, and puborectalis muscles is then performed, using interrupted prolene sutures giving support to the posterior rectal wall. These sutures should be tied in a tension-free manner to avoid necrosis of the puborectalis muscle. The skin is closed in a V–Y fashion, and a suction drain is left in situ for one to two postoperative days. This operation has never gained popularity in the United States due to poor functional results, reportedly only 59% among the published series (Table 13) (158–168).

Matsuoka et al. (168) reported a series of 21 incontinent patients who underwent postanal repair after a median of 6.8 years of incontinence prior to that operation. After a mean follow-up of 22 months, only 35% of patients considered their surgery to be successful. Similarly, previous reports analyzing this operation in a long-term period concluded that successful rates are achieved in only 33% of patients (167). Despite these suboptimal results, postanal repair can be a low-risk procedure for patients who have failed other conservative measures or previous repairs and wish to avoid a permanent stoma.

A recent evaluation of the structural and functional results of postanal repair using dynamic MRI concluded that there is no difference in static pelvic floor measurements when patients remaining symptomatic after postanal repair are compared with those who are improved (169). In contrast, dynamic measurements may predict failure in those who demonstrate excessive posterior pelvic floor mobility.

Total Pelvic Floor Repair

This technique was proposed for patients with disappointing results after postanal repair and consists of a combination of anterior external sphincter plication with levatorplasty and postanal repair (170). As with postanal repair, clinical improvement does not correlate with anorectal angle changes, and widespread acceptance of this technique has never been achieved. One randomized trial undertaken by Deen et al. (171) compared three methods of pelvic floor repair for neuropathic fecal incontinence. They compared postanal repair, anterior levatorplasty, and total pelvic floor reconstruction in 36 female patients, 12 in each group. They concluded that total pelvic floor reconstruction is a viable option for idiopathic incontinence. However, their results do not seem to reflect the reality in terms of functional outcome because physiologic investigation was not performed in any of the patients. Because PNTML assessment was not performed in any patients in this trial, it is possible that the superior results in the total pelvic floor repair group were due to pudendal neuropathy in patients in the anterior sphincteroplasty-alone group. Another randomized trial comparing postanal and total pelvic floor repair for neurogenic incontinence concluded that these procedures produce no consistent changes in anatomy or physiology, and that clinical improvement is caused by creation of a local stenosis or by the placebo effect rather than by any actual improvement in muscle function (172).

Neosphincter Operations

Severe damage to the anal sphincter muscles, with multiple defects in different quadrants of the anal circumference, is usually amenable to direct repair. Insufficient muscle mass may

Table 13 Postanal Repair Series

Author	Year	Patients (*N*)	Good to excellent outcome (%)
Parks et al. (158)	1966	–	–
Browning et al. (159)	1983	140	86
Keighley (160)	1984	114	32
van Vroonhaven et al. (161)	1984	16	70
Ferguson (162)	1984	9	67
Henry and Simpson (163)	1985	204	58
Womack et al. (21)	1988	16	88
Yoshioka et al. (164)	1988	–	–
Scheuer et al. (165)	1989	39	43
Rainey et al. (166)	1990	42	31
Orrom et al. (167)	1991	17	59
Matsuoka et al. (168)	1997	15	40

be the result of a congenital defect, trauma, or neurogenic injury and may account for severe dysfunction despite an intact sphincter muscle. In these situations, a number of neosphincter operations are available. These are complex operations with very high morbidity rates related mainly to infection, technical problems with the device, and disrupted muscle wraps, among other problems (173–175). Despite this high morbidity, dynamic gracioplasty is still thought to play a role in selected cases of end-stage fecal incontinence when undertaken by an experienced team, as demonstrated by a multicenter trial (176).

Free Muscle Transplantation

Free transplantation of the palmaris longus or a portion of the sartorius muscle was popularized by Hakelius and Olsen (177) mainly for the treatment of severe incontinence resulting from congenital absence or traumatic injury to the puborectalis muscle. Successful transplantation depends on reinnervation of the transplanted muscle following transplantation into the functional position of the puborectalis muscle. After reinnervation has taken place, the muscle becomes integrated as part of the reflex mechanism.

Gluteus Maximus Transposition

This operation was initially described by Chetwood in 1902 (178). The gluteus maximus was the most commonly used muscle for transposition operations during the first half of the 20th century. Transposition of this muscle is facilitated due to the proximity to the anal canal, thin belly, and proximal single innervation. One advantage of using the gluteus maximus muscle instead of the gracilis is that it is a large and strong muscle whose proximity to the perianal area eliminates the need for thigh incisions. Anal canal encirclement using this muscle allows voluntary contraction and is indicated for patients with neurogenic incontinence, multiple failed previous repairs, and severe sphincter defects with good functional outcomes. One of the most common complications after gluteus maximus transposition is infection of the wound that, generally, can be locally managed without the need for fecal diversion. The series in the literature involve small number of patients, and overall rates of complete and partial restoration of continence are 60% and 36%, respectively (Table 14) (178–191).

In one publication, 11 patients with longstanding fecal incontinence, who underwent augmented unilateral gluteoplasty, were followed for 6 to 18 months (192). Improvement was demonstrated in almost 73% of patients with less incidence of morbidity. A prospective randomized trial comparing total pelvic floor repair and gluteus maximus transposition demonstrated that both procedures significantly improved continence in 24 women with neuropathic incontinence (193). However, when compared with gracioplasty, the results of a multicenter prospective trial demonstrated that the results of gluteoplasty were less successful and should be limited to investigational purposes (194).

Table 14 Unstimulated Bilateral Gluteoplasty Series

Author	Year	Patients (*N*)	Results	
			Good	Fair
Chetwood (178)	1902	1	1	–
Schoemaker (179)	1909	6	6	–
Bistrom et al. (180)	1944	3	2	1
Bruining et al. (181)	1981	1	2	–
Prochiantz and Gross (182)	1982	15	9	1
Hentz (183)	1982	5	4	–
Skef et al. (184)	1983	1	1	–
Iwai et al. (185)	1985	1	1	–
Chen and Zhang (186)	1987	6	3	1
Onishi et al. (187)	1989	1	1	–
Pearl et al. (188)	1991	7	4	2
Christansen et al. (189)	1995	7	0	3
Devesa et al. (190)	1992	10	6	3
Devesa et al. (191)	1997	17	9	1

In 1997, a larger series was reported in the literature by Devesa et al. (191). Their results in 20 incontinent patients were not as remarkable as those described by Pearl et al. (188), and failures were related to suture disruption, poor muscular contraction, and intractable constipation. Reviewing the experience of gluteoplasty in a group of six children aged five to six years, improvement was achieved in four (71%) (190). The patients who remained incontinent were unable to sense rectal distention.

Gracilis Muscle Transposition

Gracilis transposition was initially created in an attempt to treat children with fecal incontinence due to neurological and congenital anomalies (195). The gracilis muscle is wrapped around the anus and fixed to the contralateral ischial tuberosity (Fig. 20). The basic concept of this technique was to create a natural barrier to the passage of stool similar to the Thiersch repair. However, it offers the advantage that the anal encirclement is performed with autologous viable tissue, rather than foreign material. In order to harvest the gracilis muscle, both legs are prepared and draped free to allow repositioning during the operative procedure. The superficial medial location of the gracilis muscle in the thigh and the muscle's proximal blood supply allow division of the distal insertion site and proximal mobilization of the muscle without compromising viability. The position of the muscle is first traced on the surface of the thigh from the pubic arch to the upper medial tubercle of the tibia. Several small incisions overlying the gracilis muscle in the upper and middle-third of the thigh, and over the knee joint, are made. The tendon of the gracilis muscle is identified distally and severed from its insertion on the tibia. The muscle is then carefully mobilized until the neurovascular bundle is encountered in the proximal-third of the muscle. The neurovascular bundle is carefully preserved and defines the cephalad limit of the gracilis muscle dissection. Two incisions approximately 1.5 to 2 cm from the anal verge are made on the right and left sites. A tunnel is fashioned between the two perianal incisions and the proximal dissection of the gracilis muscle. The distal tendinous portion of the gracilis muscle is then passed through this tunnel and under the anterior and posterior raphe to encircle the anus in the ischioanal space. The leg is then fully adducted to minimize tension on the gracilis, and the tendinous end of the muscle is anchored to the contralateral tibial tuberosity with a strong nonabsorbable suture. When complete, the anal canal should allow one finger to pass snugly. Incisions are closed primarily without the use of drains. Immediate postoperative care consists of bed rest for 48 hours, followed by gradual ambulation. Although considered a "living Thiersch" procedure, the gracilis muscle can sometimes be relaxed purposely at the time of defecation, by assuming the squatting position and avoiding abduction of the thigh. Suppositories or enemas can be used to help establish a regular pattern of defecation and to promote complete evacuation of the rectum. Functional results are not as good as expected, because most patients can only control solid stool. Selected patients may benefit from gracilis transposition when other means have failed, or inadequate sphincter muscle is available for a classic sphincter repair. If graciloplasty alone is insufficient to restore anal continence, the addition of electrostimulation may improve sphincter pressures. However, patients should not have evacuatory dysfunction.

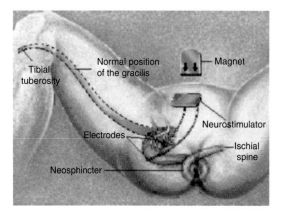

Figure 20   Gracilis neosphincter procedure.

Stimulated Gracilis Neosphincter

In 1953, Pickrell (195) first used the gracilis muscle transposition in an attempt to function as a dynamic Thiersch sling around the anal canal. However, because skeletal muscles become easily fatigued, Salmons and Henriksson (196) introduced a new technique, whereby fatigable muscles could be transformed into nonfatigable muscles: the stimulated gracilis neosphincter operation. This operation has been used for the treatment of incontinence secondary to trauma, neurologic causes, or patients with anorectal agenesis. Contraindications include patients with a damaged sphincter muscle, Crohn's disease, perineal sepsis, and a cardiac pacemaker.

Firstly, two or three incisions are made in the leg, and the gracilis muscle is dissected with long scissors. The tendon is cut as close to the end as possible and exteriorized. With two incisions around the anus at the 3 o'clock and 9 o'clock positions, the perianal area is dissected and controlled with red rubber catheters, creating a tunnel to transpose the muscle. The transposition can be performed using three wrap configurations: alpha, gamma, or epsilon (Fig. 21). The tendon is sutured to the ischial tuberosity with nonabsorbable sutures, and two suction drains are placed before finishing the procedure.

The second stage of the operation is performed six weeks after the first, provided that all wounds have healed with no infection. The upper incision in the thigh is reopened, the edges of the muscle dissected, and the area of the nerve is located with the nerve stimulator. Two leads are then implanted; the higher serial numbered lead is implanted first and sutured to the distal aspect of the nerve. The second lead is then sutured to the proximal aspect of the nerve. The position of the lead is assured at the entrance and exit sites of the muscle (Fig. 22). Lastly, an incision is made at the lower quadrant of the abdomen where a pocket is made to implant the battery, and a subcutaneous tunnel is used to connect the leads to the battery. After the muscle is transposed, it is left unstimulated for two weeks after which low voltage low frequency electrical stimulation commences. Over this 8- to 12-week period, the stimulation time is gradually increased.

In the last several years, a number of retrospective and prospective trials have been published to assess the safety and efficacy of dynamic gracloplasty. Although adverse events are common, significant changes in quality of life have encouraged the performance of this operation in adequately selected patients. However, due to the complexity of this procedure, it is generally recommended that it should only be performed in specialized surgical centers (175,197,198).

In a study analyzing the cost-effectiveness of dynamic gracloplasty, the total direct costs of lifelong dynamic gracloplasty, lifelong conventional treatment, and the associated costs of colostomy including lifelong stoma care were \$31,733, \$12,180, and \$71,576, respectively (199). Although dynamic gracloplasty is initially more expensive than conventional treatment, it is much more attractive than stoma creation and stoma care relative to both cost and outcome. Moreover, stimulated gracloplasty results in a significantly improved quality of life compared to conventional treatment and stoma creation.

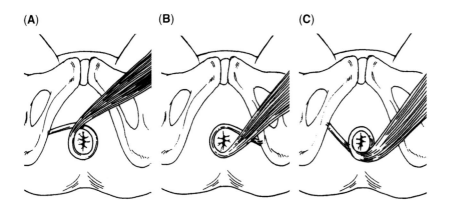

(A) **(B)** **(C)**

Figure 21 Gracilis muscle wrap configurations: (**A**) alpha, (**B**) gamma, and (**C**) epsilon around the anus in the gracilis neosphincter procedure.

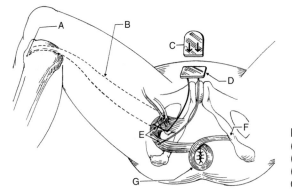

Figure 22 Lead implantation: (**A**) tibial tuberosity; (**B**) normal position of gracilis muscle; (**C**) magnet; (**D**) neostimulator; (**E**) electrodes; (**F**) ischial ramus (spine); (**G**) neosphincter. *Source*: From W. B. Saunders, London, U.K.

One of the more recent publications was a two-year follow-up after dynamic graciloplasty in 200 consecutive patients, wherein the overall success rate was 72% (200). Although complications were frequent, the majority were treatable, although disturbed evacuation remained a problem in 16% of these patients. The results of various series in the literature of gracilis transposition are shown in Table 15 (195,196,201–214). Currently, however, the stimulated graciloplasty is not offered in the United States for the treatment of fecal incontinence.

Artificial Bowel Sphincter

The initial experience with artificial sphincter for anal incontinence was undertaken by using an inflatable prosthesis in animal models (215). Subsequent clinical studies have led to the development of a subcutaneous cuff that is placed around the anal canal. The indications are usually related to neurogenic incontinence or severe traumatic anal sphincter injury. This prosthesis is an implantable, fluid-filled, solid silicone elastomer device, consisting of three components: a cuff, control-pump, and pressure-regulating balloon attached by a kink-resistant tube (Fig. 23). The artificial bowel sphincter simulates normal sphincter function by opening and closing the anal canal, controlled by the patient.

The operation is relatively simple, beginning with the implantation of the occlusive cuff around the anal canal. For this purpose, a variety of cuff sizes are available. Next, the

Table 15 Gracilis Transposition Series

Author	Year	Patients (*N*)	Successful outcome (%)	Infection
Pickrell et al. (195)	1952	34	100	–
Salmons and Henriksson (196)	1981	–	–	–
Williams et al. (201)	1991	6	0	–
Baeten et al. (202)	1988	–	–	–
Cavina et al. (203)	1987	–	–	–
Konsten et al. (204)	1993	–	–	–
Seccia et al. (205)	1994	75	71	–
Baeten et al. (206)	1995	52	73	–
Korsgen and Keighley (207)	1995	–	–	–
Kumar (208)	1995	–	–	–
Wexner et al. (209)	1996	17	60	–
Altomare et al. (173)	1996	–	–	–
Lubowski et al. (210)	1996	–	–	–
Geerdes et al. (211)	1996	67	78	12
Adang et al. (199)	1998	–	–	–
Mander et al. (212)	1999	64	56	–
Madoff et al. (194)	1999	128	66	–
Baeten et al. (214)	2000	123	50	–
Matzel et al. (213)	2001	93	87	31
Wexner et al. (197)	2002	115	62	–
Bresler et al. (174)	2002	24	79	25
Ronger et al. (200)	2003	200	72	–

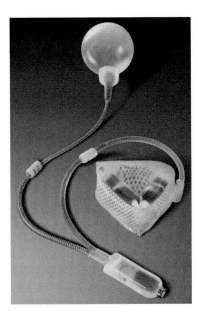

Figure 23 Artificial bowel sphincter. *Source*: From W. B. Saunders, London, U.K.

pressure-regulating balloon is implanted in the prevesical space, controlling the amount of pressure exerted by the occlusive cuff. Finally, the control pump is implanted in the soft tissue of the scrotum or vaginal greater labium. The upper part of the control pump contains the resistor and valves needed to transfer fluid to and from the cuff as well as the deactivation button. The patient squeezes and releases the bulb at the bottom-half of the control pump to transfer fluid within the device. A septum at the bottom of the control pump is designed to allow insertion of a small amount of fluid, if needed, in the postoperative period.

The first publication of the initial experience with an artificial sphincter for anal incontinence was by Christiansen and Lorentzen in 1987 (216). This series included five patients with neurogenic incontinence treated by implantation of an 800 American Medical Systems (AMS) urinary sphincter around the anus. Subsequently, these authors reported their experience with 12 patients; only 10 of these patients were available for follow-up longer than six months, five of whom reported excellent results (217). In 1996, Wong et al. (218) reported their experience with the implantation of 12 artificial sphincters with complications in four patients (33%) and successful outcome in nine (75%). In the same year, Lehur et al. (219) described their experience with 13 patients at a mean follow-up of 20 months; three patients required device explanation due to infection, and 9 of 10 patients were continent. Subsequently, a number of small series of patients who underwent implantation of an artificial bowel sphincter were published in the literature (220–223) including an updated series from Christiansen (222) that included 17 patients and a longer follow-up.

The largest personal series published to date reports the implantation of 53 artificial bowel sphincters followed-up for a mean period of 26 months (224). In this series, two-thirds of the patients achieved virtually normal continence, with a significant improvement in quality of life. Infection and skin erosion were the most common causes of explanation.

Of the series reported in the literature, improved continence was achieved in the majority of patients. Infectious complications, mechanical problems, and difficulty in evacuation were the main problems reported (Table 16) (217–230). A consensus statement regarding the current status of anal sphincter replacement was published in 2000, including an interesting guideline for the use of this new technique for fecal incontinence (221). Some of the most important conclusions related by this working included (i) strict attention to sterile technique; (ii) routine use of intravenous and local antibiotics; (iii) limited number of centers with an experienced team; (iv) assessment of functional results using the American Society of Colon and Rectal Surgeons (ASCRS) FIQL scale; (v) deep venous thrombosis prophylaxis; and (vi) immediate ambulation after surgery. Moreover, the eligibility criteria for sphincter replacement by artificial bowel sphincter should be (i) severe incontinence (level III or IV on the incontinence scale utilized

Table 16 Artificial Anal Sphincter Series

Author	Year	Patients (*N*)	Successful outcome (%)	Infection	Explanation
Cristiansen and Lorentzen (215)	1987	2	–	–	–
Cristiansen and Lorentzen (216)	1992	12	50	–	–
Wong et al. (218)	1996	12	75	–	–
Lehur et al. (219)	1996	13	70	–	–
Lehur et al. (225)	1998	13	–	–	–
Cristiansen et al. (222)	1999	17	21	3	–
Savoye et al. (223)	2000	12	–	–	–
Madoff et al. (221)	2000	–	–	–	–
Altomare et al. (226)	2001	28	–	–	–
Lehur et al. (225)	2002	16	–	–	–
Devesa et al. (220)	2002	53	–	–	–
Ortiz et al. (227)	2002	22	–	–	–
Michot et al. (228)	2003	37	–	–	–
Romano et al. (229)	2003	8	–	–	–
Parker et al. (230)	2003	45	–	–	–

by the working party); (ii) fecal incontinence not amenable to standard therapy or failure of previous therapy; (iii) patient in good health and excellent functional status; and (iv) minimum age of 16 years. All the exclusion criteria are outlined in Table 17.

At the present stage of development and clinical experience, some questions may be raised regarding the implantable artificial bowel sphincter: (i) How long does an artificial sphincter last? (ii) Will this device become acceptable for younger patients? (iii) Should the artificial bowel sphincter be used for both primary and secondary anal reconstruction after rectal cancer excision?

Despite these unanswered questions, the artificial bowel sphincter seems to be a viable option for severe cases of fecal incontinence with severe impact in quality of life where other simpler options have failed.

However, randomized, prospective and long-term follow-up trials are certainly required to provide adequate evidence-based data to support the use of this device as a standard procedure for fecal incontinence.

Synthetic Encirclement Procedures

Several investigators have attempted to correct damaged nonfunctioning sphincter musculature by encirclement procedures using synthetic material. In 1895, Thiersch originally described synthetic encirclement of the anus for the treatment of rectal prolapse associated with fecal incontinence. Thiersch hypothesized that circumanal wiring would support the anus and contain the prolapse, while tissue reaction to the foreign material would create a fibrosis, thereby providing additional support to the wire. However, due to a high incidence of wire breakage, various types of materials have been proposed to overcome this complication, such as steel wire, nylon, and Dacron-impregnated silastic. Clearly, synthetic material cannot be expected to function as normal muscle, and to date, the results have been suboptimal. Improvement in continence using this procedure appears to rely on stenosis of the anal canal as a result of postoperative scarring. Although a silastic sling is not free of infection and erosion, it appears to be the most reasonable material because the static properties of

Table 17 Exclusion Criteria for Implantation of Artificial Bowel Sphincter

Psychological instability
Low mental capacity
Significant comorbidity
Poor functional status
Neuromuscular disease
Severe arthritis
Chronic diarrheal states
Patients with impaired rectal emptying

Source: From Ref. 221.

wire can be overcome by the elasticity of this material, thereby allowing defecation. The operative procedure involves incision over both the ischioanal fossae and the development of a tunnel deep enough to accommodate a 2-cm strip of silastic material, which is encircled around the anus. The Dacron sheet is tightened around the tip of an index finger and secured with staples. The wounds are closed in layers, and the patient is discharged home following the first bowel movement. Unfortunately, due to reportedly high incidences of infection and extrusion related to the implant, this operation has little to offer the patient and should be performed only in very highly select circumstances.

Continent Colonic Conduit

In some cases, patients with fecal incontinence sustain simultaneous disorders of rectal evacuation. For this reason, a technique was developed, whereby regular antegrade irrigation of the colon is employed to achieve evacuation. The use of antegrade evacuation through a reversed appendicostomy was initially developed for the treatment of infants with fecal incontinence and later applied to adults with evacuatory disorders (231). The surgical technique involves division of the hepatic flexure of the colon, creation of a colonic conduit with the proximal transverse colon, and construction of an intussuscepted valve that allows introduction of a Foley catheter that is left "in situ" for one month (Fig. 24). The antegrade irrigation starts on postoperative day eight, and patients are clearly instructed to perform daily self-irrigations using a median of one to two liters of tap water.

A recent evaluation of a group of 62 children who underwent an antegrade continence enema procedure due to a variety of diagnoses demonstrated that, although this procedure is an option for intractable incontinence and constipation, it is not universally successful (232). Hence, selection of surgical candidates should be stringent, and perhaps other continence restoring strategies should first be considered.

Sacral Nerve Stimulation

The first sacral nerve stimulators implanted by Tanago and Schmidt (232) were performed for urinary symptoms. The use of neuromodulation for fecal incontinence in patients with a structurally intact sphincter mechanism seems a promising option.

Initially, patients undergo a temporary percutaneous stimulation or percutaneous neuromodulation test because this is the only method available to determine if a given patient will have an acceptable response to the implantation of a sacral stimulator.

Under local anesthesia, a spinal needle is percutaneously placed bilaterally into the S3 foramen (Fig. 25). The needle is electrically stimulated with an external electrical stimulator; once the S3 root is stimulated, a contraction of the perineal musculature should be appreciated. A subchronic stimulation wire is then placed through the needle, and the spinal needle

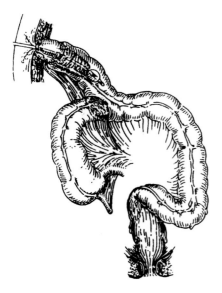

Figure 24 Continent colonic conduit. *Source*: From W. B. Saunders, London, U.K.

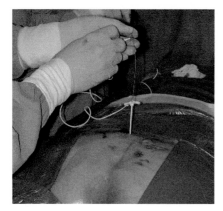

Figure 25 Sacral nerve stimulation. A spinal needle is percutaneously placed into the S3 foramen.

is removed. The wire is secured in place and the pacer wire is connected to a pulse generator to stimulate a constant and comfortable perineal muscle contraction for three to seven days (Fig. 26). General contraindications include spina bifida, pilonidal cysts, inflammatory bowel disease, cardiac disease, age over 75 years, and pregnancy.

The first publication of sacral modulation for fecal incontinence was in 1995 by Matzel et al. (234) who described an improvement in fecal incontinence and anal pressures in three patients who underwent a permanent implant. The report of short-term effects of sacral nerve stimulation in 12 patients demonstrated an increase in squeeze pressures, a decrease in rectal contractility, and possible stabilization of the anal resting pressures. The same institution reported their medium-term results of permanent sacral stimulation for fecal incontinence in 2002 (235). Fifteen consecutive patients underwent temporary and subsequent permanent stimulation. At a follow-up period of 24 months, all patients had an improvement in continence, and 11 patients were fully continent. Other small series from various institutions have been encouraging the use of this novel technique in a selected group of patients, mainly due to its safety and ability to improve quality of life in patients who are unsuitable candidates for or have failed other treatment options (236,237).

Stoma Creation

The creation of an intestinal stoma is usually the last option in the treatment of patients with fecal incontinence. Specifically, these include patients who have failed to improve after a number of anal sphincter reconstructive techniques, those who lack the motivation required to deal with complex procedures, elderly hospitalized, mentally incapacitated or neurologically impaired patients, or those in whom complex neosphincter procedures would confer little or no benefit due to poor general health.

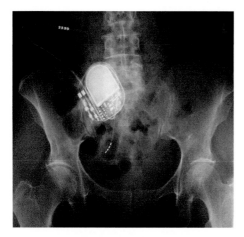

Figure 26 Sacral nerve stimulation. The wire is connected to a pulse generator.

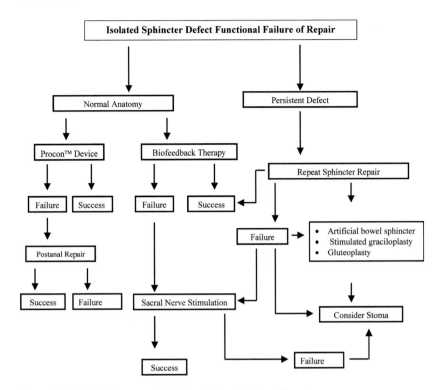

Figure 27 Algorithmic approach to the treatment of fecal incontinence.

In the past, most of the ostomies created were proximal or distal colostomies. These procedures were well tolerated and easily performed. However, long-term follow-up has revealed a number of later complications, including hernia formation and colostomy prolapse, which are not specifically related to the surgical technique. In addition, due to the nature of the ostomy output, odor and gas formation poses a problem.

It has already been demonstrated that loop ileostomy is a safe method of fecal diversion (238). This procedure is easy to perform and due to the small size of the ostomy, appliances are easily managed. In addition, this type of ostomy is much better tolerated by patients because the problem of odor is minimized. A number of ileostomy supplies have been developed to avoid peristomal skin problems. However, enterostomal therapist supervision is an important aspect and should always be strongly recommended.

Ileostomy and colostomy creation can be easily performed laparoscopically. A series of 32 patients who underwent laparoscopic fecal diversion demonstrated that this method is safe, feasible, and effective. In addition, the laparoscopic method provides complete visualization of the abdominal cavity, and correct identification of the best bowel segment to be used as a stoma (239).

CONCLUSION

Given the plethora of options for the treatment of fecal incontinence, the treatment must be matched to the patient. Figure 27 is an algorithmic approach to aid in this decision-making process.

REFERENCES

1. Thomas TM, Egan M, Walgrave A, Meade TW. The prevalence of faecal and double incontinence. Community Med 1984; 6:216–220.
2. Thomas TM, Egan M, Meade TW. The prevalence and implications of faecal (and double) incontinence. Br J Surg 1985; 72(suppl):S141.

3. Enck P, Bielefeldt K, Rathamann W, et al. Epidemiology of faecal incontinence in selected patients groups. Int J Colorectal Dis 1991; 6:143–146.
4. Johansen JF, Lafferty J. Epidemiology of fecal incontinence: the silent affliction. Am J Gastroenterol 1996; 91:33–36.
5. Drossman DA, Zhming L, Andruzzi E, et al. US householder survey of functional gastrointestinal disorders. Dig Dis Sci 1993; 38:1569–1580.
6. Henry MM. Pathogenesis and management of fecal incontinence in the adult. Gastroenterol Clin North Am 1987; 16:35–45.
7. Perry S, Shaw C, McGrother C, Matthews RJ, et al. Prevalence of faecal incontinence in adults aged 40 years or more living in the community. Gut 2002; 50(4):480–484.
8. Cheskin LJ, Schuster MM. Fecal incontinence. In: Hazzard WR, Andres R, Bierman EL, Blass JP, eds. Principles of Geriatric Medicine and Gerontology. 2nd ed. New York: McGraw-Hill, 1990:1143–1145.
9. Lahr CJ. Evaluation and treatment of incontinence. Practical Gastroenterol 1988; 12:27–35.
10. Mellgren A, Jensen LL, Zetterstrom JP, Wong WD, Hofmeister JH, Lowry AC. Long term cost of fecal incontinence secondary to obstetric injuries. Dis Colon Rectum 1999; 42(7):857–865.
11. Oliveira L, Wexner SD. Anal Incontinence. In: Beck DE, Wexner SD, eds. Fundamentals of Anorectal Surgery. 2nd ed. London: WB Saunders, 1998:115–152.
12. Kelly JH. Cinedefecography in anorectal malformation. J Pediatr Surg 1968; 4:538.
13. Parks AG. Anorectal incontinence. J R Soc Med 1975; 68:21–30.
14. Lane RN. Clinical application of anorectal physiology. Proc Soc Med 1975; 68:28–30.
15. Rudd WW. The transanal anastomosis: a sphincter-saving operation with improved continence. Dis Colon Rectum 1979; 22:102–105.
16. Holschneider AM. Treatment and functional results of anorectal continence in children with imperforate anus. Acta Chir Belg 1983; 3:191–204.
17. Keighley MR, Fielding WL. Management of faecal incontinence and results of surgical treatment. Br J Surg 1983; 70:463–468.
18. Corman M. Gracilis muscle transposition for anal incontinence. Late results. Br J Surg 1985; 72: S21–S22.
19. Hiltunen KNM, Matikainen M, Auvinen O, Hietanen P. Clinical and manometric evaluation of anal sphincter function in incontinent patients. Am J Surg 1986; 151:489–492.
20. Broden G, Dolk A, Holmstroem B. Recovery of the internal anal sphincter following rectopexy: a possible explanation for continence improvement. Int J Colorectal Dis 1988; 3:23–28.
21. Womack NR, Morrison JF, Williams NS. Prospective study of the effects of postanal repair in neurogenic fecal incontinence. Br J Surg 1988; 75:48–52.
22. Rainey JB, Donaldson DN, Thomson JP. Postanal repair: which patients derive most benefit? J R Coll Surg Edinb 1990; 35:101–105.
23. Miller R, Bartolo DC, Lock-Edminds JC, Mortensen NJ. Prospective study of conservative and operative treatment for faecal incontinence. Br J Surg 1988; 75:101–105.
24. Pescatori M, Anastasio G, Bottini C, Mentasti A. New grading and scoring for anal incontinence. Evaluation of 335 patients. Dis Colon Rectum 1992; 35:482–487.
25. Rockwood TH, Church J, Fleshman JW, et al. Fecal incontinence quality of life scale. Quality of life instrument for patients with fecal incontinence. Dis Colon Rectum 2000; 43:9–17.
26. Jorge JMN, Wexner SD. Etiology and management of fecal incontinence. Dis Colon Rectum 1993; 36:77–97.
27. Rothbarth J, Bemelman WA, Meijerink WJHJ, et al. What is the impact of fecal incontinence on quality of life? Dis Colon Rectum 2001; 44:67–71.
28. Rockwood TH, Church JM, Fleshman JW, et al. Patient and surgeon ranking of the severity of symptoms associated with fecal incontinence. Dis Colon Rectum 1999; 42:1525–1532.
29. Ware L, Snow K, Kosinski M, Gandek B. SF-36 Health survey. Manual and interpretation guide. Boston: The Health Institute, New England Medical Center, 1993.
30. Jorge JMN, Wexner SD. Anorectal manometry: techniques and clinical applications. South Med J 1993; 86:924–931.
31. Law PJ, Bartram CI. Anal endosonography: technique and normal anatomy. Gastrointest Radiol 1989; 14:349–353.
32. Law PJ, Kamm MA, Bartram CI. Anal endosonography in the investigation of faecal incontinence. Br J Surg 1991; 78:312–314.
33. Rieger NA, Sweeney JL, Hoffmann DC, Young JF, Hunter A. Investigation of fecal incontinence with endoanal ultrasound. Dis Colon Rectum 1996; 39(8):860–864.
34. Cheong DMO, Vaccaro CA, Salanga VD, et al. Electrodiagnostic evaluation of fecal incontinence. Muscle Nerve 1995; 18:612–619.
35. Burnett SJ, Speakman CT, Kamm MA, Bartram CI. Confirmation of endosonographic detection of external anal sphincter defects by simultaneous electromyographic mapping. Br J Surg 1991; 78:448–450.
36. Tjandra JJ, Milson JW, Schroeder T, Fazio VW. Endoluminal ultrasound is preferable to electromyography in mapping anal sphincter defects. Dis Colon Rectum 1993; 36:689–692.
37. Enck P, Von Giesen HJ, Schafer A. Comparison of anal sonography with conventional needle electromyography in the evaluation of anal sphincter defects. Am J Gastroenterol 1996; 91:2539–2543.

38. Wexner SD, Marchetti F, Jagelman D. The role of sphincteroplasty for fecal incontinence reevaluated: a prospective physiologic and functional review. Dis Colon Rectum 1991; 34:22–30.
39. Sangwan YP, Coller JA, Barret RC, et al. Unilateral pudendal neuropathy: impact on outcome of anal sphincter repair. Dis Colon Rectum 1996; 39:686–689.
40. Londono-Schimmer EE, Garcia-Duperly R, Nicholls RJ, Thomson JPS, Hawley PR. Overlapping anal sphincter repair for faecal incontinence due to sphincter trauma: fiveyear follow-up of functional results. Int J Colorectal Dis 1994; 9:110–113.
41. Gilliland R, Altomare DF, Moreira H Jr., Oliveira L, Gilliland JE, Wexner SD. Pudendal neuropathy is predictive of failure following anterior overlapping sphincteroplasty. Dis Colon Rectum 1998; 41:1516–1522.
42. Rociu E, Stoker J, Eijkemans MJC, Schouten WR, Laméris JS. Fecal incontinence: endoanal US versus endoanal MR imaging. Radiol 1999; 212:453–458.
43. Malouf AJ, Williams AB, Halligan S, Bartram CI, Dhillon S, Kamm MA. Prospective assessment of accuracy of endoanal MR imaging and endosonography in patients with fecal incontinence. AJR 2000; 175:741–745.
44. Harford WV, Krejs GJ, Santa Ana CA, Fordtran JS. Acute effect of diphenoxylate with atropine (lomotil) in patients with chronic diarrhea and fecal incontinence. Gastro 1980; 78:440–443.
45. Hallgren T, Fasth S, Delbro DS, Nordgren S, Oresland T, Hulten L. Loperamide improves anal sphincter function and continence after restorative proctocolectomy. Dig Dis Sci 1994; 39:2612–2618.
46. Hopkinson BR, Lightwood R. Electrical treatment of anal incontinence. Lancet 1966; 1:297.
47. Pescatori M, Pavesio R, Anastasio G, Daini S. Transanal electrostimulation for fecal incontinence: clinical, psychologic and manometric prospective study. Dis Colon Rectum 1991; 34:540–545.
48. Hosker G, Norton C, Brazzelli M. Electrical stimulation for fecal incontinence in adults. Cochrane Database Syst Rev 2000; (2):CD001310.
49. Takahashi T, Garcia-Osogobio S, Valdovinos MA, et al. Radiofrequency energy delivery for the treatment of fecal incontinence. Dis Colon Recum 2001; 44(4):A37.
50. Takahashi T, Garcia-Osogobio S, Valdovinos MA, Belmonte C, Barr C, Velasco L. Extended two-year results of radiofrequency energy delivery for the treatment of fecal incontinence the secca procedure. Dis Colon Rectum 2003; 46:711–715.
51. Efron J, Corman ML, Fleshman J, et al. Safety and effectiveness of temperature-controlled radiofrequency energy delivery to the anal canal secca procedure for the treatment of fecal incontinence. Dis Colon Rectum 2003; 46:1606–1618.
52. Weiss EG, Wexner SD, Efron J, Nogueras J. Submucosal injection fo carbon coated beads is a successful and safe office based treatment for fecal incontinence. Colorectal Dis 2002; 4(suppl 1):34.
53. Giamundo P, Welber A, Weiss EG, Vernava AM III, Nogueras JJ, Wexner SD. The procon incontinence device: a new nonsurgical approach to preventing episodes of fecal incontinence. Am J Gastroenterol 2002; 97(9):2328–2332.
54. Norton C, Hosker G, Brazzelli M. Biofeedback and/or sphincter exercises for the treatment of faecal incontinence in adults. Cochrane Database Syst Rev 2000; (2):CD002111.
55. Haskell B, Rovner H. Electromyography in the management of the incompetent anal sphincter. Dis Colon Rectum 1967; 10:81–84.
56. Engel BT, Nikoomanesh P, Schuster MM. Operant conditioning of rectosphincteric responses in the treatment of fecal incontinence. N Engl J Med 1974; 290:646–649.
57. Cerulli MA, Nikoomanesh P, Schuster MM. Progress in biofeedback conditioning for fecal incontinence. Gastroenterology 1979; 76:742–746.
58. Goldenberg DA, Hodges K, Hersh T, et al. Biofeedback for fecal incontinence. Am J Gastro 1980; 74:342–345.
59. Wald A. Biofeedback therapy for fecal incontinence. Ann InterN Med 1981; 99:146–149.
60. MacLeod JH. Biofeedback in the management of partial anal incontinence. Dis Colon Rectum 1983; 26:244–246.
61. Wald A. Biofeedback for neurogenic fecal incontinence: rectal sensation is a determinant of outcome. J Pediatr Gastroenterol Nutr 1983; 2:302–306.
62. Latimer PR, Campbell D, Kasperski J. A component analysis of biofeedback in the management of fecal incontinence. Biofeedback Self-Reg 1984; 9:311–324.
63. Wald A, Tunuglunta K. Anorectal sensorimotor dysfunction in fecal incontinence and diabetes mellitus. N Engl J Med 1984; 310(20):1282–1287.
64. Whitehead WE, Burgio KL, Engel BT. Biofeedback treatment of fecal incontinence in geriatric patients. J Am Geriatr Soc 1985; 33:320–324.
65. Buser WD, Miner DB. Delayed rectal sensation with fecal incontinence: successful treatment using ano-rectal manometry. Gastroenterology 1986; 91:1186–1191.
66. Whitehead WE, Parker L, Basmajian L, et al. Treatment of fecal incontinence in children with spina bifida: comparison of biofeedback and behaviour modification. Arch Phys Med Rehab 1986; 67:218–224.
67. MacLeod JH. Management of anal incontinence by biofeedback. Gastroenterology 1987; 93:291–294.
68. Berti Riboli E, Frascio M, Pittio G, et al. Biofeedback condition for fecal incontinence. Arch Phys Med Rehab 1988; 69:29–31.

69. Loening-Baucke V. Efficacy of biofeedback training in improving fecal incontinence and anorectal physiological function. Gut 1990; 31:1395–1402.
70. Miner PB, Donnelley TC, Read NW. Investigation of mode of action of biofeedback in treatment of fecal incontinence. Dig Dis Sci 1990; 35:1291–1298.
71. Chiarioni G, Scattolini C, Bonfante F, et al. Liquid stool incontinence with severe urgency: anorectal function and effective biofeedback treatment. Gut 1993; 34:1576–1580.
72. Salomon MC, Ferrara A, Larach SW, et al. Early improvement of rectal sensation and anal canal responsiveness after biofeedback treatment for fecal incontinence. Dis Colon Rectum 1993; 36:21.
73. Jensen LL, Lowry AC. Are pudendal latencies a predictive factor in the success of biofeedback for fecal incontinence? [abstr]. Dis Colon Rectum 1993; 26:30.
74. Souza A, Araujo AS, Damico FM, et al. Manometric findings prior to and after biofeedback for anal incontinence [abstr]. Dis Colon Rectum 1994; 36:37–24.
75. Arhan P, Faverdin C, Devroede G, et al. Biofeedback re-education of fecal incontinence in children. Int J Colorectal Dis 1994; 9:128–133.
76. Keck JO, Staniunas RJ, Coller YES, et al. Biofeedback training is useful in fecal incontinence but disappointing in constipation. Dis Colon Rectum 1995; 37:1271–1276.
77. Enck P, Daublin G, Lubke HJ, Strohmeyer G. Long-term efficacy of biofeedback training for fecal incontinence. Dis Colon Rectum 1994; 37:997–1001.
78. Ferrara A, Lord SA, Larach SW, et al. Biofeedback with home trainer program is effective for both incontinence and pelvic floor dysfunction[abstr]. Dis Colon Rectum 1995; 38:A17.
79. Sangwan YP, Coller JA, Barret RC, et al. Can manometrric parameters predict response to biofeedback therapy in fecal incontinence? Dis Colon Rectum 1995; 38:1021–1025.
80. Guillemot F, Bouche B, Gower-Rousseau C, et al. Biofeedback for the treatment of fecal incontinence. Long-term clinical results. Dis Colon Rectum 1995; 38:393–397.
81. Van Tets WF, Kuijpers JHC, Bleijenberg G. Biofeedback treatment is ineffective in neurogenic fecal inontinence. Dis Colon Rectum 1996; 39:992–994.
82. Rao SSC, Welcher KD, Pelsang RE. Effects of biofeedback therapy on anorectal function in obstructed defecation. Dis Dig Sci 1997; 42:2197–2205.
83. Ko CY, Tong J, Lehman RE, Shelton AA, Schrock TR, Welton ML. Biofeedback is effective therapy for fecal incontinence and constipation. Arch Surg 1997; 132:829–834.
84. Guilliland R, Heymen S, Vickers D, Wexner SD. Biofeedback in the treatment of fecal incontinence [abstr]. Br J Surg 1997; 12:183.
85. Karlboum U, Hallden M, Eeg-Olofsson KE, et al. Results of biofeedback in constipated patients. Dis Colon Rectum 1997; 40:1149–1155.
86. Rieger NA, Wattchow DA, Sarre FG, et al. Prospective study of biofeedback for treatment of constipation. Dis Colon Rectum 1997; 40:1143–1148.
87. Patankar SK, Ferrera A, Levy Jr., Larach SW, Williamson PR, Perozo SE. Biofeedback in colorectal practice. A multicenter, statewide, three-year experience. Dis Colon Rectum 1997; 40:827–831.
88. Patankar SK, Ferrera A, Larach SW, et al. Electromyographic assessment o biofeedback training for fecal incontinence and chronic constipation. Dis Colon Rectum 1997; 40:907–911.
89. Glia A, Gylin M, Akerlund JE, Lindfors U, Lindberg G. Biofeedback training in patients with fecal incontinence. Dis Colon Rectum 1998; 41:359–364.
90. Pager CK, Solomon MJ, Rex J, Roberts RA. Long-term outcomes of pelvic floor exercise and biofeedback treatment for patients with fecal incontinence. Dis Colon Rectum 2002; 45:997–1003.
91. Mc Leod JH. Fecal incontinence. A practical program of management. Endosc Rev 1988:45–56.
92. Kegel A. The nonsurgical treatment of genital relaxation. Ann West Med Surg 1948; 2:213.
93. Kegel A. Progressive resistance exercise in the functional restoration of the perineal muscles. Am J Obstet Gynecol 1948; 56:242–245.
94. McHugh S, Walma K, Diamant NE. Fecal incontinence. A controlled trial of biofeedback. Gastroenterology 1990:91–1060.
95. Oliveira L, Mello AV. Biofeedback therapy for fecal incontinence. Is it a valuable interrogation [abstr]. Dis Colon Rectum 2003; 46(5):A37.
96. Shafik A. Perianal injection of autologous fat for treatment of sphincteric incontinence. Dis Colon Rectum 1995; 38:583–587.
97. Bernardi C, Favetta U, Pescatori M. Autologous fat injection for treatment of fecal incontinence: manometric and ecographic assessment. Plast Reconstr Surg 1998; 102:1626–1628.
98. Shafik A. Polytetrafluroethylene injection for the treatment of partial faecal incontinence. Int Surg 1993; 78:159–161.
99. Kumar D, Benson M. Glutaraldehyde cross-linked collagen in the treatment of faecal incontinence. Br J Surg 1998; 85:978–979.
100. Kenefick NJ, Vaizey CJ, Malouf AJ, Norton CS, Marshall A, Kamm MA. Injectable silicone biomaterial for faecal incontinence due to internal anal sphincter dysfunction. Gut 2002; 51:225–228.
101. Cheetham MJ, Kamm MA, Phillips RK. Topical phenylephrine increases anal canal resting pressure in patients with incontinence. Gut 2001; 48:356–359.
102. Santoro GA, Eitan BZ, Pryde A, Bartolo DC. Open study of low-dose amitriptyline in the treatment of patients with idiopathic fecal incontinence. Dis Colon Rectum 2000; 43:1676–1682.

103. Belmonte-Montes C, Hagerman G, Vega-Yepez PA, Hernandez-de-Anda E, Fonseca-Morales V. Anal sphincter injury after vaginal delivery in primiparous females. Dis Colon Rectum 2001; 44(9): 1244–1248.

104. Oliveira L, Pfeifer J, Wexner SD. Physiological and clinical outcome of anterior sphincteroplasty. Br J Surg 1996; 83:1244–1251.

105. Briel JW, De Boer LW, Hop WC, Southern WR. Clinical outcome of anterior overlapping external sphincter repair with internal anal imbrication. Dis Colon Rectum 1998; 41:209–214.

106. Cook TA, Mortensen NJ. Management of faecal incontinence following obstetric trauma. Br J Surg 1998; 85:293–299.

107. Engel AF, Kamm AM, Sultan AH, Bartram CI, Nicholls RJ. Anterior sphincter repair in patients with obtetric trauma. Br J Surg 1994; 81:1231–1234.

108. Londono-Schimmer EE, Garcia-Duperly R, Nicholls RJ, Thomson JPS, Hawley PR. Overlapping anal sphincter repair for faecal incontinence due to sphincter trauma: five year follow-up of functional results. Int J Colorcetal Dis 1994; 9:110–113.

109. Ganio E, Luc AR, Clerico G, Trompetto M. Sacral nerve stimulation for treatment of fecal incontinence: a novel approach for intractable fecal incontinence. Dis Colon Rectum 2001; 44(5):619–629.

110. Wexner SD, Beck DE. Sepsis prevention in colorectal surgery. In: Fielding LP, Goldberg SM, eds. Robb and Smiths Operative Surgery: Colon Rectum and Anus. 5th ed. Oxford: Butterworth-Heinemann:41–46, 2004.

111. Vernava AM III, Stratton MD. Preoperative and postoperative management. In: Beck DE, Wexner SD, eds. Fundamentals of Anorectal Surgery. 2nd ed. London: WB Saunders, 1998:70–78.

112. Oliveira L, Wexner SD, Daniel N, et al. Mechanical bowel preparation for elective colorectal surgery. A prospective randomized surgeon-blinded trial comparing sodium phosphate and polyethylene glycol-based oral lavage solutions. Dis Colon Rectum 1997; 40:585–591.

113. Sorensen SM, Bondesen H, Ister O, et al. Perineal rupture following vaginal deliveries. Long-term consequences. Acta Obstet Gynaecol Scand 1988; 67:315–318.

114. Bek KM, Laurberg S. Risks of anal incontinence from subsequent vaginal delivery after a complete obstetric anal sphincter tear. Br J Obstet Gynaecol 1992; 99:724–726.

115. Leigh RJ, Turnberg LA. Fecal incontinence: the unvoiced symptoms. Lancet 1982; 1:1349–1351.

116. Schofield PF, Grace R. Faecal incontinence after childbirth. Clin Risk 1999; 5:201–204.

117. Sultan AH, Kamm MA, Hudson CN, Bartram CI. Third degree obstetric anal sphincter tears: risk factors and outcome after primary repays. BMJ 1994; 308:887–891.

118. Tetzschner T, Sorenson M, Lose G, Christiansen J. Anal and urinary incontinence in women with obstetric anal sphincter rupture. Br J Obstet Gynaecol 1996; 103:1034–1040.

119. Oberwalder M, Connor J, Wexner SD. Meta-analysis to determine the incidence of obstetric anal sphincter damage. Br J Surg 2003; 90(11):1333–1337.

120. Fernando RJ, Sultan AH, Radley S, Jones PW, Johanson RB. Management of obstetric anal sphincter injury: a systematic review and national practice survey. BMC Health Serv Res 2002; 2(1):9.

121. Sultan AH. Obstetrical perineal injury and anal incontinence. Clin Risk 1999; 5:193–196.

122. Haadem K, Dahlostrom A, Ling L, Ohrlander AS. Anal sphincter function after delivery rupture. Obstet Gynecol 1987; 70:53–70.

123. Vencatesh SK, Ramanujam PS, Larson DM, Haywood MA. Anorectal complications of vaginal delivery. Dis Colon Rectum 1989; 32:1039–1041.

124. Jacobs PP, Scheuer M, Kuijpers JHC. Obstetric fecal incontinence: role of pelvic floor denervation and results of delayed sphincter repair. Dis Colon Rectum 1990; 33:494–497.

125. Christianson LM, Bovbjerg VE, McDavitt EC, Hullfish KL. Risk factors for perineal injury during delivery. Am J Obstet Gynecol 2003; 189(1):255–260.

126. Eason E, Labrecque M, Marcoux S, Mondor M. Anal incontinence after childbirth. CMAJ 2002; 166(3):326–330.

127. Hueston WJ. Factors associated with the use of episiotomy during vaginal delivery. Obstet Gynecol 1996; 87:1001–1005.

128. Poen AC, Felt-Bersma RJ, Dekker GA, Deville W, Cuesta MA, Meuwissen SG. Third degree obstetric perineal tears: risk factors and the preventive role of mediolateral episiotomy. Br J Obstet Gynaecol 1997; 104(5):563–566.

129. De Leeuw JW, Struijk PC, Vierhout ME, Wallenburg HC. Risk factors for third degree perineal ruptures during delivery. BJOG 2001; 108(4):383–387.

130. Kettle C, Johanson RB. Absorbable synthetic versus catgut suture material for perineal repair. Oxford: The Cochrane Library, update software 2001, issue 4.

131. Nessim A, Wexner SD, Agachan F, Alabaz O, Weiss EG, Nogueras JJ. Is bowel confinement necessary after anorectal reconstructive surgery? Dis Colon Rectum 1999; 42:16–23.

132. Hasegawa H, Yoshioka K, Keighley MRB. Randomised trial of faecal diversion for sphincter repair. Dis Colon Rectum 2000; 43:961–965.

133. Klosterhalfen B, Offner F, Topf N, Vogel P, Mittermayer C. Sclerosis of the internal anal sphincter-a process of aging. Dis Colon Rectum 1990; 33(7):606–609.

134. Gardner E. Decrease in human motor neurones with age. Anat Rec 1940; 77:529–536.

135. Nikiteas N, Korsgen S, Kumar D, Keighley MR. Audit of sphincter repair. Factors associated with poor outcome. Dis Colon Rectum 1996; 39:1164–1170.

136. Korsgen S, Deen KI, Keighley MR. Long-term results of total pelvic floor repair for postobstetric fecal incontinence. Dis Colon Rectum 1997; 40:835–839.

137. Simmang C, Birbaum EH, Kodner IJ, Fry RD, Fleshman JW. Does advancing age affect outcome? Dis Colon Rectum 1994; 37:1065–1069.

138. Laurberg S, Swash M, Henry M. Delayed external sphincter repair for obstetric tear. Br J Surg 1988; 75:786–788.

139. Sitzler PJ, Thomson JP. Overlap repair of damaged anal sphincter. A single surgeon's series. Dis Colon Rectum 1996; 39:1356–1360.

140. Jackson SL, Weber AM, Hull TL, Mitchinson AR, Walters MD. Fecal incontinence in women with urinary incontinence and pelvic organ prolapse. Obstet Gynecol 1997; 89:423–427.

141. Donnelly VS, O'Connel PR, O'Herlihy C. The influence of oestrogen replacement on faecal incontinence in post-menopausal women. Br J Obstet Gynaecol 1997; 104:311–315.

142. Pinedo G, Vaizey CJ, Nicholls RJ, et al. Results of repeat anal sphincter repair. Br J Surg 1999; 86:66–69.

143. Giordano P, Renzi A, Efron J, et al. Previous sphincter repair does not affect the outcome of repeat repair. Dis Colon Rectum 2002; 45:635–640.

144. Blaisdell PC. Repair of the incontinent sphincter ani. Surg Gynecol Obstet 1940; 70:692–697.

145. Moskowitz I, Rotholtz N, Wexner SD, et al. Overlapping sphincteroplasty: does preservation of scar influence the immediate outcome? Dis Colon Rectum 2000; 43:A11.

146. Fang DT, Nivatgongs S, Vermeulen FD, et al. Overlapping sphincteroplasty for acquired anal incontinence. Dis Colon Rectum 1984; 27:720–722.

147. Yoshioka K, Keighley MRB. Sphincter repair for fecal incontinence. Dis Colon Rectum 1989; 32:39–42.

148. Fleshman JW, Peters WR, Shemesh EI, et al. Anal sphincter reconstruction: anterior overlapping muscle repair. Dis Colon Rectum1991; 34:739–743.

149. Engel AF, Baal SJV, Brummelkamp WH. Late results of anterior sphincter plication for traumatic fecal incontinence. Eur J Surg 1994; 160:633–636.

150. Engel AF, Kamm MA, Sultan AH, et al. Anterior anal sphincter repair in patients with obstetric trauma. Br J Surg 1994; 81:1231–1234.

151. Felt-Bersma RJF, Cuesta MA, Koorevar M. Anal sphincter repair improves anorectal function and endosonographic image. Dis Colon Rectum 1996; 39:878–885.

152. Roche B, Savioz D, Marti MC. Is there age limit to susscessful sphincteroplasty? [abstr]. Int J Colorectal Dis 1997; 12:156.

153. Ternent CA, Shashidharan M, Blatchford GJ, et al. Transanal ultrasound and anorectal physiology findings affecting continence after sphincteroplasty. Dis Colon Rectum 1997; 40:462–467.

154. Halverson AL, Hull TL. Long-term outcome of overlapping anal sphincter repair. Dis Colon Rectum 2002; 43:813–820.

155. Briel JW, De Boer LW, Hop WC, Southern WR. Clinical outcome of anterior overlapping external sphincter repair with internal anal imbrication. Dis Colon Rectum 1998; 41:209–214.

156. Deen KI, Kumar D, Willians JG, et al. Randomized trial of internal anal sphincter plication with pelvic floor repair for neuropathic fecal incontinence. Dis Colon Rectum 1995; 38:14–18.

157. Leroi AM, Kamm MA, Weber J, et al. Internal anal sphincter repair. Int J Colorectal Dis 1997; 12:243–245.

158. Parks AG. Anorectal incontinence. J Roy Soc Méd 1975; 68:21–30.

159. Browning GGP, Parks AG. Postanal repair for neuropathic faecal incontinence: correlation of clinical results and anal canal pressures. Br J Surg 1983; 70:101–104.

160. Keighley MRB. Postanal repair for faecal incontinence. J Royal Soc Med 1984; 77:285–288.

161. van Vroonhaven TJ, Schouten WR. Postanal repair in the treatment of anal incontinence. Neth J Surg 1984; 36:160–162.

162. Ferguson EF Jr. Puborectalis sphincteroplasty for anal incontinence. South Med J 1984; 77:423–425.

163. Henry MM, Simpson JNL. Results of postanal repair. A prospective study. Br J Surg 1985; 72:17–19.

164. Yoshioka K, Hyland G, Keighley MRB. Physiological changes after postanal repair and parameters predicting outcome. Br J Surg 1988; 75:1220–1224.

165. Scheuer M, Kuijpers HC, Jacobs PP. Postanal repair restores anatomy rather than function. Dis Colon Rectum 1989; 32:960–963.

166. Rainey JB, Donaldson DR, Thomson JPS. Postanal repair: which patients derive most benefit? Jr Coll Surg Edinb 1990; 35:101–115.

167. Orrom WJ, Miller R, Cornes H, et al. Comparison of anterior sphincteroplasty and postanal repair in idiopathic fecal incontinence. Dis Colon Rectum 1991; 34:305–310.

168. Matsuoka H, Mavrantonis C, Wesner SD, et al. Long-term results of postanal repair for neurogenic faecal incontinence. Br J Surg 1994; 81:140–144.

169. Healy JC, Halligan S, Bartram CI, Kamm MA, Phillips RK, Reznek R. Dynamic magnetic resonance imaging evaluation of the structural and functional results of postanal repair for neuropathic fecal incontinence. Dis Colon Rectum 2002; 45:1629–1634.

170. Keighley MR. Results of surgery in idiopathic faecal incontinence. A Afr J Surg 1991; 29:87–93.

171. Deen KI, Oya M, Ortiz J, Keighley MR. Randomised trial comparing three forms of pelvic floor repair for neuropathic fecal incontinence. Dis Colon Rectum 1993; 80:794–798.

172. Osteberg A, Edebol Eeg-Olofsson K, Graf W. Results of surgical treatment for fecal incontinence. Br J Surg 2000; 87:1546–1552.

173. Altomare DF, Rinaldi M, Pannarale OC, Memeo V. Electrostimulated gracilis neosphincter for faecal incontinence. Int J Colorectal Dis 1997; 12:308–312.

174. Bresler L, Riebel N, Brunaud L, et al. Dynamic graciloplasty in the treatment of severe fecal incontinence. French multicentric retrospective study. Ann Chir 2002; 127:520–526.

175. Chapman AE, Geerdes B, Hewett P, et al. Systematic review of dynamic graciloplasty in the treatment of fecal incontinence. Br J Surg 2002; 89:138–153.

176. Baeten CG, Bailey HR, Bakka A, et al. Safety and efficacy of dynamic graciloplasty for fecal incontinence: report of a prospective multicenter trial. Dynamic graciloplasty therapy study. Dis Colon Rectum 2000; 43:743–751.

177. Hakelius L, Olsen L. Free autologus muscle transplantation in children. Eur J Pediatr Surg 1991; 1:353–357.

178. Chetwood CH. Plastic operation of the sphincter ani: report of a case. Med Rec 1902; 61:529.

179. Schoemaker J. Un nouveau procede operatoire pour la reconstitution du sphincter anal. Semin Med 1909; 29:160.

180. Bistrom O. Plastichesarzatz des m: sphincter ani. Acta Chir Scand 1944; 90:431–438.

181. Bruining HA, Bos KE, Colthoff EG, et al. Creation of an anal sphincter mechanism by bilateral proximaly based gluteal muscle transposition. Plast Reconstr Surg 1981; 67:70–73.

182. Prochiantz A, Gross P. Gluteal myoplasty for sphincter replacement: principles, results and prospects. J Pediatr Surg 1982; 17:25–30.

183. Hentz VR. Construction of rectal sphincter using the origin of the gluteus maximus muscle. Plast Reconst Surg 1982; 70:82–85.

184. Skef Z, Radhakrishnan J, Reyes HM. Anorectal continence following sphincter reconstruction utilizing the gluteus maximus muscle: a case report. J Pediatr Surg 1983; 18:779–781.

185. Iwai N, Kaneda H, Tsuto T, Yanagihara J, Takahashi T. Objective assessment of anorectal function after sphincter reconstruction using the gluteus maximus muscle. Report of a case. Dis Colon Rectum 1985; 28:973–977.

186. Chen YL, Zhang XH. Reconstruction of rectal sphincter by transposition of gluteus muscle for fecal incontinence. J Pediatr Surg 1987; 22:62–64.

187. Onishi K, Maruyama Y, Shiba T. A wrap-around procedure using gluteus maximus muscle for the functional reconstruction of the sphincter in a case of anal incontinence. Acta Chir Plast 1989; 31:56–63.

188. Pearl RK, Prasad ML, Nelson RL, Orsay CP, Abcarian H. Bilateral gluteus maximus transposition for anal incontinence. Dis Colon Rectum 1991; 34:478–481.

189. Christiansen J, Hansen CR, Rassmussen O. Bilateral gluteus maximus transposition for anal incontinence. Br J Surg 1995; 82:903–905.

190. Devesa JM, Vicente E, Enriquez JM, et al. Total fecal incontinence-new method of gluteus maximus transposition: preliminary results and report of previous experience with similar procedures. Dis Colon Rectum 1992; 35:339–349.

191. Devesa JM, Madrid JM, Gallego BR, Vicente E, Nuno J, Enriquez JM. Bilateral gluteoplasty for fecal incontinence. Dis Colon Rectum 1997; 40:883–888.

192. Farid M, Moneim HA, Mahdy T, Omar W. Augmented unilateral gluteoplasty with fascia lata grat in fecal incontinence. Tech Coloproctol 2003; 7:23–28.

193. Yoshioka K, Ogunbiyi OA, Keighley MR. A pilot study of total pelvic floor repair or gluteus maximus transposition for postobstetric neuropathic fecal incontinence. Dis Colon Rectum 1999; 43:1635–1636.

194. Madoff RD, Rosen HR, Baeten CG, et al. Safety and efficacy of dynamic muscle plasty for anal incontinence: lessons from a prospective multicenter trial. Gastroenterology 1999; 116:549–556.

195. Pickrell KL, Broadbent TR, Masters FW, Metzger JT. Construction of a rectal sphincter and restoration of anal continence by transplanting the gracilis muscle. Report of four cases in children. Ann Surg 1952; 135:853–862.

196. Salmons S, Henriksson J. The adaptive response of skeletal muscle to increased use. Muscle Nerve 1981; 4:94–105.

197. Wexner SD, Baeten C, Bailey R, et al. Long-term efficacy of dynamic graciloplasty for fecal incontinence. Dis Colon Rectum 2002; 45:809–818.

198. Herman RM, Walega P, Richter P, Grylewski A, Poliela T. Preliminary results of dynamic graciloplasty in the treatment of fecal incontinence. Przegl Lek 2001; 58:1047–1051.

199. Adang EM, Engel GL, Rutten FF, Geerdes BP, Baeten CG. Cost-effectiveness of dynamic graciloplasty in patients with fecal incontinence. Dis Colon Rectum 1998; 41:725–733.

200. Rongen MJ, Uludag O, El Naggar K, Geerdes BP, Konsten J, Baeten CG. Long-term follow-up of dynamic graciloplasty for fecal incontinence. Dis Colon Rectum 2003; 46:716–721.

201. Williams NS, Patel J, George BD, et al. Development of an electrically stimulated neoanal sphincter. Lancet 1991; 338:1166–1169.

202. Baeten CG, Spaans F, Fluks A. An implanted neuromuscular stimulator for fecal incontinence following previously implanted gracilis muscle: report of a case. Dis Colon Rectum 1988; 31:134–137.

203. Cavina E, Seccia M, Evangelista G, et al. Construction of a continent perineal colostomy by using electrostimulated gracilis muscle after abdominoperineal resection: personal technique and experience with 32 cases. Ital J Surg Sci 1987; 17:305–314.

204. Konsten J, Baeten CG, Spaans F, et al. Follow-up of anal dynamic graciloplasty or fecal incontinence. World J Surg 1993; 17:404–408.

205. Seccia M, Menconi C, Balestri R, Cavina E. Study protocols and functional results in 86 electrostimulated graciloplasties. Dis Colon Rectum 1994; 37:897–904.

206. Baeten CG, Geerdes BP, Adang EM, et al. Anal dynamic graciloplasty in the treatment of intractable fecal incontinence. N Engl J Med 1995; 332:1600–1605.

207. Korsgen S, Keighley MRB. Stimulated gracilis neosphincter-not as good as previously thought. Dis Colon Rectum 1995; 38:1331–1333.

208. Kumar D, Hutchinson R, Grant E. Bilateral gracilis neosphincter construction for treatment of faecal incontinence. Br J Surg 1995; 82:1645–1647.

209. Wexner SD, Gonzales-Padron A, Rius J, et al. Stimulated gracilis neosphincter operation. Initial experience pitfalls and complications. Dis Colon Rectum 1996; 39:957–964.

210. Lubowski DZ, Kennedy H, Nguyen H. Clinical outcome of stimulated gracilis neosphincter. Int J Colorectal Dis 1996; 11:134.

211. Geerdes BP, Heineman E, Konsten J, et al. Dynamic graciloplasty. Complications and management. Dis Colon Rectum 1996; 39:912–917.

212. Mander BJ, Wexner SD, Williams NS, et al. Preliminary results of a multicentre trial of the electrically stimulated gracilis neoanal sphincter. Br J Surg 1999; 86:1543–1548.

213. Matzel KE, Madoff RD, LaFontaine LJ, et al. Complications of dynamic graciloplasty. Dis Colon Rectum 2001; 44:1427–1435.

214. Baeten CG, Bailey HR, Bakka A, et al. Graciloplasty for fecal incontinence. Report of a prospective multicenter trial. Dis Colon Rectum 2000; 43:743–751.

215. Christiansen J, Lorentzen M. Implantation of artificial sphincter for anal incontinence. Lancet 1987; 1:244–245.

216. Christiansen J, Lorentzen M. Implantation of artificial sphincter for anal incontinence: report of five cases. Dis Colon Rectum 1989; 32:432–436.

217. Christiansen J, Sparso B. Treatment of anal incontinence by implantable prosthetic anal sphincter. Ann Surg 1992; 215:383–386.

218. Wong WD, Jensen LL, Bartolo DCC, Rothenberger DA. Artificial anal sphincter sphincter. Dis Colon Rectum 1996; 39:1352–1355.

219. Lehur PA, Michot F, Denis P, et al. Results of artificial sphincter in severe anal incontinence. Report of 14 consecutive implantations. Dis Colon Rectum 1996; 39:1352–1355.

220. Devesa JM, Rey A, Hervas PL, et al. Artificial anal sphincter: complications and functional results of a large personal series. Dis Colon Rectum 2002; 45:1154–1163.

221. Madoff RD, Baeten CG, Christiansen J, et al. Standards for anal sphincter replacement. Dis Colon Rectum 2000; 43:135–141.

222. Christiansen J, Rasmussen OO, Lindorff-Larsen K. Long-term results of artificial anal sphincter implantation for severe anal incontinence. Ann Surg 1999; 230:45–48.

223. Savoye G, Leroi AM, Denis P, Michot F. Manometric assessment of an artificial bowel sphincter. Br J Surg 2000; 87:586–589.

224. Lehur PA, Glemain P, Bruley Des Varannes S, Buzelin JM, Leborgne J. Outcome of patients with an implanted artificial anal sphincter for severe faecal incontinence. A single institution report. Int J Colorectal Dis 1998; 13:88–92.

225. Lehur PA, Zerbib F, Neunlist M, Glemain P, Bruley Des Varannes S. Comparison of quality of life and anorectal function after artificial sphincter implantation. Dis Colon Rectum 2002; 45:508–513.

226. Altomare DF, Dodi G, La Torre F, et al. Multicenter retrospective analysis of the outcome of artificial anal sphincter implantation for severe faecal incontinence. Br J Surg 2001; 88:1481–1486.

227. Ortiz H, Armendariz P, De Miguel M, et al. Complications and functional outcome following artificial anal sphincter implantation. Br J Surg 2002; 89:877–881.

228. Michot F, Costaglioli B, Leroi AM, Denis P. Artificial anal sphincter in severe fecal incontinence: outcome of prospective experience with 37 patients in one institution. Ann Surg 2003; 237:52–56.

229. Romano G, La Torre F, Cutini G, et al. Total anorectal reconstruction with the artificial bowel sphincter: report of eight cases. A quality-of-life assessment. Dis Colon Rectum 2003; 46:730–734.

230. Parker SC, Spencer MP, Madoff RD, et al. Artificial bowel sphincter: long term experience at a single institution. Dis Colon Rectum 2003; 46:722–729.

231. Malone PS, Ransley PG, Kiely EM. Preliminary report: the antegrade continence enema. Lancet 1990; 336:1217–1218.

232. Dey R, Ferguson C, Kenny SE, Shankar KR, et al. After the honeymoon-medium-term outcome of antegrade continence enema procedure. J Pediatr Surg 2003; 38:65–68.

233. Tanago EA, Schmidt RA. Bladder pacemaker: scientific basis and clinical future. Urology 1982; 20:614–619.

234. Matzel KE, Stadelmaier U, Hohenfellner M, Gall FP. Electrical stimulation of sacral spinal nerves for the treatment of faecal incontinence. Lancet 1995; 346:1124–1127.

235. Kenefick NJ, Vaizey CJ, Cohen RC, Nicholls RJ, Kamm MA. Medium-term results of permanent sacral nerve stimulation for faecal incontinence. Br J Surg 2002; 89:896–901.
236. Ripetti V, Caputo D, Ausania F, Esposito E, Bruni R, Arullani A. Sacral nerve neuromodulation improves physical psychological and social quality of life in patients with fecal incontinence. Tech Coloproctol 2002; 6:147–152.
237. Ratto C, Orelli U, Paparo S, Parello A, Doglietto GB. Minimally invasive sacral neuromodulation implant technique: modifications to the conventional procedure. Dis Colon Rectum 2003; 46:414–417.
238. Wexner SD, Taranow DA, Johansen OB, et al. Loop ileostomy is a safe option for fecal diversion. Dis Colon Rectum 1993; 36:349–354.
239. Oliveira L, Reissman P, Wexner SD. Laparoscopic creation of stomas. Surg Endosc 1997; 11:19–23.

4 | Rectal Prolapse

Kelli Bullard Dunn
Division of Surgical Oncology, Roswell Park Cancer Institute, and the State University of New York at Buffalo, Buffalo, New York, U.S.A.

Robert D. Madoff
Division of Colon and Rectal Surgery, Department of Surgery, University of Minnesota, Minneapolis, Minnesota, U.S.A.

HISTORY

Rectal prolapse has been recognized since antiquity. The first description of this condition can be found in the Ebers Papyrus from 1500 B.C. (1). Through the ensuing centuries, understanding of rectal prolapse focused on the perineum, and therapy was designed to hide the prolapse, tighten the anus, or scar the rectum to prevent protrusion (2). Modern understanding of the pathophysiology and treatment of prolapse began with Moschowitz's description in 1912. Moschowitz emphasized the abdominal component of prolapse and its similarity to other abdominal wall hernias. The repair that bears his name is based upon these principles (3). Since 1912, our understanding of rectal prolapse has improved. Preoperative evaluation now includes anorectal physiology testing and evaluation of bowel function. Dozens of surgical approaches have been described with variable success. Finally, evaluation of postoperative success has shifted to include not only anatomic recurrence, but also assessment of function.

ANATOMY AND PATHOPHYSIOLOGY

Rectal prolapse refers to a circumferential, full-thickness protrusion of the rectum through the anus and has also been called "first degree" prolapse, "complete" prolapse, or procidentia. The majority of surgical procedures designed to treat rectal prolapse focus upon full-thickness prolapse. Internal prolapse occurs when the rectal wall intussuscepts but does not protrude, and is probably more accurately described as internal intussusception. Controversy exists over the necessity for treatment and optimal procedure for internal intussusception. Mucosal prolapse is a partial thickness protrusion often associated with hemorrhoidal disease, and is usually treated with hemorrhoidectomy (2,4).

The cause of rectal prolapse remains incompletely understood. Most patients share a number of anatomic characteristics: a redundant sigmoid colon, deep cul-de-sac, diastasis of the levator ani muscles, loss of posterior rectal fixation, loss of the usual anorectal angle, and a patulous anus (5). As a result of these common findings, many surgeons, beginning with Moschowitz, have thought of rectal prolapse as a form of sliding hernia (3). Others have suggested that rectal prolapse is the last stage of progressively worsening intussusception. These authors cite the similarities in manometric findings among patients with prolapse, internal intussusception, and solitary rectal ulcer syndrome (SRUS) (6). Studies of the natural history of internal intussusception, however, dispute this. Both Mellgren and Ihre have shown that the vast majority of patients with internal intussusception do not progress to frank prolapse (7,8). Perineal descent and stretching of the pudendal nerves has also been suggested as a cause of prolapse (9). Given the anatomic and physiologic complexity of the pelvis, it is likely that each of these processes contributes to rectal prolapse to some degree.

EPIDEMIOLOGY

The true incidence of rectal prolapse is unknown. In adults, this condition is far more common among women, with a female:male ratio of 6:1. Prolapse becomes more prevalent with age in women and peaks in the seventh decade of life. In men, prevalence is unrelated to age. It was long thought that childbearing contributed to the pelvic laxity associated with rectal prolapse. However, the epidemiology of prolapse does not support this assertion because half of women with rectal prolapse are nulliparous (1). Rectal prolapse has been associated with a number of other conditions including constipation, diarrhea, and polyps, or other neoplasms (2). Unusual causes include trauma (10,11) and parasitic infection (2,12,13). Rectal prolapse has been variably associated with psychiatric illness (2).

PRESENTATION

As with many anorectal disorders, many patients with full-thickness rectal prolapse come to the office complaining of "hemorrhoids." Symptoms include a sensation of tissue protruding from the anus, which may or may not spontaneously reduce, tenesmus, and sensation of incomplete evacuation. Mucus discharge and leakage may accompany the protrusion. Occasionally, patients experience bleeding or pain which results from ulceration of the mucosa or rarely from incarceration. Differentiating mucosal prolapse (partial thickness) from true rectal prolapse (full thickness) can sometimes be problematic. Mucosal prolapse and/or hemorrhoidal prolapse have characteristic radial folds in the protruding mucosa. Prolapse of the full-thickness rectal wall produces circumferential folds (Fig. 1). Full-thickness rectal prolapse also produces a palpable sulcus between the rectal wall and anus, which is not present with mucosal prolapse.

Patients with rectal prolapse also present with myriad functional complaints, from incontinence and diarrhea to constipation and outlet obstruction. Up to two-thirds of patients report constipation (14,15), which is variably described as infrequent bowel movements, need to strain at stool, or a sensation of incomplete evacuation. Colonic dysmotility may cause infrequent bowel movements in half of these patients (16). A smaller proportion may have paradoxic puborectalis contraction (17,18). In some patients, the intussusceptum itself may produce outlet obstruction (19). Preoperative functional studies can often differentiate these problems.

Paradoxically, an equal number of patients with rectal prolapse report incontinence (15). The mechanism underlying prolapse-induced incontinence is incompletely understood. Chronic stretch of the sphincters by the prolapsed rectum may reduce resting internal anal sphincter pressure (20,21). Similarly, chronic stretch of the pudendal nerves is thought to produce a neuropathy that weakens the external sphincter (9,22). Occult sphincter defects may also play a role. As with constipation, preoperative physiologic evaluation can better define these abnormalities.

EVALUATION

A thorough preoperative evaluation is crucial for patients with rectal prolapse. Obviously, patients should undergo a complete medical examination with special focus on identifying factors that predispose the patient to prolapse. The colon should be evaluated by colonoscopy

(A)   **(B)**

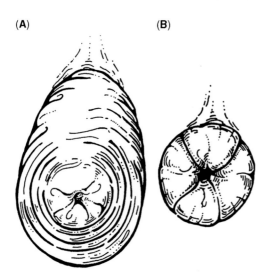

Figure 1 (**A**) Full-thickness rectal prolapse (concentric folds). (**B**) Rectal mucosal prolapse (radial folds). *Source*: From Ref. 2.

or air-contrast barium enema to exclude neoplasms or diverticular disease. Cardiopulmonary condition should be thoroughly evaluated as well because comorbidities may influence the choice of surgical procedure.

All patients with constipation should undergo colonic transit studies to detect slow transit constipation. In addition, anal manometry and electromyography can identify paradoxical puborectalis contraction. Pudendal nerve terminal motor latency (PNTML) studies have largely replaced needle electromyography, and should also be performed to identify neuropathy that may impact postoperative function. Cinedefecography is useful in patients in whom the prolapse is not immediately obvious and may identify internal intussusception or incomplete relaxation of the puborectalis muscle.

Patients with incontinence should undergo a similar evaluation. Anal manometry can identify low resting and squeeze pressures and pudendal nerve assessment can identify neuropathy. In some patients, endoanal ultrasound may be useful in identifying occult sphincter injury.

TREATMENT

Nonoperative therapy has occasionally been suggested for rectal prolapse, especially in high-risk patients. Approaches have included biofeedback, buttock taping, bowel regimens to decrease straining, and injection of sclerosants to fix the rectum in place (2). In adults these methods have been largely unsuccessful, therefore, the primary therapy for rectal prolapse remains surgical. Over one hundred different procedures have been described to treat this condition. These operations can be categorized as either abdominal or perineal. Abdominal operations have taken three major approaches: (i) reduction of the perineal hernia and closure of the cul-de-sac, (ii) fixation of the rectum, or (iii) resection of redundant bowel (or some combination of these). Perineal approaches have focused upon (i) tightening the anus, (ii) reefing the rectal mucosa, or (iii) resecting the prolapsed bowel from the perineum.

ABDOMINAL PROCEDURES

Moschowitz believed that rectal prolapse was a form of abdominal wall herniation, and the Moschowitz repair is based upon this premise. The goal in this operation is to obliterate the pouch of Douglas using a series of horizontal purse-string sutures between the anterior wall of the rectum and vagina (or prostate capsule) (Fig. 2) (2,3,23). The Moschowitz–Graham procedure is a modification of this technique in which the levator muscles are plicated to strengthen the pelvic floor (2). While this approach is anatomically appealing, recurrence rates approach 50%, and it has therefore fallen out of favor as a primary operation (24). Modifications have been proposed including the addition of rectal fixation and/or resection, and have met with greater success (25,26); however, most surgeons believe that obliteration of the cul-de-sac per se adds little to strengthen the repair. The one exception to this may be in patients with an associated enterocele in which this approach may be useful.

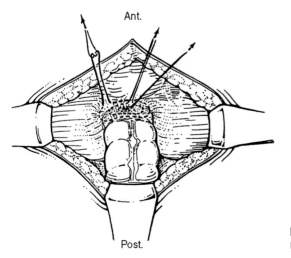

Figure 2 Obliteration of the cul-de-sac (Moschowitz repair). *Source*: From Ref. 2.

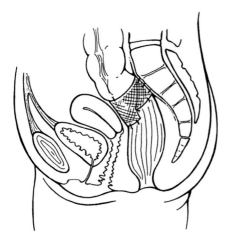

Figure 3 Anterior (Ripstein) rectopexy. *Source*: From Ref. 2.

A number of different operations have been proposed to fix the rectum in the pelvis. Initial experience with fixation to the anterior abdominal wall, uterus, or pelvic brim was largely unsuccessful, and prolapse recurred in one-third of patients (27,28). Anterior colpopexy had better results, but failed to gain wide acceptance (29). Most fixation procedures currently performed are based upon fixation of the rectum to the presacral fascia—presacral rectopexy. Ripstein described an anterior sling created from a fascia lata graft, which was placed around the rectum then sutured to the sacrum (Fig. 3) (30–32). The Wells rectopexy uses a posterior sling to attach the rectum to the sacrum (Fig. 4) (33). A number of modifications to both the Ripstein and Wells procedures have been described using different materials or points of attachment; all have excellent results with low recurrence rates (2–10%) and few complications (34,35). The final modification of this approach is suture rectopexy. In this operation, the posterior sling is abandoned, and the lateral rectal attachments are sutured directly to the sacrum, thus avoiding the need for mesh or other foreign material (Fig. 5). Long-term follow-up indicates that suture rectopexy is equally durable (recurrence in less than 5% of patients) and has few associated complications (20). An operation combining abdominal rectopexy with colpopexy has also been described for treating patients with both rectal prolapse and vaginal prolapse, and may be useful in patients with prolapse of multiple pelvic organs (36,37).

The existence of multiple modifications of these rectopexy procedures reflects a longstanding debate over the best technique and material for rectal suspension. Rectopexy has been performed using autologous fascia lata, various types of prosthetic mesh, and a variety of suture materials (33,34,38,39). Regardless of the material utilized, results have been good, and recurrence rates are consistently reported to be less than 10% (Table 1). Controversy has also existed regarding the optimal placement of the sling. The Ripstein anterior sling has been criticized on the grounds that it contributes to outlet obstruction, and therefore may increase postoperative constipation. This opinion, however, is based upon historical data in which preoperative function

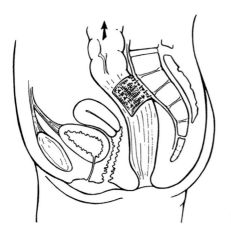

Figure 4 Posterior (Wells) rectopexy. *Source*: From Ref. 2.

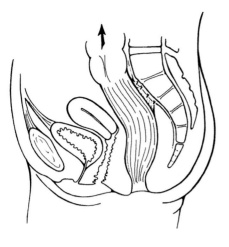

Figure 5 Presacral suture rectopexy. *Source*: From Ref. 2.

was not assessed. More recent studies have reported good functional results using a loose circumferential sling (56). Because there is no prospective data to support any one technique over another in terms of either recurrence or postoperative function, the choice of rectal suspension technique is largely based upon individual patient characteristics and surgeon preference.

Anterior resection has also been suggested for treating rectal prolapse based upon two premises: (i) resection of the redundant colon allows the rectum to be suspended from the splenic flexure, and (ii) an anastomosis in the pelvis results in scarring that fixes the rectum to the sacrum. Several authors have reported low recurrence rates after this procedure (7–9%); however, 10% to 20% of patients with incontinence had deterioration in function, probably because of the loss of the rectal reservoir. Moreover, an anastomosis below the peritoneal reflection increased morbidity (57–59). This risk of incontinence along with risk of an anastomotic leak make anterior resection alone a poor choice for repair of rectal prolapse.

Frykman first described an approach that combines sigmoid colectomy with rectopexy (resection rectopexy) (60). This combined procedure has a low recurrence rate (between 2% and 9%), and few anastomotic complications (approximately 4%) (14,61–63). There are few studies that compare resection rectopexy to rectopexy alone. Luukkonen et al., however, did compare 15 patients who underwent resection and sutured rectopexy to 15 patients who underwent mesh rectopexy alone. In this study, there were no recurrences and functional results were similar (64). Several small studies have also demonstrated an improvement in preexisting constipation after resection rectopexy (16,64,65). Preoperative evaluation is crucial;

Table 1 Abdominal Suspension/Fixation Techniques

Authors	References	Procedure	Material	Number of patients recur/operated	Recurrence (%)
Ripstein	(30,40)	Anterior sling	Teflon®/Marlex®	2/500	0
Morgan	(41)	Anterior sling	Teflon	1/64	2
Holmstom et al	(42)	Anterior sling	Marlex	4/97	4
Roberts et al	(43)	Anterior sling	Teflon	13/130	10
Tjandra et al	(44)	Anterior sling	Teflon	10/129	8
Anderson et al	(45)	Posterior sling	Ivalon®	1/40	3
Atkinson & Taylor	(46)	Posterior sling	Ivalon	4/40	10
Kuijpers & de Morree	(47)	Posterior sling	Teflon	3/30	10
Arndt & Pircher	(39)	Posterior sling	Vicryl®/Dexon®	4/62	6
Yoshioka et al	(48)	Posterior sling	Marlex	2/135	2
Novell et al	(49)	Posterior sling	Ivalon	1/31	3
Goligher	(50)	Suture rectopexy	–	0/40	0
Carter	(51)	Suture rectopexy	–	1/32	3
Graham et al	(52)	Suture rectopexy	–	0/23	0
Ejerblad & Krause	(53)	Suture rectopexy	–	2/48	4
Blatchford et al	(54)	Suture rectopexy	–	1/42	2
Khanna et al	(55)	Suture rectopexy	–	0/65	0

Source: From Ref. 4.

however, because a few patients with severe slow transit constipation may benefit from a subtotal colectomy and rectopexy (14). Given the low recurrence rate and relative safety of this operation, many surgeons favor combining resection with rectopexy, especially in patients with a very redundant sigmoid colon and/or preoperative constipation.

PERINEAL PROCEDURES

Perineal operations for rectal prolapse avoid the morbidity of an abdominal procedure. Some of the first described perineal approaches for treating prolapse involved rectal encirclement. Thiersch described encirclement of the anus with silver wire in 1891 (66,67), and this procedure was subsequently modified to make use of fascia, tendon, and various types of mesh with varying levels of encirclement around the anus and distal rectum (2,68). The Angelchik prosthesis, developed for the treatment of esophageal reflux, was also briefly proposed as an anorectal encirclement device (69). The advantage of these procedures is their relative simplicity and the ability to perform the operation with minimal anesthesia. However, the high recurrence rate and risk of local complications related to placement of a foreign body make these operations less appealing than other perineal approaches (70).

At the turn of the century, Delorme proposed a procedure that involves rectal mucosal stripping and plication of the underlying muscle (Fig. 6) (71). This operation can be performed with minimal anesthesia and, unlike perineal rectosigmoidectomy (described below), does not involve entry into the peritoneal cavity. While this approach may be ideal for mucosal prolapse or a small full-thickness prolapse, recurrence rates as high as 37% make it less ideal for large, full-thickness rectal prolapse (Table 2) (72).

The perineal procedure most often recommended for treatment of full-thickness rectal prolapse is rectosigmoidectomy. This procedure was first described by Mickulicz in 1889 (83), and subsequently popularized by Altemeier in 1971 (84). In this operation, the prolapsed rectum is divided approximately 2 cm proximal to the dentate line. The cylinder of prolapsed rectum is then placed on traction, and the mesorectal vessels ligated and divided. When the prolapsed bowel can no longer be delivered any further through the anus, it is divided and an anastomosis is created between the end of the proximal bowel and the distal rectum. The anastomosis can be created using either a hand-sewn technique or a circular stapler (Fig. 7) (85,86). This procedure is generally well tolerated, even among patients with multiple medical problems, and complications related to the operation are rare (approximately 3%) (87). Recurrence, however, is more common than recurrence after abdominal rectopexy, ranging from 0% to 60% (although most recent studies report recurrence rates between 10% and 15%) (Table 3) (24,63,72,84,87–97). For this reason, perineal rectosigmoidectomy may be best suited for high-risk patients in whom the risk of a laparotomy exceeds the risk of recurrent prolapse.

LAPAROSCOPIC PROCEDURES

Technological advances over the past two decades have triggered a proliferation of operations performed with minimally invasive techniques. It has been suggested that abdominal

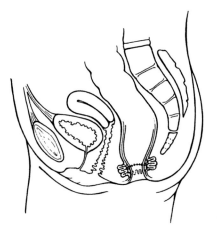

Figure 6 Resection of mucosal sleeve and plication of the rectal wall (Delorme procedure). *Source*: From Ref. 2.

Table 2 Delorme Procedure Results

Authors	References	Number of patients recur/operated	Recurrence (%)
Uhlig and Sullivan	(73)	3/44	7
Christiansen and Kirkegaard	(74)	1/12	17
Gundersen and Cogbill et al.	(75)	1/18	6
Monson et al.	(76)	2/27	7
Houry et al.	(77)	3/18	17
Graf et al.	(78)	3/14	21
Tobin and Scott	(79)	11/43	26
Oliver et al.	(80)	9/41	22
Senapati et al.	(81)	4/32	13
Plusa et al.	(82)	26/104	17
Agachan et al.	(72)	3/8	37

Source: From Ref. 4.

rectopexy may be an ideal procedure for laparoscopy. The operation is performed for benign disease, and if it is performed without resection, there is no specimen to remove and no anastomosis to create. As surgeons have become more experienced with laparoscopic bowel resection, laparoscopic rectopexy with resection has also become possible because the redundant sigmoid colon can be resected and removed through a small extended port site incision and either an intra- or extracorporeal anastomosis performed. As with all new technology, data assessing the safety, efficacy, and durability of this approach is relatively lacking; however, a number of authors are addressing these questions.

Several retrospective series have addressed the feasibility of laparoscopic rectopexy using either a suture or mesh technique. Initial reports showed that this procedure is technically feasible and safe, with few perioperative complications (98–103). With short follow-up, recurrences

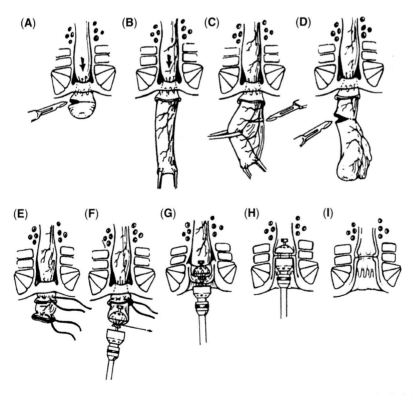

Figure 7 Perineal rectosigmoidectomy. With the rectum prolapsed, the outer rectal tube is incised circularly (**A**) and unfolded (**B**). The mesorectum is serially ligated and divided (**C**). When all the redundancy has been removed, the inner tube is divided, which completes the resection (**D**). The anastomosis may be performed with an intraluminal stapling device or may be hand sewn (**E–I**). *Source*: From Ref. 2.

Table 3 Perineal Rectosigmoidectomy Results

Authors	References	Number of patients recur/operated	Recurrence (%)
Hughes	(89)	65/108	60
Porter	(90)	55/110	50
Gabriel	(91)	16/131	12
Theuerkauf et al.	(24)	3/13	39
Altemeier et al.	(84)	3/106	3
Friedman et al.	(92)	12/27	44
Gopal et al.	(93)	1/18	6
Prasad et al.	(94)	0/25	0
Williams et al.	(87)	11/114	10
Thorne and Polglase	(95)	2/16	13
Johansen et al.	(96)	0/20	0
Ramanujam	(97)	4/72	6
Agachan et al.	(72)	5/53	10
Kim et al.	(63)	29/183	16

Source: From Ref. 4.

are rare and functional outcome also appears to be equivalent to outcome reported after open procedures (99,101,104). Recently, Solomon et al. performed a prospective randomized trial to compare laparoscopic rectopexy to the traditional open technique (105). In this study, 39 patients were randomized to either laparoscopic mesh rectopexy or open mesh rectopexy. The authors found that the laparoscopic approach improved time to regular diet and length of stay. They also found less need for pain medication and fewer pulmonary complications in the laparoscopic group. Finally, these investigators evaluated biochemical markers of physiologic stress (urinary catecholamines, interleukin-6, serum cortisol, and C-reactive protein) and found lower levels in the patients in the laparoscopic group than in the patients in the open surgery group, suggesting that the laparoscopic approach may be less physiologically injurious to patients. The only advantage to an open procedure in this series was decreased operative time (102 minutes in the open group versus 153 minutes in the laparoscopic group). With mean follow-up of 24 months, there has been one recurrence in the open surgery group (105). While this group will need longer follow-up to accurately assess long-term functional outcome and durability, these results suggest that laparoscopic rectopexy may be preferable to open rectopexy for some patients.

Laparoscopic rectopexy with resection is a more complicated procedure and adds operative time; however, several authors have shown that this procedure is equally safe. Benoist et al. compared 16 patients who underwent laparoscopic rectopexy with sigmoid resection to 32 patients who underwent either laparoscopic suture rectopexy or laparoscopic mesh rectopexy (106). They showed equivalent perioperative morbidity among the three groups (11% in the resection rectopexy group versus 14% in the mesh rectopexy group versus 19% in the suture rectopexy group) and no anastomotic leaks. Their data also suggested an improvement in constipation among the resection rectopexy group (106). Other authors report similar results, with morbidity ranging from 9% to 24% (major morbidity 9–10%), anastomotic leak rate of 0% to 6%, and recurrence rate of 0% to 7% after two years (99,107,108). The one consistent disadvantage of laparoscopic resection rectopexy was increased operative time.

Although the majority of these studies are small and have short follow-up, initial experience with laparoscopic rectopexy either with or without resection suggests that this approach is a safe and effective treatment for rectal prolapse. Larger series and longer follow-up will be necessary to determine if laparoscopy is superior to open rectopexy and to assess long-term durability. In the meantime, laparoscopic rectopexy offers an attractive option for surgeons well versed in this technology.

TREATMENT OF INCARCERATED RECTAL PROLAPSE

Incarcerated rectal prolapse is rare, but when it does occur it represents a surgical emergency. If the prolapsed segment is irreducible but appears viable, an attempt should be made to reduce the prolapse. Various techniques have been described including the use of ice packs, injection of dilute epinephrine and hyaluronidase (109), and sedation plus manual pressure (110).

One simple and effective technique adapted from veterinary practice is the application of table sugar to osmotically shrink the prolapsed bowel and allow reduction (111). If these maneuvers are unsuccessful, a final attempt at reduction under anesthesia should be attempted. If reduction is successful, the patient should undergo an elective evaluation to rule out malignancy, then be offered elective abdominal rectopexy or perineal rectosigmoidectomy if there are no medical contraindications to surgery.

If attempts at reduction are unsuccessful, or if the bowel appears gangrenous, emergent bowel resection should be performed. Emergent perineal rectosigmoidectomy is probably the procedure of choice, because it poses less operative risk than an abdominal procedure in patients who are invariably frail. However, the risk of an anastomotic dehiscence is greater than with elective resection, and some patients may ultimately require a colostomy (109).

RECTAL PROLAPSE IN CHILDREN

Rectal prolapse in infants and children is a unique disease with a different pathogenesis, natural history, and treatment than rectal prolapse in adults. Most pediatric patients present before three years of age and there is an equal gender distribution. Most cases of pediatric rectal prolapse are idiopathic; however, predisposing conditions include constipation, diarrhea, straining, vomiting, and chronic cough. In addition, rectal prolapse may occasionally be the presenting symptom of cystic fibrosis and any child presenting with rectal prolapse should be evaluated by sweat chloride analysis to rule out this disorder (112). Parasitic infection may also cause prolapse, and stool should be examined for ova and parasites. Less common predisposing factors include Hirschsprung's disease, Ehlers-Danlos syndrome, and congenital hypothyroidism. Malnutrition is a common cause of rectal prolapse in developing nations (2).

Many of these children have mild, intermittent prolapse. Treatment of any underlying disorder frequently cures these patients. In addition, an aggressive bowel regimen to prevent the child from straining at stool may be helpful. Maneuvers such as avoiding squatting, defecating in the recumbent position, and taping the buttocks between bowel movements have occasionally been advocated. The vast majority of these patients will respond to medical therapy, and require no further intervention (2,113).

Despite the success of medical therapy in most children, some will have pronounced, recurrent prolapse, which may cause bleeding and pain. Injection sclerotherapy is an effective treatment for many of these patients. A sclerosing agent (D50W, 70% ethyl alcohol, 30% saline, or 5% phenol in olive oil) is injected into the submucosa and perirectal tissues with the child under general anesthesia. Using this approach, success rates of 64% to 94% after one injection and 93% to 100% after two injections have been reported. The procedure is technically simple to perform and complications are rare (114–118). Linear cauterization is another procedure designed to induce scarring and fix the rectum in place. Under general anesthesia, the child is placed in the prone position, an anoscope is introduced through the anal canal, and the rectal mucosal is cauterized for a 3 to 4 cm distance above the dentate line in four to six tracts equally spaced around the rectum. Success rate with this procedure has been reported to be 92% after one operation, and 99% after two operations (119).

In the rare patient who fails injection sclerotherapy or linear cauterization, a more extensive surgical procedure may be required. Multiple techniques have been proposed and both abdominal rectopexy and perineal rectosigmoidectomy as described in the adult may be appropriate solutions. In addition, mucosal resection, levatoroplasty, presacral packing with gauze or gelfoam sponges (Upjohn Company, Kalamazoo, Michigan, U.S.A.), silastic or catgut encirclement, and transsacral rectopexy have been described (120). Ekehorn's rectopexy in which a U-shaped suture is passed through the skin, into the rectum, around the sacrococcygeal junction, then back through the skin and tied over gauze, has been reported to have excellent results (121,122). Fortunately, the majority of children with rectal prolapse will improve without the need for these more complex procedures.

RECTAL PROLAPSE IN MEN

Rectal prolapse is uncommon in men, and there are few studies that address this disorder in the male population. Unlike incidence in women, incidence of rectal prolapse in men does not increase with age, but instead remains constant throughout all decades of life. In the Middle

East, schistosomiasis has been reported to cause rectal prolapse in young men (12), but similar associations have not been identified in the United States. At the University of Minnesota, a retrospective review of all patients treated for rectal prolapse between 1987 and 1999 identified 55 men. This population was relatively young, with a mean age of 47 years (range 15–91 years). Many of these patients had neurologic disorders (13%), developmental delay or psychiatric illness (20%), or were nursing home residents (13%). Preoperative incontinence was reported by 27% of these patients, and preoperative constipation by 29%. Most of these men underwent a perineal rectosigmoidectomy (64%). Fifteen percent underwent a Delorme's procedure, and the remainder (21%) underwent abdominal rectopexy. Recurrence rates did not differ between perineal and abdominal approaches (17% vs. 19%), although patients with neurologic conditions did have a higher rate of recurrence regardless of the choice of operation (43%). Functional results were variable and long-term follow-up was available for only 37% of patients. Of note, this study identified three patients who developed ejaculatory dysfunction, two of whom had undergone a perineal procedure, suggesting that a perineal approach does not protect against this complication. This small series suggests that rectal prolapse in men may be treated equally well by either an abdominal or a perineal operation; however, definitive conclusions will require a larger series of patients (2).

TREATMENT OF RECURRENT PROLAPSE

The reported incidence of recurrent prolapse varies widely. Most authors report the fewest recurrences after abdominal procedures (recurrence rate ~10%) (14,20,61–63). Controversy exists over the cause of recurrence in these patients; however, technical aspects of the original operation may contribute. The extent of rectal mobilization is thought to be key, and most authorities recommend posterior mobilization to the level of the coccyx. The necessary extent of the lateral and anterior dissections is more controversial. Although one study has shown a higher rate of recurrence if the lateral ligaments are left intact (123), another showed equivalent risk of recurrence (124). The anterior dissection is generally carried to the level of the upper third of the vagina, but there is no data to support this approach (2).

Results after a perineal operation are more variable, with recurrences reported in 0% to 60% of patients after perineal rectosigmoidectomy (24,63,72,84,87,89,90,92–97,125–127), 7% to 37% of patients following the Delorme procedure (72–82), and 0% to 44% of patients after an anal encirclement procedure (66–70). Inadequate bowel resection is a major cause of recurrence in these patients; however, guidelines for the extent of resection are vague. In general, the dissection of the rectosigmoid colon is carried out until the surgeon feels that the proximal bowel is on tension. The proximal extent of the mucosal dissection during a Delorme procedure is guided by a similar principle. The addition of levatoroplasty might also be expected to improve the durability of the repair, but this remains unproven (2).

Small, asymptomatic recurrent mucosal prolapse may not require treatment; however, full-thickness recurrence will almost always require a second operation. Because abdominal rectopexy (with or without resection) has the lowest risk of recurrence, this approach is probably best for treating recurrence. However, patient factors may influence the operative plan, and comorbid medical conditions may preclude a laparotomy. One cautionary note for reoperative procedures involves bowel resection. If the patient has undergone a prior resection, it is crucial to consider the blood supply to the distal bowel before proceeding with another resection from either the abdominal or perineal approach. If resection is performed, the intervening bowel segment may become ischemic if care is not taken to carefully preserve the blood supply. Although, the risk of ischemia may be minimized by dividing vessels very close to the bowel wall, the possibility of bowel necrosis always exists in this setting, and it is probably best to avoid reresection if at all possible (2). In patients with severe incontinence, resection of the remaining rectosigmoid colon and end colostomy is also a reasonable alternative for treating recurrent prolapse.

As expected, morbidity and mortality are higher after reoperation. One series reports 14% morbidity and 7% mortality after a second operation for prolapse (128). Re-recurrence is not uncommon, and has been reported in 15% to 50% of patients. Functional results, however, are similar for a second operation, and the majority of patients will have improvement in either incontinence or constipation (2,129,130).

FUNCTIONAL RESULTS

In addition to rate of recurrence, functional outcome is crucial in evaluation of the success of any operation designed to cure rectal prolapse. A large proportion of patients with prolapse suffer from preoperative incontinence and postoperative improvement can be expected in many. The Ripstein procedure has been associated with improved continence in 52% to 57% of patients (42–44). Posterior sling procedures are associated with improvement in 10% to 83% (although most authors report improvement in 75–80%) (20,48,49,64,65,131). Suture rectopexy without resection improves continence in 50% to 93% of patients (20,49,52–54,61), while rectopexy with resection has more variable results (improvement in 38–94%) (14,16,61,62, 64,132). Results after the perineal procedures is more variable; however, many patients also have improvement in continence. Multiple studies have reported that 23% to 83% of patients report improvement in continence after a Delorme procedure, while 25% to 100% of patients report improvement after perineal rectosigmoidectomy (61,87,92,94–97). Clearly patient selection impacts these results, and the multiple factors contributing to preoperative incontinence may impact the functional result of the repair. However, taken together, the data suggest that postoperative continence is equivalent after either an abdominal or perineal approach (15).

The mechanism responsible for improved continence after repair of rectal prolapse is as poorly understood as the mechanisms responsible for preoperative incontinence. Some patients have improved anal resting (21,56,69,133–137), and/or squeeze pressures (137) after surgery; however, most patients have persistently low-sphincter pressures. Interestingly, several studies have shown that there is little correlation between improved manometric parameters and continence (48,138). Removal of the chronic rectoanal inhibitory reflex produced by the prolapsed bowel has also been suggested as a mechanism that may improve continence (21). Additionally, improved rectal sensation, and improved overall rectal function may contribute (20,123). In one study, preexisting pudendal neuropathy predicted poor functional outcome (139). Given the multifactorial causes of incontinence in patients with rectal prolapse, it is not surprising than many of these factors contribute to postoperative outcome. However, it is generally agreed that patients with severe preoperative incontinence rarely have dramatic improvement after repair.

The effect·on constipation is more difficult to measure, in part because there is no universal definition of what constitutes constipation. Two-thirds of patients report some degree of constipation preoperatively (14,15), and postoperative function is highly variable. Preoperative evaluation is crucial to differentiate patients with outlet obstruction, paradoxical contraction of the puborectalis, and slow transit constipation. It has been argued that the addition of sigmoid resection to rectopexy may improve constipation or prevent the onset of postoperative constipation in some patients (14,16,64). In addition, some patients with proven slow transit constipation may benefit from subtotal colectomy and rectopexy (14,140).

Division of the lateral ligaments during rectal mobilization has been implicated in the development of postoperative constipation. Speakman et al performed a prospective randomized trial to evaluate the effect of division of the lateral ligaments on both recurrence and postoperative function. In this study, division of the lateral ligaments was associated with an increased risk of postoperative constipation; however, nondivision led to a higher risk of recurrence (123). Scaglia et al. reported similar functional results, noting that patients who underwent division of the lateral ligaments had significantly more evacuation problems than those who did not. These authors, however, did not find a higher rate of recurrence in patients who did not undergo lateral stalk division (124). However, it is important to note that precise anatomic definition of these structures is difficult, and some surgeons have even questioned their existence. With this in mind, it is probably prudent to avoid division of the distal lateral rectal attachments, especially in patients with preexisting constipation.

INTERNAL INTUSSUSCEPTION AND SRUS

Internal intussusception can be detected radiographically in a significant proportion of the population (141). Because the majority of people with this finding are asymptomatic, it is unclear if it represents true pathology or is simply a normal anatomic variant. While internal intussusception was once thought to be a precursor to full-thickness prolapse, studies of the natural history of internal prolapse have shown that this condition rarely progresses to full-thickness prolapse (7,8). In a small proportion of patients, however, internal intussusception can be associated with disordered defecation, outlet obstruction, or incomplete evacuation. Anorectal manometric studies are likely to identify paradoxic contraction of the puborectalis and/or abnormally high-sphincter pressures in many of these individuals. In these patients, treatment should focus upon correction of the underlying pelvic floor disorder rather than correction of the intussusception (4).

SRUS and colitis cystica profunda (CCP) are associated with internal intussusception in 30% to 80% of patients (142–144). In a smaller number of patients, this finding may accompany full-thickness prolapse (145,146). Patients with SRUS and CCP may present with outlet obstruction, pain, bleeding, and/or mucus discharge. In SRUS, one or more ulcers are present in the distal rectum, usually on the anterior wall. In CCP, nodules or a mass may be found in a similar location. Both lesions may be mistaken for malignancy, and biopsy is required to confirm the diagnosis. Pathologic findings include hypertrophy of the muscularis mucosa and fibromuscular obliteration of the lamina propria (SRUS) as well as dilated mucus-filled glands in the submucosa (CCP) (147). Because symptoms and treatment are identical, SRUS and CCP are generally considered to be variants of the same disorder.

The therapeutic approach to symptomatic internal intussusception and SRUS/CCP remains controversial. Evaluation should include anorectal manometry, defecography, and either colonoscopy or barium enema to exclude other diagnoses. Biopsy of an ulcer or mass is mandatory to exclude malignancy. Most authors agree that an initial attempt at nonoperative therapy is indicated in these patients. Up to 75% of patients will heal with a regimen of high-fiber diet, defecation training to avoid straining, and laxatives or enemas (148,149). For the few patients who do not respond to medical therapy, a number of surgical approaches have been described including abdominal rectopexy (mesh or suture rectopexy) (148,150,151), Ripstein procedure (152), and Delorme procedure (153–155). Results have been highly variable, but are generally poor for patients without full-thickness rectal prolapse. As a result, nonoperative therapy should be the mainstay of treatment for internal intussusception, with surgery reserved for highly symptomatic patients who have failed all medical interventions.

CONCLUSION

Our understanding of rectal prolapse has increased dramatically over the past century. However, the wide variety of surgical procedures designed to correct this problem and the variability of outcome attest to the complexity of rectal prolapse. A thorough preoperative evaluation, including colonic transit studies, anorectal manometry, tests of PNTML, and cine-defecography, is crucial. Abdominal rectopexy with or without sigmoid resection is safe, and has very low risk of recurrence. Perineal rectosigmoidectomy has a higher rate of recurrence, but avoids a major abdominal procedure and may be preferable in high-risk patients. Laparoscopy holds promise and may increase the number of patients who can safely undergo an abdominal procedure. Functional results are variable; however, the majority of patients can expect improvement in either incontinence or constipation after surgery.

REFERENCES

1. Mann CV. Rectal prolapse. In: Morson BC, ed. Diseases of the Colon, Rectum, and Anus. New York: Appleton-Century-Crofts, 1969:238–250.
2. Karulf RE, Madoff RD, Goldberg SM. Rectal prolapse. Current Prob Surg 2001; 38:757–832.
3. Moschowitz AV. The pathogenesis, anatomy and cure of prolapse of the rectum. Surg Gynecol Obstet 1912; 15:7–21.
4. Madoff RD. Rectal prolapse and intussusception. In: Beck DE, Wexner SD, eds. Fundamentals of Anorectal Surgery. Philadelphia, PA: W. B. Saunders, 1998:99–114.
5. Goldberg SM, Gordon PH, Nivatvongs S. Essentials of Anorectal Surgery. Philadelphia: JB Lippincott Co, 1980.
6. Sun WM, Read NW, Donnelly TC, Bannister JJ, Shorthouse AJ. A common pathophysiology for full thickness rectal prolapse, anterior mucosal prolapse and solitary rectal ulcer. Br J Surg 1989; 76:290–295.
7. Mellgren A, Schultz I, Johansson C, Dolk A. Internal rectal intussusception seldom develops into total rectal prolapse. Dis Colon Rectum 1997; 40:817–820.

8. Ihre T, Seligson U. Intussusception of the rectum-internal procidentia: treatment and results in 90 patients. Dis Colon Rectum 1975; 18:391–396.
9. Parks AG, Swash M, Urich H. Sphincter denervation in anorectal incontinence and rectal prolapse. Gut 1977; 18:656–665.
10. Kram HB, Clark SR, Mackabee JR, Melendez R, Shoemaker WC. Rectal prolapse caused by blunt abdominal trauma. Surgery 1989; 105:790–792.
11. Debeugny P, Bonnevalle M, Besson R, Basset T. A recto-sigmoid lesion due to trans-anal aspiration. Apropos of a case. Chir Pediatr 1990; 31:191–194.
12. Hussein AM, Helal SF. Schistosomal pelvic floor myopathy contributes to the pathogenesis of rectal prolapse in young males. Dis Colon Rectum 2000; 43:644–649.
13. Abul-Khair MH. Bilhariziasis and prolapse of the rectum. Br J Surg 1976; 63:891–892.
14. Madoff RD, Williams JG, Wong WD, Rothenberger DA, Goldberg SM. Long-term functional results of colon resection and rectopexy for overt rectal prolapse. Am J Gastroenterol 1992; 87:101–104.
15. Madoff RD, Mellgren A. One hundred years of rectal prolapse surgery. Dis Colon Rectum 1999; 42:441–450.
16. McKee RF, Lauder JC, Poon FW, Aitchison MA, Finlay IG. A prospective randomized study of abdominal rectopexy with and without sigmoidectomy in rectal prolapse. Surg Gynecol Obstet 1992; 174:145–148.
17. Agachan F, Pfeifer J, Wexner SD. Defecography and proctography. Results of 744 patients. Dis Colon Rectum 1996; 39:899–905.
18. Kuijpers HC, Bleijenberg G. Assessment and treatment of obstructed defecation. Ann Med 1990; 22:405–411.
19. Hoffman MJ, Kodner IJ, Fry RD. Internal intussusception of the rectum. Diagnosis and surgical management. Dis Colon Rectum 1984; 27:435–441.
20. Duthie GS, Bartolo DC. Abdominal rectopexy for rectal prolapse: a comparison of techniques. Br J Surg 1992; 79:107–113.
21. Farouk R, Duthie GS, Bartolo DC, MacGregor AB. Restoration of continence following rectopexy for rectal prolapse and recovery of the internal anal sphincter electromyogram. Br J Surg 1992; 79: 439–440.
22. Neill ME, Parks AG, Swash M. Physiological studies of the anal sphincter musculature in faecal incontinence and rectal prolapse. Br J Surg 1981; 68:531–536.
23. Quenu E, Duval P. Technique de la colopexie pour prolapsus du rectum. Rev Chir Paris 1910; 41:135.
24. Theuerkauf FJ Jr., Beahrs OH, Hill JR. Rectal prolapse. Causation and surgical treatment. Ann Surg 1970; 171:819–835.
25. Goligher JC. The treatment of complete prolapse of the rectum by the Roscoe Graham operation. Br J Surg 1958; 45:323.
26. Palmer JA. Prolapse of the rectum: treatment by the Moschowitz–Graham operation. Can J Surg 1969; 12:116–123.
27. Pemberton JH, Stalker LK. Surgical treatment of complete rectal prolapse. Ann Surg 1939; 109: 799–808.
28. Beahrs OH, Vandertoll DJ, Baker NH. Complete rectal prolapse: an evaluation of surgical treatment. Ann Surg 1965; 161:221.
29. Moore HD. The results of treatment of complete prolapse of the rectum in the adult patient. Dis Colon Rectum 1977; 145:75–76.
30. Ripstein CB. Treatment of massive rectal prolapse. Am J Surg 1952; 83:68–71.
31. Morgan CN, Porter NH, Klugman DJ. Ivalon (polyvinyl alcohol) sponge in the repair of complete rectal prolapse. Br J Surg 1972; 59:841–846.
32. Gordon PH, Hoexter B. Complications of the Ripstein procedure. Dis Colon Rectum 1978; 21: 277–280.
33. Wells C. New operation for rectal prolapse. J R Soc Med 1959; 52:602–603.
34. Orr TG. A suspension operation for prolapse of the rectum. Ann Surg 1947; 126:833–840.
35. Nigro ND. Restoration of the levator sling in the treatment of rectal procidentia. Dis Colon Rectum 1958; 1:123–127.
36. Collopy BT, Barham KA. Abdominal colporectopexy with pelvic cul-de-sac closure. Dis Colon Rectum 2002; 45:522–526; discussion 526–529.
37. Barham K, Collopy BT. Posthysterectomy rectal and vaginal prolapse, a commonly overlooked problem. Aust N Z J Obstet Gynaecol 1993; 33:300–303.
38. Cutait D. Sacro-promontory fixation of the rectum for complete rectal prolapse. J R Soc Med 1959; 52:105.
39. Arndt M, Pircher W. Absorbable mesh in the treatment of rectal prolapse. Int J Colorectal Dis 1988; 3:141–143.
40. Ripstein CB. Procidentia: definitive corrective surgery. Dis Colon Rectum 1972; 15:334–336.
41. Morgan B. The teflon sling operation for repair of complete rectal prolapse. Aust N Z J Surg 1980; 50:121–123.
42. Holmstrom B, Broden G, Dolk A. Results of the Ripstein operation in the treatment of rectal prolapse and internal rectal procidentia. Dis Colon Rectum 1986; 29:845–848.

43. Roberts PL, Schoetz DJ Jr., Coller JA, Veidenheimer MC. Ripstein procedure. Lahey Clinic experience: 1963–1985. Arch Surg 1988; 123:554–557.

44. Tjandra JJ, Fazio VW, Church JM, Milsom JW, Oakley JR, Lavery IC. Ripstein procedure is an effective treatment for rectal prolapse without constipation. Dis Colon Rectum 1993; 36:501–507.

45. Anderson JR, Kinninmonth AW, Smith AN. Polyvinyl alcohol sponge rectopexy for complete rectal prolapse. J R Coll Surg Edinb 1981; 26:292–294.

46. Atkinson KG, Taylor DC. Wells procedure for complete rectal prolapse. A ten-year experience. Dis Colon Rectum 1984; 27:96–98.

47. Kuijpers JH, de Morree H. Toward a selection of the most appropriate procedure in the treatment of complete rectal prolapse. Dis Colon Rectum 1988; 31:355–357.

48. Yoshioka K, Heyen F, Keighley MR. Functional results after posterior abdominal rectopexy for rectal prolapse. Dis Colon Rectum 1989; 32:835–838.

49. Novell JR, Osborne MJ, Winslet MC, Lewis AA. Prospective randomized trial of Ivalon sponge versus sutured rectopexy for full-thickness rectal prolapse. Br J Surg 1994; 81:904–906.

50. Goligher JC. Surgery of the Anus, Rectum and Colon. New York: Macmillan, 1980.

51. Carter AE. Rectosacral suture fixation for complete rectal prolapse in the elderly, the frail and the demented. Br J Surg 1983; 70:522–523.

52. Graham W, Clegg JF, Taylor V. Complete rectal prolapse: repair by a simple technique. Ann R Coll Surg Engl 1984; 66:87–89.

53. Ejerblad S, Krause U. Repair of rectal prolapse by rectosacral suture fixation. Acta Chir Scand 1988; 154:103–105.

54. Blatchford GJ, Perry RE, Thorson AG, Christensen MA. Rectopexy without resection for rectal prolapse. Am J Surg 1989; 158:574–576.

55. Khanna AK, Misra MK, Kumar K. Simplified sutured sacral rectopexy for complete rectal prolapse in adults. Eur J Surg 1996; 162:143–146.

56. Schultz I, Mellgren A, Dolk A, Johansson C, Holmstrom B. Continence is improved after the Ripstein rectopexy. Different mechanisms in rectal prolapse and rectal intussusception? Dis Colon Rectum 1996; 39:300–306.

57. Muir KG. Treatment of complete rectal prolapse in the adult. Proc R Soc Med 1962; 55:1056.

58. Schlinkert RT, Beart RW Jr., Wolff BG, Pemberton JH. Anterior resection for complete rectal prolapse. Dis Colon Rectum 1985; 28:409–412.

59. Cirocco WC, Brown AC. Anterior resection for the treatment of rectal prolapse: a 20-year experience. Am Surg 1993; 59:265–269.

60. Frykman HM. Abdominal proctopexy and primary sigmoid resection for rectal procidentia. Am J Surg 1955; 90:780–789.

61. Watts JD, Rothenberger DA, Buls JG, Goldberg SM, Nivatvongs S. The management of procidentia. 30 years' experience. Dis Colon Rectum 1985; 28:96–102.

62. Husa A, Sainio P, von Smitten K. Abdominal rectopexy and sigmoid resection (Frykman-Goldberg operation) for rectal prolapse. Acta Chir Scand 1988; 154:221–224.

63. Kim DS, Tsang CB, Wong WD, Lowry AC, Goldberg SM, Madoff RD. Complete rectal prolapse: evolution of management and results. Dis Colon Rectum 1999; 42:460–466; discussion 466–469.

64. Luukkonen P, Mikkonen U, Jarvinen H. Abdominal rectopexy with sigmoidectomy vs. rectopexy alone for rectal prolapse: a prospective, randomized study. Int J Colorectal Dis 1992; 7:219–222.

65. Sayfan J, Pinho M, Alexander-Williams J, Keighley MR. Sutured posterior abdominal rectopexy with sigmoidectomy compared with Marlex rectopexy for rectal prolapse. Br J Surg 1990; 77: 143–145.

66. Gabriel WB. Thiersch's operation for anal incontinence. Proc R Soc Med 1948; 41:467–468.

67. Gabriel WB. Thiersch's operation for anal incontinence and minor degrees of rectal prolapse. Am J Surg 1953; 86:583–590.

68. Notaras MJ. The use of Mersilene mesh in rectal prolapse repair. Proc R Soc Med 1973; 66:684–686.

69. Ladha A, Lee P, Berger P. Use of Angelchik anti-reflux prosthesis for repair of total rectal prolapse in elderly patients. Dis Colon Rectum 1985; 28:5–7.

70. Vongsangnak V, Varma JS, Smith AN. Reappraisal of Thiersch's operation for complete rectal prolapse. J R Coll Surg Edinb 1985; 30:185–187.

71. Delorme R. Sur le traitement des prolapssu du rectum totaux pour l'excision de la musqueuse rectale ou rectocolique. Bull Mem Soc Chir Paris 1900; 26:498–499.

72. Agachan F, Pfeifer J, Joo JS, Nogueras JJ, Weiss EG, Wexner SD. Results of perineal procedures for the treatment of rectal prolapse. Am Surg 1997; 63:9–12.

73. Uhlig BE, Sullivan ES. The modified Delorme operation: its place in surgical treatment for massive rectal prolapse. Dis Colon Rectum 1979; 22:513–521.

74. Christiansen J, Kirkegaard P. Delorme's operation for complete rectal prolapse. Br J Surg 1981; 68:537–538.

75. Gundersen AL, Cogbill TH, Landercasper J. Reappraisal of Delorme's procedure for rectal prolapse. Dis Colon Rectum 1985; 28:721–724.

76. Monson JR, Jones NA, Vowden P, Brennan TG. Delorme's operation: the first choice in complete rectal prolapse? Ann R Coll Surg Engl 1986; 68:143–146.

77. Houry S, Lechaux JP, Huguier M, Molkhou JM. Treatment of rectal prolapse by Delorme's operation. Int J Colorectal Dis 1987; 2:149–152.
78. Graf W, Ejerblad S, Krog M, Pahlman L, Gerdin B. Delorme's operation for rectal prolapse in elderly or unfit patients. Eur J Surg 1992; 158:555–557.
79. Tobin SA, Scott IH. Delorme operation for rectal prolapse. Br J Surg 1994; 81:1681–1684.
80. Oliver GC, Vachon D, Eisenstat TE, Rubin RJ, Salvati EP. Delorme's procedure for complete rectal prolapse in severely debilitated patients. An analysis of 41 cases. Dis Colon Rectum 1994; 37:461–467.
81. Senapati A, Nicholls RJ, Thomson JP, Phillips RK. Results of Delorme's procedure for rectal prolapse. Dis Colon Rectum 1994; 37:456–460.
82. Plusa SM, Charig JA, Balaji V, Watts A, Thompson MR. Physiological changes after Delorme's procedure for full-thickness rectal prolapse. Br J Surg 1995; 82:1475–1478.
83. Mickulicz J. Zur operativen behandlung dis prolapsus recti et coli invaginati. Arch Klin Surg 1889; 38:74–97.
84. Altemeier WA, Culbertson WR, Schowengerdt C, Hunt J. Nineteen years' experience with the one-stage perineal repair of rectal prolapse. Ann Surg 1971; 173:993–1006.
85. Vermeulen FD, Nivatvongs S, Fang DT, Balcos EG, Goldberg SM. A technique for perineal rectosigmoidectomy using autosuture devices. Surg Gynecol Obstet 1983; 156:84–86.
86. Bennett BH, Geelhoed GW. A stapler modification of the Altemeier procedure for rectal prolapse. Experimental and clinical evaluation. Am Surg 1985; 51:116–120.
87. Williams JG, Rothenberger DA, Madoff RD, Goldberg SM. Treatment of rectal prolapse in the elderly by perineal rectosigmoidectomy. Dis Colon Rectum 1992; 35:830–834.
88. Agachan F, Reissman P, Pfeifer J, Weiss EG, Nogueras JJ, Wexner SD. Comparison of three perineal procedures for the treatment of rectal prolapse. South Med J 1997; 90:925–932.
89. Hughes ESR. In discussion on rectal prolapse. Proc Roy Soc Assoc Med 1949; 42:1007–1011.
90. Porter NH. Collective results of operations for rectal prolapse. Proc Roy Soc Assoc Med 1962; 55:1090.
91. Gabriel WB. Prolapse of the rectum. In: Thomas CC, ed. Principles and Practice of Rectal Surgery. Illinois: Springfield, 1963:165–217.
92. Friedman R, Muggia-Sulam M, Freund HR. Experience with the one-stage perineal repair of rectal prolapse. Dis Colon Rectum 1983; 26:789–791.
93. Gopal KA, Amshel AL, Shonberg IL, Eftaiha M. Rectal procidentia in elderly and debilitated patients. Experience with the Altemeier procedure. Dis Colon Rectum 1984; 27:376–381.
94. Prasad ML, Pearl RK, Abcarian H, Orsay CP, Nelson RL. Perineal proctectomy, posterior rectopexy, and postanal levator repair for the treatment of rectal prolapse. Dis Colon Rectum 1986; 29:547–552.
95. Thorne MC, Polglase AL. Perineal proctectomy for rectal prolapse in elderly and debilitated patients. Aust N Z J Surg 1992; 62:791–794.
96. Johansen OB, Wexner SD, Daniel N, Nogueras JJ, Jagelman DG. Perineal rectosigmoidectomy in the elderly. Dis Colon Rectum 1993; 36:767–772.
97. Ramanujam PS, Venkatesh KS, Fietz MJ. Perineal excision of rectal procidentia in elderly high-risk patients. A ten-year experience. Dis Colon Rectum 1994; 37:1027–1030.
98. Graf W, Stefansson T, Arvidsson D, Pahlman L. Laparoscopic suture rectopexy. Dis Colon Rectum 1995; 38:211–212.
99. Kessler H, Jerby BL, Milsom JW. Successful treatment of rectal prolapse by laparoscopic suture rectopexy. Surg Endosc 1999; 13:858–861.
100. Berman IR. Sutureless laparoscopic rectopexy for procidentia. Technique and implications. Dis Colon Rectum 1992; 35:689–693.
101. Himpens J, Cadiere GB, Bruyns J, Vertruyen M. Laparoscopic rectopexy according to Wells. Surg Endosc 1999; 13:139–141.
102. Boccasanta P, Venturi M, Reitano MC, et al. Laparotomic vs. laparoscopic rectopexy in complete rectal prolapse. Dig Surg 1999; 16:415–419.
103. Heah SM, Hartley JE, Hurley J, Duthie GS, Monson JR. Laparoscopic suture rectopexy without resection is effective treatment for full-thickness rectal prolapse. Dis Colon Rectum 2000; 43:638–643.
104. Poen AC, de Brauw M, Felt-Bersma RJ, de Jong D, Cuesta MA. Laparoscopic rectopexy for complete rectal prolapse. Clinical outcome and anorectal function tests. Surg Endosc 1996; 10:904–908.
105. Solomon MJ, Young CJ, Eyers AA, Roberts RA. Randomized clinical trial of laparoscopic versus open abdominal rectopexy for rectal prolapse. Br J Surg 2002; 89:35–39.
106. Benoist S, Taffinder N, Gould S, Chang A, Darzi A. Functional results two years after laparoscopic rectopexy. Am J Surg 2001; 182:168–173.
107. Bruch HP, Herold A, Schiedeck T, Schwandner O. Laparoscopic surgery for rectal prolapse and outlet obstruction. Dis Colon Rectum 1999; 42:1189–1194; discussion 1194–1185.
108. Kellokumpu IH, Vironen J, Scheinin T. Laparoscopic repair of rectal prolapse: a prospective study evaluating surgical outcome and changes in symptoms and bowel function. Surg Endosc 2000; 14:634–640.

109. Ramanujam PS, Venkatesh KS. Management of acute incarcerated rectal prolapse. Dis Colon Rectum 1992; 35:1154–1156.
110. Harrison BP, Cespedes RD. Pelvic organ prolapse. Emerg Med Clin North Am 2001; 19:781–797.
111. Myers JO, Rothenberger DA. Sugar in the reduction of incarcerated prolapsed bowel. Report of two cases. Dis Colon Rectum 1991; 34:416–418.
112. Stern RC, Izant RJ Jr., Boat TF, Wood RE, Matthews LW, Doershuk CF. Treatment and prognosis of rectal prolapse in cystic fibrosis. Gastroenterology 1982; 82:707–710.
113. Siafakas C, Vottler TP, Andersen JM. Rectal prolapse in pediatrics. Clin Pediatr (Phila) 1999; 38:63–72.
114. Chan WK, Kay SM, Laberge JM, Gallucci JG, Bensoussan AL, Yazbeck S. Injection sclerotherapy in the treatment of rectal prolapse in infants and children. J Pediatr Surg 1998; 33:255–258.
115. Kay NR, Zachary RB. The treatment of rectal prolapse in children with injections of 30 per cent saline solutions. J Pediatr Surg 1970; 5:334–337.
116. Malyshev YI, Gulin VA. Our experience with the treatment of rectal prolapse in infants and children. Am J Proctol 1973; 24:470–472.
117. Dutta BN, Das AK. Treatment of prolapse rectum in children with injections of sclerosing agents. J Indian Med Assoc 1977; 69:275–276.
118. Wyllie GG. The injection treatment of rectal prolapse. J Pediatr Surg 1979; 14:62–64.
119. Hight DW, Hertzler JH, Philippart AI, Benson CD. Linear cauterization for the treatment of rectal prolapse in infants and children. Surg Gynecol Obstet 1982; 154:400–402.
120. Qvist N, Rasmussen L, Klaaborg KE, Hansen LP, Pedersen SA. Rectal prolapse in infancy: conservative versus operative treatment. J Pediatr Surg 1986; 21:887–888.
121. Schepens MA, Verhelst AA. Reappraisal of Ekehorn's rectopexy in the management of rectal prolapse in children. J Pediatr Surg 1993; 28:1494–1497.
122. Sander S, Vural O, Unal M. Management of rectal prolapse in children: Ekehorn's rectosacropexy. Pediatr Surg Int 1999; 15:111–114.
123. Speakman CT, Madden MV, Nicholls RJ, Kamm MA. Lateral ligament division during rectopexy causes constipation but prevents recurrence: results of a prospective randomized study. Br J Surg 1991; 78:1431–1433.
124. Scaglia M, Fasth S, Hallgren T, Nordgren S, Oresland T, Hulten L. Abdominal rectopexy for rectal prolapse. Influence of surgical technique on functional outcome. Dis Colon Rectum 1994; 37:805–813.
125. Boccasanta P, Rosati R, Venturi M, et al. Surgical treatment of complete rectal prolapse: results of abdominal and perineal approaches. J Laparoendosc Adv Surg Tech A 1999; 9:235–238.
126. Takesue Y, Yokoyama T, Murakami Y, et al. The effectiveness of perineal rectosigmoidectomy for the treatment of rectal prolapse in elderly and high-risk patients. Surg Today 1999; 29:290–293.
127. Kimmins MH, Evetts BK, Isler J, Billingham R. The Altemeier repair: outpatient treatment of rectal prolapse. Dis Colon Rectum 2001; 44:565–570.
128. Fengler SA, Pearl RK, Prasad ML, et al. Management of recurrent rectal prolapse. Dis Colon Rectum 1997; 40:832–834.
129. Hool GR, Hull TL, Fazio VW. Surgical treatment of recurrent complete rectal prolapse: a thirty-year experience. Dis Colon Rectum 1997; 40:270–272.
130. Pikarsky AJ, Joo JS, Wexner SD, et al. Recurrent rectal prolapse: what is the next good option? Dis Colon Rectum 2000; 43:1273–1276.
131. Boulos PB, Stryker SJ, Nicholls RJ. The long-term results of polyvinyl alcohol (Ivalon) sponge for rectal prolapse in young patients. Br J Surg 1984; 71:213–214.
132. Huber FT, Stein H, Siewert JR. Functional results after treatment of rectal prolapse with rectopexy and sigmoid resection. World J Surg 1995; 19:138–143; discussion 143.
133. Poole GV Jr., Pennell TC, Myers RT, Hightower F. Modified Thiersch operation for rectal prolapse. Technique and results. Am Surg 1985; 51:226–229.
134. Earnshaw JJ, Hopkinson BR. Late results of silicone rubber perianal suture for rectal prolapse. Dis Colon Rectum 1987; 30:86–88.
135. Hunt TM, Fraser IA, Maybury NK. Treatment of rectal prolapse by sphincteric support using silastic rods. Br J Surg 1985; 72:491–492.
136. Madden MV, Kamm MA, Nicholls RJ, Santhanam AN, Cabot R, Speakman CT. Abdominal rectopexy for complete prolapse: prospective study evaluating changes in symptoms and anorectal function. Dis Colon Rectum 1992; 35:48–55.
137. Sainio AP, Voutilainen PE, Husa AI. Recovery of anal sphincter function following transabdominal repair of rectal prolapse: cause of improved continence? Dis Colon Rectum 1991; 34:816–821.
138. Williams JG, Wong WD, Jensen L, Rothenberger DA, Goldberg SM. Incontinence and rectal prolapse: a prospective manometric study. Dis Colon Rectum 1991; 34:209–216.
139. Birnbaum EH, Stamm L, Rafferty JF, Fry RD, Kodner IJ, Fleshman JW. Pudendal nerve terminal motor latency influences surgical outcome in treatment of rectal prolapse. Dis Colon Rectum 1996; 39:1215–1221.
140. Piccirillo MF, Reissman P, Wexner SD. Colectomy as treatment for constipation in selected patients. Br J Surg 1995; 82:898–901.
141. Shorvon PJ, McHugh S, Diamant NE, Somers S, Stevenson GW. Defecography in normal volunteers: results and implications. Gut 1989; 30:1737–1749.

142. Mackle EJ, Manton Mills JO, Parks TG. The investigation of anorectal dysfunction in the solitary rectal ulcer syndrome. Int J Colorectal Dis 1990; 5:21–24.

143. Mahieu PH. Barium enema and defaecography in the diagnosis and evaluation of the solitary rectal ulcer syndrome. Int J Colorectal Dis 1986; 1:85–90.

144. Kuijpers HC, Schreve RH, ten Cate Hoedemakers H. Diagnosis of functional disorders of defecation causing the solitary rectal ulcer syndrome. Dis Colon Rectum 1986; 29:126–129.

145. Martin CJ, Parks TG, Biggart JD. Solitary rectal ulcer syndrome in Northern Ireland. 1971–1980. Br J Surg 1981; 68:744–747.

146. Halligan S, Nicholls RJ, Bartram CI. Evacuation proctography in patients with solitary rectal ulcer syndrome: anatomic abnormalities and frequency of impaired emptying and prolapse. Am J Roentgenol 1995; 164:91–95.

147. Lowry AC, Goldberg SM. Internal and overt rectal procidentia. Gastroenterol Clin North Am 1987; 16:47–70.

148. van den Brandt-Gradel V, Huibregtse K, Tytgat GN. Treatment of solitary rectal ulcer syndrome with high-fiber diet and abstention of straining at defecation. Dig Dis Sci 1984; 29:1005–1008.

149. Keighley MR, Shouler P. Clinical and manometric features of the solitary rectal ulcer syndrome. Dis Colon Rectum 1984; 27:507–512.

150. Nicholls RJ, Simson JN. Anteroposterior rectopexy in the treatment of solitary rectal ulcer syndrome without overt rectal prolapse. Br J Surg 1986; 73:222–224.

151. Briel JW, Schouten WR, Boerma MO. Long-term results of suture rectopexy in patients with fecal incontinence associated with incomplete rectal prolapse. Dis Colon Rectum 1997; 40:1228–1232.

152. Schultz I, Mellgren A, Dolk A, Johansson C, Holmstrom B. Long-term results and functional outcome after Ripstein rectopexy. Dis Colon Rectum 2000; 43:35–43.

153. Berman IR, Manning DH, Dudley-Wright K. Anatomic specificity in the diagnosis and treatment of internal rectal prolapse. Dis Colon Rectum 1985; 28:816–826.

154. Christiansen J, Hesselfeldt P, Sorensen M. Treatment of internal rectal intussusception in patients with chronic constipation. Scand J Gastroenterol 1995; 30:470–472.

155. Orrom WJ, Bartolo DC, Miller R, Mortensen NJ, Roe AM. Rectopexy is an ineffective treatment for obstructed defecation. Dis Colon Rectum 1991; 34:41–46.

5 | Constipation—Including Sigmoidocele and Rectocele

J. Marcio N. Jorge
Division of Colorectal Surgery, Department of Gastroenterology, University of São Paulo, São Paulo, Brazil

INTRODUCTION

Despite its common nature, constipation can be one of the most difficult problems to manage; this is reflected in a relatively high failure rate both with medical and with surgical treatment (1). Many factors contribute to this challenge. First, definitions vary among patients and professionals, which partly explains the tremendous differences among epidemiological studies and clinical trials (2). Second, constipation has a multifactorial and complex etiology, including not only anatomical and functional, but also dietary, psychological, and cultural factors. Third, this symptom is still surrounded by misconceptions and taboos, which hamper an objective evaluation and determine self-medication, not always innocuous to the patient. Finally, the patient may either be labeled as having a psychiatric disorder or undergo more aggressive medicamentous therapy by the physician without previous physiologic investigation.

DEFINITION

Before addressing the prevalence of constipation, one must first define the symptom. Although physicians often rely on the infrequency of bowel movements to define constipation, the definition of constipation can vary tremendously among patients. When adults not seeking health care were asked to define constipation, their most frequent definitions included "straining" (52%), "hard stools" (44%), "infrequent stools" (32%), and also terms such as "abdominal discomfort," and sense of incomplete evacuation (3). Conversely, patients may associate the symptom of constipation with what they perceive to be less than desirable frequency of bowel movements; they may report constipation if they fail a daily bowel movement or a bowel movement at their usual time each day. In fact, one survey found that 62% of the general population believes that a bowel movement each day is necessary to good digestive health (4). Therefore, the definition of self-reported constipation is much broader. Constipation is a frequent complaint when the patient feels the situation to be unsatisfactory.

Traditionally, physicians have looked for more objective definitions such as stool frequency and colonic transit times (2). Based on the study from Connell et al. (5), 99% of the otherwise healthy population of Great Britain had between three bowel movements a week and three bowel movements a day, and therefore constipation has been defined on the basis of less than three bowel movements per week. A normal total colonic transit time, which is defined as the 95th percentile for healthy controls, is approximately 68 hours (6). However both definitions do not take into account patients with normal transit or frequency, but with symptoms of difficult evacuation, which is more subjective. Therefore, the Rome criteria have been accepted as the more comprehensive definition for constipation (2). These criteria are based on the presence of at least two of the following four symptoms without the use of laxatives for at least 12 months: (i) straining on greater than 25% of bowel movements, (ii) sensation of incomplete evacuation on greater than 25% of bowel movements, (iii) hard or pellet-like stools on greater than 25% of bowel movements, and (iv) less than three bowel movements per week. In addition, if fewer than two bowel movements per week on a regular basis is reported, even in the absence of any other symptom, the criteria for definition of constipation is fulfilled.

PREVALENCE AND RISK FACTORS

Constipation is a common symptom in the medical practice. In the general population, constipation has been reported in the range of 2% to 34%, depending on demographic factors, the sampling situation, and, more importantly, the definition used (2). This symptom accounts for approximately 50% of the patients' complaints at specialists' offices (7,8). Fortunately, most people who seek medical care for constipation do not have a life-threatening or disabling disorder, and the primary need is for control of symptoms.

The prevalence of constipation is three times more common in women and most studies have shown a marked increase after the age of 65 years (3,9). Accordingly, in a longitudinal survey of self-reported bowel habits of 14,407 adults in the United States, Everhart et al. (10) found that women were more likely to report constipation than men, 20.8% compared to 8.0%, and infrequent defecation (9.1% compared to 3.2%, respectively). In addition, older respondents reporting constipation were more likely to use laxatives or stool softeners than younger respondents. Stewart et al. (11), in a survey data on 10,018 adults, found an overall prevalence of constipation of 14.7%. By subtype, prevalence was 4.6% for functional constipation, 2.1% for irritable bowel syndrome, 4.6% for outlet obstruction, and 3.4% for the association of outlet obstruction and irritable bowel syndrome. Outlet obstruction alone or associated with irritable bowel syndrome was the most common subtype among women, with a female to male ratio of 1.65:2.27.

Constipation is a common and serious problem in women of childbearing age, and the reason for this preponderance has not been explained (12,13). It has been suggested that progesterone may decrease levels of the polypeptide motilin, which may influence progression of food through the bowel (14). Preston et al. (15) reported elevated prolactin levels in young constipated women, although this has not been observed by others (16). In addition, gynecological surgery, particularly hysterectomy, has been associated with constipation (17,18). The precise link between slow transit constipation and hysterectomy remains obscure; possible factors include hormone variation, postoperative depression, and, most probably, damage to the pelvic parasympathetic and hypogastric nerves and pelvic plexus during resection of the ligament of the uterus (17). In fact, denervation hypersensitivity to carbachol provocation test in the rectosigmoid has been demonstrated in some patients with severe constipation after hysterectomy, suggesting dysfunction in the autonomic innervation of the hindgut (19). The association of urinary and sexual dysfunction in patients undergoing pelvic surgery seems to support this theory (20,21).

Based on cross-sectional studies, other risk factors for constipation include inactivity, low caloric intake, low income, low education level, depression, and sexual abuse (11,22–26). However, interpretation of these factors is not simple, and data from trials regarding the results after modification of these risk factors are still lacking.

HISTORY

The clinical presentation of constipation includes a broad spectrum of symptoms, therefore obtaining an adequate history is often difficult and time consuming; an extensive questionnaire is recommended. In any event, questioning must be specific and emphasize which symptom the patient considers as most distressing. It is important to distinguish if the main complaint is infrequent bowel movements per se, straining, hard stools, unsatisfactory defecation, or symptoms suggesting irritable bowel syndrome such as bloating or abdominal pain.

The onset of constipation is an important question. Most patients who have constipation due to congenital disorders such as Hirschsprung's disease or meningocele have this symptom from birth. When constipation occurs later in life, the symptom may be of chronic or recent onset. Constipation of recent onset, specifically if less than two years, is frequently related to secondary causes, and exclusion of organic colonic and extracolonic disorders, including malignancy, is mandatory (27).

A constipation scoring system (Cleveland Clinic Score) has been proposed by Agachan et al. (28) in order to achieve uniformity in the assessment of the severity of symptoms. This scoring system is based upon eight parameters: frequency of bowel movements, difficult or painful evacuation effort, completeness of evacuation, abdominal pain, time in minutes per attempt for evacuation, type of assistance (laxatives, digitation, or enema), number of unsuccessful attempts for evacuation per 24 hours, and duration (years) of constipation. Based on the questionnaire, scores range from 0 to 30, with 0 indicating normal and 30 indicating severe constipation. According to the author's experience with 232 patients, the proposed scoring system correlated well with objective physiologic findings. Recently, another symptom-scoring questionnaire was validated for chronic constipation by Knowles et al. (29). The questionnaire is composed of 11 questions and, in a study of 71 patients and 20 asymptomatic controls, a strong correlation was found with the Cleveland Clinic Score.

In the assessment of patients with constipation, it is imperative to ask if the patient has experienced episodes of incontinence of gas or stool. Anal incontinence is frequently an underreported condition and, in fact, many constipated patients have symptoms related to denervation of the sphincter and pelvic muscles due to chronic straining. In this situation, the questionnaire should also assess the frequency and type of incontinence and its effects on the patient's quality of life (30).

PHYSICAL EXAMINATION

Physical examination must be thorough and complement the history in order to rule out systemic etiology. Evidence of systemic illness, including neurologic or muscular deterioration, and endocrine or metabolic disorders, should be sought. In addition, special attention should be directed to the abdomen and anorectal regions.

The abdominal examination may detect excessive stool or gaseous distension, presence of surgical scars, and evidence for neoplasic or inflammatory bowel diseases. Palpation may reveal a soft mass in patients with a dilated rectosigmoid filled with stool, a tender mass in the left lower quadrant, suggestive of a diverticular disease or a hard mass, more characteristic of a neoplasm. Percussion can differentiate gaseous distension from ascites. Finally, auscultation may show hyperactive waves in patients with abdominal distension, which can be visualized in the relaxed patient, characteristic of partial bowel obstruction or hypoactive or absent sounds, in ileus.

The anorectal examination should begin by inspection of the patient's undergarment and perineal skin for evidence of fecal soiling. Soiling may result from overflow incontinence associated with fecal impaction ("overflow or paradoxical fecal incontinence"), especially in elderly patients. This situation must be differentiated from true incontinence, due to sphincter dysfunction and "humid anus" or pseudoincontinence, which is caused by hemorrhoidal prolapse, pruritus ani, perianal fistula, rectal mucosal prolapse, and anorectal venereal diseases. Perineal examination will exclude anatomical causes of constipation such as tumors, stenosis, and fissures.

Both the lateral decubitus (Sims) and the prone jackknife positions are used for routine anorectal examination. Although the prone position is purported to provide better exposure, the left lateral decubitus is a good alternative and better accepted by patients, particularly the elderly or those otherwise incapacitated. Occasionally, in order to reveal a rectal prolapse, the patient needs to be examined in the squatting position.

Patients with constipation may have signs of anal incontinence during physical examination due to progressive neural injury related to chronic injury, or an associated neuromuscular lesion due to childbirth. Occasionally, incontinence is suspected only during physical examination or even during physiological testing. This may occur due to the patient's embarrassment and unwillingness to seek medical therapy, or as a subclinical finding. Descent of the perineum can be easily recognized during physical examination; with the buttocks separated, descent and elevation of the perineum can be seen during simulated defecation and squeeze. During simulated defecation, the anal verge should be observed for any patulous opening or rectal prolapse. Cutaneous sensation around the anus may be absent in patients with neurogenic disorders and may also indicate the level and side of the lesion. An intact bilateral anal reflex, as tested by a light pinprick or scratch, demonstrates that innervation of the external sphincter mechanism is present.

The next step is gentle palpation with a well-lubricated gloved index finger to evaluate resting tone. Fecal impaction is often noted in children and the elderly, with symptoms of severe constipation and soiling (paradoxical fecal incontinence). Constipated patients will often have hard stool in the rectal vault. Patients with Hirschsprung's disease usually have an empty, contracted distal rectum.

The lower rounded edge of the internal anal sphincter can be felt on physical examination, at approximately 1.2 cm distal to the dentate line. In patients with spinal lesions, the return of the anal resting tone after digital examination is characteristically very slow. The groove between the internal and external anal sphincter (intersphincteric sulcus) can be visualized or easily palpated. The entire circumference of the anorectum should be palpated by gentle circumanal rotation of the examining finger to assess the integrity of the anorectal ring. This is a strong muscular ring that represents the upper end of the anal sphincter, more precisely the puborectalis, and the upper border of the internal anal sphincter, around the anorectal junction. During dynamic palpation, the examiner should note both the increase in anal canal tone and the mobility of the posterior loop of the puborectal muscle during squeeze. Acute localized pain triggered by pulling or compressing the border of the puborectalis muscle is a feature of levator spasm syndrome.

To assess the presence of paradoxical puborectalis syndrome, the patient is asked to strain, while the examiner's finger is kept in the rectum. Patients with paradoxical puborectalis syndrome will squeeze and some will have intermittent contractions. Prior to diagnosing paradoxical contraction, this procedure should be repeated several times to ensure that the Valsalva maneuver could not be accomplished due to true paradoxical contraction and not to the patient's misunderstanding or embarrassment.

The presence of a rectocele can be assessed during physical examination by curving the examining finger and pressing it against the anterior rectal wall until it appears in the vagina, on the other side of the perineal body. Bulging of the rectum as a result of an internal prolapse may be confounded as a rectocele. Internal prolapse can be palpated by the examining finger as a descending mass during straining on digital examination. However, at times, the differential diagnosis can only be made by defecography. Defecography can assist in determining the size of the rectocele. Moreover, by providing data on rectal emptying, defecography will allow differentiation of a secondary finding from a clinically relevant rectocele. An overt rectal prolapse or procidentia can be diagnosed by examining the patient while straining on a commode.

A combined vaginal digital examination can be very helpful; with the patient in a standing position, the examiner's index finger is inserted into the rectum and the thumb is inserted into the vagina. During this examination, the patient should be asked to strain. A peritoneal sac, containing omentum or a loop of bowel dissecting the rectovaginal septum, can be palpable between the thumb and the index finger, indicating the presence of peritoneocele or enterocele. This examination can be an effective method of distinguishing between enterocele, prolapse of the vaginal vault, rectocele, or a combination of these weakened conditions. Again, defecography is crucial in order to confirm these findings and evaluate their role in the dynamics of defecation.

Both anoscopy and proctosigmoidoscopy are useful to exclude anorectal diseases such as neoplasms, rectoanal intussusception, solitary rectal ulcer syndrome, and inflammatory bowel. Rigid proctosigmoidoscopy is a more accurate method of measuring distance from the anal verge; however, the average reached length is approximately 20 cm. Flexible sigmoidoscopy has a three to six times higher yield and is more comfortable to the patient. In patients with anthraquinone laxative abuse, the rectal mucosa may present a characteristic aspect of pseudomelanosis coli; however, the mucosa can be normal in these patients, and the diagnosis may be revealed only after rectal biopsy. This procedure is also required in the diagnosis of Hirschsprung's disease and amyloidosis.

DIFFERENTIAL DIAGNOSIS

Constipation is a disorder and not a disease and can be secondary to several diseases, including colonic diseases (stricture, cancer, anal fissure, proctitis), metabolic and endocrine disturbances (hypercalcemia, hypothyroidism, and diabetes mellitus), and neurologic disorders (Parkinson's disease and spinal cord lesions) or pharmacologic (antidepressive) (Table 1). Therefore, exclusion of both intestinal and systemic organic etiologies is an imperative step prior to referring the patient with functional symptoms to the physiology laboratory. Barium enema and/or colonoscopy are usually indicated, and the primary pathology treated. Additional

Table 1 Etiology of Constipation

Poor habits	Low fiber diet, inadequate fluid intake, inadequate exercise, ignoring call to stool, situational factors (travel, illness)	
Intrinsic bowel disease	Mechanical obstruction	Neoplasm, inflammation, volvulus, infection, incarceration, intussusception, ischemia
	Collagen vascular disease	Scleroderma, amyloidosis
	Anorectal disease	Anal stenosis, fissure, inflammation
Pharmacologic agents	Antidepressants	Amoxapine, bupropion, clomipramine, fluoxetine, maprotiline, mirtazepine, paroxetine, sertraline, venlafaxine
	Tranquilizers	Alprazolam, clozapine, olanzapine, risperidone
	Neurological drugs	Bromocriptine, felbamate, pergolide, valproic acid
	Narcotics	Burtorphanol, codeine, fentanyl, morphine
	Nonsteroidal anti-inflammatories	Diclofenac, indomethacin, nabumetone, naproxen, salicylates, sulindac
	Muscle relaxants and other analgesics	Baclofen, carisoprodol, tizanidine, tramadol
	Calcium channel blockers	Nifedipine, verapamil
	Antiarrhythmic drugs	Amiodarone, flecainide, mexiletine, propafenone
	Lipid-lowering agents	Cholestyramine, colestipol, lovastatin, provachol
	Antihypertensives	Diuretics, acebutolol, clonidine, guanfacine
	Antiplatelet	Anagrelide
	Hematological/oncological drugs	Iron therapy, carboplatin, erythropoetin, filgrastim, vinblastine
	Gastrointestinal drugs	Aluminum- and calcium-containing antacids, mesalamine, pancreatin, octreotide
	Heavy metal intoxication	Arsenic, lead, mercury, phosphorus
	Miscellaneous agents	Barium sulphate, thalidomide, alendronate, interferon alfa-2b, leuprolide, levofloxacin, ondansetron, pamidronate
Neurologic disorders	Cerebral	Parkinson's disease, stroke, tumor
	Spinal	Cauda equina tumor, meningocele, spinal cord injury, tabes dorsalis, multiple sclerosis, paraplegia
	Peripheral	Chagas' disease, Hirschsprung's disease, surgical disruption of nervi erigentes, senna toxicity, Von Recklinghausen's disease, autonomic plexus neuropathy, multiple endocrine neoplasia ii-b, hypoganglionosis
Endocrine causes	Hypothyroidism, hypopituitarism, diabetes mellitus, pheochromocytoma	
Metabolic causes	Dehydration, uremia, hypercalcemia, porphyria, pregnancy, hypokalemia	

tests, dictated by history and physical examination, may be necessary to exclude the above-mentioned diseases.

Barium enema has been replaced by colonoscopy in screening and evaluation of many diseases, including diverticular disease and colorectal cancer. Barium enema is usually not useful in the diagnosis of chronic constipation (31). However, it has the advantage of providing a permanent record, available for future evaluations, of the size, length, and anatomical abnormalities of the colon. In this sense, barium enema is probably superior to colonoscopy. In addition, colonic redundancy in constipation is frequently a reason for an incomplete colonoscopy. High-quality double-contrast technique and inclusion of the lateral views of the rectum are essential in a good study. A large, dilated (megacolon) and elongated (dolichocolon) colon is frequently found in patients with constipation; however, these findings have also been noted in healthy individuals and are therefore insufficient surgical indicators.

Colonoscopy is a complementary study to a barium enema for exclusion of colonic pathology. Compared to barium enema, colonoscopy has a higher risk of complications, it is more expensive, and both are probably comparable in the diagnosis of lesions associated with constipation (32,33).

MEDICAL TREATMENT: GENERAL RECOMMENDATIONS

Because the most common causes of constipation are related to misconceptions of normal bowel function and inadequate diet and habits, the initial approach should include careful assessment, reassurance, and simple guidance. Thus, this initial therapeutic schema should include the following:

1. Evaluation of the patient's expectations and concept of normal bowel frequency, in order to understand the complaints and reassure the patient.
2. Dietary assessment including fiber supplementation, increased fluid intake, and balanced meals. Meals should be balanced, at regular intervals, and contain generous portions of vegetables and fruits. Excessive ingestion of processed carbohydrates should be discouraged. Likewise, omission of breakfast may contribute to abnormal bowel function due to inadequacy in elicitation of the gastrocolic reflex. Recommended empirical fiber therapy should include 20–40 g of dietary fiber or 10–20 g of crude fiber per day (34,35). The most inexpensive cereal with the highest concentration of crude fiber is bran. Unprocessed bran, particularly coarser preparations, has high hydrophilic properties that soften the stool and increase its volume, which stimulates peristalsis. In addition, an increase in daily intake of fluids will increase the efficacy of a high fiber diet.
3. Physical exercise is encouraged; a simple walk in the morning may be effective.
4. Attention to the call to stool. Environmental factors such as work or school schedule are often difficult to change. Patients should be advised that neglecting the call to stool will, through the mechanisms of rectal capacity and compliance, lead to fecal stasis.
5. Use of a defecation diary (frequency and consistency of stool) and association of symptoms. This is important because symptoms often vary with time, and the severity of constipation may be related to associated events in the patient's life (35).
6. Psychological evaluation should be done, whenever indicated (36,37).

This initial trial of empirical therapy is recommended, unless alarm symptoms such as rectal bleeding, abdominal distension, or weight loss are present (34). These measures will permit better evaluation of the severity of the symptom, and patients should be reevaluated by a defecation and symptoms diary. Furthermore, symptoms may improve if they are dietary or psychologically related. If symptoms disappear during this trial, no further evaluation is necessary and treatment should be maintained. If symptoms persist, patients should be referred to the physiology lab for investigation. Patients referred for colorectal physiologic testing, therefore, present with refractory and severe idiopathic symptoms (38).

PHYSIOLOGICAL INVESTIGATION

The mechanisms responsible for both anal continence and defecation are complex and maintained by the interaction of multiple factors. These factors include stool consistency and delivery of colonic contents to the rectum, rectal capacity and compliance, anorectal sensation, the function of the anal sphincter mechanism, and the pelvic floor muscles and nerves. In order to adequately evaluate these different aspects, a combination of physiologic studies is usually required, including colonic transit time study, anorectal manometry, defecography, electromyography (EMG) and pudendal nerve latency, and small-bowel transit study (38,39). No single test is pathognomonic; thus, final diagnosis of functional disorders must be based on collective interpretation of these studies. According to Rantis (40), the mean cost to investigate chronic constipation in the United States is $2752 (range, $1150–4792) and includes colonoscopy, barium enema, transit times, defecography, electromyography (EMG), and rectal biopsy. However, most studies have shown that physiologic testing adds significant information, leading to a specific diagnosis in 50% to 75% of patients (41–43). Furthermore, physiologic testing permits objective assessment and reliable post-therapeutic follow-up of subjective functional colorectal disorders.

Colonic Transit Time

Patient complaints of stool frequency are subjective; thus an objective method for measuring colonic transit time is desirable to evaluate patients with chronic and "idiopathic" symptoms of constipation. The colon, through segmentation, mass, and retrograde movements, accounts for approximately 90% of the total digestive transit time (6). Therefore, since 1907, colonic transit time has been primarily evaluated as the total digestive transit through the elimination of different markers in the feces: contrast medium (barium sulphate) (44), dyes (carmine and charcoal) (45), particles (seeds and colored glass beads) (46), chemical substances (copper thiocyanate) (47), and radioisotopes (48,49). These methods, however, have been abandoned due to the lack of use, difficulty in interpretation, or inaccuracy. In 1969, Hinton (50) proposed markers, initially prepared by cutting radiopaque Levine tubes into circular or cylindrical shapes. These later became commercially available, enclosed in gelatine capsules that ensure their arrival in bolus into the gastric lumen. The simplest and most practical method of evaluating colonic transit requires ingestion of 24 radiopaque markers and quantification of these markers on abdominal radiographs. Normal total intestinal transit time involves elimination of at least 80% of markers on the fifth day of study (50).

Subsequently, segmental colonic transit time study was proposed as the ideal assessment of colonic transit (51,52). Rather than measuring the elimination or clearance of markers, the index of transit time of this method was the actual number of retained markers on each colonic segment. The spinal processes and imaginary lines from the fifth lumbar vertebra to the pelvic outlet have been used to recognize the three segments of the large bowel (right colon, left colon, and rectosigmoid) on the radiographs (51). The classical technique of measuring segmental transit time consisted of a single ingestion of 20 or 24 markers, followed by serial radiographs taken at 24-hour intervals until total elimination of markers occurred. When using 24 markers, the sum of the retained markers in each colonic segment on the successive radiographs represents the value, in hours, for each segmental transit time. In order to reduce irradiation exposure and achieve more use, subsequent technical modifications included multiple ingestion of markers, rather than multiple radiographs and the use of markers of different shapes. The rationale behind segmental colonic transit time study is that embryological, anatomical, and functional differences exist among the right colon, left colon, and rectosigmoid. Therefore, all three segments may be affected independently in motility disorders. In fact, with the advent of this method of study, the motility patterns of colonic inertia, outlet obstruction, and left colon delay could be demonstrated (53). However, although proven useful, the value of this assessment remains a controversial issue. Accurate assessment of segmental transit times still involves either multiple ingestion of markers or multiple abdominal radiographs.

For practical purposes, however, the technique involving two radiographs taken on days 3 and 5 after a single day ingestion of 24 radiopaque markers may suffice. Prior to testing, a digital examination and, if necessary, a simple abdominal radiograph are indicated to ensure that the colon is cleared of any contrast material from previous studies and that there is no fecal impaction in the rectum. In addition, the use of enemas, laxatives, or any other medication known to affect gastrointestinal motility should be discontinued for three days prior to ingestion of the markers until completion of the study. Markers should be taken at a specified time, usually at 8 A.M. Patients are oriented to maintain their normal diet; however, supplemental fiber such as bran or psyllium can be helpful to exclude dietary causes. The use of a diary of bowel frequency and related symptoms during the period of the study is also helpful, as symptoms can be better evaluated; the study may be repeated if the patient reports that the frequency during the study is not representative of his usual bowel habits. The abdominal radiograph should include the diaphragm and the pubis to yield identification of all markers in the colon.

In normal individuals, markers reach the cecum within eight hours after their ingestion. The mean and maximal values for normal individuals for the total colonic transit time are 36 and 55 hours, respectively (54). The mean segmental transit times are 12, 14, and 11 hours for right colon, left colon, and rectosigmoid, respectively; the maximal values for the segmental transit times are 22, 34, and 27 hours for right colon, left colon, and rectosigmoid, respectively (54). The mean value of normal total colonic transit time is about 32 hours for men and 41 hours for women. This difference is even greater when the right colon transit time is analyzed separately. Age, however, does not seem to affect total colonic transit times. In children, although the rectosigmoid transit time is more prolonged, the total colonic transit time is similar to that in the adult, probably due to the proportional reduction of segmental transit times for the right and left colons (52).

Several factors including diet, physical activity, and psychologic and hormonal factors may affect digestive transit time results; therefore significant variation is expected. However, segmental colonic transit time study using radiopaque markers has proven reproducible when analyzed in the same individual within a mean interval of three months (55). When colonic transit times are evaluated using two different methods, specifically single ingestion and multiple ingestion of markers, the mean difference between the two measurements are 2.1 hours, 0.34 hours, and 1.54 hours for the right colon, left colon, and rectosigmoid, respectively (56). Recently in a study of reproducibility of colonic transit time in patients with chronic constipation, Nam et al. (57) have shown this test to be ideal for patients with idiopathic constipation and worst for colonic inertia; therefore according to these authors consideration should be given to repeat colonic transit studies before colectomy, in order to secure the diagnosis and improve outcome.

Colonic transit time assessment provides a definition for constipation by converting an otherwise hopelessly subjective symptom to an objective part of the medical record. Therefore, its most important role lies in excluding factitious constipation. Additionally, segmental transit times can help to uncover causative diagnoses, by stratifying motility disorders into two main patterns: colonic inertia and outlet obstruction. Colonic inertia is characterized by diffuse stasis of markers throughout the colon, usually more markedly in the right colon (Fig. 1). Outlet obstruction is characterized when the stasis of markers is limited to the rectosigmoid (Fig. 2). In this condition, the association of other tests, particularly cinedefecography, anorectal manometry, and anal EMG, is of importance to diagnose the causative disorder. A third abnormal pattern found during segmental colonic transit time assessment is the isolated delay of markers in the left colon (Fig. 3). However, this pattern is of uncertain physiopathology and usually representative of patients with less severe and dietary-related symptoms.

Colonic Myoelectrical and Motor Function

Based on colonic manometric findings in a study by Adler (58), three types of colonic motor patterns were classically described in humans: Type I contractions are monophasic waves of low amplitude (5–10 cmH$_2$O) and short duration (5–10 seconds) of a mean frequency of 10/min. Type II contractions represent about 90% of all normal manometric recording activity and correspond to combined contraction/relaxation haustral movements. These contractions occur in bursts of two per minute, and they are of longer duration (25–30 seconds) and of higher amplitude (15–30 cm H$_2$O). Type III contractions are of low amplitude (less than 10 cm H$_2$O), overimpose Type I or II contractions, and represent a change in basal pressure. Subsequently, two other phenomena were recognized: giant motor contractions and migrating motor complex (59). Giant motor contractions are high amplitude, rapidly propagated

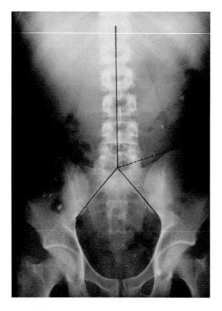

Figure 1 Colonic transit time study on fifth day of study, showing stasis of colonic markers in right colon.

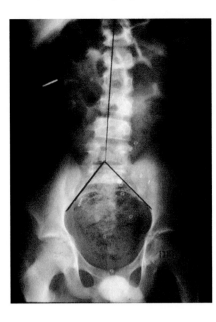

Figure 2 Colonic transit study on fifth day of study showing retention of markers in the rectosigmoid colon.

contraction waves, usually seen on walking and following meals, and frequently accompanied by an urge to defecate. The migrating motor complex is a periodic motor activity, represented by rhythmic bursts of activity, usually with aboral migration. This activity has been described only in canines; in the human, this activity has been found only in the stomach and small bowel (60).

Two types of activity have been detected in colonic EMG recordings, rhythmic slow waves and spike bursts (61). Slow waves originate in the circular muscle of the colon; they represent the basal electrical activity. Spike bursts are associated with short- and long-type contractions, which last three to four seconds and 10 to 11 seconds, respectively. Long spike burst activity increases for two hours after each meal and is significantly reduced during sleep. However, to date, colonic myoelectrical activity has not been accurately correlated with colonic organized movements.

Colonic motility studies are of limited use due to the relative inaccessibility of the proximal colon, and fidelity of manometric recordings may be compromised by colonic manipulation and dilatation. Furthermore, although it was initially suggested in initial manometric and

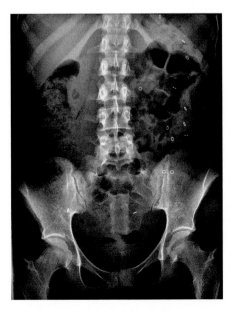

Figure 3 Colonic transit time study showing left colon delay.

electomyographic studies that it may be possible to determine patterns of colonic motility pathognomonic of underlying pathophysiologic processes, this has not been confirmed (62).

Videodefecography

Standard propedeutic examinations such as colonoscopy and barium enema detect essentially anatomic abnormalities, whereas functional disorders will require a radiographic study that demonstrates the physiological process involved during rectal evacuation. The basic concept of defecography, radiographic imaging of the pelvic dynamic changes during defecation, was introduced half a century ago when in a comprehensive study, Walldén (63) studied the relationship between deep rectovaginal pouches, enterocele, and obstructed defecation.

Despite the apparent simplicity in the technique of defecography, several difficulties have to be overcome in order to achieve methodologic standardization: adequacy of the contrast medium consistency, conciliation between seated position and quality of obtained imagery, and incorporation of an effective recording device (64–67). Defecography is now considered an important test in patients with chronic idiopathic constipation to exclude causes of obstructed defecation. In patients with idiopathic fecal incontinence, especially if a history of chronic straining at stool is reported, defecography can be helpful to exclude an internal rectal prolapse. Furthermore, in patients with solitary rectal ulcer and chronic idiopathic rectal pain, this exam may also uncover a causative disorder.

The current patient preparation regimen for cinedefecography includes a disposable phosphate enema 30 minutes prior to the procedure that will yield a more standardized examination and provide comfort for both patient and investigator. The patient is placed in the left lateral decubitus position. A small amount (50 mL) of barium suspension is injected into the rectum in order to coat the rectal mucosa and enhance the contrast imagery. After initial barium instillation, air is insufflated to outline the rectal mucosa. Contrast medium consistency affects the rectal emptying rate; the ideal contrast material should simulate stool in weight and consistency (68). Commercially available thick media preparations, easily assembled into a caulking gun to facilitate injection, have been developed; usually 250 cc (500 g) of a thick barium paste (Anatrast^{TM}, E-Z-EM, Westbury, New York, U.S.A.) is introduced, or less if the patient experiences rectal fullness prior to that point. Injection is continued while the injector is withdrawn in order to outline the entire anal canal (69). The X-ray table is tilted upright to a 90°angle, and the patient is comfortably seated on a water-filled radiolucent commode. Lateral films of the pelvis are then taken at rest and during both squeeze and push. The patient is then asked to evacuate the rectal contents and, with the aid of fluoroscopy, the process of defecation is recorded on videotape. In order to effectively study all phases of defecation, the use of video recording is crucial in defecography, and the reason for the widespread use of appellations such as cinedefecography, videodefecography, or videoproctography. By replaying the examination, the entire process of defecation can be reviewed, and the effects of abnormalities such as rectocele, intussusception, and nonrelaxing puborectalis in rectal emptying can be better evaluated, not only by the investigator but also by the referring physician. In addition, "spot" films may not register enterocele and sigmoidocele, because a deep cul de sac may contain bowel only intermittently, usually after prolonged straining (63). If necessary, the test may be performed one to three hours after ingestion of barium-contrast medium to delineate small-bowel loops (70). Other technical modifications recommended include the association of colpocystography, the so-called four-contrast defecography (oral, vaginal, bladder, and rectal constrast) and peritoneography (71,72).

Specifically, defecography provides pelvic measurements at rest and during both squeeze and pushing, which are used to assess evacuation dynamics, anatomical detail, and rectal emptying. Pelvic measurements, including the anorectal angle, perineal descent, and puborectalis length, are taken at rest and during both squeeze and pushing, on static proctography. A wide range of normal values for each of these parameters is observed (65,67). However, the exact value of any of these isolated parameters is of relatively little consequence, and comparison of an absolute measurement in a patient against a group of controls is frequently frustrating. Instead, the role of static proctography is to provide a basis for relative comparison among resting, squeezing, and pushing values in a single patient. Evaluation of both absolute and dynamic (evacuation–rest) values of anorectal angle, perineal descent, and puborectalis length allows diagnosis of excessive perineal descent and paradoxical puborectalis syndrome.

The anorectal angle, the most quoted measurement on defecography, is better defined as the angle between the axis of the anal canal and the distal half of the posterior rectal wall (65,67,68). The resting anorectal angle ranges from 70° to 140° with a mean of 92° to 114°. During evacuation, this angle becomes more obtuse, 110° to 180°, and more acute during squeeze, ranging from 75° to 90°.

Perineal descent is quantitatively defined by measuring the vertical distance between the position of the anorectal angle and a fixed plane relating the levator ani muscle to the pelvis, represented by the pubococcygeal line. The normal pelvic floor position is up to 1.8 cm below the pubococcygeal line at rest and up to 3.0 cm below the pubococcygeal line during maximal push effort; therefore, abnormally increased perineal descent has been classically defined as descent of more than 3.0 cm during evacuation when compared to the value measured at rest (65,70). However, the dynamic changes in the pelvic floor during straining may not account for the diagnosis of abnormal perineal descent in all cases. Patients may present a flaccid and non-contractile pelvic floor. In this situation, although little change is seen during straining, an abnormally increased perineal descent is already observed at rest. This so-called "fixed increased perineal descent," considered when perineal descent exceeds 4.0 cm at rest, has been particularly associated with advancing age (73).

The puborectalis length is measured as the distance between the anorectal angle and the pubic symphysis. The resting puborectalis length ranges from 14 to 16 cm. During squeeze, the puborectalis length is shorter (12–15 cm), and during evacuation, the muscle length increases, 15 to 18 cm (39,70). Comparison of these measurements, along with the anorectal angle, corroborates with the diagnosis of paradoxical puborectalis syndrome.

Causative or associated "anatomical" abnormalities such as nonrelaxing puborectalis (puborectalis indentation), rectocele, internal rectal prolapse, sigmoidocele, and enterocele can all be diagnosed by defecography (Figs. 4–7). These findings, particularly a small rectocele, and an intussusception, may be found in 25% to 77% of asymptomatic individuals (70). Failure to recognize these variants of normal can easily lead to overdiagnosis and overtreatment (43). Therefore, decision should be made based upon both clinical history and evaluation of rectal emptying during cinedefecography.

During defecography, most individuals evacuate their rectum within 15 to 20 seconds (74). A variety of detailed techniques to quantitate rectal emptying have been described, including weight transducers to plot the contrast expelled against time (75), planimetrical evaluation of the retained contrast media area, digital subtraction defecography, and scintigraphic studies (68,76,77). Paradoxical contraction of the pelvic floor during attempted defecation may represent either an embarrassed reaction of the patient or a true functional disorder. Patients must be reassured and fully informed, regarding the importance of the cinedefecographic findings in their therapeutic approach. In this situation, a valuable technique is to ask the patient to evacuate in the privacy of a bathroom and fluoroscopically reassess the rectum.

Anorectal Manometry

Anorectal manometry is an objective method of studying the physiologic apparatus of defecation provided by the anorectal sphincter. Sensing devices include microballoons,

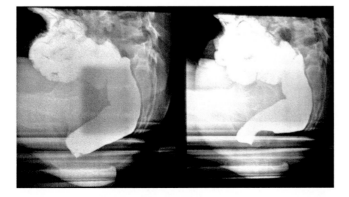

Figure 4 Paradoxical puborectalis syndrome. The puborectalis impression can be seen during the attempted defecation.

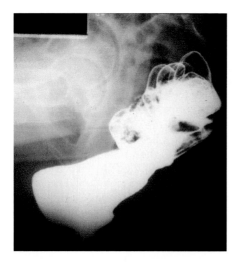

Figure 5 Anterior rectocele.

microtransducers, and water-perfused catheters. Microballoon devices do not provide information about radial variations in pressure; instead, a single pressure value is measured, based on collective forces. Although microtransducers may have a promising future, plastic multichannel catheters, perfused with water by a microperfusion system, are the most commonly used sensing devices. The principle of this technique is the measurement of the resistance in terms of pressure that the sphincters offer to a constant flow of water through the port. A constant perfusion rate, usually 0.3 mL per channel per minute, is required to adequately measure the outflow from the tube(78,79). The most important advantage of perfused catheters is that multiple channels, more commonly four to eight channels, can be set on a single

(A)   **(B)**

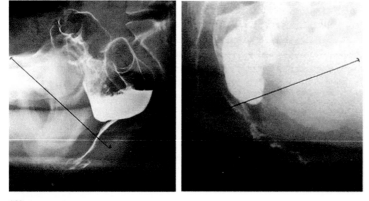

(C)

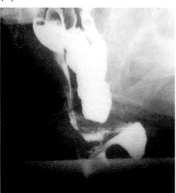

Figure 6 Sigmoidocele classification. (**A**) First degree sigmoidocele.
(**B**) Second degree sigmoidocele. (**C**) Third degree sigmadocele.

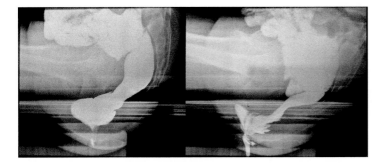

Figure 7   Rectoanal intussusception.

catheter. Depending on the purpose of the study, catheters may have their channel ports displayed in either a radial or a stepwise fashion. The technique of manometric measurement also varies. The catheter can be left at one position (stationary technique), can be manually moved at continuous intervals (manual or station pull-through technique), or can be continuously withdrawn (continuous pull-through). Theoretically, the manual pull-through provides a more accurate pressure at a single point, because a stabilization period is obtained before each interval recording. Conventional anorectal manometry enables measurement of resting and squeeze pressures as well as the high-pressure zone or functional anal canal length. Adjunct studies, using an intrarectal balloon, include assessment of the rectoanal inhibitory reflex, rectal sensory threshold, rectal capacity, and rectal compliance.

The mean anal canal resting tone in healthy adults is generally in the range of 50 to 70 mmHg, and tends to be lower in women and in the elderly (79). In the composition of the resting tone, the internal anal sphincter is responsible for 50% to 85%, the external anal sphincter accounts for 25% to 30%, and the remaining 15% is attributed to expansion of the anal cushions (80–82). A gradual increase in pressures is noted from proximal to distal in the anal canal; the highest resting pressures are usually recorded 1 to 2 cm cephalad to the anal verge. This high-pressure zone or functional anal canal length, which corresponds anatomically to the condensation of the smooth muscle fibers of the internal anal sphincter, is shorter in women (2.0–3.0 cm) compared to men (2.5–3.5 cm) (79,83). Interestingly, although parity may contribute to this difference, nulliparous women still have a significantly shorter functional anal canal than men (83). The anal canal is also relatively asymmetric on its radial profile (84). The normal values for the radial asymmetry index are <10%; however, these values are subject to the technique and equipment used (83,85). This functional asymmetry is found for both resting and squeeze pressures profiles; it follows the inherent anatomic asymmetry in the arrangement of the sphincter muscles. In the upper-third of the anal canal, higher pressures are found posteriorly due to the activity of the puborectalis along with the deep portion of the external anal sphincter, whereas in the lower-third, pressures are higher anteriorly, due to the posteriorly directed superficial loop of the external anal sphincter.

During maximal voluntary contraction or squeeze efforts, intra-anal pressures usually reach two or three times their baseline resting tone (100–180 mmHg). However, due to muscular fatigue, maximal voluntary contraction of the external anal sphincter and levator ani can be sustained for only 40 to 60 seconds. More recently, the fatigue rate index has been proposed by Marcello et al. (86) as a new manometric parameter to evaluate the voluntary component of the anal sphincter function. This parameter is a calculated measure, in minutes, of the time necessary for the sphincter to be completely fatigued to a pressure equivalent to the resting tone. According to their results, the mean fatigue rate index was 3.3 minutes for volunteers, 2.8 minutes for constipated patients, 2.3 minutes for patients with seepage, and 1.5 minutes for incontinent patients. In fact, in patients with incontinence, and some with constipation, despite an initial normal squeeze pressure, a rapid decrease in values can be noted, and therefore, this inability of sustaining the voluntary contraction may represent either an initial or different mechanism of lesion. Further studies are needed to solve this question.

Anal manometry is often of no "diagnostic value" in idiopathic constipation in adults, except in the rare cases of segmental Hirschsprung's disease (Figs. 8A and B). In these cases,

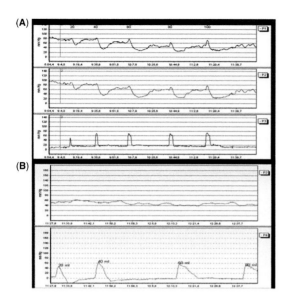

Figure 8 Manometric tracings show rectoanal inhibitory reflex present (**A**) and absent (**B**) in an adult patient with Hirschsprung's disease.

and more often in children and adolescents with constipation and encopresis, the absence of the rectoanal inhibitory reflex should be correlated with rectal biopsy (87,88). More often, anal manometry provides supportive data for pelvic floor dysfunction; for example, high resting tone with an elongated functional anal canal and little voluntary augmentation suggest paradoxical puborectalis contraction. In addition, high rectal capacity and compliance may suggest outlet obstruction. Anal manometry may also be helpful to preoperatively assess the functional status of the anal sphincter prior to colectomy for constipation. In fact, as mentioned before, occult incontinence may be diagnosed only during physiologic testing, particularly during manometry.

Electromyography

Anal EMG is the recording of myoelectrical activity from the striated sphincter at rest, during voluntary and reflex contraction and simulated defecation. EMG can be performed using needle, wire, or cutaneous patch electrodes. The concentric needle EMG has achieved more widespread acceptance in North America than other techniques (89). Patients are given a single disposable phosphate enema prior to the examination. They are then placed in the left lateral decubitus position with maximum flexion of the knees. The sphincter muscle halves are independently examined both at rest and during activity, using a bipolar disposable concentric needle electrode, with a diameter of 0.64 mm, length of 75 mm, and a recording area of 0.07 mm². Activity consists of squeezing (prevention of bowel evacuation), coughing (to evaluate reflex sphincteric activity), and pushing (attempted evacuation (90). A normal study is defined as the recruitment of an ample number of motor units with normal amplitude and duration while squeezing and coughing, and either electrical silence or a marked decrease in motor unit potentials during pushing (91,92).

Conventional concentric needle EMG is especially valuable in the assessment of fecal incontinence by providing quantification of motor unit potentials, mapping external anal sphincter defects, and assessing reinnervation patterns. In patients with idiopathic constipation, EMG may corroborate the diagnosis of nonrelaxing puborectalis syndrome, if doubt persists after cinedefecography. Failure to achieve a significant decrease in the electrical activity of the external anal sphincter and puborectalis during attempted evacuation is considered as a criteria for the electromyographic diagnosis of nonrelaxing puborectalis syndrome. For this particular purpose, the surface electrodes may be of use (93). Both EMG and cinedefecography have comparable sensitivity and specificity, but are individually suboptimal (94). Cinedefecography should be initially performed because it is pain-free and provides useful data on rectal emptying.

Pudendal Nerve Terminal Motor Latency

Pudendal nerve terminal motor latency (PNTML) measurement is a simple method of assessing pudendal nerve function that confirms the integrity of the distal motor innervation of the pelvic floor musculature. This assessment is of paramount importance in the evaluation of neurogenic fecal incontinence. PNTML is performed by transrectal stimulation of the pudendal nerve with the patient placed in the left lateral decubitus position. The sensor consists of two stimulating electrodes located at the tip of the index finger of a glove and two surface recording electrodes incorporated into its base (St. Mark's electrode) (95). Stimuli of 22 mV of amplitude and 0.1 msec duration are applied to the nerves at one-second intervals. Using the ischial tuberosities as landmarks, the tip of the finger is gradually moved until the sphincter is felt to contract around the base of the finger, and the motor unit action potential achieves a maximal amplitude. The latency from each stimulus to the evoked muscle action potential in the external anal sphincter is recorded on each side. The mean PNTML is calculated from the best amplitude measured. The normal value of the mean PNTML is 2.0 + 0.2 msec (87,96). Latencies greater than 2.2 msec are considered excessive and representative of pudendal neuropathy.

PNTML is particularly important in suspected neurogenic incontinence and in parous women prior to sphincter repair. This test is the most important predictor of functional outcome after sphincter repair as neuropathy, even when unilateral, is associated with poor postoperative functional results (97,98). However, PNTML is not a quantitative method; it is a measurement of the most rapid motor conduction in the pudendal nerve (99). Although normal PNTML does not exclude partial damage, when prolonged, pudendal latencies seem to be reliably related to neuropathy. Despite the substantial anatomic overlapping of the pudendal innervation on both sides of the external anal sphincter, asymmetrical pudendal neuropathy is not an uncommon finding.

Abnormally prolonged pudendal latency is usually found in patients with other pelvic floor disorders such as constipation with chronic straining, rectal prolapse, solitary rectal ulcer, and descending perineal syndrome (100). Neuropathy due to stretching of the pudendal nerve has been implicated, in theory, to explain the prolonged latencies in those patients with chronic straining at stool (101). This entrapment/stretch theory is also thought to be the mechanism of pudendal lesion during vaginal delivery (102). However, a lack of correlation between perineal descent measurements and pudendal latencies has been recently demonstrated, and, therefore, other mechanisms may be involved (103).

Small-Bowel Transit

The need to investigate the contribution of the small bowel to motility gastrointestinal disorders, including constipation, diarrhea, and malabsorption syndromes, led to the advent of several methods. Studies using the traditional method of barium sulfate–containing meal have shown that 83% of asymptomatic subjects have small-bowel transit of two hours or less (104). This method, however, requires radiation exposure, and interference of barium sulphate with small-bowel transit has been demonstrated (46). Intubation techniques have been shown to inhibit gastric emptying and to accelerate small-bowel transit (105). Isotope-labeled test meals represent technologically advanced and attractive methods; however some radiation exposure is necessary. Moreover, superposition of radioactivity often obscures the area of interest (106). The widespread availability of these various techniques is testimony to the failure of any one of them to be proven as the ideal method.

Bond and Levitt (107) in 1975 described the breath hydrogen test as a measure of orocecal transit time. This alternative approach is provided by the bacterial metabolism in the colon. Fermentation of lactulose by colonic flora results in hydrogen and short-chain fatty acid production. Hydrogen is considered the most diffusible gas and due to its low molecular weight and relative insolubility in water, it is rapidly absorbed into the blood, transported to the lungs, and exhaled in the breath. Pulmonary excretion of hydrogen occurs within eight minutes after the carbohydrate reaches the cecum.

Preparation for the test includes a 24-hour period of abstinence from alcohol and food rich in nonutilizable sugars or fiber (108). Patients must fast for six hours prior to the study and abstain from tobacco on the day of the study. The breath hydrogen analysis is performed on end-expiratory breath specimens using an electrochemical technique. The equipment includes a Microlizer gas chromatograph analyzer (Quintron Inc., Milwaukee, Wisconsin, U.S.A.), breath sampling device, and collection bags. The gas chromatograph analyzer is calibrated each day using a known source of hydrogen. The breath hydrogen baseline value is determined as a mean of two samples taken at a 10-minute interval (109). After collection of the baseline samples, lactulose syrup is given in a dose of 10 g of solution diluted in 100 mL of water. The hydrogen excretion curve is obtained by taking breath samples at 10-minute intervals for a minimum of two hours. Values equal to or more than 3 ppm above the baseline in three consecutive measurements have been shown to reliably define hydrogen production (110). If any consistent increase of breath hydrogen is observed within two hours, the period of study can be extended to three hours. In the literature, the mean orocecal transit times measured by hydrogen breath test using 10 g of lactulose for normal subjects is of $94 + 15$ minutes (107,111). The mean coefficient of variation is 8% within subjects and 18% and 38% between subjects (110,111).

The breath hydrogen test in the assessment of constipated patients permits differentiation of isolated colonic inertia from generalized intestinal hypomotility (112,113). Marzio et al. (114) reported more prolonged orocecal transit time in constipated patients compared to controls. They also observed that, after the administration of fiber, these patients reversed the pattern to the normal range. Prolonged orocecal transit time in constipated patients may theoretically be a primary disturbance in the small bowel or a secondary phenomenon due to retarded colonic transit. However, because prolonged orocecal transit time cannot be reversed after emptying the colon with enemas, this pattern in constipation is probably a consequence of a disordered small bowel (13).

As in any other method of indirect measurement of small-bowel transit, the breath hydrogen test has its limitations. Approximately 5% to 20% of healthy individuals do not show any significant (>2 ppm) or sustained (three or more consecutive measurements) increases in breath hydrogen concentration over a three-hour period (115,116). Therefore, in these "hydrogen nonproducers," small-bowel transit cannot be assessed. This phenomenon has been attributed to either lack of hydrogen-producing bacteria in the gut or presence of an active hydrogen-utilizing methanogenic flora (116). The prevalence of "nonproducers" is not affected by gender; however, it is two to four times higher in constipated patients compared to controls (110,114). This finding may be related to modification of the colonic flora due to the frequent use of enemas and laxatives. Ideally, patients must abstain from any assistance in bowel movements for a minimum period of 15 days prior to evaluation (117). However, longer periods of abstinence from laxatives and enemas are frequently impractical.

The breath hydrogen test does not measure the rate of gastric emptying. Moreover, no significant correlation between orocecal and duodenocecal transit time has been demonstrated. Thus, different control mechanisms of gastric emptying and intestinal transit appear to exist (118). Although isolated measurement of small-bowel transit is attractive, doing so requires selective infusion of lactulose into the descending part of the duodenum via an oroduodenal tube. Intubation has been shown to inhibit gastric emptying and to accelerate small-bowel transit (105). For this reason, breath hydrogen orocecal transit time is actually superior to a lactulose tube infusion–measured duodenocecal transit test. If there is clinical indication, gastric emptying should be evaluated by a separate study.

Although the breath hydrogen test has its limitations, the test is simple, noninvasive, and reproducible. To achieve maximal reliability, a small and sustained rise in breath hydrogen should be used as criteria. The lactulose breath test may be of great value in the assessment of patients with constipation, particularly in those with colonic inertia, to help differentiate generalized hypomotility from colonic inertia.

TREATMENT
Conservative Therapy

Traditionally the mainstay of conservative treatment of constipation has included laxatives, suppositories, and enemas. In addition, agents with presumed effect in colonic neuromuscular function or prokinetic drugs have been developed and included in the conservative treatment of constipation (Table 2).

Table 2 Classification of Drugs Used in the Treatment of Constipation

Bulking or hydrophilic agents	Lubricating agent
Dietary fiber	Mineral oil
Psyllium (plantago)	Neuromuscular agents
Polycarbophil	Cholinergic agonists
Methylcellulose, carboxymethylcellulose	Bethanecol
Osmotic agents	Neostigmine
Poorly absorbed ions	5-HT$_4$ agonists
Magnesium: sulphate (epson salt), hydroxide (Milk of Magnesia), citrate	Cisapride
Sodium: phosphate, sulphate (Glauber's salt)	Prucalopride
Potassium soium tartrate (Rochelle salt)	Tegaserod
Poorly absorbed disaccharides, sugar alcohols	Prostaglandin agonist
Lactulose	Misoprostol
Sorbitol, mannitol	Colchicine
Glycerin	Opiate antagonists
Polyethylene glycol	Naloxone
Stimulant laxatives	Naltrexone
Surface-active agents	
Docusates (dioctyl sulfosuccinate)	
Bile acids	
Diphenylomethane derivatives	
Phenolphtalein	
Bisacodyl	
Sodium picosulphate	
Rinoleic acid (castor oil)	
Anthaquinones	
Senna	
Cascara sagrada	

Source: Adapted from Ref. 34.

Laxatives

Laxatives are drugs that facilitate the passage and elimination of feces from the colon and rectum, either by modifying stool consistency or inducing defecation. The consumption of laxatives, based on the tenet that nonprescription medication is safe and without adverse effects, creates an economic and health problem of tremendous proportions. After a massive bowel movement induced by a laxative, it may take several days before enough stool is present to be evacuated. Thus, in an attempt to maintain a daily bowel movement, a vicious cycle develops with more use of the same laxative or a more potent one. Such longstanding use of laxatives generates a substantial onus to the patient, due to both the costs of medication and their potential side effects. The number of laxatives currently available are countless; there are more than 700 proprietary laxative preparations available in almost every dosage form (119). Classification of these drugs becomes very important but correspondingly difficult. The most meaningful method of classification is based on their mechanisms of action and chemical properties (Table 2).

Bulking or hydrophilic laxatives are dietary or medicinal fiber supplements that add both solid material and water to the stool, increasing stool weight and softening feces. Fiber supplements should be prescribed, because a high fiber diet may be unpalatable and less tolerable to many patients. Fermentation of fiber in the colon produces gas, which accounts for the side effects of bloating and excess flatus.

Osmotic laxatives provide poorly absorbed osmotically active substances that hold additional water intraluminally, increasing water content in the stool. Lactulose is available in syrup form that contains $10 \, g/15 \, mL$ and as powder for solution. It is a synthetic disaccharide, which cannot be hydrolyzed by lactase in the small bowel, but is fermented by bacteria, producing gas as a byproduct. It has been estimated that 10 g of lactulose can produce up to 1 L of hydrogen and carbon dioxide gas; much of this is absorbed into the blood stream and exhaled (34). Standard doses of lactulose, 10 to 20 g per day, produce only mild laxation. Higher doses may limit its use due to distension, bloating, and flatulence.

Polyethylene glycol solutions are isotonic and poorly absorbed when ingested at a rapid rate and have been widely used for bowel preparation before colonoscopy or colorectal surgery. Rapidly passing through the gastrointestinal tract, these solutions do not induce water or electrolyte absorption or secretion. Powdered polyethylene glycol has been recently proposed as a laxative. It is tasteless and odorless and can be mixed in noncarbonated beverages to increase acceptance. Randomized, placebo-controlled studies have shown that 17 g of polyethylene glycol per day, ingested with 250 mL of water, increase stool consistency and frequency and facilitates evacuation (120,121). Large doses may increase delivery of nutrients to the colon and produce abdominal distension due to bacterial fermentation. However, powdered polyethylene glycol is apparently the best osmotic laxative, especially, for patients with renal dysfunction or problems with absorption of sulphate, phosphate, or magnesium from other agents.

Administered either orally or by retention enema, lubricants such as mineral oil and paraffin alter the physical characteristics of stool by forming a slippery layer around fecal pellets, thus softening and lubricating the passage of stool. Side effects include lipoid pneumonitis due to aspiration, malabsorption of fat-soluble vitamins, and foreign body reactions in intestinal mucosa and regional lymph nodes. Because mineral oil retains its fluidity at body temperature, anal seepage may occur, even in patients with normal anal sphincter tone.

Stimulant laxatives act by directly irritating the intestinal mucosa, or by selective stimulation of the enteric nervous system or intestinal smooth muscle. These drugs inhibit intestinal absorption, promote intestinal secretion, or stimulate motility and reduce transit time, thus determining an increase in unabsorbed water in the stool. They can cause abdominal cramps, increased mucous secretion, and excessively rapid evacuation in some patients. Therefore, stimulant laxatives are useful in the treatment of acute constipation caused by prolonged bed rest and bowel preparation for radiological studies. However, prolonged use should be discouraged. Current preparations of anthraquinones are impure and contain a mixture of chemicals, including usually senna or cascara sagrada. They have in common the tricyclic anthracene nucleus and are large molecules that pass unchanged to the colon, thus converted by bacterial metabolism to active forms. Some of these metabolites are absorbed and its urinary excretion provides a useful diagnostic test of laxative abuse. Laxative abuse is not uncommon but clinically important to cause diarrhea; the diagnosis can be difficult and includes a high index of suspicion, a comprehensive history, and detection of laxative metabolites in the stool or urine. Anthraquinones (senna glycosides and danthron) and diphenolic (phenolphthalein, biscodyl, and oxyphenizatin) are the most commonly abused groups of laxatives, with some specific effects (122).

Melanosis coli, a well-known characteristic side effect of anthranoid-containing laxatives, is due to apoptosis of colonic epithelial cells. The damaged organelles form the lipofuscin, a brownish pigment, which is incorporated into the lysosomes of macrophages found in the lamina propria and, in severe cases, in the submucosa (123). Melanosis coli is also a reliable and specific parameter of chronic use (longer than 9–12 months) of anthraquinones. A relative risk for colorectal carcinoma as a result of anthraquinone abuse has been initially estimated at 3.04; this risk has been calculated based on studies that have shown a significantly higher incidence of melanosis coli in patients with colorectal carcinoma, when compared to patients with no abnormality, on colonoscopy (119). However, epidemiological and animal studies have not supported this theory (123–126). Similarly, development of the so-called cathartic colon with chronic abuse of anthraquinones, because the classic findings of this entity are rarely seen, is somewhat controversial (127,128). However, recent data suggest that some of the effects of anthraquinones are due to mucosal cell damage, with consequent release of mediators that affect enteric nervous function (129). Nonetheless, stimulant laxatives should be used with caution, under medical supervision, and no more often than twice per week to minimize the risk of tolerance (2).

Suppositories and Enemas

Suppositories are useful for promoting reflex evacuation of the lower bowel. Although not as effective as enemas, suppositories are more acceptable to both patient and nursing personnel. Glycerin is well absorbed in the small bowel and therefore cannot be taken orally as a laxative, but is not as well absorbed in the colon. Therefore, glycerin is commonly used as a suppository or enema in order to draw water into the rectum and promote defecation, usually within 30 minutes. Other preparations include bisacodyl, senna, or dioctyl sodium sulfosuccinate.

Enemas usually work within five minutes by two mechanisms—distension and osmotic activity. In order to prevent cramps, enemas should be introduced slowly, with the patient in the lateral decubitus position. Warm tap water or warm saline enemas are preferred because they are less irritating to the mucosa. Complications include electrolyte depletion, particularly with hypertonic solutions, water intoxication, and colon or rectal perforation.

Prokinetic Agents

Prokinetic agents are drugs that act through diverse mechanisms to enhance motility of the gastrointestinal tract. Pharmacologic stimulation of colonic transit in the treatment of refractory idiopathic constipation has been an area of active research. However, the main obstacle is still an incomplete understanding of the normal and altered gastrointestinal motility (130).

Because decreased cholinergic nerve activity has been demonstrated in some patients with slow transit constipation, presumably due to damage to the enteric nervous system, cholinergic agonists such as bethanecol and neostigmine have been used in a few series. Bethanecol in doses of 25–50 mg three or four times per day has been deemed helpful to treat constipation related to the use of tricyclic antidepressants (131). Neostigmine in a single dose of 2.0–2.5 mg intravenously has proven effective to treat acute colonic pseudo-obstruction; side effects include bradycardia, abdominal pain, increased salivation, and vomiting (132,133). In more chronic types of constipation, although not formally tested, neostigmine at doses of 15 mg orally three to four times daily may be helpful (34).

The benzamides, including metoclopramide, cisapride, and prucalopride, are prokinetics that act via serotonin [5-hydroxytryptamine (5-HT)]. They activate $5-HT_4$ receptors on myenteric cholinergic nerves with consequent increased acetylcholine release in the intramural plexuses and smooth muscle contraction. Metoclopramide is effective in gastroparesis but not in the treatment of postoperative ileus or colonic motility disorders (124,130). Cisapride was also developed as a prokinetic primarily directed to the upper gut. Subsequently, several studies using cisapride in constipated patients, including placebo-controlled randomized clinical trials and studies in pediatric groups, have demonstrated an increased stool frequency and a decreased colonic transit time; results, however, are inconsistent (134–137). Although in clinical trials cisapride appears to be effective, the results have been disappointing in clinical practice (138). Moreover, safety concerns regarding an association between the use of cisapride and prolonged QT syndrome and fatal arrhythmia has led to its withdrawal from commercial distribution (139).

In an effort to identify other prokinetics that affect colonic serotonin $5-HT_4$ receptors, prucalopride has recently been shown to speed colonic transit time in volunteers (140,141). However its role in the treatment of chronic constipation is still under evaluation by clinical trials. Tegaserod, a partial $5-HT_4$ receptor agonist, is also under investigation; however, preliminary data suggest that this drug accelerates orocecal transit in patients with constipation-predominant irritable bowel syndrome (142).

Macrolide antibiotics, particularly erythromycin, may act as motilin agonists; they seem to inhibit the binding of motilin, a gastrointestinal peptide hormone, to its receptors on gastrointestinal smooth muscle membranes. Erythromycin seems to be effective in the treatment of gastroparesis and colonic pseudo-obstruction, but its role in the treatment of chronic constipation remains unclear (130,143). The major problems are related to the side effects inherent to the prolonged use of antibiotics.

More recently, in a randomized double-blind placebo-controlled crossover trial of 16 patients who received colchicines in doses of 0.6 mg t.i.d. for four weeks for chronic constipation showed an increased frequency of bowel movements and a hastening of colonic transit (144). The main side effect is abdominal pain, which tends to decrease during the treatment period. Colchicine may be an effective agent to treat a subset of patients with refractory chronic constipation; however, more experience with this drug is needed.

Surgical Treatment

The role of surgery in the treatment of chronic constipation has been regarded with skepticism by many surgeons. In fact, constipation is a multifactorial condition in which both psychological and psychiatric disorders are often recognized, particularly, in young females. Considering the high cost of the medical treatment of constipation and the uncontrolled use of laxatives, patients with a proven diagnosis of a treatable causative disorder should be

offered operative treatment. Only a small group of patients with chronic refractory constipation is suitable for surgical treatment, and a comprehensive physiologic investigation is
crucial to achieve successful results (145).

After completing diagnostic evaluation, "functional" causes of chronic refractory constipation can be stratified into the following: (i) colonic cause: slow transit constipation (colonic
inertia), idiopathic megacolon, and adult Hirschsprung's disease; (ii) pelvic outlet obstruction: paradoxical puborectalis contraction, rectocele, sigmoidocele and enterocele, rectoanal
intussusception, and perineal descent syndrome; (iii) combined colonic inertia with outlet
obstruction; and (iv) normal transit constipation.

Colonic Inertia (Slow Transit Constipation)

Colonic inertia is characterized by diffuse stasis of markers throughout the colon, usually more
markedly in the right colon. This condition typically affects young women as a severe and incapacitating symptom (146). The etiopathogeny of colonic inertia remains unclear. Lesions of the
myenteric plexus have been demonstrated in patients with colonic inertia, but most of these are
either primary or related to chronic use of laxatives (147). Histopathologic alterations include a
reduction of argyrophilic neurons in myenteric ganglia (112), oligoneuronal hypoganglionosis
in myenteric plexus (148), hypertrophic nerve fibers, and giant ganglia (intestinal neuronal
dysplasia) (149). Abnormalities in content and distribution of neurotransmitters include
increased serotonin and 5-hydroxyindolacetic acid and enterochromaffin cells in the sigmoid
(150), changes in nitric oxide synthetase and vasoactive intestinal peptide (VIP) distribution
(151), and somatostatin and pancreatic glucagons (152). Colonic inertia can also be associated
with other symptoms of visceral stasis; therefore a hypothesis of a systemic disorder has been
proposed (16). Immunohistochemic studies have supported this theory, revealing a lack of
myenteric nerve fibers immunoreactive for neurofilaments (153) and a significant increase of
the myenteric plexus fraction immunoreactive for protein S-100 (154). Further studies in this
field may contribute to a better understanding of the pathophysiology of colonic inertia, and
hopefully point to new prokinectics that are effective for this condition.

Colectomy for constipation was first proposed by Lane (146) almost one century ago, and
was subsequently abandoned due to both high complication rates and poor success rates.
During the last two decades, however, with more accurate patient selection through physiologic testing, the interest for total colectomy with ileorectal anastomosis to treat colonic inertia
has been renewed. This procedure may alleviate symptoms in 70% to 90% of cases, although
careful patient selection is strongly mandated (Table 3) (113,145,155–165). In spite of the
excellent results in the literature, postoperative morbidity remains a discouraging problem.
Small-bowel obstruction, the most frequent complication, occurs in 7% to 50% of patients, some
of whom may require reoperation (161,164,166–169). In a study of 30 patients who underwent
colectomy for colonic inertia, Pikarsky et al. (163) reported that all patients considered the outcome of surgery as "excellent" at a long-term follow-up of 106 months. The mean frequency of
bowel movements was 2.5 (range, 1–6). During the follow-up period, six (20%) patients

Table 3 Results of Total Abdominal Colectomy and Ileorectal Anastomosis for Colonic Inertia

Authors/Year	No.	Female (%)	Mean age (yr)	Follow-up (yr)	Success (%)
Barnes et al. (155) 1986	6	43	38	5	67
Walsh et al. (156) 1987	19	86	–	3.2	65
Vasilevsky et al. (113) 1988	51[a]	94	45	4	81
Yoshioka and Keighley (157) 1989	40[b]	98	35	3	58
Zenilman et al. (158) 1989	12	100	35	2	100
Pemberton et al. (159) 1991	38	84	40	–	100
Wexner et al. (145) 1991	16	92	45	1.2	94
Mahendrarajah et al. (160) 1994	9	100	38	1.3	88
Piccirillo et al. (161) 1995	54	78	49	2.2	94
Redmond et al. (162) 1995	34	92	43	7.5	90
Pikarsky et al. (163) 2001	30	70	60	8.9	100
Mollen et al. (164) 2001	21	86	43	5.2	76
Glia et al. (165) 2004	17	94	46	5	86

[a]Ileorectal anastomosis or ileosigmoid anastomosis.
[b]34 ileorectal anastomosis, 5 cecorectal anastomosis, and 1 ileosigmoid anastomosis.
Source: Adapted from Ref. 163.

required admission for small-bowel obstruction, three of whom (10%) required laparotomy. All obstructions occurred within two years of the operation. Four patients complained of mild postoperative pelvic pain, three of whom also had preoperative pain. Two patients (6%) required assistance with bowel movements by laxatives or enemas, and two (6%) required antidiarrheal medications to reduce bowel frequency. In this study, which had a mean follow-up of approximately 10 years, some issues relating to the adaptive process of the alimentary tract to colectomy could be more comprehensively addressed. There was a slight decrease in bowel frequency from 3.7 per day at 27 months to 2.5 per day at up to 10 years. In addition to the change in stool consistency in 16% of patients from semiliquid to semisolid form, the incidence of incontinent episodes decreased from 24% to 17%, and the use of antidiarrheal medications decreased from 24% to 17%. Bloating, present in 60% of patients preoperatively, remained unchanged at 27 months and decreased to 23% at up to 10 years. The authors concluded total abdominal colectomy could be recommended to patients with well-established colonic inertia with expectations of sustained benefit of up to 10 years after surgery.

Selection criteria for colonic inertia include reassessment of severity of symptoms (history, transit times, and response to trials of therapy with laxatives and prokinetics), exclusion of small-bowel dysmotility (lactulose and H2 breath test), and exclusion of pelvic floor dysfunction. If dyspeptic symptoms such as nausea, vomiting, heartburn, and bloating are present, gastric emptying studies are indicated in order to exclude a generalized gastrointestinal stasis. In a recent study, Glia et al. (165) found a trend toward better long-term results after colectomy for slow transit constipation in patients with a normal preoperative antroduodenal manometry. Unsatisfactory results are frequently due to inadequate selection of patients with generalized dysmotility, underdetected evacuation disorders (including outlet obstructive causes or weakened sphincters), or a significant psychological overlay (164,165).

Segmental resection of the colon is rarely effective, usually resulting in recurrent constipation and dilation of the remaining colon. Reported overall success rates of 89% after total abdominal colectomy decrease to only 68% after segmental colectomy (166). In a very small carefully and selected subgroup of patients, isolated left-sided colectomy with low colorectal or coloanal anastomosis may be successful (170). Similarly, subtotal colectomy either with preservation of the cecum (cecorectal anastomosis) or the sigmoid (ileosigmoid anastomosis) are also fated to persistent postoperative constipation (171,172). Conversely, if the ileorectal anastomosis is performed at the level below 7 to 10 cm from the anal verge, an unacceptably high frequency of bowel movements or incontinence may occur.

Although total colectomy with ileorectal anastomosis is the best option for colonic inertia, there remain approximately 10% of patients who will have persistent symptoms of constipation. Therefore, it is crucial to review functional studies in order to exclude pelvic floor dysfunction in these patients. If studies are positive for any such disorders, a completion proctectomy and an ileoanal pouch procedure (although a very radical surgical approach) may be offered as an alternative to a stoma to this very small, highly selected group of patients (173,174).

Colostomy allows the possibility of colonic irrigation; however, results are frequently unsatisfactory due to persistent colonic inertia proximal to the site of the ostomy or a more generalized disorder of motility. Creation of a continent colonic conduit has also been proposed for these patients (175). After being shown how to intubate and irrigate the colonic conduit, patients recount an increased number of bowel movements, and less time required to evacuate the rectal contents. More recently, a cecal access for antegrade colon enemas has been proposed by Rongen et al. (176) to treat 12 patients with refractory slow transit constipation. In the long term, four patients required subtotal colectomy, two of whom needed an ileostomy due to persistent symptoms. Overall, the constipation score dropped from a median of 21.5 to 5.5. The authors concluded that the procedure is promising, and, because it is a minimally invasive procedure, the need for future surgery due to failure is not compromised.

Megabowel

In patients with dilation of the bowel, universal (megacolon), segmental (megasigmoid, megarectum), or a combination of both, anorectal manometry is an important diagnostic tool. The absence of the rectoanal inhibitory reflex is characteristic of congenital (Hirschsprung's disease) or acquired (Chagas' disease) megabowel. Patients with megabowel with an intact anorectal inhibitory reflex are considered as an idiopathic megabowel.

Adult Hirschsprung's Disease

In Hirschsprung's disease, the diagnosis can be established by the absence of ganglia in a full-thickness biopsy and by anorectal manometry. Short- or ultrashort-segment Hirschsprung's disease can be successfully treated by posterior anorectal myectomy (177,178). The technique includes removal of a long strip of internal anal sphincter and circular muscle at least 6 × 1-cm wide, starting from 2 cm above the dentate line. Abdominal procedures for the treatment of adult Hirschsprung's disease include the Duhamel retrorectal transanal anastomosis, Soave endorectal pull-through, and Swenson abdominoperineal pull-through. Good-to-excellent functional results are in the range of 90% to 100%, and complications include persistent constipation and incontinence (179–181).

Chagasic Megacolon

Chagas'disease is endemic in certain rural areas of Brazil and other neighboring South American countries. It is caused by a parasite, *Trypanosoma cruzi*, transmitted to humans by the hematophagic *Triatominae* insect. Patients with megacolon, the most common clinical presentation of intestinal trypanosomiasis, present with severe constipation and are prone to develop fecaloma and sigmoid volvulus. Diagnosis is confirmed by a complement-fixation test (Machado Guerreiro's test). Colonic transit times are significantly prolonged in Chagasic megacolon, and left colon delay is the most common pattern. Rectoanal inhibitory reflex is absent in approximately 90% of these patients (182,183). Removal or exclusion of the dyskinetic rectum, which acts as a functional obstacle to the progression of the fecal bolus, is the principle of surgical treatment of this disabling disease. Pull-through operations, particularly the Duhamel-Haddad, have yielded satisfactory results, although disturbances of fecal incontinence do occur. In fact, experience with this technique for Hirschsprung's disease has shown perfect fecal control in only 60.4% of patients; 31.3% have occasional staining and/or gas incontinence, 8.3% constant fecal soiling, and 10.4% persistent constipation (184). More recently, abdominal rectosigmoidectomy with end-to-side colorectal anastomosis has been proposed as a modified Duhamel's technique for surgical treatment of Chagasic megacolon, with the advantage of being a one-stage technique (185). The rectum is sectioned and closed at the level of the peritoneal reflection, and the end of the descending colon is anastomosed with an intraluminal stapler to the posterior surface of the rectum, as distal as possible. Functional results with this technique are reportedly better; however a longer follow-up is required to evaluate its actual effectiveness.

Neuronal Intestinal Dysplasia

Neuronal intestinal dysplasia is a dysganglionosis, a specific congenital denervation of the intestinal wall. It is estimated to account for approximately 20% of colonic denervation (186). Intestinal dysplasia Type A is characterized by aplasia or hypoplasia of the sympathetic innervation and seen exclusively in children, whereas Type B is characterized by dysplasia of the submucous plexus, and occurs in both children and adults. Neuronal intestinal dysplasia type B is characterized by weak propulsive motility of the colon and may be evident in adults with idiopathic chronic constipation and colonic diverticulosis (187). Diagnosis is confirmed by histopathologic findings of hyperplasia and giant ganglia and enzyme histochemical findings of increased acetylcholinesterase activity in the parasympathetic plexus. Surgery—subtotal colectomy—is usually necessary.

Idiopathic Megacolon

Exclusion of Hirschsprung's disease is an important diagnostic step, especially in children and adolescents because these patients can often be successfully managed conservatively. Megarectum and associated encopresis can be effectively treated by habit retraining in which the patient is required to attempt to defecate at a set time during the day, rather than in response to urge. A few controlled trials in children with chronic constipation and encopresis have shown that biofeedback does not seem to increase long-term recovery rates above those achieved with conventional treatment alone, results are conflicting (188,189). Functional megarectum is also common in the elderly (22). Most patients will respond to empiric measures, including modification of dietary habits, mobilization, and bowel habit retraining. In others, the condition can be difficult to treat, which may be related to underlying physiological abnormalities. Prolonged transit times, particularly outlet obstructive patterns, reduced anal sphincter pressures, and increased rectal sensory threshold are common findings in elderly patients with constipation (190). It has been suggested that a neurogenic deficit of the sacral spinal cord may be responsible for this impairment of rectal motor and sensory function (190).

Treatment options for idiopathic megacolon are similar to those for colonic inertia; surgery is indicated only if conservative treatment fails, and colectomy with ileorectal anastomosis is the best option for patients with a moderately or extensively dilated megacolon or with dilation of the left colon (166). Similar to colonic inertia, if the cecal reservoir is maintained, dilation follows and constipation recurs; likewise, if any part of the sigmoid colon is left in place, constipation may occur. The only exception is probably patients with isolated megasigmoid. Success rates of 75% to 100% have been achieved with sigmoid resection in these patients (168,169,191–193).

PELVIC FLOOR DYSFUNCTION

Nonrelaxing puborectalis syndrome, paradoxical puborectalis syndrome, nonrelaxing or paradoxical contraction puborectalis syndrome, or pelvic floor dyssynergia or spastic pelvic floor are all terms attributed to a complex and not well understood entity characterized by contraction, rather than relaxation of the puborectalis and other striated pelvic floor muscles during attempted evacuation (194). The term "anismus" by analogy from "vaginismus" also has been applied to depict this syndrome; however, the former terms are more applicable because they describe the phenomenon without implying a psychosomatic etiology.

The etiology of this dysfunction is obscure; proposed theories include voluntary suppression of the normal inhibitory reflex, muscular dystonia, abuse of cathartics and sympathetic nerve abnormalities, spastic contraction due to local inflammatory perianal and pelvic conditions, partial denervation of the pelvic floor, generalized pelvic floor disorder, and psychologic factors (194). The behavioral disorder theory, based upon lack of coordinated relaxation of the striated anal sphincters during defecation, is supported by the improvement in nonrelaxing puborectalis syndrome noted after biofeedback therapy (195,196).

Although the exact incidence of nonrelaxing puborectalis syndrome remains unknown, it apparently represents an important etiologic factor in constipation, especially in obstructed defecation. In a series of 180 patients with idiopathic chronic constipation, nonrelaxing puborectalis syndrome was found twice as often as was colonic inertia (33% vs. 17%, respectively) (43). Typical clinical manifestations of nonrelaxing puborectalis syndrome include symptoms of obstructed evacuation such as straining, tenesmus, and the sensation of incomplete evacuation, as well as the frequent need of suppositories, enemas, or digitation. Frequently, these patients have a history of previous treatment for other anorectal conditions associated with straining such as rectocele, descending perineal syndrome, solitary rectal ulcer syndrome, rectoanal intussusception, or prolapse.

Although the physical examination may be suggestive of paradoxical contraction of the external anal sphincter and puborectalis, the patient's embarrassment may cause a "paradoxical reaction," and the diagnosis is usually reached only after thorough anorectal physiology investigation. Segmental colonic transit time may suggest the diagnosis by demonstrating an outlet obstruction pattern; however, this is not a specific test. EMG and defecography provide the most accurate assessment of puborectalis muscle function. EMG provides data on external anal sphincter and puborectalis neuromuscular activity while cinedefecography allows measurement of the anorectal angle, which is directly related to sphincter muscle activity. Defecographic criteria of nonrelaxing puborectalis syndrome includes failure to open the anorectal angle, persistence of the puborectalis impression during attempted defecation, an overly capacious rectum, a long and persistently closed anal canal, ballooning of the rectum, and the presence of compensatory anterior and posterior rectoceles. These findings can be associated with nonemptying, incomplete emptying, or even total evacuation after a prolonged and difficult attempt.

Both defecography and EMG have their own limitations. Voluntary contraction of the pelvic floor due to embarrassment may simulate a functional disorder on defecography. Similarly, the inability to relax the sphincter may occur during pushing as a response to fear or pain during the electromyographic assessment. These factors may result in false-positive findings of nonrelaxing puborectalis syndrome in patients without symptoms of obstructed evacuation. Sensitivity, specificity, and predictive values of both EMG and defecography are suboptimal, and the association of these tests can be necessary to permit optimal data accrual (94). However, defecography is probably superior on the basis that it can detect associated abnormalities and demonstrate both the dynamics of evacuation and the rectal emptying. It has been suggested that false-positive results may ensue due to the patient's embarrassment of evacuating in front of other people. However, if this issue is truly preventing evacuation, the patient can be offered the privacy of a bathroom for evacuation, followed by fluoroscopic reassessment of the evacuated rectum. The diagnosis of nonrelaxing puborectalis syndrome should be given only to patients whose clinical symptoms of pelvic outlet obstruction are supported by physiologic confirmation of their significance.

To date, biofeedback therapy represents the most appealing resource in the management of patients with paradoxical puborectalis syndrome. Rectal massage, progressive boogie dilation, intrarectal diathermy, and antispasmodic agents have all been tried and not proven beneficial (97). Surgery for paradoxical puborectalis syndrome is deemed to low success rates and high morbidity due to postoperative incontinence. Posterior partial V-shaped resection of the puborectalis muscle has been reported initially with a rate 75% of success (194,197,198). However, subsequent reports with division of this muscle have reported success rates of 24% with incontinence of gas and liquid stool in approximately 55% (199,200).

For patients who fail biofeedback therapy, botulin toxin type-A injection has been considered a valid alternative. In 1988, Hallan et al. (201) used the British form of BTX-A (Dysport, Porton, U.K.) and reported some concerns with postinjection complications, particularly fecal incontinence. Some years later, the interest in this technique was renewed and a less potent, presumably, safer form was developed in the United States (Botox, Allergan). Although techniques vary, 10 to 30 units of Botox-A can be injected by palpation to each side of the puborectalis, or 20 units injected to the posterior angle of the muscle; both electromyography and anal ultrasound have been used to locate the site of injection (202,203). Experience with this technique is still limited and to date, no controlled studies to assess the role of botulin toxin type-A in paradoxical puborectalis syndrome have been reported. In a study of four patients, Maria et al. (202) demonstrated a decreased resting tone from $96.2 + 12$ mmHg to $42.5 + 13$ mmHg at four weeks and $63.2 + 22$ mmHg at eight weeks. Defecography performed at eight weeks after treatment showed an increase in the anorectal angle, from $94 + 11°$ to $114 + 13°$, and evacuation of barium paste. One patient had recurrent symptoms at 16 weeks after treatment and was successfully treated with 50 units, and again eight months later, with a further 60 units. This patient reported unassisted normal bowel movements at seven months after the last injection. The authors concluded that the use of a higher dosage and a more precise method of toxin injection under anal ultrasound-guidance accounted for the higher long-term success rate. However, because the effects of toxin wane within three months of administration, repeated injections may be necessary to maintain clinical improvement. According to Ron et al. (203), although manometric relaxation was achieved after the first injection in 18 patients (75%) and no other complications other than pain during injections were observed, only 37.5% of patients were satisfied with the overall results.

BIOFEEDBACK

Indications for biofeedback for constipation are more stringent than for incontinence, and careful patient selection is crucial. In fact, it has been demonstrated that biofeedback has little therapeutic effect in the management of intractable constipation when heterogeneous etiology are grouped (204). On the contrary, biofeedback therapy has proven particularly valuable in the treatment of paradoxical puborectalis syndrome.

Biofeedback techniques vary considerably among institutions, which have been previously described in detail (205). The principle of treatment is to retrain pelvic floor and external anal sphincter muscles under electromyography monitoring, either alone or synchronized with rectal distension. Patients are generally seen in an office setting for three to four weekly sessions. More often, biofeedback is performed with a noninvasive anal surface EMG plug, connected to a computer to provide visual output of the patient's effort. The patient is first asked to contract the sphincter and then is made aware of the degree of external sphincter contraction. To properly contract and relax the external anal sphincter, instructions are given to focus on isolation of the muscle. In a second phase, a rectal balloon is inserted, and volumes large enough to be perceived by the patient are used, along with visual and verbal feedback. The patient is trained to recognize smaller distension volumes and to synchronize and increase external sphincter contractions. Patients are instructed to exercise at home by squeezing and holding the contraction for a count of 10 seconds, then relaxing for an equal amount of time. A high fiber diet and a self-observation diary, including frequency of defecation and related symptoms, are very helpful during the treatment in order to better evaluate patient symptoms.

The methodology of biofeedback for constipation differs in some aspects to that for fecal incontinence. First, a sensation of muscular relaxation is more poorly appreciated by constipated patients. Second, manometry provides precise measurement of contraction of the external anal sphincter, although it does not accurately reflect puborectalis relaxation. Therefore, for patients with anismus, the electromyographic method of biofeedback is preferred. Although the benefit of a single training session has been reported in up to 69% of patients, a variable number of sessions are generally required (196).

Psychotherapy has been used in addition to biofeedback to treat women with anismus (206,207). Several factors, including dietary manipulations and the effect on the patient's well-being and confidence, have been listed as mechanisms responsible for improving symptoms after biofeedback (208). However, others have found no clinical improvement using only relaxation techniques such as yoga (209,210).

Most studied factors do not seem to determine the results after biofeedback, including patient age, gender, duration of symptoms, presence of rectal pain, anal pressures, and abnormalities of rectal sensation (211,212). Others, however, have found that a long history of difficult and prolonged defecation is related to a poor outcome after biofeedback training (212,213). Interestingly, recent reports have shown a better response to biofeedback in patients with both prominent puborectalis impression and less perineal descent on cinedefecography (213,214). Park et al. (214) demonstrated that based on cinedefecographic findings, anismus can be subdivided into two types: type A with a flattened anorectal angle without definite puborectalis indentation, but with anal canal hypertonia and type B, with clear persistent puborectalis indentation, narrow anorectal angle, and a closed anal canal. Biofeedback was successful in the treatment of 86% of patients with type B anismus and only in 25% of patients with type A anismus. Accordingly Weber et al. (215) found biofeedback to be ineffective in 16 patients with anal canal hypertonia and ultraslow waves.

Biofeedback therapy has been associated with an overall success rate of 68.5% for constipation attributable to paradoxical puborectalis contraction (211–216). More recently, Gilliland et al. (211) observed that biofeedback was completely successful in only 35% of patients. However, the success rate improved significantly after five or more sessions, and complete success was achieved by 63% of patients who finished the prescribed treatment course, compared with 25% of those who self-discharged. Karlbom et al. (213) have demonstrated a success rate of biofeedback of 43% in patients with paradoxical puborectalis contraction, with a treatment effect lasting at least one year. In a study of five women with anismus treated with biofeedback associated to psychotherapy, Turnbull and Ritvo (206) found continued improvement in bowel function and abdominal symptomatology in a follow-up of 2 to 4.5 years post-therapy.

Although most studies report positive results using biofeedback to treat constipation, studies comparing its efficacy over other treatment modalities are needed. In addition, there are inconsistencies in the literature regarding patient selection criteria, technique, and definition of a successful outcome. Definitions of success vary considerably among series and include an overall increase in stool frequency (213,217–219), reduction of laxative use (218,220), and a decrease in associated symptoms such as pain, bloating, and straining (206). The use of more stringent criteria such as defining complete success as a return to the patient's normal bowel habits has been adopted with resultant success rates of 50% to 60% with follow-up of six months or more (211,220). The use of a constipation-scoring system may contribute in establishing uniformity when assessing these results.

The patient's willingness to expend time and effort to alleviate their symptoms may be the most important predictor of success. Therefore, all efforts should be made to ensure complete patient cooperation. It may be helpful to review the cinedefecography tapes with the patients in order to better acquaint them with their disorder and, subsequently, to improve cooperation. The use of booster sessions of biofeedback also has been proposed to maintain success (216,220). No correlation has been found between successful outcome and physiologic tests. Karlbom et al. (213) found that improvement in balloon expulsion after biofeedback training was not statistically significant in the group who improved clinically (56%) compared to the nonimproved group (46%). Similarly, electromyographic values do not correlate with improvement after biofeedback treatment (221).

Recently, a comprehensive meta-analysis was undertaken to compare the outcome of various biofeedback protocols for treating constipation and reviewed both the pediatric and the adult literature from 1970 to 2002 (222). The authors reviewed 38 studies; 10 of those that used a parallel treatment design were evaluated in detail, including seven that randomized subjects to treatment groups. The mean success rate of studies using pressure biofeedback (78%) was superior to the mean success rate for studies using EMG biofeedback (70%). However, the mean success rates comparing studies using intra-anal EMG sensors to studies using perianal EMG sensors were 69% and 72%, respectively. Thus, no advantages for one type of EMG protocol over the other were noted and no anatomic, physiologic, or demographic variables were identified, which would assist in predicting successful outcome. Associated psychological symptoms may influence treatment outcome; however, this requires further study. According to the authors, recommendations for future investigations include improvement of experimental design, definition of treatment protocol according to different types of subjects, adequate evaluation of etiology and severity of symptoms, assessment of the role of psychopathology in this population, a clear definition of outcome measures, and the inclusion of long-term follow-up data of an adequate sample size.

RECTOCELE

Rectoceles represent herniations of the rectal wall, with the anterior site much more common than the posterior. This condition is more prevalent in females, and factors such as multiparity and traumatic vaginal delivery that weakens the rectovaginal septum are usually implicated. The clinical history can be highly suspicious when patients refer to the need to either press the posterior vaginal wall or rectal digitation in order to assist defecation.

Prior to initiating treatment of a rectocele, it is crucial to assess both its clinical significance and its concomitant functional disorders (223). Rectoceles are found in up to 70% of asymptomatic women; therefore, care must be taken to avoid overtreatment whether found during physical examination or on videodefecography. Larger rectoceles (>3.0 cm in diameter) with prolonged or even absent emptying are more likely to cause symptoms of constipation (70). In patients with difficult, prolonged, incomplete, or assisted (rectal or vaginal digitation) defecation, these findings represent the best criteria for surgery. Rectocele repair can be accomplished by a transrectal, transvaginal, combined rectovaginal, or perineal approach, with success rates ranging from 84% to 98% (224–227). According to some authors, transvaginal repair does not provide sufficient relief and, moreover, may lead to dyspareunia (225,226). Transrectal repair is probably the most common technique among colorectal surgeons yielding excellent or good results in approximately 90%, as well as lower infection rates compared to combined transrectal, transvaginal, or transperineal approaches (226–228). However, transvaginal repair with posterior perineorrhaphy and colporrhaphy has gained increased acceptance because it is technically easier and offers satisfactory results in 84% of patients. Selection of one of these approaches will depend on the type of rectocele, association of other disorders (colpocystocele, enterocele, and sigmoidocele), and the surgeons's experience and preference.

Common associated abnormalities include excessive perineal descent, enterocele, colonic inertia, and nonrelaxing puborectalis syndrome. Rectoceles can be found in up to 45% of patients with emptying disorders due to nonrelaxing puborectalis syndrome (229,230). This type of rectocele usually represents a compensatory mechanism due to the functional closure of the anal canal during attempted defecation and consequent high intrarectal pressure. This finding is of primary importance because under these circumstances, surgical treatment of rectocele will fail; instead biofeedback should be indicated.

CUL-DE-SAC HERNIAS: ENTEROCELE AND SIGMOIDOCELE

The cul de sac or pouch of Douglas can eventually extend caudally between the rectum and vagina in varying degrees, even as far as the perineum, and result in a cul de sac or vaginal hernia. Hernia contents can include omentum, small bowel, and, occasionally, an elongated loop of sigmoid (63). A hernia is named according to its location and not to its contents; therefore, strictly speaking, the term cul de sac hernia is more adequate than enterocele or sigmoidocele. However, this terminology seems more discriminative and has gained wide acceptance among both colorectal surgeons and gynecologists. Cul-de-sac hernias have been classified as primary, when factors such as multiparity, advanced age, general lack of elasticity, obesity, constipation, or increased abdominal pressure are present, and secondary when enteroceles followed prior gynecologic procedures especially vaginal hysterectomy. The incidence of enterocele at one year or more following vaginal hysterectomy ranges from 6% to 25%; however, it can be significantly reduced by obliteration of the cul de sac by suturing the uterosacral ligaments (231). The pathophysiology of sigmoidocele in obstructed defecation is complex, and several mechanisms may be involved including rectal infolding, direct compression by the hernia contents, and sigmoid stasis. The contents of a cul-de-sac hernia split the fascia of Denonvilliers and weaken the rectovaginal septum. Consequently, in these patients, the anterior rectal wall is exposed to the direct action of the abdominal pressure. Therefore, a collapse of the rectal ampulla, which is also influenced by factors such as the gradient of pressure and rate of flow, occurs during straining. In addition to a deep rectogenital pouch and slackening of the supporting structures of the uterus, intraoperative findings in these patients frequently include a long sigmoid loop and eventual elongation of a proximal mesorectum.

Sigmoidocele is similar to an enterocele but is usually part of a complex entity known as pelvic laxity or pelvic relaxation; this occurs as a result of weakened-supporting vaginal tissue and pelvic diaphragm. Several defects may coexist, including an anterior rectocele, rectoanal intussusception or overt rectal prolapse, cystocele, and vaginal or uterine prolapse. Therefore, the clinical relevance of a sigmoidocele or enterocele in this complex syndrome is an important issue to be considered when planning treatment of these disorders. Although more pronounced cul-de-sac hernias can be diagnosed during physical examination as a prolapse of the upper posterior vaginal wall during Valsalva's maneuver, more accurate assessment of this entity, especially sigmoidocele, became possible only after the advent of defecography.

Technical variants have been proposed in an attempt to enhance the diagnostic capability of defecography, especially to assist delineation of deep cul de sac pouches, enteroceles, and sigmoidoceles. In addition to the use of videorecording (videoproctography), systematic instillation of air, barium suspension, and a substantial amount of barium paste, oral ingestion of 150 mL of barium contrast one to three hours prior to the examination may assist in the delineation of pelvic small-bowel loops. More recently, intraperitoneal instillation of 50 mL of nonionic contrast has been proposed; despite the potential risk of complications, peritoneography combined with dynamic proctography can provide better assessment of pelvic floor disorders, particularly peritoneocele with or without enterocele (72). The use of a tampon soaked in iodine-contrast medium placed in the posterior fornix of the vagina, either as an isolated method or combined with a voiding cystography (colpocysto-defecography), assists in the assessment of the depth of the rectogenital fossa and the eventual interposition of intra-abdominal content between the rectum and vagina (71). More recently, dynamic anorectal endosonography by measuring the change in peritoneal-anal distance during evacuation has been proposed to evaluate enterocele; however, further studies are warranted to prove its sensitivity for screening of this disorder (232). Dynamic pelvic resonance imaging has also been proposed to investigate complex pelvic disorders, particularly in the diagnosis of cul de sac hernias and their contents (233,234). Matsuoka et al. (235) compared dynamic pelvic magnetic resonance imaging and videoproctography in patients with constipation and revealed that, despite a cost of approximately 10 times more for dynamic pelvic resonance imaging than for videoproctography, no clinical changes ensued as a result of this study. The routine application of dynamic pelvic magnetic resonance imaging is not supported, and further studies are necessary to establish the exact role of this method.

Despite advances in the diagnosis of sigmoidocele, this entity has been generally regarded as an incidental finding on defecography. More definite criteria are required to differentiate an incidental sigmoidocele from an obstructing sigmoidocele. One proposed classification was based on the degree of descent of the lowest portion of the sigmoid during maximum straining in relation to the following pelvic anatomic landmarks: pubis, coccyx, and ischium (236). First-degree sigmoidocele was considered when an intrapelvic loop of sigmoid was observed on cinedefecography, but the sigmoid did not surpass the pubococcygeal line (Figure 6A) second-degree sigmoidocele, when the sigmoid loop was situated below the pubococcygeal line but remained above the ischiococcygeal line (Figure 6B) and third degree if the sigmoid loop transcended the ischiococcygeal line (Figure 6C). In a study to assess the incidence and clinical significance of sigmoidocele as a finding during defecography, 24 sigmoidoceles were noted in a total of 463 cinedefecographic studies (5.2%). In this study, symptoms of constipation were present in 20 of the 24 (83%) patients. The most common symptoms were incomplete evacuation, straining, bloating, sensation of rectal pressure or fullness, infrequent bowel movements, and abdominal pain; 67% of these patients reported assisted defecation, including the use of laxatives, enemas, digitations, and suppositories. One patient reported the need to press the lower abdomen in the left-lower quadrant and suprapubic areas in order to achieve a bowel movement. Nine patients had first-degree sigmoidocele, seven had second-degree, and eight had third-degree sigmoidoceles. This proposed classification system yielded excellent correlation between the mean level of the sigmoidocele, the degree of sigmoid redundancy, and the clinical symptoms. The clinical significance of third-degree sigmoidocele is supported by the fact that all eight patients of this group were females with severe disturbances of defecation, and seven (87%) had impaired rectal emptying on cinedefecography. Furthermore, all five third-degree sigmoidocele patients who underwent colonic resection reported symptomatic improvement at a follow-up ranging from 14 to 60 months. Therefore, sigmoidocele may account for symptoms of obstructed defecation, and the staging of sigmoidocele is useful in determining both clinical significance and an objectively planned therapy.

According to gynecologists, enterocele repair techniques include excision of redundant cul de sac peritoneum, approximation of uterosacral ligaments, and obliteration of the distal part of the cul de sac. Obliteration of the cul de sac can be performed by either an abdominal approach (Moschowitz) or transvaginally, and sutures can be longitudinally or circumferentially applied (Marion–Moschowitz); abdominal colposacropexy has also been advocated by some gynecologists. The transvaginal approach is associated with a risk of dyspareunia caused by scarring and narrowing of the vaginal lumen. In any event, assessment of results with these techniques is subjective, and there is concern that obliteration of the distal part of the cul de sac does not restore pelvic anatomy. Obliteration of the pelvic inlet with a U-shaped Mersilene® mesh has been used to treat patients with symptomatic enterocele with good results (237).

In contrast to the small bowel, the herniated sigmoid, due to its larger diameter and more solid contents, is more prone to stasis. Consequently, symptoms of pelvic discomfort, sensation of incomplete evacuation, and prolonged straining can be more severe in patients with sigmoidocele. Colonic resection (sigmoidectomy) in these patients is followed by symptomatic improvement (236).

INTUSSUSCEPTION

Intrarectal and rectoanal intussusception represent initial phases of rectal prolapse whereby a fold develops in the rectal wall during push, prolapsing into the rectum; subsequently, the intussusception descends to obstruct the anal canal, which finally becomes an external prolapse. Internal intussusception can be difficult to diagnosis during cinedefecography. McGee and Bartram (238) reported that intra-anal intussusception may be missed in 33% of patients undergoing routine defecography; furthermore, these authors claim that during defecography, the posteroanterior rectum should be screened to validate this diagnosis. Firstly, prolapse of the anal cushions and variations of fold patterns due to some degree of rectal asymmetry during its emptying may confuse interpretation. Secondly, as with rectocele, intussusception can represent a mere cinedefecographic finding or be the cause of obstructed defecation. Criteria of clinical importance includes the presence of transverse or oblique infolding of >3 mm of thickness, formed by invagination of the rectal wall and causing subsequent obstructed rectal evacuation. These findings must be interpreted in light of the clinical history. More advanced degrees of intussusception can cause rectal pain or even lead to solitary rectal ulcer syndrome; the latter is characterized by the triad of rectal discharge of blood and mucus, a lower-anterior benign rectal ulcer, and disordered defecation. Apparently, the nature of the ulcer is traumatic due to excessive straining. Defecography will demonstrate intussusception or paradoxical puborectalis syndrome in most of these patients and is therefore the method of choice to uncover its causative defecation disorder (239).

PERINEAL DESCENT SYNDROME

The "syndrome of the descending perineum" was first observed by Porter in 1962 (240) and subsequently recognized as a definite entity by Parks and colleagues in 1966 (241). This syndrome is considered as a component of a vicious cycle, involving excessive and repeated straining, protrusion of the anterior rectal wall into the anal canal, sensation of incomplete evacuation, weakness of the pelvic floor musculature, more straining and further pelvic floor weakness.

Increased dynamic perineal descent is diagnosed during defecography when, during maximal push effort, perineal descent exceeds values of 3 cm from those measured at rest, whereas increased fixed perineal descent is considered when perineal descent exceeds 4 cm at rest (70). Increased perineal descent can also be estimated during physical examination by observing of the position of the perineum during Valsalva's maneuver and by the use of a perineometer, which consists of a freely moving graduated cylinder within a steel frame positioned on the patient's ischial tuberosities. However, both methods are not physiologically appropriate as evaluation is performed with the patient in the lateral decubitus position and during feigned rather than actual expulsion of intrarectal contents.

Based on the fact that excessive perineal descent and pudendal neuropathy are commonly present in patients with defecatory disturbances, Parks et al. (241) proposed the entrapment-stretch theory in which pelvic floor descent during childbirth or secondary to chronic prolonged difficult evacuation can result in stretch injury of the pudendal nerves because they are tightly bound by connective tissue in the pudendal canal. This often espoused relationship between increased perineal descent, and pudendal neuropathy was not supported by a prospective study of 213 consecutive patients with pelvic floor disorders (73). A lack of any relationship was noted for the entire group, regardless of gender or diagnosis, as well as for those patients with either neuropathy or increased perineal descent. Although increased perineal descent and prolonged PNTML are frequently observed in patients with pelvic floor functional disorders, they may represent independent findings. Therefore, unlike abnormally prolonged pudendal nerve latency, the isolated radiographic finding of increased perineal descent should not be considered as a predictive factor of pelvic neuromuscular function.

Excessive perineal descent is a physical sign indicative of pelvic floor weakness; however, it may also merely represent one facet in a constellation of a myriad of symptoms and findings. Patients with abnormally increased perineal descent may present with rectal prolapse, partial or major incontinence, obstructed evacuation, solitary rectal ulcer syndrome, or vague symptoms of incomplete evacuation or rectal pain. Potentially surgical disorders such as large nonemptying rectocele, enterocele, or sigmoidocele may also coexist. However, there is no surgical option for isolated perineal syndrome. Symptomatic improvement may be achieved with biofeedback or an artificial device, consisting of a polycarbonate plate that is placed under the toilet seat in order to support the perineum during defecation (242). Biofeedback is still the most common therapeutic option; however, success is only approximately 50% (7).

COMBINED COLONIC INERTIA WITH OUTLET OBSTRUCTION

Failure of subtotal colectomy has been frequently attributed to concomitant paradoxical puborectalis syndrome. Therefore, if a combined pattern of colonic inertia with outlet obstruction is diagnosed, a conservative approach such as biofeedback therapy is indicated in order to first treat the outlet obstruction. After successful treatment of outlet obstruction, physiologic tests should be repeated and if colonic inertia is still confirmed, patients should be offered surgery.

NORMAL EVALUATION

Most patients with constipation and normal physiologic investigation have either irritable bowel syndrome or psychiatric disorders.

Psychiatric Disorders

The correlation between psychologic factors and constipation is a well-known fact, both in clinical practice and in the literature (36,37). Patients with the greatest psychologic problems tend to have the lowest tolerance for abdominal pain and tend to seek surgical treatment (243). Moreover, in a study using a more objective instrument, the Minnesota Multiphasic Personality Inventory, revealed significantly higher scores for the "neurotic triad" (hypochondria, depression, and hysteria) in patients with constipation, when compared to those with anal incontinence and rectal pain (244). Organic causes of constipation, however, must not be overlooked in psychiatric patients. When a psychiatric disorder is diagnosed in a patient with symptoms of constipation, there are three possibilities: (i) the patient developed both simultaneously; (ii) the presence of chronic constipation affected the patient's behavior; and (iii) the psychiatric disorder–precipitated fixation on bowel function symptoms (245). Psychological therapy includes one or more of the following methods: psychotherapy, judicious use of antidepressant and anxiolytic drugs, hypnotherapy, and behavior modification therapy (246,247).

Spinal Cord Injury

Constipation is a major problem in the management of patients with spinal cord injury. The mechanisms involved are lack of the conscious urge to defecate, body immobilization, motor paralysis of abdominal and pelvic muscles, and possible motor alterations at the colon, rectum, and anus. In most spinal cord injuries, the foregut and midgut, which are innervated by parasympathetic fibers in the vagus and sympathetic fibers from T6 to T12, remain normally innervated, whereas the hindgut, innervated by parasympathetic fibers from the sacral plexus and sympathetic fibers from the lumbar vertebrae, loses input from the cerebral and spinal cord (248). Accordingly, colonic transit times in these patients are characteristically more prolonged in the left colon and rectum (249). The loss of regulation of the anorectal reflex activity from cerebral input results in fecal impaction and incontinence. Because the rectum spontaneously evacuates its contents after stimulation by distention, these patients benefit from a bowel retraining regimen in which the defecation reflex is initiated at fixed time intervals. A high fiber diet, laxatives, suppositories, enemas, or anal digital evacuation are used as part of this retraining program. In more severe cases, a colostomy or a cecostomy with anterograde lavage may be indicated.

SUMMARY

Anorectal physiological testing does not reveal the cause in 25% to 50% of patients who complain of chronic constipation. Reasons for this include transient symptoms, misperceptions of the normal range of bowel patterns, or psychological causes of the symptoms. However, in the majority of patients, a causative diagnosis can be made by these investigations. A small group of patients may be suitable for surgical treatment, and a comprehensive physiologic investigation is crucial in order to successfully treat these challenging disorders.

REFERENCES

1. Stark ME. Challenging problems presenting as constipation. Am J Gastroenterol 1999; 94:567–574.
2. Whitehead WE, Chaussade S, Corazziari E, Kumar D. Report of an international workshop on management of constipation. Gastroenterology Intl 1991; 4:99–113.
3. Sandler RS, Drossman DA. Bowel habits in young adults not seeking for health care. Dig Dis Sci 1987; 32:841–845.
4. Ruben BD. Public perceptions of digestive health and disease. Survey findings and communications implications. Pract Gastroenterol 1986; 10:35–42.
5. Connell AM, Hilton C, Irvine G, Lennard-Jones JE, Misiewicz JJ. Variation of bowel habit in two population samples. BMJ 1965; 2:1095–1099.
6. Metcalf AM, Phillips SF, Zinsmeister AR, MacCarty RL, Beart RW, Wolff BG. Simplified assessment of segmental colonic transit time. Gastroenterology 1987; 92:40–47.
7. American Gastroenterological Association medical position statement: guidelines on constipation. Gastroenterology 2000; 119:1761–1778.
8. Sonnenberg A, Koch TR. Physician visits in the United States for constipation: 1958 to 1986. Dig Dis Sci 1989; 34:606–611.

9. Sonnenberg A, Koch TR. Epidemiology of constipation in the United States. Dis Colon Rectum 1989; 32:1–8.

10. Everhart JE, Go VLW, Johanes RS, Fitzsimmons SC, Roth HP, White LR. Dig Dis Sci 1989; 34: 1153–1162.

11. Stewart WF, Liberman JN, Sandler RS, et al. Epidemiology of Constipation Study in the United States: relation of clinical subtypes to socioeconomic features. Am J Gastroenterol 1999; 94:3530–3539.

12. Read NW, Timms JM, Barfield LJ, Donnelly TC, Bannister JJ. Impairment of defecation in young women with severe constipation. Gastroenterology 1986; 90:53–60.

13. Bannister JJ, Timms JM, Barfield LJ, Donnelly TC, Read NW. Physiological studies in young women with chronic constipation. Int J Colorect Dis 1986; 1:175–182.

14. Christofides ND, Ghatei MA, Bloom SR, Borberg C, Gillmer MDG. Decreased plasma motilin concentrations in pregnancy. Br Med J 1982; 285:1453–1454.

15. Preston DM, Rees LH, Lennard Jones JE. Gynecological disorders and hyperprolcatinemia in chronic constipation. Gut 1983; Vol. 24. A480.

16. Watier A, Devroede G, Duranceau A, et al. Constipation with colonic inertia. A manifestation of sistemic disease? Dig Dis Sci 1983; 28:1025–1033.

17. Taylor T, Smith AN, Fulton PM. Effect of hysterectomy on bowel function. Br Med J 1989, 299: 300–301.

18. Roe AM, Bartolo DC, Mortensen NJ. Slow transit constipation. Comparison between patients with or without previous hysterectomy. Dig Dis Sci 1988; 33:1159–1163.

19. Smith NA, Varma JS, Binnie NR, Papachrysostomou M. Disordered colorectal motility in intractable constipation following hysterectomy. Br J Surg 1990; 77:1361–1366.

20. Ferghaly AS, Hindmarsh JR, Worth PHL. Post-hysterectomy urethral dysfunction: evaluation and management. Br J Urol 1986; 58:299–302.

21. Long DM, Bernstein WC. Sexual dysfunction as a complication of abdomino-perineal resection of the rectum in male: an anatomic and physiologic study. Dis Colon Rectum 1959; 2:540–548.

22. Talley NJ, Fleming KC, Evans JM, et al. Constipation in an elderly community: a study of prevalence and potential risk factors. Am J Gastroenterol 1996; 91:19–25.

23. Campbell AJ, Busby WJ, Horwarth CC. Factors associated with constipation in an elderly community: a study of prevalence abd potential risk factors. Am J Gastroenterol 1996; 91:19–25.

24. Sandler RS, Jordan MC, Shelton BJ. Demographic and dietary determinants of constipation in the us population. Am J Public Health 1990; 80:185–189.

25. Whitehead WE, Drinkwater D, Cheskin LJ, Heller BR, Schuster MM. Constipation in the elderly living at home. Definition, prevalence, and relationship to lifestyle and health status. J Am Geriatr Soc 1989; 37:423–429.

26. Leroi AM, Bernier C, Watier A, et al. Prevalence of sexual abuse among patients with functional disorders of the lower gastrointestinal tract. Int J Colorectal Dis 1995; 10:200–206.

27. Kruis W, Thieme C, Weinzierl M, Schussles P, Holl J, Paulus W. A diagnosis score for irritable bowel syndrome. Its value in the exclusion of organic disease. Gastroenterology 1984; 87:1–7.

28. Agachan F, Chen T, Pfeifer J, Reissman P, Wexner SD. A constipation scoring system to simplify evaluation and management of constipated patients. Dis Colon Rectum 1996; 39:681–685.

29. Knowles CH, Eccersley AJ, Scott SM, Walker SM, Reeves B, Luniss PJ. Linear discriminant analysis of symptoms in patients with chronic constipation: validation of a new scoring system (KESS). Dis Colon Rectum 2000; 43:1419–1426.

30. Jorge JMN, Wexner SD. Etiology and management of fecal incontinence. Dis Colon Rectum 1993; 36:77–97.

31. Patriquin H, Martelli H, Devroede G. Barium enema in chronic constipation: is it meaningful? Gastroenterology 1978; 75:619–622.

32. Beck DE. Initial evaluation in constipation. In: Wexner SD, Bartolo DCC, eds. Constipation: Etiology, Evaluation and Management. Oxford: Butterworth-Heinemann, 1995:31–38.

33. Wexner SD, Jagelman DG. Chronic constipation. Postgrad Adv Colorect Surg 1989; 1:1–22.

34. Schiller LR. Review article: the therapy of constipation. Aliment Pharmacol Ther 2001; 15:749–763.

35. Devroede G. Constipation:. In: Sleisenger MH, Fordtran JS, eds. Gastrointestinal Disease: Pathophysiology, Diagnosis and Treatment. Philadephia: WB Saunders, 1989:331–368.

36. Devroede G, Girard G, Bouchoucha M, et al. Idiopathic constipation by colonic dysfunction: relationship with personality and anxiety. Dig Dis Sci 1989; 34:1428–1433.

37. Fisher SE, Breckon K, Andrews HA, Keighley MRB. Psychiatric screening for patients with faecal incontinence or chronic constipation referred for surgical treatment. Br J Surg 1989; 76: 352–355.

38. Jorge JMN, Wexner SD. A practical guide to basic anorectal physiology. Contemp Surg 1993; 43: 214–224.

39. Jorge JMN, Wexner SD. Physiologic evaluation. In: Wexner SD, Vernava AM, eds. Clinical Decision Making In Colorectal Surgery. Igaku-Shoin: New-York, 1995:11–22.

40. Rantis PC Jr., Vernava AM III, Daniel GL, Longo WE. Chronic constipation—is the work-up worth the cost? Dis Colon Rectum 1997; 40:280–286.

41. Halverson AL, Orkin BA. Which physiologic tests are useful in patients with constipation? Dis Colon Rectum 1998; 41:735–739.
42. Glia A, Lindberg G, Nilsson LH, Minocsa L, Åkerlund JE. Constipation assessed on the basis of colorectal physiology. Scand J Gastroenterol 1998; 33:1273–1279.
43. Wexner SD, Jorge JMN. Colorectal physiological tests: use or abuse of technology? Eur J Surg 1994; 160:167–174.
44. Hertz AF, Morton CJ, Cook F, et al. The passage of food along the human alimentary canal. Guys Hosp Rep 1907; 61:389–427.
45. Labayle D, Modigliani R, Matuchansky C, Rambaud JC, Bernier JJ. Diarrhee avec acceleration du transit intestinal. Gastroenterol Clin Biol 1977; 1:231–242.
46. Alvarez WC, Freedlander BL. The rate of progress of food residues through the bowel. JAMA 1924; 23:576–580.
47. Dick M. Use of cuprous thiocyanate as a short-term continuous marker for faeces. Gut 1969; 10: 408–412.
48. Kirwan WO, Smith AN. Gastrointestinal transit estimated by an isotope capsule. Scand J Gastroenterol 1974; 9:763–766.
49. Krevsky B, Malmud LS, D'ercole F, Maurer AH, Fisher RS. Colonic transit scintigraphy. A physiologic approach to the quantitative measurement of colonic transit in humans. Gastroenterology 1986; 91:1102–1112.
50. Hinton JM, Lennard-Jones JE, Young AC. A new method for studying gut transit times using radiopaque markers. Gut 1969; 10:842–847.
51. Martelli H, Devroede G, Arhan P, Duguay C, Dornic C, Faverdin C. Some parameters of large bowel motility in normal man. Gastroenterology 1978; 75:612–618.
52. Arhan P, Devroede G, Jehannin B, et al. Segmental colonic transit time. Dis Colon Rectum 1981; 24:625–629.
53. Martelli H, Devroede G, Arhan P, Duguay C. Mechanisms of idiopathic constipation: outlet obstruction. Gastroenterology 1978; 75:623–631.
54. Jorge JMN, Habr-Gama A. Tempo de transito colonico total e segmentar: analise critica dos metodos e estudo em individuos normais com marcadores radiopacos. Rev Bras Colo Proct 1991; 11: 55–60.
55. Cohen S, Vaccaro C, Kaye M, Wexner S. Can segmental colonic transit times be reproduced with reliable results? Presented as a poster. 93rd Annual Meeting of the American Society of Colon and Rectal Surgeons, Orlando, Florida, 1994.
56. Bouchoucha M, Devroede G, Arhan P, et al. What is the meaning of colorectal transit time measurement? Dis Colon Rectum 1992; 35:773–782.
57. Nam YS, Pikarsky AJ, Wexner SD, et al. Reproducibility of colonic transit study in patients with chronic constipation. Dis Colon Rectum 2001; 44:86–92.
58. Adler HF, Atkinson AJ, Ivy AC. Supplementary and synergistic action of stimulating drugs on motility of human colon. Surg Gynecol Obstet 1942; 74:809–813.
59. Kumar D, Wingate DL. Colorectal motility. In: Henry MM, Swash M, eds. Coloproctology and the Pelvic Floor. Oxford: Butterworth-Heinemann, 1992:72–85.
60. Sarna SK, Condon R, Cowles V. Colonic migrating and non-migrating motor complexes in dogs. Am J Physiol 1984; 246:G355–G360.
61. Goligher J. Surgery of the Anus, Rectum And Colon. London: BaillièreTindall, 1984:1–47; Frantzides CT. Physiology of the colon. In: Zuidema GD, ed. Shackelford's Surgery of the Alimentary Tract. Philadelphia: WB Saunders, 1991:16–21.
62. Camilleri M, Thompson G, Fleshman JW, Pemberton JH. Clinical management of intractable constipation. Ann Intern Med 1994; 121:520–528.
63. Walldén L. Defecation block in cases of deep rectogenital pouch. A surgical, roentgenological and embryological study with special reference to morphological conditions. Acta Chir Scand 1952; 165:121–122.
64. Broden B, Snellman B. Procidentia of the rectum studied with cineradiography: a contribution to the discussion of causative mechanism. Dis Colon Rectum 1968; 11:330–347.
65. Mahieu P, Pringot J, Bodart P. Defecography: I. Description of a new procedure and results in normal patients. Gastrointest Radiol 1984; 9:247–251.
66. Mahieu P, Pringot J, Bodart P. Defecography: II. Contribution to the diagnosis of defecation disorders. Gastrointest Radiol 1984; 9:253–261.
67. Bartram CI, Turnbull GK, Lennard-Jones JE. Evaluation proctography: an investigation of rectal expulsion in 20 subjects without defecatory disturbance. Gastrointest Radiol 1988; 13:72–80.
68. Ambroze WL, Pemberton JH, Bell Am, Brown ML, Zinsmeister AR. The effect of stool consistency on rectal and neorectal emptying. Dis Colon Rectum 1990; 34:1–7.
69. Jorge JMN, Wexner SD, Marchetti F, Rosato GO, Sullivan ML, Jagelman DG. How reliable are currently available methods of measuring the anorectal angle? Dis Colon Rectum 1992; 35:332–338.
70. Finlay IG, Bartolo DCC, Bartram CI, et al. Symposium: proctography. Int J Colorectal Dis 1988; 3: 67–89.
71. Hock D, Lombard R, Jehaes C, et al. Colpocystodefecography. Dis Colon Rectum 1993; 36:1015–1021.

72. Bremmer S, Ahlbäck SO, Udén R, Mellgren A. Simultaneous defecography and peritoneography in defecation disorders. Dis Colon Rectum 1995; 38:969–973.
73. Jorge JMN, Ger GC, Gonzalez L, Wexner SD. Patient position during cinedefecography. Influence on perineal descent and other measurements. Dis Colon Rectum 1994; 37:927–931.
74. Turnbull GK, Bartram CI, Lennard-Jones JE. Radiologic studies of rectal evacuation in adults with idiopathic constipation. Dis Colon Rectum 1988; 31:190–197.
75. Kamm MA, Bartram CI, Lennard-Jones. Rectodynamics-quantifying rectal evacuation. Int J Colorect Dis 1989; 4:161–163.
76. Ting KH, Mangel E, Eibl-Eibesfeldt B, Muller-Lissner SA. Is the volume retained after defecation a valuable parameter at defecography? Dis Colon Rectum 1992; 35:762–767.
77. Hutchinson R, Mostafa AB, Grant EA, et al. Scintigraphic defecography: quantitative and dynamic assessment of anorectal function. Dis Colon Rectum 1993; 36:1132–1138.
78. Coller JA. Clinical application of anorectal manometry. Gastroenterol Clin North Am 1987; 16: 17–33.
79. Jorge JMN, Wexner SD. Anorectal manometry: techniques and clinical applications. South Med J 1993; 86:924.
80. Frenckner B, Euler CV. Influence of pudendal block on the function of the anal sphincters. Gut 1975; 16:482–489.
81. Lestar B, Penninckx F, Kerremans R. The composition of anal basal pressure. An in vivo and in vitro study in man. Int J Colorect Dis 1989; 4:118–122.
82. Gibbons CP, Trowbridge EA, Bannister JJ, Read NW. Role of anal cushions in maintaining continence. Lancet 1986; 1:886–887.
83. Jorge JMN, Habr-Gama A. The value of sphincteric asymmetry index analysis in anal incontinence. Int J Colorectal Dis 2000; 15:303–310.
84. Taylor BM, Beart RW, Phillips SF. Longitudinal and radial variations of pressure in the human anal sphincter. Gastroenterology 1984; 86:693–697.
85. Braun JC, Treutner KH, Dreuw B, Klimaszewski M, Schlumpelick V. Vectormanometry for differential diagnosis of fecal incontinence. Dis Colon Rectum 1994; 37:989–996.
86. Marcello PW, Barrett RC, Coller JÁ, et al. Fatigue rate index as a new measurement of external sphincter function. Dis Colon Rectum 1998; 41:336–343.
87. Stuphen J, Borowitz S, Ling W, Cox DJ, Kovatchev B. Anorectal manometric examination in encopretic-cosntipated children. Dis Colon Rectum 1997; 40:1051–1055.
88. Ricciardi R, Counihan TC, Banner BF, Sweeney WB. What is the normal aganglionic segment of anorectum in adults? Dis Colon Rectum 1999; 42:380–382.
89. Beck A. Electromyographische untersuchungen am sphinkter ani. Arch Physiologie 1930; 224: 278–292.
90. Wexner SD, Marchetti F, Salanga VD, Corredor C, Jagelman DG. Neurophysiologic assessment of the anal sphincters. Dis Colon Rectum 1991; 34:606–612.
91. Stalberg E, Trontelj J. Single fibre electromyography. In: Mirvalle Press Ltd. Old Walking, Surrey. U.K.: Mirvalle, 1979:69.
92. Rosato GO, Miguel MA. Anal sphincter electromyography and pudendal nerve terminal motor latency. Sem Colon Rectal Surg 1992; 3:68–74.
93. Binnie NR, Kawimbe BM, Papachrysostomou M, Clare N, Smith AN. The importance of the orientation of the electrode plates in recording the external anal sphincter EMG by non-invasive anal plug electrodes. Int J Colorect Dis 1991; 6:5–8.
94. Jorge JMN, Wexner SD, Ger GC, Jagelman DG. Cinedefecography and EMG in the diagnosis of non-relaxing puborectalis syndrome. Dis Colon Rectum 1993; 36:668.
95. Kiff ES, Swash M. Normal proximal and delayed distal conduction in the pudendal nerves of patients with idiopathic (neurogenic) faecal incontinence. J Neurol Neurosurg Psych 1984; 47:820–823.
96. Snooks SJ, Swash M. Nerve stimulation techniques. In: Henry MM, Swash M, eds. Coloproctology and the Pelvic Floor. London: Butterworth-Heinemann, 1985:112–128.
97. Laurberg S, Swash M, Henry MM. Delayed external sphincter repair for obstetric tear. Br J Surg 1988; 75:786–788.
98. Wexner SD, Marchetti F, Jagelman DG. The role of sphincteroplasty for fecal incontinence reevaluated: a prospective physiologic and functional review. Dis Colon Rectum 1991; 34:22.
99. Jones PN, Lubowski DZ, Swash M, Henry MM. Relation between perineal descent and pudendal nerve damage in idiopathic faecal incontinence. Int J Colorect Dis 1987; 2:93–95.
100. Kiff E, Barnes PH, Swash M. Evidence of pudendal neuropathy in patients with perineal descent and chronic straining at stool. Gut 1984; 25:1279–1282.
101. Parks AG, Swash M, Urich H. Sphincter denervation in anorectal incontinence and rectal prolapse. Gut 1977; 18:656–665.
102. Snooks SJ, Swash M, Mathers SE, Henry MM. Effect of vaginal delivery on the pelvic floor: 5-year follow-up. Br J Surg 1990; 77:1358–1360.
103. Jorge JMN, Wexner SD, Ehrenpreis ED, Noqueras JJ, Jagelman DG. Does perineal descent correlate with pudendal neuropathy? Dis Colon Rectum 1993; 36:475–483.
104. Kim SK. Small intestine transit time in the normal small bowel study. Am J Radiol 1968; 104:522–524.

105. Read NW, Al-Janabi MN, Edwards CA, Barber DC. Relationship between postprandial motor activity in the human small intestine and the gastrointestinal transit of food. Gastroenterology 1980; 79:1276–1282.

106. Caride VJ, Prokop EK, Troncale FJ, Buddoura W, Winchenbach K, McCallum RW. Scintigraphic determination of small intestinal transit time: comparison with the hydrogen breath technique. Gastroenterology 1984; 86:714–720.

107. Bond JH, Levitt MD. Investigation of small bowel transit time in man utilizing pulmonary hydrogen (H2) measurements. J Lab Clin Med 1975; 85:546–555.

108. Bond JH, Levitt MD. Effect of dietary fiber on intestinal gas production and small bowel transit time in man. Am J Clin Nutr 1978; 31:S169–S174.

109. Staniforth DH, Rose D. Statistical analysis of the lactulose/breath hydrogen test in the measurement of orocaecal transit: its variability and predictive value in assessing drug action. Gut 1989; 30: 171–175.

110. Jorge JMN, Wexner SD, Ehrenpreis ED. The lactulose hydrogen breath test as a measure of orocaecal transit time. Eur J Surg 1994; 160:409–416.

111. La Brooy SJ, Male PJ, Beavis AK, Misiewicz JJ. Assessment of the reproducibility of the lactulose H2 breath test as a measure of mouth to caecum transit time. Gut 1983; 24:893–896.

112. Krishnamurthy S, Schuffler MD, Rohrmann CA, Pope CE II. Severe idiopathic constipation is associated with a distinctive abnormality of the colonic myenteric plexus. Gastroenterology 1985; 88:26–34.

113. Vasilevsky CA, Nemer FD, Balcos EG, Christenson CE, Goldberg SM. Is subtotal colectomy a viable option in the management of chronic constipation? Dis Colon Rectum 1988; 31:679–681.

114. Marzio L, Del Bianco R, Donne MD, Pieramico O, Cuccurullo F. Mouth-to-cecum transit time in patients affected by chronic constipation: effect of glucomannan. Am J Gastroenterol 1989; 84:888–991.

115. King CE, Toskes PP. Comparison of the 1 gram [14C] xylose, 10 gram lactulose–H2, and 80 gram glucose–H2 breath tests in patients with small intestine bacterial overgrowth. Gastroenterology 1986; 91:1447–1451.

116. Bjorneklett A, Jensen E. Relationship between hydrogen H2 and Methane CH4 production in man. Scand J Gastroenterol 1983; 17:985–992.

117. Gilat T, Ben Hur H, Gelman-malachi E, Terdiman R, Peled Y. Alterations of the colonic flora and their effect on the hydrogen breath test. Gut 1981; 19:602–605.

118. Read NW, Cmamack J, Edward C, Holgate AM, Cann PA, Brown C. Is the transit time of a meal through the small bowel related to the rate at which it leaves the stomach? Gut 1982; 23:824–828.

119. Schouten WR, Gordon PH. Constipation. In: Gordon PH, Nivatvongs S, eds. Principles and Practice Of Surgery For The Colon, Rectum and Anus. St. Louis: Missouri: Quality Medical Publishing, Inc. 1999:1181–1231.

120. Badiali D, Corazziari E. Use of low dose polyethylene glycol solutions in the treatment of functional constipation. Ital J Gastroenterol Hepatol 1999; 31(Suppl 3):S253–S254.

121. DiPalma JA, DeRidder PH, Orlando RC, Kolts BE, Cleveland MBA. Randomized placebo-controlled, multicenter study of the safety and efficacy of a new polyethylene glycol laxative. Am J Gastroenterol 2000; 95:446–450.

122. Baker EH, Sandle GI. Complications of laxative abuse. Annu Rev Med 1996; 47:127–134.

123. Balazs M. Melanosis coli: ultrastructural study of 45 patients. Dis Colon Rectum 1986; 29:839–844.

124. Van Gorkom BA, Karrenbeld A, Van Der Sluis T, Koudstaal J, De Vries EG, Kleibeuker JH. Influence of a highly purified senna extract on colonic epithelium. Digestion 2000; 61:113–120.

125. Nusgo G, Schneider B, Schneider I, Wittekind C, Hahn EG. Antranoid laxative use is not a risk for colorectal neoplasia: results of a case control study. Gut 2000; 46:651–656.

126. Mascolo B, Mereto E, Borrelli F, et al. Does senna extract promote growth of aberrant crypt foci and malignant tumors in rat colon? Dig Dis Sci 1999; 44:2226–2230.

127. Muller-Lissner S. What has happened to the cathartic colon? Gut 1996; 39:486–488.

128. Wald A. Is chronic use of stimulant laxatives harmful to the colon? J Clin Gastroenterol 2003; 36: 386–389.

129. Van Gorkom BA, De Vries EG, Karrenbeld A, Kleibeuker JH. Review article: anthranoid laxatives and their potential carcinogenic effects. Aliment Pharmacol Ther 1999; 13:443–452.

130. Longo WE, Vernava AM III. Prokinetic agents for lower gastrointestinal motility disorders. Dis Colon Rectum 1993; 36:696–708.

131. Everett HC. The use of bethanecol chloride with tricyclic antidepressants. Am J Psychiatry 1975; 132:1202–1204.

132. Ponec RJ, Saunders MD, Kimmey MB. Neostigmine for the treatment of acute colonic pseudo-obstruction. N Engl J Med 1999; 341:137–141.

133. Paran H, Silverberg D, Mayo A, Schwartz I, Neufeld D, Freund U. Treatment of acute colonic pseudo-obstruction with neostigmine. J Am Coll Surg 2000; 190:315–318.

134. Van Daele L, DeCuypere A, Van Kerckhove M. Routine radiological follow-through examination shows effect of cisapride on gastrointestinal transit: a controlled study. Curr Ther Res 1984; 36: 1038–1044.

135. Nurko S, Garcia-Aranda JA, Worona LB, Zlochisty O. Cisapride for the treatment of constipation in children: a double-blind study. J Pediatr 2000; 136:35–40.

136. Muller-Lissner AS, The Bavarian Constipation Study Group. Treatment of chronic constipation with cisapride and placebo. Gut 1987; 28:1033–1038.

137. Krevsky B, Maurer AH, Malmud LS, Fisher RS. Cisapride accelerates colonic transit in constipated patients with colonic inertia. Am J Gastroenterology 1989; 84:882–887.

138. Ehrenpreis ED, Jorge JMN, Wexner SD, et al. Cisapride: an open label trial in patients with colonic inertia. Coloproctology 1995; 17:258–262.

139. Walker AM, Szneke P, Weatherby LB, et al. The risk of serious cardiac arrhytmias among cisapride users in the United Kingdon and Canada. Am J Med 1999; 107:356–362.

140. Poen AC, Felt-Berma RJ, Dongen PA, Meuwissen SG. Effect of prucalopride, a new enterokinetic agent, on gastrointestinal transit and anorectal function in healthy volunteers. Aliment Pharmacol Ther 1999; 13:1493–1497.

141. Sloots CEJ, Poen AC, Kerstens R, et al. Effects of prucalopride on colonic transit, anorectal function and bowel habits in patients with chronic constipation. Aliment Pharmacol Ther 2002; 16:759–767.

142. Prather CM, Camilleri M, Burton DD, McKinzie S, Thamforde G. Tegaserod accelerates orocecal transit in patients with constipation-predominant irritable bowel syndrome. Gastroenterology 2000; 118:463–468.

143. Armstrong DN, Ballantye GH, Modlin IM. Erythromycin for reflex ileus in Ogilvie's syndrome. Lancet 1991; 337:378.

144. Verne GN, Davis RH, Robinson ME, Gordon JM, Eaker EY, Sninksy CA. Treatment of chronic constipation with colchicine: randomized, double–blind, placebo-controlled, crossover trial. Am J Gastroenterol 2003; 98:1112–1116.

145. Wexner SD, Daniel N, Jagelman DG. Colectomy for constipation: physiologic investigation is the key to success. Dis Colon Rectum 1991; 34:851–856.

146. Lane WA. The results of operative treatment of chronic constipation. BMJ 1908; 1:1125–1128.

147. Smith B. Effect of irritant purgatives on the myenteric plexux in man and the mouse. Gut 1968; 9:139–143.

148. Wedel T, Roblick UJ, Ott V, et al. Oligoneuronal hypoganglionosis in patients with idiopathic slow-transit constipation. Dis Colon Rectum 2002; 45:54–62.

149. Meier-Ruge WA, Bronnimann PB, Gambazzi F, Schmid PC, Schmidt CP, Stoss F. Histopathological criteria for intestinal neuronal dysplasia of the submucosal plexus (type B). Virchows Arch 1995; 426:549–556.

150. Lincoln J, Crowe R, Kamm MA, Burnstock G, Lennard-Jones JE. Serotonin and 5-hydroxyindoleacetic acid are increased in the sigmoid colon in severe idiopathic constipation. Gastroenterology 1990; 98:1219–1225.

151. Cortesini C, Cianchi F, Infantino A, Lise M. Nitric oxide synthase and VIP distribution in enteric nervous system in idiopathic chronic constipation. Dig Dis Sci 1995; 40:2450–2455.

152. Van Der Sijp JR, Kamm MA, Nightingale JM, et al. Circulating gastrointestinal hormone abnormalities in patients with severe idiopathic constipation. Am J Gastroenterol 1998; 93:1351–1356.

153. Schouten WR, ten Kate FJ, de Graaf EJ, Gilberts EC, Simons JL, Kluck P. Visceral neuropathy in slow transit constipation: an immunohistochemical investigation with monoclonal antibodies against neurofilament. Dis Colon Rectum 1993; 36:1112–1117.

154. Park HJ, Kamm MA, Abbasi AM, Talbot IC. Immunohistochemical study of the colonic muscle and innervation in idiopathic chronic constipation. Dis Colon Rectum 1995; 38:509–513.

155. Barnes PR, Lennard-Jones JE, Hawley PR, Todd IP. Hirschsprung's disease and idiopathic megacolon in adults and adolescents. Gut 1986; 27:534–541.

156. Walsh PV, Peebles-Brown DA, Watkinson G. Colectomy for slow transit constipation. Ann R Coll Surg Engl 1987; 69:71–75.

157. Yoshioka K, Keighley MR. Clinical results of colectomy for severe constipation. Br J Surg 1989; 76:600–604.

158. Zenilman ME, Dunnegan DL, Sopen NJ, Becker JM. Successful surgical treatment of idiopathic colonic dymotility. The role of preoperative evaluation of coloanal motor function. Arch Surg 1989; 124:947–951.

159. Pemberton JH, Rath DM, Ilstrup DM. Evaluation and surgical treatment of severe chronic constipation. Ann Surg 1991; 214:403–413.

160. Mahendrarajah K, Van der Schaff A, Lovegrove FT, Mendelson R, Levitt MD. Surgery for severe constipation: the use of a radioisotope transit scan and barium evacuation proctography in patient selection. Aust N Z J Surg 1994; 64:183–186.

161. Piccirilo MF, Reissman P, Wexner SD. Colectomy as a treatment for constipation in selected cases. Br J Surg 1995; 82:898–901.

162. Redmond JM, Smith GW, Barofsky I, Ratych RE, Goldsborough DC, Schuster M. Physiological tests to predict long-term outcome of total abdominal colectomy for intractable constipation. Am J Gastroenterol 1995; 90:748–753.

163. Pikarsky AJ, Singh JJ, Weiss EG, Nogueras JJ, Wexner SD. Long-term follow-up of patients undergoing colectomy for colonic inertia. Dis Colon Rectum 2001; 44:179–183.

164. Mollen RM, Kuijpers HC, Claasen AT. Colectomy for slow transit constipation: preoperative functional evaluation is important but not a guarantee for a successful outcome. Dis Colon Rectum 2001; 44:577–580.

165. Glia A, Akerlund JE, Lindberg G. Outcome of colectomy for slow-transit constipation in relation to presence of small-bowel dysmotility. Dis Colon Rectum 2004; 47:96–102.
166. Pfeifer J, Agachan F, Wexner SD. Surgery for constipation: a review. Dis Colon Rectum 1996; 39: 444–460.
167. Lane RH, Todd IP. Idiopathic megacolon: a review of 42 cases. Br J Surg 1977; 64:305–310.
168. McCready RA, Beart RW Jr. The surgical treatment of incapacitating constipation associated with idiopathic megacolon. Mayo Clin Proc 1979; 54:779–783.
169. Belliveau P, Goldberg SM, Rothengerger DA, Nivatvongs S. Idiopathic acquired megacolon: the value of subtotal colectomy. Dis Colon Rectum 1982; 25:118–121.
170. Kamm MA, Van der Sijp JR, Hawley PR, Phillips RK, Lennard-Jones JE. Left hemicolectomy with rectal excision for severe idiopathic constipation. Int J Colorectal Dis 1991; 6:49–51.
171. Fasth S, Hedlund H, Svaninger G, Öresland T, Hulten L. Functional results after subtotal colectomy and caecorectal anastomosis. Acta Chir Scand 1983; 149:623–627.
172. Preston DM, Hawley PR, Lennard Jones JE, Todd IP. Results of colectomy for severe idiopathic constipation in women. Br J Surg 1984; 71:547–552.
173. Nicholls RJ, Kamm MA. Proctocolectomy with restorative ileoanal reservoir for severe idiopathic constipation: report of two cases. Dis Colon Rectum 1988; 31:968–969.
174. Hosie KB, Kmiot WA, Keighley. Constipation: another indication for restorative proctocolectomy. Br J Surg 1990; 77:801–802.
175. William NS, Hughes SF, Stuchfield B. Continent colonic conduit for rectal evacuation in severe constipation. Lancet 1994; 343:1321–1324.
176. Rongen MJ, van der Hoop AG, Baeten CG. Cecal access for antegrade colon enemas in medically refractory slow transit constipation: a prospective study. Dis Colon Rectum 2001; 44:1644–1649.
177. Hamdy MH, Scobie WG. Anorectal myectomy in adult Hirschsprung's disease: a report of six cases. Br J Surg 1984; 71:611–613.
178. Fishbein RH, Handelsman JC, Schuster MM. Surgical treatment of hirschsprung's disease in adults. Surg Gynecol Obstet 1986; 163:458–464.
179. Elliot MS, Todd IP. Adult Hirschsprung's disease: results of the Duhamel procedure. Br J Surg 1985; 72:884–885.
180. Luukkonen P, Heikkinen M, Huikuri K, Jarvinen H. Adult's Hirschsprung's disease: clinical features and functional outcome after surgery. Dis Colon Rectum 1990; 33:65–69.
181. Wheatley MJ, Wesley JR, Coran AG, Polley TZ Jr. Hirschsprung's disease in adolescents and adults. Dis Colon Rectum 1990; 33:622–629.
182. Habr-Gama A, Raia A, Netto AC. Motility of the sigmoid colon and rectum: contribution to the physiopathology of megacolon in Chagas' disease. Dis Colon Rectum 1971; 14:291–304.
183. Jorge JMN, Habr-Gama A, Yusuf AS, Bocchini SF, Araujo SE. Physiologic investigation of constipated patients with Chagas' disease. Colorectal Dis 2001; 3:86.
184. Bjornland K, Diseth TH, Emblem R. Long-term functional, manometric, and ensosonographic evaluation of patients operated upon with the Duhamel technique. Pediatr Surg Int 1998; 13:24–28.
185. Habr-Gama Kiss DR, Bocchini SF, Teixeira MG, Pinotti HW. Megacolon chagásico: tratamento pela retossigmoidectomia abdominal com anastomose mecânica término-lateral-resultados preliminares. Rev Hosp Clin Fac Med Sao Paulo 1994; 49:199–203.
186. Meier-Ruge W. Epidemiology of congenital innervation defects of the distal colon. Virchows Archiv A Pathol Anat 1992; 420:171–177.
187. Stoss F, Meier-Ruge W. Experience with neuronal intestinal dysplasis (NID) in adults. Eur J Pediatr 1994; 4:298–302.
188. Loening-Baucke V. Biofeedback treatment for chronic constipation and encopresis in childhood: long term outcome. Pediatrics 1995; 96:105–110.
189. Van der Plas RN, Benninga MA, Redekop WK, Taminiau JA, Buller HA. Randomised trial of biofeedback training for encopresis. Arch Dis Child 1996; 75:367–374.
190. Varma JS, Bradnock J, Smith RG, Smith NA. Constipation in the elderly. A physiologic study. Dis Colon Rectum 1988; 31:111–115.
191. Hughes ES, McDermott FT, Johnson WR, Polglase AC. Surgery for constipation. Aust N Z J Surg 1981; 51:144–148.
192. Coremans GE. Surgical aspects of severe chronic non-Hirschsprung constipation. Hepatogastroenterology 1990; 37:588–595.
193. Stabile G, Kamm MA, Hawley PR, Lennard-Jones JE. Colectomy for idiopathic megarectum and megacolon. Gut 1991; 32:1538–1540.
194. Wasserman IF. Puborectalis syndrome (rectal stenosis due to anorectal spasm). Dis Colon Rectum 1964; 7:87–98.
195. Wexner SD, Cheape JD, Jorge JMN, Heymen S, Jagelman DG. Prospective assessment of biofeedback for the treatment of paradoxical puborectalis contraction. Dis Colon Rectum 1992; 35: 145–150.
196. Lestàr B, Penninckx F, Kerremans R. Biofeedback defaecation training for anismus. Int J Colorect Dis 1991; 6:202–207.

197. Wallace WC, Madden WM. Experience with partial resection of the puborectalis muscle. Dis Colon rectum 1969; 12:196–200.
198. Yoshioka K, Keighley MR. Anorectal myectomy for outlet obstruction. Br J Surg 1987; 74:373–376.
199. Keighley MR. Surgery for constipation. Br J Surg 1988; 75:625–626.
200. Barnes PR, Hawley PR, Presto DM, Lennard-Jones JE. Experience of posterior division of the puborectalis muscle in the management of chronic constipation. Br J Surg 1985; 72:475–477.
201. Hallan RI, Williams NS, Melling J, Waldron DJ, Womack NR, Morrison JF. Treatment of anismus in intractable constipation with botulinum A toxin. Lancet 1988; 2:714–717.
202. Maria G, Brisinda G, Bentivoglio AR, Cassetta E, Albanese A. Botulinum toxin in the treatment of outlet obstruction constipation caused by puborectalis syndrome. Dis Colon Rectum 2000; 43: 376–380.
203. Ron Y, Avni Y, Lukovetski A, et al. Botulinum toxin type-a in therapy of patients with anismus. Dis Colon Recum 2001; 44:1821–1826.
204. Rieger NA, Wattchow DA, Sarre RG, et al. Prospective study of biofeedback for treatment of constipation. Dis Colon Rectum 1997; 40:1143–1148.
205. Jorge JMN, Habr-Gama A, Wexner SD. Biofeedback therapy in the colon and rectal practice. Appl Psychophysiol Biofeedback 2003; 28:47–61.
206. Turnbull GK, Ritvo PG. Anal sphincter biofeedback relaxation treatment for women with intractable constipation symptoms. Dis Colon Rectum 1992; 35:530–536.
207. Leroi AM, Duval V, Roussignol C, Berkelmans I, Peninque P, Denis P. Biofeedback for anismus in 15 sexually abused women. Int J Colorectal Dis 1996; 11:187–190.
208. Miner PB, Donelly TC, Read NW. Investigation of mode of action of biofeedback in treatment of fecal incontinence. Dig Dis Sci 1990; 35:1291–1298.
209. Brodén G, Dolk A, Frostell C, Nilsson B, Holmstrom B. Voluntary relaxation of the external anal sphincter. Dis Colon Rectum 1989; 32:376–378.
210. Dolk A, Holmstrom B, Johansson C, Frostell C, Nilsson BY. The effect of yoga on puborectalis paradox. Int J Colorect Dis 1991; 6:139–142.
211. Gilliland R, Heymen S, Altomare DF, Park UC, Vickers D, Wexner SD. Outcome and predictors of success of biofeedback for constipation. Br J Surg 1997; 84:1123–1126.
212. Beninga MA, Buller HA, Taminiau JAA. Biofeedback training in chronic constipation. Arch Dis Child 1993; 68:126–129.
213. Karlbom U, Hallden M, Eeg-Olofsson KE, Pahlman L, Graf W. Results of biofeedback in constipated patients: a prospective study. Dis Colon Rectum 1997; 40:1149–1155.
214. Park UC, Choi SK, Piccirillo MF, Verzaro R, Wexner SD. Patterns of anismus and the relation to biofeedback therapy. Dis Colon Rectum 1996; 39:768–773.
215. Weber J, Ducrotte Ph, Touchais JY, Roussignol C, Denis PH. Biofeedback training for constipation in adults and children. Dis Colon Rectum 1987; 30:844–846.
216. Siproudhis L, Dautreme S, Ropert A, et al. Anismus in biofeedback: who benefits? Eur J Gastroenterol Hepatol 1995; 7:547–552.
217. Bleijenberg G, Kuijpers HC. Treatment of spastic pelvic floor syndrome with biofeedback. Dis Colon Rectum 1987; 30:108–111.
218. Fleshman JW, Dreznik Z, Meyer K, Fry RD, Carney R, Kodner IJ. Outpatient protocol for biofeedback therapy of pelvic floor outlet obstruction. Dis Colon Rectum 1992; 35:1–7.
219. Glia A, Gylin M, Gullberg K, Lindberg G. Biofeedback retraining in patients with functional constipation and paradoxical puborectalis contraction: comparison of anal manometry and sphincter electromyography for feedback. Dis Colon Rectum 1997; 40:889–895.
220. Dahl J, Lindquist BL, Tysk C, Leissner P, Philipson L, Jarnerot G. Behavioral medicine treatment in chronic constipation with paradoxical anal sphincter contraction. Dis Colon Rectum 1991; 34: 769–776.
221. Ko CY, Tong J, Lehman RE, Shelton AA, Schrock TR, Welton ML. Biofeedback is effective therapy for fecal incontinence and constipation. Arch Surg 1997; 132:829–834.
222. Heymen S, Jones KR, Scarlett Y, Whitehead WE. Biofeedback treatment of constipation: a critical review. Dis Colon Rectum 2003; 46:1208–1217.
223. Van Dam JH, Ginai AZ, Gosselink MJ, et al. Role of defecography in predicting clinical outcome of rectocele repair. Dis Colon Rectum 1997; 40:201–207.
224. Capps WF Jr. Rectoplasty and perineoplasty for the symptomatic rectocele: a report of fifty cases. Dis Colon Rectum 1975; 18:237–243.
225. Marks MM. The rectal side of the rectocele. Dis Colon Rectum 1967; 10:287–288.
226. Sehapayak S. Transrectal repair of rectocele: an extended armamentarium of colorectal surgeons: a report of 355 cases. Dis Colon Rectum 1985; 28:422–433.
227. Sullivan ES, Laeverton GH, Hardwick CE. Transrectal perineal repair: na adjunct to improve function after anorectal surgery. Dis Colon Rectum 1968; 11:106–114.
228. Mellgren A, Anzen B, Nilson B-Y, et al. Results of rectocele repair: a prospective study. Dis Colon Rectum 1995; 38:7–13.
229. Janssen LW, van Dijke CF. Selection criteria for anterior rectal wall repair in symptomatic rectocele and anterior rectal wall prolapse. Dis Colon Rectum 1994; 37:1100–1107.

230. Johansson C, Nilsson BY, Holmstrom B, Dolk A, Mellgren A. Association between rectocele and paradoxical sphincter response. Dis Colon Rectum 1992; 35:503–509.
231. Hawksworth W, Roux JP. Vaginal hysterectomy. J Obstet Gynecol 1958; 63:214–228.
232. Karaus M, Neuhaus P, Wiedenmann B. Diagnosis of enteroceles by dynamic anorectal endosonography. Dis Colon Rectum 2000; 43:1683–1688.
233. Lienemann A, Anthuber C, Baron A, Reiser M. Diagnosing enteroceles using dynamic magnetic resonance imaging. Dis Colon Rectum 2000; 43:205–213.
234. Rentsch M, Paetzel CH, Lenhart M, Feuerbach S, Jauch KW, Fürst A. Dynamic magnetic resonance imaging defecography: a diagnostic alternative in the assessment of pelvic disorders in proctology. Dis Colon Rectum 2001; 44:999–1007.
235. Matsuoka H, Wexner SD, Desai MB, et al. A comparison between dynamic pelvic resonance imaging and videoproctography in patients with constipation. Dis Colon Rectum 2001; 44:571–576.
236. Jorge JMN, Yang Y-K, Wexner SD. Incidence and clinical significance of sigmoidoceles as determined by a new classification system. Dis Colon Rectum 1994; 37:1112–1117.
237. Gosselink MJ, Van Dam JH, Huisman WM, Ginai AZ, Schouten WR.s. Treatment of enterocele by obliteration of the pelvic inlet. Dis Colon Rectum 1999; 42:940–944.
238. McGee SG, Bartram CI. Intra-anal intussusception: diagnosis by posteroanterior stress proctography. Abdom Imaging 1993; 18:136–140.
239. Kerremans R. Radio-cinematographic examination of the rectum and the anal canal in cases of rectal constipation. A radio-cinematographic and physical explanation of dyschezia. Acta Gastroent Belg 1968; 31:561–570.
240. Porter NH. A physiological study of the pelvic floor in rectal prolapse. Ann Roy Coll Surg 1962; 31:379–404.
241. Parks AG, Porter NH, Hardcastle J. The syndrome of the descending perineum. Proc Roy Soc Med 1966; 59:477–482.
242. Lesaffer LPA. Perineal support device. In: Smith LE, ed. Practicel Guide to Anorectal Testing. New York: Igaku-Shoin, 1990:205–208.
243. Kamm MA. Role of surgical treatment in patients with severe constipation. Ann Med 1990; 22:435–444.
244. Heymen S, Wexner SD, Gulledge AD. MMPI assessment of patients with functional bowel disorders. Dis Colon Rectum 1993; 36:593–596.
245. Creed F, Guthrie E. Psychological factors in the irritable bowel syndrome. Gut 1987; 28:1307–1318.
246. Pace F, Coremans G, Dapoigny M, et al. Therapy of irritable bowel syndrome—an overview. Digestion 1995; 56:433–442.
247. Whitehead WE, Crowell MD. Psychologic considerations in irritable bowel syndrome. Gastroenterol Clin North Am 1991; 20:249–267.
248. Longo WE, Ballantyne GH, Modlin IM. The colon anorectum and spinal cord patient. A review of the functional alterations of the denervated hindgut. Dis Colon Rectum 1989; 32:261–267.
249. Menardo G, Bausano G, Corazziari E, et al. Large-bowel transit in paraplegic patients. Dis Colon Rectum 1987; 30:924–928.

6 | Colonoscopy

John K. DiBaise
*Division of Gastroenterology and Hepatology, Mayo Clinic Scottsdale, Scottsdale,
Arizona, U.S.A.*

Jon S. Thompson
Department of Surgery, University of Nebraska Medical Center, Omaha, Nebraska, U.S.A.

INTRODUCTION

The development of a means to accurately and safely visualize the entire colon endoscopically
has revolutionized the diagnosis and management of colonic diseases and, indeed, the clinical
practice of gastroenterologists and colorectal surgeons alike. While instruments to examine
the anus and rectum had been available since antiquity, it was not until the advent of flexible
fiberoptic technology in the late 1950s that total colonoscopy became more than a dream (1).
The adaptation of fiberoptics to the colon was more difficult compared to esophagogastroduodenoscopy due to the tortuous colonic lumen. Nevertheless, the first commercially available
fiberoptic colonoscope, developed by Overholt, appeared in the late 1960s (2). The early acceptance of colonoscopy into clinical practice was slow because of limited tip deflection and field
of view, unfamiliarity with the technique, and reluctance to use sedation and analgesia to
reduce patient discomfort. Subsequent advances in instrument development and colonoscopy
technique in the 1970s and the demonstration of safe colonoscopic biopsy and snare polypectomy (3) led to more widespread application of colonoscopy by clinicians. Further advances
in colonoscope development, techniques for instrument manipulation, incorporation of
other diagnostic and therapeutic applications of colonoscopy, and the development of more
effective and tolerable means of bowel preparation and patient sedation have currently made
colonoscopy the primary method of imaging the colon. Indeed, with recent guidelines and
recommendations endorsing colonoscopy as a screening option for colorectal cancer (4–6),
the demand for colonoscopy is likely to increase substantially. While the feasibility of this
strategy remains problematic due to concerns of the high demand for colonoscopy and an
inadequate number of colonoscopists and infrastructure (7), it also highlights the importance
of fully trained, competent colonoscopists.

    In this chapter, the principles of the technique of colonoscopy will be reviewed, as will
the major indications for its use. The intent is not to serve as a comprehensive guide to the
colonoscopist. For this, other excellent sources are available (8,9), including specific discussions elsewhere in this textbook.

COLON EMBRYOLOGY AND ENDOSCOPIC ANATOMY

To facilitate learning of colonoscopy technique, a basic understanding of colonic embryology
and endoscopic anatomy is important, and is discussed in greater detail elsewhere (10), as well
as in Chapter 1 of this book. Briefly, the fetal intestine and colon lengthen into a U shape and
rotate on a longitudinal mesentery within an umbilical hernia outside the abdominal cavity,
from about five weeks to three months of gestation. By the third month of development,
the small and large intestine return to the peritoneal cavity with the result that the colon is
rotated such that the cecum lies in the right upper quadrant and the descending colon on
the left side of the abdomen. With further elongation, the cecum migrates inferiorly to the right

iliac fossa. At this point, the mesentery of the transverse colon is free but the mesenteries of the descending and ascending colon fuse against the posterior abdominal wall so that the ascending and descending colon become retroperitoneal.

Incomplete fusion of the mesocolon and posterior abdominal wall may occur, resulting in a variable amount of original mesocolon remaining and, thus, in variable degrees of mobility of the right and left colon. A persistent descending mesocolon may be present in up to 36% of the population—a finding that may explain many of the strange configurations caused by the colonoscope in the left colon and splenic flexure regions.

The colonic mucosa is smooth and shiny and displays a fine vascular pattern that is composed of parallel pairs of vessels comprising a venule and an arteriole. The vessel pattern visualized colonoscopically depends upon the transparency of the mucosa as the vessels run in the submucosa. Decreased visualization of these vessels, for example, is an early sign of mucosal edema. There is a wide range of size of normal submucosal vessels; unless the vessels are extraordinarily tortuous or serpentine, they should not generally be thought of as abnormal. The colonic musculature develops as three fused external longitudinal muscle bundles or teniae coli, arranged roughly 120° apart, and within these lie the circular muscle fibers. The teniae coli, which bulge visibly into the ascending and transverse colon, are less evident in the left colon due to their thicker muscular layer; haustral folds segment the lumen of the colon.

The anatomic anal canal is about 3 cm in length, ends at the squamocolumnar junction or dentate line, and is lined by squamous epithelium. The surgical anal canal extends from the anal verge to the anorectal ring, the palpable upper border of the anal sphincter complex, about 1 to 2 cm above the dentate line. Sensory innervation to the anus may extend a few centimeters into the distal rectum. Around the anal canal are the internal and external anal sphincters. The rectum extends about 15 cm proximal to the dentate line. Three or more prominent folds (valves of Houston) may create blind spots for endoscopists (Fig. 1). A prominent mucosal vascular pattern is typically seen in the rectum. The rectum is extraperitoneal for its distal 10 cm; proximal to this, it enters the peritoneal cavity.

While the sigmoid colon may stretch up to 70 cm during insertion of the colonoscope, it is generally only 30 to 35 cm long when the instrument is fully straightened. This point underscores the importance of inspection during both insertion and withdrawal of the colonoscope in this region. The teniae coli are less evident in the left colon, giving this segment a circular appearance (Fig. 2). The sigmoid colon loops anteriorly and then passes up into the left paravertebral gutter. An understanding of the spiral loops that can develop during colonoscope insertion through the sigmoid colon forms the basis for the rotational movements and other techniques used to successfully negotiate this area while causing the least amount of discomfort to the patient.

The descending colon is generally fixed retroperitoneally and runs in a straight line for about 20 cm, making it easy to traverse its length quickly with the colonoscope. The descending colon joins the sigmoid colon at an acute bend, however, which can be very difficult to

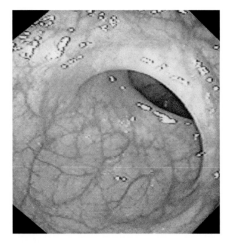

Figure 1 Prominent rectal folds, also referred to as valves of Houston, may present "blind spots" for the endoscopist. Note also the typical colonic mucosal vascular pattern.

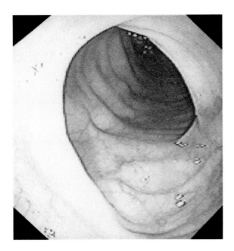

Figure 2 The semilunar folds, characteristic of the sigmoid colon, give this segment a circular appearance and are responsible for its tortuous path.

negotiate for the endoscopist. Occasionally, when the sigmoid colon is long, an alpha loop, which is in essence an iatrogenic volvulus, occurs. This helps avoid the angulation at the sigmoid-descending junction. The formation of the alpha loop depends upon the anatomical fact that the base of the sigmoid mesocolon, on its short inverted "V" at the pelvic brim, allows easy rotation. One clue to endoscopic localization within the descending colon occurs when a large-volume, fluid-electrolyte bowel preparation has been used. When in the left lateral decubitus position, the descending colon is often fluid filled, while the sigmoid colon and transverse colon are not.

Upon passing the splenic flexure, which is commonly identified by the endoscopic visualization of a bluish splenic "shadow," the transverse colon is usually easily identified by the characteristic triangular outline resulting from the relative thickness of the three longitudinal teniae coli that act as tethers for air distribution compared to the circular muscle layer (Fig. 3). The transverse mesocolon, which originates from the posterior abdominal wall, varies considerably in length, resulting in a transverse loop of varying length. Women seem to have a longer transverse loop compared to men. This longer transverse colon length, despite the smaller stature of women, may contribute to the increased difficulty colonoscopists occasionally encounter in women. The localization of the hepatic flexure is usually readily apparent by the presence of a bluish hue resulting from the proximity of the liver surface to the colon (Fig. 4). The hepatic flexure, a nearly 180° hairpin bend, is similar to the sigmoid-descending colon junction from an anatomical standpoint and in difficulty negotiating with the colonoscope.

Once proximal to the hepatic flexure, the characteristic notch of the superior lip of the ileocecal valve is commonly seen (Fig. 5). The ileocecal valve may appear yellowish and

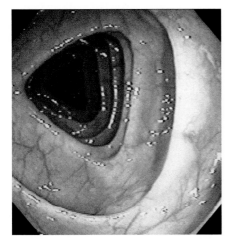

Figure 3 The transverse colon is usually easily recognized by the characteristic triangular outline.

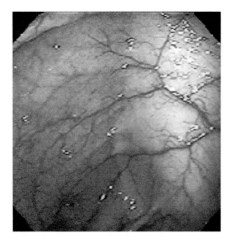

Figure 4 (*See color insert*) The hepatic flexure is frequently identified by the bluish hue resulting from its close proximity to the liver.

thickened due to fat accumulation ("lipomatous" valve). The opening into the ileum is on the inferior side of the fold and may frequently be seen only on a retroflexed view in the cecum. The appendiceal orifice is typically seen as a crescent-shaped slit at the cecal pole (Fig. 6). Multiple, small erythematous halos are commonly present near the appendiceal orifice and represent lymphoid aggregates. The terminal ileal mucosa has a granular appearance with scattered areas of nodularity resulting from the individual villi and presence of Peyer's patches.

ROLE OF SIGMOIDOSCOPY

Before discussing colonoscopy in greater detail, it is appropriate to briefly comment on the role of sigmoidoscopy in the evaluation of the colon (11). Sigmoidoscopy continues to play a role in the evaluation of complaints suspected to be due to distal colonic disease when there is no indication for total colonoscopy, and for colon cancer screening in average-risk individuals and those with a family history of familial adenomatous polyposis (12). A recent multidisciplinary panel of experts has recommended that if a polyp at least 1 cm in diameter is found during screening sigmoidoscopy, colonoscopy with polypectomy should be performed (4). Alternatively, if a polyp less than 1 cm is found, biopsy is suggested and colonoscopy is only recommended if the polyp is adenomatous (4). Importantly, the use of electrocautery for polyp removal is contraindicated during flexible sigmoidoscopy unless a complete bowel preparation has been performed, because there is a risk of igniting explosive gas mixtures.

Other potential indications for sigmoidoscopy include the evaluation of the entire colon in conjunction with a barium enema when colonoscopy is not possible, surveillance of anastomotic recurrence in those with a history of rectosigmoid cancer, and evaluation of lower gastrointestinal bleeding after an upper gastrointestinal source has been ruled out and colonoscopy is not indicated, and for therapeutic purposes when a colonoscopy is not indicated and

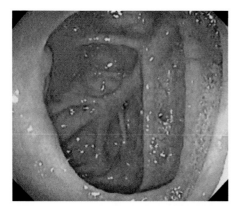

Figure 5 (*See color insert*) The characteristic notch of the superior lip of the ileocecal valve is demonstrated. The opening to the ileum lies on the inferior aspect of the fold.

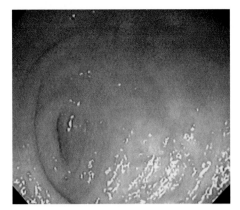

Figure 6 (*See color insert*) The appendiceal orifice is typically seen as a crescent-shaped slit as shown here but may have other appearances. Multiple, small erythematous halos are commonly seen near the appendiceal orifice.

a proper bowel preparation has been performed (12). Advantages of sigmoidoscopy over colonoscopy include the lack of need of sedation-analgesia, the lower complication risk, and the less intensive bowel preparation.

While rigid sigmoidoscopy has been shown to be of value in screening asymptomatic, average-risk adults over the age of 50 (13), its use has not been widely adopted due to the higher yield and greater patient acceptance of flexible sigmoidoscopy. Indeed, comparative studies indicate that flexible sigmoidoscopy detects an average of three times as many polyps and cancers and has greater patient and physician acceptability than rigid sigmoidoscopy (14,15). Nevertheless, cost-effectiveness comparisons between flexible sigmoidoscopy and rigid sigmoidoscopy have not been made. Lastly, it should be remembered that anoscopy is the preferred method for evaluating anal canal pathology, which are frequently poorly visualized upon retroflexion of the flexible sigmoidoscope.

COLONOSCOPY
Training and Competence

Objectives of colonoscopy training include an understanding of its indications, contraindications, and diagnostic and therapeutic alternatives, the ability to perform it safely, completely, and expeditiously, the ability to recognize and interpret findings and proceed with the appropriate action, an understanding of its risks and how to minimize and manage complications, and, lastly, the ability to acknowledge limits and know when to stop or request assistance (16). The amount of time and experience required to learn the safe and effective performance of colonoscopy varies considerably between individuals (17). Realistic computerized endoscopic simulators are now commercially available. While designed to enhance the acquisition of endoscopic skills, their utility in accomplishing this goal has yet to be established (18,19). For instance, it remains unclear whether competency on the simulator will predict competency in humans, and vice versa; important validation studies are ongoing. Other potential applications of the simulators include standardization of training and the ability to perform objective assessment of endoscopic skills (18).

Factors that constitute competency in colonoscopy remain highly contentious but should include both cognitive and technical abilities. It has been suggested that experts should be expected to perform at a technical success rate of 95% or greater (20) while competency has been suggested at a minimum of 80% (21,22). Clearly, the number of procedures performed provides only a rough benchmark for guiding competency and few studies of the rate at which proficiency is attained have been performed (21,23). Other factors such as cecal intubation rate, adherence to safe patient monitoring and sedation, complication rate, response to complications, time of procedure, interpretive skills, knowledge of what to do if something is encountered, and the ability to incorporate endoscopic findings into the overall patient care are more important (24). Until recently, there had been considerable variability among professional societies in the threshold number of procedures required before assessing trainee competency (25,26). However, a joint consensus statement agreed upon by the governing bodies of the American Society of Colon and Rectal Surgeons (ASCRS), the American Society for Gastrointestinal Endoscopy (ASGE), and the Society of American Gastrointestinal and Endoscopic Surgeons (SAGES) and published in the respective journals of the three societies concluded that it is the endoscopy training director's opinion and recommendation, based upon the training experience rather than an absolute number of procedures performed, and observed level of competency that are of utmost importance in determining a trainee's competence in gastrointestinal endoscopy (27).

Certainly, documented competence in colonoscopy should precede the granting of hospital privileges (27). The assurance of adequate training has implications with respect to both quality of care and legal liability (28). This point is assuming increasing importance in the present day because of the rising demand for colonoscopy and the desire of non–gastroenterology or colorectal surgery-trained physicians and even nonphysicians to perform colonoscopy. While colonoscopy is far more demanding cognitively and technically, this situation is somewhat analogous to the training of nongastroenterologists to perform screening flexible sigmoidoscopy more than a decade ago.

Patient Preparation
Patient Education and Informed Consent
Colonoscopy is an invasive test that causes considerable anxiety for most people. For many, the rigorous bowel preparation that precedes colonoscopy serves to accentuate this anxiety and dislike of colonoscopy. To reduce anxiety, it is helpful to carefully explain to the patient the nature of the procedure and its goal. It is useful to discuss the bowel preparation, the use of sedative-analgesic medications, and the monitoring of vital signs, which occurs during the test and the postprocedural recovery period. Commercially available videotapes that review these areas can be useful preprocedural tools to reduce patient anxiety and improve compliance. If the videotapes are not readily available or the patient does not wish to view a videotape, a handout of bowel preparation instructions given to the patient is valuable and may result in improved compliance and colonoscopy performance. Similarly, a handout describing the test and its potential discomforts and the risks associated with its performance may be helpful.

Prior to performing colonoscopy, informed consent must be obtained from the patient. This allows an opportunity for the endoscopist and the patient to interact and develop trust and mutual respect and allows patients to make a reasoned decision regarding their welfare (29,30). When adequately undertaken, the disclosure process also shifts a portion of the risk and burden of potential complications to the patient. If consent is unobtainable from the patient, the next of kin or legal guardian may substitute. A written form should be used to document the consent process, but by itself, a signed consent form does not constitute the entirety of the discussion and disclosure that adequate consent entails. A witness to the process can be invaluable. This form should be incorporated into the patient's permanent medical record and should include the following essential elements: (i) indication for the test, (ii) nature of the procedure, (iii) risk of potential complications including diagnostic error (limitations of the exam), (iv) potential benefits, and (v) relevant alternative diagnostic studies.

Bowel Preparation
Removal of fecal material from the colon is essential in order to allow adequate visualization of the entire mucosa. Several satisfactory regimens are available for bowel preparation prior to colonoscopy; however, few data exist regarding the ideal form (31–33). It is important to keep in mind that some patients, such as those with chronic constipation or who have recently undergone a barium enema, may require a more prolonged preparation. Additionally, patients with severe diarrhea and those with a surgically defunctionalized bowel usually require a complete bowel preparation prior to colonoscopy because the mucosa may be obscured by a coating of fecal material. Full bowel preparation is also useful when performing colonoscopy in persons with suspected acute lower gastrointestinal bleeding. This can usually be accomplished rapidly and without deleterious hemodynamic consequences. Bowel preparation is usually not possible before colonoscopy in patients with acute colonic pseudo-obstruction requiring decompression. Bowel preparation is contraindicated in the face of suspected bowel obstruction or perforation.

Bowel preparation should be preceded by a low-residue or liquid diet, usually for a period of about 24 to 48 hours before the procedure. Oral iron supplements should be stopped four or five days before colonoscopy because they tend to combine with certain dietary substances, resulting in black, sticky fecal material that is difficult to clear. Constipating agents such as narcotic analgesics and antidiarrheals should be discontinued at least 12 hours before the procedure.

Purgative regimens remain the most commonly used form of bowel preparation. There are currently two widely accepted forms and both seem to be of equivalent efficacy. The first uses a 4-L polyethylene glycol–based balanced electrolyte solution usually given over two to four hours the evening before the procedure. This solution has been available since the early 1980s (34) and does not alter the circulating blood volume and is, therefore, safe even in patients with systemic illness. Tolerance to the large volume ingested is the major disadvantage of this method of bowel preparation. It has been suggested that a prokinetic, given 30 minutes before beginning ingestion of the solution, may decrease abdominal distension, the sensation of fullness, and the development of nausea and vomiting. Different flavors of the solution are also available to enhance tolerance. A nasogastric tube may be used to infuse the solution if the patient is unable to orally ingest this volume.

The second form of bowel preparation is sodium phosphate-based. Due to its smaller volume, this form of preparation seems to be better tolerated. Indeed, a recent meta-analysis of all eight randomized controlled trials comparing the two preparations concluded that sodium phosphate is as effective and less costly than polyethylene glycol (32). Typically, a 45-mL dose of sodium phosphate solution is taken orally the evening before and again four hours prior to the procedure. The major disadvantages of this preparation are that abdominal cramping and fluid and electrolyte shifts may occur, resulting in electrolyte abnormalities and dehydration. Therefore, increased attention to fluid balance and electrolytes is necessary in patients sensitive to sudden volume changes, such as the elderly and those with cardiopulmonary and renal disease and those susceptible to enhanced sodium absorption, such as patients with intestinal dysmotility. The sodium phosphate preparation has also been associated with endoscopic and histologic findings of colitis (35)—an important point to recognize as the changes could be confused with other forms of colitis. Recently, a preparation using sodium phosphate tablets ingested orally the evening before and the morning of the procedure has become commercially available and has been demonstrated to be safe and to have equal cleansing efficacy and improved patient tolerance compared to both the liquid sodium phosphate and polyethylene glycol–based regimens (36).

Ultimately, the regimen chosen will depend upon the clinical situation and patient and physician preference. Certainly, none of the existing regimens is universally efficacious and well tolerated; thus, advances are still needed both in the administration of bowel preparation and in the type of preparation used. It is important to keep in mind that some patients, such as the elderly, seriously ill, incontinent or chronically constipated, may require a modified bowel preparation.

Antibiotic Prophylaxis

The risk of infection from most gastrointestinal endoscopic procedures is very low; nevertheless, both the American Heart Association and the ASGE have developed detailed guidelines regarding antibiotic prophylaxis prior to endoscopy (37,38). There has been no prospective, randomized study investigating antibiotic prophylaxis in the setting of any endoscopic procedure. Indeed, current recommendations are based mainly on limited studies and anecdotal experience. Guidelines for antibiotic prophylaxis characterize the need for prophylaxis on the basis of both the risk of the underlying condition and the procedure being performed. High-risk patient conditions include a history of endocarditis, prosthetic heart valve replacement, complex cyanotic congenital heart disease, surgically constructed systemic pulmonary shunts, or synthetic grafts less than one year old. Antibiotic prophylaxis is not recommended in patients with other forms of heart disease, those with cirrhosis and ascites, immunocompromised patients, or those with prosthetic joints or implanted pacemakers/ defibrillators.

Colonoscopy with or without polypectomy is a low-risk procedure for inducing bacteremia as compared to other endoscopic procedures, such as dilation or sclerotherapy, and, even when performed in patients with the aforementioned high-risk conditions, there is insufficient data to strongly recommend prophylactic antibiotics. Indiscriminate use of antibiotics in association with endoscopy adds unnecessary cost and potential for adverse drug reactions and is discouraged. Ultimately, the options should be discussed with the patient and/or the consulting cardiologist and the mutual decision documented. If antibiotics are deemed necessary, several oral and parenteral regimens have been proposed (37,38). Typically, parenteral ampicillin 1 g and gentamicin 1.5 mg/kg is given within 30 minutes of the procedure. Vancomycin 1 g intravenously can be substituted in penicillin-allergic patients. The most recent American Heart Association recommendation forgoes the use of postprocedural dosing.

Anticoagulant and Antiplatelet Medication Use

Chronic anticoagulation is commonly used in patients with various medical conditions, most notably cardiac, such as chronic atrial fibrillation and prosthetic valves. In general, a biopsy can be performed safely in these individuals if their international normalization ratio (INR) is within the therapeutic range, generally, 1.5 to 2.5 (39). Anticoagulants should be discontinued prior to high-risk procedures, such as polypectomy, laser ablation/coagulation, and stricture dilation. In those with a condition associated with higher risk for a thromboembolic event related to interruption of anticoagulant therapy, such as atrial fibrillation with valvular disease, mechanical valve in the mitral position or mechanical valve and prior thromboembolic event, it may be prudent to begin continuous intravenous unfractionated heparin while their INR is subtherapeutic. The outpatient use of subcutaneous injections of low-molecular-weight heparin seems to be a reasonable, safe, and effective alternative, although extensive data are still lacking. These agents should be discontinued several hours prior to the procedure and, in general, may be resumed afterward.

In addition, mucosal biopsies may be performed safely in patients receiving aspirin or nonsteroidal anti-inflammatory drugs. In the absence of a preexisting bleeding disorder, discontinuation of these medications is unnecessary prior to colonoscopy regardless of whether a biopsy or polypectomy is performed (40). Whether the newer antiplatelet agents, such as ticlopidine, dipyridamole, and clopidogrel, confer a higher risk of bleeding and, therefore, require temporary discontinuation prior to colonoscopy with polypectomy remains unclear at present. A cautious approach is recommended until additional data become available.

There are no data on the benefit of routine laboratory testing prior to endoscopy, even before high-risk procedures such as polypectomy. In general, the history and physical examination should be used to screen the individual's bleeding status and coagulation studies only performed selectively, for example, in patients with a history of bleeding, those with liver or renal disease, and those on anticoagulants (41,42).

COLONOSCOPY PROCEDURE
Equipment

Before performing colonoscopy, a thorough familiarity with the endoscopic equipment and accessories is necessary. Modern flexible endoscopes consist of an umbilical cord that attaches the endoscope to a light source and air/water pump, a control head/hand grip, and an insertion tube of varying length. Running through this apparatus are a suction channel, an air/water channel, a biopsy shaft, control wires for tip deflection, and fiberoptic bundles (fiberoptic instruments only).

Fiberoptic instruments are based upon optical viewing bundles that contain thousands of very fine glass fibers each coated with glass of a different density that does not transmit light. Light focused onto the face of each fiber is transmitted by repeated internal reflections. The image is relayed from the distal tip to the control head where the endoscopist focuses on an eyepiece image using one eye. A teaching head attachment is available for training purposes. Similarly, a video head converter attachment is available whereby the image is relayed to a video monitor. Disadvantages of the fiberoptic compared to the video endoscope include a smaller image with poorer definition, the need for a teaching head attachment to allow others to view the image, more difficult photography capabilities, and increased potential for contamination given the proximity of the endoscopist's face to the controls and the patient.

Video instruments are mechanically similar to fiberoptic instruments; however, a video or charge-coupled device (CCD) "chip" and supporting electronics replace the fiberoptic bundles, and the image is relayed onto a video monitor instead of an eyepiece. Video endoscopes require a video processor, a light source/air pump, suction, and a color monitor. Hard copy images can be generated using a video printer and can be stored on hard disk. A computer is needed to create a patient database and image management system. The obvious hygienic advantage coupled with a higher resolution and magnified image that multiple people can view simultaneously has resulted in video instruments generally superceding the fiberoptic system. A distinct disadvantage of the video systems is their cost.

In addition to its previously mentioned attributes, the increased flexibility of modern videocolonoscopes along with a tip angulation of greater than 180° allows increased maneuverability and minimizes the risk of failing to detect significant lesions "hidden" in difficult-to-view areas. The control head consists of separate up/down and right/left dials with locking levers, separate air/water and suction buttons, and additional buttons to freeze an image and take photographs. Optional CO_2 insufflation capabilities are also incorporated into most colonoscopes. The length of the standard colonoscope is 168 cm while the shaft diameter ranges from about 10 mm for the pediatric colonoscope up to 17 cm for the adult instrument. A recent study suggests there is no difference between the standard colonoscope length and a shorter (133 cm) colonoscope with regard to procedural efficiency as determined by the rate of success and time required for cecal intubation (43).

A colonoscope with a mechanism to vary the shaft stiffness has recently become commercially available. While the initial studies demonstrated more rapid cecal intubation compared to a standard colonoscope (44), this has not been confirmed in subsequent evaluations conducted in the United States (45). Another technological innovation that has recently become commercially available involves magnetic electronic imaging (46–48). This device allows the contour of the colonoscope to be displayed so that the presence and shape of loops can be identified. Insufficient data exist regarding improvement of insertion efficiency using this technology. High-resolution, utilizing a high-pixel CCD, and magnification (1.5–150×) endoscopes are also now commercially available and offer the theoretical ability to differentiate neoplasia from other pathology by endoscopic characterization of mucosal surface detail (49,50). Both systems are designed to be used in conjunction with chromoendoscopy (51,52). Currently, there are insufficient data to recommend the routine use of either of these colonoscopes.

Endoscopic accessories available for colonoscopy include biopsy forceps, hot-biopsy (monopolar cautery) forceps, retrieval devices, cytology brushes, guidewires, washing/spraying catheters, sclerotherapy needles, band ligators, dilating balloons, polypectomy snares, stents, and long decompression tubes. An overtube is also available to use as a stiffening device to control looping in the sigmoid colon and facilitate cecal intubation. Lastly, bipolar electrocoagulation, the heater probe, argon plasma coagulation, and laser can be applied to the colon through the colonoscope much like their utilities in the upper gastrointestinal tract.

Colorectal endoscopic ultrasound (EUS), discussed in more detail elsewhere in this book, (Chapter 10) combines endoscopic visualization and ultrasound, which permits delineation of the individual colonic wall layers, and allows locoregional staging of neoplasms and the origin of submucosal lesions, and differentiation of other gut wall abnormalities (53). Fine needle aspiration can be performed using linear array echoendoscopes, thus allowing tissue diagnosis of extraluminal lesions and lymph nodes. Extensive training is needed to perform these studies due to the image interpretation required. Currently, EUS of the lower gastrointestinal tract has been mainly restricted to the rectum; however, the development of high-frequency ultrasound probes that can be passed through the instrument channel of a standard colonoscope (54) and a colonoscope that incorporates an ultrasound probe on the tip may increase the use of this imaging modality in the colon.

Finally, a number of promising optical imaging techniques, that have the potential to obviate the need for tissue sampling, are being evaluated for clinical application and include tissue spectroscopy and optical coherence tomography (55). The ultimate role of such "optical biopsy" technology in clinical practice remains to be determined.

Role of the Colonoscopy Assistant

While not essential for endoscopic procedures performed without conscious sedation, an assistant is necessary for colonoscopy. Before the procedure, they can assist with patient preparation and counseling, set up the endoscopy suite, and ensure that all accessories are available, if needed. During the procedure, their main role is to continuously monitor the patient's well-being and provide reassurance and comfort to the patient. The assistant's appropriate attention to patient monitoring, in particular, clinical observation, before, during, and after the procedure is essential to help minimize complications by early recognition of signs of distress, so that appropriate early resuscitation can be initiated. During the procedure, they can also assist with diagnostic and therapeutic maneuvers, advance the colonoscope (two-person technique), and assist with abdominal compression and changes in patient position. After the procedure, the assistant can process the endoscopic photographs and biopsy specimens, clean the endoscopy suite, and assist with patient recovery, as well as patient education and disposition. Finally, the assistant is also responsible for maintenance of the emergency "crash" cart and the cleaning, care, and proper maintenance of the endoscopy equipment.

Sedation-Analgesia and Monitoring During Colonoscopy

Sedation-analgesia, previously referred to as conscious sedation, is routinely used during colonoscopy to reduce patient anxiety, discomfort, and gastrointestinal secretions and motility. While colonoscopy may be performed successfully without sedation-analgesia (56), clinical experience suggests that the use of sedation-analgesia enhances patient tolerance, an important consideration if colonoscopy is to be accepted as a primary means of screening for colorectal cancer. Most endoscopists also seem to prefer to use sedation-analgesia during endoscopy because it results in perceived improved patient comfort and overall satisfaction (57). Because nearly one-half of procedure-related morbidity and mortality may be due to the use of sedation-analgesia (58), the ability to provide it safely and effectively and ensure the patient's stability by appropriate monitoring are essential skills for colonoscopy (59–61). The amount of medication required varies considerably depending upon the patient's age, comorbidities, body habitus, history of routine sedative and opiate use, preprocedural anxiety level, and the procedure to be performed (59). Certainly, using less sedation allows for easier changes in the patient's position, if needed, and greater safety. Recently, the addition of relaxation music before and during colonoscopy was shown to reduce the dose of sedative medications required and may be a useful adjunct (62). The use of deep sedation and general anesthesia is generally discouraged during elective colonoscopy because the patient is no longer able to protect his/her airway with the former method and feedback from the patient relating to pain from looping or therapeutic procedures is lost with both methods (63).

Medications used for sedation-analgesia usually consist of an opioid analgesic, such as meperidine or fentanyl, and a benzodiazepine, such as midazolam or diazepam. A synergistic effect resulting from using a combination of these two classes of medications has been demonstrated to result in improved efficacy of conscious sedation compared to that achieved when either agent is used alone (64). These medications should be administered intravenously immediately prior to the procedure. Initial bolus dosing of these agents followed by additional dosing as needed has recently been shown to be a safe, effective, and efficient alternative to the traditional dose-titration method (65). While there have been suggestions that the use of reversal agents such as naloxone and flumazenil either at the end of the procedure or when the cecum is reached may shorten the recovery time and, thus, improve the efficiency of the endoscopy unit, there currently remain insufficient data to recommend their use.

Evidence supporting the use of propofol sedation by gastroenterologists and nurses acting under supervision without the assistance of an anesthesiologist or nurse anesthetist has been accumulating (66,67). Advantages of propofol sedation include the more rapid induction of sedation and reduced recovery time, potentially resulting in improved patient satisfaction and patient flow through the endoscopy center. However, given its narrow therapeutic window and the potential for causing severe respiratory depression, this agent should only be used by those properly trained and experienced in the use of propofol, monitoring the patient, and advanced airway management.

Sedation-analgesia should only be used by personnel experienced in the administration of conscious sedation, the cardiopulmonary monitoring needed during and after the procedure, and the cardiopulmonary resuscitation techniques that may be required (59–61). In addition, sedation-analgesia should only be administered after obtaining informed consent from the patient, which specifically includes a discussion of this component of the procedure. Devices for cardiopulmonary resuscitation should be available nearby when sedation-analgesia is used. In addition to the mechanical monitoring techniques, such as pulse oximetry, automated blood pressure monitoring, electrocardiography, and respirometery, it is essential for an endoscopy assistant to closely observe the patient for signs of distress during the procedure. The use of supplemental oxygen during colonoscopy should be considered in those patients who develop sustained oxygen desaturation during the procedure, those with significant cardiopulmonary disease, and the elderly. Care must be taken to avoid suppression of the hypoxic ventilatory drive resulting in profound hypercapnia. Despite its theoretical advantages of early detection of respiratory depression and prevention of hypoxemia, hypercapnia, hypotension, and dysrhythmia, there is insufficient data to support the routine use of expiratory or transcutaneous CO_2-monitoring or capnography (68) at this time. This may change as the data supporting the routine use of propofol by gastroenterologists without the assistance of an anesthesiologist accumulate.

Infection Control and Colonoscope Disinfection

Both the colonoscopist and the assistant must adhere to universal precautions regarding exposure to blood and body fluids at all times during the exam. Although the risk of acquiring hepatitis B from a patient is small, immunization of all personnel should be considered. Suggested protective gear to be worn at all times during the exam includes a gown, gloves, facemask, and protective eye wear (69).

The colonic lumen contains millions of bacteria and other potentially pathogenic organisms, and endoscopes have potential sites for microorganisms to accumulate. Since the publication of guidelines on endoscope reprocessing, very few cases of infections transmitted during endoscopy have been reported (70,71). The greatest risk of infection results from improperly cleaned and disinfected endoscopes. Indeed, proper cleaning and disinfection of the endoscope is more important than antibiotic prophylaxis to decrease the risk of endoscope-related infections. The risk of transmitting infection from properly reprocessed endoscopes is estimated to be 1 in 1.8 million procedures (72). Most episodes of infection can be traced to errors in cleaning, disinfection, or storage of the endoscope or accessories, emphasizing the need for strict and compulsive adherence to reprocessing guidelines for endoscopes and accessories (73). The clinical spectrum of infection can range from asymptomatic colonization to death. The organisms most commonly implicated are salmonellae and pseudomonads. Viruses, in general, are quite sensitive to disinfection. The Centers for Disease Control and Prevention states that currently recommended cleaning and disinfection procedures are adequate for endoscopes contaminated with hepatitis B virus and human immunodeficiency virus (74,75).

Endoscope reprocessing protocols are categorized by their anticipated microbial resistance. Pertinent to endoscopes and their accessories, "sterilization" refers to the complete elimination of all forms of microbial life, while "high-level disinfection" destroys all microorganisms except for some spores when found in high concentration. The prevention of infection transmission by endoscopes requires high-level disinfection, which consists of proper mechanical cleaning, complete immersion in an effective disinfectant for at least 20 minutes (76,77), further rinsing, proper drying and storage and, perhaps most importantly, proper training and compliance of personnel performing these techniques. The biopsy forceps and other reusable accessories should be cleaned and sterilized. There are currently insufficient data to recommend the routine use and reuse of disposable endoscopic accessories on the basis of efficacy, safety, or cost-effectiveness (78,79).

Recently, the sheathed endoscope system, which includes permanent, detachable, and disposable portions, was developed as a semidisposable unit to avoid the risks of exposure to infectious material and disinfectants and to decrease reprocessing time. While theoretically beneficial, this system has yet to be shown to be superior to conventional endoscopes with regard to patient outcomes or cost-effectiveness (80,81).

Colonoscope Insertion, Withdrawal, and Localization

Before every exam, the equipment should be checked to make sure that all functions are in working order. At the beginning of the procedure, the patient usually lies in the left lateral decubitus (Sims') position. The patient should be positioned on his/her left side with the hips and knees flexed with the right knee slightly above the left knee and the head comfortably positioned so as to relax the abdominal musculature. Changes in patient position, such as to the prone, supine, or right lateral decubitus positions, may be useful during difficult insertions to aid tip advancement and in the bleeding patient to allow inspection of previously obscured mucosa.

It is important to examine the perianal region prior to inserting the colonoscope for potential pathology such as condylomata, skin tags, external hemorrhoids, prolapsed internal hemorrhoids, fissures, and fistulae. The digital rectal exam is an essential part of the preliminary evaluation as it serves to lubricate the anal canal and relax the anal sphincter, allows for the detection of pathology in the distal rectum including the prostate gland, and provides an initial assessment of the effectiveness of the bowel preparation (82). Inquiry about a latex allergy should be accomplished before beginning the procedure. The pad of a well-lubricated, gloved index finger is generally gently "rolled" into the rectum at a 90° angle. In cases of painful anal pathology, an anesthetic lubricant may decrease discomfort. Having the patient perform the Valsalva maneuver may relax the sphincter and allow easier entry of the finger into the rectum.

Next, the lubricated colonoscope tip, in an unlocked and neutral position, is inserted into the rectum in a manner similar to the digital rectal exam by flexion of the right index finger guiding the instrument into the rectum from a 90° angle. Alternatively, the tip may be directly inserted into the rectum. Initially, a "red-out" is seen because of the close positioning of the instrument tip to the rectal mucosa. Simultaneous withdrawal of the endoscope and insufflation of the rectum with air is necessary to obtain a view of the rectal lumen. A "red-out may" occur numerous times during any given colonoscopic examination. When this occurs, the colonoscope should be withdrawn slightly and the lumen position reassessed. A "white-out" suggests that pressure is being applied to the mucosa by the colonoscope tip, resulting in mucosal blanching. If this occurs, the colonoscope should be immediately withdrawn slightly and the lumen position reassessed as further insertion and pressure may result in perforation. There may be a considerable amount of liquid material in the rectum; nevertheless, because most of the examination of the mucosa occurs upon withdrawal of the endoscope following its initial maximal insertion, suctioning of this material may be deferred during the initial advancement.

There are two methods of colonoscope advancement: the one- and the two-person techniques. With the one-person technique, the colonoscopist's left hand is used to manipulate the control head while the right hand guides the insertion tube. In contrast, with the two-person technique, the colonoscopist's left and right hands are used to manipulate the control head while an assistant advances the insertion tube. This technique has the obvious disadvantage of requiring a second person; however, it may be easier for the inexperienced colonoscopist. While only a limited number of maneuvers can be performed with the colonoscope, it is the coordinated use of these options that forms the basis for a complete, accurate, and safe exam with minimal patient discomfort. The options include inserting or withdrawing the instrument, torquing the shaft, insufflating or removing air, using the tip controls, and using abdominal pressure and/or changes in patient body position to reduce loops. The colonoscope should be advanced by steady, slow insertion, with the lumen always in view and without sharp tip angulation. The least amount of air insufflation possible is advised during insertion to prevent undue patient discomfort and lengthening of the bowel loops. Alternatively, it has been suggested that the routine use of CO_2 insufflation rather than air may reduce patient discomfort due to gas retention and would also allow for electrocautery use in a poorly prepared colon (83).

After passing the three rectal valves of Houston, the rectosigmoid junction is encountered, approximately 15 to 20 cm from the anal verge. Colonoscope advancement across this sharp angulation may pose a challenge. If pelvic surgery fixes the sigmoid loop in front of the rectum, advancement will be even more difficult and painful. In general, after advancing the colonoscope tip beyond the last rectal valve, it is oftentimes helpful to deflect the tip upward and, while simultaneously twisting, or torquing, the insertion tube with the right hand, advance the instrument with the lumen in view. Once the endoscope is around this turn, the tip deflection controls can be used to straighten the tip.

The sigmoid colon is made up of a series of semilunar valves. As the lumen may be partially hidden by the semilunar valves, gentle torquing combined with forward motion may help, along with the use of the up/down tip deflection by the left thumb. Continuing to advance the instrument when the lumen cannot be seen rarely results in tip advancement, frequently causes patient discomfort due to looping, and is a risk for perforation. The "slide-by" technique describes the appearance when the instrument tip is closely apposed to the colonic wall and pushed forward, resulting in the mucosal vessels visibly sliding across the lens. While occasionally used to maneuver around sharply angulated corners, its use should be limited to short distances and only when the colonoscopist is certain of the correct direction of the lumen; tactile assessment of resistance to insertion is an important form of feedback to the colonoscopist as well.

Diverticular disease frequently presents a challenge to the colonoscopist when negotiating the sigmoid colon. The distortions and angulations resulting from myochosis coli and pericolic adhesions can result in difficulty identifying the lumen and advancing the instrument. Additionally, if many diverticula are present, determining the true lumen can be very difficult. In general, the true lumen will be found in the presence of haustral folds. In situations where operative or peridiverticular adhesions fix the pelvic colon so as to make passage of a standard colonoscope through the sigmoid colon impossible, use of a different diameter or length of endoscope, a change in patient position, a different endoscopist, or a repeated attempt on another day may be helpful (44,84–86).

Other tips to aid colonoscope insertion include noting that the lumen will be in the direction of the darker mucosa, that is, the point farthest from tip illumination, the lumen will be behind a curvilinear mucosal fold, and, when concave arcs representing haustral folds are found, the lumen will be in the center of an imaginary circle formed by these arcs (9). Lastly, when in doubt, the skilled colonoscopist's instinct will always be to pull the colonoscope back and reassess the lumen, rather than advance blindly.

Traversing the sigmoid colon usually results in the formation of a sigmoid loop. A characteristic sign of loop formation is paradoxical endoscope movement in which further shaft insertion results in either no tip advancement or withdrawal of the colonoscope tip. When the sigmoid-descending colon junction is in view, it is helpful to remove the rectosigmoid loop in order to complete the remainder of the exam with minimal discomfort for the patient and effort for the colonoscopist. Indeed, difficulty passing the hepatic flexure and reaching the cecum is usually related to failure to reduce the sigmoid loop formed earlier. To reduce the loop, the tip of the colonoscope should be hooked behind a mucosal fold and slowly withdrawn while simultaneously torquing the insertion tube in a clockwise manner. Another technique that may be helpful involves utilizing short forward and withdrawal motions, sometimes combined with clockwise torquing, resulting in telescoping of the bowel over the sigmoidoscope. This is referred to as "jiggling." Occasionally, these maneuvers are unsuccessful and require the colonoscopist to "push" through the loop, although attention to the resistance encountered is critical to safety. Finally, if spasm is encountered, patience is necessary to allow the spasm to spontaneously relax before advancing further.

After maneuvering through the elbow-type turn at the sigmoid-descending colon junction, the descending colon will be entered. Advancing the endoscope through the descending colon is generally done without difficulty, because it is essentially a straight tube. The splenic flexure may be identified by a bluish hue due to the splenic shadow. The transverse colon is readily identified by its characteristic triangular appearance. Maneuvering the instrument across the splenic flexure is usually not difficult as long as a sigmoid loop can be reduced. Using a combination of gentle advancement with torquing the shaft and applying abdominal pressure over the sigmoid area is usually successful (87). If this is unsuccessful, rotating the patient into the right lateral decubitus position will generally allow the colonoscope to pass across the splenic flexure. A change back to the left lateral decubitus position is usually necessary in the middle to proximal portion of the transverse colon in order to allow successful completion of the procedure. Withdrawal of air is extremely useful to aid in passing the hepatic flexure and advancing to the cecum. Aspiration of air acts to both shorten and decrease the diameter of the colon. Reduction of loops is also frequently needed to maneuver across the hepatic flexure and down to the cecum.

In cases of extreme difficulty reaching the cecum, where the previously described options have been unsuccessful, a variety of other methods have been shown to be useful (86). These include the use of deeper sedation such as propofol, use of a pediatror colonoscope or upper endoscope to overcome narrowing, use of variable stiffness colonoscope or enteroscope, use of fluoroscopic or magnetic imaging of the colonoscope, use of overtube, or other straightening device (88), and guidewire exchange. Interestingly, the only factor recently shown to predict incomplete colonoscopy was women with low body mass index ($\leq 22.1 \, \text{kg/m}^2$) (89). Similarly, another recent study showed that factors associated with prolonged insertion time (over

10 minutes) included inadequate bowel preparation, advanced age, and constipation, while female gender was the only factor associated with significant discomfort during colonoscopy (90).

With patience and attention to technique, the cecum is usually reached with only between 60 and 80 cm of the colonoscope inserted. Visualizing the appendiceal orifice and the ileocecal valve clearly identifies the cecum. The "crow's foot" appearance of the teniae coli converging in the cecum can be a misleading landmark because a similar appearance can be seen at an angulated hepatic flexure. Certainly, intubating the terminal ileum leaves no doubt that the cecum has been reached. Documentation of cecal intubation by photography or videotape is important for obvious patient care, quality assurance, and medicolegal reasons. Due to anatomical variation among individuals, a combination of cecal photographs has been shown to be more convincing than a single photograph (91). Ileal intubation can be difficult, requiring skill and patience. While terminal ileal inspection is not needed in all examinations, a skilled colonoscopist can intubate the ileocecal valve in about 80% of cases. Failures usually occur because of scarring or deformity of the ileocecal valve, poor bowel preparation, or difficulty controlling the instrument tip because of looping. The view of the terminal ileum is typically limited to the most distal 10 cm, although depths of up to 50 cm can sometimes be accomplished. Acute angulations in the small bowel is the usual limiting factor.

Colonoscope withdrawal is the most important part of the examination (92). It is essential to be meticulous and patient and examine all parts of the mucosa, remembering to check behind folds, particularly in the sigmoid colon and rectum, and at areas of angulation such as the hepatic and splenic flexures. It has been suggested that the withdrawal phase should average at least 6 to 10 minutes, excluding the time spent for biopsy and polypectomy, to ensure adequate detection rates. A circular or "cork-screwing" motion of the instrument tip is helpful and is best accomplished by using coordinated movements of the up/down dial with the left thumb and rotary torquing of the insertion tube by the right hand. During colonoscope withdrawal, and often during its initial insertion, it is useful to lock the right/left dial on the control head in order to "stiffen" the colonoscope tip and allow improved control of the colonoscope. During withdrawal is the best time to suction pools of residual liquid material. While it is important to use sufficient air to distend the lumen for adequate visualization, it is also important to suction air as each portion of the bowel has been examined, because this will reduce patient discomfort.

Prior to the removal of the colonoscope from the rectum, a retroflexion of the instrument tip should be performed to inspect the distal rectum, an area that may easily be missed on the forward view (Fig. 7) (93,94). To perform this maneuver, the colonoscope tip should be positioned approximately 10 cm from the anal verge. While deflecting the tip maximally upward, the colonoscope should be advanced slightly. The right/left dial should then be turned maximally in either direction and locked. The use of rotary torquing with the right hand along with air insufflation should allow examination of the entire circumference of the anorectal junction. When completed, the tip control dials should be placed back into their neutral positions, air removed, and the colonoscope withdrawn. It should be remembered that the best view of the anal canal is obtained using an anoscope.

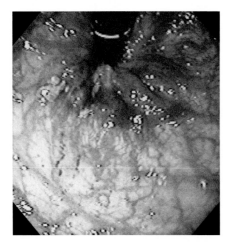

Figure 7 (*See color insert*) Prior to the removal of the colonoscope from the rectum, a retroflexion of the instrument tip should be performed to inspect the distal rectum, an area that may easily be missed on the forward view.

Accurate anatomic localization of the instrument tip and, therefore, of pathological lesions identified during colonoscopy is difficult. Judgments that rely on landmarks, transabdominal illumination, or palpation can be mistaken while those that rely on the length of the instrument inserted are fraught with error as a consequence of potential instrument looping. The only definitive landmark is the ileum seen through the ileocecal valve. Even experienced colonoscopists can mistake the location of lesions, thereby misleading surgeons as to the site requiring resection (95). The use of fluoroscopy or barium enema to assist in localization may also be inaccurate. As a consequence, lesions seen during colonoscopy, which require surgical resection or colonoscopic follow-up, should be marked for subsequent localization. The use of sterilized India ink injected through a sclerotherapy needle passed via the working channel of the colonoscope has proven to be a simple, safe, inexpensive, and permanent means of identifying the site of such lesions (96,97).

In the absence of prior tissue staining to mark lesion location for subsequent surgical resection, intraoperative colonoscopy is occasionally performed (98–100). Intraoperative colonoscopy may also be useful to locate acute and chronic bleeding sites and may be performed after an unsuccessful conventional colonoscopy. Typically, this procedure is accomplished with the patient in a position to allow easy access of the colonoscope and the surgeon. Following the initiation of general anesthesia, a laparotomy is performed and routine inspection performed. Next, a noncrushing clamp is placed across the terminal ileum to prevent small bowel distension. The colonoscope is then inserted and advanced, with the assistance of the surgeon, to the cecum using minimal air insufflation. The usual colonoscope withdrawal technique and any necessary therapy are then applied. When a stenosing lesion has blocked passage of the colonoscope, a cleaned colonoscope can be introduced via a colotomy at the proximal margin of planned resection (99). Intraoperative colonoscopy should be viewed as an adjunct to conventional colonoscopy, rather than as a substitute (100).

Procedure Report

After the procedure, the patient is allowed to recover, with continued monitoring of vital signs and physical well-being until awake and alert. Prior to discharge from the recovery area, it is important to provide the patient with exam findings, education, and disposition instructions including recommendations for subsequent care, usually accomplished by an assistant. It is helpful to provide these instructions both verbally and in writing. It is essential to instruct the patient to call if any unusual symptoms develop after discharge and to inform the patient given intravenous sedation that no driving or potentially dangerous activity is allowed for a reasonable time period, usually the remainder of the day.

A procedure report should always be completed and signed shortly after each examination and placed into the patient's permanent record (101). The procedure report may be written and/or dictated. There seems to be an increasing use of computerized endoscopic medical record systems (102). In addition to simply providing information regarding the procedure, these systems can incorporate administrative functions, pathology reports, and photographs. The development of databases using these systems allows the information to be used for clinical outcomes research and quality assurance measures, while network connectivity allows the sharing of this information with other institutions. Ultimately, these systems promote completeness of the medical record and their use is encouraged (103).

The procedure report should systematically include the date, patient identification data, endoscopist and assistants, procedure being performed, indication, brief history and pertinent physical exam with relevant laboratory and X-ray data, informed consent, instrument used, and medications and monitoring devices used. The report of the examination should also include information concerning the depth of insertion, any difficulty arising during either insertion or withdrawal, the quality of the bowel preparation, description of findings, tissue or fluid samples taken, photographs taken, a list of any complications that may have arisen, and outcome. Finally, the report should include an impression with differential diagnosis based on the findings, recommendations for future management, disposition, and follow-up.

Indications

As its availability has increased and its benefits more readily recognized, the indications of colonoscopy have broadened (12). Certainly, colonoscopists should know the appropriate indications for colonoscopy and the interval at which it should be repeated for any given indication (4,5,104). Indications for colonoscopy, summarized in Table 1, can be divided into diagnostic and therapeutic. Because most of the diagnostic indications will be discussed in other chapters of this book, this discussion will instead focus on the therapeutic indications of colonoscopy. It is worthwhile mentioning that diagnostic colonoscopy is generally not indicated in patients with chronic, stable irritable bowel syndrome or abdominal pain, acute diarrhea, metastatic adenocarcinoma of unknown primary site in the absence of colonic signs or symptoms when it will not influence management, routine follow-up of inflammatory bowel disease, and melena with a demonstrated upper gastrointestinal source (12). Contraindications to colonoscopy are discussed in a later section of this chapter.

Colonoscopy allows for the performance of a number of therapeutic interventions (Table 1). Polypectomy was described shortly following the introduction of total colonoscopy (3) and was a major impetus for its successful acceptance into clinical practice. Prior to performing polypectomy, an understanding of the different electrical waveforms and the clinical effects of electrosurgery is necessary. It is also important to be aware that, at this time, there is no evidence that the use of electrosurgical equipment for endoscopic therapy should not be used in patients with pacemakers and implantable cardioverter/defibrillators (ICD) (105). However, to minimize theoretical risks, it is advised to continuously monitor the cardiac rhythm, use a grounding pad, deactivate ICD, use bipolar electrosurgical instruments (106), if available, and use short, repetitive bursts of energy rather than long bursts. Polypectomy is performed by placing the open loop of a snare device, passed through the accessory channel of the colonoscope, around the stalk or base of the polyp making sure not to snare the polyp itself or contiguous tissue, and applying low electrical power while slowly constricting the snare. This technique has proven to be an efficient and safe means of removing polyps. The amount of power and duration delivered and the use of pure coagulation versus blended current depends upon the thickness of the stalk and the experience of the colonoscopist. Except for

Table 1 Indications for the Performance of Colonoscopy

Colorectal cancer screening and surveillance
  Average-risk individuals
  Personal history of adenomatous colon polyps or colorectal cancer
  Family history of adenomatous colon polyps or colorectal cancer
  Hereditary nonpolyposis colorectal cancer syndrome
  Personal history of endometrial or ovarian cancer diagnosed at age <50
Unexplained diarrhea and bleeding
  Chronic diarrhea
  Positive fecal occult blood test
  Iron deficiency anemia
  Hematochezia if distal source is excluded by anoscopy/sigmoidoscopy
  Melena or moderate-to-severe hematochezia after an upper gut source has been excluded
Previously detected abnormality
  Abnormality seen on barium enema or other imaging study, which is likely to be clinically significant, such as
    a filling defect, stricture or, colon wall thickening
  Evaluation of remainder of colon and removal of polyp seen on sigmoidoscopy
Inflammatory bowel disease
  Surveillance of dysplasia in long-standing inflammatory bowel disease
  Determination of extent of inflammatory bowel disease
Intraoperative colonoscopy
  Location of previous polypectomy site, bleeding site, or nonpalpable lesion requiring surgical resection
  Inability to complete preoperative colonoscopy
  Assistance with colonoscopic polypectomy
  Assistance with the identification of strictures or extent of disease in Crohn's disease
Therapeutic colonoscopy
  Polypectomy
  Treatment of bleeding lesions (e.g., electrocoagulation, injection, heater probe, laser, argon plasma coagulation)
  Foreign body removal
  Colonic decompression
  Balloon dilatation of stenotic lesions
  Palliation of stenosing or bleeding neoplasms (e.g., laser, argon plasma coagulation, stent)
  Placement of stent in partially obstructing colon cancer to allow bowel prep/primary anastomosis

very broad-based polyps, almost all benign-appearing polyps can be removed via colonoscopy. In general, colonoscopic removal should be considered for benign-appearing lesions that occupy more than 30% of the circumference and do not cross two haustral folds (104). Saline-assisted polypectomy, where large sessile polyps receive submucosal injections of saline thereby elevating the polyp off the muscularis, provides the ability for safe and complete polypectomy of these lesions (107). For very large polyps, piecemeal resection may be successfully accomplished.

In some instances, usually depending upon the patient's age and health status, surgical resection of these large lesions may be advisable. In these situations, the preoperative use of India ink to tattoo the area may help the surgeon localize the lesion, thus obviating the need for intraoperative colonoscopy, and may also assist the colonoscopist at follow-up exams if the piecemeal resection approach is chosen. Alternatively, laparoscopy-assisted colonoscopic polypectomy allows patients to undergo removal of polyps that are too large or in an inaccessible location for safe conventional colonoscopic polypectomy (108). The use of laparoscopy to mobilize the pertinent portion of the bowel, straighten the sigmoid, and push the polyp base to an optimal position for conventional polypectomy, along with the ability to directly observe the serosa for complication during the polypectomy, allows this technique to be a safe and effective means of removing polyps that would otherwise require segmental colonic resection.

Effort should be made to retrieve all polyps removed and submit them for histologic review. Sometimes this can be difficult, especially with polyps removed piecemeal. A number of techniques have been described to assist polyp retrieval, including the use of grasping devices such as forceps, baskets, or mesh bags passed through the accessory channel of the endoscope, aspirating the polyp through the endoscope into a suction trap and sucking the polyp against the tip of the colonoscope and then slowly removing the instrument while suction is maintained.

While small polyps can also be removed using a snare, oftentimes without electrocautery (109), for convenience, a "hot" biopsy is often done instead. This technique was initially described in 1973 (110–112) and can be used to remove small sessile polyps, treat small angiodysplasia, and fulgurate residual tissue following snare polypectomy. To perform this procedure, the tissue is grasped, tented, and electrosurgical current is applied, resulting in a visible whitening of the base of the tissue. A potential limitation of this technique is the lesser quality of the biopsy specimen on histology due to coagulation artifact. There may be an increased risk of bleeding after hot biopsy, particularly delayed bleeding involving lesions treated in the right side of the colon (113). Finally, it is worth recognizing that it has been suggested that snare removal is more effective than hot or cold forceps removal for the treatment of small polyps.

Electrocoagulation can also be applied to the treatment of bleeding lesions as can injection therapy using dilute epinephrine or saline, laser photocoagulation, and the argon plasma coagulator (APC). These latter two therapies also offer the ability to debulk tumors in order to maintain lumen patency, ablate sessile polyps if conventional means are inappropriate, and fulgurate residual tissue remaining at the base of large polyps removed piecemeal. APC is a relatively new monopolar device that delivers thermal energy in a noncontact fashion through ionized argon gas. Advantages of the APC over laser therapy include its decreased cost, portability, and lower risk to the endoscopist and assistants (114,115). Nonetheless, complications can occur and have included abdominal distension, rectal pain, tenesmus, transmural coagulation, submucosal emphysema, and perforation.

Colonoscopy is occasionally used in patients with acute colonic pseudo-obstruction to decompress the colon and prevent ischemic injury and perforation (116,117). The presence of stool in the colon usually makes this procedure difficult and increases the risk of complication. While immediate decompression is the rule, because of the frequent occurrence of colonic redilation, many experts recommend the placement of a decompressive tube to at least the level of the hepatic flexure (118). This is usually accomplished without the need of fluoroscopy by passing the tube over a colonoscopically placed guidewire.

Dilation of colonic and anastomotic strictures can typically be accomplished without the need for prior guidewire placement using through-the-scope balloons inserted through the accessory channel of the colonoscope. A single dilation can be effective for a variable period of time depending upon the etiology of the stricture (e.g., Crohn's or postoperative anastomotic) (119). The degree of dilation also depends upon the etiology of the stricture and the initial lumen size. Occasionally, delivery of electrocoagulation via a needle-knife can be used to incise thin, short stenotic lesions.

Another endoscopic therapy that has recently been applied to the colon involves the placement of a self-expanding metal stent for nonsurgical palliation of left-sided colonic obstruction (120). This therapy may also allow for temporary relief of obstruction so that subsequent colonic resection can be performed under elective conditions following a proper bowel preparation, often allowing for a single-stage colonic anastomosis rather than diverting ostomy and subsequent closure. Placement of the stent may be accomplished using either a through-the-scope delivery system or over a guidewire placed by colonoscopy.

Endoscopic mucosal resection (EMR) is a promising technique that may allow the endoscopist to resect lesions not previously amenable to standard excisional techniques (121). EMR may be curative for superficial neoplasms without lymph node involvement or metastases. While most of the experience with EMR comes from its use in the upper gastrointestinal tract, this technique has been applied to the colon. A variety of EMR techniques have been described, and perforation and bleeding are the main complications reported. Long-term outcome data and cost analyses comparing EMR to surgical resection are currently lacking. Recently, successful use of a transmural resection device in a porcine model was described (122), and study of its clinical use in humans is planned.

Finally, the endoscopic treatment of symptomatic internal hemorrhoids using a band ligation system attached to the tip of the endoscope, identical to that used to treat esophageal varices, has also been shown to be safe and effective (123). This band ligation system has also been used to successfully treat bleeding colonic lesions. Clearly, this is an exciting time for colonoscopy, with rapid advances in both its diagnostic and therapeutic uses.

Contraindications, Complications, and Limitations

While colonoscopy is technically demanding for the endoscopist, it is also physiologically demanding on the patient undergoing the procedure. From the bowel preparation, which may cause electrolyte imbalance and dehydration, to the cardiorespiratory effects of the sedative-analgesic medications and the "sometimes strong" vagal stimulus caused by bowel distension related to colonoscope insertion, colonoscopy can produce dysrhythmias and other electrocardiographic abnormalities, hypotension, and hypoxia. While these effects are usually minor, they can rarely be catastrophic. As a consequence, there are a number of contraindications to the performance of colonoscopy (Table 2) (12). Nevertheless, depending upon the need for the information to direct medical or surgical therapy, colonoscopy is occasionally undertaken in each of these settings. Clearly, when the risks to the patient's health exceed the potential benefit of the procedure, colonoscopy should not be performed.

Colonoscopy is an invasive procedure and, as such, complications will sometimes occur despite the competent colonoscopist's technical abilities and good judgment. There are relatively few published articles prospectively reporting the incidence of such complications and because most are from centers with extensive experience, they may not accurately reflect the true risk in the general population (124–127). As would be expected, therapeutic colonoscopy is associated with a higher risk of complication than diagnostic colonoscopy. Fortunately, complications of colonoscopy occur infrequently and generally during the endoscopist's learning phase. An awareness of potential complications and avoidance of pain during colonoscopy will result in increased patient safety and tolerance (124).

Table 2 Contraindications to the Performance of Colonoscopy

Absolute	Relative
Acute peritonitis	Recent myocardial infarction
Suspected bowel perforation	Serious cardiac arrhythmia
Acute diverticulitis	Other serious medical conditions
Fulminant colitis	Late stages of pregnancy
Toxic megacolon	Recent colon resection
Suspected colonic obstruction	Poor colon preparation
Uncooperative patient	
Refusal of consent by a mentally competent patient	

Perforation is the most dreaded complication of colonoscopy, with an estimated incidence of 0.04% to 0.9% and 0.06% to 0.7% for diagnostic and therapeutic procedures, respectively (124). Recent reports suggest a decreased incidence of perforations—a finding that may be related to improvements in endoscopist training and equipment performance. Perforation can occur secondary to pressure from the instrument tip or a loop formed along the shaft, air pressure, or biopsies or therapeutic maneuvers such as polypectomy and stricture dilation. Perforation occurs most commonly in the sigmoid colon during diagnostic colonoscopy and the right colon for therapeutic colonoscopy. Possible risk factors for perforation include an uncooperative patient, poor bowel preparation, adhesions, diverticulosis, radiation, and ischemic colitis and obstruction (128,129). While old age does not seem to be a risk factor for perforation (130), a recent study suggests that female gender is a risk factor (125). While in most instances, the occurrence of a perforation is immediately recognized, many times the diagnosis is delayed. It has been suggested that in the absence of clinical evidence of peritonitis, regardless of the degree of pneumoperitoneum, and in the setting of a well-prepped colon, delayed presentation and therapeutic perforation, conservative management with nothing by mouth intravenous antibiotics, and nasogastric suction should be provided initially (131). If the patient's condition worsens, and in all other instances of perforation, urgent surgery is needed. Certainly, a surgeon should be a part of the decision-making in all instances of perforation.

The most common complication of colonoscopy is bleeding with an estimated incidence of 0.02% to 0.03% and 0.31% to 2.7% for diagnostic and therapeutic procedures, respectively (124). Bleeding after polypectomy, which is most commonly related to an imbalance of thermal and transectional forces, usually occurs immediately. Nevertheless, delayed bleeding also occurs, typically within two weeks of the polypectomy, and can be massive. Potential risk factors for bleeding include the removal of polyps greater than 2 cm in size, particularly large sessile lesions and pedunculated polyps with thick stalks, old age, and the presence of coagulation defects (124). Most immediate and delayed bleeding episodes stop spontaneously and require no intervention. In cases where intervention is needed, a number of injection, thermal, and mechanical therapies are available. If unsuccessful, angiography or surgery may be necessary. Saline-assisted polypectomy of large sessile lesions and the injection of dilute epinephrine into the stalk of thick-stalked pedunculated polyps may prevent bleeding. Furthermore, the use of cold snare polypectomy (i.e., without the use of electrocoagulation) of polyps lesser than 1 cm in size appears to be a safe and effective technique and may reduce the risks of both perforation and hemorrhage.

Two complications generally seen only after the performance of polypectomy include the postpolypectomy distension and the postpolypectomy coagulation syndromes (124). The former refers to the development of significant pain and abdominal distension in the absence of evidence of perforation occurring as a result of excessive air insufflation during colonoscopic polypectomy. While various maneuvers have been tried to decompress the patient, none have been consistently successful. Prevention of this complication is possible by limiting the amount of air insufflated, removing air at appropriate times, and remaining vigilant to the degree of abdominal distension (124). While the use of CO_2 instead of air insufflation has been advocated by some, its use has not been widely adopted. The postpolypectomy coagulation syndrome results from full-thickness thermal injury to the colonic wall and causes localized pain, fever, and leukocytosis up to 24 hours after polypectomy. Although the damage is self-limited, it is important to exclude perforation. Treatment is conservative (bowel rest and antibiotics) and the symptoms generally resolve within 48 hours. Nevertheless, close observation is necessary because progressive necrosis and perforation can occur.

As previously mentioned, the cardiorespiratory effects of the sedative-analgesic medications administered during colonoscopy and the vagal stimulus caused by bowel distension related to colonoscope insertion may cause dysrhythmias and other electrocardiographic abnormalities, hypotension, and hypoxia (132). Indeed, it has been estimated that 50% to 60% of endoscopic procedure–related morbidity and mortality is due to the use of sedation-analgesia (58). While these effects are usually minor, they can be catastrophic (133). The risk of cardiorespiratory complications is increased in patients with higher American Society of Anesthesiology (ASA) classes. Therefore, consideration should be given to reduced sedation doses, increased monitoring, and performing procedures in a hospital-based endoscopy unit in patients with higher ASA classes (104). Other reported complications of intravenous sedation include local thrombophlebitis and other local injection site reactions and, rarely, pulmonary embolism and cerebrovascular accident.

Endoscopy-related infection might occur from patient to patient by contaminated equipment, from the gut to the bloodstream and then to susceptible tissues or prostheses, or from patient to endoscopy personnel and vice versa (72,73). Clearly, the greatest risk of infection results from improperly cleaned and disinfected endoscopes. The risk of transmitting infection from properly reprocessed endoscopes is estimated to be 1 in 1.8 million procedures. Transient bacteremia, as detectable at 5 but not 15 minutes following a procedure, has an estimated incidence of 4% to 17% after colonoscopy and appears to be clinically insignificant. Furthermore, the organisms responsible for the bacteremia are not typical organisms associated with bacterial endocarditis. The addition of biopsy or polypectomy does not increase the risk. The recommendations for appropriate use of prophylactic antibiotics prior to colonoscopy, colonoscope reprocessing, and universal precautions have been discussed previously.

Complications related to bowel preparation are uncommon (33). The major problem related to the polyethylene glycol solution is the need to ingest a large volume over a relatively short time interval. To prevent excessive sodium absorption, abstinence from carbohydrate-containing food/fluid before and during ingestion of the solution is advised. A significant minority of patients develops nausea, vomiting, or other gastrointestinal complaints that may preclude their completion of bowel preparation or leave them with a poor bowel preparation at the time of colonoscopy (82). Hypothermia, gastrointestinal bleeding from a Mallory–Weiss tear, angioedema, and pulmonary complications following aspiration have also been reported with the use of this form of bowel preparation. The major disadvantages of sodium phosphate preparation are that abdominal cramping and fluid and electrolyte shifts may occur, resulting in electrolyte abnormalities and dehydration. Cases of fatal electrolyte abnormalities have been reported, but are extremely rare (134). Therefore, increased attention to fluid balance and electrolytes is necessary in patients sensitive to sudden volume changes, such as the elderly, dehydrated, or debilitated. Its use should be avoided in those with megacolon, ascites, renal disease, congestive heart failure, or bowel obstruction. It should be used with caution in those susceptible to electrolyte abnormalities, such as patients with other significant cardiac or renal diseases and intestinal dysmotility, and those on medications that affect electrolytes. The sodium phosphate preparation has also been associated with endoscopic and histologic findings of colitis (35). Lastly, a possible association between sodium phosphate tablets and tonic–clonic seizures has recently been described (135).

Death occurring directly as a result of colonoscopy is extremely uncommon, with an estimated mortality incidence of lesser than 0.02%. This is usually related to oversedation or operative complications following surgery for a colonoscopy-related complication.

Finally, there have been a number of uncommon complications of colonoscopy reported in the literature (124,136). Some of these include electrocautery-induced colonic explosion, appendicitis, diverticulitis, snare wire entrapment, ruptured spleen, lacerated liver, pneumatosis coli, pneumomediastinum, impaction of the colonoscope in a hernia sac, glutaraldehyde-induced colitis, dissecting aortic aneurysm, and superior mesenteric artery thrombosis. They will not be individually discussed here further.

Elements useful to minimize the complication risk include carefully selecting patients, having a constant awareness of the colonic lumen location, minimizing air insufflation, withdrawing the sigmoidoscope slightly if severe patient discomfort or "white-out" occurs, and above all, knowing when to stop and when to ask for help.

Occasionally, cancer will be identified shortly after a clearing colonoscopy. While generally considered the most sensitive test to image the colon, colonoscopy is not 100% accurate in detecting polyps or cancer (137–139). Indeed, there is an inherent miss rate of colonoscopy, which has been demonstrated in so-called tandem colonoscopy studies (140–142). Fortunately, most of these misses occur with adenomas 10 mm or less in diameter, where the likelihood of progression to invasive carcinoma is low. Nevertheless, this point underscores the need for vigilance when examining the colon and documentation of the limitations of the procedure. Given the obvious medicolegal implications of a "missed" cancer identified shortly after a clearing colonoscopy, a recent report suggests a number of measures to reduce the risks to the colonoscopist (143). These include educating the patient during the informed consent process that colonoscopy can occasionally miss significant lesions, documentation of cecal intubation, examination time, adequacy of bowel preparation and any difficulty that arose during the procedure, and vigilance during colonoscope withdrawal, with particular attention to subtle lesions such as flat or depressed lesions. Certainly, those with inadequate bowel preparation should undergo a repeat exam at an interval earlier than would normally be chosen on the basis of an adequate prep. There is insufficient evidence to support the routine use of chromoendoscopy to aid in the identification of subtle lesions at present.

AIR-CONTRAST BARIUM ENEMA AND VIRTUAL COLONOSCOPY

Colonoscopy has overtaken the air-contrast barium enema (ACBE), discussed in more detail in the radiology, Chapter 7, of this text, as the diagnostic test of choice in the evaluation of the colon, given its superior diagnostic accuracy combined with the ability to obtain biopsies and provide therapy at the time of the procedure (144). Clearly, ACBE is inferior to colonoscopy in assessing fine mucosal detail and small polyps and early cancers (145,146) and its interpretation may be further hindered by poor bowel preparation, diverticulosis, air bubbles, and bowel spasm. In addition, colonoscopy seems to be preferred by patients over ACBE (147). However, colonoscopy is more difficult to perform, is more expensive, generally requires intravenous sedation-analgesia, and is associated with a higher incidence of complications. Additionally, colonoscopy is occasionally unsuccessful in reaching the cecum. In these circumstances, ACBE is useful to evaluate the remainder of the colon (148). Of note is the fact that colonic biopsy, and probably hot biopsy and snare polypectomy of small lesions, can be performed safely before ACBE (149). ACBE is also useful when evaluating colon configuration and structural abnormalities such as strictures, fistulae, megacolon, and Hirschsprung's disease. ACBE may be preferable in the debilitated patient where colonoscopy may be too hazardous. A modified enema study, usually with a water-soluble contrast agent, may be preferred when evaluating possible colonic obstruction and computed tomographic (CT) imaging is indeterminate. This modified enema study may also be useful therapeutically to aid the evacuation of stool in severely obstipated patients or in decompressing a volvulus. Therefore, colonoscopy and ACBE can be seen as complementary tests particularly when a skilled colonoscopist is not available or the colonoscopy proves to be too difficult, incomplete, or too high risk.

In its relative infancy, virtual colonoscopy, also discussed in Chapter 7, refers to the use of helical CT scanning and advanced imaging software to produce both two- and three-dimensional images of the colon (150–152). A similar technique using magnetic resonance imaging has also been described. This technique has the obvious advantage of absence of radiation but the disadvantage of increased cost. Virtual colonoscopy is viewed as a safe and noninvasive test that may prove to be an alternative to barium enema and diagnostic colonoscopy—an increasingly important point as the demand for colonoscopy, particularly screening colonoscopy, increases. This technique still requires bowel cleansing and pneumocolon but not patient sedation. Colonoscopy is still required when abnormalities are detected or findings are indeterminate. This is a particularly important point that patients should be aware of (153). Recent studies have demonstrated good but not excellent rates of polyp detection, and only for lesions at least 8 mm in diameter. Its cost-effectiveness has also recently been questioned (154). Nevertheless, with advances in imaging software and scanning technique and the development of a contrast agent that allows computer subtraction of stool and, thus, obviates the need for bowel preparation, the potential of virtual colonoscopy is substantial and unmistakable.

CONCLUSION

Advances in colonoscope development, techniques for instrument manipulation, incorporation of diagnostic and therapeutic applications of colonoscopy, and the development of more effective and tolerable means of bowel preparation and patient sedation have made colonoscopy the primary method of imaging the colon. Further advances in these areas along with the development of additional diagnostic and therapeutic techniques are sure to keep the practice of colonoscopy thriving.

REFERENCES

1. Modlin IM. A Brief History of Endoscopy. Milano: Multimed, 2000.
2. Overholt BF. Clinical experience with the fiber sigmoidoscoope. Gastrointest Endosc 1968; 15:27.
3. Wolff WI, Shinya H. A new approach to colon polyps. Ann Surg 1973; 178:367–378.

4. Winawer SJ, Fletcher RH, Miller L, et al. Colorectal screening guidelines and rationale. Gastroenterology 1997; 112:594–642.

5. Smith RA, von Eschenbach AC, Wender R, et al. American Cancer Society guidelines for the early detection of cancer: update of early detection guidelines for prostate, colorectal and endometrial cancers. CA Cancer J Clin 2001; 51:38–75.

6. Rex D, Johnson D, Lieberman DA, Burt RA, Sonnenberg A. Colorectal cancer prevention 2000: screening recommendations of the American College of Gastroenterology. Am J Gastorenterol 2000; 95:868–877.

7. Rex DK, Lieberman DA. Feasibility of colonoscopy screening: discussion of issues and recommendations regarding implementation. Gastrointest Endosc 2001; 54:662–667.

8. Hunt RH, Waye JD, eds. Colonoscopy: Techniques, Clinical Practice and Colour Atlas. London: Chapman and Hall, 1981.

9. Cotton PB, Williams CB. Practical Gastrointestinal Endoscopy. 4th ed. Cambridge: Blackwell Science Ltd, 1996.

10. Moore KL. Essentials of Human Embryology. Philadelphia: BC Decker Inc., 1988.

11. ASGE. Flexible sigmoidoscopy. Gastrointest Endosc 1998; 48:695–696.

12. ASGE. Appropriate use of gastrointestinal endoscopy. Gastrointest Endosc 2000; 52:831–837.

13. Gilbertson VA. Proctosigmoidoscopy and polypectomy in reducing the incidence of rectal cancer. Cancer 1974; 34:936–939.

14. Marks G, Goggs HW, Castro AF, Gathright JB, Ray JE, Salvati E. Sigmoidoscopic examinations with rigid and flexible fiberoptic sigmoidoscopes in the surgeon's office: a comparative prospective study of effectiveness in 1,012 cases. Dis Colon Rectum 1979; 22:162–168.

15. Winnan G, Berci G, Panish J, Talbot TM, Overholt BF, McCallum RW. Superiority of the flexible to the rigid sigmoidoscope in routine proctosigmoidoscopy. N Engl J Med 1980; 302:1011–1012.

16. ASGE. Principles of training in gastrointestinal endoscopy. Gastrointest Endosc 1999; 49:845–853.

17. Marshall JB. Technical proficiency of trainees performing colonoscopy: a learning curve. Gastrointest Endosc 1995; 42:287–291.

18. ASGE. Endoscopy simulators. Gastrointest Endosc 2000; 51:790–792.

19. Hochberger J, Maiss J, Magdeburg B, Cohen J, Hahn EG. Training simulators and education in gastrointestinal endoscopy: current status and perspectives in 2001. Endoscopy 2001; 33:541–549.

20. Cass OW, Freeman ML, Peine CJ, Zera RT, Onstad GR. Objective evaluation of endoscopy skills during training. Ann Intern Med 1993; 118:40–44.

21. Cass OW, Freeman ML, Cohen J, et al. Acquisition of competency in endoscopic skills (ACES) during training: a multicenter study. Gastrointest Endosc 1996; 43:A308.

22. Chak A, Cooper GS, Blades EW, Canto M, Sivak MV. Prospective assessment of colonoscopic intubation skills in trainees. Gastointest Endosc 1996; 44:54–57.

23. Hawes R, Lehman GA, Hast J, et al. Training resident physicians in fiberoptic sigmoidoscopy: how many supervised examinations are required to achieve competence? Am J Med 1986; 80:465–470.

24. Bond JH. Evaluation of trainee competence. Gastrointest Endosc Clin N Am 1995; 5:337–346.

25. ASGE. Methods of granting hospital privileges to perform gastrointestinal endoscopy. Gastrointest Endosc 2002; 55:780–783.

26. Health and Public Policy Committee, ACP. Clinical competence in colonoscopy. Ann Intern Med 1987; 107:772–774.

27. ASGE. Principles of privileging and credentialing for endoscopy and colonoscopy. Gastrointest Endosc 2002; 55:145–147.

28. Shapiro M. Granting hospital privileges to perform endoscopies. Hosp Med Staff 1982; 11:3.

29. ASGE. Preparation of patients for gastrointestinal endoscopy. Gastrointest Endosc 1998; 48:691–694.

30. ASGE. Informed consent for gastrointestinal endoscopy. Gastrointest Endosc 1988; 34 (suppl 3): S26–S27.

31. ASGE. Colonoscopy preparations. Gastrointest Endosc 2001; 54:829–832.

32. Hsu CF, Imperiale TF. Meta-analysis and cost comparison of polyethylene glycol lavage versus sodium phosphate for colonoscopy preparation. Gastrointest Endosc 1998; 48:276–282.

33. Wexner SD, Beck DE, Baron TH, et al. A consensus document on bowel preparation before colonoscopy: prepared by a task force from the American Society of Colon and Rectal Surgeons (ASCRS), the American Society for Gastrointestinal Endoscopy (ASGE), and the Society of American Gastrointestinal and Endoscopic Surgeons (SAGES). Dis Colon Rectum. 2006; 49:792-809.

34. Davis GR, Santa Ana CA, Morawski SG, Fordtran JS. Development of a lavage solution associated with minimal water and electrolyte absorption or secretion. Gastroenterology 1980; 78:991–995.

35. Watts DA, Lessells AM, Penman ID, Ghosh S. Endoscopic and histologic features of sodium phosphate bowel preparation-induced colonic ulceration: case report and review. Gastrointest Endosc 2002; 55:584–587.

36. Aronchick CA, Lipshultz WH, Wright SH, Dufrayne F, Bergman G. A novel tableted purgative for colonoscopic preparation: efficacy and safety comparisons with Colyte and Fleet Phospho-Soda. Gastrointest Endosc 2000; 52:346–352.

37. ASGE. Antibiotic prophylaxis for gastrointestinal endoscopy. Gastrointest Endosc 1995; 42:630–635.

38. Dajani AS, Taubert KA, Wilson W, et al. Prevention of bacterial endocarditis: recommendations by the American Heart Association. JAMA 1997; 277:1794–1801.

39. ASGE. Guidelines on the management of anticoagulation and platelet therapy for endoscopic procedures. Gastrointest Endosc 2002; 55:775–779.
40. Shiffman ML, Farrel MT, Yee YS. Risk of bleeding after endoscopic biopsy or polypectomy in patients taking aspirin or other NSAIDs. Gastrointest Endosc 1994; 40:458–462.
41. ASGE. The recommended use of laboratory studies before endoscopic procedures. Gastorintest Endosc 1994; 39:892–894.
42. Van Os EC, Kamath PS, Gostout CJ, Heit JA. Gastroenterological procedures among patients with disorders of hemostasis: evaluation and management recommendations. Gastrointest Endosc 1999; 50: 536–543.
43. Dickey W, Garrett D. Colonoscope length and procedure efficiency. Am J Gastroenterol 2002; 97: 79–82.
44. Brooker JC, Saunders BP, Shah SG, Williams CB. A new variable stiffness colonoscope makes colonoscopy easier: a randomized controlled trial. Gut 2000; 46:801–805.
45. Shumaker DA, Zama A, Katon RM. A randomized controlled trial in a training institution comparing a pediatric variable stiffness colonoscope, a pediatric colonoscope, and an adult colonoscope. Gastrointest Endosc 2002; 55:172–179.
46. Shah SG, Saunders BP, Brokker JC, Williams CB. Magnetic imaging of colonoscopy: an audit oflooping, accuracy and ancillary maneuvers. Gastrointest Endosc 2000; 52:1–8.
47. Shah SG, Brooker JC, Williams CB, Thapar C, Saunders BP. Effect of magnetic endoscope imaging on colonoscopy performance: a randomized controlled trial. Lancet 2000; 356:1718–1722.
48. Shah SG, Brooker JC, Thapar C, Suzuki N, Williams CB, Saunders BP. Effect of magnetic endoscope imaging on patient tolerance and sedation requirements during colonoscopy: a randomized controlled trial. Gastrointest Endosc 2002; 55:832–837.
49. ASGE. High resolution and high-magnification endoscopy. Gastrointest Endosc 2000; 52:864–866.
50. Tung SY, Wu CS, Su MY. Magnifying colonoscopy in differentiating neoplastic from nonneoplastic colorectal lesions. Am J Gastroenterol 2001; 96:2628–2632.
51. Eisen GM, Kim CY, Fleischer DE, et al. High-resolution chromoendoscopy for classifying colonic polyps: a multicenter study. Gastrointest Endosc 2002; 55:687–694.
52. Fujii T, Hasegawa RT, Saitoh Y, et al. Chromoscopy during colonoscopy. Endoscopy 2001; 33: 1036–1041.
53. ASGE. Role of endoscopic ultrasonography. Gastrointest Endosc 2000; 52:852–859.
54. Saitoh Y, Obara T, Einami K, et al. Efficacy of high-frequency ultrasound probes for the preoperative staging of invasion depth in flat and depressed colorectal tumors. Gastrointest Endosc 1996; 44: 34–39.
55. Pasricha PJ, Motamedi M. Optical biopsies, "bioendoscopy," and why the sky is blue: the coming revolution in gastrointestinal imaging. Gastroenterology 2002; 122:571–575.
56. Seow-Choen F, Leong A, Tsang C. Selective sedation for colonoscopy. Gastrointest Endosc 1994; 40:661–664.
57. Daneshmind TK, Bell GD, Logan RFA. Sedation for upper gastrointestinal endoscopy: results of a nationwide survey. Gut 1991; 32:12–15.
58. Silvis SE, Nebel O, Rogers G, Sugawa C, Mandelstam P. Endoscopic complications: results of the 1974 American Society for Gastrointestinal Endoscopy survey. JAMA 1976; 235:928–930.
59. ASGE. Guidelines for training in patient monitoring and sedation and analgesia. Gastrointest Endosc 1998; 48:669–671.
60. Freeman M. Sedation and monitoring for gastrointestinal endoscopy. Gastrointest Endosc Clin N Am 1994; 4:475–499.
61. American Society of Anesthesiologists. Practice guidelines for sedation and analgesia by non-anesthesiologists. Anesthesiology 1996; 84:459–471.
62. Lee DWH, Chan K-W, Poon C-M, et al. Relaxation music decreases the dose of patient-controlled sedation during colonoscopy: a prospective randomized controlled trial. Gastrointest Endosc 2002; 55:33–36.
63. Jimenez-Perez J, Pastor G, Aznarez R, Carral D, Rodriguez C, Borda F. Iatrogenic perforation in diagnostic colonoscopy related to the type of sedation. Gastrointest Endosc 2000; 51:AB68.
64. Frehlich F, Horens J, Schwizer W, et al. Sedation and analgesia for colonoscopy: patient tolerance, pain, and cardiorespiratory parameters. Gastrointest Endosc 1997; 45:1–9.
65. Morrow JB, Zuccaro G, Conwell DL, et al. Sedation for colonoscopy using a single bolus is safe, effective, and efficient: a prospective, randomized, double-blind trial. Am J Gastroenterol 2000; 95: 2242–2247.
66. Sipe BW, Rex DK, Latinovich D, et al. Propofol versus midazolam/meperidine for oupatient colonoscopy: administration by nurses supervised by endoscopists. Gastrointest Endosc 2002; 55:815–822.
67. Rex DK, Overley C, Kinser K, et al. Safety of propofol administered by registered nurses with gastroenterologist supervision in 2000 endoscopic cases. Am J Gastroenterol 2002; 97:159–1163.
68. Vargo JJ, Zuccaro G, Dumot JA, Conwell DL, Morrow JB, Shay SS. Automated graphic assessment of respiratory activity is superior to pulse oximetry and visual assessment for the detection of early respiratory depression during therapeutic upper endoscopy. Gastrointest Endosc 2002; 55:826–831.
69. ASGE Technology Assessment Position Paper. Personal protective equipment. November 1998.
70. ASGE. Reprocessing of flexible gastrointestinal endoscopes. Gastrointest Endosc 1996; 43:540–546.

71. Alvarado CJ, Mark R. APIC guidelines for infection prevention and control in flexible endoscopy. Am J Infect Control 2000; 28:138–155.
72. ASGE Technology Assessment Position Paper. Transmission of infection by gastrointestinal endoscopy. April 1993.
73. Spach DH, Silverstein FE, Stamm WE. Transmission of infection by gastrointestinal endoscopy and bronchoscopy. Ann Intern Med 1993; 118:117–128.
74. Muscarella LF. High-level disinfection or "sterilization" of endoscopes? Infect Control Hosp Epidemiol 1996; 17:183–187.
75. ASGE. Infection control during gastrointestinal endoscopy. Gastrointest Endosc 1999; 49:836–841.
76. Cronmiller JR, Nelson DK, Salman G, et al. Antimicrobial efficacy of endoscopic disinfection procedures: a controlled, multifactorial investigation. Gastrointest Endosc 1999; 50:152–158.
77. Kovacs BJ, Chen YK, Kettering JD, Aprecia PM, Roy I. High-level disinfection of gastrointestinal endoscopes: are current guidelines adequate? Am J Gastroenterol 1999; 94:1546–1550.
78. ASGE Technology Assessment Position Paper. Disposable endoscopic accessories. September 1994.
79. Turk DJ, Kozarek RA, Botoman VA, Patterson DJ, Ball TJ. Disposable endoscopic biopsy forceps: comparison with standard forceps of sample size and adequacy of specimen. J Clin Gastroenterol 1991; 13:76–78.
80. ASGE. Sheathed endoscopes. Gastrointest Endosc 1999; 49:862–864.
81. Sardinha TC, Wexner SD, Gilliland J, et al. Efficiency and productivity of a sheathed fiberoptic sigmoidoscope compared with a conventional sigmoidoscope. Dis Colon Rectum 1997; 40:1248–1253.
82. Galia A, Niv Y. Predictors of inadequate colonic preparation for colonoscopy. Am J Gastroenterol 2002; 97:216.
83. Stevenson GW, Wilson JA, Wilkinson J, Norma G, Goodacre RL. Pain following colonoscopy: elimination with carbon dioxide. Gastrointest Endosc 1992; 38:564–567.
84. Marshall JB, Perez RA, Madsen RW. Usefulness of a pediatric colonoscope for routine colonoscopy in women who have undergone hysterectomy. Gastrointest Endosc 2002; 55:838–841.
85. Kozarek RA, Botoman VA, Patterson DJ. Prospective evaluation of a small caliber upper endoscope for colonoscopy after unsuccessful standard examination. Gastrointest Endosc 1989; 35:333–335.
86. Rex DK, Goodwine BW. Method of colonoscopy in 42 consecutive patients presenting after prior incomplete colonoscopy. 2002; 97:1148–1151.
87. Waye JD, Yessayan SA, Lewis BS, Fabry TL. The technique of abdominal pressure in total colonoscopy. Gastrointest Endosc 1991; 37:147–151.
88. Catalano F, Catanzaro R, Branciforte G, et al. Colonoscopy technique with an external straightener. Gastrointest Endosc 2000; 51:600–604.
89. Anderson JC, Gonzalez JD, Messina CR, Pollack BJ. Factors that predict incomplete colonoscopy: thinner is not always better. Am J Gastroenterol 2000; 95:2784–2787.
90. Kim WK, Cho YJ, Park JY, Min PK, Kang JK, Park IS. Factors affecting insertion time and patient discomfort during colonoscopy. Gastrointest Endosc 2000; 52:600–605.
91. Rex DK. Still photography versus videotaping for documentation of cecal intubation: a prospective study. Gastrointest Endosc 2000; 51:451–459.
92. Rex DK. Colonoscopic withdrawal technique is associated with adenoma miss rates. Gastrointest Endosc 2000; 51:33–36.
93. Hanson JM, Atkin WS, Cunliffe WJ, et al. Rectal retroflexion: an essential part of lower gastrointestinal endoscopic examination. Dis Colon Rectum 2001; 44:1706–1708.
94. Cutler AF, Pop A. Fifteen years later: colonoscopic retroflexion revisited. Am J Gastroenterol 1999; 94:1537–1538.
95. Hancock JH, Talbot RW. Accuracy of colonoscopy in localization of colorectal cancer. Int J Colorectal Dis 1995; 10:140.
96. ASGE. Endoscopic tattooing. Gastrointest Endosc 2002; 55:811–814.
97. Nizam R, Siddiqi N, Landas SK, Kaplan DS, Holtzapple PG. Colonic tattooing with India ink: benefits, risks, and alternatives. Am J Gastroenterol 1996; 91:1804–1808.
98. Saclarides TJ, Wolff BG, Pemberton JH, Devine RM, Nivatvongs S, Dozois RR. Clean sweep of the colon. The use of intraoperative colonoscopy. Dis Colon Rectum 1989; 32:864–866.
99. Brullet E, Montane JM, Bombardo J, Bonfill X, Nogue M, Bordas JM. Intraoperative colonoscopy in patients with colorectal cancer. Br J Surg 1992; 79:1376–1378.
100. Whelan RL, Buls JG, Goldberg SM, Rothenberger DA. Intra-operative endoscopy. University of Minnesota experience. Am Surg 1989; 55:281–286.
101. ASGE. Quality improvement of gastrointestinal endoscopy. Gastrointest Endosc 1999; 49:842–844.
102. ASGE Technology Status Evaluation Report. Computerized endoscopic medical record systems. November 1999.
103. Gouveia-Oliveira A, Raposos VD, Salgado NC, Almeida I, Nobre-Leitao C, de Melo FG. Longitudinal comparative study on the influence of computers on reporting of clinical data. Endoscopy 1991; 23:334–337.
104. Rex DK, Bond JH, Winawer S, et al. Quality in the technical performance of colonoscopy and the continuous quality improvement process for colonoscopy: recommendations of the U.S. multisociety task force on colorectal cancer. Am J Gastroenterol 2002; 97:1296–1308.

105. ASGE Technology Assessment. Electrocautery use in patients with implanted cardiac devices. Gastrointest Endosc 1994; 40:794–795.
106. ASGE Technology Assessment Status Evaluation. Bipolar and multipolar accessories. February 1996.
107. Shirai M, Nakamura T, Matsuura A, Ito Y, Kobayashi S. Safer colonoscopic polypectomy with local submucosal injection of hypertonic saline-epinephrine solution. Am J Gastroenterol 1994; 89: 334–338.
108. Franklin ME Jr., Diaz-E JA, Abrego D, Parra-Davila E, Glass JL. Laparascopic-assisted colonoscopic polypectomy: the Texas endosurgery institute experience. Dis Colon Rectum 2000; 43:1246–1249.
109. Uno Y, Obara K, Zheng P, et al. Cold snare excision is a safe method for diminutive colorectal polyps. Tohoku J Exp Med 1997; 183:243–249.
110. Williams CB. Diathermy-biopsy: a technique for the endoscopic management of small polyps. Endoscopy 1973; 5:215–218.
111. ASGE. Status evaluation: hot biopsy forceps. Gastrointest Endosc 1992; 38:753–756.
112. Woods A, Sanowski RA, Wadas DD, Manne RK, Friess SW. Eradication of diminutive polyps: a prospective evaluation of bipolar electrocoagulation versus conventional biopsy removal. Gastrointest Endosc 1989; 35:536–539.
113. Dyer WS, Quigley EMM, Noel SM, Camacho KE, Manela F, Zetterman RK. Major colonic hemorrhage following electrocoagulating (hot) biopsy of diminutive colon polyps: relationship to colonic location and low-dose aspirin therapy. Gastrointest Endosc 1991; 37:361–363.
114. ASGE. The argon plasma coagulator. Gastrointest Endosc 2002; 55:807–810.
115. Wahab PJ, Mulder CJJ, den Hartog G, Thies JE. Argon plasma coagulation in flexible gastrointestinal endoscopy: pilot experiences. Endoscopy 1997; 29:176–181.
116. Bode WE, Beart RWJ, Spencer RJ, Culp CE, Wolff BG, Taylor BM. Colonoscopic decompression for acute pseudoobstruction of the colon (Ogilvie's syndrome): report of 22 cases and review of the literature. Am J Surg 1984; 147:243–245.
117. Martin FM, Robinson AM, Thompson WR. Therapeutic colonoscopy in the treatment of colonic pseudo-obstruction. Am Surg 1988; 54:519–522.
118. Geller A, Petesen BT, Gostout CJ. Endoscopic decompression of acute colonic pseudo-obstruction. Gastrointest Endosc 1996; 44:144–150.
119. Breysem Y, Janssens JF, Coremans G, Vantrappen G, Hendrickx G, Rutgeerts P. Endoscopic balloon dilation of colonoic and ileo-colonic Crohn's strictures: long-term results. Gastrointest Endosc 1992; 38:142–147.
120. Law WL, Chu KW, Ho JWC, Tung HM, Law SYK, Chu KM. Self-expanding metallic stent in the treatment of colonic obstruction caused by advanced malignancies. Dis Colon Rectum 2000; 43: 1522–1527.
121. ASGE. Endoscopic mucosal resection. Gastrointest Endosc 2000; 52:860–863.
122. Rajan E, Gostout CJ, Burgart LJ, et al. First endoluminal system for transmural resection of colorectal tissue with a prototype full-thickness resection device in a porcine model. Gastrointest Endosc 2002; 55:915–920.
123. Trowers EA, Ganga U, Rizk R, Ojo E, Hodges D. Endoscopic hemorrhoidal ligation: preliminary clinical experience. Gastrointest Endosc 1998; 48:49–52.
124. Waye JD, Kahn O, Auerbach ME. Complications of colonoscopy and flexible sigmoidoscopy. Gastrointest Endosc Clin North Am 1996; 6:343–377.
125. Nelson DB, McQuaid KR, Bond JH, Lieberman DA, Weiss DG, Johnston TK. Procedural success and complications of large-scale screening colonoscopy. Gastrointest Endosc 2002; 55:307–314.
126. Dafnis G, Ekbom A, Pahlman L, Blomqvist P. Complications of diagnostic and therapeutic colonoscopy within a defined population in Sweden. Gastrointest Endosc 2001; 54:302–309.
127. Zubarik R, Fleischer DE, Mastropietro C, et al. Prospective analysis of complications 30 days after outpatient colonoscopy. Gastrointest Endosc 1999; 50:322–328.
128. Anderson ML, Pasha TM, Leighton JA. Endoscopic perforation of the colon: lesions from a 10-year study. Am J Gastroenterol 2000; 95:3418–3422.
129. Orsoni P, Berdah S, Verrier C, et al. Colonic perforation due to colonoscopy: a retrospective study of 48 cases. Endoscopy 1997; 29:160–164.
130. DiPrima RE, Barkin JS, Blinder M, Goldberg RI, Phillips RS. Age as a risk factor in colonoscopy: fact versus fiction. Am J Gastroenterol 1988; 2:123–125.
131. Ecker MD, Goldstein M, Hoexter B, Hyman RA, Naidich JB, Stein HL. Benign pneumoperitoneum after fiberoptic colonoscopy: a prospective study of 100 patients. Gastroenterology 1977; 73:226–230.
132. Fennerty MB, Earnest DL, Hudson PB, Sampliner RE. Physiologic changes during colonoscopy. Gastrointest Endosc 1990; 36:22–25.
133. Cappell MS. Safety and clinical efficacy of flexible sigmoidoscopy and colonoscopy for GI bleeding after myocardial infarction. Dig Dis Sci 1994; 39:473.
134. Ullah N, Yeh R, Ehrinpreis M. Fatal hyperphosphatemia from a phosphosoda bowel preparation. J Clin Gastroenterol 2002; 34:457–458.
135. Mackey AC, Shaffer D, Prizant R. Seizure associated with the use of Visicol for colonoscopy. N Engl J Med 2002; 346:2095.
136. Rice E, DiBaise JK, Quigley EMM. Superior mesenteric artery thrombosis after colonoscopy. Gastrointest Endosc 1999; 50:706–707.

137. Haseman JH, Lemmel GT, Rahmani EY, Rex DK. Failure of colonoscopy to detect colorectal cancer: evaluation of 47 cases in 20 hospitals. Gastrointest Endosc 1997; 45:451–455.

138. Ee HC, Semmens JB, Hoffman NE. Complete colonoscopy rarely missed cancer. Gastrointest Endosc 2002; 55:167–171.

139. Shehadeh I, Rebala S, Kumar R, Markert RJ, Barde C, Gopalswamy N. Retrospective analysis of missed advanced adenomas on surveillance colonoscopy. Am J Gastroenterol 2002; 97:1143–1147.

140. Rex DK, Cutler CS, Lemmel GT, et al. Colonoscopic miss rates of adenomas determined by back-to-back colonoscopies. Gastroenterology 1997; 112:24–28.

141. Bensen S, Mott LA, Dain B, Rothstein R, Baron J. The colonoscopic miss rate and true one-year recurrence of colorectal neoplastic polyps. Polyp Prevention Study Group. Am J Gastroenterol 1999; 94:194–199.

142. Hixson LJ, Fennerty MB, Sampliner RE, Garewal HS. Prospective blinded trial of the colonoscopic miss-rate of large colorectal polyps. Gastrointest Endosc 1991; 37:125–127.

143. Rex DK, Bond JH, Feld AD. Medical-legal risks of incident cancers after clearing colonoscopy. Am J Gastroenterol 2001; 96:952–957.

144. Lindsay DC, Freeman JG, Cobden I. Should colonoscopy be the first investigation for colonic disease? Br Med J 1988; 296:167–168.

145. Rex DK, Rahmani EY, Haseman JH, Lemmel GT, Kaster S, Buckley JS. Relative sensitivity of colonoscopy and barium enema for detection of colorectal cancer in clinical practice. Gastroenterology 1997; 112:17–23.

146. Winawer SJ, Stewart ET, Zauber AG, et al. A comparison of colonoscopy and double contrast barium enema for surveillance after polypectomy. N Engl J Med 2000; 342:1766–1772.

147. Kim LS, Koch J, Yee J, Halvorsen R, Cello JP, Rockey DC. Comparison of patients' experiences during imaging tests of the colon. Gastrointest Endosc 2001; 54:67–74.

148. Mark DG, Rex DK, Lappas JC. Quality of air contrast barium enema performed the same day as incomplete colonoscopy with air insufflation. Gastrointest Endosc 1992; 38:693–695.

149. Harned RK, Consigny PM, Cooper NB, Williams SM, Wottjen AJ. Barium enema examination following biopsy of the rectum or colon. Radiology 1982; 145:11–16.

150. ASGE. Virtual colonoscopy. Gastrointest Endosc 1998; 48:708–710.

151. Johnson CD, Hara AK, Reed JE. Computed tomographic colonography (virtual colonoscopy): a new method for detecting colorectal neoplasms. Endoscopy 1997; 29:454–461.

152. Yee J. Virtual colonoscopy (CT and MR colonography). Gastrointest Endosc 2002; 55(suppl):S25–S32.

153. Akerkar GA, Yee J, Hung R, McQuaid K. Patient experience and preferences toward colon cancer screening: a comparison of virtual colonoscopy and conventional colonoscopy. Gastrointest Endosc 2001; 54:310–315.

154. Sonnenberg A, Delco F, Bauerfeind P. Is virtual colonoscopy a cost-effective option to screen for colorectal cancer? Am J Gastroenterol 1999; 94:2268–2274.

7 | Radiology of the Colon

Ruedi F. Thoeni and Raymond Thornton
Department of Radiology, University of California–San Francisco, San Francisco, California, U.S.A.

INTRODUCTION

Within less than 10 years of the discovery of X rays by Roentgen in 1895, examinations of the colon with opaque contrast material were pioneered and later became part of the routine clinical service that radiology could provide in assessing colonic disease (1,2). Over almost 100 years, the barium enema has undergone many changes and refinements and, in skilled hands, remains at the forefront of radiologic examinations of the large bowel. This technique has evolved from the single-contrast barium enema examination to double-contrast techniques that provide excellent mucosal detail in patients with inflammatory changes, particularly in patients with idiopathic inflammatory bowel disease and in patients at risk for colonic neoplasms. Although the barium enema examination is no longer the most important method of examining patients with suspected inflammatory bowel disease, it does aid in reaching the correct diagnosis in conjunction with the clinical history and examination, laboratory tests, and colonoscopy. The introduction of fiberoptic endoscopic methods has markedly reduced the number of barium enemas performed in the United States. Colonoscopy has the advantage of directly visualizing the colonic mucosa and enables determining the extent of disease, obtaining tissue specimens through biopsies, cauterizing sources of colonic hemorrhage, obliterating small polyps, or decompressing a markedly distended colon. In short, diagnostic as well as therapeutic options are available with colonoscopy.

To the technique of directly visualizing the lumen of the large bowel, endoscopic ultrasound (EUS) has been added. EUS permits assessment of the entire thickness of the large bowel wall and differentiation of the various layers within the colonic wall. However, with this method, determining the depth of involvement by an inflammatory or neoplastic process is limited, and other techniques are still needed to ascertain the extent of disease beyond the confines of the bowel wall to local and distant sites. Cross-sectional imaging with computed tomography (CT) and magnetic resonance (MR) can achieve this goal and has a major role in assessing patients with inflammatory disease of the large bowel and in the preoperative staging of patients to assess both locally advanced and distal disease. It also can be used to determine the presence or absence of recurrent disease. To this armamentarium of imaging methods, positron emission tomography (PET) has been more recently added, which can provide information on the metabolism of primary and metastatic lesions. Its role has increased in recent years. Overall, radiology of the colon has a pivotal role in the diagnosis of colonic disease. The following chapter will address the various techniques, their results, and their roles.

PLAIN FILMS

Plain film radiography remains a quick and powerful tool for the assessment of the patient with abdominal symptoms. Familiarity with the normal pattern of abdominal bowel gas distribution and the normal appearances of visible soft tissues permits specific diagnoses to be made. While a review of abdominal plain film radiography is beyond the scope of this chapter, key points relating to colon imaging are reviewed below.

Pneumoperitoneum

Abdominal radiographs provide a quick means to assess for the presence of extraluminal air in the peritoneal cavity, indicative of a perforated viscus. Left lateral decubitus and upright lateral chest films are the most sensitive plain film examinations for the detection of

(A)   **(B)**

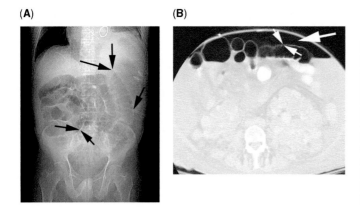

Figure 1 (**A**) Plain film of the abdomen in patient with ischemia. The small bowel wall can be seen outlined by air on both sides (*arrows*), indicative of perforation with free air in the abdomen (Rigler's sign). (**B**) CT of the abdomen in the same patient as (**A**) clearly demonstrates a significant amount of free air underneath the abdominal wall. The wall of the small bowel (*arrows*) is highlighted by air in the lumen and by free air in the peritoneal cavity.

pneumoperitoneum, with free air identified along nondependent surfaces—the surface of the liver and beneath the hemidiaphragm, respectively. Equally important, however, is the perception of signs of pneumoperitoneum on the supine radiograph. These features include sharp outlines of both the inner and the outer walls of the bowel by intraluminal and extraluminal gas (Rigler's sign) (Figs. 1A and B); sharp visualization of the falciform ligament; and, the so-called "football sign," wherein gas outlines the entire peritoneal cavity. Perforations of the ascending colon, descending colon, and rectum, however, produce air in the retroperitoneum. Linear, streaky gas collections may be seen tracking along retroperitoneal fascial boundaries, even possibly dissecting into the mediastinum. The interpretive imperative is to ensure that all visualized gas collections are contained within the bowel lumen.

Other Extraluminal Gas Collections

Lucent, bubbly, or linear gas collections may rarely occur in the bowel wall in a condition referred to as pneumatosis. In the context of an inflammatory, infectious, or ischemic cause, the presence of intramural gas is considered alarming, and a further search for air in mesenteric and portal veins is undertaken. Benign causes of pneumatosis are well known, however, and include obstructive pulmonary disease and various connective tissue disorders. In this context, even development of a so-called balanced pneumoperitoneum may occur without clinical consequence.

Amorphous collections of gas, collections associated with gas–liquid levels, and unexplainable soft tissue and gas densities raise suspicion for abdominal abscesses. While these collections may occur anywhere within the abdomen, air collections in the right lower quadrant related to perforated appendicitis and lesser sac collections related to perforated ulcer disease are examples of diagnoses often first suggested by plain film findings.

Normal Intraluminal Distribution of Bowel Gas

A trained observer, integrating a wide range of possible normal appearances, can almost instantaneously make the visual impression of a normal bowel gas pattern. However, several principles do routinely apply. Gas–liquid levels, while common in the stomach and not infrequent in the small bowel, should not be observed distal to the hepatic flexure in a normal patient. Under normal circumstances, the vast majority of gas should be colonic. Aerophagia, whether due to habit or iatrogenic (recent passage of a nasogastric tube, recent intubation), may substantially alter this pattern, causing a temporary preponderance of small bowel gas. Alterations in intestinal caliber must be interpreted within the global context of bowel gas distribution. Normal small bowel loops, for example, do not exceed 2.5 cm in transverse diameter, and normal colon may range in maximal transverse diameter to 6 or 8 cm. Isolated, segmental dilation, or dilation associated with thickening of the viscus wall should never be attributed to normal variation. Finally, interpretation of bowel gas distribution requires knowledge of the patient's position. Upright, colonic gas collects at the flexures. Supine, gas distributes more uniformly throughout nondependent colonic segments. Prone, gas routinely fills the rectum.

Colonic Obstruction

Abrupt change in caliber from a distended, gas-filled segment to a collapsed, gasless segment should raise suspicion for an obstructing mass. Close inspection may reveal the soft tissue density of the culprit lesion. When no gas refluxes through the ileocecal valve, dilatation of the colon is seen. With high-grade obstructions and colonic dilation, however, reflux of gas through the ileocecal valve often produces a pattern of mixed small bowel and colon dilation. When the apparent transition point from the distended to collapsed bowel occurs in the distal sigmoid or rectal region, prone radiography is of particular use. The pattern of gas distribution will not change in high-grade obstructing lesions. The causes of low-grade obstruction and colonic ileus, however, permit passage of gas into the nondependent rectal vault. A pseudo-obstruction at the splenic flexure can occur in pancreatitis when pancreatic fluid extends to the phrenocolic ligament and causes spasm in the colon. This finding has been referred to as the "colon-cut-off" sign (3).

Volvulus

The ascending colon, descending colon, and rectum are retroperitoneal structures. The transverse colon, while intraperitoneal, is firmly anchored at each of its ends by the retroperitoneal continuation of the colon. Variability in the degree of peritoneal fixation, however, potentiates cecal motion; likewise, the sigmoid colon may torse on its intraperitoneal mesentery. In both cases, characteristic alterations in bowel gas pattern are noted. In cecal volvulus, a gas-distended loop with an inverted U-shape can be seen rising out of the right lower quadrant into the left upper quadrant. In sigmoid volvulus, the gas-distended loop with an inverted U-shape can be seen rising out of the left lower quadrant into the right upper quadrant (coffee bean sign) (Figs. 2A and B) (4). Barium examination in either case reveals a beak-like termination of the barium column at the point of twisting.

Toxic Megacolon

Fulminant inflammatory, infectious, or ischemic colitis leading to loss of bowel tone and colon dilation is referred to as toxic megacolon (5). Many different inflammatory processes can cause a toxic megacolon (Table 1). The key radiographic observation is transverse colon dilation greater than 6.5 cm in the presence of bowel wall abnormalities. Bowel wall abnormalities include focal thickening, polypoid densities, and nodularity. Barium enema is absolutely contraindicated in this setting, due to the risk of perforation.

Ischemic Colitis

Colon ischemia may result from global hypoperfusion injury or, more uncommonly, thromboembolic occlusion of arteries or veins. The watershed territory between the superior and

(A)   **(B)**

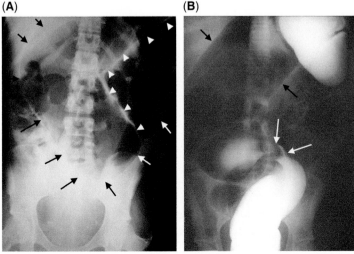

Figure 2 (**A**) The classic sign of a markedly distended sigmoid colon [proximal limb of sigmoid colon (*white arrows*); distal limb of sigmoid colon (*black arrows* and *white arrowheads*)] with no air in the rectum is suggestive of a sigmoid volvulus. (**B**) The barium study reveals the twist of the sigmoid colon (*white arrows*) typical in a sigmoid volvulus. The sigmoid colon above the twist (*black arrows*) is markedly distended and partially filled with barium.

Table 1 Etiology of Toxic Megacolon

Ulcerative colitis
Crohn's colitis
Pseudomembranous colitis
Ischemia
Infectious colitis
   Amebiasis
   Campylobacter colitis
   Strongyloidiasis
   Cytomegalovirus colitis
   Bacillary dysentery
   Typhoid fever

the inferior mesenteric arterial supply typically occurs at the splenic flexure and descending colon or mid- to distal transverse colon, making these regions most susceptible to ischemia. Nonspecific colon wall thickening may be seen in addition to "thumbprinting" (Fig. 3), which is caused by multiple mass-like mounds of soft tissue, which impress upon the colon lumen as the result of accumulated edema in the bowel wall. Similar findings can be seen in pseudomembranous colitis and some other infectious types of colitis (6).

Appendicitis

In inflammation of a retrocecal appendix, infiltration of properitoneal fat can lead to a focal loss of visualization of this fine line of fat on a supine film of the abdomen. Also, a mass between properitoneal fat and ascending colon, gas in the appendix, or a coprolith above the anterior superior iliac spine combined with haustral irregularity of the ascending colon can bear witness to appendicitis on plain films. Perforation may be visualized as retrocecal extraperitoneal gas (7).

Conclusion

Plain film radiography remains a key component in the early radiographic assessment of patients with abdominal pain. Specific diagnoses can be inferred from skillful interpretation, directing further clinical and radiographic investigation.

BARIUM ENEMA

For a long time, a controversy existed as to the role of single- versus double-contrast barium enema. Today, the single-contrast technique is no longer recommended except in suspected colonic

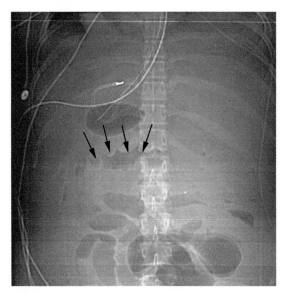

Figure 3 In this patient with pseudomembranous colitis, thumbprinting (*arrows*) is clearly seen on the plain film, indicative of edema in the bowel wall.

obstruction, in the very young, the very old, the disabled, and the very ill patient. Even in these instances, water-soluble contrast media is preferable to barium. Many patients with symptoms attributable to the colon first undergo a barium enema, sigmoidoscopy, or colonoscopy. While the use of barium enemas has experienced a steady decline since 1982 in favor of colonoscopy (8,9), many barium enemas are still performed today and with the restriction on health-care costs, demonstration of its cost-effectiveness has increased, more recently, the interest in its use (10).

Preparation

Residual feces in the colon can prevent accurate detection of polyps, cancer, and the presence and extent of inflammatory changes and could be confused with a neoplasm. A good bowel preparation, therefore, is essential. This preparation consists of dietary restrictions as described for colonoscopy, initial removal of solid material by a laxative, and final removal of small particles by liquid flushing through oral administration as used in colonoscopy or through rectal administration in the form of water enemas. This approach should result in an optimally clean colon in 95% of the patients while the remaining 5% of individuals need to be rescheduled for another examination.

Most centers use saline cathartics such as magnesium citrate or sodium phosphate or irritant cathartics such as castor oil or bisacodyl. Some radiologists have advocated a combination of the two types of cathartics (11). The combination of dietary restrictions and cathartics is used as the sole preparation for barium enemas in many centers. Some radiologists prefer to add the liquid flushing to the preparatory regimen because they think it helps achieve superior cleansing to cathartics alone.

Choice of Contrast Agent
Barium
For double-contrast examinations, high-density (75–95% weight per volume) barium, $BaSO_4$, is used which assures optimal coating of the colonic mucosa. Initially, this barium is administered followed by a large amount of air to achieve optimal distention of the colon. Once the cecum is reached and all colonic segments are well distended, multiple radiographs of the colon are obtained with the patient placed into different positions. This approach achieves optimal visualization and coating of the rectum, sigmoid colon, descending, transverse and ascending colon, and cecum. Barium may or not reflux into the terminal ileum during the procedure. For the single-contrast technique, low-density barium (15–20% weight per volume) is used to allow a see-through effect, which is combined with compression during the examination.

Water-Soluble Contrast Agents
In patients with suspected perforation or leaks into the peritoneal cavity, with fistulas and/or sinus tracts, and with abdominal stab wounds that might communicate with the colon, barium is contraindicated and hyperosmolar water-soluble contrast agents are recommended. These hyperosmolar contrast agents can absorb water and become dilute, thus easily passing through the intestine and readily demonstrating fistulas and sinus tracts. In the United States, we usually use Hypaque (diatrizoate, Amersham Health, Princeton, New Jersey, U.S.A.) or Gastrografin (sodium and meglumine amidotrizoate, Schering AG, Germany). Hyperosmolar agents could lead to severe dehydration, shock, and even death in hypovolemic infants and in very old or very ill patients. Therefore, the fluid and electrolyte status in patients at risk should be carefully monitored before administering a hyperosmolar rectal contrast agent. In infants and in any hypovolemic patient, nonionic contrast agents can be safely used, such as Omnipaque 200 (iohexol, Amersham Health, Princeton, New Jersey, U.S.A.). These nonionic agents provide excellent image quality but their higher cost must be considered.

Adjuvant Drugs
Adjuvant drugs are not frequently used. Glucagon [Eli Lilly and Company, Indianapolis, Indiana, U.S.A. (given as a dose of 0.5 to 1.0 mg)] or Buscopan® [N-butylscopolaminiumbromide, Boehringer Ingelheim, Germany, Pharma KG, Ingelheim, (given as a dose of 10 mg (plus) or 20 mg)] are used to relax the colon. Buscopan is currently not available in the United States. Most centers use one of these drugs only if the patient has cramps but they may be used to render the patient more comfortable (12–14). Glucagon is contraindicated in patients with pheochromocytomas and insulinomas. Buscopan should not be used in patients who are

suffering from eye (glaucoma) or cardiac problems, as well as patients who are taking beta blockers, had a recent myocardial infarction, are suffering from heart failure, or are on cardiac medication. In these cases, Glucagon should be used unless also contraindicated.

Contraindications for a Barium Enema

Patients with a suspected perforation, toxic megacolon, severe acute inflammatory bowel disease, peritonitis, and recent deep rectal or colonic biopsy should not undergo a barium enema. A barium enema may be performed without delay following a superficial biopsy of non-diseased colon, but should not be performed until at least six days after a deep biopsy unless obtained from a large mass. Transcolonoscopic biopsies are likely to be superficial, while trans-proctoscopic biopsies have the potential to be deep. A barium enema should be delayed at least six days following polypectomy or polyp biopsy performed with electrosurgery (15–17). Relative contraindications for a double-contrast examination include infants, limited mobility and/or cooperation, acute diverticulitis, and fistulas. The single-contrast examination is not indicated in a mobile patient, when searching for inflammatory bowel disease or in patients with a history of rectal bleeding or a personal or family history of colorectal polyps or cancer.

Performance of Barium Enemas
Single-Contrast Barium Enema
As previously discussed, the single-contrast barium enema is performed in very ill patients, in very old, and very young patients, in patients who are unable to cooperate, in patients with complete obstruction, suspected fistula, diverticulitis and volvulus, and in any patient who is unable to retain the barium. The single-contrast barium enema is an examination that is primarily based on fluoroscopy with skilled compression, an art that must be mastered by the radiologist for accurate diagnosis. Because the rectum and lower rectosigmoid colon cannot be adequately compressed, the single-contrast barium enema is not accurate in these areas.

Initially a plain film of the abdomen is obtained to assess for residual stool and to find any possible abnormalities. Depending on the size of the patient, approximately 1600–2400 mL of a 15% to 20% weight per volume barium solution is prepared using lukewarm water. It is advisable to use a soft tip with inflatable balloon unless the patient is very young and/or is able to easily retain the barium. Glucagon (1 mg, given intravenously) should only be used if the patient has spasms, experiences cramps, or has great difficulty in retaining the barium. However, if a distal fistula is suspected, then a balloon-tipped catheter should not be employed because it may occlude the internal fistulous opening. In these cases, a cone-tip placed against the anus is preferable.

With the patient in a slight left posterior oblique (LPO) and 20° upright position, barium is instilled. The flow of barium is carefully observed and the barium column constantly compressed in search of polyps and lesions. Most stool particles can be distinguished from real lesions by the fact that stool can be moved. Spot films are liberally taken, particularly in the sigmoid area, which later in the study may be obscured by barium refluxing into the terminal ileum. An attempt is made to fill the terminal ileum at the end of the examination. If barium refluxes freely into the small bowel, the patient should be moved into the prone position. This maneuver frequently prevents further reflux of barium into the small bowel due to the fact that the majority of ileocecal valves are located toward the retroperitoneum. Overhead films of the entire abdomen and pelvis are then obtained and include supine, prone, and oblique views of the abdomen and pelvis as well as a prone-angled view and lateral view of the rectum. A postevacuation film is always taken to determine emptying function of the colon and presence or absence of haustral edema. Every attempt is made not to force barium beyond a point of marked narrowing or incomplete obstruction in order to avoid inspissation of barium. In the case of partial obstruction, the colonic mucosa absorbs water out of the barium column that was forced beyond the point of narrowing. This can lead to a complete obstruction. Water absorption does not occur in the small bowel and therefore it is safe to use barium for a suspected small bowel obstruction as long as colonic obstruction can be excluded.

Double-Contrast Barium Enema
If a barium enema is to be performed, a double-contrast barium rather than a single-contrast barium enema should always be obtained in patients with suspected or previously established

inflammatory bowel disease, suspected polyps, family history of polyps, previously demonstrated or resected polyps, and cancer (suspected, high-risk group, guaiac-positive stools). Initially, approximately 500 mL of high-density barium (75–95% weight per volume) is administered. If a patient has a redundant colon, which has taken up a large amount, it is important to release some of that barium. Following this procedure, air is instilled in various positions. It is useful to obtain some films of the sigmoid colon before all of the barium reaches the cecal tip. More spot films are then obtained and overhead films are added that include supine, prone, and left oblique views of the abdomen and pelvis followed by the right and left decubitus projections, and finally prone-angled and lateral views of the rectum.

In patients in whom colonic perforation, obstruction, or colitis is not suspected and in whom it is not important to observe the flow of barium such as in patients with suspected fistula, a simplified version, the so-called "7 pump" methods can be employed (18). This method employs the same approach as the conventional method of performing a double-contrast barium enema; however, no fluoroscopy is used until the entire colon is filled with barium and air. Five pumps of air are insufflated starting with the patient in the left lateral decubitus position. For each 45-degree turn to the left (counter clockwise), five to seven more puffs of the air balloon are given until the patient is turned onto his back and finally to the LPO position. Fluoroscopy is then used to obtain spot films of the different areas: rectum and sigmoid, both flexures, cecum, and terminal ileum. No more than 350 to 450 mL of barium should be used. This method may not render optimal results in patients with a redundant colon. It is the best method for the work-up of guaiac-positive stools or lower gastrointestinal (GI) bleeding. It is particularly useful for young patients of childbearing age in whom the amount of radiation given should be limited to a bare minimum.

Other Methods
Water-Soluble Contrast Enema

A Gastrografin or Hypaque enema is performed for suspected perforation, leak, fistula, or constipation. At times, the surgeon does not want to have barium in the colon when colonic surgery is imminent and in these instances, water-soluble contrast material can be very helpful (19). Patients with fistulae, leaks, or perforation often are quite ill and the examination needs to be tailored to the individual clinical question; e.g., for demonstrating a fistula, a higher concentration of the water-soluble contrast agent is used than for proximal leaks or obstruction. For rectovaginal fistula, contrast is administered slowly with the patient in the lateral position and spot films are obtained in frequent succession to assure that the abnormal anatomy can be sorted out. Overflooding of the rectum with contrast agent will not permit an accurate diagnosis; an inflated balloon will obviously obscure the fistula and render the study useless.

When leaks or perforation are suspected more proximally, Hypaque or Gastrografin can be used until the splenic flexure is reached. Introduction of water per rectum will displace the dense contrast material and fill the right colon and cecum whereas the sigmoid colon will be cleared from the dense material and appear translucent, thus allowing better visualization of the proximal colon. This is helpful in patients with redundant sigmoid and transverse colons and reduces the cost of the examination, as Gastrografin is relatively expensive. A water-soluble agent should be used for any postoperative study such as in a patient who has had either a coloanal or ileoanal anastomosis. Again, an intrarectal inflated balloon should not be employed in these cases.

In patients with severe constipation, a small bowel obstruction may develop and oral laxatives may only make matters worse rather than help in these situations. The examination needs to be performed slowly so that the contrast can creep around the impacted stool. The hyperosmolar contrast agent needs to reach the cecum for maximum effect. The patient needs to be encouraged not to immediately evacuate as the hyperosmolar contrast agent pulls fluid into the colon and thus facilitates expulsion of the impacted feces. At times, it is necessary to repeat the enema to clear the colon. Such enemas may be particularly of help in patients with cystic fibrosis and inspissation in colon and distal small bowel.

Colostomy Examinations

Upstream colostomy studies are done after abdominoperineal resection for cancer or before reanastomosis when a colostomy was placed for bowel rest such as in patients with severe diverticulitis or with a perforation. Following cancer surgery, evaluation of the remaining colon for recurrent or metachronous tumors initially should be performed by colonoscopy and if negative, follow-up studies can be obtained with double-contrast barium enemas through the colostomy. Because these studies are done to search for small neoplasms, either study must be performed with meticulous technique and after thorough colonic cleansing. For these studies, a Foley catheter can be inserted through a nipple device that is held against the stoma or a cone-tipped catheter can be placed against the stoma after careful digital examination to avoid disruption of the stoma (20). Alternatively, a balloon catheter can be inserted and the balloon inflated but only after some barium was administered to assure proper placement of the catheter that would not lead to disruption of the stoma by balloon inflation. Towels are placed around the stoma to absorb leaking material. In difficult cases, Glucagon or Buscopan may be helpful to relax the colon.

In cases where reanastomosis is considered, the anatomy of the distal colon has to be evaluated. For this purpose, it is often helpful to perform a downstream colostomy study as the anal sphincter tone permits better distention of the lower colon and rectum than when the contrast agent is introduced through the rectum and flows out through the colostomy.

Examination for Intussusception

Intussusception occurs when a proximal segment of bowel passes into the lumen of a more distal segment of bowel. It is seen most commonly in children between three months and three years of age, with male predominance and no obvious leading cause. Children outside of this range have a leading point in about 30% (21). A plain film is not essential provided the clinical diagnosis is clear. Sonography can be used for diagnostic purposes but, in most instances, barium, water-soluble contrast medium or more recently, gas, air, or carbon dioxide have been used for diagnosing and treating suspected intussusception. Consultation with the surgeons should always precede the procedure, as they may be involved if a perforation occurs. The incidence of perforation with a hydrostatic enema is about 6 in 1000 (22).

The hydrostatic or pneumatic pressure of the enema is employed to drive the infolded segment of bowel in a retrograde fashion to its normal position. For the hydrostatic enema, the contrast medium is instilled with relatively low pressure (at about a height of 1 m) until the intussusception is met. Then while maintaining a good seal, administration of the contrast agent is continued with constant hydrostatic pressure until clear reflux is noted into the terminal ileum and distal small bowel. Resistance is usually encountered at the ileocecal valve, which can be overcome with perseverance and constant pressure. For the pneumatic enema, gas or air is introduced with an electrical or hand pump at a pressure of between 85 and 120 mmHg, similar to the hydrostatic enema (23). This method is effective, easy, fast and uses lower radiation doses and is successful in about 85% of cases (24). Recurrence of intussusception after enema reduction occurs in about 8%, after surgical reduction in about 4%, and after surgical reduction and resection in 1% (25).

Absolute contraindications for a hydrostatic enema include fever, elevated white blood cell count, peritoneal signs, and marked systemic toxicity because they suggest bowel perforation and/or possibly gangrenous bowel. Relative contraindications include very young or very old patients, small bowel obstruction, and/or persistence of symptoms for over 24 hours.

Common Errors and Interpretation Problems

One of the most common reasons for a failed pneumocolon is the failure to deliver thick barium to the cecum, thereby obtaining poor or no coating of the mucosa. One study showed that with careful technique, double-contrast barium enema could provide additional information in cases where the colonoscope could not reach the ileocecal valve (26). However, optimal visualization of the entire colon is only possible with meticulous technique. Often rotating the patient 360° and placing him/her in an upright position can facilitate coating of the right colon and cecal tip with barium. Sometimes, too much barium is instilled, and not enough drained out. This can lead to obscuring lesions. Inadequate overhead films also can lead to interpretative errors. The focus must be on the air column for best visualization of polyps and other mass lesions. All lines and contour features have to be accounted for. It takes much longer to thoroughly evaluate a pneumocolon with a single-contrast barium enema, which relies on displacement of the barium column by masses or contour defects such as apple-core lesions in the case of a malignant neoplasm (Fig. 4) or filling of outpouchings with barium in the case of diverticula.

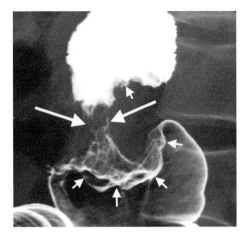

Figure 4 This double-contrast barium enema demonstrates an area of narrowing with irregular margins in the descending colon, a so-called apple-core lesion that is highly suggestive of an adenocarcinoma.

Results with Barium Enema
Inflammatory Disease of the Colon
Diverticular Disease and Appendicitis
The radiological diagnosis of early-stage diverticulitis based on barium enema is not very accurate where a CT is very successful (see below). A barium enema can demonstrate deformed sacs or diverticula in an otherwise fully distended segment. Microperforation and formation of a small abscess that deforms the smooth outline of the diverticulum cause this abnormality. However, fecal particles retained in the diverticulum or scarring can mimic this appearance. Another sign of acute early diverticulitis is a mass effect on the colon caused by an abscess. It is entirely possible to miss a small abscess on a barium enema. Such abscesses or extrinsic pressure defects may be caused by other etiologies such as foreign body perforation, stercoral ulceration, ischemia, tumoral implants, and endometriosis. CT usually can establish the source of the colonic defect. Extravasation is the most reliable sign but also can occur in perforated colon carcinoma. In these cases, a track of barium or water-soluble contrast material may be seen; usually such a perforation is contained. The accuracy of the barium enema has been listed as 60% (27), which was surpassed by CT (63%) in the same investigation. Today, the accuracy of CT should range from 84% to 99%, with the best sensitivity achieved by multirow helical CT (28–30). If because of financial or equipment constraints a CT cannot be accomplished, then a contrast enema may be appropriate. However, a water-soluble contrast agent and not barium should be utilized in case a perforation is present.

Plain films of the abdomen reveal abnormalities in 50% of patients with appendicitis. These findings include appendicolith, sentinel loop (dilated atonic ileum containing fluid), dilated cecum, medial displacement of cecum, cecal edema, and effacement of extraperitoneal fat line. A combination of these findings is of greater value than an individual sign. Once the value of CT in diagnosing appendicitis had been shown, a barium enema is rarely performed. Signs of appendicitis during a barium enema include a mass indenting the cecum, displacement of the cecum, enlargement of haustra and partial or nonfilling of the appendix. On its own, nonfilling of the appendix has little diagnostic significance. The sensitivity of CT for appendicitis should range from 94% to 98% (see below) (31–33).

Idiopathic Inflammatory Bowel Disease
The barium enema examination is indicated in patients with suspected inflammatory bowel disease when it is necessary to establish the diagnosis or the extent of disease and to assess complications such as stricture formation, fistula, or carcinoma. If a toxic megacolon is present, a barium enema is contraindicated because of the risk of perforation and bacteremia (34). It is also advisable to delay a barium enema in patients with fulminant disease and perform the examination in a less active phase of the disease.

Ulcerative Colitis. Ulcerative colitis and Crohn's disease form the group of idiopathic inflammatory bowel diseases that may involve the colon. In ulcerative colitis, the disease is contiguous

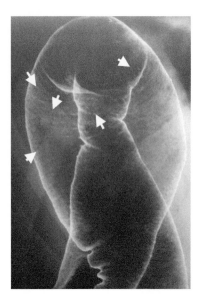

Figure 5 In this patient with ulcerative colitis, the colonic mucosa has lost its smooth texture and demonstrates a granular appearance interspersed with small flecks of barium (*arrows*) indicative of superficial erosions.

and uniformly involves the left colon but pancolitis may be seen. Because the rectum is always involved, the diagnosis is usually established by sigmoidoscopy or colonoscopy. In the early phase of ulcerative colitis, the mucosa loses its even smooth texture and the barium enema demonstrates an amorphous or finely stippled appearance, called "granularity" (Fig. 5) (35). At times, only blunting of the acute angles of the rectal valves is seen. When the disease progresses, superficial erosions that appear as small flecks of barium on the background of granular mucosa can be seen. In the chronic stages, granulation tissue develops, which leads to a coarse granular pattern. If an acute attack occurs in chronic disease, ill-defined collections of barium that represent ulcerations are seen. They are best visualized in profile because they are linear in relation to the tenial attachment and undermine the mucosa. These ulcers are referred to as collar-button ulcers (Fig. 6) because of their T-shaped appearance (36). While these ulcers have been described originally with ulcerative colitis, they are not diagnostic of ulcerative colitis and can be seen in tuberculous colitis, shigellosis, amebiasis, and even ischemic colitis. Polyps may be seen at any stage and range from pseudopolyps that represent inflamed islands of mucosa on a background of denuded mucosa, inflammatory polyps that are areas of inflamed mucosa that result in polypoid elevations on a background of granular mucosa, and postinflammatory polyps that are seen in the quiescent phase and represent polypoid changes that are a result of epithelization in the reparative phase (37,38). Some of them

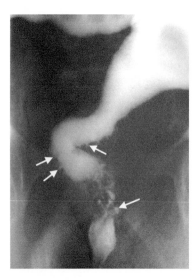

Figure 6 In another patient with a chronic phase of ulcerative colitis, ill-defined collections of barium are seen that in profile assume a T-shaped appearance representative of the so-called "collar button" ulcers (*arrows*). Also, the rectosigmoid colon appears diffusely narrowed.

have a filiform appearance (39,40). In patients with pancolitis, the terminal ileum may be involved. This back-wash ileitis consists of a gaping ileocecal valve and a dilated terminal ileum that can be easily confused with the cecum. Often granular mucosa is observed in this segment of the ileum. Back-wash ileitis can usually be distinguished from Crohn's ileitis by a contracted or strictured ileocecal valve and the string sign that consists of irregular narrowing of the terminal ileum, often associated with fistulae.

Secondary changes consist of foreshortening of the colon, lack of haustration, and tubular narrowing that gives the colon the appearance of a garden hose or stove pipe (Fig. 7). Complications with ulcerative colitis include toxic megacolon that is diagnosed on plain films based on a diameter of more than 6.5 cm in the transverse colon and abnormal mucosa (thickened, irregular-appearing walls with polypoid protrusion into the air column). Toxic megacolon can occur in other inflammatory conditions (Table 1). Perforation rarely occurs in ulcerative colitis, but when it does, is usually associated with toxic megacolon. Strictures are in seen in 7% to 11% (41). If multiple strictures are present, cathartic colon needs to be excluded. Cathartic colon usually involves the cecum and right colon but may be diffuse (42). It is characterized by bizarre colonic contractions. Patients with long-standing disease or pancolitis have an increased risk of developing colon cancer (43,44). The risk of developing cancer begins approximately 10 years after the onset of acute disease but may be earlier (45). Because of this increased cancer risk, patients with long-standing and severe disease or patients with pancolitis often undergo total colectomy with creation of an ileoanal pouch (46,47). Therefore, the chronic changes of ulcerative colitis are less commonly seen today.

Crohn's Disease.   Crohn's disease is a disease that most commonly involves the terminal ileum, the remainder of the small bowel and cecum, and various segments of the colon. The incidence of Crohn's colitis and ileocolitis is higher for adult-onset and/or late-onset whereas young patients are more prone to develop jejunoileitis.

On a barium enema, the earliest findings are tiny elevations that represent inflamed lymphoid follicles. In many of these elevations, superficial ulcers develop centrally, which are called "aphthous ulcers" (Fig. 8). Radiographically, they are tiny collections of barium with a halo around them, which are seen on a background of normal-appearing mucosa (48). Such ulcers can also be identified in Yersinia enterocolitis, amebic colitis, and other nonspecific inflammatory conditions.

In the intermediate phase, asymmetric involvement is another typical feature, with the mesenteric side becoming stiff and spiculated whereas the antimesenteric side shows scalloping (49). In advanced disease, skip areas or discontinuous disease is present in 90% of all patients with Crohn's colitis (50). While skip areas may be seen with amebiasis or pseudomembranous colitis, they are not a feature of ulcerative colitis. Strictures, pseudosacculations,

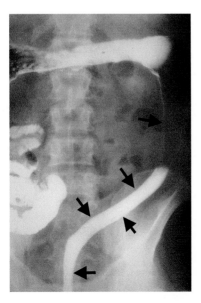

Figure 7   A diffusely narrowed rectum and descending colon (*arrows*) is identified in this patient with burned-out ulcerative colitis. The colon assumes the appearance of a lead pipe. Acute changes are seen in the transverse colon.

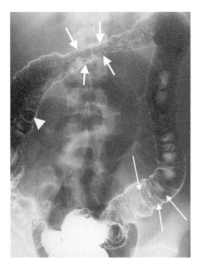

Figure 8 In this patient with active Crohn's disease, aphthous ulcers are seen (*thin arrows*) and areas of severe narrowing and inflammatory changes (*thick arrows*) alternate with normal or near-normal appearing bowel segments. Pseudosacculation (*arrowhead*) is also apparent due to the asymmetry of the disease.

fistulae, and sinuses may also develop. Pseudosacculations (Fig. 8) can also be encountered in ischemia and scleroderma.

Marked thickening of the bowel wall and mesentery develops over time that is best appreciated by CT. The classical feature of advanced Crohn's disease is the so-called cobblestoning of bowel loops, which is created by deep longitudinal and transverse ulcerations that crisscross the wall of the large or small bowel and surround edematous mucosa. Inflammatory polyps may also develop. The so-called string sign of the terminal ileum originally described reversible spasm (Fig. 9). However, strictures are frequently present in the colon and in the terminal ileum. Intramural or paracolonic fistula tracts may be seen. If the rectum is involved (approximately in 50%), the disease is patchy and not uniform (51).

Crohn's disease is reversible to a certain degree but in the colon some type of scarring usually remains (asymmetry, narrowing). Crohn's disease frequently recurs after resection, and recurrent disease always spreads in an oral direction from the anastomosis of the colon with the small bowel (52). Separation of bowel loops commonly seen in Crohn's disease may be caused by fibrofatty proliferation, mesenteric phlegmon, or fistulas with abscess formation. While fistulas are well demonstrated by a barium study, CT is much better suited to ascertain the underlying cause of the bowel loop separation. A late complication of Crohn's disease also is the development of a carcinoma but it seems to occur less frequently than in ulcerative colitis (53).

Infectious Colitis

Most infectious types of colitis have an appearance that mimics ulcerative colitis on a barium enema and clinical history and thus laboratory tests are needed to make a specific diagnosis. Some of the infectious types have a more suggestive pattern and are described below.

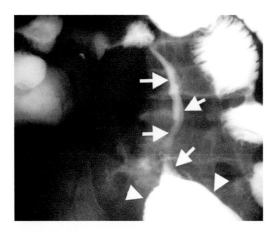

Figure 9 The string sign (*arrows*) is well demonstrated in this patient with Crohn's disease. The ileum proximal to the area of stenosis (*arrowheads*) is dilated.

Pseudomembranous colitis is encountered with increasing frequency, usually complicating antibiotic therapy. It is caused by overgrowth of *Clostridium difficile* and the subsequent release of cytotoxic enterotoxin, which produces ulcerations of the mucosa and formation of pseudomembranes that consist of fibrin, sloughed epithelial cells, and leukocytes. Early cases may not be detectable by barium enema but in advanced cases, haustral thickening (thumb printing or accordion pattern), shaggy walls, and mucosal plaques can be visualized. The accordion pattern is created when barium gets trapped between thickened haustral folds that are aligned in a parallel fashion. Usually, the entire colon is involved but the rectum may be spared and skip areas can be seen (54). Toxic megacolon and perforation may occur if the disease is not recognized (55). Therefore, a water-soluble contrast agent may be preferable to barium in some cases.

Tuberculous colitis mimics all the features that have been described for Crohn's disease (56). In the United States, it is a disease that is diagnosed by exclusion. Tuberculous colitis also shares many features described for amebiasis below. It seldom involves extensive areas of the colon. It may show skip areas but fistulas or perforation are not very common. The barium enema outlines the constricted area that simulates the string sign of Crohn's disease but at times it assumes an apple-core appearance and may be difficult to distinguish from a malignancy. The diagnosis of tuberculosis of the colon is not made with great accuracy by barium enema.

Amebic colitis, like many of the other infectious types of colitis, appears similar to ulcerative colitis and even toxic megacolon can be seen in this type of colitis (57). Usually the small bowel is spared. In chronic cases, the right colon may be involved with skip lesions. At times, an inflammatory mass or ameboma develops, which can produce obstruction. The conical shape of the cecum described for the chronic form of amebiasis is only rarely encountered.

AIDS-related infectious colitis includes cytomegalovirus (CMV) colitis and cryptosporidiosis. Patients with a CD4 lymphocyte count of $200 \, \text{mm}^3$ or less are at greatest risk. In both diseases, only the right colon may be involved but more typically the entire colon is abnormal. The colon usually reveals marked haustral thickening and shaggy walls not unlike pseudomembranous colitis or ulcerative colitis (58). The correct diagnosis is suggested by the patient's clinical history and lab values. Pneumatosis and intramural hemorrhage may be present.

Because of the increased risk of bowel perforation, a barium enema in critically ill patients with suspected typhlitis should not be performed and CT is the diagnostic method of choice. Typhlitis (or neutropenic enterocolitis) is an inflammatory process of the cecum and ascending colon, often associated with involvement of the terminal ileum. It can be seen in severely immunosuppressed and neutropenic patients including patients with AIDS, organ transplants, acute leukemia under chemotherapy, aplastic anemia, multiple myeloma, and bone marrow transplantation (59,60).

Ischemic Disease

Ischemic colitis presents clinically with acute onset of abdominal pain with or without bloody diarrhea depending on the severity of involvement. Laboratory tests may reveal a metabolic acidosis, although they are often normal early in the disease. Ischemic colitis is caused by vascular insufficiency and bleeding into the bowel wall. It preferentially affects the splenic flexure, descending colon, and sigmoid colon, usually in the vascular distribution of the inferior mesenteric artery (IMA) (61). It is most commonly seen in middle-aged to elderly patients, often with underlying vascular and/or cardiac disease. Occasionally only the sigmoid colon is involved. On plain films, thumbprinting and dilated bowel loops are seen. Often the right side of the colon is markedly distended because the affected area acts as a functional obstruction. The thumbprinting is caused by submucosal hemorrhage and bleeding. There is a transient type and a chronic stricturing type that reflects transmural disease (62). When a barium enema is performed, thumbprinting is seen in 75% and mucosal ulceration in 60%. In one serial study, eccentric deformity was found in 19 of 40 patients (48%), sacculation in 12 (30%), and transverse ridging in 5 (13%) (63). Today, barium enemas are only rarely performed because CT can assess the extent and degree of bowel wall thickening much better than barium enema. It can also demonstrate that the involved areas follow a vascular distribution pattern.

Neoplastic Disease of the Colon

Colonoscopy and more recently CT colonography (CTC) have substantially altered the diagnosis and management of colonic polyps. Colonoscopy not only allows direct visualization of polyps and cancers but also permits histologic diagnoses through biopsies and therapeutic excision of polyps under certain favorable circumstances that are discussed in the relevant chapters.

Polyps

A polyp is shown as a radiolucent defect, a contour defect, or a ring shadow because it represents a mass protruding into the lumen of the colon. Another lesion that manifests itself primarily as an alteration of the surface texture has been called a "carpet" lesion and represents a tubular adenoma with varying degrees of villous change (64).

Cancer

Radiologically, early detection of colorectal cancer means early detection of polyps. As a general rule of thumb, most polyps smaller than 5 mm in diameter do not harbor a malignancy. The incidence of cancer in polyps of size 5 to 10 mm is approximately 1%. This incidence increases to 50% for polyps larger than 2 cm. Rapid growth over time favors malignancy as does an irregular, lobulated surface and a broad short stalk. In general, a long thin stalk is a sign of a benign polyp. Most symptomatic colorectal carcinomas are annular or polypoid lesions that are visualized during the barium enema as contour defects (Fig. 4). Plaque-like lesions may be seen only as abnormal lines in the barium column. Often synchronous lesions are present in the form of polyps or cancer (65). This emphasizes the importance of a thorough examination of the entire colon. Carcinomas located in an area of extensive diverticulosis can be difficult to detect. In equivocal cases of a barium enema, flexible sigmoidoscopy should be performed for definitive evaluation. Advanced carcinomas may have an atypical appearance and linitis plastica type of lesions have predominantly submucosal infiltration and a strong fibrous reaction. This type of tumor is predominantly seen in patients with long-standing ulcerative colitis.

Complications with colon cancer include bleeding (usually manifested as occult blood in stool or chronic anemia), bowel obstruction, perforation, and fistula formation. When perforation is present, extracolonic gas and/or barium may be seen.

Results with Barium Enema

A recent retrospective study in the United Kingdom demonstrated that barium enemas reached a sensitivity of 96% for polyps larger than 1 cm and a sensitivity of 97% for carcinomas (66). A Canadian study revealed a sensitivity of 100% and a specificity of 82% for a combination of flexible sigmoidoscopy and double-contrast barium enema for polyps larger than 5 mm and cancers (67). Using the same combination of examinations, this study missed four polyps measuring less than 5 mm in diameter. In yet another study from Norway, barium enema (sensitivity 90%) compared favorably with colonoscopy. In this later study, it was noteworthy that colonoscopy was incomplete in 13.9% and in all these cases, a lesion was present in the nonvisualized area (68). However, most recent studies have demonstrated at least a 94% to 95% incidence of completion of colonoscopy (69,70). Barium enemas can be helpful in patients who had an incomplete colonoscopy. In a recent study, five of six lesions measuring more than 1 cm in the right colon were correctly identified by barium enema but not demonstrated by colonoscopy (71). Two were annular carcinomas and three were polyps with a high grade of dysplasia. The sixth lesion was a false-positive result by barium enema. This study emphasizes the complementary role of barium enema and colonoscopy. Even colonoscopy can miss lesions and in one study, 15% of lesions detected radiologically with barium enema were not seen on colonoscopy (72). However, comparable results between colonoscopy and double-contrast enema can only be achieved with meticulous attention to technique and by a radiologist well trained in performing and interpreting this examination. Even the best barium enema remains a diagnostic examination whereas a colonoscopy can also be a therapeutic procedure. In experienced hands, the double-contrast barium enema remains a very cost-effective examination (73). Virtually every abnormality seen on barium enema requires colonoscopic verification, thus necessitating a second bowel preparation and a second procedure. Barium enema is suited to patients in whom colonoscopy has been incomplete.

DEFECOGRAPHY

Among functional GI complaints, perhaps none is more anxiety-provoking or socially stigmatizing than anorectal dysfunction. Dynamic rectal examination, also known as cinedefecography,

defecography, videoproctography, or evacuation proctography, offers unique diagnostic information regarding the function of the anorectum and pelvic floor at rest, during squeezing maneuvers, and during defecation. Such information is valuable in the evaluation of patients with complaints of disordered defecation, including severe constipation (74–83).

Technique

After the rectum is opacified with a contrast agent simulating stool in weight and consistency, the patient sits on a radiolucent commode and video- or cinefluoroscopic images of the anorectum are obtained in lateral projection during rest, squeeze maneuver, and evacuation (Fig. 10). Careful attention to patient history permits further tailoring of the examination. In patients who must compress the low anterior abdominal wall or support the vagina in order to defecate, additional images demonstrating the effect of these maneuvers should be included. Abnormalities in the lateral projection should be further scrutinized in the abdominoperoneal (AP) projection.

Evacu-Paste 100 (E-Z-EM, Westbury, New York, U.S.A.) and Anatrast (E-Z-EM, Westbury, New York, U.S.A.) are examples of commercially available defecography pastes. Contrast medium may be injected into the rectum using a specially prepared caulking gun. Although patient tolerance may dictate a smaller volume, 250 cc of contrast is generally instilled.

Triple-contrast defecography refers to simultaneous opacification of anorectum, small bowel, and vagina. Prior to the examination, the small bowel may be opacified with a typical suspension of thin barium. Opacification of the vagina can also provide useful information and may be achieved by injection of amidotrizoic acid (50% gel) or a 60% barium sulfate suspension (84,85). A gauze square can be folded and placed at the introitus to assist in retention of this contrast. Various manufacturers offer radiolucent commodes for the examination. The use of dynamic rectal examination has been shown to significantly increase diagnostic confidence among clinicians when the clinical diagnosis and radiographic findings are in accordance. Alternatively, results may alter the diagnosis and planned therapy for this group of patients (86).

Normal Findings

The puborectal sling encircles the anorectal junction and attaches to the pubis. Tonic contraction of the sling at rest produces an angle of 90° to 110° between the anus and longitudinal axis of the distal rectum (the anorectal angle). Normal defecation requires inhibition of the sling, opening the anorectal angle to 130° to 140°, permitting passage of stool. The position of the anorectal junction relative to the AP plane of the ischial tuberosities provides information regarding perineal descent. At maximal strain, there should be less than 2 cm inferior translation of the anorectal junction. At maximal squeeze, anterosuperior translation of the

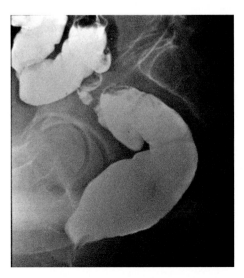

Figure 10 During defecography, the rectum is opacified with a contrast agent simulating stool in weight and consistency; images of the anorectum are obtained in lateral projection during rest, squeeze maneuver (*shown*), and evacuation.

anorectal junction, decrease in the anorectal angle, and increased conspicuity of the posterior puborectalis impression confirm the patient's ability to voluntarily contract the pelvic floor, a necessary condition for volitional continence.

Abnormal Findings

Abnormalities that may be discovered during defecography include rectocele, enterocele, sigmoidocele, rectal intussusception and prolapse, paradoxical contraction of the puborectalis, and perineal descent.

Rectocele

A rectocele is an outpouching of the anterior rectal wall, usually more pronounced with straining, and possibly due to weakness of the rectovaginal septum. Rectoceles are far more common in women than in men, and not all are symptomatic. Trapping of fecal residue within the rectocele may lead to a pattern of defecating in stages, sometimes requiring digital support of the vagina for complete evacuation. Most women have a rectocele, although few are clinically relevant.

Enterocele and Sigmoidocele

An enterocele is a peritoneal sac containing loops of small bowel, which has herniated inferiorly to lie immediately anterior to the rectal wall in the pouch of Douglas. A sigmoidocele similarly occurs with prolapse of a sigmoid loop into the pouch of Douglas, anterior to the rectum. Both conditions are classified in degrees. First degree refers to loops situated above the pubococcygeal line. Second degree refers to loops situated between the pubococcygeal and ischiococcygeal lines. Third degree refers to loops displaced inferior to the ischiococcygeal line.

Rectal Intussusception and Prolapse

Intussusception of the rectal wall is classified according to the caudal extent of the process. Grade 1 intussusceptions are intrarectal. Grade 2 refers to rectal intussusceptions which have passed into the anus. Grade 3 refers to rectal prolapse, with protrusion beyond the anus.

Paradoxical Contraction of the Puborectalis

Tonic contraction of the puborectalis permits continence. Likewise, failure of muscle relaxation inhibits defecation and is considered a functional abnormality of defecation. The diagnosis can be made during defecography by noting intermittent or persistent conspicuous posterior impression of the puborectalis during defecation and diminished or absent opening of the anorectal angle.

Perineal Descent

Descent of the pelvic floor is diagnosed when, during defecation or straining, the anorectal junction descends more than 2 cm.

CROSS-SECTIONAL IMAGING
Computed Tomography

CT has been extensively employed for assessing inflammatory and ischemic changes in the colon and to determine the level and cause of obstruction. CT also has been applied to detect and stage many tumors, including primary and recurrent colorectal neoplasms.

Technique

CT of the colon consists of an examination of the abdomen and pelvis. Whenever possible, intravenous contrast material (e.g. Omnipaque 300^{TM}, Amersham Health, Cork Ireland) is administered at a rate of 3 to 4 mL/sec for a total of 150 cc. With multi-detector row CT (16- or 64-slice scanners), multiple sections are then obtained through the abdomen and pelvis at a slice thickness of 2.5 to 0.625 mm. Thin sections are needed for optimal multiplanar reconstructions. This is particular important for best assessment of the rectum, its relationship to the levator ani muscles and mesorectal fascia. With thin sections, reconstructions are possible in any desired plane at optimal resolution. The axial slices usually are reconstructed at 5 mm slice thickness for ease of interpretation. Oral and rectal contrast is also administered unless a contraindication exists for their use. For faster opacification of the entire GI tract, we administer metoclopramide (Reglan, A. H. Robbins, Richmond, Virginia, U.S.A.) with the first 450 mL of oral contrast material (87). There is some evidence that optimal distention of the small bowel can be achieved by obtaining an enteroclysis study first followed by a helical CT (88). Using a neutral oral contrast agent (VoLumen™, E-Z-EM, Westbury, NY, 11590) that contains sorbitol and 0.1% barium solution can achieve similar results without being invasive and time consumimg as CT enteroclysis is. We prefer water for rectal contrast unless a leak or fistula is suspected. For best results in the colon, a colonic preparation should be obtained.

Non-neoplastic Diseases of the Colon
Idiopathic Inflammatory and Infectious Diseases of the Colon
Crohn's Disease
Crohn's disease produces changes in the wall of the small and/or the large bowel and in the tissue surrounding the involved bowel loops. The changes in the pericolonic area are best assessed by CT. Features suggesting Crohn's disease include marked wall thickening (1–2 cm) with or without the target sign, skip areas, increased fat ("creeping" fat) and/or stranding of fat (fibrofatty proliferation), enlarged lymph nodes near the involved bowel segments, fistulas, and sinus tracts with or without abscesses (89).

In many cases of idiopathic inflammatory disease, infectious enterocolitis, and ischemia of the bowel, an outer ring of enhancement (corresponding to the muscularis propria) and inner ring (corresponding to the mucosa) can be distinguished, which are separated by a ring of low density (corresponding to submucosal edema) (Fig. 11) This appearance has been called the target sign, but can be seen only when a fast scan series is obtained during a large and rapidly delivered pulse. In Crohn's disease, identification of these various rings indicates that the changes are inflammatory in nature and do not represent fibrotic changes that are irreversible. Such a distinction is important for the decision whether surgical intervention is needed. In most cases of Crohn's disease, wall thickening is due to edema and occurs in up to 83% of cases (90).

Complications associated with Crohn's enterocolitis are abdominal or pelvic abscesses, fistulas, stricture formation with or without obstruction, phlegmonous reaction in mesentery, bowel perforation, and even perforation with free intraperitoneal air and neoplasm. At times, the inflammatory process may cause matting of bowel loops and contiguous inflammation of the abdominal wall. All these findings can be readily seen on CT. Increased fat surrounding involved bowel loops in Crohn's disease (creeping fat), local lymph adenopathy, and increased density within the fat (fibrofatty proliferation) are features that favor the diagnosis of Crohn's disease in the differential diagnosis of marked bowel wall thickening. All of these findings may be present or only a few, but the most common features seen in Crohn's disease are marked bowel wall thickening lymph nodes and fibrofatty proliferation. The presence of significant bowel wall enhancement and mesenteric changes allow differentiating patients in the active phase from those patients in remission where enhancement and mesenteric changes are minimal (91).

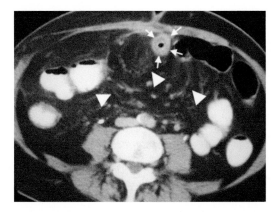

Figure 11 In this patient with Crohn's disease, the concentric rings (*arrows*) are clearly identified. Fibrofatty proliferation is also seen (*arrowheads*).

In patients with Crohn's disease, CT can assess the degree of thickening of the bowel wall or mesentery, permit differentiation of fibrofatty proliferation, phlegmonous reaction of mesentery, and abscess, and detect fistulous tracts between bowel loops and sinus tracts into mesentery and soft tissue near bowel loops, around a stoma, or in the perineum (92). Many of these abscesses or fistulas cannot be detected by conventional studies. In patients with idiopathic bowel disease, separation of bowel loops seen on a small bowel follow through or enteroclysis often leads to a CT that can distinguish among abscess, phlegmonous reaction, and increased fatty tissue. This distinction is important for management of these patients. However, in patients with thickened colonic wall and pericolonic abscess in the absence of fibrofatty proliferation, CT cannot distinguish among diverticulitis with abscess formation, Crohn's disease with abscess, and colon cancer with perforation.

Ulcerative Colitis

Ulcerative colitis involves the colon in a continuous fashion, i.e., the wall is moderately thickened and there is no evidence of fibrofatty proliferation and rarely pericolonic stranding. CT can easily demonstrate all these changes. Layering of the bowel wall can also be seen. Similar to the "target sign" of Crohn's disease, the inner enhanced layer represents the mucosa whereas the outer enhanced ring represents the serosa and muscularis propria separated by a nonenhancing layer of submucosal edema fat (Fig. 12). Fat is more often encountered in the submucosa of patients with ulcerative colitis than in patients with Crohn's disease (93). In patients with bowel wall thickening and soft tissue stranding, the differential diagnosis is quite extensive and often additional data such as clinical history and laboratory tests are necessary for a definitive diagnosis. Because CT detection of wall thickening in small or large bowel is a nonspecific finding, various etiologies must be considered (Table 2) (94). The most pronounced wall thickening of the colon is seen in Crohn's disease, pseudomembranous colitis, CMV colitis, ischemic changes, and hemorrhage into the bowel wall (see below). Most infectious types of colitis produce wall thickening that is less severe.

In comparison to Crohn's disease, uncomplicated ulcerative colitis usually shows less prominent wall thickening, absence of increased peri-intestinal or pericolonic fat, and lack of fistulous tracts. Ulcerative colitis may be associated with sinus tracts in the perineum, but phlegmonous reactions surrounding the colon are rarely seen in ulcerative colitis unless perforation has occurred. Often, the target sign can be seen in ulcerative colitis as an expression of acute inflammation, but this is not seen in chronic or "burned-out" ulcerative colitis.

CT is particularly helpful in patients with a suspected pelvic floor abscess because it can distinguish between a supralevator and infralevator process. It is important to differentiate a perianal or supralevator abscess from one that is located below the levator in the ischiorectal fossa, a so-called ischiorectal abscess. Failure to recognize extension of an infralevator abscess into the space above the levator ani can lead to inadequate surgical drainage and recurrence of an abscess. CT is also useful in suspected postoperative complications related to ileoanal pouches that were created for patients with ulcerative colitis or familial adenomatous polyposis (47). These patients may show pouchitis, fistulae, sinus tracts, or leakage of contrast material

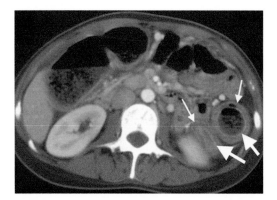

Figure 12 In this patient with ulcerative colitis, computed tomography reveals the "target" sign in the colon. The inner enhanced layer (*thick arrows*) represents the mucosa whereas the outer enhanced ring (*thin arrows*) represents the serosa and muscularis propria separated by a nonenhancing layer of submucosal fat.

Table 2 Differential Diagnosis of Bowel Wall Thickening (Diffuse or Focal)

Diffuse Processes:	Focal Processes:
Idiopathic inflammatory bowel disease	*Focal Colitis*
Crohn's disease	Diverticulitis
Ulcerative colitis	Appendicitis
Infectious colitis	Pelvic inflammatory disease with contiguous
Bacterial colitis	colorectal inflammation
Viral colitis	Rectal perforation and inflammation
Parasitic colitis	Prostatitis, abscess, and contiguous inflammation
Fungal colitis	Pancreatitis extending to transverse colon or
Noninfectious Colitis	splenic flexure
Typhlitis	Peritonitis with infected fluid in the pouch of
Eosinophilic colitis	Douglas
Graft versus host disease	*Neoplasm*
Ischemic colitis (also post-radiation colitis)	Adenocarcinoma
Vasculitis (usually focal)	Lymphoma
Traumatic (focal hematoma)	Cloacogenic carcinoma
Amyloidosis	Metastases
Generalized edema (uremia, heart failure, etc.)	Giant condyloma accuminata
Hemolytic-uremic syndrome	
Exogenous causes of colitis	
Pseumembranous colitis	
Drug-induced colitis	
Caustic colitis	
Endometriosis	

administered into the pouch. In these cases, instituting the appropriate treatment and monitoring the success of therapy often can be based on CT. A combination of barium examination and CT for determining the extent of disease and complications is also often useful (95).

Diverticulitis

The use of CT in patients with suspected diverticulitis is very effective, particularly in the early stages of the disease. Barium enemas, which frequently have been used for evaluating patients with suspected diverticulitis, cannot detect early and mild changes of this disease or assess extraluminal disease. CT can diagnose such changes based on wall thickening and pericolonic stranding. These findings may be associated with an abscess in more advanced stages. Care must be taken not to confuse muscular hypertrophy with wall thickness due to inflammation. In most of these patients, diverticula can be identified.

For suspected diverticulitis, we prefer to administer all three contrast materials—oral, rectal, and intravenous contrast agents. The intravenous contrast material facilitates the demonstration of hyperemia in mesenteric vessels, leading to the involved bowel segment as well as recognition of increased enhancement of the inflamed bowel wall.

Signs of diverticulosis include muscular hypertrophy visualized as wall thickening without stranding and diverticula. Pericolonic standing can be the earliest sign of diverticulitis, a feature that cannot be detected by a barium enema. It is seen in 96% of patients (30). In addition to the above-mentioned features, signs of diverticulitis include increased wall thickness, thickened or displaced diverticula, abscess (Fig. 13), contiguous inflammation of surrounding structures such as bladder and ureters, and fistula to bowel loops, bladder and vagina (28,29).

Similar to idiopathic inflammatory bowel disease, demonstration of wall thickening is nonspecific and a colon cancer with perforation can mimic diverticulitis with or without an abscess. The presence of local lymphadenopathy favors cancer over diverticulitis if Crohn's disease can be excluded. Also, the presence of diverticula and preservation of enhancement of the colonic wall on thin sections was shown to strongly favor diverticulitis over carcinoma in the right colon. Diverticulitis of the right colon is less common than in the sigmoid colon in Western individuals, but is more common in Asian patients. Diverticulitis tends to involve a long segment (often >10 cm) whereas colon cancer tends to involve a short segment with or without adenopathy. Patients with a suspected or presumptive diagnosis of acute diverticulitis should undergo colonoscopy once the acute inflammation has resolved to exclude a malignancy (96).

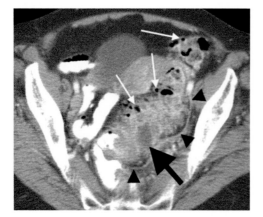

Figure 13 Computed tomography in this patient with diverticulitis demonstrates diverticula (*thin white arrows*); wall thickening, fascial thickening, and stranding (*arrowheads*); and an abscess (*black arrow*).

In a recent study (30), the most frequent sign of diverticulitis were bowel wall thickening (96%) followed by fat stranding (91%). Highly specific but less frequently found signs included fascial thickening (45%), free fluid (43%), and inflamed diverticula (30%). Interestingly enough, diverticula were demonstrated on CT in only 50%. The overall accuracy for CT assessment of diverticulitis was 99%. In comparison to a water-soluble enema, CT outperformed the enema (97) in most aspects, particularly in the assessment of pericolonic findings including phlegmon and abscess where accurate assessment permits appropriate triage of these patients.

Appendicitis

The typical findings associated with acute appendicitis include an appendix greater than 6 mm in diameter, presence of inflammatory changes in the periappendiceal area combined with a dilated and thickened appendix, thickening of the right lateral conal fascia next to the inflamed appendix, retrocecal inflammatory changes extending to the psoas, calcified appendicolith associated with inflammatory changes (30–70% of all cases), fluid collection with enhancing rim suggesting abscess near the suspected location of the appendix, thickened cecal tip and terminal ileum associated with detection of an abnormal appendix and periappendiceal fat stranding, air in the wall of the appendix, in the retroperitoneum, or abdomen associated with inflammatory changes in the periappendiceal area, and arrowhead sign in cecum pointing to an inflamed appendix (Fig. 14) (98). It should be noted here that air in the lumen of the appendix may be normal.

A solid or ring-like calcification in the right lower quadrant, which often is close to the cecum, suggests an appendicolith and, combined with inflammatory changes in the periappendiceal area, implies a high likelihood of appendicitis. This combination of findings may represent acute appendicitis even if the actual appendix is not well demonstrated. Patients with appendicoliths have a higher incidence of perforation and gangrene of the appendix. If the appendix and an appendicolith are not visualized, only a differential diagnosis can be offered.

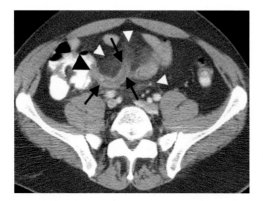

Figure 14 Computed tomography in this patient with appendicitis demonstrates a dilated and thick-walled inflamed appendix (*black arrows*). The black arrowhead points to the origin of the inflamed appendix at the cecal tip. The white arrowheads highlight soft tissue stranding.

The most common location of the appendix is retrocecal (60–66%). Many are located in the pelvis (32%). Atypical locations can lead to erroneous diagnoses and an atypical clinical picture. Entities that can mimic appendicitis include mesenteric adenitis, sigmoid diverticulitis, cecal diverticulitis, perforating cecal carcinoma, ileocecal Crohn's disease, ischemic bowel, appendagitis (inflamed appendix epiploicum), and neutropenic colitis. Tubo-ovarian abscess (pelvic inflammatory disease), ovarian torsion, corpus luteum cyst, and ectopic pregnancy in the female patient also need to be considered. Occasionally a rare lymphoma of the appendix can mimic appendicitis but in these cases the appendiceal wall is unusually thick (over 1.5 cm).

Appendagitis presents similar to appendicitis or diverticulitis but, usually, the white blood cell count is not or only mildly elevated. The radiographic appearance is highly suggestive of appendagitis (99). Fat stranding in a well-encapsulated area of oval to round shape is seen adjacent to the colon. The mass often impresses the colon but does not cause wall thickening and the treatment for appendagitis usually is conservative.

Appendiceal abscesses appear as a well-demarcated fluid collection in the right lower quadrant of the abdomen or right pelvis with or without tissue stranding in the periappendiceal fat. The inflammatory changes may extend up to the liver if the appendix is retrocecal in location. Occasionally, only thickening of the appendiceal wall is noted, which on axial images can appear as three concentric rings or more often as a single thick ring of enhancement, frequently associated with periappendiceal soft tissue stranding.

CT has a reported sensitivity of 79% to 98% (100–102). Most recent studies list a sensitivity and specificity of approximately 95% (100–111). In a comparative study of contrast-enhanced unfocused appendiceal CT versus unenhanced focused appendiceal CT, the sensitivity for appendicitis was significantly higher for the enhanced study (88–97% vs. 71–83%) but the specificity was not significantly different (103). Therefore, the diagnostic accuracy for appendicitis improves significantly with intravenous contrast material. In a comparative study of CT and graded compression ultrasound (US) in acute childhood appendicitis, CT had sensitivity of 97%, an accuracy of 95%, and a negative predictive value (NPV) of 92% (104). US had a sensitivity of 80%, an accuracy of 89%, and an NPV of 88% (104).

Based on the available evidence, US should be used in young women of childbearing age, in pregnant women, and in children. Children may be particularly difficult to examine ultrasonographically because of the pain associated with acute appendicitis (98). For the remainder of the patients, it is best to proceed directly to CT, especially in men, in obese patients, or in patients with an ileus or extensive bowel gas. CT is particularly useful in the differential diagnosis of appendicitis. Some controversy still exists as to which of the two methods is best. A study in the pediatric population showed that CT was more reliable in reducing negative appendectomies (105). Without imaging, the negative appendectomy rate was 14% but increased to 17% for ultrasound and decreased to 2% with CT (105). This study also showed that the perforation rate without imaging was similar to results after CT or US. A combination of CT and US had the highest perforation rare but this may have been due to selection bias because the surgeons requested both methods in clinically difficult cases. This study concluded that the use of CT leads to significant reduction of negative appendectomies without the danger of increased perforation rates if a negative CT result was accepted as the truth. In questionable cases, the decision was based on the severity of the clinical presentation. A more recent study in children showed that a combination of CT and US can be reliably used by experienced hands but in inconclusive cases, CT can improve the diagnostic accuracy rate (104). Nonetheless, one has to keep in mind that US is more operator dependent and may fail in obese patients. CT does not have such limitations but does expose the patient to radiation.

Infectious Colitis

Infectious changes in the colon can be grouped into those that involve only the colon and those that demonstrate inflammatory changes in the colon and terminal ileum (Table 3) (106). Infectious colitis can produce diffuse or localized wall thickening, which may be associated with thumb printing.

A previously mentioned, one of the diseases that causes significant wall thickening is pseudomembranous colitis (Fig. 15) (107–110). In these patients, the wall thickening appears similar to that seen in Crohn's disease; however, fibrofatty proliferation or fistulae are not present. Skip areas may be shown in pseudomembranous colitis, which makes distinction from Crohn's disease even more challenging. Another infectious type of colitis, which causes

Table 3 Colitis With and Without Small Bowel Involvement

Colitis	Left-sided or pancolitis	Small bowel involved
Cytomegalovirus, pseudomembranous (PM)	+++ (R > L)	+ (TI)
Tuberculosis	++	+ (TI)
Campylobacter	++	+ (TI)
Typhlitis	++ (R only)	+ (TI)
Yersinia	(+)	++ (TI)
Salmonellosis	+	++
Shigellosis	++	− − −
Amebiasis	++ (R)	− − −
Schistosomiasis	++ (ca^{++}, polyps)	− − −
Strongyloidiasis	++ (fistulae)	− − −
E. coli 0157: H7	++ (transverse)	− − −

Abbreviation: TI, terminal ileum.

marked thickening of the colonic wall, is CMV infection of the colon (111). This type of colitis is seen in immunosuppressed patients such as in patients with cancer, in patients with AIDS, or in patients undergoing chemotherapy. Marked wall thickening is usually present but the radiographic diagnosis is not specific for CMV colitis (58). Ischemic changes of the colon or small bowel with their extensive wall thickening can also mimic Crohn's disease. Distinction between ischemic and inflammatory etiology of bowel wall thickening can only be made if a typical vascular distribution pattern is detected or if the clinical history strongly suggests a vascular compromise (see below).

CT may be helpful in patients with neutropenic colitis, also called typhlitis or necrotizing enteropathy, which is a condition associated with severe neutropenia (112). It is a complication of acute leukemia, aplastic anemia, or cyclic neutropenia. Usually, only the cecum is involved, but other portions of the colon or even terminal ileum may show similar changes. In patients with typhlitis, CT shows thickening of the cecal wall with areas of low density caused by edema, hemorrhage, necrosis, or even pneumatosis (113). Often stranding in the pericolonic fat is associated with the abnormalities of the colonic wall. Thickening of the cecal wall is caused by mucosal ulcerations produced by distention of the bowel alone or by intramural hemorrhage, the effects of steroids or antimetabolites and folic acid antagonists. Bacteriae, viruses, and fungi, which profusely grow in the absence of neutrophils, invade the damaged mucosa. All of these changes lead to the CT feature of wall thickening. Often, the remaining bowel loops are distended related to a paralytic ileus. CT is helpful in patients with leukemia and nonspecific symptoms, abdominal pain, nausea, and vomiting that can be considered side effects of chemotherapy because in these instances, the detection on CT of a thickened cecal wall can expedite effective medical and possibly surgical treatment. Findings similar to those features described above for neutropenic typhlitis can also be seen in patients with renal, hepatic, or cardiac transplants and in patients with bone marrow transplants. Findings similar to those observed for Crohn's disease in the rectum and perirectal space can also be seen in patients after corrective surgery for Hirschsprung's disease, after subtotal colectomy and

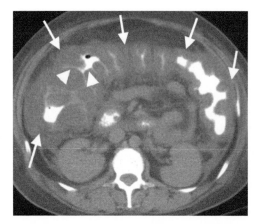

Figure 15 Marked wall thickening (*arrows*) is seen in this patient with pseudomembranous colitis. Thumbprinting is also seen (*arrowheads*).

reanastomosis, and in patients with perforated rectal neoplasms such as seen in advanced adenocarcinoma or rectal lymphoma. Occasionally, traumatic proctitis with perforation can be encountered, which manifests itself on barium enema as narrowing of the lumen due to edema in the wall with or without perforation and abscess formation.

Ischemic Disease of the Colon

Imaging is an indispensable part of the diagnostic evaluation in patients with suspected ischemic bowel disease because the definitive clinical diagnosis often is difficult to make for both acute and chronic disease. Certain radiographic features are highly suggestive of this disease and can lead to an accurate diagnosis when plain film radiography, CT scanning, or angiography detects them. In most instances of suspected ischemia when a patient presents with severe abdominal pain and distention, an abdominal series will be obtained. If thumb-printing (bowel wall thickening) and air in the bowel wall is seen without or with portal venous gas, the diagnosis of ischemia is highly suggestive, especially if the patient also has metabolic acidosis. If the abdominal series is not conclusive, the patient should undergo a CT examination as rapidly as possible. With the advent of multi-detector row CT scanners and the ease of three dimensional (3-D) reconstructions, CT angiograms that are of very high quality can be obtained. The success with CT angiography has largely eliminated the need for conventional angiography in assessing patients with acute mesenteric arterial and venous occlusive disease (114).

Technique

A special CT protocol should be performed for suspected ischemic disease with intravenous contrast material delivered at a high injection rate (4–5 mL/sec) for a total of 150 mL. At the University of California San Francisco, we prefer a rate of 5 mL and start scanning with a scan delay of 15 to 20 seconds. If needed, a test bolus can be used to settle on the best timing of the bolus. Based on precontrast scans, the location of the superior mesenteric artery (SMA) to celiac axis is determined and scans are obtained over a segment of about 5 cm with very thin slices (subcentimeter slice thickness, varying from 0.33 mm to 0.625 mm depending on scanners). Postprocessing permits 3-D reconstruction of the celiac axis, superior mesenteric artery, and IMA with their branches. Once the CT angiogram portion of the study has been completed, the rest of the abdomen can be examined with a slice thickness of 5 to 7 mm.

As far as the bowel is concerned, either no oral contrast material or a neutral oral contrast material such as VoLumen™ (E-Z-EM, Westbury, NY, 11590) or water should be used, which allows for better assessment of the bowel wall and avoids interference with 3-D reconstruction. In this fashion, lack of perfusion of the bowel wall also can be better determined. The use of positive (opaque) contrast may be beneficial in patients with chronic ischemia.

Features in Acute Mesenteric Occlusive Disease

Acute ischemia due to occlusion of major vessels is the most severe form of intestinal ischemia that is often life threatening. Furthermore, it is the cause of intestinal ischemia in about one-third of patients with bowel ischemia (115) and may be due to thrombosis or emboli in large arteries such as the SMA or IMA. It could be caused by occlusion of small arteries due to vasculitis from lupus, periarteritis nodosa, diabetes, or radiation (Fig. 16). Another cause of intestinal ischemia could be due to venous occlusion seen in hypercoaguable states, portal hypertension, and inflammation or infection in the abdomen and pelvis. Occlusion of arteries and veins can occur in patients with marked mechanical bowel obstruction and distention such as closed loop, volvulus, or internal hernia.

In the early and mild form of bowel ischemia, the bowel may be normal on CT. The most common findings on CT include dilation of the bowel and/or bowel wall thickening, which are nonspecific, but in combination, are suggestive of intestinal ischemia. Bowel wall thickening has a CT sensitivity of 38% and a specificity of 78% in suspected ischemic disease (116). Bowel wall thickening and/or dilation also can occur in intestinal infection or inflammation, hypoproteinemia, intestinal hemorrhage, and immunosuppression. Either increased or decreased (sensitivity of 48% and specificity of 100%) enhancement of the bowel wall is suggestive of intestinal ischemia (116). Occasionally, a thrombus may be seen in one of the mesenteric vessels. When the ischemic event is moderate to severe, peri-intestinal or pericolonic stranding with or without fluid may be seen. Distribution of the abnormalities in a vascular

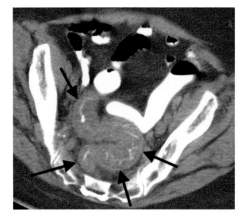

Figure 16 Marked thickening of the wall of the rectum and sigmoid (*black arrows*) is present in this patient who received radiation to the pelvis. The radiographic changes represent an ischemic event caused by radiation-induced proliferation of the arterial intima.

pattern strongly favors ischemia as the underlying cause. Lack of enhancement of the bowel wall, air in the bowel wall, and demonstration of a thrombus have been shown to be highly reliable predictors of ischemic bowel disease with a specificity of 90% (117).

Air in the bowel wall is also a suggestive sign (Fig. 17), which may indicate a graver prognosis particularly if portal venous gas is present (Fig. 18). In a study in 23 patients with pneumatosis or portomesenteric venous gas, these findings were associated with transmural bowel infarction in 78% and 81%, respectively (118). Fifty-six percent of these patients with portomesenteric venous gas died. Of seven patients with infarction limited to one bowel segment (jejunum, ileum, or colon), only one patient (14%) died, whereas of the 10 patients with infarction of two or three bowel segments, 8 patients (80%) died. The authors concluded that CT findings of pneumatosis intestinalis and portomesenteric venous gas due to bowel ischemia do not generally allow prediction of transmural bowel infarction, because they may be observed in patients with only partial ischemic bowel wall damage. The clinical outcome of patients with bowel ischemia with these CT findings seems to depend mainly on the severity and extent of their underlying disease. Portal venous gas may be detected by Doppler ultrasound in the absence of CT findings (119).

In venous intestinal thrombosis, the onset of symptoms is more gradual or chronic, with slowly increasing abdominal pain. The plain film and CT findings may be similar to arterial occlusive disease. Occasionally, a thrombus is seen in the superior mesenteric vein (SMV), which may extend into the portal and/or splenic vein. This finding usually is associated with an enhancement of the wall of the SMV and multiple venous collaterals.

Features in Nonocclusive Mesenteric Ischemia
Nonocclusive intestinal ischemia is more common and is seen in about 60% of patients with intestinal ischemia (115). Nonocclusive intestinal ischemia presenting with abdominal pain is often encountered in patients at risk, such as in patients with cardiovascular disease or

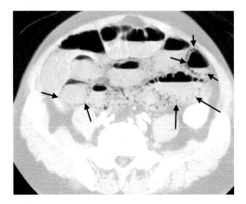

Figure 17 A string of air bubbles (*arrows*) is seen in the bowel wall in a patient with severe ischemia.

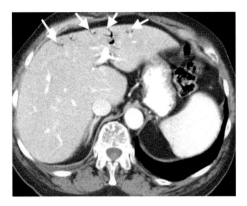

Figure 18 Air (*arrows*) is seen in portal veins in the periphery of the liver. The patient suffered from bowel infarction.

arrhythmias and in patients who suffer from severe blood loss, dehydration, shock, or sepsis. The plain film and CT findings in nonocclusive mesenteric ischemia are similar to those described for the occlusive type; however, thrombi or emboli in the mesenteric vessels are not present. Again, bowel thickening with or without thumbprinting and an ileus pattern is evident on plain films and on CT. Early in the ischemic process, severe narrowing of the smaller vessels can be seen. Abnormal small-beaded peripheral arteries may be identified, which are due to spasm; usually poor filling of the mesenteric veins can also be found.

Sensitivity of CT for Intestinal Ischemia

A diagnosis of ischemia was made at surgery in 24 of 144 patients with bowel obstruction examined by CT (116). CT diagnosis was correct in 23 patients (96% sensitivity) while there were 9 false-positive diagnoses (93% specificity); the negative predictive value of CT was 99%. In this study, mesenteric fluid had a sensitivity of 88% and a specificity of 90%, congestion of mesenteric veins had a sensitivity of 58% and specificity of 79%, and ascites had a sensitivity of 75% and specificity of 76%. As this data represents a subset of patients who developed ischemia secondary to bowel obstruction, these later signs may be more specific in patients with, than in patients without, bowel obstruction. Balthazar reported a sensitivity of 83%, specificity of 93%, accuracy of 91%, a positive predictive value (PPV) of 79%, and NPV of 95% of CT for bowel ischemia (120). The authors of this study also concluded that CT enables accurate detection of bowel ischemia, particularly when small bowel obstruction is present. Exploratory laparotomy should be performed when unexplained disparities exist between equivocal CT findings and a deteriorating clinical condition in patients with possible small bowel obstruction or mesenteric infarction. The same authors also looked at 54 cases of proved ischemic colitis and found that in 30% ischemia was clinically not suspected but seen on CT (121). They found complications such as abscess formation in 24%. In yet another study of 20 patients with ischemia proximal to an obstructing colon cancer, CT was able to distinguish between ischemic segment and tumor extension in 75% of the cases (122).

Based on the available data and the experience of the authors, CT can be used to confirm the clinical suspicion of ischemic events in the colon and small bowel, to suggest ischemia when it is unsuspected, and to diagnose complications. Helical CT is a highly sensitive method particularly to diagnose or rule out intestinal ischemia in the context of acute small-bowel or colonic obstruction. In cases of disparities between CT findings that are suggestive but not diagnostic of ischemia and a clinically deteriorating patient, exploratory laparotomy should be performed.

Colonic Obstruction

Colonic obstruction is diagnosed in many instances on plain films but CT is often used to determine the cause of obstruction. CT serves well in distinguishing between an obstruction caused by inflammation and that caused by scarring or adhesions. It also can determine that a neoplastic process is the underlying cause and permits one to accurately stage advanced neoplastic disease (T3 and higher). In cases of pancreatitis, CT can demonstrate that the so-called colon-cut-off sign is caused by pancreatic fluid extending to the phrenocolic ligament. CT can diagnose sigmoid and cecal volvulus or cecal bascule but often a barium enema is used to confirm the diagnosis suspected on plain films. Processes that cause colonic obstruction by an extrinsic source can also be readily determined, such as endometriosis, hernias, tubo-ovarian abscess, or even appendiceal abscess. Colonic obstruction associated with a vascular phenomenon including intra- or extramural hematomas (123) has been addressed in the previous section. Finally, CT also can readily image fecal impaction, bezoars, foreign bodies, and intussusception.

Technique

A routine CT examination of the abdomen and pelvis is performed but the administration of rectal contrast is important. Water as rectal contrast allows for better evaluation of the colonic wall, especially if a fast bolus of intravenous contrast material is delivered. If intra- or extra-peritoneal abscesses or fistula are suspected, opaque rectal contrast is of greater advantage to allow for distinction between bowel loops filled with positive contrast material and extracolonic fluid collections that are of water density.

Sensitivity of Computed Tomography for Colonic Obstruction

In one study, CT successfully diagnosed colonic obstruction with a sensitivity of 96% and correctly identified pseudo-obstruction (specificity of 93%) (124). CT correctly localized the point of obstruction in 44 of 47 patients (94%). In the same study, barium enema successfully diagnosed obstruction in only 20 of 25 patients (80% sensitivity). In this study, CT proved to be a satisfactory modality in evaluating patients with suspected colonic obstruction. CT may in certain circumstances be preferable to the traditional barium enema in evaluating these patients.

Preoperative Staging of Colorectal Tumors

For general screening after the age of 50, a flexible sigmoidoscopy combined with a well-performed barium enema often is used in place of a colonoscopy alone for safe, cost-effective, complete, and accurate examination of the colon (125). Colonoscopy and/or barium enema is recommended in patients with suspected or known colorectal carcinoma or for screening of patients with a family history of hereditary nonpolyposis colorectal cancer. However, even though these methods can detect tumor with a sensitivity of over 90%, they cannot assess local, regional, and distant extent to enable staging of a neoplasm. High sensitivity and high specificity for tumor extent and nodal involvement are essential for any imaging method to provide useful information on the stage of tumor. Debate continues as to which imaging method or combination of methods should be used for the most effective preoperative staging. For preoperative staging, CT remains the best method combined with PET for assessing metastatic disease (M) and for detecting extensive local disease that might benefit from preoperative radiation. EUS frequently is used for local extent of disease (T) and local nodes (N) although T and N staging generally are based on surgical and pathologic results (Table 4).

CT together with transrectal ultrasonography (for rectal lesions) allows evaluation of tumor stage beyond manual examination, barium enema, and fiberoptic techniques. Both

Table 4 Computed Tomographic Staging of Primary or Recurrent Colorectal Tumor with Tumor Node Metastasis Correlation (TNM)

Computed tomographic staging	Tumor node metastasis correlation	Description
I	(T1)	Intraluminal mass without thickening of wall
II[a]	(T2)	Thickened large bowel wall (>0.6 cm) or pelvic mass; no extension beyond bowel wall
IIIa[a]	(T3)	Thickened large bowel wall or pelvic mass with invasion of adjacent tissue but not to pelvic sidewalls or abdominal wall
IIIb[a]	(T4a and b)	Thickened large bowel wall or pelvic mass with perforation or invasion of adjacent organs or structures with or without extension to pelvic/abdominal walls but without distant metastases
IV[a]	(Any T, M1)	Distant metastases with or without local abnormality

[a]With or without lymph adenopathy (N0 or N1).
Source: From Ref. 126.

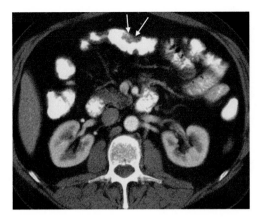

Figure 19 A sessile lesion with irregular margins (*arrows*) is seen in the transverse colon representing an early adenocarcinoma. Computed tomography cannot assess the depth of infiltration within the bowel wall.

CT and ultrasonography may image a colorectal cancer as a discrete mass (Fig. 19) or focal wall thickening, but this is a nonspecific finding and requires further exploration (126). Extent of tumor beyond the bowel wall is diagnosed as a mass in the bowel wall with irregular outer margins without or with soft tissue stranding extending from the outer rectal–colonic margin into the perirectal or pericolonic fat (Fig. 20). Image reconstructions in coronal or sagittal planes can be helpful (Fig. 21). Extracolonic tumor spread is also suggested by loss of tissue fat planes between the large bowel and surrounding muscles—levator ani, obturator internus, piriformis, coccygeal, and gluteus maximus or surrounding structures such as female or male reproductive organs, bladder, stomach, spleen, or liver. However, invasion is definite only when a tumor mass extends directly into an adjacent muscle, obliterating the fat plane and enlarging the individual muscle. Metastases to liver, spleen, adrenal glands, lung, and peritoneum can be readily diagnosed based on the presence of discrete soft tissue masses. The pathologic nature of node enlargement cannot be determined absolutely by CT, although asymmetry, irregularity of outer margins, and increased size (shorter diameter $>1\,cm$) can be used to establish lymph node abnormality (127). Size alone is not a reliable indicator of malignant lymphadenopathy as reactive hyperplasia can also enlarge lymph nodes.

CT is not sensitive enough to detect microscopic invasion of the fat surrounding the colon or rectum and tends to understage these patients. Spread to contiguous organs in the pelvis can be simulated by absence of tissue planes between the viscera and the tumor mass without actual invasion. Vascular or lymphatic congestion, inflammation, or actual absence of fat because of severe cachexia can cause obliteration of fat planes. Therefore, invasion should be cautiously diagnosed and considered definite only if an obvious mass clearly involves an adjacent organ. Distinction between tumor infiltration of adjacent muscle and simple absence of fat separating normal structures is particularly difficult in the area of lower rectum and anal verge. Because radiation induces fibrosis as well as acute inflammatory responses in the radiated area, it is recommended to stage patients before radiation treatment to avoid overstaging of tumor. A follow-up CT may be obtained to establish reduction in size of the tumor extent.

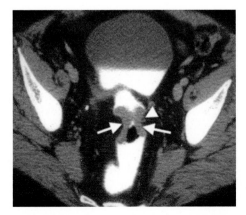

Figure 20 Computed tomography demonstrates an apple-core lesion (*arrows*) with subtle invasion of the pericolonic fat (*arrowhead*), indicative of an invasive colon carcinoma.

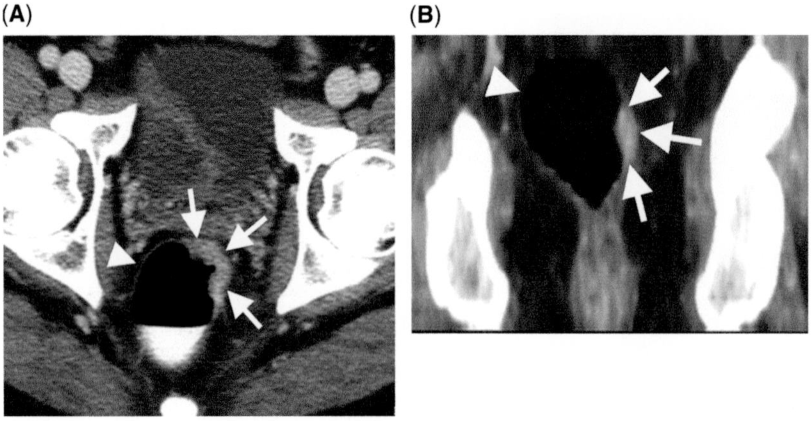

(A)   **(B)**

Figure 21   (**A**) Wall thickening is present in the anterior and lateral wall (*arrows*) of the rectum in a patient with adenocarcinoma of the rectum. The normal wall (*arrowhead*) measures less than 3 mm in diameter. (**B**) Coronal reconstruction shows no evidence of extension beyond the bowel wall (*arrows*). The right lateral wall of the rectum is normal (*arrowhead*).

Early reports suggested that CT findings for local extent and regional spread of tumor correlated well with surgical and histopathologic findings, and accuracy rates between 77% and 100% were reported (126,128–131). Because of the high accuracy rates, these early studies suggested CT should be used routinely as a preoperative staging procedure (130–133). Later studies showed much lower accuracy rates (41–64%), largely due to low sensitivity for detection of lymph node metastases (22–73%) and low sensitivity of local tumor extent (53–77%) (132–138). The use of different scanners and the lack of information on the amount and modus of administering the contrast material make a direct comparison of these variable results very difficult. Nevertheless, most errors in interpretation result from the inability to determine extent of tumor within the bowel wall, microscopic invasion of perirectal or pericolonic fat, and presence or absence of metastatic foci in normal-sized lymph nodes. Lymph node metastases were not separately analyzed in some of the earlier studies, which tended to have more advanced stages in their series. One study demonstrated that staging accuracy increased from 17% for Dukes' B lesions to 81% for Dukes' D lesions (137), reflecting the fact that advanced local and distant disease is diagnosed well with CT. Tumors in the rectosigmoid area are more accurately diagnosed than tumors in the other areas of the colon. This is due to the fixed position of the rectosigmoid colon in relation to the pelvis.

Refinements of CT techniques such as multi-detector row helical CT, colonic preparation, prone positioning of the patient, and air-distention of the rectum have increased the accuracy of assessing local tumor extent by CT (139–141). Also, the threshold for diagnosing lymph node metastases could be lowered, but such an approach, while increasing sensitivity, decreases specificity for detecting absence of lymph node metastases. However, in the perirectal area, any visible adenopathy should be considered abnormal.

Imaging of Recurrent Colorectal Tumor

Several investigations have shown that the stage, histology, and site of primary tumor at the time of diagnosis are most predictive of eventual relapse (142,143). In one study, the incidence of recurrence for initial Duke A and B1 was 10%, for B2, 33%, for C1, 35%, and for C2, 50% (144). Rectosigmoid tumors appeared to have a higher recurrence rate (30%) than right colon lesions (20%) or transverse and left colon tumors (10%) (145), likely due to a less aggressive resection margin. Local recurrence alone was found in 33% to 66%, local and distant metastases in 14% to 19%, and distant metastases alone in 26% to 46%. Anastomotic recurrence occurs mostly after anterior resection and is usually related to residual tumor outside the colorectal wall, which grows into the suture site. Because recurrence may be seen in 30% to 50% of patients with apparently curative resection and in at least 80% of these patients within the first two years (146), early and frequent follow-up studies have been recommended. The most commonly recommended sequence of follow-up studies consists of a baseline CT (or MRI study, see below) at two to four months with repeat imaging examinations at six-month intervals for two years and then at yearly intervals for up to five years. Nonetheless, earlier detection of recurrent colorectal cancer by intensified follow-up does not lead to either significantly increased reresectability or improved five-year survival.

Following resection of the primary tumor and anastomosis, a locally recurrent tumor can be diagnosed when a mass is seen at the site of anastomosis. This mass often has an extrinsic component. Following AP resection, a soft tissue mass in the pelvis can be suggestive of tumor recurrence. The appearance of such a mass must be compared to a baseline CT study to avoid confusion of scar tissue with tumor recurrence. The search for recurrent disease must include evaluation of possible distant sites such as liver, adrenal glands, lung, peritoneal cavity, and lymph nodes. In patients who underwent abdominoperineal resection, some studies suggested that streaky densities or a clean operative bed suggest fibrosis while the presence of a mostly globular mass favors the diagnosis of tumor recurrence as long as unopacified small bowel loops or relocated pelvic structures (such as vesicles or uterus) as source of the presacral mass can be excluded (127). However, several other studies indicated that one could expect to see a mass of soft tissue density in the early postoperative period due to granulation tissue, hemorrhage, edema, and/or fibrosis (126). Also post-radiation changes can produce the appearance of streaky densities or a presacral mass. Serial CT scans obtained within 28 months of operation established that persistence of a mass for up to at least 24 months after AP resection might be normal (147). Obtaining a baseline CT study two to four months after surgery frequently demonstrates the presence of a mass. A study at four to nine months often reveals decrease in size and better definition of margins, often associated with at least partial separation from the sacrum, and possible change into a thin sliver of soft tissue density indicates benign changes. In the absence of symptoms and raised carcinoembryonic antigen (CEA) titers, such a change of a mass should not result in concern for local tumor recurrence. However, any increase in size of a mass, with or without invasion of adjacent structures and with or without appearance of lymphadenopathy or perineal soft tissue density, should be considered suggestive of recurrence and percutaneous biopsy is indicated (148–150).

CT has been used extensively to detect the presence or absence of recurrent colorectal cancer, and a general consensus has been reached that either MR (see below) or CT have merit inasmuch as each enables detection of recurrence at a time when CEA titers are normal and/or symptoms are absent (151,152). As with CT results for primary tumors, initially very high sensitivity rates of 93% to 95% were reported for detecting locally recurrent tumor and metastases to lymph nodes, liver, peritoneal cavity, and the retroperitoneum (153,154), but more recent investigations indicate accuracy rates ranging from 69% to 88% (155–158). Similar to primary tumor sites, these results are markedly improved by combining CT and PET (see below under PET). PET has an even larger role in patients with suspected recurrent disease.

The value of cross-sectional imaging is particularly great in patients with total AP resection and colostomies. In male patients with total AP resection, manual examination or colonoscopy cannot provide information whether local recurrent tumor is present whereas in female patients, a vaginal examination can provide some information on possible local tumor recurrence. In either case, extensive fibrosis after surgery, with or without radiation, often renders such assessment impossible and lymphadenopathy and other metastases cannot be detected with the clinical or endoscopic examination. Colonoscopy in patients following curative resections and ileocolonic or colorectal anastomoses has been shown to be successful for the detection of recurrence at the anastomosis. Follow-up studies in these patients with potentially curative resection of recurrence have demonstrated an average of 38 months without symptoms compared to an average survival of eight months in patients without resection of recurrent tumor (159,160). While today, CT and MRI are both accepted methods for detection of recurrent colorectal tumor, the debate on the appropriate timing of these imaging tests is ongoing and has gained even more importance due to the high cost of frequent imaging in these patients. Moreover, by the time any recurrence is radiographically apparent, it may no longer be resectable for cure.

Magnetic Resonance
Non-neoplastic Disease of the Colon
CT is the preferred imaging method in patients with inflammatory bowel disease whether idiopathic or infectious, suspected diverticulitis, appendicitis ischemia, colonic obstruction or

anomalies. It has the advantage of short examination time, high spatial resolution, and, with state-of-the-art multislice technique, superb reconstructions in any plane. However, in patients with Crohn's disease, when fistulas are suspected, MR often is best in delineating these tracts (161).

Neoplastic Disease of the Colon

Preoperative Staging of Colorectal Tumors

Similar to CT, for accurate visualization of the intraluminal component of tumors, particularly smaller ones, preparation of the colon to avoid confusion with feces, air insufflation, gadolinium enhancement, and often prone positioning are necessary (162,163). On T1-weighted spin echo images, tumors appear as wall thickening with signal intensity similar to or slightly higher than that of skeletal muscle (long T1) (Fig. 22). Because perirectal fat has a short T1 and therefore high signal intensity, air no signal intensity, and tumor a long T1 and moderate signal intensity, tumors are shown with high contrast on T1-weighted sequences. For the same reason, extension of tumor beyond the colon wall is seen well on T1-weighted images. The signal intensity of tumor on T2-weighted spin echo images increases relative to that of muscle; however, the contrast between tumor and perirectal fat decreases because both tissues have long T2 relaxation times. Therefore, T2-weighted images are not as useful as T1-weighted images for determining extracolonic tumor extension. However, T2-weighted sequences are useful if uterine or pelvic sidewall invasion is suspected because of the differences in signal intensity between muscle, tumor, and muscle invaded by tumor. Invasion of adjacent organs is best demonstrated on transverse or coronal MR images, and MR is superior to CT in demonstrating invasion of levator ani or internal and external sphincter muscles. Lateral extension of tumor is difficult to detect on sagittal MR images. Extension into prostate, seminal vesicles, vagina, and cervix can be shown well by MRI, but extension into bladder may be missed if the bladder is not well distended.

MR imaging has difficulty to distinguish among the various layers of the colonic wall unless a rectal coil is used. Therefore tumors localized to the mucosa and tumors that infiltrate the entire colon wall cannot be correctly identified. Also, microinvasion into surrounding fat cannot be detected by MR. As with CT, the MR diagnosis of lymph node abnormality is based on the size of the nodes (129,164), and tumor deposits within normal-sized nodes may not be detected (165). For demonstration of liver and adrenal metastases, MR and CT are comparable if an optimal CT bolus technique is used. MR imaging with a liver-specific contrast agent [e.g., manganese dipyridoxyl-ethylenediamine-diacetate-(bis)phosphate, Teslascan™ (Nycomed Inc., Princeton, New Jersey, U.S.A.) or iron oxide particles, Feridex™ (Berlex, Wayne, New Jersey, U.S.A.)] may render MR superior to CT, particularly for small lesions (166,167) but larger series are needed to prove this point.

At present, MRI appears to have overall the same limitations as CT, but multiplanar imaging offers special advantages (Fig. 23). This advantage of MRI is largely eliminated by the multiplanar reconstruction possibilities offered by multi-detector row helical CT. An early investigation showed CT and MRI were equally effective in staging. MRI may better show direct invasion of tumor into bone or muscles such as the levator ani. However, depth of tumor infiltration in the wall of bowel and presence of metastatic foci in lymph nodes cannot

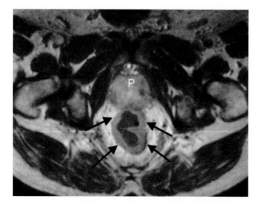

Figure 22 On the T1-weighted magnetic resonance sequence, the diffusely thickened rectal wall represents tumor (*arrows*) and is of slightly higher signal intensity than muscle. *Abbreviation*: P, prostate.

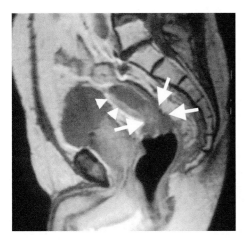

Figure 23 The sagittal view of the pelvis demonstrates an apple-core tumor in the upper rectum (*arrows*) with submucosal extension (*arrowheads*).

be accurately determined by MRI. An overall staging accuracy of 74% to 79% was found, but only small MRI series have been reported (165,168–170). If involvement of the urinary bladder and the uterus cannot be ruled out using CT, MR is helpful due to its higher soft tissue contrast resolution and multiplanar capability (171). Preoperative radiation with subsequent edema and fibrosis can lead to overstaging by MR (172). Results with endorectal coils have shown great promise for assessment of local tumor extension, but detection of lymphadenopathy, even though superior to MRI with a body coil, is limited (173,174). Nevertheless, the use of endorectal coils has not gained wide popularity for staging rectal cancers. Rectal ultrasound remains the gold standard. It is less expensive, portable, and more widely available than abdominal coil MRI.

Imaging of Recurrent Colorectal Tumor

It is possible to detect and stage presacral masses with MRI. Initial reports suggested that fibrosis after surgery with or without radiation had low signal intensity on both T1- and T2-weighted sequences whereas tumor recurrence had high signal intensity on T2-weighted images. It was concluded that MRI was superior to CT at distinguishing between fibrosis and recurrent tumor, and the hope was raised that MRI could eliminate the need for percutaneous biopsies. However, more recent studies have demonstrated that it is doubtful whether MRI can distinguish among recurrent tumor, fibrosis, and inflammation (175,176).

One study, using long repetition time (TR), long echo time (TE) (T2-weighted) sequences, examined the value of MRI in distinguishing among early fibrosis (one to six months after first treatment), tumor or late fibrosis (more than 12 months), and recurrent tumor (175). On T2-weighted images, tumor recurrence is diagnosed on the basis of high signal intensity (Fig. 24) whereas scar or fibrosis remains of low signal intensity (Fig. 25). The authors found that early fibrosis after treatment had higher signal intensity values than late fibrosis, probably due to increased vascularity, edema, and the presence of immature mesenchymal cells in granulation tissue. Radiation-induced necrosis and postsurgical inflammatory reaction can also contribute to an increase in signal intensity on T2-weighted images. It is the increase in tissue fluids seen in granulation tissue and necrosis due to radiation that renders distinction between early fibrosis and tumor recurrence so difficult or even impossible. However, late fibrosis and tumor recurrence could be clearly distinguished from one another (175). Other studies found similar results (176–179), but one study showed that the MRI accuracy for differentiating between radiation damage and residual/recurrent tumor varied with the primary site (180). It was excellent for cervical carcinoma but suboptimal for rectal carcinoma. The best investigation yet to appear on this topic was published by de Lange et al. who compared MRI results with histologic sections from tissue obtained during radical pelvic exenteration or extensive partial resection of a mass in patients with suspected recurrent rectosigmoid carcinoma (181). They found that the signal intensities on T2-weighted images do not permit prediction of the histologic diagnosis of the lesion in question. High signal intensity was found in areas of viable tumor, tumor necrosis, benign inflammation, and edematous tissue.

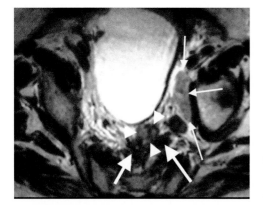

Figure 24 Recurrence of tumor after abdominoperoneal resection is visualized on T2-weighted magnetic resonance sequence as an area of higher signal intensity (*arrowheads*). Malignant adenopathy along the pelvic wall (*thin arrows*) has similar signal intensity. Scar tissue remains dark (*large arrows*).

Because desmoplastic reaction is a common host response to many benign and malignant processes including tumors of the colon and rectum, areas of low signal intensity on T2-weighted images were also nonspecific, and the differential diagnosis included tumor-induced fibrosis and non-neoplastic, benign fibrotic tissue. However, MRI can depict a presacral mass accurately and demonstrate its extent well. If such a mass consists mainly of desmoplastic tissue with only small strands of tumor tissue interspersed, even a percutaneous biopsy may show only fibrous tissue and no malignant cells. In these cases, a definitive diagnosis needs to be obtained by surgical removal of the mass or by biopsy at laparotomy.

Like CT, MRI is a sensitive method for detecting masses after colorectal surgery, but its specificity is not improved over that of CT. While CT cannot distinguish a benign from a malignant process based on attenuation coefficients and morphologic appearance in these patients, MRI is unable to base such a distinction on signal intensity. Studies with endorectal coils and contrast enhancement after rectal surgery and/or radiation have shown improved results (182). For overall screening to detect distant recurrence, CT may be more valuable than MRI, but more studies are needed to determine the efficacy of these procedures and their possibly complementary natures. A multi-institutional prospective study on the use and effectiveness of these imaging techniques is eagerly awaited.

Conclusions for Cross-Sectional CT and MR in Neoplastic Disease

Based on the presently available results, routine CT staging is not recommended for primary colorectal tumors except for assessing metastatic disease (M) and for detecting extensive local disease that might benefit from preoperative radiation. Whether MRI may offer other advantages over CT in patients with primary colorectal cancer is uncertain and more comprehensive studies are needed. CT should be reserved for those patients suspected of having locally extensive or widespread disease. If CT shows extensive local spread of tumor, these patients can

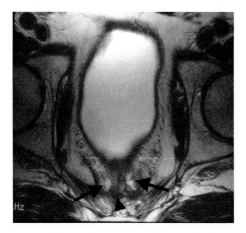

Figure 25 Scar tissue (*arrowhead*) but no recurrence of tumor is present in an elderly man with a total abdominal personal resection. The high signal intensity areas in the presacral space represent the seminal vesicles (*large arrows*).

be treated with radiation therapy alone or can be radiated and later undergo tumor resection, if feasible. While presence or absence of lymphadenopathy is not a significant clinical problem, if a colonic resection is planned, the decision on local tumor excision by surgery or colonoscopy cannot be based on CT or MR due to poor sensitivity for possible adenopathy. CT may be used to guide fine-needle aspirates of suspected metastases and assess complications such as perforation with abscess formation. Transrectal ultrasonography should be employed to determine local tumor extent. The differences between T1 and T2 lesions have significant consequences relative to selection of surgical procedure. Patients with T1 tumors may be candidates for transanal excision whereas T2 lesions generally warrant an extirpative approach. Similarly, and although less accurate than depth of penetration, nodal status is critical. Patients with T3 or N1 disease may be considered for preoperative neoadjuvant therapy. Rectal ultrasound remains the gold standard to assess both depth of tumor extension and local nodal involvement but has limited depth penetration. MRI with coronal views and gadolinium-enhanced images may be beneficial in determining involvement of the levator ani and with endorectal coils may gain valuable information regarding the presence of sphincteral invasion and the surrounding structures in patients with cancers in the lower third of the rectum (183). It is possible that endorectal coils and contrast-enhanced MRI, particularly MRI lymphangiography, could improve staging of colorectal tumors.

Advances in CT with multislice helical scanners and their ability to optimize contrast bolus timing (140) and to reconstruct in any plane and MRI with contrast-enhanced sequences, endoluminal coils, phase-array coils, and fast imaging have improved results with these modalities. Newer techniques such as monoclonal antibody imaging and PET with fluorodeoxyglucose F-18, especially if combined with CT, demonstrate very promising results and may prove to hold the key to accurate detection of tumor stage and distinguishing of recurrent rectal cancer from scar. Based on currently available results, PET has more value in suspected recurrent disease than in primary staging but prospective studies with large numbers of patients are needed for definitive evaluation.

CT Colonography

Carcinoma of the colon is the second leading cause of cancer mortality in the United States, with 135,4000 new cases in 2001 and 56,700 deaths attributable to the disease (184). Strong evidence supports the theory that most carcinomas arise from preexisting, benign adenomatous polyps. If detected and removed during the dwell time prior to malignant transformation, colon carcinoma may be prevented. Recognizing the importance of early detection, many medical societies including the American Cancer Society and the American Gastroenterological Association have published guidelines for colon cancer screening.

There is to date no clear consensus regarding the optimal method for screening. Fecal occult blood testing and flexible sigmoidoscopy have been used together, but neither provides a total colon examination. Colonoscopy, the current reference standard examination, is more invasive and costly, requires colon preparation and patient sedation, and carries a very small but definite risk of complications. When polyps are discovered, however, they can be biopsied or removed immediately. Until recently, the only radiologic alternative was the double-contrast barium enema (185). The development of CTC, better known to the general public as virtual colonoscopy, has added a significant new diagnostic tool in the detection of abnormalities of the colon wall. CTC may be defined as a CT examination of the colon wall, made possible by colon distention and the absence or digital subtraction of colon contents. However, because CTC is not yet a reimbursable procedure, it is more expensive to the patient than is colonoscopy.

Patient Preparation
Currently, most protocols require thorough colon cleansing, achieved by a combination of a low residue diet and some combination of polyethylene glycol electrolyte solution (Go-Lytely, Braintree Laboratories, Braintree, Massachusetts, U.S.A.), magnesium citrate, bisacodyl tablets, suppositories, and cleansing enemas depending upon local practice (186). Research efforts are currently under way to identify successful protocols for labeling stool and colon contents with barium. Preliminary results indicate that taking small quantities of barium with meals for several days preceding the examination can label colon contents with high density. Such fecal

residue labeled with barium can be digitally subtracted from the colon lumen, potentially obviating the necessity and inconvenience of bowel cleansing.

Examination Technique

When collapsed, haustral folds and other mucosal surfaces coapt, obscuring large segments of mucosa. Appropriate colon distention is achieved for CTC by the insufflation of room air or carbon dioxide via a rectal tube. The distending gas may be administered by 50 to 60 manual bulb compressions or by automated delivery through a system calibrated to maintain constant colonic pressure. In either case, careful attention to patient comfort is the rule, and the mild abdominal crampiness associated with adequate colon distention is generally well tolerated. Spasmolytics, though commonly used in some centers, have been shown not to significantly improve the degree of colon distention (187). A CT scout radiograph prior to scanning confirms the adequacy of colon distention, and additional gas may be instilled if necessary.

CT scanning is performed in a single breath-hold both supine and prone, permitting the redistribution of gas and retained fluid so that every portion of the colon mucosa can be inspected when it is outlined by gas. The combination of colon anatomy and gravitational redistribution of gas and retained liquid results in optimal distention for differing colon segments in supine and prone positions. Using a single detector CT scanner, 5 mm collimation is usually employed, with reconstruction at 2 to 3 mm intervals. Using multidetector CT scanners, smaller collimation is possible but may not be necessary for detection of clinically relevant polyps (188). Lower tube currents (100 to 140 mA) may be employed in CTC compared to conventional abdominal CT (250 mA) due to the high inherent contrast between gas and colon wall (189).

Interpretation

The resulting set of conventional two-dimensional (2-D) axial images displays the familiar anatomy of the abdomen and pelvis, permitting detection of significant extracolonic disease when it is present. Review of these images in both soft tissue and lung windows is the basis for CTC interpretation. The normal colon wall appears 1 to 2 mm thin and is sharply demarcated by luminal gas and extracolonic fat. Normal haustra appear as regular, thin circumferential rings about the colon lumen. More complex haustral patterns, potentially confusing to inexperienced readers, are primarily found near flexures. Polyps are seen as rounded protrusions into the colon lumen and should be sought on both colon wall and haustral surfaces (Figs. 26A and B). Polyps 10 mm or larger are usually considered clinically significant, as smaller excrescences are more likely to represent non-neoplastic, hyperplastic polyps. Carcinomas are larger, irregular intraluminal masses—some associated with luminal constriction (Fig. 26C).

The CTC data set can be postprocessed into a variety of formats. Multiplanar reformats of the original axial data produce coronal and sagittal images, permitting simultaneous

(A)   **(B)**   **(C)**

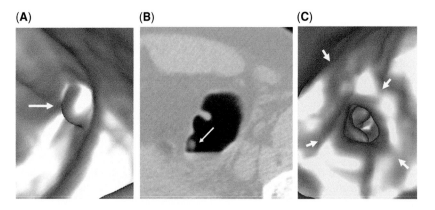

Figure 26 **(A)** Three-dimensional (3-D) computed tomography colonography (CTC) demonstrates a sessile polyp (*arrow*) in the sigmoid colon. **(B)** An axial view of the lower pelvis demonstrates a polyp with a small stalk (*arrow*) in the sigmoid colon. **(C)** 3-D CTC demonstrates an annular adenocarcinoma (*arrows*) with nodular surface. *Source:* Courtesy of Dr. Judy Yee, Veterans Administration Hospital, San Francisco, California, U.S.A.

scrutiny of any finding in three planes. Volume-rendered 3-D displays facilitate endoluminal navigation or "fly-through," producing the radiographic equivalent of the colonoscopic view. Additionally, however, the ability to navigate the colon lumen in reverse direction reveals portions of the colon mucosa—the backsides of haustra, for example, which are blind spots to the colonoscopist. While numerous possible projections and display options have been developed, conventional axial images and multiplanar reformats remain the cornerstone of interpretation.

Diagnostic Performance of CTC

We await the results of prospective, multicenter trials, currently under way to determine the diagnostic efficacy of CTC. Dachman, summarizing reported cohorts in the literature, showed that the by-patient sensitivity for patients with polyps 10 mm and larger ranges from 75% to 100% and was 100% in the two largest series to date (190). Improvements in technology and accumulating experience suggest that CTC is a potentially powerful tool in the detection of precancerous colon polyps.

CTC is a promising technique with tremendous potential for colorectal cancer screening. However, concerns about diagnostic interpretation times with experienced radiologists reporting average interpretation times as long as 30 minutes (191) and reimbursement issues must be resolved before CTC becomes an effective tool for screening. Therefore, for the present, the double-contrast barium enema examination remains the established and available radiologic test for colorectal cancer screening (192).

MR Colonography

MR colonography is a feasible alternative to CTC with similar indications. Although fast acquisition times and availability have favored the development of CTC, MR colonography offers the advantages of no radiation and the potential to distinguish layers of the colon wall, yielding staging information. As experience accrues, direct comparisons between these techniques will be possible.

Two general techniques, called bright lumen and dark lumen, are in use for MR colonography. The bright lumen technique involves administration of a water enema containing paramagnetic contrast, generally as a 10 mM solution of gadolinium. 3-D gradient recalled echo (GRE) and 2-D half-Fourier, single-shot, turbo spin echo/single shot, fast spin echo (HASTE/SSFSE) without fat saturation sequences are obtained. The dark lumen technique uses either a water or gaseous (room air, carbon dioxide, or hyperpolarized helium) enema, followed by acquisition of 2-D HASTE/SSFSE without fat saturation and 3-D GRE sequences before and after the administration of intravenous gadolinium. Intravenous contrast serves to delineate the enhancing mucosa in these protocols (193). In contrast to CTC, Glucagon is routinely administered prior to MR colonography in order to minimize image artifacts from bowel motion. As in CTC, bowel preparation is necessary. Stool-labeling techniques are evolving as a means to obviate this inconvenience. Stool can be rendered dark on MR images by barium taken with meals for several days prior to the examination or bright by gadolinium taken the same way (194).

Endoscopic Ultrasound

Although transabdominal ultrasonography may be used to assess the presence or absence of liver metastases, transrectal ultrasound is increasingly used to detect the depth of tumor infiltration and local adenopathy in patients with rectal carcinomas. Its advantage lies in its ability to distinguish the normal layers of the bowel wall and to visualize disruption of one or more of these layers by tumor. With this method, sensitivities of 67% to 96% have been reported for assessing perirectal spread, but the presence of regional lymph node metastases is less well detected (sensitivity 50–57%) (168,169,195–197). The broad range of sensitivities of transrectal ultrasound for detection of tumor extent in and through bowel wall emphasizes the operator dependence of this method. EUS has expanded the application of ultrasonographic methods to the entire colon. While ultrasonography of colon and rectum appears promising, valid and comprehensive clinical trials remain necessary.

Endosonographic examination of the colon and rectal ultrasound will be discussed in a separate chapter in greater detail. This discussion serves only to place EUS in the context

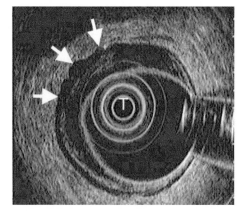

Figure 27 Endoscopic ultrasound demonstrates rectal wall thickening with extension of tumor into the perirectal fat (T3, arrows). *Abbreviation*: T, tumor.

with cross-sectional imaging by CT and MR. While CT and MR are the methods of choice for assessing large tumors with possible extension to pelvic sidewalls or clear infiltration of surrounding structures ("fixed masses"), EUS is superior in distinguishing the various layers of the colonic/rectal wall and in determining minimal perirectal infiltration (Fig. 27) (198). As CT and MR cannot distinguish the various layers in the bowel wall, they cannot discern between tumor stages T1, T2, and T3 with microscopic invasion of the fat. For local adenopathy, both cross-sectional imaging and endosonography are not accurate enough to determine early malignant involvement from reactive changes. CT and MR use size and irregular margins as diagnostic features, both of which are not specific enough. However, in the perirectal area, the diagnosis is more accurately made because in this anatomical location, hyperplastic nodes are not present.

For rectal tumors, endosonography can accurately assess small (<3 cm) well-differentiated tumors for possible local resection. It also can determine if the tumor has penetrated the bowel wall and if any local nodes are present. T2 and/or N1 disease generally preclude local resection. Endosonography also can be used to assess whether a large villous adenoma is invading the muscularis propria. Such invasion would preclude submucosal resection of the mass (199). Endosonography also may serve as a diagnostic tool for deciding on invasion of neighboring structures such as the prostate, vagina, or cervix and establishing the presence or absence of local recurrence at the level of reanastomosis following resection for a malignant lesion. It can also resolve where any palpable mass is located within the gut wall and determine the depth of penetration if any is present.

Overall, it is apparent from a multicenter prospective study (200) that transrectal ultrasound and EUS of the colon are most reliable in experienced hands at high-volume centers. Therefore, best results are achieved if suspected cases are referred to a subspecialized center with physicians with special training in EUS.

POSITRON EMISSION TOMOGRAPHY

PET is used for oncologic imaging and, since its introduction, has shown great promise for assessing the colon. PET provides a functional metabolic map of glucose uptake in the body when 2-[18F]fluoro-2-deoxy-D-glucose (F-18 FDG) is used. F-18FDG is a glucose analogue labeled with fluorine-18 and PET scanning measures F-18 FDG transport across cell membranes and intracellular accumulation. Neoplasms show increased metabolic rates, which results in increased uptake of F-18 FDG, and areas of tumor deposits demonstrate increased tracer localization.

Technique

Imaging is performed with a whole-body scanner (e. g., ECAT 953, Siemens, Knoxville, Tennessee, U.S.A.). The scanner parameters include an in-plane and transverse spatial resolution of 6 mm full width half maximum and a 10.5 cm field of view. Patients are instructed to fast overnight before the day of the imaging study or for at least four hours. The patient should not receive intravenous dextrose solutions for a minimum of four hours prior to the study. A urinary catheter may be placed if imaging of the pelvic region is required. Whole-body PET is performed 45 to 60 minutes following intravenous administration of F-18 FDG. All nonattenuation-corrected images are reconstructed by using a conventional filtered back-projection algorithm and reviewed in transverse, sagittal, and coronal planes. Length of study is one to four hours depending on how much of the body is to be included in the survey. Increased tracer localization may be present in the primary tumor site or in the surgical bed in cases with recurrent disease and throughout the liver, adrenal gland, lung, lymph nodes, or bone consistent with metastases. Also abnormal uptake in implants may be found through-out the abdominal and pelvic cavity.

Primary Colorectal Cancer

One study demonstrated that adenomatous polyps measuring 13 mm or larger could be detected by (F-18-FDG)-PET in 90%; however, the number of polyps of that size was small ($n = 10$) (201). There is little evidence for supporting the use of F-18 FDG-PET in screening asymptomatic individuals, and current modalities appear better suited for detection of symp-tomatic primary colorectal cancers. More recently, there is evidence of increased accuracy for F-18 FDG-PET in staging primary disease, but this area remains controversial and larger stud-ies are necessary. In patients with mucinous adenocarcinomas, false-negative results can be encountered. One study found a positive correlation between tumor FDG uptake and cellular-ity but a negative correlation with the amount of mucin (202). Therefore, F-18 FDG-PET is limited in the evaluation of mucinous tumors, particularly in hypocellular lesions with abun-dant mucin. For liver metastases, results have been excellent, and PET is currently considered the most reliable imaging technique for preoperative assessment of liver metastases from GI cancer (203) (Fig. 28). Our meta-analysis of patients with liver metastases from GI cancer demonstrated, at a specificity of 85% or more, a sensitivity of 90% for PET (95% CI 80–97%), compared to a sensitivity of 72% for CT (95% CI 63–80%), 76% for MR (95% CI 57–91%), and 55% for ultrasound (95% CI 41–68%) (203).

Recurrent Colorectal Cancer

For imaging of suspected recurrent colorectal neoplasms with F-18 FDG-PET, the situation is quite the reverse to imaging for initial staging of primary tumors. F-18 FDG PET is more sensi-tive and specific than conventional techniques. F-18 FDG-PET is capable of demonstrating

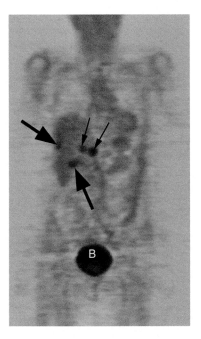

Figure 28 Positron emission tomography with F18-deoxy-glucose demonstrates two metastases in the liver (*large arrows*) and extrahepa-tic adenopathy (*small arrows*) in a patient with recurrent colon carcinoma. *Abbreviation:* B, bladder.

disease that mimics normal structures on conventional imaging, as well as finding disease in otherwise normal-sized lymph nodes. Abnormal areas of F-18 FDG uptake in the setting of known colorectal cancer are almost always due to recurrent disease. CT and MR can have difficulty in distinguishing conclusively between scar tissue following resection and/or radiation and recurrent tumor but PET can resolve the diagnostic dilemma in most instances. The major benefit of PET comes from its ability to alter patient management and results in cost savings. PET also appears to have a specific place in the evaluation of patients undergoing radiotherapy and chemotherapy where the success of treatment can be successfully monitored. This role likely will expand, particularly as more targeted therapies become available. The evidence suggests that PET may eventually become incorporated into patient management algorithms for suspected recurrent colorectal cancer in routine clinical oncology practices. It has been shown that PET is far superior to serial CEA level determinations (204). Technological improvements and introduction of novel tracers should improve this technique even further.

Sensitivity of PET

The usefulness of PET for recurrent colorectal cancer has been evaluated in retrospective studies (205,206) and confirmed in prospective studies (204,207). In Johnson's retrospective study, PET was found to be more sensitive than CT when compared with actual operative findings in the liver (100% vs. 69%, $p = 0.004$), extrahepatic region (90% vs. 52%, $p = 0.015$), and the abdomen as a whole (87% vs. 61%, $p < 0.001$). Sensitivities of PET and CT were not significantly different in the pelvic region (87% vs. 61%, $p = 0.091$). In each case, specificity was not significantly different between the two examinations. In Kalff's prospective study (207), PET influenced management in 60% of 102 patients who had no evidence of unresectable disease on conventional staging imaging studies including CT. In 57 patients, in whom results were discrepant; PET was correct in 91%. There was one false-positive result in one patient because of a pelvic abscess and the extent of metastatic disease was underestimated in four (7%). Relapse was confirmed in 98% of 50 patients with positive PET findings. Significantly, planned surgery was abandoned in 60% of 43 patients because of incremental PET findings. This prospective study confirmed the high impact, suggested by previous retrospective analyses (205,206), of (18) F-FDG PET on management of patients with suspected recurrent colorectal cancer. The major benefit of PET is the fact that inappropriate local therapies can be avoided by documenting widespread disease.

Because the limited availability of PET scanners precludes (22) F-FDG assessment of many patients for whom the study is indicated, the SPECT system in coincidence mode [dual-head camera (18) F-FDG coincidence imaging (DHC) (22) F-FDG] has been suggested as an alternative for assessing patients with recurrent colorectal cancer. In one study, the sensitivity was 88%, specificity was 80%, PPV was 98%, NPV was 42%, and accuracy was 87%. For CT, the sensitivity was 63%, specificity was 10%, PPV was 85%, NPV was 3%, and accuracy was 57%. While DHC (18) F-FDG did not achieve the sensitivity and specificity of PET, it can be considered an adequate readily available technique for assessing recurrent colorectal cancer (208).

Conclusion

Insufficient data are currently available to support the recommendation that F-18 FDG PET should be routinely used in the initial staging of colorectal cancer. PET can provide excellent results for detecting metastases in the liver (Figs. 28 and 29). However, for assessing recurrent colorectal cancer, F-18 FDG PET has been found to be more accurate than CT, MR, or serial CEA level determinations. It can be successfully used to determine resectability of recurrent disease and to monitor the success of treatment.

NUCLEAR STUDIES FOR BLEEDING

Hemorrhage from the lower GI tract occurs in a variety of conditions, most commonly colonic diverticulosis, angiodysplasia of the bowel wall, ischemia, and neoplasms, both benign and malignant. While endoscopy routinely identifies the source of upper GI hemorrhage, it is of lesser value during active colonic bleeding. The source of bleeding in these cases may be

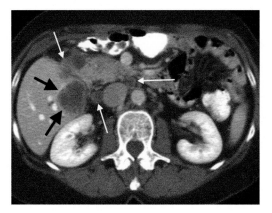

Figure 29 Computed tomography in the same patient as in Figure 24 demonstrates one of the two liver metastases (*black arrows*) and perihepatic and retroperitoneal l adenopathy (*white arrows*).

localized using nuclear medicine techniques or catheter angiography. Usual practice is to perform a nuclear medicine bleeding scan as a road map for definitive intervention, whether by surgery or transcatheter angioembolization.

Scintigraphic Technique

The choice of radiotracer for use in GI bleeding studies will usually be based on local practice. Red blood cells or sulfur colloid labeled with technicium-99-m may be used. Tc-99-m is used to label autologous red blood cells in a whole-blood specimen. Once the radiolabeled red blood cells have been reinjected into the patient, imaging commences using a large field-of-view gamma camera with the abdomen and pelvis in view, obtaining flow images as 60 one-second frames followed by 60 to 90 one-minute static frames. When no active bleeding is demonstrated, further images may be acquired in two to four hours, or anytime within 24 hours of tracer injection when there is clinical evidence of acute hemorrhage.

Alternatively, Tc-99-m–labeled sulfur colloid may be chosen as the radiotracer. After injection, the agent is cleared from the bloodstream by the reticuloendothelial system causing the disappearance of activity from the vascular system. During GI bleeding, however, activity accumulates within the bowel lumen. Flow images are obtained as one-second frames for one minute following injection, and subsequent static images are acquired every one to two minutes for twenty minutes.

Tc-labeled red blood cells offer the advantage of optional repeat imaging up to 24 hours after the initial injection. Misinterpretation of normal variants, the presence of free Tc-99m pertechnetate, or misinterpretation of delayed images are potential disadvantages (209). Tc-labeled sulfur colloid offers the advantage of shorter imaging time and high target-to-background ratios. However, Tc-labeled sulfur colloid can detect bleeding only during the relatively brief imaging period. High levels of activity accumulated in the liver and spleen may complicate diagnosis of bleeding at hepatic and splenic flexures. Studies defending the superiority of either technique abound (210,211).

Image Interpretation

Extravasation of radiolabeled red blood cells or sulfur colloid into the bowel is detected as radiotracer activity conforming to the bowel lumen. Bleeding rates as low as 0.1 mL/min can be detected, whereas detection by conventional angiography requires bleeding rates 5 to 10 times higher. Initial flow images provide a nuclear angiogram. Subsequent static images may be viewed in cinematic fashion. Abnormal activity within the bowel lumen, accumulating over time and passing through the gut, is the usual scintigraphic finding of GI hemorrhage (Fig. 30). Noting where the activity first appears in the lumen and the course it takes as it is conducted along the intestinal tract localizes the source of bleeding.

Using these techniques, identification of the locus of bleeding yields crucial diagnostic information for patient therapy. When a site of hemorrhage can be demonstrated, the patient may be spared total or subtotal colectomy in favor of segmental resection (212) or superselective transcatheter angioembolization (213) where appropriate.

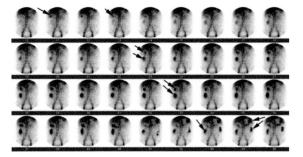

Figure 30 Patient with dark stools and low hematocrit. Abnormal activity within the large bowel lumen is the usual scintigraphic finding of a colonic hemorrhage. Increased activity (*arrows*) is first seen at the hepatic flexure, then accumulates over time in the right colon and eventually fills most of the large bowel. *Source*: Courtesy of Dr. Robert Lull, SFGH Nuclear Medicine Services University of California–San Francisco, San Francisco, California, U.S.A.

ANGIOGRAPHY AND TRANSCATHETER TECHNIQUES FOR GI BLEEDING

The role of catheter angiography has evolved in recent years to include both diagnosis and therapy in the setting of GI bleeding. Most often, GI bleeding is diagnosed and localized to either the upper or lower GI tract on the basis of other tests such as nasogastric aspiration, endoscopic visualization, or nuclear medicine bleeding scans. Often colorectal surgeons are unwilling to perform a segmental colonic resection based solely on a Tc-labeled red blood cells scan because of fear of false-positive results. Colonoscopic or angiographic localization of the bleeding site can then be followed by either transcatheter coil embolization or vasopressin infusion.

Coil embolization is performed after superselective catheterization of the bleeding vessel. This method is preferred for angiographic control of upper GI tract bleeding, where abundant collateral circulation significantly decreases the likelihood of ischemic injury to bowel distal to the embolization.

There is growing evidence in the literature that superselective microcoil embolization for colonic hemorrhage is an effective and well-tolerated procedure (Figs. 31A and B) (214). The risk for ischemic damage to the colon is approximately 10% when embolization is proximal to the mesenteric border of the colon (215). Subselection and embolization of distal arteries smaller than 1 mm appears to minimize this risk.

Many experts still advocate transcatheter vasopressin infusion for treatment of lower GI bleeding. Such therapy can be administered by catheters placed in the main trunk of the SMA orIMA, significantly diminishing technical difficulty (Figs. 32A and B).

Finally, in those patients who are candidates for immediate surgical therapy, a 3 Fr catheter placed into the bleeding vessel can serve as a useful surgical marker. At surgery, methylene blue injection into the catheter can delineate the area of bowel for resection (216).

(A)   **(B)**

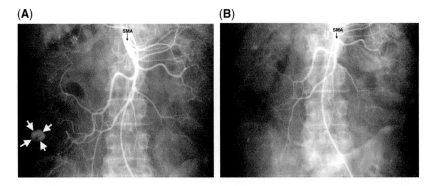

Figure 31   (**A**) This angiogram with selective injection of the SMA demonstrates a bleeding diverticulum (*arrows*) in the right colon. (**B**) Same patient as in (**A**). Following embolization of the distal artery that fed the diverticulum, extravasation of contrast material is no longer seen. *Abbreviation*: SMA, superior mesenteric artery. *Source*: Courtesy of Dr. Ernie Ring, University of California–San Francisco, San Francisco, California, U.S.A.

(A) **(B)**

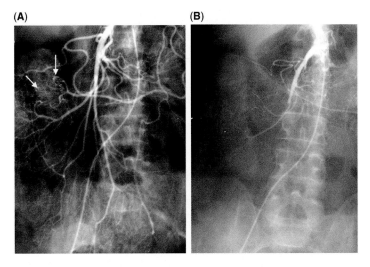

Figure 32 (**A**) Selective catheterization of the superior mesenteric artery (SMA) for lower gastrointestinal bleeding shows small telangiectasias (*arrows*) near the hepatic flexure. (**B**) Following excessive transfusion of the SMA with vasopressin, only the most proximal branches are filled. *Source:* Courtesy of Dr. Ernie Ring, University of California–San Francisco, San Francisco, California, U.S.A.

SUMMARY

When faced with an abdominal diagnostic challenge, plain films may be initially obtained if an obstruction, ileus, or perforation is suspected. In some instances, depending on the clinical history and laboratory tests, CT is the next best diagnostic procedure. However, in many cases, CT is the initial imaging method. especially in patients with suspected obstruction, inflammatory diseases of the bowel, or abscess formation. It is the primary method for assessing ischemia of the colon and its extent. CT has the advantages of being universally available and acquiring images in a very short time. It also can provide images of superb resolution and state-of-the-art scanners permit reconstruction in multiple planes that can be helpful in delineating the anatomy, particularly for staging of tumors. A CT angiogram with 3-D reconstruction can obviate the need for an invasive conventional angiogram. In trauma cases, it can provide a road map for embolization and quick assessment of blunt or invasive injuries to the colon.

In neoplastic disease, CT is helpful in patients with suspected advanced disease and metastases to distant sites. However, for local disease within the bowel wall, EUS provides superior results because CT, similar to MR, cannot visualize the various layers of the bowel wall. MR can provide information on extension into bone or muscle, and with an endorectal coil may improve staging of low rectal cancers where a decision on local resection versus extensive surgery needs to be made. In most cases, results with MR and CT for the colon are similar but MR examinations are longer and some patients may experience claustrophobia. For functional abnormalities, for reduction of intussusception, and in screening for polyps and cancer, the double-contrast barium enema still has a role. Its low cost makes it a viable alternative to colonoscopy in our cost-conscious health environment. The role of screening for polyps and cancer may be replaced by CTC in the future but not enough data are currently available to reach any definitive conclusions. For optimal staging of colorectal tumors, particularly for recurrent colorectal tumors, PET is the emerging technique that, in combination with CT, permits full assessment of primary site or scar versus recurrence as well as metastases to nodes and other local or distant sites. Scintigraphy is occasionally used in patients with an unknown source of bleeding.

REFERENCES

1. Schuele A. Ueber die sondierung und radiographie des dickdarms. Arch Verdauungskr 1904; 10:111.
2. Haenisch GF. The roentgen examination of the large intestine. Arrch Roentgen Ray 1912; 17:208.

3. Pickhardt PJ. The colon cutoff sign. Radiology 2000; 215:387–389.

4. Feldman D. The coffee bean sign. Radiology 2000; 216:178–179.

5. Levine CD. Toxic megacolon: diagnosis and treatment challenges. AACN Clin Issues 1999; 10: 492–429.

6. Stanley RJ, Melson GL, Tedesco FJ, Saylor JL. Plain-film findings in severe pseudomembranous colitis. Radiology 1976; 118:7–11.

7. Vaudagna S, McCort JJ. Plain film diagnosis of retrocecal appendicitis. Radiology 1975; 117:533–536.

8. Thoeni RF, Margulis AR. The current state of radiologic technique in the examination of the colon: a survey. Radiology 1978; 127:317–323.

9. Margulis AR, Thoeni RF. The present status of the radiologic examination of the colon. Radiology 1988; 167:1–5.

10. Glick S, Wagner JL, Johnson CD. Cost-effectiveness of double-contrast barium enema in screening for colorectal cancer. Am J Roentgenol 1998; 170:629–636.

11. Gelfand DW, Chen MYM, Ott DJ. Preparing the colon for the barium enema examination. Radiology 1991; 178:609–613.

12. Thoeni RF, Vandeman F, Wall S. The effect of glucagon on diagnostic accuracy of double-contrast barium enema examinations. Am J Roentgenol 1984; 142:111–114.

13. Miller RE, Chernish SM, Skucas J, Rosenak BD, Rodda BE. Hypotonic colon examination with glucagon. Radiology. 1974; 113:555–562.

14. Simpkins KC. Radiology now. the colon pacified. Br J Radiol 1976; 49:303–305.

15. Harned RK, Williams SM, Maglinte DD, Hayes JM, Paustian FF, Consigny PM. Clinical application of in vitro studies for barium-enema examination following colorectal biopsy. Radiology 1985; 154:319–321.

16. Harned RK, Consigny PM, Cooper NB, Williams SM, Woltjen AJ. Barium enema examination following biopsy of the rectum or colon. Radiology 1982; 145:11–16.

17. Maglinte DD, Strong RC, Strate RW, et al. Barium enema after colorectal biopsies: experimental data. Am J Roentgenol 1982; 139:693–697.

18. Miller RC, Maglinte DD. Barium Pneumocolon: technologist–performed "7 pump" method. Am J Roentgenol 1982; 139:1230–1232.

19. Wexner SD, Daly TH. The initial management of left lower quadrant peritonitis. Dis Colon Rectum 1986; 29:635–638.

20. Goldstein HM, Miller RH. Air contrast colon examination in patients with colostomies. AJR 1976; 127:607–610.

21. Ong NT, Beasley SW. The leadpoint in intussusception. J Pediatr Surg 1990; 25:640–643.

22. Humphrey A, Ein SH, Mok PM. Perforation of the intussuscepted colon. Am J Roentgenol 1981; 137:1135–1138.

23. Shiels WE 2nd, Maves CK, Hedlund GL, Kirks DR. Air enema for diagnosis and reduction of intussusception: clinical experience and pressure correlates. Radiology 1991; 181:169–172.

24. Palder S, Ein SH, Stringer DA, Alton D. Intussusception: barium or air? J Pediatr Surg 1991; 26: 271–274.

25. Ein SH, Shandling B, Reilly BJ, Stringer DA. Hypostatic reduction of intussusceptions caused by lead points. J Pediatr Surg 1986; 21:883–886.

26. Thoeni RF, Petras A. Double–contrast barium enema examination and endoscopy in the detection of polypoid lesion in the cecum and ascending colon. Radiology 1982; 144:257–260.

27. Morris Tl, Tudor RG. The management of inflammatory complications of colonic diverticular disease. Br J Hosp Med 1987; 37:36–41.

28. Pradel JA, Adell JF, P Taourel P, Djafari M, Monnin–Delhom E, Bruel JM. Acute colonic diverticulitis: prospective comparative evaluation with US and CT. Radiology 1997; 205:503–512.

29. Rao PM, Rhea JT, Novelline RA, Dobbins JM, Lawrason JN, Sacknoff R, Stuk JL. Helical CT with only contrast material of diagnosing diverticulitis: prospective evaluation of 150 patients. ATR 1998; 170:1445–1449.

30. Kircher MF, Rhea JT, Kihiczak D, Novelline RA. Frequency, sensitivity, and specificity of individual signs of diverticulitis on thin–section helical CT with colonic contrast material: experience with 312 cases. AJR 2002; 178:1313–1318.

31. Balthazar EJ. Appendicitis: prospective evaluation with high–resolution CT. Radiology 1991; 180: 21–24.

32. Rao PM, Rhea JT, Novelline RA, Mostafavi AA, Lawrason JN, McCabe CJ. Helical CT combined with contrast material administered only through the colon for imaging of suspected appendicitis. Am J Roentgenol 1997; 169:1275–1280.

33. Raman SS, Lu DSK, Kadell BM, Vodopich DJ, Sayre J, Cryer H. Accuracy of nonfocused helical CT for the diagnosis of acute appendicitis: a 5-year review. Am J Roentgenol 2002; 178:1319–1325.

34. Ritchie JK. Results of surgery for inflammatory bowel disease, a further survey of one hospital region. Br Med J 1974; 1:264–268.

35. Fraser GM, Findlay JN. The double contrast enema inulcerative Crohn's colitis. Clin Radiol 1976; 27:103–112.

36. Lichtenstein JE, Madewell JE, Feigin DS. The collar button ulcer. Gastrointest Radiol 1979; 4:79–84.

37. Bartram CI, Walmsley K. A radiological and pathological correlation of the mucosal changes in ulcerative colitis. Clin Radiol 1978; 29:323–328.
38. Buck JL, Dachman AH, Sobin LH. Polypoid and pseudopolypoid manifestations of inflammatory bowel disease. Radiographics 1991; 11:293–304.
39. Hammerman AM, Shatz BA, Sussman N. Radiographic characteristics of colonic "mucosal bridges," sequelae of inflammatory bowel disease. Radiology 1978; 127:611–614.
40. Zegel H, Laufer L. Filiform polyposis. Radiology 1978; 127:615–619.
41. Hunt RH, Teague RH, Swarbrick ET, Williams CB. Colonoscopy in management of colonic strictures. Br Med J 1975; 3:360–361.
42. Urso FP, Urso MI, Lee CM. The cathartic colon: pathological findings and radiological–pathological correlation. Radiology 1975; 116:557–559.
43. Butt JH, Lennard-Jones JE, Ritchie JK. A practical approach to the risk of cancer in inflammatory bowel disease. Reassure, watch, or act? Med Clin North Am 1980; 64:1203–1220.
44. Rosenstock E, Farmer RG, Petras R, Sivak MV Jr., Rankin GB, Sullivan BH. Surveillance for colonic carcinoma in ulcerative colitis. Gastroenterology 1985; 89:1342–1346.
45. Cook MG, Path MRC, Goligher JC. Carcinoma and epithelial dysplasia complicating ulcerative colitis. Gastroenterology 1975; 68:1127–1136.
46. Hillard AE, Mann FA, Becker JM, Nelson JA. The ileoanal J pouch: radiographic evaluation. Radiology 1985; 155:591–594.
47. Thoeni RF, Fell SC, Engelstad D, Schrock TB. Ileoanal pouches: comparison of CT, scintigraphy and contrast enemas for diagnosing postsurgical complications. Am J Roentgenol 1990; 154:73–78.
48. Thoeni RF. Idiopathic inflammatory disease of the large and small bowel. In: Stevenson G, Freeny P, eds. Alimentary Tract Radiology. 5th ed. St. Louis Missouri: C.V Mosby Co, 1994:564–626.
49. Pringot J, Goncette L, Van Heuverzwyn R, Bodart P. The features of granulomatous colitis in double contrast radiography. J Belge Radiol 1977; 60:25–35.
50. Laufer I, Hamilton JD. The radiologic differentiation between ulcerative and granulomatous colitis by double contrast radiology. Am J Gastroenterol 1976; 66:259–269.
51. Korelitz BI, Sommers SC. Differential diagnosis of ulcerative and granulomatous colitis by sigmoidoscopy, rectal biopsy and cell counts of rectal mucosa. Am J Gastroenterol 1974; 61:460–469.
52. Hildell J, Lindstrom C, Wenckert A. Radiographic appearances in Crohn's disease. III. Colonic lesions following surgery. Acta Radiol Diagn 1980; 21:71–78.
53. Hamilton SR. Colorectal carcinoma in patients with Crohn's disease. Gastroenterology 1985; 89:398–407.
54. Rubesin SE, Levine MS, Glick SN, Herlinger H, Laufer I. Pseudomembranous colitis with rectosigmoid sparing on barium studies. Radiology 1989; 170:811–813.
55. Trudel JL, Deschenes M, Mayrand S, Barkun AN. Toxic megacolon complicating pseudomembranous enterocolitis. Dis Colon Rectum 1995; 38:1033–1038.
56. Han JK, Kim SH, Choi BI, Yeon KM, Han MC. Tuberculous colitis. Findings at double–contrast barium enema examination. Dis Colon Rectum 1996; 39:1204–1209.
57. Matsui T, Iida M, Tada S, Fuchigami T, Iwashita A, Sakamoto K, Fujishima M. The value of double-contrast barium enema in amebic colitis. Gastrointest Radiol 1989; 14:73–78.
58. Balthazar EJ, Megibow AJ, Fazzini E, Opulencia JF, Engel I. Cytomegalovirus colitis in AIDS: radiographic findings in 11 patients. Radiology 1985; 155:585–588.
59. Abramson SJ, Berdon WE, Baker DH. Childhood typhlitis: its increasing association with acute myelogenous leukemia. Report of five cases. Radiology 1983; 146:61–64.
60. Del Fava RL, Cronin TG Jr. Typhlitis complicating leukemia in an adult: barium enema findings. Am J Roentgenol 1977; 129:347–348.
61. Wittenberg J, Athanasoulis CA, Williams LF Jr., Paredes S, O'Sullivan P, Brown B. Ischemic colitis. radiology and pathophysiology. Am J Roentgenol 1975; 123:287–300.
62. Reeders JW, Tytgat GN. Ischemic colitis: serial changes in double–contrast barium enema examination. Radiology 1987; 162:583.
63. Iida M, Matsui T, Fuchigami T, Iwashita A, Yao T, Fujishima M. Ischemic colitis: serial changes in double-contrast barium enema examination. Radiology 1986; 159:337–341.
64. Rubesin SE, Sul Sh, Laufer I. Carpet lesions of the colon. Radiographics 1985; 5:537–552.
65. Fischel RE, Dermer R. Multifocal carcinoma of the large intestine. Clin Rad 1975; 26:495–498.
66. Law RL, Longstaff AJ, Slack N. A retrospective 5-year study on the accuracy of the barium enema examination performed by radiographers. Clin Radiol 1999; 54:80–83.
67. Hough DM, Malone DE, Rawlinson J, et al. Colon cancer detection: an algorithm using endoscopy and barium enema. Clin Radiol 1994; 49:170–175.
68. Strom E, Larsen JL. Colon cancer at barium enema examination and colonoscopy: a study from the county of Hordaland, Norway. Radiology 1999; 211:211–214.
69. Wexner SD, Forde KA, Sellers G, et al. How well do surgeons perform colonoscopy? Surg Endosc 1998; 12:1410–1414.
70. Wexner SD, Garbus J, Singh JJ. SAGES Colonoscopy Outcomes Study Group. A prospective analysis of 13, 580 colonoscopies: reevaluation of credentialing guidelines. Surg Endosc 2001; 15:251–261.

71. Chong A, Shah JN, Levine MS, et al. Diagnostic yield of barium enema examination after incomplete colonoscopy. Radiology 2002; 223:620–624.
72. Gelfand DW, Chen MY, Ott DJ. Benign colorectal neoplasms undetected by colonoscopy. Gastrointest Radiol 1992; 17:344–346.
73. McMahon PM, Bosch JL, Gleason S, Halpern EF, Lester JS, Gazelle GS. Cost–effectiveness of colorectal cancer screening. Radiology ; 219:44–50.
74. Mahieu PHG. Defecography. In: Margulis AR, Burhenne HJ, eds. Alimentary Tract Radiology. 4th ed. St. Louis, MO: CV Mosby, 1989:933–941.
75. Agachan F, Pfeifer J, Wexner SD. Defecography and proctography: results of 744 patients. Dis Colon Rectum 1996; 39:899–905.
76. Jorge JMN, Ger GC, Gonzalez L, Wexner SD. Patient positioning during cinedefecography. Influence on perineal descent and other measurements. Dis Colon Rectum 1994; 37:927–931.
77. Jorge JMN, Habr–Gama A, Wexner SD. Clinical applications and techniques of cindefecography. Am J Surg 2001; 182:93–101.
78. Matsuoka H, Wexner SD, Desai MB, et al. A comparison between dynamic pelvic MRI and video-proctography in patients with constipation. Dis Colon Rectum 2001; 44:571–576.
79. Moreira H Jr., Wexner SD. Anorectal physiology testing. In: Beck DE, Wexner SD, eds. Fundamentals of Anorectal Surgery. 2nd ed. London: WB Saunders, 1998:37–53.
80. Pfeifer J, Oliveira L, Park UC, Gonzalez AR, Agachan F, Wexner SD. Are interpretations of video defecographies reliable and reproducible? Int J Colorectal Dis 1997; 12:67–72.
81. Takao Y, Okano H, Gilliland R, Wexner SD. Cindefecographic evidence of difficult evacuation in constipated patients with complex symptoms. Int J Colorectal Dis 2000; 14:291–296.
82. Wexner SD, Gilliland R. Setting up a colorectal physiology laboratory. In: Corman M, ed. Colon and Rectal Surgery. 4th ed. Philadelphia: Lippincott–Raven, 1998:106–140.
83. Wexner SD, Jorge JMN. Defecography. Sem Colon Rectal Surg 2002; 13:176–186.
84. Wiersma TjG, Mulder CJJ, Reeders JWAJ. Dynamic rectal examination: its significant clinical value. Endoscopy 1997; 29:462–471.
85. Ho LM, Low VHS, Freed KS. Vaginal opacification during defecography: utility of placing a folded gauze square at the introitus. Abdomin Imag 1999; 24:562–564.
86. Harvey CJ, Halligan S, Bartran CI, Hollings N, Sahdev A, Kingston K. Evacuation proctography: a prospective study of diagnostic and therapeutic effects. Radiology 1999; 211:223–227.
87. Thoeni RF, Filson RG. Abdominal and pelvic CT: use of oral metoclopramide to enhance bowel opacification in abdominal and pelvic CT examinations. Radiology 1988; 169:391–393.
88. Turetschek K, Schober E, Wunderbaldinger P, et al. Findings at helical ct–enteroclysis in symptomatic patients with Crohn's disease: correlation with endoscopic and surgical findings. J Comput Assist Tomogr 2002; 26:488–492.
89. Gore RM, Marn CS, Kirby DF, Vogelzang RL, Neiman HL. CT findings in ulcerative, granulomatous, and indeterminate colitis. Am J Roentgenol 1984; 143:279–784.
90. Raptopoulos V, Schwartz RK, McNicholas MM, Movson J, Pearlman J, Joffe N. Multiplanar helical CT enterography in patients with Crohn's disease. Am J Roentgenol 1997; 169:1545–1550.
91. Del Campo L, Arribas I, Valbuena M, Mate J, Moreno-Otero R. Spiral CT findings in active and remission phases in patients with Crohn's disease. J Comput Assist Tomogr 2001; 25:792–797.
92. Horton KM, Corl FM, Fishman EK. CT of nonneoplastic diseases of the small bowel: spectrum of disease. J Comput Assist Tomogr 1999; 23:417–428.
93. Philpotts LE, Heiken JP, Westcott MA, Gore RM. Colitis: use of CT findings in differential diagnosis. Radiology 1994; 190:445–449.
94. Jacobs JE, Birnbaum BA. CT of inflammatory disease of the colon. Semin Ultrasound CT MR 1995; 16:91–101.
95. Carucci LR, Levine MS. Radiographic imaging of inflammatory bowel disease. Gastroenterol Clin North Am 2002; 31:93–117.
96. Stollman NH, Raskin JB. Related articles, links no abstract diagnosis and management of diverticular disease of the colon in adults. Ad Hoc Practice Parameters Committee of the American College of Gastroenterology. Am J Gastroenterol 199; 94:3110–3121.
97. Ambrosetti P, Becker C, Terrier F. Colonic diverticulitis: impact of imaging on surgical management—a prospective study of 542 patients. Eur Radiol 2002; 12:1145–1149.
98. Birnbaum BA, Wilson SR. Appendicitis at the millennium. Radiology 2000; 215:337–348.
99. Son HJ, Lee SJ, Lee JH, et al. Clinical diagnosis of primary epiploic appendagitis: differentiation from acute diverticulitis. J Clin Gastroenterol 2002; 34:435–438.
100. Rao PM, Rhea JT, Novelline RA. CT signs of appendicitis: sensitivity, specificity and diagnostic value. J Comput Assist Tomogr 1997; 21:686–692.
101. Lane MJ, Liu DM, Huynh MD, Jeffrey RB Jr., Mindelzun RE, Katz DS. Suspected acute appendicitis: nonenhanced helical CT in 300 consecutive patients. Radiology 1999; 213:341–346.
102. Rhea JT, Halpern EF, Ptak T, Lawrason JN, Sacknoff R, Novelline RA. The status of appendiceal CT in an urban medical center 5 years its introduction: experience with 753 patients. AJR 2005; 184:1802–1808.
103. Jill E. Jacobs, Bernard A. Birnbaum, Michael Macari, et al. Acute Appendicitis: comparison of helical ct diagnosis-focused technique with oral contrast material versus nonfocused technique with oral and intravenous contrast material. Radiology 2001; 220:683–690.

104. Kaiser S, Frenckner B, Jorulf HK. Suspected appendicitis in children: US and CT—a prospective randomized study. Radiology 2002; 223:633–638.
105. Applegate KE, Sivit CJ, Salvator AE, et al. Effect of cross-sectional imaging on negative appendectomy and perforation rates in children. Radiology 2001; 220:103–107.
106. Horton KM, Corl FM, Fishman EK. CT evaluation of the colon: inflammatory disease. Radiographics 2000; 20:399–418.
107. Fishman EK, Kavuru M, Jones B, et al. Pseudomembranous colitis: CT evaluation of 26 cases. Radiology 1991; 180:57–60.
108. Boland GW, Lee MJ, Cats AM, Ferraro MJ, Matthia AR, Mueller PR. Clostridium difficile colitis: correlation of CT findings with severity of clinical disease. Clin Radiol. 1995; 50:153–156.
109. Kawamoto S, Horton KM, Fishman EK. Pseudomembranous colitis: spectrum of imaging findings with clinical and pathologic correlation. Radiographics 1999; 19:887–897.
110. Kirkpatrick ID, Greenberg HM. Evaluating the CT diagnosis of *Clostridium difficile* colitis: should CT guide therapy? Am J Roentgenol 2001; 176:635–639.
111. Knollmann FD, Grunewald T, Adler A, et al. Intestinal disease in acquired immunodeficiency: evaluation by CT. Eur Radiol 1997; 7:1419–1429.
112. Frick MP, Maile CW, Crass JR, Goldberg ME, Delaney JP. Computed tomography of neutropenic colitis. AJR Am J Roentgenol 1984; 143:763–765.
113. Wu CM, Davis F, Fishman EK. Radiologic evaluation of the acute abdomen in the patient with acquired immunodeficiency syndrome (AIDS): the role of CT scanning. Semin Ultrasound CT MR 1998; 19:190–199.
114. Bradbury MS, Kavanagh PV, Chen MY, Weber TM, Bechtold RE. Noninvasive assessment of portomesenteric venous thrombosis: current concepts and imaging strategies. J Comput Assist Tomogr 2002; 26:392–404.
115. Endean ED, Barnes SL, Kwolek CJ, Minion DJ, Schwarcz TH, Mentzer RM Jr. Surgical management of thrombotic acute intestinal ischemia. Ann Surg 2001; 233:801–808.
116. Zalcman M, Sy M, Donckier V, Closset J, Gansbeke DV. Helical CT signs in the diagnosis of intestinal ischemia in small-bowel obstruction. Am J Roentgenol 2000; 175:1601–1607.
117. Taourel PG, Deneuville M, Pradel JA, Regent D, Bruel JM. Acute mesenteric ischemia: diagnosis with contrast-enhanced CT. Radiology 1996; 199:632–636.
118. Wiesner W, Mortele KJ, Glickman JN, Ji H, Ros PR. Pneumatosis intestinalis and portomesenteric venous gas in intestinal ischemia: correlation of CT findings with severity of ischemia and clinical outcome. Am J Roentgenol 2001; 177:1319–1323.
119. Maher MM, Tonra BM, Malone DE, Gibney RG. Portal venous gas: detection by gray–scale and Doppler sonography in the absence of correlative findings on computed tomography. Abdom Imaging 2001; 26:390–394.
120. Balthazar EJ, Liebeskind ME, Macari M. Intestinal ischemia in patients in whom small bowel obstruction is suspected: evaluation of accuracy, limitations, and clinical implications of CT in diagnosis. Radiology 1997; 205:519–522.
121. Balthazar EJ, Yen BC, Gordon RB. Ischemic colitis: CT evaluation of 54 cases. Radiology 1999; 211:381–388.
122. Ko GY, Ha HK, Lee HJ, et al. Usefulness of CT in patients with ischemic colitis proximal to colonic cancer. Am J Roentgenol 1997; 168:951–956.
123. Whittick WF, Viamonte M Jr. Splenic hematoma causing colonic obstruction. Am J Roentgenol 1994; 163:224.
124. Frager D, Rovno HD, Baer JW, Bashist B, Friedman M. Prospective evaluation of colonic obstruction with computed tomography. Abdom Imaging 1998; 23:141–146.
125. Winawer S, Fletcher R, Rex D, et al. Colorectal cancer screening and surveillance: clinical guidelines and rationale-update based on new evidence. Gastroenterology 2003; 124(2):544–560.
126. Thoeni RF, Moss AA, Schnyder P, et al. Detection and staging of primary rectal and rectosigmoid cancer by computed tomography. Radiology 1981; 141:135–138.
127. Lee KT, Stanley RJ, Sagel SS, et al. Accuracy of CT in detecting intra-abdominal and pelvic lymph node metastases from pelvic cancers. AJR 1978;131:675–679.
128. Zaunbauer W, Haertel M, Fuchs WA. Computed tomography in carcinoma of the rectum. Gastrointest Radiol 1981; 6:79–84.
129. Dixon AK, Fry IK, Morson BC, et al. Preoperative computed tomography of carcinoma of the rectum. Br J Radiol 1981; 54:655–659.
130. Grabbe E, Lierse W, Winkler R. The perirectal fascia: morphology and use in staging of rectal carcinoma. Radiology 1983; 149:241–246.
131. Van Waes PF, Koehler PR, Feldberg MA. Management of rectal carcinoma: impact of computed tomography. Am J Roentgenol 1983; 140:1137–1142.
132. Cohan RH, Silverman PM, THompson WM, et al. Computed tomography of epithelial neoplasms of the anal canal. Am J Roentgenol 1985; 145:569–573.
133. Adalsteinsson B, Gimelius B, Graffman S, et al. Computed tomography in staging rectal carcinoma. Acta Radiol Diagn 1985; 26:45–50.
134. Freeny PC, Marks WM, Ryan JA, et al. Colorectal carcinoma evaluation with CT: preoperative staging and detection of postoperative recurrence. Radiology 1986; 158:347–353.

135. Thompson WM, Halvorsen RA, Foster WL, et al. Preoperative and postoperative CT staging of rectosigmoid carcinoma. Am J Roentgenol 1986; 146:703–710.

136. Holdsworth PJ, Johnston D, Chalmers AG, et al. Endoluminal ultrasound and computed tomography in the staging of rectal cancer. Br J Surg 1988; 75:1019–1022.

137. Balthazar EJ, Megibow AJ, Hulnick D, et al. Carcinoma of the colon: detection and preoperative staging by CT. AJR 1988; 150:301–306.

138. Rifkin MD, Ehrlich SM, Marks G. Staging of rectal carcinoma: prospective comparison of endorectal US and CT. Radiology 1989; 170:319–322.

139. Gazelle GS, Saini, S, Shellito P. Staging of colon carcinoma using water enemas CT. J Comput Assist Tomogr 1995; 19:87–91.

140. Matsuoka H, Nakamura A, Masaki T, et al. Preoperative staging by multidetector-row computed tomography in patients with rectal carcinoma. Am J Surg 2002; 184:131–1315.

141. Ng CS, Doyle TC, Pinto EM, et al. Caecal carcinomas in the elderly: useful signs in minimal preparation CT. Clin Radiol 2002; 57:359–364.

142. Buhler H, Seefeld U, Dehyle P, et al. Endoscopic follow–up after colorectal cancer surgery. Cancer 1984; 54:791–793.

143. Butch RJ, Wittenberg J, Mueller PR, et al. Presacral masses after abdominoperineal resection for colorectal carcinoma: the need for needle biopsy. Am J Roentgenol 1985; 144:309–312.

144. Nauta R, Stablein D, Holyoke D. Survival of patients with stage B2 colon carcinoma: the gastrointestinal tumor study group experience. Arch Surg 1989; 124:180–182.

145. Olson RM, Perencevich P, Malcolm AW, et al. Patterns of recurrence following curative resection of adenocarcinoma of the colon and rectum. Cancer 1980; 45:2969–2974.

146. Cass AW, Million RR, Pfaff W. Patterns of recurrence following surgery alone for adenocarcinoma of the colon and rectum. Cancer 1976; 37:1861–1865.

147. Kelvin FM, Korobkin M, Heaston DK, et al. The pelvis after surgery for rectal carcinoma: serial CT observations with emphasis on nonneoplastic features. Am J Roentgenol 1983; 141:959–964.

148. Reznek RH, White FE, Young JW, et al. The appearances on computed tomography after abdomino-perineal resection for carcinoma of the rectum: a comparison between the normal appearances and those of recurrence. Br J Radiol 1983; 56:237–240.

149. Koelbel G, Schmiedl U, Majer MC, et al. Diagnosis of fistulae and sinus tracts in patients with Crohn's disease: value of MR imaging. Am J Roentgenol 1989; 152:999–1003.

150. Schnall MD, Furth EE, Rosato EF, Kressel HY. Rectal tumor stage: correlation of endorectal MR imaging and pathologic findings. Radiology 1994; 190:709–714.

151. Thoeni RF, Moss AA. The gastrointestinal tract. In: Moss AA, Gamsu G, Genant H, eds. Computed Tomography of the Body. Philadelphia: WB Saunders, 1992:643–734.

152. Kelvin FM, Korobkin M, Breiman RS, et al. Recurrent rectal carcinoma in an asymptomatic patient. J Comput Assist Tomogr 1982; 6:186–188.

153. Husband JE, Hodson NJ, Parsons CA. The use of computed tomography in recurrent rectal tumors. Radiology 1980; 134:677–682.

154. Ellert J, Kreel L. The value of CT in malignant colonic tumors. J Comput Tomogr 1980; 4:225–240.

155. Moss AA, Thoeni RF, Schnyder P, et al. Value of computed tomography in the detection and staging of recurrent rectal carcinomas. J Comput Assist Tomogr 1981; 5:870–874.

156. Adalsteinsson B, Glimelius B, Graffman S, et al. Computed tomography of recurrent renal carcinoma. Acta Radiol Diagn 1981; 22:669–672.

157. Bachmann G, Pfeifer T, Bauer T. (MRT and dynamic CT in the diagnosis of a recurrence of rectal carcinoma). Rofo. Fortschritte auf dem gebiete der Rontgenstrahlen und der Neuen. Bildgebenden Verfahren 1994; 161:214–219.

158. Chen YM, Ott DJ, Wolfman N. Recurrent colorectal carcinoma evaluation with barium enema examination and CT. Radiology 1987; 163:307–310.

159. Barkin JS, Cohen ME, Flaxman M, et al. Value of routine follow-up endoscopy program for the detection of recurrent colorectal carcinoma. Am J Gastroenterol 1984; 88:1355–1360.

160. Stulc JP, Petrelli NJ, Herrera L, et al. Anastomotic recurrence of adenocarcinoma of the colon. Arch Surg 1986; 121:1077–1080.

161. Meyenberger C, Wildi S, Külling D, et al. Tumor staging and follow-up care in rectosigmoid carcinoma: colonoscopic endosonography compared to CT, MRI and endorectal MRI. Rundschau Medizin Praxis 1996; 85:622–631.

162. Lomas DJ, Sood RR, Graves MJ, Miller R, Hall NR, Dixon AK. Colon carcinoma: MR imaging with CO2 enema—pilot study. Radiology 2001; 219:558–562.

163. Wallengren NO, Holtas S, Andren-Sandberg A, Jonsson E, Kristoffersson DT, McGill S. Rectal carcinoma: double-contrast MR imaging for preoperative staging. Radiology 2000; 215:108–114.

164. Dooms GC, Hricak H, Crooks LE, et al. Magnetic resonance imaging of the lymph nodes: comparison with CT. Radiology 1984; 153:710–738.

165. Butch RJ, Stark DD, Wittenberg J, et al. Staging rectal cancer by MR and CT. Am J Roentgenol 1986; 146:1155–1160.

166. Birnbaum BA, Weinreb JC, Fernandez MP, Brown JJ, Rofsky NM, Young SW. Comparison of contrast enhanced CT and Mn-DPDP enhanced MRI for detection of focal hepatic lesions. Initial findings. Clin Imaging 1994; 18:21–27.

167. Schwartz LH, Seltzer SE, Tempany CM, et al. Superparamagnetic iron oxide hepatic MR imaging: efficacy and safety using conventional and fast spin-echo pulse sequences. J Magn Reson Imaging 1995; 5:566–570.

168. Thaler W, Watzka S, Martin F, et al. Preoperative staging of rectal cancer by endoluminal ultrasound vs. magnetic resonance imaging. Preliminary results of a prospective, comparative study. Dis Colon Rectum 1994; 37:1189–1193.

169. Guinet C, Buy JN, Ghossain MA, et al. Comparison of magnetic resonance imaging and computed tomography in the preoperative staging of rectal cancer. Arch Surg 1990; 125:385–388.

170. de Lange EE, Gechner RE, Edge SB, et al. Preoperative staging of rectal carcinoma with MR imaging: surgical and histopathologic correlation. Radiology 1990; 176:623–628.

171. Zagoria RJ, Schlarb CA, Ott DJ, et al. Assessment of rectal tumor infiltration utilizing endorectal MR imaging and comparison with endoscopic rectal sonography. J Surg Oncol 1997; 64:312–317.

172. Torricelli P, Lo Russo S, Pecchi A, Luppi G, Cesinaro AM, Romagnoli R. Endorectal coil MRI in local staging of rectal cancer. Radiol Med (Torino) 2002; 103:74–83.

173. Blomqvist L, Holm T, Nyren S, Svanstrom R, Ulvskog Y, Iselius L. MR imaging and computed tomography in patients with rectal tumours clinically judged as locally advanced. Clin Radiol 2002; 57:211–218.

174. Blomqvist L, Machado M, Rubio C, et al. Rectal tumour staging: MR imaging using pelvic phased-array and endorectal coils vs. endoscopic ultrasonography. Eur Radiol 2000; 10:653–660.

175. Ebner F, Kressel HY, Mintz MC, et al. Tumor recurrence versus fibrosis in the female pelvis: differentiation with MR imaging at 1.5T. Radiology 1988; 166:333–340.

176. Rafto SE, Amendola MA, Gefter WB. MR imaging of recurrent colorectal carcinoma versus fibrosis. J Comput Assist Tomogr 1988; 12:521–523.

177. Johnson RH, Jenkins JPR, Isherwood I, et al. Quantitative magnetic resonance imaging in rectal carcinoma. Br J Radiol 1987; 60:761–764.

178. Gomberg JS, Friedman AC, Radecki PD. MRI differentiation of recurrent colorectal carcinoma from postoperative fibrosis. Gastrointest Radiol 1986; 11:361–363.

179. Glazer HS, Lee JKT, Levitt RG, et al. Radiation fibrosis: differentiation from recurrent tumor by MR imaging. Radiology 1985; 156:721–726.

180. Sugimura K, Carrington BM, Quivey JM, et al. Postirradiation changes in the pelvis: assessment with MR imaging. Radiology 1990; 175:805–813.

181. De Lange EE, Fechner RE, Wanebo HJ. Suspected recurrent rectosigmoid carcinoma after abdomino-perineal resection: MR imaging and histopathologic findings. Radiology 1989; 170:323–328.

182. Pegios W, Hunerbein M, Schroder R, et al. Comparison between endorectal MRI (EMRTI) and endorectal sonography (ES) after surgery or therapy for rectal tumors to exclude recurrent or residual tumor. Rofo Fortschr Geb Rontgenstr Neuen Bildgeb Verfahr 2002; 174:731–737.

183. Urban M, Rosen HR, Holbling N, et al. MR imaging for the preoperative planning of sphincter-saving surgery for tumors of the lower third of the rectum: use of intravenous and endorectal contrast materials. Radiology 2000; 214:503–508.

184. American Cancer Society. Cancer Facts and Figures, 2001. Last accessed May 29, 2001. Available from: http://www3.cancer.org/cancerinfo/

185. Glick SN, Ralls PW, Balfe DM, et al. Screening for colorectal cancer. ACR Appropriateness Criteria. Radiology 2000; 215(suppl):231–237.

186. Yee, J. CT colonography: examination prerequisites. Abdom Imaging 2002; 27:244–252.

187. Yee J, Hung RK, Steinauer-Gebauer AM, et. al. Colonic distention and prospective evaluation of colorectal polyp detection with and without glucagons during CT colonography [abstr]. Radiology 1999; 213(suppl):341.

188. McCollough CH. Optimization of multidetector array CT acquisition parameters for CT colonography. Abdom Imaging 2002; 27:253–259.

189. Johnson CD, Reed JE, et al. Reducing data size and radiation dose for CT colonography. Am J Roentgenol 1997; 168:1181–1184.

190. Dachman AH. Diagnostic performance of virtual colonoscopy. Abdom Imaging 2002; 27:260–267.

191. Yee J, Akerkar GA, Hung RK, Steinauer-Gebauer AM, Wall SD, McQuaid KR. Colorectal neoplasia: performance characteristics of CT colonography for detection in 300 patients. Radiology 2001; 219:685–692.

192. Marc S. Levine, Seth N. Glick, Stephen E. Rubesin, Laufer I. Double-contrast barium enema examination and colorectal cancer: a plea for radiologic screening. Radiology 2002; 222:313–315.

193. Luboldt W, Morrin MM. MR colonography: status and perspective. Abdom Imaging 2002; 27: 400–409.

194. Lauenstein TC, Goehde SC, Debatin JF. Fecal tagging: MR colonography without colonic cleansing. Abdom Imaging 2002; 27:410–417.

195. Tio TL, Coene PPL, Van Delden OM, et al. Colorectal carcinoma: preoperative TNM classification with endosonography. Radiology 1991; 179:165–170.

196. Herzog U, von Flue M, Tondelli P, et al. How accurate is endorectal ultrasound inthe pre-operative staging of rectal cancer? Dis Colon Rectum 1993; 36:127–134; Harewood GC, Wiersema MJ, Nelson H, et al. A prospective, blinded assessment of the impact of preoperative staging on the management of rectal cancer. Gastroenterology 2002; 123:24–32.

197. Harewood GC, Wiersma MJ, Nelson H, et al. A prospective blinded assessment of the impact of pre-operative staging on the management of rectal cancer. Gastroenterology 2002; 123:24–32.

198. Kruskal JB, Sentovich SM, Kane RA. Staging of rectal cancer after polypectomy: usefulness of endor-ectal US. Radiology 1999; 211:31–35.

199. Pikarsky AJ, Wexner SD, Lebensari P, etal. The use of rectal ultrasound for the correct diagnosis and treatment of rectal villous tumors Am J Surg 2000;17:261–265.

200. Marusch F, Koch A, Schmidt U, et al. Routine use of transrectal ultrasound in rectal carcinoma: results of a prospective multicenter study. Endoscopy 2002; 34:385–390.

201. Yasuda S, Fujii H, Nakahara T, et al. 18F–FDG PET detection of colonic adenomas. J Nucl Med 2001; 42:989–992.

202. Berger KL, Nicholson SA, Dehdashti F, Siegel BA. FDG PET evaluation of mucinous neoplasms: correlation of FDG uptake with histopathologic features. Am J Roentgenol 2000; 174:1005–1008.

203. Kinkel K, Lu Y, Both M, Warren RS, Thoeni RF. Detection of hepatic metastases from cancers of the gastrointestinal tract by using noninvasive imaging methods (US, CT, MR Imaging, PET): a meta-analysis. Radiology 2002; 224:748–756.

204. Libutti SK, Alexander HR Jr, Choyke P, et al. A prospective study of 2–[18F] fluoro–2–deoxy–D–glucose/positron emission tomography scan, 99mTc–labeled arcitumomab (CEA–scan), and blind second–look laparotomy for detecting colon cancer recurrence in patients with increasing carci-noembryonic antigen levels. Ann Surg Oncol 2001; 8:779–786.

205. Arulampalam TH, Costa DC, Bomanji JB, Ell PJ. The clinical application of positron emission tom-ography to colorectal cancer management. Q J Nucl Med 2001; 45:215–230.

206. Johnson K, Bakhsh A, Young D, Martin TE Jr., Arnold M. Correlating computed tomography and positron emission tomography scan with operative findings in metastatic colorectal cancer. Dis Colon Rectum 2001; 44:354–357.

207. Kalff V, Hicks RJ, Ware RE, Hogg A, Binns D, McKenzie AF. The clinical impact of (18) F–FDG PET in patients with suspected or confirmed recurrence of colorectal cancer: a prospective study. J Nucl Med 2002; 43:492–499.

208. Even-Sapir E, Lerman H, Figer A, et al. Role of (18) F-FDG dual-head gamma-camera coincidence imaging in recurrent or metastatic colorectal carcinoma. J Nucl Med 2002; 43:603–609.

209. Thrall JH, Ziessman HA. Nuclear Medicine. In: The Requisites. St. Louis, MO: Mosby-Year Book, Inc, 1995:241–248.

210. Siddiqui AR, Schauwecker DS, Wellman HN, Mock BH. Comparison of technetium-99m sulfur colloid and in vitro labeled technetium-99m RBCs in the detection of gastrointestinal bleeding. Clin Nucl Med 1985; 10:546–549.

211. Ponzo F, Zhuang H, Liu FM, et al. Tc-99m sulfur colloid and Tc-99m tagged red blood cell methods are comparable for detecting lower gastrointestinal bleeding in clinical practice. Clin Nucl Med 2002; 27:405–409.

212. Schuetz A, Jauch KW. Lower gastrointestinal bleeding: therapeutic strategies, surgical techniques and results. Langenbecks Arch Surg 2001; 386:17–25.

213. Luchtefeld MA, Senagore AJ, Szomstein M, Fedeson B, Van Erp J, Rupp S. Evaluation of transarterial embolization for lower gastrointestinal bleeding. Dis Colon Rectum 2000; 43:532–534.

214. Funaki B, Kostelic JK, Lorenz J, et al. Superselective microcoil embolization of colonic hemorrhage. Am J Roentgenol 2001; 177:829–836.

215. Rosenkrantz H, Bookstein JJ, Rosen RJ, Boff WB II, Healy JF. Postembolic colonic infarction. Radiology 1982; 142:47–51.

216. LaBerge JM. Management of gastrointestinal bleeding. In: LaBerge JM, ed. Interventional Radiology Essentials. Philadelphia: Lippincott, Williams and Wilkins, 2000:303–314.

8 | Laparoscopic Surgery of the Colon

Shmuel Avital
Department of Surgery, Tel-Aviv Sourasky Medical Center and the Sackler Faculty of Medicine, Tel-Aviv University, Tel-Aviv, Israel

Dana R. Sands
Department of Colorectal Surgery, Cleveland Clinic Florida, Weston, Florida, U.S.A.

Raul Rosenthal
Bariatric Institute, Cleveland Clinic Florida, Weston, Florida, U.S.A.

INTRODUCTION

Laparoscopy, the visualization of the abdominal cavity, has been utilized as a diagnostic tool by gastroenterologists, gynecologists, and surgeons for more than a century. Rapid advances in fiberoptic technology and stapling instrumentation as well as refined insufflation techniques in the late 1980s, have brought laparoscopy to the mainstream surgeons' armamentarium in both diagnostic and therapeutic endeavors (1,2).

The first therapeutic laparoscopic procedure extensively performed and accepted by both surgeons and patients was laparoscopic cholecystectomy. When compared to more than 100 years of experience with traditional open cholecystectomy, laparoscopy demonstrated clear advantages over the open approach by avoiding a large incision. Retrospective and prospective reviews documented faster postoperative recovery and earlier return to daily activities due to decreased pain, and less pulmonary and wound complications. Additionally, there was an obvious improvement in cosmesis resulting in greater patient acceptance.

During the last 10 years, laparoscopic techniques have reached the same high standards of care achieved with open surgery. This has replaced the traditional approach to accessing the abdominal cavity for many procedures including cholecystectomy, appendectomy, inguinal and ventral hernia, donor nephrectomy, adrenalectomy, and bariatric surgery (3–9). Other surgical subspecialties such as pediatric surgery, cardiothoracic surgery, plastic surgery, and gynecology have also embraced the laparoscopic approach as the standard for many disease processes (10–14).

The implementation of therapeutic laparoscopy in the management of colorectal diseases has been slower to evolve and still remains controversial. The first laparoscopic colorectal procedure was performed in the early 1990s (15). Several factors have been responsible for preventing rapid acceptance of laparoscopy in colorectal surgery. Aside from the inherent technical demands of the procedure, as in any laparoscopic abdominal operation, laparoscopic colorectal surgery frequently involving all four abdominal quadrants, control of large blood vessels, extraction of friable and inflamed specimens, and identification of extraperitoneal structures such as the ureters. Furthermore, reconstruction of bowel continuity adds to the complexity of the procedure.

The spectrum of surgical procedures accomplished laparoscopically in the field of colorectal surgery is expanding, and can be categorized from a pathological standpoint. Inflammatory conditions, functional pelvic disorders, and neoplasia are the three main areas. Inflammatory processes such as Crohn's disease, ulcerative colitis, and diverticulitis may present a hostile environment for the laparoscopic surgeon due to distorted anatomy, particularly if approached in the acute phase. Pelvic disorders such as rectal prolapse are challenging, as they may require the advanced laparoscopic skills of intracorporeal suturing to achieve proper fixation of the rectum. Finally, successful laparoscopic colorectal surgery for neoplastic diseases is contingent upon the surgeon's ability to perform an oncologically sound resection.

Laparoscopic Resection for colorectal malignancy is currently a less controversial issue. In the early days of laparoscopy, numerous reports of port-site metastasis following laparoscopic resection for colon cancer were published. These raised concern as to the adequacy of the laparoscopic approach for cancer. Recently, there are fewer reports on port-site metastasis and more showing acceptable long-term survival rates for patients after laparoscopic resection of colonic tumors (16,17). Currently, there are several ongoing multicenter prospective randomized studies comparing open to laparoscopic procedures for colonic cancer that hopefully will resolve this issue more definitively (18).

Although the postoperative benefits of laparoscopic versus open colorectal procedures have been demonstrated in many reports, they are not as dramatic as those seen in other intra-abdominal procedures. This finding may be partly related to the fact that most laparoscopic colorectal procedures are performed as laparoscopic-assisted procedures, with an additional abdominal incision that cannot be standardized. Furthermore, the standardization of postoperative care for both laparoscopic and open surgery has resulted in less dramatic benefits with respect to postoperative ileus and length of hospitalization in the laparoscopic setting. Patients undergoing open surgery could enjoy the same nutritional and psychological benefits achieved with early dietary advancement, as those who had laparoscopic resection (19).

Laparoscopic colorectal surgery has grown in popularity for both benign and malignant indications. Laparoscopic skills continue to be acquired and perfected by yet more surgeons, stressing the postoperative benefits of the procedure over open approaches and most likely reflecting patients' preference.

RECTAL PROLAPSE

An increasingly large number of reports have demonstrated the feasibility and the potential benefits of the laparoscopic approach for repair of rectal prolapse (20–22). Full-thickness rectal prolapse repaired by fixation rectopexy is well suited to laparoscopy, as no specimen is removed and no anastomosis is necessary; thus, most reports have focused on laparoscopic rectopexy.

A number of studies have retrospectively compared the outcome of laparoscopy to historical results of open surgery (23,24). There is only one prospective randomized trial comparing laparoscopic and open repair for rectal prolapse (25). This study included 40 patients randomly assigned to either one of the methods. The surgical technique included full-rectal mobilization to the anorectal junction and a posterior incomplete mesh wrap with fixation to the sacral promontory (Fig. 1).

Postoperative pain, postoperative oral intake, cardiorespiratory morbidity, and hospital length of stay (3.9 vs. 6.6 days) were all in favor of the laparoscopic group. All objective stress response measurements such as serum cortisol, C-reactive protein, and urine catecholamines signified less physiological stress in the laparoscopic group. Apart from the operating time (199 vs. 148 minutes) there were no subjective or objective measures favoring the open group. During a follow-up of two years, comparable results in terms of incontinence and constipation were demonstrated.

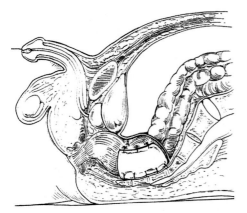

Figure 1   Laparoscopic rectopexy; fixation of the mesh to the sacrum and presacral fascia. *Source*: From Ref. 25.

A retrospective study comparing the functional results in 20 patients with rectal prolapse and fecal incontinence (23) demonstrated a similar significant improvement in fecal incontinence in the two groups. Baseline anal sphincter resting pressure, squeezing pressure, and rectoanal reflex similarly improved in the two groups. The authors concluded that laparoscopic posterior rectopexy has the same clinical and functional results as the open technique, with a shorter hospital stay and decreased costs.

Functional results one year after laparoscopic Well's rectopexy were studied in a series of 29 patients (26). Anal resting and squeeze pressures improved significantly, and were associated with clinical improvement in continence. Overall, 77% of patients were satisfied with the operative result and recurrence was detected in only one patient (3.8%). These results were comparable to the results obtained after open rectopexy in patients with rectal prolapse and associated incontinence (27,28).

Suture rectopexy has also demonstrated a good outcome using the laparoscopic approach (29,30). Heah et al. (30) published a prospectively collected series of 25 patients treated by laparoscopic suture rectopexy for full-thickness rectal prolapse, with no prolapse recurrence after a median follow-up of 26 months. Although laparoscopic resection rectopexy is a more challenging procedure involving resection with an anastomosis (Fig. 2), it is feasible and should be considered in patients with associated constipation if an abdominal approach is considered (31,32).

Baker et al. (31) retrospectively compared a matched series of patients who underwent laparoscopic-assisted resection rectopexy with those who underwent laparotomy. The operative time for the laparoscopic group was substantially longer than the open group; however, this was compensated by a better postoperative recovery with earlier resumption of oral intake and a shorter hospital stay. Long-term outcome revealed good results in both groups with a subjective improvement in constipation for all patients who had preoperative constipation. A larger case series (32) of 30 patients who had laparoscopic-assisted resection rectopexy demonstrated good short- and long-term outcomes. Table 1 shows a summary of the perioperative results.

Complication rates from laparoscopic procedures for rectal prolapse range from 9% to 19%, and may include urinary tract infection, port-site hematoma, and trocar-site hernia. Closure of port sites, as in other laparoscopic procedures, is important to prevent trocar-site complications. Mortality is extremely rare with only one reported case of a patient who died due to aspiration pneumonia (32).

The operative time using the laparoscopic approach is generally longer than the open approach (24,32,34) in keeping with the additional operating time required for most laparoscopic colorectal procedures. A history that reflects dense lower abdominal adhesions may render the laparoscopic approach much more difficult, with increased complications and a higher conversion rate (30,32).

Table 2 summarizes functional results and recurrence after laparoscopic procedures for rectal prolapse that are comparable to that for open procedures (35,36). As in the open approach, patients should be carefully evaluated preoperatively, as constipation may be worsened after rectopexy procedures, regardless of the approach (30,37).

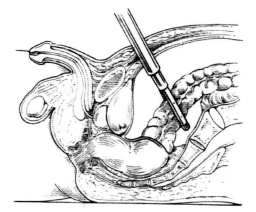

Figure 2 Laparoscopic sigmoid colectomy with rectopexy; transection of the rectum at or just below the sacral promontory. *Source*: From Ref. 25.

Table 1 Laparoscopic Repair of Rectal Prolapse—Operative Results

Authors/year	Patients (*N*)	Laparoscopic approach	Conversion (%)	Mean operative time (minutes)	Hospital stay (days)	Complications (no. of patients)
Darzi et al. 1995 (33)	29	Posterior rectopexy	1 (3.4%)	95	5	1-Urinary tract infection
						1-Trocar-site hernia
						1-Port-site hematoma
Solomon and Eyers 1996 (24)	21	Posterior rectopexy	3 (14%)	198	6.3	3-Port-site hematoma
						1-Pseudomembranous colitis
Bruch et al. 1999 (34)	71	Suture rectopexy (31) + resection rectopexy (40)	1 (1.4%)	227, 258	15	5-Postoperative hemorrhage with reintervention
						1-Anastomotic leak
						1-Port-site hernia
Heah et al. 2000 (30)	25	Suture rectopexy	4 (16%)	96	7	1-Deep vein thrombosis + trocar-site hernia
						1-Rectal perforation
						1-Hematoma
						1-Wound infection
Stevenson et al. 1998 (32)	30	Laparoscopic resection rectopexy	0	185	5	1-Urinary tract infection
						1-Anastomotic bleeding
						1-Small bowel obstruction
						1-Pneumonia
						1-Death due to pneumonia

An original technique of laparoscopic-assisted perineal rectosigmoidectomy was described by Reissman et al. (38) and entailed delivery of a sufficiently long segment of rectum through the anus, followed by introduction of the laparoscope parallel to the prolapsed segment for evaluation of any remaining redundancy, tension, and adhesions, which could be lysed using laparoscopic scissors.

In summary, laparoscopic repair for rectal prolapse is feasible, safe, has short-term benefits in postoperative recovery, acceptable complication rates, and comparable long-term results to the open approach. However, it seems that many surgeons prefer to perform laparoscopic rectopexy rather than laparoscopic resection rectopexy, due to the lesser technical difficulty, shorter operative time, and improved cosmetic and postoperative recovery.

This approach may compromise the patient's functional outcome in constipated patients. Several prospective randomized studies have demonstrated a significant advantage for

Table 2 Functional Results and Recurrence Following Laparoscopic Procedures for Rectal Prolapse

Author/year	No. of pts.	Laparoscopic approach	Follow-up (months)	Recurrence rate *N* (%)	Postoperative incontinence	Postoperative constipation
Darzi et al. 1995 (33)	29	Posterior rectopexy	8	1 (3.3%)	NA	NA
Bruch et al. 1999 (34)	71	Suture rectopexy (32) + resection rectopexy (40)	24	0	64% (improved/ resolved)	76% (improved/ resolved)
Zittel et al. 2000 (26)	29	Posterior rectopexy	22	1 (4.5%)	76% improved	No increase
Heah et al. 2000 (30)	25	Suture rectopexy	26	0	60% improved/ unchanged	Increased to 11 patients from 9
Stevenson et al. 1998 (32)	30	Resection rectopexy	18	2 (7%)	70% improved	64% improved

resection rectopexy compared to rectopexy alone regarding postoperative exacerbation or onset of constipation (39,40). Thus, patients should be carefully evaluated preoperatively, and the decision to use a perineal or abdominal approach and either laparoscopy or laparotomy with or without sigmoid resection should be tailored to each patient. Constipated patients who have a redundant sigmoid colon and deemed suitable for an abdominal repair should be offered resection rectopexy regardless of the surgical approach (laparoscopy vs. laparotomy). Patients with prolapse and colonic inertia or megacolon may benefit from a total abdominal colectomy with ileoproctostomy and rectopexy.

DIVERTICULAR DISEASE

The laparoscopic approach for diverticular disease has been reported in numerous series and mostly include elective patients undergoing laparoscopic sigmoid resections. However, a laparoscopic intervention in acute complicated diverticulitis has also been reported (41–48).

Although a total laparoscopic technique was utilized in colonic resection for diverticular disease (41), and may even augment the postoperative benefits seen after laparoscopic-assisted procedures (42), the technique most often used is the laparoscopic-assisted approach. This offers the postoperative benefits of minimally invasive surgery coupled with facilitation of the specimen extraction as well as anastomotic formation (43–45).

The surgical technique utilizes three to four ports, and a complete mobilization of the sigmoid and left colon. While some authors advocate routine mobilization of the splenic flexure (49), others have demonstrated the possibility of achieving a tension-free anastomosis, with a selective approach for splenic flexure mobilization (45). The ureter and retroperitoneal vessels are identified and resection is performed. The distal resection at the level of the sacral promontory, and division of the mesenteric vessels is accomplished with the use of a linear stapler (Fig. 3). The mobilized specimen is then exteriorized through a small incision in the left lower abdomen, transected, and the anvil of a circular stapler inserted. The end-to-end anastomosis is subsequently accomplished by passing the stapling device through the anus to the apex of the rectal stump. Laparoscopic dissection may be difficult due to dense pericolic and mesenteric inflammation after recurrent and complicated diverticulitis that can distort the normal anatomic planes. Prospective randomized studies comparing laparoscopic and open procedures for diverticular disease are not yet available; however, other forms of comparison (50,51) and large case series (52–54) have demonstrated the feasibility and potential benefits of this approach.

Liberman et al. (55) compared 14 patients who underwent laparoscopic resection for diverticulitis with 14 patients who underwent laparotomy, and demonstrated significantly less intraoperative blood loss (171 vs. 321 mL, respectively), earlier return to oral diet (2.9 vs. 6.1 days, respectively), and shorter hospital stay (6.3 vs. 9.2 days, respectively) in the

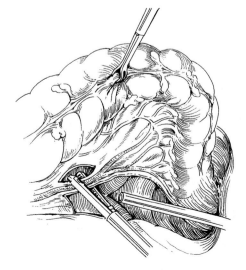

Figure 3 Laparoscopic sigmoidectomy; transection of the interior mesenteric vessels with a linear stapling device. *Source*: From Ref. 22.

laparoscopic group. The operative time did not significantly differ between the two groups (192 vs. 182 minutes, respectively), a finding that has not been reported in other published series (50,56,57). Despite calculated increased operating room costs in the laparoscopic group, the overall hospital charges were not significantly different.

The postoperative benefits after laparoscopic surgery for diverticular disease were demonstrated in a retrospective study comparing 25 patients who underwent laparoscopic resection versus 17 patients who underwent laparotomy (56). Patients tolerated regular diet after a mean of 3.2 days in the laparoscopic group compared to 5.7 days in the open group. Hospital stay was 4.2 days in the laparoscopic group versus 6.8 in the open group. A trend toward decreased perioperative complications was demonstrated in favor of the laparoscopic group, and the operative time was substantially longer in the laparoscopic group (397 vs. 115 minutes); this finding was partly attributed to the fact that, in the laparoscopic group, there were twice as many patients who had previously undergone a laparotomy. In contrast to previously published studies (55), the overall charges were significantly higher in the laparoscopic group.

Tuech et al. (50) studied the benefits of laparoscopy for diverticular disease in a subgroup of elderly patients. They conducted a prospective nonrandomized comparative study in patients aged greater than or equal to 75 years, undergoing laparoscopy versus those having laparotomy. The laparoscopic procedures were substantially longer; however, the patients enjoyed a better postoperative course with a decreased need for parenteral analgesia (5.4 vs. 8.2 days), and a shorter hospital stay. Data from those comparative studies is summarized in Table 3.

Although the results of these nonrandomized comparative studies should be carefully evaluated, they consistently show a better postoperative outcome in favor of the laparoscopic groups, with an earlier return to an oral diet, a shorter hospital stay, and comparable morbidity to the open approach, but are generally associated with longer operative times. In addition to these trials, numerous case series have been published as well (Table 4).

Sher et al. (58) studied the impact of the severity of diverticulitis, as classified by a modified Hinchey classification, on the conversion and complication rates, and compared it to patients who underwent laparotomy. Patients with Hinchey I disease had no postoperative morbidity or conversion to a laparotomy, and had a shorter median hospital stay than patients with Hinchey I disease who underwent laparotomy (five vs. seven days, respectively). Patients with Hinchey IIA or IIB diverticulitis had a 50% conversion and a 33% complication rate, respectively. However, when excluding the very first laparoscopic patients, even patients with Hinchey II diverticulitis had a shorter hospital stay when compared to the equivalent laparotomy group.

Vargas et al. (45) reported a 14% conversion rate for uncomplicated diverticulitis. Conversion rates as high as 61% were reported for patients with diverticulitis associated with fistula or previous diverticular abscess and a significantly longer paralytic ileus and hospital stay in the converted group. However, a general trend toward fewer conversions over time was also demonstrated.

Intermediate-term follow-up results after laparoscopic sigmoid resection for diverticular disease have been evaluated in various studies (45,49,54). Generally, recurrent disease following surgery depends on accurate identification and transection at the rectosigmoid level

Table 3 Comparative Studies of Laparoscopic Versus Open Sigmoid Resection for Diverticular Disease

Author	Study	Procedure	No. of patients	Operative time (minutes)	Conversion (%)	Morbidity (%)	Diet (days)	Hospital stay (days)
Faynsod et al. (51)	Case control	Laparoscopy	20	251	30	10	1[a]	4.8[a]
		Laparotomy	20	243		10	5[a]	7.8[a]
Tuech et al. (50)	Prospective Non-randomized	Laparoscopy	22	234[a]	9	18[a]		13.1[a]
		Laparotomy	24	136[a]		50[a]		20.2[a]
Liberman et al. (55)	Case control	Laparoscopy	14	192		14	2.9[a]	6.3[a]
		Laparotomy	14	182		14	6.1[a]	9.2[a]
Bruce et al. (56)	Retrospective comparison	Laparoscopy	25	397[a]	12	16	3.2[a]	4.2[a]
		Laparotomy	17	115[a]		23	5.7[a]	6.8[a]

[a]Statistically significant difference.

Table 4 Case Series of Laparoscopic Surgery for Diverticular Disease

Author	No. of patients	Operative time (minutes)	Conversion (%)	Complications	Death (%)	Diet (days)	Hospital stay (days)
Kockerling et al. (1999) (52)	304	164	7.2	14.8	1.1		
Vargas et al. (45)	69	155	26	10.1	0	3.5	4.2
Siriser et al. (54)	65		4.6	17	0	2.6	7.6
Smadja et al. (57)	54	298	9.2	14	0	2.3	6.4
Stevenson et al. (49)	100	180	8	21	0	2	4

(59). In a mean follow-up of 48 months, only 1 of 69 patients who underwent laparoscopic colectomy for diverticulitis had recurrent disease (45). Another report of 100 patients (49) found no recurrent diverticulosis-related symptoms at a 37-month follow-up.

Applying a laparoscopic approach during acute phase of diverticulitis is more controversial, and is less frequently reported than is laparoscopic treatment of diverticular disease in the elective setting (60). Laparoscopic intervention in acute diverticulitis ranges from resection with primary anastomosis to Hartmann's procedure (Fig. 4) to laparoscopic lavage with drainage (46–48).

Schlachta et al. (46) reported their experience with one-stage laparoscopic procedures in 22 patients with acute diverticulitis. Patients were considered to have acute diverticulitis if the surgery was performed in the same hospital admission as an acute attack, and there was evidence of acute inflammation such as fever, leukocytosis and abdominal tenderness. However, surgery was performed only after abdominal tenderness had resolved; patients with purulent or feculent peritonitis were excluded. Conversion to open surgery was required in 14% of patients compared to only a 4% conversion rate in patients who underwent the same procedure in an elective setting. Despite this selection, neither the perioperative complication rate nor the postoperative recovery parameters significantly differed between the two groups. The authors concluded that laparoscopic resection for acute and chronic diverticulitis had equivalent outcomes in these settings.

A more heterogeneous group of patients laparoscopically treated was reported by Fine (47). This group of patients had undrained abscesses, refractory acute diverticulitis, colovesical fistula, obstruction, and free perforation. In most cases, resection with primary anastomosis was performed with repair of colovesical fistula when needed. Three of the 16 patients underwent laparoscopic Hartmann's procedures, and two underwent irrigation with drainage or colostomy; conversion was required in three patients (17%). The postoperative recovery was uneventful, except for one patient who developed necrotizing fascitis and eventually recovered.

Several authors have demonstrated the feasibility of laparoscopic lavage and drainage in cases of generalized peritonitis associated with perforated sigmoid diverticulitis, obviating the need for a stoma creation in these patients (48,60,61). Faranda et al. (48) laparoscopically

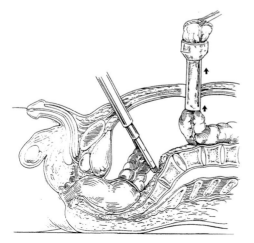

Figure 4 Laparoscopic Hartmann's procedure; withdrawal of the proximal bowel through the 33-mm port placed at the preoperatively selected stoma site is optional. *Source*: From Ref. 25.

treated 18 patients with acute presentation of perforated diverticulitis. All patients underwent laparoscopic lavage of the peritoneal cavity, the infected sigmoid lesion was sealed with biologic glue and drains were inserted; no colostomies were performed. Fourteen of the patients subsequently underwent elective laparoscopic sigmoid resection. This approach was associated with low morbidity (three patients with lymphangitis/pulmonary disease, and no patient with wound abscess or abdominal collection), short hospital stay, and improvement in the patients' quality of life as colostomy was avoided. Similarly, favorable results have been reported by other authors (60,61).

In summary, laparoscopic-assisted elective sigmoid colectomy for diverticular disease is feasible and safe. Apart from the longer operative time, laparoscopic resection has resulted in less postoperative pain, earlier return to a normal diet, a shorter hospital stay, and comparable or lower morbidity. Conversion is generally related to the complexity of the pathological process, and should be considered in difficult cases to prevent surgical complications. With sufficient experience in minimally invasive colon and rectal surgery, acute diverticulitis with complications that mandate emergent surgery can be laparoscopically managed with potential significant benefit to the patient.

LAPAROSCOPY AND INFLAMMATORY BOWEL DISEASE
Crohn's Disease

Laparoscopy may be utilized in many commonly performed operations for Crohn's disease (CD) including diagnostic laparoscopy, lysis of adhesions, ileocolic or segmental bowel resection, proctectomy, total proctocolectomy, stoma creation and reversal and strictureplasty (62–65). Crohn's disease is often marked by a thick and inflamed mesentery, inflammatory phlegmons and adhesions, and possible abscesses and fistulas that may present a difficult and complicated environment (66,67). Generally, the surgeon's laparoscopic skills and experience, the specific procedure to be performed, and proper patient selection play an important role in the successful completion of any laparoscopic intervention.

Diagnostic Laparoscopy

Diagnostic laparoscopy may serve as a useful and simple method of assessment in cases of persistent unclear diagnosis and when the standard evaluations for suspected Crohn's disease failed to achieve a definitive diagnosis. It can also be performed as an initial assessment of the abdomen to determine the feasibility of laparoscopic resection (62).

Fecal Diversion

Fecal diversion (Fig. 5) may be indicated in Crohn's disease for severe rectal or perianal disease. Laparoscopic stoma creation in these cases can offer the laparoscopic benefits of better cosmetic results, earlier return of bowel function, and shorter hospital stay compared to laparotomy (68). Moreover, as opposed to other laparoscopic colorectal procedures, stoma formation is not associated with longer operative times compared to laparotomy and may average 55 minutes in patients who have had no prior abdominal surgery (68,69).

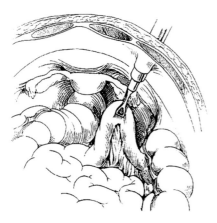

Figure 5 Laparoscopic ileostomy creation; the bowel is manipulated to the stomal opening using the laparoscopic Babcock grasper; the grasper, port, and the bowel are withdrawn as a unit. *Source*: From Ref. 22.

Bowel Resection

Ileocolic resection is the most frequently performed surgical procedure in patients with Crohn's disease. Approximately half of the patients with Crohn's disease eventually require surgical resection and almost half will require a subsequent operation (70). Laparoscopic ileocolic resection has become the most common laparoscopic procedure in patients with Crohn's disease, and is usually performed in a laparoscopic-assisted fashion. Guidelines for laparoscopy are the same as for laparotomy; the entire length of the small bowel should be inspected and evaluated in a sequential manner, any additional diseased segments should be marked, exteriorized, and evaluated for resection or strictureplasty as indicated.

The first report of laparoscopic ileocolic resection in Crohn's disease was published in 1993 (71). This report included nine patients with terminal ileitis who underwent laparoscopic-assisted resection. Three were converted to laparotomy and no complications were encountered.

Since this initial report, several other studies have demonstrated the feasibility and potential benefits of the laparoscopic approach in patients with Crohn's disease mostly performed for terminal ileitis (63,67,72).

Experience with both advanced laparoscopic techniques and conventional surgery for inflammatory bowel disease has allowed the successful management of patients with complicated Crohn's disease with comparable complication rates to open surgery.

Canin-Endres et al. (63) reported their experience with 88 patients with Crohn's disease who underwent laparoscopic intestinal resection. Seventy patients underwent ileocolic resection, while the others underwent small bowel resection or segmental colectomy. Despite the considerable number of patients with previous abdominal surgery (42%), and intraoperative findings of inflammatory masses (19%), abscesses (12%), and fistulas (18%), only one patient was converted to a formal laparotomy. The operative time averaged 183 minutes, return of bowel function occurred at an average time of three days, length of stay averaged two to four days, and complications occurred in only 12 patients.

Subtotal colectomy for Crohn's colitis may also be laparoscopically performed, although it is a far more extensive and challenging procedure. Hamel et al. (72) compared 109 laparoscopic ileocolic resections to 21 laparoscopic subtotal colectomy in CD patients. In 19 (17%) patients with ileocolic resection and five (24%) with subtotal colectomy, the procedure had to be converted to a laparotomy. As expected, the total operative time was shorter for ileocolic resection (167 vs. 231 min), but the hospital length of stay was similar in both groups (8.8 days). There were more intraoperative complications associated with subtotal colectomy, but the overall postoperative morbidity was the same in both groups.

Comparative Studies

A clear advantage for laparoscopy over laparotomy is cosmesis and body image (73,74). In young patients with Crohn's disease, better cosmesis may prove to be a most important and lasting advantage for choosing a laparoscopic approach (73).

Several studies that compared laparoscopy to laparotomy revealed comparable morbidity, and a trend toward faster recovery, reflected mainly in shorter hospital stay for patients who underwent laparoscopy (Table 5). A better short-term recovery for laparoscopic-assisted patients was also demonstrated by less pain medication requirements, quicker return to normal activity including return to work and to social and sexual interactions (73), and faster postoperative recovery of pulmonary functions (76). Furthermore, in a long-term comparison follow-up averaging 30 months, the incidence of symptomatic small bowel obstruction was higher in the conventional group as compared to the laparoscopic-assisted group (31% vs. 7.6%, respectively) (73).

In summary, laparoscopy for the treatment of Crohn's disease is becoming the preferred approach for terminal ileal disease and stoma creation. There seems to be less value in cases of colectomy, proctectomy, and stoma reversal.

LAPAROSCOPIC COLECTOMY FOR ULCERATIVE COLITIS AND FAP

The surgical treatment of ulcerative colitis is greatly affected by the patient's condition at the time of intervention. As the experience with laparoscopy for colorectal diseases increases, surgeons

Table 5 Comparative Studies of Laparoscopy Versus Open Surgery for Crohn's Disease

Author	Study	No. of patients open procedure	No. of patients laparoscopic-assisted procedure	Operative time (minutes)	Conversion (%)	Morbidity (%)	Early diet (days)	Hospital stay (days)
Bemelman et al. (75)	Retrospective comparative (ileocolic resection)	48	30	104[a] 138[a]	6.6	14.6 10	5.1 4.3	10.2[a] 5.7[a]
Alabaz et al. (73)	Retrospective comparative (ileocolic resection)	48	26	90.5[a] 150[a]	11.5	16.6 15.3	NA	9.6[a] 7[a]
Milsom et al. (76)	Prospective randomized (ileocolic resection)	29	31	85[a] 140[a]	6.4	Major–3.4 Minor–27.5[a] Major–3.2 Minor–12.7[a]	4 (BM) 4 (BM)	5 6

[a]Statistically significant difference.
Abbreviation: BM, bowel movement.

have been increasingly able to treat mucosal ulcerative colitis in both the chronic and acute settings with a laparoscopic approach. From a technical standpoint, the treatment of ulcerative colitis is perhaps the most demanding of the colorectal maladies approached with the laparoscope. The need for maneuvering in all quadrants of the abdomen, the mobilization of both flexures, and the large and often friable specimen create unique challenges, which can lead to increased operative times and surgeon frustration. Given similarities in the surgical procedures performed, the surgical treatment of Familial Adenomatous Polyposis (FAP) will also be addressed. The mainstay of treatment for both diseases involves the removal of the entire colon and, depending on the disease severity at the time of the initial intervention, removal of the rectum with construction of an ileoanal J pouch or permanent ileostomy in those patients with poor sphincter function. Patients with severe disease and systemic illness will typically have the first operation limited to a total abdominal colectomy with end ileostomy, deferring the pelvic dissection to a later time when overall status has improved. Similarly, surgeons treating young patients with FAP who have relative rectal sparing may elect to leave the rectum in place and perform an ileorectal anastomosis, thereby avoiding the morbidity of a pelvic dissection.

Early experience with laparoscopic total abdominal colectomy was discouraging. In 1992, the Cleveland Clinic Florida preliminary experience compared five patients who underwent laparoscopic-assisted total abdominal colectomy with five laparoscopic-assisted proctocolectomies and five open total abdominal colectomies. They showed that the laparoscopic approach was associated with an increased operative time and a prolonged ileus (77). At the time of that study, all mesenteric division was extracorporeally performed. In a larger series from 1994, 22 patients were treated with laparoscopic proctocolectomy, and were compared to 20 patients who had open surgery (78). There was no difference noted in the time to resolution of ileus or length of hospital stay between the two groups. With results such as these, many pioneers of laparoscopic colorectal surgery were reluctant to treat mucosal ulcerative colitis and FAP using the laparoscopic method. These same surgeons, however, continued to gain experience with the more en vogue segmental resections for other benign diseases. Bennett et al. (79) questioned the influence of the learning curve on patient outcome after laparoscopic surgery. In an analysis of almost 1200 laparoscopic colectomies performed by 114 surgeons, they found that surgeons who had performed at least 40 cases had a lower probability of both intraoperative and postoperative complications. More recently, the Laparoscopic Colorectal Surgery Study Group evaluated the outcome of 1658 patients who underwent laparoscopic colectomy between 1995 and 1999 (80). This retrospective review found that there was no difference in morbidity between patients who underwent surgery at a center that performed over 100 cases, and those whose surgery was performed by centers with less experience. There were, however, significantly lower conversion rates (4.3% vs. 6.9%, respectively) and a higher percentage of rectal procedures (26.7 vs. 9.5, respectively) performed at the more experienced centers. Additionally, they found that laparoscopic-assisted restorative proctocolectomy was not a frequently performed procedure.

As the importance of the learning curve associated with laparoscopy became more significant, and surgeons continued to routinely perform segmental colonic resections for benign disease, many have revisited the more complex procedures of total abdominal colectomy and total proctocolectomy. Araki et al. (81) compared 21 patients who underwent laparoscopic total proctocolectomy with 11 patients treated by laparotomy. They found no differences relative to operative time, blood loss, or mortality. The laparoscopic group had a shortened postoperative ileus, decreased time to the formation of more solid stool, and a trend toward decreased morbidity. The Canadian experience with laparoscopic total abdominal colectomy has also shown promising results (82). When comparing 37 laparoscopic to 36 open total abdominal colectomies, Seshadri and colleagues (82) found that while the patients laparoscopically treated had longer operative times, there was a lower incidence of both short-term (wound infection and pneumonia) and long-term (hernias and stoma problems) complications. The experience with elective resection for ulcerative colitis from the Cleveland Clinic Foundation in Ohio showed that, while the operative times remained longer, the return of bowel function was faster and hospital stay was shorter; although morbidity was decreased, this did not reach statistical significance (83).

During the infancy of laparoscopic colectomy, acute colitis was considered a contraindication to this approach. A more recent review of 10 laparoscopic total colectomies for acute colitis in The Netherlands revealed longer operative times, shorter hospital stays, and no difference in the rate of complications. This led Dunker and colleagues (84) to conclude that the approach is both safe and feasible.

More recent results in a larger series from the Lahey Clinic revealed that the laparoscopic approach for acute colitis was safe, feasible, and associated with faster recovery (85). However, the caveat in these studies is that the surgeons and their teams were highly skilled, and had significant experience with complex laparoscopic colorectal surgery. This result may not be achieved in every setting.

In the young patient population, Milsom et al. (86) showed that there was minimal disability in those patients who underwent laparoscopic colectomy for FAP, with 75% of patients returning to normal activity within one month and two-thirds of these patients not having to miss school. Cosmesis may be a relatively unimportant consideration for patients with ulcerative colitis and FAP. However, in this typically young patient population, cosmesis can play an important role in the postoperative psychological recovery. This principle was aptly demonstrated in a group of young patients with Crohn's disease. A cosmetic grading scale was significantly improved in patients undergoing laparoscopic resection. There was also a significant correlation with the level of self-confidence in the postoperative period. Approximately two-thirds of the patients would have preferred a laparoscopic resection even when faced with a 5% risk of ureteral injury, and 25 of the 34 patients were willing to pay up to $500 for a smaller incision. It can be demonstrated that laparoscopic total abdominal colectomy and proctocolectomy are feasible and safe procedures and, in a more varied setting, patient preference may be an important driving force for laparoscopy in the treatment of inflammatory bowel disease (74).

Realistically, regardless of patient requests, the decision may be impacted by consideration of finances and rendered not by the surgeon or patient, but by the administrator of the hospital or the health plan. While the early experience with laparoscopy for ulcerative colitis and FAP may not have shown all of the touted benefits, several recent studies have demonstrated that laparoscopy for ulcerative colitis and FAP is both feasible and safe. Whereas, previously it was reserved for the elective patient, expert surgeons have shown it to be safe in a few patients with acute colitis. There is still an association with longer operative times; however, more consistently, laparoscopic resection offers shorter hospital stay, improved pulmonary function, presumably from decreased postoperative pain associated with the midline laparotomy. The benefits of improved cosmesis, not to be easily dismissed in this patient population, are an important secondary consideration. Current investigations into the effect on adhesion formation and immunologic status will hopefully add more support to the laparoscopic approach for ulcerative colitis and FAP.

LAPAROSCOPIC RESECTION FOR COLORECTAL CANCER

The feasibility and safety of the laparoscopic approach for benign diseases led to its subsequent use in the treatment of colorectal cancer (87,88). In benign diseases, the immediate postoperative benefits play an important role in the selection of the surgical approach. However, in cancer, this issue becomes secondary to the primary goal of achieving long-term cure. In applying the minimally invasive surgical approach to colorectal malignancy, it is important to demonstrate that laparoscopy does not compromise oncological principles or jeopardize outcome. While it is easier to demonstrate that with acceptable technical skills it is possible to resect colonic tumors with adequate margins and adequate number of lymph nodes (89), evaluation of long-term oncological outcome needs a large number of patients with long-term follow-up.

Perioperative Outcome After Laparoscopic Resection of Colorectal Cancer—Recovery and Complications
Postoperative Recovery
The benefits observed after laparoscopic colorectal surgery are not as dramatic as after other laparoscopic procedures. Some studies have shown only minimal differences in analgesic requirements, reflecting the associated abdominal incision required even in the laparoscopic approach and the magnitude of the intra-abdominal operation (90).

New protocols of early feeding and early discharge were used successfully in patients following laparoscopic colorectal surgery (91). However, the same protocols were well tolerated in open surgery as well (92,93).

Most study results suggest a shorter hospital stay following laparoscopic colorectal cancer surgery, this difference is somewhat modest. In a review of several studies, the mean hospital stay after laparoscopic surgery was 9.2 days compared to 10.8 days after laparotomy (90).

The largest and most comprehensive prospective randomized study evaluating short-term quality of life outcomes following laparoscopic-assisted colectomy versus laparotomy for colon cancer has reported the outcome of 428 patients in the two groups (94). Analysis was based on an intent-to-treat basis, thus the 25% of patients whose procedures were converted to a laparotomy were analyzed as part of the laparoscopic group. The duration of postoperative in-hospital analgesic use, length of hospital stay, and three various validated quality of life and pain indices were used to assess the patients two days, two weeks, and two months after surgery. The laparoscopic group demonstrated a better postoperative outcome in some of the measured parameters. Clinical outcome revealed shorter durations of both oral and parenteral analgesic therapy and a mean of 0.8 days shorter hospital stay (5.6 vs. 6.4 days) for the laparoscopic group. Only minimal short-term quality of life benefits were found with laparoscopic-assisted surgery for colon cancer compared with standard open colectomy.

The drawbacks of this recent study were related to the fact that this is a multicenter study, which may represent varying degrees of laparoscopic expertise across the different centers, reflected in the relatively high conversion rate. It can be argued that, with more experienced surgeons the conversion rate would decrease and the postoperative benefits would become more pronounced. In addition, a total laparoscopic technique may yield a better outcome in terms of postoperative recovery and pain (95).

Complications, Conversion, and Operative Time

Death rate, perioperative complications, conversion, and operative time are measurable end point parameters that are reported in the vast majority of studies. A recent meta-analysis reviewed 42 studies with a total number of 3430 patients in which 1903 had malignant colorectal disease treated laparoscopically (90) and found an average 30-day mortality rate of 1.64% (0–5.1%). There were no data to indicate that laparoscopy was related to a greater incidence of intraoperative complications. Nevertheless, precautions, which include the marking of vital structures, location of viscera, and the use of atraumatic instruments placed within camera view, remain essential. The morbidity rate for malignant cases was comparable to open series averaging 15% with a 4.6% anastomotic leak rate, and an 18.4% wound infection rate. The relatively high wound infection rates for laparoscopy represents the 5–8 cm incision required for specimen retrieval in the laparoscopic-assisted approach.

Length of surgery was significantly higher for laparoscopic cases in comparable series. The mean operative time was 174 minutes in mixed case series, and 196 minutes for series reporting only malignant conditions. The mean conversion rate was 17.2%, which rose to 28% in series representing only malignant cases. This slightly higher conversion rate may be attributed to reasons related to the tumor itself such as advanced disease or positive margins (94). Interestingly, there was no correlation found between conversion and total patient volume or complexity of the procedure (90).

Port-Site Metastasis and Long-Term Outcome

Several published reports have described the phenomenon of tumor recurrence in port sites following laparoscopic resection for colon cancer (96–98). These reports, together with the same phenomenon described with other malignancies (99,100), promoted concern over the adequacy of laparoscopy in the management of cancer in general and particularly in colorectal cancer. The significance of any postoperative benefits of laparoscopy such as reduced postoperative pain and faster recovery would be insignificant if the chance for cure was jeopardized.

The actual incidence of port-site metastasis was not determined; however, its existence was quite evident. In a small series from 1994, 14 patients underwent laparoscopic resection for colorectal cancer, three (21%) of whom developed wound recurrence (101). Moreover, laparoscopic wound recurrence has been reported for early stage tumors such as T1 and T2

(102). These reports have led to extensive research proposing two main mechanisms for possible port-site cancer cell implantation: pneumoperitoneum-related and tissue handling factors (103).

Results regarding the pneumoperitoneum effect have been controversial. Several studies demonstrated an aerosolization phenomenon of tumor cells through the port sites during pneumoperitoneum (104–107). Others found no effect of pneumoperitoneum on port-site cell implantation, and even proposed that pneumoperitoneum has a protecting effect from wound tumor cells implantation (108–111). Other mechanisms associated with pneumoperitoneum and were postulated to increase tumor cell wound implantation included the use of carbon dioxide (112) and the intra-abdominal pressure itself generated by pneumoperitoneum (105,113). Mechanisms related to tissue handling have been proposed as well. Extraction of the specimen through a small incision may cause a direct contact of tumor cells with the abdominal wall and lead to cell implantation. However, this theory does not explain the findings of port-site metastasis in remote trocar sites. Another issue is the difference in tissue handling and manipulation during laparoscopy. Some authors have demonstrated, in an animal model, that laparoscopic manipulation is associated with higher rates of wound metastasis compared to open manipulation regardless of the pneumoperitoneum (114,115). Mechanisms related to trocar-site trauma (116) and laparoscopic instrument contamination (106,108) have also been proposed.

The controversial results of the various studies were attributed to several research limitations. Investigations differ widely in many research aspects such as study design, animal and tumor cell type, methods for tumor establishment, tumor dose inocula, and pressure and duration of pneumoperitoneum. Additionally, crucial variables of the clinical circumstances such as tumor load and the specific biological behavior of tumor cells, could not be reproduced in many research settings (113).

Following early reports on port-site recurrence and the related extensive research, some preventative measurements have been proposed. Wound protectors such as endo-bags or plastic wound protectors, are probably the most commonly used preventive measure. Although there is no clear evidence that wound protectors play a role in preventing wound recurrence, they are simple to use and relatively inexpensive. Other proposed preventative measures are less frequently employed and include gasless laparoscopy, different types of gas, wound excision, and peritoneal and wound irrigation (16).

Incidence of Port-Site Metastasis

Along with the extensive laboratory research, efforts have been made more recently to reevaluate the phenomenon of port-site recurrence, and define its true incidence. One of the first large series addressing this issue was published in 1996 (117). In this study, 372 patients who underwent laparoscopic-assisted colectomy for cancer before 1994 were retrospectively evaluated. The overall three-year survival rate was comparable to reported data for open surgery and only 1.1% (four patients) had wound recurrence. In concordance with this study, port-site metastases are now rarely reported.

Assessment of several reports that included at least 50 patients in each series, comparing a total of 1737 patients, revealed a port-site recurrence incidence of 0.62% (16). This rate compares favorably to wound recurrence rates after open laparotomy for colorectal cancer reportedly in the range of 0.6% to 0.8% (118,119).

Available results of prospective randomized studies, though limited in size and follow-up (17,120,121), showed no difference in wound recurrence between laparoscopy and open surgery in colorectal cancer patients. In one study, port-site recurrence was not detected in the laparoscopy group, while two patients in the open group (121) had wound recurrence associated with widespread disease. These accumulated recent data suggest that after ascending the learning curve, the actual incidence of port-site metastasis is much lower than initially reported, and is comparable to open surgery. This lower incidence is probably technique-related, and may reflect increased surgeons' experience and the adoption of some precautions when performing the procedure in patients with colorectal cancer. Nevertheless, the fact that these port-site metastases are not always associated with advanced disease and may develop after a relatively short time and in remote ports from the specimen retrieval port still raises a concern.

Long-Term Follow-Up

Until recently most of the data on long-term survival following laparoscopy for colorectal cancer came from unstructured observational studies limited in number of patients and follow-up time that included colon and rectal cancer patients together in different stages of disease. However, in all of these studies (Table 6) and in other two small prospective randomized comparative studies (120,121) the long term out come following laparoscopy was comparable to the traditional open approach. The two most important studies, which were recently published, are the single center study reported by Lacy et al (17) and the intermediate results reported by the Clinical Outcomes of Surgical Therapy Study Group (COST) (128). These studies have finally lead to an approved statement by the American Society of Colon and Rectal Surgeons (ASCRS) endorsed by the Society of American Gastointestinal Endoscopic Surgeons (SAGES) in 2004 on the oncological safety of the laparoscopic approach in colon cancer patients. It is important to note that these studies did not include rectal cancer patients.

Lacy et al. (17) reported the outcome of 101 patients who underwent open colectomy for nonmetastatic colon cancer compared to 105 patients who underwent laparoscopic-assisted colectomy. At a median follow-up of 43 months, the rate of tumor recurrence as well as overall survival was not significantly different between the two groups. Interestingly, patients with Stage III disease who underwent laparoscopic surgery had a better long-term survival. The authors suggested that this finding may be related to the fact that laparoscopic surgery results in less immunosuppression than does laparotomy.

In the COST study (128), 872 patients with adenocarcinoma of the colon were randomly assigned to undergo open or laparoscopically assisted colectomy in a multi center study. At three years, the rates of recurrence were similar in the two groups: 16 percent among patients in the laparoscopic assisted group and 18 percent among patients in the open-colectomy group. Recurrence rates in surgical wounds were less than 1 percent in both groups. The overall survival rate at three years was very similar as well (86 percent in the laparoscopic-surgery group vs. 85 percent in the open-colectomy group). No significant differences in survival were found when comparing the two groups by the disease stage. Based on this data, it is suggested that long-term survival in colon cancer patients undergoing laparoscopic resection is comparable to laparotomy when performed by experienced surgeons. In addition, adherence to standard cancer resection techniques is crucial.

Since the large prospective randomized studies mentioned earlier did not include rectal cancer the role of laparoscopy in rectal cancer and specifically in mid and low tumors is yet to be concluded.

COMPLICATIONS AND CONVERSIONS IN LAPAROSCOPIC COLONIC SURGERY

Laparoscopic colorectal surgery is a technically demanding procedure utilized in a large variety of pathological conditions and involving difficult laparoscopic maneuvers. Evaluating the complications related to laparoscopic colorectal surgery reveals some uniquely laparoscopic complications along with known complications associated with laparotomy.

Intraoperative Complications and Their Prevention

Most recent series have suggested that the rate of intraoperative complications associated with laparoscopic colorectal surgery ranges from 5% to 7% (79,129–132). The two most common intraoperative surgical complications are bleeding, both at intra-abdominal and at the port site, and bowel injury. Port-site bleeding can be minimized by placing the trocars in the midline or well lateral to the rectus muscle, therefore reducing the risk of injuring the inferior epigastric or smaller rectus muscle vessels.

In an attempt to avoid bleeding from large mesenteric vessels, complete dissection and visualization of the vascular pedicle prior to clipping, stapling, or irrigating should be performed to achieve a more precise and secure hemostasis. Gentle handling of the bowel with atraumatic graspers and avoiding bowel grasping in diseased segments minimizes bowel injury. Less frequent complications include instrument failure (stapling device failure), visceral injuries such as ureteral tears, subcutaneous emphysema due to trocar dislocation, rotated anastomosis and missed small colonic lesions that were not preoperatively marked (130,131).

Table 6 Intermediate-Term Follow-Up in Laparoscopy for Colorectal Cancer

Author	Study type	No. of patients	Procedures included	Follow-up (months)	Survival	P-value
Leung et al. (122)	Case control study	28–LAC, 56–open	Right colectomy	Median LAC–21.4, open–23.5	(5-year DFS by Kaplan-Meier) LAC–94%, open–75%	NS
Franklin et al. (123)	Prospective case series	50 only Stage III patients	All forms of colectomy and rectal resections	Median–24	(5-year DFS by Kaplan-Meier) 49%	
Hartley et al. (124)	Comparison to a matched open group single surgeon	Attempted LAP–42 (completed–22), open–22	Anterior resection and APR with TME	Median–38	Crude survival lap–71%, open–77%	NS
Lord et al. (125)	Case series	41	All procedures	Mean 16.7	Disease-free survival 97%	
Fleshman et al. (117)	Retrospective multicenter study (COST)	372	All procedures	Mean 22.6	3-year by Kaplan-Meier Stage I–93%, Stage II–72% DFS, Stage III–53%	
Schiedeck et al. (126)	Multicenter	399	All procedures	Mean 30	DFS, Stage I–98%, Stage II–86%, Stage III–89%	
Poulin et al. (127)	Case series–prospective	135		Median 24	Observed 2-year survival, Stage I–100%, Stage II–88.7%, Stage III–80.6%	

Abbreviations: LAC, laparoscopic assisted colectomy; LAP, laparoscopy; APR, abdomino perineal resection; TME, total mesorectal excision; DFS, disease-free survival; NS, non significant.

Early diagnosis and immediate treatment is the key for decreasing the consequences of such surgical complications. An enterotomy, for instance, may have no adverse sequelae if diagnosed and repaired intraoperatively, but may have severe consequences if missed during surgery and left untreated. As with other laparoscopic procedures, nonsurgical complications may result from the intraoperative elevated intra-abdominal pressure and CO_2 insufflation (130,132). Conversion may be indicated when retention of carbon dioxide or decreased cardiac output are encountered during the procedure (129,133).

Conversion

Conversion to open surgery can be followed either by a preemptive decision or a reactive decision to either avoid or respond to an intraoperative complication. However, conversion outside of these parameters is not considered a complication. Approximately 25% of conversions are associated with intraoperative complications (130,131,134,135). In some cases, it serves as an important tool in avoiding unnecessary complications. Conversion should be considered in cases of unclear anatomy such as in patients with dense adhesions or failure to identify important structures such as the ureters, in obese patients, and in cases of severe inflammation. Timely abandonment of the laparoscopic approach should be regarded as good surgical judgment rather than as failure.

Postoperative Complications

The 30-day mortality rate reported for laparoscopic colorectal surgery ranges from 0% to 2% (130,131,133,134,136,137), which is comparable to the 1% to 5% reported for open colonic surgery (138–140). The rate of overall postoperative morbidity ranges from 6% to 30% (130,131,134,136,141–144) that is also comparable to the 10% to 30% reported complication rate after open surgery (140,145,146).

Postoperative medical morbidity includes known complications as for open surgery such as pulmonary, urinary, cardiac, and thromboembolic complications. However, some postoperative medical complications occur less frequently after laparoscopic colorectal surgery than after open procedures. Specifically, laparoscopic surgery causes less disturbance to pulmonary function as reflected in a decreased rate of postoperative pneumonia for all laparoscopic procedures (147–149). This advantage has been reflected in laparoscopic colorectal surgery with the incidence of postoperative pneumonia as low as 1% to 2% (132,150) compared to 5% to 14% is open colorectal surgery (151,152). Urinary tract infection may be seen after any type of colonic surgery. The urinary tract infection rate found after laparoscopic colorectal surgery is in the range of 0.3% to 5% (136,150). Data from open colonic surgery reveal a slightly higher rate ranging from 4% to 9% (152–154). This difference may be explained by a more liberal approach toward early removal of the urinary catheter after laparoscopic colorectal surgery.

Postoperative surgical complications include the same as those after open colonic surgery, in addition to more laparoscopic-specific complications such as bleeding and port-site hernias. In laparoscopy, as in open surgery, anastomotic leaks are usually associated with technical failure or tension at the anastomosis with compromised blood supply. Therefore, a tension-free anastomosis and adequate blood supply are essential and, if this cannot be achieved laparoscopically, the procedure should be converted to a laparotomy. The overall anastomotic leak rate in recent laparoscopic surgery series is 0% to 4.5% (121,136,150). These figures are comparable to open colonic surgeries with a leak rate of 3% to 7% (155,156). As in open colonic resections, clinical leaks are most frequently seen with anastomoses of the rectum, ranging from 12.7% to 20% (136,143,157), and similar to the rates in open surgery (158,159). In a large series reporting 949 laparoscopic colonic resections, the majority of the anastomoses were performed extracorporeally, the overall clinical leak rate was 4.25%; with 2.9% in the colon and 12.7% in the rectum. Approximately, one-fourth of the patients who developed leaks had to be reoperated (136). A lower leak rate was seen in patients who underwent surgery for benign colonic diseases (150).

Intra-abdominal abscesses may result from various factors related to technical problems, location of anastomosis (rectal vs. non-rectal), or associated medical conditions. The rate of intraoperative abscesses after laparoscopic colonic surgery is relatively lower or equal to that reported for open series, and is in the range of 1% (150).

One of the benefits of laparoscopic surgery is a decreased wound infection rate. This has been demonstrated in several reports where the wound infection rate is reportedly in the range of 2% to 7.2% (130,136,143,150) compared to an average of 11% in open colorectal resections (160). However, a one report (161) demonstrated that the extraction site for laparoscopic colonic resection could be associated with an even higher incidence of infection and incisional hernia, compared to open colectomy. Therefore, strategies to alter operative technique should be considered to reduce the incidence of these potential complications.

Although small bowel obstruction due to adhesion formation should theoretically develop less frequently after laparoscopic procedures, there have been reported incidences of this postoperative complication. Another cause of small bowel obstruction with laparoscopic colorectal surgery is internal hernia, suggesting the need to close the mesenteric defect after colorectal resections.

Complications Unique to Laparoscopic Colorectal Surgery

There are a few postoperative complications unique to laparoscopic colorectal surgery. Missed or insecure bleeding sources during laparoscopy may present postoperatively and may necessitate abdominal exploration. This problem can be avoided by meticulous homeostasis during the laparoscopic procedure. However, this is not a common complication, and is reported in only 1% of laparoscopic colorectal procedures (130). Another potential and much more common complication is port-site hernia, which can manifest early in the postoperative period as either an incarcerated hernia or an incisional hernia. An incarcerated trocar-site hernia may go unrecognized and develop into ischemic bowel with associated morbidity and mortality (132). Port-site hernias can be almost completely avoided by ensuring routine secure closure of the fascial opening (131).

Intraoperative iatrogenic complications such as bleeding, bowel injury, or ureteral tears, which may go undetected during the procedure may manifest postoperatively, thereby causing substantial morbidity. Therefore, intraoperative diagnosis and immediate treatment is the key to avoiding late and potentially devastating sequelae.

Surgeon Experience and Procedure Complexity

Several studies have demonstrated that surgeon experience and the complexity of the procedure have an impact on the incidence of complications (79,131,134). Studies addressing the issue of surgeon experience in laparoscopic colorectal surgery have demonstrated a substantial decrease in the complication rate when comparing surgeon experience. In an analysis comparing high-volume surgeons to low-volume surgeons, the probability of intraoperative and postoperative complications was lower for surgeons who had performed more than 40 laparoscopic procedures. The intraoperative, as well as postoperative complication rates were almost double in patients who were treated by less experienced surgeons (6.3% vs. 3.7% for intraoperative complications, and 18.6% vs. 9.9% for postoperative complications) (79). Another study showed that a significant decrease in intraoperative complications could be achieved after a surgeon had performed 55 laparoscopic procedures (134). However, other important factors may influence the learning curve of an individual surgeon including prior experience in other laparoscopic procedures as well as colorectal procedures.

Laparoscopic colorectal surgery encompasses a wide variety of various operations with different pathologies. Complex laparoscopic procedures may increase the risk for intraoperative complications. Low-anterior resection, sigmoid resection for diverticulitis, and more extensive procedures such as subtotal abdominal colectomy and total proctocolectomy are more difficult to perform laparoscopically and may harbor a greater risk for intraoperative complications (132–134). It is important to note that, in most series, previous abdominal operations were not found to increase the risk of intraoperative complications (79,131,132,134).

Surgeon experience may signify better technical skills, better patient selection, and often an improvement in technology. The most important factors in avoiding potential complications are careful patient selection, and adequate training in laparoscopic instrumentation and stapling devices. Timely conversion is a crucial factor in avoiding complications and should be considered without hesitation, when necessary. Despite these precautions, complications may occur; early identification and treatment is the key for minimizing their consequences.

CONCLUSIONS

The laparoscopic revolution had an enormous impact in almost all surgical fields including colorectal surgery. Compared to the excellent and obvious advantages in cholecystectomy, laparoscopic colorectal surgery has had more modest proven benefits. This is due to the fact that colorectal procedures are technically more challenging, require good laparoscopic skills, and a large experience. Nevertheless, laparoscopy in colorectal surgery has gained a wider acceptance, and with experience in the various procedures, the postoperative benefits have become more pronounced and the cosmetic results more appealing to both the surgeon and the patient. There is still an association with longer operative times; however, this approach generally offers shorter hospital stay, improved pulmonary function, decreased postoperative pain, and the benefits of improved cosmesis. The controversy regarding the use of laparoscopy for colon cancer was recently resolved. Recent data indicate that this procedure is oncologically safe.

For the future, it is reasonable to assume that laparoscopy will have a broader role and will be adopted by increasingly more colorectal surgeons. For the new generations of surgeons who are trained in the laparoscopic era, it will be more natural to approach these patients laparoscopically. Technological developments and public demand will most likely contribute to this evolution.

REFERENCES

1. Semm K. New methods of pelviscopy (gynecologic laparoscopy) for myomectomy, varicectomy, tubectomy, and adenectomy. Endoscopy 1979; 11(2):85–93.
2. Mouret P. Celioscopic surgery. Evolution or revolution? Chirurgie 1990; 116(10):829–832; discussion 832–833.
3. Rappaport WD, Gordon P, Warneke JA, Neal D, Hunter GC. Contraindications and complications of laparoscopic cholecystectomy. Am Fam Physician 1994; 50(8):1707–1711, 1714.
4. Fischer CP, Castaneda A, Moore F. Laparoscopic appendectomy: indications and controversies. Semin Laparosc Surg 2002; 9(1):32–39.
5. Schwab JR, Beaird DA, Ramshaw BJ, et al. After 10 years and 1903 inguinal hernias, what is the outcome for the laparoscopic repair? Surg Endosc 2002; 16(8):1201–1206.
6. Rawlins MC, Hefty TL, Brown SL, Biehl TR. Learning laparoscopic donor nephrectomy safely: a report on 100 cases. Arch Surg 2002; 137(5):531–534.
7. Pillinger SH, Bambach CP, Sidhu S. Laparoscopic adrenalectomy: a 6-year experience of 59 cases. ANZ J Surg 2002; 72(7):467–470.
8. Gentileschi P, Kini S, Catarci M, Gagner M. Evidence-based medicine: open and laparoscopic bariatric surgery. Surg Endosc 2002; 16(5):736–744.
9. Trus TL, Hunter JG. Minimally invasive surgery of the esophagus and stomach. Am J Surg 1997; 173(3):242–255.
10. Telsey JI, Caldamone AA. Laparoscopy in pediatric urology. Curr Urol Rep 2001; 2(2):132–137.
11. Kaiser LR, Shrager JB. Video-assisted thoracic surgery: the current state of the art. AJR Am J Roentgenol 1995; 165(5):1111–1117.
12. Matarasso A. Minimal-access variations in abdominoplasty. Ann Plast Surg 1995; 34(3):255–263.
13. Dargent DF. Laparoscopic surgery in gynecologic oncology. Surg Clin North Am 2001; 81(4):949–964.
14. Montz FJ. Managed care in benign gynecology. Curr Opin Obstet Gynecol 1997; 9(4):267–269.
15. Jacobs M, Verdeja JC, Goldstein HS. Minimally invasive colon resection (laparoscopic colectomy). Surg Laparosc Endosc 1991; 1(3):144–150.
16. Zmora O, Weiss EG. Trocar site recurrence in laparoscopic surgery for colorectal cancer. Myth or real concern? Surg Oncol Clin N Am 2001; 10(3):625–638.
17. Lacy AM, Garcia-Valdecasas JC, Delgado S, et al. Laparoscopy-assisted colectomy versus open colectomy for treatment of non-metastatic colon cancer: a randomised trial. Lancet 2002; 359(9325): 2224–2229.
18. Pikarsky AJ. Update on prospective randomized trials of laparoscopic surgery for colorectal cancer. Surg Oncol Clin N Am 2001; 10(3):639–653.
19. Sands DR, Wexner SD. Nasogastric tubes and dietary advancement after laparoscopic and open colorectal surgery. Nutrition 1999; 15(5):347–350.
20. Berman IR. Sutureless laparoscopic rectopexy for procidentia. Technique and implications. Dis Colon Rectum 1992; 35(7):689–693.
21. Cuesta MA, Borgstein PJ, de Jong D, Meijer S. Laparoscopic rectopexy. Surg Laparosc Endosc 1993; 3(6):456–458.
22. Nessim A, Wexner SD. Minimally invasive anorectal surgery. In: Beck DE, Wexner SD, eds. Fundamentals of Anorectal Surgery. 2nd ed. London: WB Saunders, 1998:510–531.

23. Boccasanta P, Rosati R, Venturi M, et al. Comparison of laparoscopic rectopexy with open technique in the treatment of complete rectal prolapse: clinical and functional results. Surg Laparosc Endosc 1998; 8(6):460–465.

24. Solomon MJ, Eyers AA. Laparoscopic rectopexy using mesh fixation with a spiked chromium staple. Dis Colon Rectum 1996; 39(3):279–284.

25. Solomon MJ, Young CJ, Eyers AA, Roberts RA. Randomized clinical trial of laparoscopic versus open abdominal rectopexy for rectal prolapse. Br J Surg 2002; 89(1):35–39.

26. Zittel TT, Manncke K, Haug S, et al. Functional results after laparoscopic rectopexy for rectal prolapse. J Gastrointest Surg 2000; 4(6):632–641.

27. Winde G, Reers B, Nottberg H, Berns T, Meyer J, Bunte H. Clinical and functional results of abdominal rectopexy with Absorbable mesh-graft for treatment of complete rectal prolapse. Eur J Surg1993; 159(5):301–305.

28. Williams JG, Wong WD, Jensen L, Rothenberger DA, Goldberg SM. Incontinence and rectal prolapse: a prospective manometric study. Dis Colon Rectum 1991; 34(3):209–216.

29. Graf W, Stefansson T, Arvidsson D, Pahlman L. Laparoscopic suture rectopexy. Dis Colon Rectum 1995; 38(2):211–212.

30. Heah SM, Hartley JE, Hurley J, Duthie GS, Monson JR. Laparoscopic suture rectopexy without resection is effective treatment for full-thickness rectal prolapse. Dis Colon Rectum 2000; 43(5):638–643.

31. Baker R, Senagore AJ, Luchtefeld MA. Laparoscopic-assisted vs open resection. Rectopexy offers excellent results. Dis Colon Rectum 1995; 38(2):199–201.

32. Stevenson AR, Stitz RW, Lumley JW. Laparoscopic-assisted resection-rectopexy for rectal prolapse: early and medium follow-up. Dis Colon Rectum 1998; 41(1):46–54.

33. Darzi A, Henry MM, Guillou PJ, Shorvon P, Monson JR. Stapled laparoscopic rectopexy for rectal prolapse. Surg Endosc 1995; 9(3):301–303.

34. Bruch HP, Herold A, Schiedeck T, Schwandner O. Laparoscopic surgery for rectal prolapse and outlet obstruction. Dis Colon Rectum 1999; 42(9):1189–1194; discussion 1194–1195.

35. Blatchford GJ, Perry RE, Thorson AG, Christensen MA. Rectopexy without resection for rectal prolapse. Am J Surg 1989; 158(6):574–576.

36. Tjandra JJ, Fazio VW, Church JM, Milsom JW, Oakley JR, Lavery IC. Ripstein procedure is an effective treatment for rectal prolapse without constipation. Dis Colon Rectum 1993; 36(5):501–507.

37. Jacobs LK, Lin YJ, Orkin BA. The best operation for rectal prolapse. Surg Clin North Am 1997; 77(1):49–70 (Review).

38. Reissman P, Weiss E, Teoh TA, Cohen SM, Wexner SD. Laparoscopic-assisted perineal rectosigmoidectomy for rectal prolapse. Surg Laparosc Endosc 1995; 5(3):217–218.

39. Luukkonen P, Mikkonen U, Jarvinen H. Abdominal rectopexy with sigmoidectomy vs. rectopexy alone for rectal prolapse: a prospective, randomized study. Int J Colorectal Dis 1992; 7(4):219–222.

40. McKee RF, Lauder JC, Poon FW, Aitchison MA, Finlay IG. A prospective randomized study of abdominal rectopexy with and without sigmoidectomy in rectal prolapse. Surg Gynecol Obstet 1992; 174(2):145–148.

41. Darzi A, Super P, Guillou PJ, Monson JR. Laparoscopic sigmoid colectomy: total laparoscopic approach. Dis Colon Rectum 1994; 37(3):268–271.

42. Bergamaschi R, Tuetch JJ, Pessaux P, Arnaud JP. Intracorporeal vs. laparoscopic-assisted resection for uncomplicated diverticulitis of the sigmoid. Surg Endosc 2000; 14(6):520–523.

43. Bernstein MA, Dawson JW, Reissman P, Weiss EG, Nogueras JJ, Wexner SD. Is complete laparoscopic colectomy superior to laparoscopic assisted colectomy? Am Surg 1996; 62(6):507–511.

44. Gellman L, Salky B, Edye M. Laparoscopic-assisted colectomy. Surg Endosc 1996; 10(11):1041–1044.

45. Vargas HD, Ramirez RT, Hoffman GC, et al. Defining the role of laparoscopic-assisted sigmoid colectomy for diverticulitis. Dis Colon Rectum 2000; 43(12):1726–1731.

46. Schlachta CM, Mamazza J, Poulin EC. Laparoscopic sigmoid resection for acute and chronic diverticulitis. An outcomes comparison with laparoscopic resection for nondiverticular disease. Surg Endosc 1999; 13(7):649–653.

47. Fine AP. Laparoscopic surgery for inflammatory complications of acute sigmoid diverticulitis. JSLS 2001; 5(3):233–235.

48. Faranda C, Barrat C, Catheline JM, Champault GG. Two-stage laparoscopic management of generalized peritonitis due to perforated sigmoid diverticula: eighteen cases. Surg Laparosc Endosc 2000; 10(3):135–138; discussion 139.

49. Stevenson AR, Stitz RW, Lumley JW, Fielding GA. Laparoscopically assisted anterior resection for diverticular disease: follow-up of 100 consecutive patients. Ann Surg 1998; 227(3):335–342.

50. Tuech JJ, Pessaux P, Rouge C, Regenet N, Bergamaschi R, Arnaud JP. Laparoscopic vs. open colectomy for sigmoid diverticulitis: a prospective comparative study in the elderly. Surg Endosc 2000; 14(11):1031–1033.

51. Faynsod M, Stamos MJ, Arnell T, Borden C, Udani S, Vargas H. A case-control study of laparoscopic versus open sigmoid colectomy for diverticulitis. Am Surg 2000; 66(9):841–843.

52. Kockerling F, Schneider C, Reymond MA, et al. Laparoscopic resection of sigmoid diverticulitis. Results of a multicenter study. Laparoscopic Colorectal Surgery Study Group. Surg Endosc 1999; 13(6):567–571.

53. Wexner SD, Moscovitz ID. Laparoscopic colectomy in diverticular and Crohn's disease. Surg Clin North Am 2000; 80(4):1299–1319.
54. Siriser F. Laparoscopic-assisted colectomy for diverticular sigmoiditis. A single-surgeon prospective study of 65 patients. Surg Endosc 1999; 13(8):811–813.
55. Liberman MA, Phillips EH, Carroll BJ, Fallas M, Rosenthal R. Laparoscopic colectomy vs. traditional colectomy for diverticulitis. Outcome and costs. Surg Endosc 1996; 10(1):15–18.
56. Bruce CJ, Coller JA, Murray JJ, Schoetz DJ Jr., Roberts PL, Rusin LC. Laparoscopic resection for diverticular disease. Dis Colon Rectum 1996; 39(suppl 10):S1–S6.
57. Smadja C, Sbai Idrissi M, Tahrat M, et al. Elective laparoscopic sigmoid colectomy for diverticulitis. Results of a prospective study. Surg Endosc 1999; 13(7):645–648.
58. Sher ME, Agachan F, Bortul M, Nogueras JJ, Weiss EG, Wexner SD. Laparoscopic surgery for diverticulitis. Surg Endosc 1997; 11(3):264–267.
59. Benn PL, Wolff BG, Ilstrup DM. Level of anastomosis and recurrent colonic diverticulitis. Am J Surg 1986; 151(2):269–271.
60. Franklin ME Jr, Dorman JP, Jacobs M, Plasencia G. Is laparoscopic surgery applicable to complicated colonic diverticular disease? Surg Endosc 1997; 11(10):1021–1025.
61. O'Sullivan GC, Murphy D, O'Brien MG, Ireland A. Laparoscopic management of generalized peritonitis due to perforated colonic diverticula. Am J Surg 1996; 171(4):432–434.
62. Gurland BH, Wexner SD. Laparoscopic surgery for inflammatory bowel disease: results of the past decade. Inflammatory Bowel Dis 2002; 8(1):46–54.
63. Canin-Endres J, Salky B, Gattorno F, Edye M. Laparoscopically assisted intestinal resection in 88 patients with Crohn's disease. Surg Endosc 1999; 13(6):595–599.
64. Hurst RD, Cohen RD. The role of laparoscopy and strictureplasty in the management of inflammatory bowel disease. Semin Gastrointest Dis 2000; 11(1):10–17.
65. Wu JS, Birnbaum EH, Kodner IJ, Fry RD, Read TE, Fleshman JW. Laparoscopic-assisted ileocolic resections in patients with Crohn's disease: are abscesses, phlegmons, or recurrent disease contraindications? Surgery 1997; 122(4):682–688.
66. Bauer JJ, Harris MT, Grumbach NM, Gorfine SR. Laparoscopic-assisted intestinal resection for Crohn's disease. Which patients are good candidates? J Clin Gastroenterol 1996; 23(1):44–46.
67. Reissman P, Salky BA, Pfeifer J, Edye M, Jagelman DG, Wexner SD. Laparoscopic surgery in the management of inflammatory bowel disease. Am J Surg 1996; 171(1):47–50.
68. Hollyoak MA, Lumley J, Stitz RW. Laparoscopic stoma formation for faecal diversion. Br J Surg 1998; 85(2):226–228.
69. Oliveira L, Reissman P, Nogueras J, Wexner SD. Laparoscopic creation of stomas. Surg Endosc 1997; 11(1):19–23.
70. Borley NR, Mortensen NJ, Jewell DP. Preventing postoperative recurrence of Crohn's disease. Br J Surg 1997; 84(11):1493–1502.
71. Milsom JW, Lavery IC, Bohm B, Fazio VW. Laparoscopically assisted ileocolectomy in Crohn's disease. Surg Laparosc Endosc 1993; 3(2):77–80.
72. Hamel CT, Hildebrandt U, Weiss EG, Feifelz G, Wexner SD. Laparoscopic surgery for inflammatory bowel disease. Surg Endosc 2001; 15(7):642–645.
73. Alabaz O, Iroatulam AJ, Nessim A, Weiss EG, Nogueras JJ, Wexner SD. Comparison of laparoscopically assisted and conventional ileocolic resection for Crohn's disease. Eur J Surg 2000; 166(3): 213–217.
74. Dunker MS, Stiggelbout AM, van Hogezand RA, Ringers J, Griffioen G, Bemelman WA. Cosmesis and body image after laparoscopic-assisted and open ileocolic resection for Crohn's disease. Surg Endosc 1998; 12(11):1334–1340.
75. Bemelman WA, Slors JF, Dunker MS, et al. Laparoscopic-assisted vs. open ileocolic resection for Crohn's disease. A comparative study. Surg Endosc 2000; 14(8):721–725.
76. Milsom JW, Hammerhofer KA, Bohm B, Marcello P, Elson P, Fazio VW. Prospective, randomized trial comparing laparoscopic vs. conventional surgery for refractory ileocolic Crohn's disease. Dis Colon Rectum 2001; 44(1):1–8.
77. Wexner SD, Johansen OB, Nogueras JJ, Jagelman DG. Laparoscopic total abdominal colectomy. A prospective trial. Dis Colon Rectum 1992; 35(7):651–655.
78. Schmitt SL, Cohen SM, Wexner SD, Nogueras JJ, Jagelman DG. Does laparoscopic-assisted ileal pouch anal anastomosis reduce the length of hospitalization? Int J Colorectal Dis 1994; 9(3):134–137.
79. Bennett CL, Stryker SJ, Ferreira MR, et al. The learning curve for laparoscopic colorectal surgery. Preliminary results from a prospective analysis of 1194 laparoscopic-assisted colectomies. Arch Surg 1997; 132(1):41–44.
80. Marusch F, Gastinger I, Schneider C, et al. Experience as a factor influencing the indications for laparoscopic colorectal surgery and the results. Surg Endosc 2001; 15(2):116–120.
81. Araki Y, Ishibashi N, Ogata Y, et al. The usefulness of restorative laparoscopic assisted total colectomy for ulcerative colitis. Kurume Med J 2001; 48(2):99–103.
82. Seshadri PA, Poulin EC, Schlachta CM, et al. Does a laparoscopic approach to total abdominal colectomy and proctocolectomy offer advantages? Surg Endosc 2001; 15(8):837–842.
83. Marcello PW, Milsom JW, Wong SK, et al. Laparoscopic restorative proctocolectomy: case-matched comparative study with open restorative proctocolectomy. Dis Colon Rectum 2000; 43(5):604–608.

84. Dunker MS, Bemelman WA, Slors JF, et al. Laparoscopic-assisted vs. open colectomy for severe acute colitis in patients with inflammatory bowel disease (IBD): a retrospective study in 42 patients. Surg Endosc 2000; 14(10):911–914.

85. Marcello PW, Milsom JW, Wong SK, et al. Laparoscopic total colectomy for acute colitis: a case control study. Dis Colon Rectum 2001; 44(10):1441–1445.

86. Milsom JW, Ludwig KA, Church JM, Garcia-Ruiz A. Laparoscopic total abdominal colectomy with ileorectal anastomosis for familial adenomatous polyposis. Dis Colon Rectum 1997; 40(6): 675–678.

87. Schlinkert RT. Laparoscopic-assisted right hemicolectomy. Dis Colon Rectum 1991; 34(11):1030–1031.

88. Guillou PJ, Darzi A, Monson JR. Experience with laparoscopic colorectal surgery for malignant disease. Surg Oncol 1993; 2(suppl 1):43–49.

89. Goh YC, Eu KW, Seow-Choen F. Early postoperative results of a prospective series of laparoscopic vs. open anterior resections for rectosigmoid cancers. Dis Colon Rectum 1997; 40(7):776–780.

90. Yong L, Deane M, Monson JR, Darzi A. Systematic review of laparoscopic surgery for colorectal malignancy. Surg Endosc 2001; 15(12):1431–1439.

91. Bardram L, Funch-Jensen P, Jensen P, Crawford ME, Kehlet H. Recovery after laparoscopic colonic surgery with epidural analgesia, and early oral nutrition and mobilisation. Lancet 1995; 345(8952): 763–764.

92. Han-Geurts IJ, Jeekel J, Tilanus HW, Brouwer KJ. Randomized clinical trial of patient-controlled versus fixed regimen feeding after elective abdominal surgery. Br J Surg 2001; 88(12):1578–1582.

93. Ortiz H, Armendariz P, Yarnoz C. Early postoperative feeding after elective colorectal surgery is not a benefit unique to laparoscopy-assisted procedures. Int J Colorectal Dis 1996; 11(5):246–249.

94. Weeks JC, Nelson H, Gelber S, Sargent D, Schroeder G. Short-term quality-of-life outcomes following laparoscopic-assisted colectomy vs. open colectomy for colon cancer: a randomized trial. JAMA 2002; 287(3):321–328.

95. Marescaux J, Rubino F, Leroy J, Henri M. Laparoscopic-assisted surgery for colon cancer. JAMA 2002; 287(15):1938–1939.

96. Alexander RJ, Jacques BC, Mitchell KG. Laparoscopically assisted colectomy and wound recurrence. Lancet 1993; 341(8839):249–250.

97. Nduka CC, Monson JR, Menzies-Gow N, Darzi A. Abdominal wall metastases following laparoscopy. Br J Surg 1994; 81(5):648–652.

98. Jacquet P, Averbach AM, Jacquet N. Abdominal wall metastasis and peritoneal carcinomatosis after laparoscopic-assisted colectomy for colon cancer. Eur J Surg Oncol 1995; 21(5):568–570.

99. Kadar N. Port-site recurrences following laparoscopic operations for gynaecological malignancies. Br J Obstet Gynaecol 1997; 104(11):1308–1313.

100. Lundberg O, Kristoffersson A. Port site metastases from gallbladder cancer after laparoscopic cholecystectomy. Results of a Swedish survey and review of published reports. Eur J Surg 1999; 165(3):215–222.

101. Berends FJ, Kazemier G, Bonjer HJ, Lange JF. Subcutaneous metastases after laparoscopic colectomy. Lancet 1994; 344(8914):58.

102. Cirocco WC, Schwartzman A, Golub RW. Abdominal wall recurrence after laparoscopic colectomy for colon cancer. Surgery 1994; 116(5):842–846.

103. Stocchi L, Nelson H. Wound recurrences following laparoscopic-assisted colectomy for cancer. Arch Surg 2000; 135(8):948–958.

104. Hewett PJ, Texler ML, Anderson D, King G, Chatterton BE. In vivo real-time analysis of intraperitoneal radiolabeled tumor cell movement during laparoscopy. Dis Colon Rectum 1999; 42(7):868–875.

105. Knolmayer TJ, Asbun HJ, Shibata G, Bowyer MW. An experimental model of cellular aerosolization during laparoscopic surgery. Surg Laparosc Endosc 1997; 7(5):399–402.

106. Hewett PJ, Thomas WM, King G, Eaton M. Intraperitoneal cell movement during abdominal carbon dioxide insufflation and laparoscopy. An in vivo model. Dis Colon Rectum 1996; 39(suppl 10): S62–S66.

107. Wittich P, Marquet RL, Kazemier G, Bonjer HJ. Port-site metastases after CO(2) laparoscopy. Is aerosolization of tumor cells a pivotal factor? Surg Endosc 2000; 14(2):189–192.

108. Allardyce RA, Morreau P, Bagshaw PF. Operative factors affecting tumor cell distribution following laparoscopic colectomy in a porcine model. Dis Colon Rectum 1997; 40(8):939–945.

109. Pauwels M, Lauwers P, Hendriks J, Hubens A, Eyskens E, Hubens G. The effect of CO2 pneumoperitoneum on the growth of a solid colon carcinoma in rats. Surg Endosc 1999; 13(10):998–1000.

110. Gutt CN, Riemer V, Kim ZG, Jacobi CA, Paolucci V, Lorenz M. Impact of laparoscopic colonic resection on tumour growth and spread in an experimental model. Br J Surg 1999; 86(9):1180–1184.

111. Southall JC, Lee SW, Allendorf JD, Bessler M, Whelan RL. Colon adenocarcinoma and B-16 melanoma grow larger following laparotomy vs. pneumoperitoneum in a murine model. Dis Colon Rectum 1998; 41(5):564–569.

112. Neuhaus SJ, Ellis T, Rofe AM, Pike GK, Jamieson GG, Watson DI. Tumor implantation following laparoscopy using different insufflation gases. Surg Endosc 1998; 12(11):1300–1302.

113. Jacobi CA, Wenger FA, Ordemann J, Gutt C, Sabat R, Muller JM. Experimental study of the effect of intra-abdominal pressure during laparoscopy on tumour growth and port site metastasis. Br J Surg 1998; 85(10):1419–1422.

114. Lee SW, Southall J, Allendorf J, Bessler M, Whelan RL. Traumatic handling of the tumor independent of pneumoperitoneum increases port site implantation rate of colon cancer in a murine model. Surg Endosc 1998; 12(6):828–834.

115. Mathew G, Watson DI, Rofe AM, Baigrie CF, Ellis T, Jamieson GG. Wound metastases following laparoscopic and open surgery for abdominal cancer in a rat model. Br J Surg 1996; 83(8):1087–1090.

116. Tseng LN, Berends FJ, Wittich P, et al. Port-site metastases. Impact of local tissue trauma and gas leakage. Surg Endosc 1998; 12(12):1377–1380.

117. Fleshman JW, Nelson H, Peters WR, et al. Early results of laparoscopic surgery for colorectal cancer. Retrospective analysis of 372 patients treated by Clinical Outcomes of Surgical Therapy (COST) Study Group. Dis Colon Rectum 1996; 39(suppl 10):S53–S58.

118. Hughes ES, McDermott FT, Polglase AL, Johnson WR. Tumor recurrence in the abdominal wall scar tissue after large-bowel cancer surgery. Dis Colon Rectum 1983; 26(9):571–572.

119. Reilly WT, Nelson H, Schroeder G, Wieand HS, Bolton J, O'Connell MJ. Wound recurrence following conventional treatment of colorectal cancer. A rare but perhaps underestimated problem. Dis Colon Rectum 1996; 39(2):200–207.

120. Stage JG, Schulze S, Moller P, et al. Prospective randomized study of laparoscopic versus open colonic resection for adenocarcinoma. Br J Surg 1997; 84(3):391–396.

121. Milsom JW, Bohm B, Hammerhofer KA, Fazio V, Steiger E, Elson P. A prospective, randomized trial comparing laparoscopic versus conventional techniques in colorectal cancer surgery: a preliminary report. J Am Coll Surg 1998; 187(1):46–54; discussion 54–55.

122. Leung KL, Meng WC, Lee JF, Thung KH, Lai PB, Lau WY. Laparoscopic-assisted resection of right-sided colonic carcinoma: a case-control study. J Surg Oncol 1999; 71(2):97–100.

123. Franklin ME, Kazantsev GB, Abrego D, Diaz-E JA, Balli J, Glass JL. Laparoscopic surgery for stage III colon cancer: long-term follow-up. Surg Endosc 2000; 14(7):612–616.

124. Hartley JE, Mehigan BJ, Qureshi AE, Duthie GS, Lee PW, Monson JR. Total mesorectal excision: assessment of the laparoscopic approach. Dis Colon Rectum 2001; 44(3):315–321.

125. Lord SA, Larach SW, Ferrara A, Williamson PR, Lago CP, Lube MW. Laparoscopic resections for colorectal carcinoma. A three-year experience. Dis Colon Rectum 1996; 39(2):148–154.

126. Schiedeck TH, Schwandner O, Baca I, et al. Laparoscopic surgery for the cure of colorectal cancer: results of a German five-center study. Dis Colon Rectum 2000; 43(1):1–8.

127. Poulin EC, Mamazza J, Schlachta CM, Gregoire R, Roy N. Laparoscopic resection does not adversely affect early survival curves in patients undergoing surgery for colorectal adenocarcinoma. Ann Surg 1999; 229(4):487–492.

128. Clinical Outcomes of Surgical Therapy Study Group. A comparison of laparoscopically assisted and open colectomy for colon cancer. N Engl J Med 2004; 350(20):2050–2059.

129. Chen HH, Wexner SD, Weiss EG, et al. Laparoscopic colectomy for benign colorectal disease is associated with a significant reduction in disability as compared with laparotomy. Surg Endosc 1998; 12(12):1397–1400.

130. Schlachta CM, Mamazza J, Seshadri PA, Cadeddu M, Poulin EC. Determinants of outcomes in laparoscopic colorectal surgery: a multiple regression analysis of 416 resections. Surg Endosc 2000; 14(3):258–263.

131. Larach SW, Patankar SK, Ferrara A, Williamson PR, Perozo SE, Lord AS. Complications of laparoscopic colorectal surgery. Analysis and comparison of early vs. latter experience. Dis Colon Rectum 1997; 40(5):592–596.

132. Kockerling F, Schneider C, Reymond MA, et al. Early results of a prospective multicenter study on 500 consecutive cases of laparoscopic colorectal surgery. Laparoscopic Colorectal Surgery Study Group (LCSSG). Surg Endosc 1998; 12(1):37–41.

133. Schwandner O, Schiedeck TH, Bruch H. The role of conversion in laparoscopic colorectal surgery: do predictive factors exist? Surg Endosc 1999; 13(2):151–156.

134. Agachan F, Joo JS, Weiss EG, Wexner SD. Intraoperative laparoscopic complications. Are we getting better? Dis Colon Rectum 1996; 39(suppl 10):S14–S19.

135. Marusch F, Gastinger I, Schneider C, et al. Importance of conversion for results obtained with laparoscopic colorectal surgery. Dis Colon Rectum 2001; 44(2):207–214; discussion 214–216.

136. Kockerling F, Rose J, Schneider C, et al. Laparoscopic colorectal anastomosis: risk of postoperative leakage. Results of a multicenter study. Laparoscopic Colorectal Surgery Study Group (LCSSG).Surg Endosc 1999; 13(7):639–644.

137. Wexner SD, Reissman P, Pfeifer J, Bernstein M, Geron N. Laparoscopic colorectal surgery: analysis of 140 cases. Surg Endosc 1996; 10(2):133–136.

138. Fingerhut A, Hay JM, Elhadad A, Lacaine F, Flamant Y. Supraperitoneal colorectal anastomosis: hand-sewn versus circular staples—a controlled clinical trial. French Associations for Surgical Research. Surgery 1995; 118(3):479–485.

139. Kessler H, Hermanek P Jr., Wiebelt H. Operative mortality in carcinoma of the rectum. Results of the German Multicentre Study. Int J Colorectal Dis 1993; 8(3):158–166.

140. West of Scotland and Highland Anastomosis Study Group. Suturing or stapling in gastrointestinal surgery: a prospective randomized study. Br J Surg 1991; 78(3):337–341.

141. Tucker JG, Ambroze WL, Orangio GR, Duncan TD, Mason EM, Lucas GW. Laparoscopically assisted bowel surgery. Analysis of 114 cases. Surg Endosc 1995; 9(3):297–300.

142. Agachan F, Joo JS, Sher M, Weiss EG, Nogueras JJ, Wexner SD. Laparoscopic colorectal surgery. Do we get faster? Surg Endosc 1997; 11(4):331–335.

143. Lacy AM, Garcia-Valdecasas JC, Delgado S, et al. Postoperative complications of laparoscopic-assisted colectomy. Surg Endosc 1997; 11(2):119–122.

144. Reissman P, Agachan F, Wexner SD. Outcome of laparoscopic colorectal surgery in older patients. Am Surg 1996; 62(12):1060–1063.

145. Kennedy HL, Rothenberger DA, Goldberg SM, et al. Colocolostomy and coloproctostomy utilizing the circular intraluminal stapling devices. Dis Colon Rectum 1983; 26(3):145–148.

146. Detry RJ, Kartheuser A, Delriviere L, Saba J, Kestens PJ. Use of the circular stapler in 1000 consecutive colorectal anastomoses: experience of one surgical team. Surgery 1995; 117(2):140–145.

147. Frazee RC, Roberts JW, Okeson GC, et al. Open versus laparoscopic cholecystectomy. A comparison of postoperative pulmonary function. Ann Surg 1991; 213(6):651–653; discussion 653–654.

148. Poulin EC, Mamazza J, Breton G, Fortin CL, Wabha R, Ergina P. Evaluation of pulmonary function in laparoscopic cholecystectomy. Surg Laparosc Endosc 1992; 2(4):292–296.

149. Katkhouda N, Hurwitz MB, Rivera RT, et al. Laparoscopic splenectomy: outcome and efficacy in 103 consecutive patients. Ann Surg 1998; 228(4):568–578 (Review).

150. Poulin EC, Schlachta CM, Seshadri PA, Cadeddu MO, Gregoire R, Mamazza J. Septic complications of elective laparoscopic colorectal resection. Surg Endosc 2001; 15(2):203–208.

151. Lau WY, Chu KW, Poon GP, Ho KK. Prophylactic antibiotics in elective colorectal surgery. Br J Surg 1988; 75(8):782–785.

152. Mendes da Costa P, Kaufman L. Amikacin once daily plus metronidazole versus amikacin twice daily plus metronidazole in colorectal surgery. Hepatogastroenterology 1992; 39(4):350–354.

153. Lumley JW, Siu SK, Pillay SP, et al. Single dose ceftriaxone as prophylaxis for sepsis in colorectal surgery. Aust N Z J Surg 1992; 62(4):292–296.

154. Jensen LS, Andersen A, Fristrup SC, et al. Comparison of one dose versus three doses of prophylactic antibiotics, and the influence of blood transfusion, on infectious complications in acute and elective colorectal surgery. Br J Surg 1990; 77(5):513–518.

155. Laxamana A, Solomon MJ, Cohen Z, Feinberg SM, Stern HS, McLeod RS. Long-term results of anterior resection using the double-stapling technique. Dis Colon Rectum 1995; 38(12):1246–1250.

156. Lazorthes F, Chiotassol P. Stapled colorectal anastomoses: preoperative integrity of the anastomosis and risk of postoperative leakage. Int J Colorectal Dis 1986; 1(2):96–98.

157. Monson JR, Darzi A, Carey PD, Guillou PJ. Prospective evaluation of laparoscopic-assisted colectomy in an unselected group of patients. Lancet 1992; 340(8823):831–833.

158. Antonsen HK, Kronborg O. Early complications after low anterior resection for rectal cancer using the EEA stapling device. A prospective trial. Dis Colon Rectum 1987; 30(8):579–583.

159. Feinberg SM, Parker F, Cohen Z, et al. The double stapling technique for low anterior resection of rectal carcinoma. Dis Colon Rectum 1986; 29(12):885–890.

160. Song F, Glenny AM. Antimicrobial prophylaxis in colorectal surgery: a systematic review of randomized controlled trials. Br J Surg 1998; 85(9):1232–1241.

161. Winslow ER, Fleshman JW, Birnbaum EH, Brunt LM. Wound complications of laparoscopic vs. open colectomy. Surg Endosc 2002; 16(10):1420–1425.

9 | Anorectal Physiology Testing

Richard E. Karulf
Division of Colon and Rectal Surgery, Department of Surgery, University of Minnesota, Minneapolis, Minnesota, U.S.A.

Jimmy S. Levine
Minnesota Gastroenterology, Minneapolis, Minnesota, U.S.A.

INTRODUCTION

Objective evaluation of the function and dysfunction of the pelvic floor and associated disorders of defecation is a relatively new trend. Improvement in equipment and information has made the pelvic floor laboratory an essential element in the practice of medicine. The individual elements of the pelvic floor laboratory vary widely based on the influence of regional experience and preferences (1). A thorough investigation of the pelvic floor, with a judiciously selected panel of tests, will provide the practitioner with the best clues to evaluate and intervene in clinical disorders associated with continence.

PELVIC FLOOR LABORATORY

Anorectal physiologic studies have become essential tools in the treatment of pelvic floor disorders. Although individual tests can be performed, the chief value of a pelvic floor laboratory is in the performance of a battery of tests that will allow a more thorough understanding of all aspects of pelvic floor function.

Staff

The staff of the modern pelvic floor center consists of specially trained technicians, nurses, and physicians who are committed to providing specialized testing in an atmosphere that protects the dignity of patients with potentially embarrassing problems. The purpose of such a unit is to centralize the unique, low volume tests that are crucial to assessing patients with pelvic floor disorders. The tests available in the center are relatively specialized and require a commitment by the staff to insure accurate, reproducible results. Patients generally prefer a pelvic floor center, because of the convenience of a single location for multiple tests. In addition to the performance of pre and postoperative testing, many pelvic floor centers serve the community by offering biofeedback training and providing information to the public on a range of topics related to disorders of the pelvic floor. This combination of skill, compassion, and education is essential in order to build a trusting relationship between patients and staff.

Standardization

Previously, one of the main complaints with the medical literature pertaining to the physiology of the pelvic floor was the lack of standardization. More recently, attempts have been made to develop uniform techniques and terminology in the evaluation of the pelvic floor. For example, the French Society of Digestive Motility published a paper documenting their attempt to standardize the terminology associated with anorectal manometry (2). Other authors have attempted to provide normal values for anorectal manometry including anal canal length, resting pressure, and squeeze pressures (3–7); other tests have received similar attention.

The term "fecal incontinence" is difficult to precisely define. In some instances, a distinction is made between patients who leak liquid stool or have solid stool smears on their undergarments from patients with true fecal incontinence (8), while others have included all of these patients in the incontinent group. In addition to defining the type of incontinence, it is important to characterize the magnitude of fecal soiling and to identify the impact of incontinence on lifestyle. A validated quality of life scale for fecal incontinence has been published, which incorporates many of these elements (9). Finally, widespread standards must be established for the treatment of incontinence, in a manner similar to those published for anal sphincter replacement with artificial anal sphincter (10).

"Constipation" is also a term that may be variably defined. Some patients refer to constipation when they have hard stools, others report difficulty with evacuation, and still others understand it to mean infrequent bowel movements. Several scoring systems exist for constipation (11,12), but none have been universally employed. Without a clear definition of terms, it is difficult to quantify improvements or compare results among studies or institutions.

VECTOR ANALYSIS OF BOWEL CONTINENCE

Understanding pelvic floor physiology relies on the basic principles of physics. A vector is a mathematical representation of a magnitude of force and the direction in which the force is applied; stool follows the laws of physics. The movement of stool through the colon and rectum can, therefore, be analyzed by examining the pressure vectors that act upon the stool. In other words, stool will remain at rest if the pressure vectors are equal in all directions or follow the path of least resistance if there are unequal forces.

When the concept of vector analysis is applied to bowel continence, two major categories of opposing forces appear (Fig. 1). Propulsive forces are those factors with a pressure vector that would result in the elimination of stool from the body. Resistive forces are factors that slow or prevent elimination of stool from the body. A patient with "normal continence" is able to consciously control the balance of propulsive forces and resistive forces. Patients with incontinence have propulsive forces that consistently exceed the resistive forces while the opposite is true of patients with constipation or outlet obstruction. When examined from this perspective, pelvic floor disorders may be considered as a complex system to be understood rather than a one-dimensional problem.

Propulsive Forces

Forces that increase the movement of stool through the colon and out of the rectum are defined as propulsive forces.

Peristalsis

The most obvious propulsive force is peristalsis of the colon and rectum. The colon exhibits both segmental contraction and mass movement peristalsis of stool and may produce forward and retrograde movement of stool. Patients infected with cholera may have such forceful peristalsis that fecal continence is impossible even with a normal sphincter complex. Although peristalsis is indirectly evaluated with transit studies, none of the conventional tests measure this factor.

Valsalva
Patients often bear down when attempting to evacuate. This Valsalva maneuver, when properly performed, increases intra-abdominal pressure and transmits pressure to the stool to

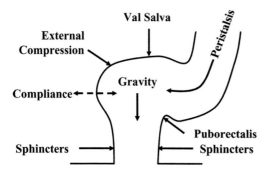

Figure 1 Concept of factors influencing defecation can be shown with pressure vectors.

assist in evacuation. However, when improperly performed, the Valsalva maneuver may hinder defecation. The effects of a Valsalva maneuver can be visualized during defecography or measured during anorectal manometry.

Gravity

While the force of gravity may be small compared to other propulsive forces, it cannot be overlooked. For example, many patients cannot reproduce a rectal prolapse when lying in the left lateral decubitus position but can readily do so when seated on a commode. This factor is rarely measured and is often negated by measuring patients while they are lying in the left lateral decubitus position.

Resistive Forces

Forces that impede the movement of stool are termed "resistive forces." The resistance may be active or passive. Active resistance is usually linked to the three sphincter muscles described below, whereas passive resistance is attributed to structures outside the rectal wall and to strictures of the rectum itself.

Primary Muscles

There are three muscles that are traditionally associated with control of stool: the puborectalis and the internal and external anal sphincters. Each of these muscles must be assessed to identify damage or dysfunction.

Puborectalis

Parks described a flap-valve theory in which the puborectalis created an acute anorectal angle to prevent rectal contents from reaching the anus (13). Intra-abdominal pressure forces were assumed to push the anterior rectal wall to occlude the top of the anal canal and prevent the escape of stool. In this theory, the primary burden of fecal control lies with the puborectalis, and its control of the anorectal angle and the sphincters provide only fine control. Studies have since shown that the anterior rectal wall does not come in contact with the upper anal canal during Valsalva, as would be expected if a flap-valve mechanism was present (14). The result is that the control of stool appears to be primarily due to the internal and external anal sphincters and the role of the anorectal angle and the puborectalis, with regard to fecal continence, is questionable. The anorectal angle and movement of the pelvic floor are best studied with defecography.

Internal Anal Sphincter

The primary component of resting tone of the anal canal is the pressure supplied by the internal anal sphincter. As smooth muscle, it is not under voluntary control and is active when the patient is asleep or distracted. Under normal circumstances, the internal anal sphincter relaxes when the rectum is distended. This rectoanal inhibitory reflex is not present in patients with Hirschsprung's disease but is present in most other forms of functional pelvic outlet obstruction. This reflex and the influence of the internal anal sphincter are best measured with anorectal manometry. Patients with anal fissures and primary anal sphincter hypertonia may have increased resting tone, which is commonly due to increased tone in the internal anal sphincter. Anatomic defects in the internal anal sphincter can be measured with endorectal ultrasound.

External Anal Sphincter

The majority of the increase in pressure noted in the anal canal during a squeeze maneuver is due to the influence of the external anal sphincter. The external sphincter may be investigated from a number of perspectives. Various forms of electromyography have been used to assess the innervation of the sphincter; ultrasound and magnetic resonance imaging (MRI) have been used to assess anatomic defects, and anorectal manometry has been used to measure the pressure generated by this muscle.

Passive Resistance

In contrast to the sphincters and levators, which actively oppose the movement of stool, other anatomic factors can provide passive resistance. These factors include strictures, angulation of the bowel, decreased compliance, and poor fixation of the rectosigmoid colon, resulting in prolapse or internal intussusception. All of these factors are best visualized using radiological techniques, including defecography. Some authors have reported increasing passive resistance as a method of treating fecal incontinence (15).

Although accessory muscles are not classically thought to be important in fecal control, they may incrementally increase the resting pressure in some patients. The use of accessory muscles is especially noted in patients with anal sphincter dysfunction and marginal continence.

CURRENT USES FOR ANORECTAL PHYSIOLOGIC TESTING

A wide range of testing options are available for the evaluation of anorectal physiology and abnormalities of evacuation (16). From this menu of tests, providers are able to select either individual tests or a panel of complementary tests based on the presenting symptoms of individual patients (Tables 1 and 2). Every patient may not require all tests; however, it is not unusual to discover multiple factors that contribute to abnormalities of evacuation.

Fecal Incontinence

There are many ways to subcharacterize patients with fecal incontinence in order to better direct treatment. A simple schema is to divide the patients into three groups: patients with sphincter defects, patients with problems associated with nerve injuries, and patients with abnormalities of transit.

Segmental Sphincter Defects

Patients with known or suspected birth injuries or with a history of anorectal surgery should be evaluated for possible segmental sphincter defects. The defect in the internal and external anal sphincters may result in decreased pressures, as determined by anorectal manometry, and an abnormal pressure vector symmetry index. The status of the pudendal nerves must be evaluated in addition to assessing the integrity of the internal and external anal sphincter with endoanal ultrasound to identify potentially correctable sphincter defects.

Neurogenic Fecal Incontinence

Nerve injury is a common cause of fecal incontinence. Use of electromyography including testing of the pudendal nerve terminal motor latency (PNTML) is important in patients with suspected nerve injury. Exclusion of other anatomic defects with endoanal ultrasound may also be beneficial.

Transit Abnormalities

Patients with very rapid transit colonic transit or with conditions that result in increased rectal compliance may have poor fecal control despite normal functioning anal sphincters and pudendal nerves. Evaluation of patients with this category of fecal incontinence usually involves defecography, endoscopy to identify the source of any increase in rectal compliance, manometry to assess the effectiveness of the sphincters, and colon or small-bowel transit studies.

Table 1 Choice of Physiology Tests Based on Symptoms or Presumed Diagnosis

	Segmental defect	Neurogenic incontinence	Slow-transit constipation	Hirschsprung's disease	Spastic puborectalis	Rectal Prolapse
Manometry	Suggested	Suggested	Suggested	Suggested	Suggested	Suggested
Balloon reflex	Optional	Optional	Suggested	Suggested	Suggested	Optional
Ultrasound	Suggested	Suggested	Optional	Optional	Optional	Optional
Electromyography recruitment	Optional	Suggested	Optional	Optional	Suggested	Optional
Pudendal nerve terminal motor latency	Suggested	Suggested	Suggested	Suggested	Suggested	Suggested
Defecography	Optional	Optional	Suggested	Suggested	Suggested	Suggested
Endoscopy	Optional	Optional	Suggested	Optional	Optional	Suggested
Marker study	Optional	Optional	Suggested	Optional	Optional	Optional

Table 2 Physiologic Tests, Factors Measured, and Common Uses

Type of physiology test	Factors measured	Common applications
Magnetic resonance imaging, positron emission tomography scan, computed tomography scan	Static pelvic anatomy	Cancer, cysts, abscesses
Endorectal ultrasonography	Distal rectal and anal anatomy	Fistulae, sphincter defects, cancer
Electromyography	Innervation and regeneration	Incontinence, Hirschsprung's disease
Colonic transit time study	Colonic motility	Constipation, outlet obstruction
Defecography	Dynamic pelvic anatomy	Rectal prolapse, rectocele, enterocele

Abbreviation: RI, .

Constipation/Pelvic Outlet Obstruction

There is a significant distinction when treating patients with obstructed defecation, slow transit constipation, and functional pelvic outlet obstruction. Patients with obstructed defecation are usually thought to have an anatomic blockage to evacuation of stool. Patients with slow transit constipation are able to evacuate stool, once it enters the rectum, but have prolonged transit through the proximal bowel. "Functional pelvic outlet obstruction" is a term reserved for patients who demonstrate an inability to pass stool even with normal colonic transit and no detectable anatomic obstruction.

The presence or absence of the rectoanal inhibitory reflex (RAIR) is useful in categorizing some forms of functional pelvic outlet obstruction. First described by Gowers, the RAIR is a reflex relaxation of the internal anal sphincter with distension of the rectum (17). Since this initial study, many centers have reported the absence of the RAIR in patients with Hirschsprung's disease. This test is usually performed with manometric assessment of the anal sphincter pressures during inflation of a small balloon inside the rectum and is sometime referred to as the balloon anorectal inhibitory reflex. Although this issue has been extensively studied, the precise nerve pathways are still a matter of debate. Several centers have reported that the spinal cord is not a major factor in the RAIR, except in patients in spinal shock, where the reflex is absent (18).

In contrast to Hirschsprung's disease, patients with paradoxical puborectalis and other forms of functional pelvic outlet obstruction have a normal RAIR. Still other patients, including those with multiple sclerosis and fecal incontinence, require a lower than normal volume of rectal distension to inhibit internal anal sphincter pressures compared with diabetic patients or normal controls (19).

Finally, patients can have constipation due to decreased sensation in the rectum. This form of constipation can be improved with biofeedback training in the absence of any other abnormality.

Rectal Prolapse/Intussusception

Many patients with rectal prolapse have associated disorders of defecation including fecal incontinence and constipation. Although there may be improvement in some or all of these disorders after surgery for prolapse, a complete evaluation of the pelvic floor is indicated before a decision is made regarding the type of treatment for prolapse. Routine evaluation would include defecography, electromyography, manometry, and, possibly, endoscopy to evaluate the colon prior to surgery. It is also not uncommon for patients with rectal prolapse to have other concomitant anatomic abnormalities such as cystocele and enterocele. If these are suspected, peritoneography and an evaluation of urinary function may be indicated.

MEASURED COMPONENTS OF NORMAL FUNCTION

Various facets of defecation can be measured. When the appropriate tests are indicated, patients can be assessed and treated based on understanding of the underlying anatomic or physiologic defect. A careful patient history and physical exam is performed in all cases, and questionnaires, bowel function diaries, and routine endoscopy are also valuable tools in many patients.

Sphincter Pressures

Anorectal manometry is used to measure the pressure of the anal canal (20). Pressure can be measured with perfused catheter systems, microtransducers, or balloon systems. In all of these systems, a panel of common parameters is routinely measured. Resting pressure refers to the pressure of the anal canal when the patient is relaxed and the rectum is empty. The main component of resting pressure is the pressure generated by the internal sphincter. Squeeze pressure is the pressure measured when the patient is voluntarily squeezing the external sphincter muscle and may be recorded as an average or as a maximum pressure. During prolonged squeeze, the external sphincter will tire, and a fatigue factor can be calculated. In multichannel perfused catheter systems, the symmetry of the anal canal can be examined, and a vector symmetry index can be calculated. Normal subjects have been measured with anorectal manometry (21) and the variation of resting pressures have been reported in normal healthy individuals, which can be used as baseline measurements (22).

Movement of the Pelvic Floor

The pelvic floor is a dynamic structure with complex movement. A number of techniques have been developed to assess pelvic floor anatomy and function. Defecography (or evacuation proctography) is performed with a fluoroscopic technique and radio-opaque contrast in the rectum. Common uses for this test include identification of rectocele, internal intussusception, and rectal prolapse, as well as testing for incomplete evacuation and perineal descent. The lack of correlation between patient symptoms and findings at defecography has been a common criticism; however, the information from this test is often helpful when supported by the results of other studies. Peritoneography can be used when an enterocele is suspected. In addition to rectal contrast, patients ingest oral contrast, and contrast is also inserted into the vagina and peritoneal cavity.

In addition to defecography, other tests measure the ability to evacuate stool from the rectum, the simplest of which is the balloon expulsion test. Some authors use this as an office-screening test for severe constipation (23). If the patient is unable to expel a water-filled balloon, the patient's complaint of constipation is felt to be verified, and further testing is indicated. A more sophisticated test employs 200 mL of isotope-labeled artificial stool, and a rectal ejection fraction may be calculated (24). This form of scintigraphy exposes the patient to a lower total dose of radiation than defecography but does not provide anatomic detail.

Integrity of the Sphincters

Disruption of the sphincter complex, due to surgical or obstetrical trauma, is the most common cause of surgically correctable fecal incontinence (25). Defects in the sphincters have been assessed by manometry (20) or with electromyography; however, the integrity of the internal and external anal sphincters is currently determined by a number of radiologic techniques (26). Anal sphincter anatomy has been investigated using intrarectal ultrasound, MRI, and positron emission tomography scan (7,27,28). The choice of tests is often made by the expertise of the individual physicians. In one series, ultrasound was the test most likely to alter management decisions regarding fecal incontinence (29). Other studies showed that 96% of sphincter muscle structural abnormalities could be identified with an MRI and an internal coil (30). Despite this information, one author has pointed out that morphologic assessment alone is unable to distinguish continent patients from incontinent patients after anorectal surgery (31).

Innervation

Electromyography may be performed to evaluate three aspects of the pelvic floor (16), map segmental sphincter defects, determine if the sphincter muscle contracts or relaxes during voluntary squeeze, and identify areas of nerve injury with reinnervation. Skeletal muscle electromyography can be performed with a surface electrode placed on the perianal skin or in the anal canal, using either concentric needles or a single-fiber electrode.

Measurement of the conduction of the pudendal nerves is important to distinguish incontinence from muscle injury from pudendal nerve injury. Stimulating and recording electrodes measure the conduction of the pudendal nerves by PNTML (32). Testing with PNTML is felt to be somewhat operator dependent with a steep learning curve (33). The PNTML is prolonged in neurogenic fecal incontinence and normal with segmental sphincter defects. While measuring sphincter integrity is important, one study showed that 8 of 22 patients with measurable sphincter defects had unsuspected pudendal neuropathy or extensive sphincter damage on anal electromyography that precluded sphincter repair (34). The damage to even one of the two pudendal nerves appears to have an impact on outcome after anal sphincter repair (35).

Bowel Motility

There is a wide range of normal results reported for human gut transit. Studies with ingested markers or radioisotopes have been used to distinguish normal from prolonged colon transit and possibly determine segments of prolonged transit (36,37). Patients with functional pelvic floor abnormalities often have delayed transit in the rectosigmoid colon. The utility of identification of prolonged segmental transit in the more proximal colon is controversial.

Sensation

Balloon inflation is used to identify sensory thresholds within the rectum (38). Authors often measure three different data points. The minimal sensory threshold is recorded as the volume of distension that can first be sensed by the patient. Values are also recorded at the volume that produces an urge to defecate and at the level that produces a sensation of pain (the maximum tolerable volume).

Rectal sensation is mediated through pelvic nerves because a pudendal block has no influence on the sensation of rectal filling. On the other hand, spinal anesthesia beginning at the L5-S1 level or transection of the pelvic nerves eliminates the sensation of rectal filling (18).

The rectum is not necessarily involved in the urge to defecate as patients with a low anastomosis are able to sense pressure. It is proposed that pressure or stretch receptors are located in the pelvic floor muscles. Inflation of a balloon near these pelvic floor muscles recreates the urge to defecate (18).

UNMEASURED COMPONENTS OF NORMAL FUNCTION

While there are many measured factors that influence defecation, those that cannot be measured are also legion, including rectal and colonic compliance, stool viscosity, dietary and pharmacologic factors, and psychological factors.

Compliance

Compliance is the measurement of the deformability or elasticity of a structure. If the colon or rectum is thickened or scarred, it is deemed to have a low compliance. Maximum tolerable volume measurements with balloon catheters in the rectum and balloon anal inhibitor reflex tests are not generally felt to accurately reflect rectal compliance. While some authors report compliance measurements, others feel that compliance cannot be measured in an open-ended system, such as the rectum (39,40). Measurements using air- or fluid-filled condoms will, at best, only approximate the compliance of the rectum. Furthermore, the caliber of the bowel being studied will affect the results obtained, making comparison of the results difficult or impossible. It is likely that compliance is an important concept in understanding the physiology of defecation, but clinical instruments for accurate measurement of rectal compliance have not yet been fully validated.

Stool Viscosity

Stool viscosity is a measure of the thickness or fluidity of the stool. If the stool is firm or hard, it will generally be easier to withhold for patients with impaired continence. Loose or liquid stool will benefit patients with strictures or other forms of functional outlet obstruction. Although the consistency of stool is considered in incontinence scoring (9), objective measurement of viscosity is rarely recorded.

Dietary Factors

The wide range of diets and the difficulty in recording foods that are consumed in the course of a week makes analysis of the effect of dietary factors on gut function difficult. Consultation with an experienced dietician may be beneficial; however, obtaining objective data will be a great challenge for most patients.

Pharmacologic Factors

Both prescription and nonprescription drugs can influence gut function (see Chapter 36). Dietary supplements, weight-loss agents, and even vitamins may contain substances that alter gut transit or viscosity. A careful review of all drugs that are taken by a patient is essential in order to try to identify causes for a change in gut function.

Psychological Factors

Toilet training is a learned behavior; therefore many authors have discussed the possible association between psychological factors and gut function. Over 50 years ago, Almy suggested an association between acute emotional stress and colonic function (41). Since that time, it has been shown that stress also alters small-bowel motility (42).

Cognitive function may also be an important factor. Patients with impaired cognitive function have been reported to have problems with rectal prolapse, incontinence, and constipation. It is unclear whether a threshold level of cognitive function required to have normal function exists.

Emotional trauma can result in alterations in continence or gut function. Although it is difficult to measure the influence of emotional or psychological factors on gut function, there is a high incidence of anxiety and depression in patients undergoing surgery for chronic constipation (43). This is also true in younger patients with chronic constipation (44). Young women with severe constipation are also reported to have a high incidence of psychosexual dysfunction and personality disorders (45).

MISCONCEPTIONS AND LIMITATIONS OF PELVIC FUNCTION TESTING

One drawback with assessing pelvic floor function is that the assumptions that such tests are based on may or may not be accurate. When these assumptions are made manifest, the possibility of exceptions becomes obvious. Unfortunately, when they remain unspoken, they may be the basis upon which clinical decisions are made. The following list details some common assumptions relevant to pelvic function testing.

Measurements Taken in a Laboratory Setting Reflect Life Outside the Laboratory

This unspoken assumption is easily overlooked. Most patients in a pelvic floor laboratory are examined when they are lying in the left lateral decubitus position. Their entire attention is turned toward the examiner and the various probes that are inserted into the anal canal. It is not unreasonable to question if data collected under these conditions reflect the values that would be collected if the patient were measured under real-life conditions such as carrying a suitcase or running to catch a bus.

Normal Numbers Imply Normal Function

In other words, if the test results are within normal limits, then the patient must be normal. Artifactual errors in performance of a test, and improperly selected tests are common reasons why patients with pelvic floor defects could have "normal results."

Abnormal Numbers Imply Abnormal Function

This is a close relative of the previous point. Experience tells us that there are many patients who have learned to live normal lives with significant pelvic floor abnormalities. The pelvic floor function of a patient is best described by a constellation of factors, rather than one or two isolated data points.

Everything that Can Be Measured Is Important

Often, all tests that are available are performed with the hope that they will identify a specific abnormality. Simply because a factor can be measured, and may be abnormal, does not guarantee its relevance to the presenting problem.

Everything that Is Important Can Be Measured

This approach assumes that the workup performed was complete and that nothing was missed. The truth of the matter is that there are many problems related to pelvic floor physiology that cannot be assessed using our existing diagnostic tools.

Averages Are Representative of True Function

In an attempt to better describe the physiologic profile of a patient, some investigators repeat a test several times to obtain an average for a patient. Although this gives the appearance of precision, it actually creates a false sense of security. Repeating an improperly performed test several times does not improve the data. Additionally, problems that cause disorders of defecation, such as fecal soiling, may not be demonstrable on demand. If a patient spends the majority of the day with complete continence and a normal physiologic profile but soils during a small time period of physiologic stress, average values may be meaningless.

Tests Can Stand Alone (Without Gold Standards)

Although improvements have been made in recent years, it was once true that testing of the pelvic floor was done only on patients with disorders of defecation, and the lack of normal ranges for common tests limited applicability. In one study, 19 patients had rectocele on clinical examination, while 18 had rectocele detected by dynamic cystocolpoproctography, and 11 had rectocele on dynamic magnetic resonance imaging (46). One could rationally ask "How many of the patients *really* had a rectocele?" Interpretation of data is difficult if there is a poorly defined normal range or the lack of a gold standard.

SUMMARY

Many patients view fecal control as a simple valve with two positions: on and off. Unfortunately, many physicians treat disorders of defecation using this same simplistic model. Although not completely understood, there are many factors that influence continence that have been investigated. The modern pelvic floor laboratory attempts to identify and measure these factors in an attempt to understand and treat disorders of continence. A long menu of test options is now available to use in the approach to such patients. Tailoring the choice of tests to the symptoms for an individual will save time and money and improve the chances of arriving at the correct diagnosis. Keeping the value of individual tests in perspective, by placing neither too much nor too little emphasis on their results, and putting the test results in the context of other available information will provide the best chance of success in treating patients with these difficult problems.

REFERENCES

1. Karulf RE, Coller JA, Bartolo DCC, et al. Anorectal physiology testing: a survey of availability and use. Dis Colon Rectum 1991; 34:464–468.
2. Meunier PD. Anorectal manometry. A collective international experience. Gastroenterol Clin Biol 1991; 15:697–702.
3. Loening-Baucke V, Anuras S. Anorectal manometry in healthy elderly subjects. Am Geriatr Soc 1984; 32:636–639.
4. Rasmussen H. Dynamic anal manometry: physiological variations and pathophysiological findings in fecal incontinence. Gastroenterology 1992; 103:103–113.
5. Pedersen IK, Christiansen J. A study of the physiological variation in anal manometry. Br J Surg 1989; 76:69–71.
6. McHugh SM, Diamant NE. Effect of age, gender, and parity on anal canal pressures. Contribution of impaired anal sphincter function to fecal incontinence. Dig Dis Sci 1987; 32:726–736.

7. Fenner DE, Kriegshauser JS, Lee HH, Beart RW. Anatomic and physiologic measurements of the internal and external anal sphincters in normal females. Obstet & Gynecol 1998; 91:369–374.

8. Sentovich SM, Rivela LJ, Blatchford GJ, Christensen MA, Thorson AG. Patterns of male fecal incontinence. Dis Colon Rectum 1995; 38:281–285.

9. Rockwood TH, Church JM, Fleshman JW, et al. Fecal incontinence quality of life scale: quality of life instrument for patients with fecal incontinence. Dis Colon Rectum 2000; 43:9–17.

10. Madoff RD, Baeten CGMI, Christiansen J, et al. Standards for anal sphincter replacement. Dis Colon Rectum 2000; 43:135–141.

11. Agachan F, Chen T, Pfeifer J, Reissman P, Wexner SD. A constipation scoring system to simplify evaluation and management of constipated patients. Dis Colon Rectum 1996; 39:681–685.

12. Knowles CH, Eccersley AJ, Scott SM, Walker SM, Reeves B, Lunniss PJ. Linear discriminant analysis of symptoms in patients with chronic constipation: validation of a new scoring system (KESS). Dis Colon Rectum 2000; 43:1419–1426.

13. Parks AG. Anorectal Incontinence. Proc R Soc Med 1975; 68:681–690.

14. Bartolo DCC, Roe AM, Locke-Edmunds JC, Mortensen NJ. Flap valve theory of anorectal continence. Br J Surg 1988; 73:1012–1014.

15. Feretis C, Benakis P, Dailianas A, et al. Implantation of microballoons in the management of fecal incontinence. Dis Colon Rectum 2001; 44:1605–1609.

16. Diamant NE, Kamm MA, Wald A, Whitehead WE. AGA technical review on anorectal testing techniques. Gastroenterology 1999; 116:735–760.

17. Gowers WR. The automatic action of the sphincter ani. Proc R Soc Lond 1878; 26:77–84.

18. Rasmussen OO. Anorectal function. Dis Colon Rectum 1994; 37:386–403.

19. Caruana BJ, Wald A, Hinds JP, Eidelman BH. Anorectal sensory and motor function in neurogenic fecal incontinence. Comparison between multiple sclerosis and diabetes mellitus. Gastroenterology 1991; 100:465–470.

20. Coller JA. Clinical application of anorectal manometry. Gastroenterol Clin North Am 1987; 16:17–33.

21. Rao SSC, Hatfield R, Soffer E, Rao S, Beaty J, Conklin JL. Manometric tests of anorectal function in healthy adults. Am J Gastroenterol 1999; 94:773–783.

22. Enck P, Eggers E, Koletzko S, Erckenbrecht JF. Spontaneous variation of anal "resting" pressure in healthy humans. Am J Physiol 1991; 261:G823–G826.

23. Pezim ME, Pemberton JH, Levin KE, Litchy WJ, Phillips SF. Parameters of anorectal and colonic motility in health and in severe constipation. Dis Colon Rectum 1993; 36:484–491.

24. Wald A, Jafri F, Rehder J, Holeva K. Scintigraphic studies of rectal emptying in patients with constipation and defecatory difficulty. Dig Dis Sci 1993; 38:353–358.

25. Stricker JW, Schoetz DJ, Coller JA, Veidenheimer MC. Surgical correction of fecal incontinence. Dis Colon Rectum 1988; 31:533–540.

26. Tjandra JJ, Milsom JW, Schroeder T, Fazio VW. Endoluminal ultrasound is preferable to electromyography in mapping anal sphincter defects. Dis Colon Rectum 1993; 36:689–692.

27. Bollard RC, Gardiner A, Lindow S, Phillips K, Duthie GS. Normal female anal sphincter: difficulties in interpretation explained. Dis Colon Rectum 2002; 45:171–175.

28. Williams AB, Bartram CI, Halligan S, Marshall MM, Nicholls RJ, Kmiot WA. Endosonographic anatomy of the normal anal canal compared with endocoil magnetic resonance imaging. Dis Colon Rectum 2002; 45:176–183.

29. Liberman H, Faria J, Ternent CA, Blatchford GJ, Christensen MA, Thorson AG. A prospective evaluation of the value of anorectal physiology in the management of fecal incontinence. Dis Colon Rectum 2001; 44:1567–1574.

30. deSouza NM, Kmiot WA, Puni R, et al. High resolution magnetic resonance imaging of the anal sphincter using an internal coil. Gut 1995; 37:284–287.

31. Zbar AP, Beer-Gabel M, Chiappa AC, Aslam M. Fecal incontinence after minor anorectal surgery. Dis Colon Rectum 2001; 44:1610–1623.

32. Kiff S, Swash M. Slowed conduction in pudendal nerves in idiopathic (neurogenic) fecal incontinence. Br J Surg 1984; 71:614–616.

33. Yip B, Barrett RC, Coller JA, et al. Pudendal nerve terminal motor latency testing: assessing the educational learning curve. Dis Colon Rectum 2002; 45:184–187.

34. Cheong DM, Salanga VD, Phillips RC. Electrodiagnostic evaluation of fecal incontinence. Muscle Nerve 1995; 18:612–619.

35. Sangwan YP, Coller JA, Barrett RC, et al. Unilateral pudendal neuropathy: impact on outcome of anal sphincter repair. Dis Colon Rectum 1996; 39:686–689.

36. Metcalf AM, Phillips SF, Zinmeister AR, MacCarty RL, Beart RW, Wolff BG. Simplified assessment of segmental colonic transit. Gastroenterology 1987; 92:40–47.

37. Stivand T, Camilleri M, Vassallo M, et al. Scintigraphic measurement of regional gut transit in idiopathic constipation. Gastroenterology 1991; 101:107–115.

38. Sun WM, Read NW, Prior A, Daly J, Chesa SK, Grundy D. Sensory and motor responses to rectal distension vary according to rate and pattern of balloon inflation. Gastroenterology 1990; 99:1008–1015.

39. Suzuki H, Matsumoto K, Amano S, Fujioka M, Honzumi M. Anorectal pressure and rectal compliance after low anterior resection. Br J Surg 1980; 67:655–657.

40. Madoff RD, Orrom WJ, Rothenberger DA, Goldberg SM. Rectal compliance: a critical reappraisal. Int J Colorectal Dis 1990; 5:37–40.
41. Almy TP, Abbot FK, Hinkle LE. Alterations in colonic function under stress. Gastroenterology 1950; 15:95–113.
42. McRae S, Younger K, Thompson DG, Wingate DL. Sustained mental stress alters human jejunal motor activity. Gut 1982; 23:404–409.
43. Fisher SE, Keighley MRB, Brecon K, Smart V, Andrews H. Do patients with disordered defaecation have a primary personality disorder?. Gut 1987; 28:A1373.
44. Abrahamian FP, Lloyd-Still JD. Chronic constipation in childhood: a longitudinal study of 186 patients. J Pediatr Gastroenterol Nutr 1984; 3:460–467.
45. Preston DM, Pfeffer J, Lennard-Jones JE. Psychiatric assessment of patients with severe constipation. Gut 1984; 25:A582–583.
46. Kaufman HS, Buller JL, Thompson JR, et al. Dynamic pelvic magnetic resonance imaging and cysto-colpoproctography alter surgical management of pelvic floor disorders. Dis Colon Rectum 2001; 44:1575–1584.

10 | Endoanal and Endorectal Ultrasound

Jorge Andres Larach and Juan J. Nogueras
Department of Colorectal Surgery, Cleveland Clinic Florida, Weston, Florida, U.S.A.

INTRODUCTION

The basis of ultrasound as an imaging technique is the interaction between transmitted sound waves and the juxtaposed different acoustic impedances of body tissues. Ultrasound probes emit pulsed sound waves of a specific frequency, usually between 1 and 30 MHz—the normal human hearing frequency range is up to 20 KHz—and a defined depth of penetration. As the sound waves penetrate through tissues of various impedances, some are reflected back towards the transducers on the probe. By calculating the time difference between transmission and reception, an image is generated through the processing of a multitude of sound waves (1,2).

The rectum is ideal for ultrasound imaging as the various layers of the wall have different acoustic impedances, thus producing good contrast. Moreover, ultrasound provides some advantages over other diagnostic techniques such as computed tomography (CT) scan or magnetic resonance imaging (MRI) in terms of length of the procedure, cost, exposure to radiation, and portability.

NORMAL ANAL CANAL ANATOMY

The ultrasonographic appearance of the anal canal has been investigated in studies using healthy volunteers and comparing the findings to anatomical models. It is easier to describe the anatomy from proximal to distal, dividing the anal canal into three segments: the upper anal canal (UAC), the middle anal canal (MAC) and the distal anal canal (DAC). The UAC is defined by the presence of the puborectalis muscle, which can be seen as a U-shaped echogenic or mixed echogenic image that slings dorsally around the rectum (Fig. 1). Anteriorly, the two limbs extend towards the pubic rami, which can be seen as hyperechogenic bright lines angling anterior to posterior as they course medial to lateral. In the central region that is void of muscle tissue, the urethra may be noted. As the probe is slowly withdrawn, the echogenic image starts to close anteriorly, showing the external anal sphincter (EAS) muscle at the level of the MAC. It is at this level that the inner hypoechogenic band, which represents the internal anal sphincter (IAS) muscle, is at its thickest. The average thickness of the internal sphincter is measured bilaterally and should be 2 mm, although it may vary with age (Fig. 2). However, the thickness is not related to gender, body mass index, or height. As the probe is further withdrawn to the DAC, the inner hypoechogenic band IAS starts thinning and ultimately disappears; the echogenic image then represents only the external sphincter. At this level, the EAS should measure between 5 and 10 mm (Fig. 3), is thinner and shorter in women, and related to body weight.

The submucosal layer may be identified as a mixed echogenic layer and its thickness increases slightly with age and the presence of internal hemorrhoids. Some authors have reported the sonographic image of the longitudinal muscle as an echogenic band between the IAS and EAS muscles that proximally fuses with the longitudinal muscle of the rectal wall. It can be delineated in the majority of males and in 40% of females. Other structures that have been described include the anococcygeal ligament, the transverse perineal muscles, and the ischiocavernous muscles.

NORMAL RECTAL WALL ANATOMY

The ultrasographic appearance of the rectum consists of a five-layer alternation of hyperechoic and hypoechoic rings (Fig. 4), although occasionally it is possible to distinguish seven

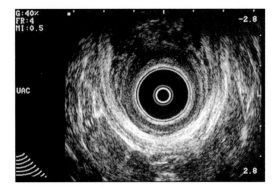

Figure 1 The upper anal canal is defined by the presence of the puborectalis muscle, which can be seen as a U-shaped echogenic or mixed echogenic image that dorsally slings around the rectum.

alternating layers (3). The interpretation of this model has been the subject of controversy among various authors. Hildebrand and Feifel (4) suggested that these five layers of alternating rings correspond to two anatomical layers and three interfaces. Similarly, Saitoh and colleagues (3) described the inner white layer as interface; however, they describe the middle white layer as the submucosa. They further interpreted the seven-layer image as the result of a split in the muscularis propria (outer black layer) into three separate layers (Fig. 5). Our preference is the five-anatomical-layer model, as described by Beynon et al. (5). This model was developed from experimental and clinical evidence in which the inner hyperechoic (white) layer represents the interface with the mucosa, while the inner hypoechoic (black) layer represents the mueosa and the muscularis mucosae. Furthermore, the middle hyperechoic line is the submucosa and the outer hypoechoic and hyperechoic lines stand for the muscularis propria and the interface with the perirectal fat, respectively (Table 1). Interestingly, consensus exists that the middle hyperechoic layer represents the submucosa or the interface of the submucosa with the muscularis and that this layer defines invasion. Similarly, widening of the outer hypoechoic layer represents a T2 tumor (Fig. 6) while a break in the outer hyperechoic layer represents a T3 lesion (Fig. 7). Thus, there is debate regarding the interpretation of ultrasound, findings that may be of academic importance but of relatively little clinical relevance.

Normal lymph nodes in the perirectal fat are not normally identified. Metastatic lymph nodes, however, are generally hypoechogenic similar to a primary tumor (Fig. 8). This fact was first described in the upper gastrointestinal tract (6) and later applied to the rectum (7). Metastasic (hypoechoic) lymph nodes must be differentiated from vessels in the perirectal fat, which also appear as hypoechoic structures. However, when followed longitudinally, they seem to extend further than the corresponding diameter and often branch and elongate in a longitudinal fashion (Fig. 8). Hyperechoic round lesions in the mesorectum are often interpreted as inflammatory lymph nodes (7).

Endorectal ultrasound (ERUS) may also provide images of adjacent organs or structures. In males, the seminal vesicles are clearly observed and must be distinguished from lymph nodes. The prostate may also be seen and tumor invasion through Denonvillier's fascia can be easily recognized (Fig. 9) (2).

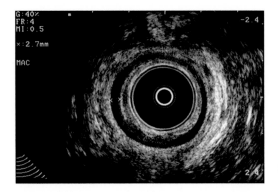

Figure 2 The inner hypoechogenic band, which represents the internal anal sphincter, is at its thickest at the middle anal canal.

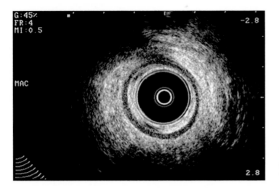

Figure 3 The internal anal sphincter, seen as the inner hypoechoic band, starts to get thinner at the level of the distal anal canal. It ultimately disappears, leaving only the echogenic image of the external anal sphincter.

ENDOANAL ULTRASONOGRAPHY
Procedure

The patient can be given two disposable sodium phosphate enemas one hour prior to the examination for bowel cleansing. However, enemas are not mandatory as the endoanal ultrasound (EAUS) probe barely enters the rectum. With the patient in left lateral position and the knees bent, the exam begins with a digital rectal examination to evaluate the anal canal musculature and any areas of stenosis or pain. For EAUS, the transducer is covered in a plastic sonolucent cap filled with water, which in turn is protected by a condom filled with ultrasound jelly to produce coupling. The probe is then inserted into the anal canal and imaging is usually undertaken from proximal to distal, defining a variety of levels as it progresses.

Indications

EAUS is particularly useful to delineate the anal sphincter anatomy; hence, its primary indication is to detect sphincter defects in incontinent patients. Although well tolerated, it is complementary to electromyography (EMG). Ultrasound demonstrates anatomy while EMG reveals function.

Ultrasonography can also be useful in patients with perianal sepsis, fistula tracts, and internal openings, especially in patients with complex and/or recurrent fistula in ano. As with rectal ultrasonography, anal ultrasonography has been used to stage anal cancer and to guide biopsy.

Evaluation of Incontinence

Endoanal ultrasonography (EAUS) has played a major role in the changes associated with the evaluation and treatment of fecal incontinece (FI). Prior to the introduction of EAUS by Law in 1989 (8), pudendal nerve damage was deemed as the main cause of FI (9,10). Endosonography

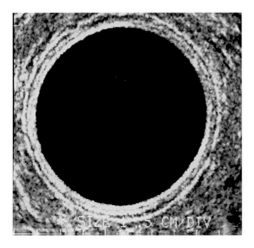

Figure 4 The ultrasonographic appearance of the normal rectum consists of a five-layer alternation of hyperechoic and hypoechoic rings.

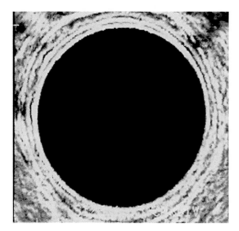

Figure 5 The seven-layer image as a result of splitting of the muscular propria (*outer black layer*) into three separate layers.

has proven that sphincter defects, usually due to obstetrical trauma, are the main etiology of FI (11–13). EAUS is capable of identifying sphincter defects with an accuracy of nearly 90% (14–18). This compares favorably to the 50% accuracy associated with clinical examination, and the 75% accuracy associated with both anorectal manometry and EMG (19), Not only is EAUS more accurate, it is also less painful than needle EMG (16,20,21). MRI of the anal canal seems to provide more accurate delineation of the EAS compared to EAUS, with an accuracy of 90% to 95% in detecting EAS lesions (22,23). Conversely, the internal anal sphinter (IAS) seems to be well represented by EAUS, which has proven superior to MRI (15,22,23). The role of MRI in the management of FI has yet to be elucidated. However, EAUS has the advantage of wider availability and lower cost and the results are reproducible. However, it is complementary to surface EMG as when combined both structure and function can be analyzed (24).

Perianal Sepsis and Fistulas

Clinical examination and probing of the fistula is often inaccurate or impossible. Therefore, other techniques have been developed to improve preoperative diagnosis. EAUS was described in 1989 by Law et al, (25). They defined the internal opening as a break in the mucosal layer. Fistula tracts create hypoechoic bands within the intersphincteric plane and usually communicate with a cavity or scar that appears as a hypoechoic area. Hypoechoic defects within the EAS were interpreted as fistula tracts. Further data from ongoing trials are promising. Although Choen et al. (26) did not find EAUS more helpful than clinical examination, other trials have reported higher accuracy rates. Deen (27) found EAUS to be accurate in 17 of 18 patients (94%) compared to surgical findings. These findings are further improved by the use of hydrogen peroxide as a contrast agent. Fistula tracts become hyperechoic with hydrogen peroxide as a result of the bubbles in the tract. This technique, originally described by Cheong et al. (28) has been verified in subsequent studies (29,30) confirming good results with accuracy nearly 90%; it is also safe and inexpensive.

Table 1 Interpretation of the Anatomical Correlations of the Five-Layer Rectal Wall Model

Series	Layer 1 (white)	Layer 2 (black)	Layer 3 (white)	Layer 4 (black)	Layer 5 (white)
Hildebrandt et al. (4)	Interface (balloon-mucosa)	Mucosa-submucosa	Interface (submucosa-muscularis propria)	Muscularis propria	Interface (rectal wall, perirectal fat)
Beynon et al. (5)	Interface (balloon-mucosa)	Mucosa-muscularis mucosae	Muscularis propria	Muscularis propria	Perirectal fat
Saitoh et al. (3)	Interface (balloon-mucosa)	Mucosa	Submucosa	Submucosa	Perirectal fat

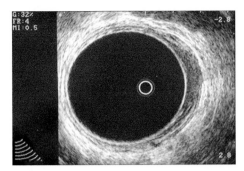

Figure 6   Widening of the outer hypoechoic layer represents a T2 tumor.

Anorectal fistulas may also be imaged using MRI. The accuracy between MRI and EAUS has been compared in several trials (31,32) although none have used hydrogen peroxide as a contrast agent in EAUS. As with FI, the advantage of EAUS over MRI is cost, availability, and the possibility of performing EAUS in the operating room.

Anal Cancer

Reports on the use of EAUS in patients with anal cancer have focused on preoperative assessment and postoperative follow-up. The majority of the trials emphasized that EAUS is easy to perform and accurate in evaluating the depth of penetration and the size of the anal cancers (33–35). Some reports have tried to establish the prognostic significance of ultrasound findings, proposing new staging systems based on the tumor penetration depth (34,35). In a multicenter prospective trial, Giovannini et al. (34) found that staging based on ultrasound assessment of penetration of the submucosa, IAS, external anal sphincter (EAS) or other structures correlates better than the size of the tumor in terms of local recurrence and patient survival. EAUS has also been described in the follow-up of patients with anal cancer, using needle guided biopsy to assess areas suspicious for recurrence (33). The precise role of EAUS in anal cancer is not yet well defined nor widely accepted, however it seems promising for staging and follow-up.

Other Indications

There are numerous sporadic reports of EAUS for other disorders of the pelvic floor. Kamm et al. (36) described a family with hereditary internal sphincter myopathy, depicted on EAUS as an extremely thickened IAS. EAUS has also been described in patients with rectal intussusception, solitary rectal ulcer syndrome (36,37), anal pain, hemorrhoids, and inflammatory bowel disease. Most of these indications have very little or no clinical significance and are of limited clinical value (38).

ENDORECTAL ULTRASONOGRAPHY
Procedure

The patient is given two disposable sodium phosphate enemas one hour prior to the exam for bowel cleansing. With the patient in left lateral position, the exam begins with a digital rectal

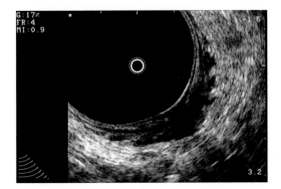

Figure 7   A break in the outer hypoechoic layer represents a T3 lesion.

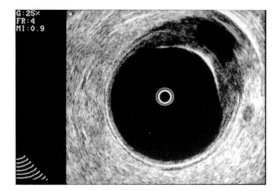

Figure 8 Metastatic lymph nodes are generally hypoechogenic, similar to a primary tumor.

examination to evaluate the anal canal musculature, size, location, morphology, and fixation of the lesion. A proctoscope is then inserted which allows visual examination of the lesion and measurement of the distance from the anal verge as well as removal of any residual stool. It is important to have a clean rectum as residual stool may distort the images. The proctoscope also facilitates passage of the ultrasound probe above the tumor, to assure complete evaluation of the rectal wall layers and the lymph node status at the superior, middle, and inferior aspects of the tumor. It is of great importance to obtain images of the entire tumor, as it is possible to have different depths of penetration at different levels.

The most commonly used probe in North America is probably the Bruel and Kjaer Type 1850 rotating endoprobe (Bruel and Kjaer, Denmark). This probe can be used with either a 7 or 10 MHz transducer that is rotated at four to six cycles per second. The 7 MHz transducer is capable of emitting sound waves that penetrate more deeply into the tissue, thus being more helpful in identifying lymph nodes in the perirectal fat, while the 10 MHz transducer is more reliable at the superficial layers due to its superior resolution. A latex balloon filled with water is used to cover the end of the probe, thus allowing contact with the rectal wall. It is important to ensure that no air bubbles are in the balloon as sound waves may be dispersed and images difficult or impossible to interpret. The balloon is filled with a minimum of 30 mL of water, but more may be used to maintain good coupling with the rectal wall. The probe with the balloon is placed inside a water-soluble gel-filled condom.

Indications

Indication for ERUS includes the evaluation of benign and malignant diseases. This exam can provide important information regarding tumor penetration through the rectal wall and the presence of lymph nodes. ERUS is crucial in the preoperative period as it helps to select the appropriate treatment option. Patient selection for local excision techniques and adequate preoperative staging for neoadjuvant therapy make ERUS the paramount preoperative test in

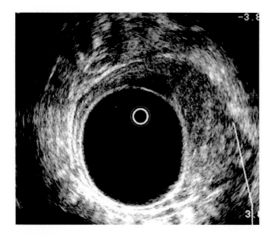

Figure 9 Tumor invasion through the Denonvillier's fascia can be easily recognized.

patients with rectal cancer. Moreover, recent studies have suggested that ERUS has a role in postoperative surveillance and detection of local and regional recurrences. In benign disease, ERUS is helpful in identifying and assessing pararectal and retrorectal masses, delineating complex supralevator fistulas, abscesses, and in some cases, evaluation of Crohn's disease.

Diagnosis and Staging
Adenomas and Carcinomas

Preoperative staging of rectal adenocarcinomas is based on a modification of the tumor node metastases classification (39), as proposed by Hildebrandt and Feifel (4). This system basically classifies lesions as uT1-4 depending on the depth of penetration of the tumor within the rectal wall (Table 2), The prefix U denotes that the stage has been assessed ultrasonographically. Note that invasiveness is sonographically defined as a compromise of the middle hyperechoic layer, a feature that is common regardless of the anatomical model used. In situ or benign lesions such as adenomas are confined to the innermost layers and are staged as uT0 (Fig. 10). In the same fashion, lymph node status is denoted as either uN0 or uNl, depending on the absence or presence of hypoechoic images in the perirectal fat, respectively.

The overall accuracy of ERUS using this classification in determining the depth of penetration of the tumor through the rectal wall is between 69% and 93% (Table 3). Overstaging ranges from 4% to 18% and understaging from 4% to 13%. These results, however, can be influenced by multiple factors.

The value of ERUS in distinguishing between adenomas (uT0) or early carcinomas (uTl) is controversial. Some authors advocate that, as it is impossible to differentiate the mucosa from the muscularis mucosa in ultrasonographic models of the rectum, adenomas and carcinomas must be grouped together as uT0/1 lesions (41). This interpretation relies on the ultrasonic layer model proposed by Hildebrandt (7). Using the Beynon model, other authors have described an accuracy rate of 87% in preoperatively differentiating T0 from T1-3 lesions (44,45). This feature is probably the only difference in clinical staging between the two interpretative models of the ultrasonographic rectal wall. Other authors have tried to differentiate adenomas from carcinomas based on the echogenic pattern of the tumor. Knutz (46), based on the premise that malignant tumors tend to be less echogenic, reached a sensitivity of 96% in differentiating adenomas from malignant disease. Adams and Wong (47), reaching a sensitivity of only 50% with this method, could not reproduce this finding.

As seen in Table 3, it is generally easier to accurately stage more advanced disease such as T3-4 than earlier stages (T1-2) (40,44,44). Overstaging is a common occurrence, particularly in uT2 lesions (40,42,44,48), probably due to the distortion of the ultrasonographic anatomy by peritumoral inflammation (42,48,49). This limitation in staging T1-2 tumors has been used by some surgeons to argue against local resection. However, the majority of understaged uTl tumors are confined to the rectal wall (T0-2) (44), thus, it is not a limiting factor for local excision, providing that the final pathological stage and not the ultrasound stage define the need for further treatment. Overstaging can also be of critical importance as it may result in potentially available unnecessarily aggressive therapy. Staging of more advanced lesions is

Table 2 Relation Between TNM T Stage, uT Stage, and Endorectal Ultrasonography Findings

TNM T stage	UT stage	Endorectal ultrasonography depth of penetration
T0: tumor confined to mucosa	UT0	Tumor does not surpass inner hypoechoic (black) layer
T1: tumor invades submucosa	UT1	Tumor breaks through middle hyperechoic (white) layer
T2: tumor invades muscularis propria	UT2	Widening of outer hypoechoic (black) layer
T3: tumor invades through the muscularis propria into the subserosa, or into nonperitonealized pericolic or perirectal tissues	UT3	Tumor breaks through outer hyperechoic layer
T4: tumor directly invades other organs or structures, and/or perforates the visceral peritoneum	UT4	Invasion of perirectal tissues (seminal vesicles, prostate, vagina) by tumor

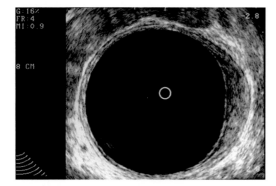

Figure 10 In situ or benign lesions such as adenomas are confined to the innermost layers.

more accurate, but also of less clinical relevance as all patients who can undergo curative surgery require radical resections (anterior resections or abdomino perineal resections). Nonetheless ERUS is a useful tool for selecting patients for neoadjuvant radiotherapy or radiochemotherapy protocols.

Accuracy in staging tumor depth by ERUS has been compared to other techniques such as clinical digital examination, CT, and MRI. ERUS appears to be more accurate at all stages, but particularly in the early stages (50–52). When compared to MRI with the use of an endo-coil, ERUS has also been proven equal to or more accurate than MRI by better differentiating between T1 and T2 lesions (53–55). There is general consensus that ERUS is less expensive and more widely available, whereas MRI has the advantage of being "operator independent" (Table 4). Moreover, the differentiation between T1 and T2-T4 lesions is the most important differentiation relative to the depth of invasion. It is this information that directs the decision between transanal and transabdominal treatment of rectal carcinoma.

Although ERUS may be useful for lymph node staging, reported results show less accuracy than staging for depth of penetration. As previously mentioned, the most commonly used criteria is identifying a spherical hypoechoic image in the perirectal fat (7,60), although some

Table 3 Percent of Accuracy, Overstaging, and Understaging for Different Levels of Depth Penetration and Different Authors

Author	N	Accuracy % uT1	Accuracy % uT2	Overstaging % / Understaging % uT3	Overstaging % / Understaging % uT4	Overall
			42	20	38	19
Sailer, 1997[a] (40)	160	98	50	77	62	78
		2	8	3	-	3
		-	0	9	0	4
Massari, 1998 (41)	75	87	89	91	100	91
		13	11	0	-	5
		-	12	10	0	8
Glaser, 1990 (42)	110	89	82	88	100	87
		11	6	2	-	5
		-	18	11	6	5
Nielsen, 1996 (43)	100	100	76	84	94	85
		0	6	5	-	10
		32	18	28	50	18
Garcia-Aguilar, 2002 (44)	545	47	68	70	50	69
		21	16	2	-	13

[a]Sailer et al. included uT0-1 tumors together in uT1.

Table 4 Depth Staging Accuracy for Different Methods

Author	N	Digital rectal exam	Computed tomography	Magnetic resonance imaging	Endorectal ultrasonography
Rifkin, 1986 (57)	85	–	59	–	93
Beynon,1989 (50)	100	58	74	–	93
Waizer, 1989 (58)	68	83	66	–	76
Milsom, 1990 (57)	52	48	–	–	83
Meyenberger, 1995 (53)	21	–	–	40	83
Kim, 1999 (54)	[a]	–	65	81	81
Hunerbein, 2000 (56)	[a]	–	–	91	84

[a]Authors have different number of patients for each group.

users have tried size (61), shape, and margins as other potentially useful criteria. The accuracy of lymph node status assessment with ERUS ranges between 79% and 83% but still compares favorably to digital rectal examination, CT, or MRI (Table 5) (63). In the last several years the possibility of ultrasound-guided biopsy has T5 emerged as a technique that may add precision in diagnosing lymph node involvement. However, its clinical value is still under scrutiny as the possibility for false-negative results may preclude optimal oncologic treatment.

It is interesting to note that, with more exhaustive pathological techniques for lymph node retrieval in resected specimens, the accuracy of ultrasound may be as low as 43%, mainly due to its low efficiency with nodes less than 5 mm (64). This drawback may be of critical importance in deciding adequate therapy as it has been suggested that 45% to 78% of metastasic lymph nodes are less than 5 mm in diameter (65,66). Regardless of the reason for any inaccuracies in staging perirectal nodes, understaging can result in failure to deliver appropriate neoadjuvant therapy whereas overstaging can cause inappropriate delivery of such chemoradiotherapy.

It has been suggested that there is a significant learning curve associated with ERUS, which may decrease accuracy. Orrom and Wong (67) reported an overall accuracy of 75% in staging penetration depth. However, when the last year and the last six months of the study duration were analyzed separately, the accuracy increased to 77% and 90%, respectively. In addition to the learning curve, ERUS has also been proven to be "operator-dependent" (44,68,69).

Napoleon et al. (71) examined the results in determination of depth of wall invasion in patients who did and did not receive radiotherapy. Invasion was correctly staged in 86% of patients without radiotherapy, but in only 47% of patients who had previous radiotherapy. Rau et al. (72) also described a low accuracy rate (50%) for wall penetration staging in patients who underwent preoperative chemoradiation. Accuracy was found to be especially low in patients who responded (29%) versus those individuals who did not respond to chemoradiation (accuracy of 82%). Although ERUS may identify tumor shrinkage in patients with neoadjuvant radiotherapy, peritumoral fibrosis makes staging unreliable (72–75). Authors have concluded that ERUS does not provide good accuracy in staging of rectal wall penetration in patients with previous radiation. Therefore, ERUS should be performed in patients prior to receiving radiotherapy to increase accuracy and its predictive value.

The location of the tumor has been a subject of controversy relative to accuracy. Sentovich and colleagues (76) suggested that a tumor more than 6 cm from the anal verge is

Table 5 Accuracy of Ultrasound, Computed Tomography, and Magnetic Resonance Imaging in Preoperative Diagnosis of Lymph Node Metastasis

Author	N	Endorectal ultrasonography	Computed tomography	Magnetic resonance imaging
Beynon, 1989 (60)	46	87	57	–
Thaler, 1994 (62)	37	80	~	60
Kim, 1999 (54)	89	64	57	63
Hunerbein, 2000 (56)	30	80	–	89
Garcia-Aguilar, 2002 (44)	238	64	–	–

harder to precisely stage than are more distal tumors. Other studies have suggested that distal tumors are actually harder to stage (48,77) while Garcia-Aguilar (44) found no difference.

Stromal Tumors

Stromal tumors represent a small proportion of primary rectal tumors (78). As such, there is little experience in the literature regarding the use of ERUS for the treatment of these tumors. Nevertheless, there are a few anecdotal reports which found ERUS to be important in treatment planning, for either local or radical resections (79–81). Stromal tumors are delineated on ERUS as hypoechoic heterogeneous masses that usually arise from the muscularis propria. ERUS is also capable of defining size, a feature that would help define treatment planning. The final treatment decision should be made once the final pathology is confirmed, as not only size but the number of mitoses per high-power field and grade of tumor differentiation have impact on local recurrence and malignant potential.

Other Tumors

Although there are no large series of patients, as with adenocarcinomas, there are numerous case reports of ERUS for conditions such as rectal endometriosis (82), colitis cystica profunda (83), retrorectal cystic hamartomas (84), retrorectal bowel duplication (85),Von Recklinghausen fibromas (86), MALT lymphoma (87), and other less frequent entities in which ERUS may be of use. ERUS guided biopsy is also possible and may aid in the diagnosis of extrarectal tumors (88).

Follow-Up and Biopsies

The role of ultrasound as part of follow-up routines in colorectal cancer has been the subject of controversy. However, it is still used in most centers and probably represents a benefit for most patients (89). Pelvic recurrence is a very morbid condition that affects not only survival but also, to a great extent, the patient's quality of life. Ultrasound may be valuable in diagnosing recurrences earlier, as it allows visualization of small lesions in scar tissue, permits time comparisons to assess growth, and with the use of specific probes, may allow accurate diagnosis of lesions as small as 5 mm. However, PET scanning may also prove accurate in this regard.

Beynon et al. (90) likened the endosonographic appearance of recurrent lesions to that of the primary lesion with disruption of the mucosa. However, recurrent lesions may also appear with intact mucosa and mixed echogenicity outside the rectal wall or as a hypoechoic area outside the rectal wall. Biopsy is important in these cases to rule out scar and granulating tissue.

Although there are no controlled trials reported in the literature, most of the existing publications suggest increased recurrence resection rates in those patients followed up by ERUS, mainly due to the possibility of detecting early asymptomatic recurrences (56,57,63, 90,92,97). Some authors suggest that this increased resection rate also translates' into an improvement in long-term survival for these patients (94,95). In the absence of bigger, controlled trials, ERUS is probably recommended for follow-up of patients with rectal cancer, as it is cost-effective and able to detect asymptomatic (early) recurrences and may imply a survival benefit for these patients.

Perirectal Sepsis

Anorectal processes such as fistula and abscesses are generally better evaluated using EAUS. Nevertheless, complex supralevator abscesses may be visualized and fluid aspirates may be obtained by ERUS ultrasound. It is not clear whether ERUS is more sensitive than MRI for this purpose, but it has the advantage of cost and the possibility of use in the operating room (96).

COLONIC ULTRASOUND

Flexible endosonography combined the advantage of proximal visualization of colonic lesions with ultrasonographic capabilities. This ability to merge a diagnostic tool with a therapeutic modality has been utilized by some investigators for the selection of patients with colonic lesions to undergo endoscopic removal. Stergiou et al. (97) described the determination of depth of penetration of a colonic polyp as one of the criteria for endoscopic excision. Hurlstone et al. (98) used the 20 mHz "mini probe" ultrasound to exclude T2 lesions prior to endoscopic mucosal resection of flat lesions, up to a depth of T1 penetration. Zhou et al. (99) described the use of endoscopic ultrasonography to characterize submucosal lesions of the colon. They reported a high accuracy in the diagnosis of these submucosal tumors. Despite these isolated reports, the application of endosonography is still limited in the evaluation of colorectal neoplasms.

SUMMARY

Anorectal ultrasound is an essential component of any colorectal practice. Its ease of use, patient tolerance, and cost make it very versatile and often employed. Its results dictate the management of fecal incontinence, rectal carcinoma, recurrent perianal sepsis, and a myriad of other conditions.

REFERENCES

1. Case TD. Ultrasound physics and instrumentation. Surg Clin N Am 1998; 73:197–217.
2. Nogueras J. Endorectal ultrasonography: technique, image interpretation, and expanding indications in 1995. Sem Colon Rectal Surg 1995; 6:70–77.
3. Saitoh N, Okui K, Sarashina H, Suzuki M, Arai T, Nunomura M. Evaluation of echographic diagnosis of rectal cancer using intrarectal ultrasonic examination. Dis Colon Rectum 1986; 29:234–242.
4. Hildebrandt U, Feifel G. Preoperative staging of rectal cancer by intrarectal ultrasound. Dis Colon Rectum 1985; 28:42–46.
5. Beynon J, Foy DM, Temple LN, Channer JL, Virjee J, Mortensen NT. The endosonic appearances of normal colon and rectum. Dis Colon Rectum 1986; 29:810–813.
6. Tio TL, Tytgat GN. Endoscopic ultrasonography in the assessment of intra- and transmural infiltration of tumours in the oesophagus, stomach and papilla of vater and in the detection of extraoesophageal lesions. Endoscopy 1984; 16:203–210.
7. Hildebrandt U, Klein T, Feifel G, Schwarz HP, Koch B, Schmitt RM. Endosonography of pararectal lymph nodes. In vitro and in vivo evaluation. Dis Colon Rectum 1990; 33:363–868.
8. Law PJ, Bartram CI. Anal endosonography: technique and normal anatomy. Gastrointest Radiol 1989; 14:349–353.
9. Snooks SJ, Setchell M, Swash M, Henry MM. Injury to innervation of pelvic floor sphincter musculature in childbirth. Lancet 1984; 2:546–550.
10. Parks AG, Swash M, Urich H. Sphincter denervation in anorectal incontinence and rectal prolapse. Gut 1977; 18:656–665.
11. Vaizey CJ, Kamm MA, Barcram CI. Primary degeneration of the internal anal sphincter as a cause of passive faecal incontinence. Lancet 1997; 349:612–615.
12. Sultan AH, Kamm MA, Hudson CN, Thomas JM, Bartram CI. Anal-sphincter disruption during vaginal delivery. N Engl J Med 1993; 329:1905–1911.
13. Kamm MA. Obstetric damage and faecal incontinence. Lancet 1994; 344:730–733.
14. Cuesta MA, Meijer S, Derksen EJ, Boutkan H, Meuwissen SG. Anal sphincter imaging in fecal incontinence using endosonography. Dis Colon Rectum 1992; 35:59–63.
15. Deen KI, Kumar D, Williams JG, Olliff J, Keighley MR. Anal sphincter defects. Correlation between endoanal ultrasound and surgery. Ann Surg 1993; 218:201–205.
16. Law PJ, Kamm MA, Bartram CI. Anal endosonography in the investigation of faecal incontinence. Br J Surg 1991; 78:312–314.
17. Meyenberger C, Bertschinger P, Zala GF, Buchmann P. Anal sphincter defects in fecal incontinence: correlation between endosonography and surgery. Endoscopy 1996; 28:217–224.
18. Nielsen MB, Hauge C, Pedersen JF, Christiansen J. Endosonographic evaluation of patients with anal incontinence: findings and influence on surgical management. AJR Am J Roentgenol 1993; 160: 771–775.
19. Sultan AH, Kamm MA, Hudson CN, Nicholls JR, Bartram CI. Endosonography of the anal sphincters: normal anatomy comparison with manometry. Clin Radiol 1994; 49:368–374.
20. Felt-Bersma RJ, Cuesta MA, Koorevaar M, et al. Anal endosonography: relationship with anal manometry and neurophysiologic tests. Dis Colon Rectum 1992; 35:944–949.
21. Enck P, von Giesen HJ, Schafer A, et al. Comparison of anal sonography with conventional needle electromyography in the evaluation of anal sphincter defects. Am J Gastroenterol 1996; 91:2539–2543.
22. Malouf AJ, Williams AB, Halligan S, Bartram CI, Dhillon S, Kamm MA. Prospective assessment of accuracy of endoanal MR imaging and endosonography in patients with fecal incontinence. AJR Am J Roentgenol 2000; 175:741–745.

23. Rociu E, Stoker J, Eijkemans MJ, Schouten WR, Lameris JS. Fecal incontinence: endoanal US versus endoanal MR imaging. Radiology 1999; 212:453–458.

24. Pfeifer J, Teoh TA, Salanga YD, Agachan F, Wexner SD. Comparative study between intra-anal sponge and needle electrode for electromyographic evaluation of constipated patients. Dis Colon Rectum 1998; 41:153–157.

25. Law PJ, Talbot RW, Bartram CI, Northover JM. Anal endosonography in the evaluation of peri-anal sepsis and fistula in ano. Br J Surg 1989; 76:752–755.

26. Choen S, Burnett S, Bartrara CI, Nicholls RJ. Comparison between anal endosonography and digital examination in the evaluation of anal fistulae. Br J Surg 1991; 78:445–447.

27. Deen Kt, Williams JG, Hutchinson R, Keighley MR, Kumar D. Fistulas in ano: endoanal ultrasonographic assessment assists decision making for surgery. Gut 1994; 35:391–394.

28. Cheong DM, Nogueras JJ, Wexner SD, Jagelman DG. Anal endosonography for recurrent anal fistulas: image enhancement with hydrogen peroxide. Dis Colon Rectum 1993; 36:1158–1160.

29. Poen AC, Felt-Bersma RJ, Eijsbouts QA, Cuesta MA, Meuwissen SG. Hydrogen peroxide-enhanced Dransanal ultrasound in the assessment of fistula-in-ano. Dis Colon Rectum 1998; 41:1147–1152.

30. Sudol-Szopinskal, Jakubowski W, Szczepkowski M, Sarti D. Usefulness of hydrogen peroxide enhancement in diagnosis of anal and ano-vaginal fistulas. Eur Radiol 2003; 13:1080–1084.

31. Maier AG, Funovics MA, Kreuzer SH, etal. Evaluation of perianal sepsis: comparison of anal endosonography and magnetic resonance imaging. J Magn Reson Imaging 2001; 14:254–260.

32. Lunniss PJ, Barker PG, Sultan AH, et al. Magnetic resonance imaging of fistula-in-ano. Dis Colon Rectum 1994; 37:708–718.

33. Magdeburg B, Fried M, Meyenberger C. Endoscopic ultrasonography in the diagnosis, staging, and follow-up of anal carcinomas. Endoscopy 1999; 31:359–364.

34. Giovannini M, Bardou VJ, Barclay R, et al. Anal carcinoma: prognostic value of endorectal ultrasound (ERUS). Results of a prospective multicenter study. Endoscopy 2001; 33:231–236.

35. Tarantino D, Bernstein MA. Endoanal ultrasound in the staging and management of squamous-cell carcinoma of the anal canal: potential implications of a new ultrasound staging system. Dis Colon Rectum 2002; 45:16–22.

36. Kamm MA, Hoyle CH, Burleigh DE, et al. Hereditary internal anal sphincter myopathy causing proctalgia fugax and constipation. A newly identified condition. Gastroenterology 1991; 100:805–810.

37. Marshall M, Halligan S, Fotheringham T, Bartram C, Nicholls RJ. Predictive value of internal anal sphincter thickness for diagnosis of rectal intussusception in patients with solitary rectal ulcer syndrome. Br J Surg 2002; 89:1281–1285.

38. Poen AC, Felt-Bersma RJ. Endosonography in benign anorectal disease: an overview. Scand J Gastroenterol Suppl 1999; 230:40–48.

39. AJCC Cancer Staging Manual. 5th ed. Lippincott-Raven Publishers, Philadelphia, PA 1997:83–90.

40. Sailer M, Leppert R, Kraemer M, Fuchs KH, Thiede A. The value of endorectal ultrasound in the assessment of adenomas, Tl- and T2-carcinomas. Int J Colorectal Dis 1997; 12:214–219.

41. Massari M, De Simone M, Cioffi U, Rosso L, Chiarelli M, Gabrielli F. Value and limits of endorectal ultrasonography for preoperaive staging of rectal carcinoma. Surg Endosc 1998; 8:438–444.

42. Glaser F, Schlag P, Herfarth C. Endorectal ultrasonography for the assessment of invasion of rectal tumours and lymph node involvement. Br J Surg 1990; 77:883–887.

43. Nielsen MB, Qvitzau S, Pedersen JF, Christiansen J. Endosonography for preoperative staging of rectal tumours. Acta Radiol 1996; 37:799–803.

44. Garcia-Aguilar J, Pollack J, Lee SH, et al. Accuracy of endorectal ultrasonography in preoperative staging of rectal tumors. Dis Colon Rectum 2002; 45:10–15.

45. Pikarsky A, Wexner S, Lebensart P, et al. The use of rectal ultrasound for the correct diagnosis and treatment of rectal villous tumors. Am J Surg 2000; 179:261–265.

46. Kuntz C, Glaser F, Buhr HJ, Herfarth C. Endorectal ultrasound in diagnosis and therapy planning of broad-base rectal adenomas. Chirurgia 1993; 64:290–294.

47. Adams WJ, Wong WD. Endorectal ultrasonic detection of malignancy within rectal villous lesions. Dis Colon Rectum 1995; 38:1093–1096.

48. Herzog V, von Flue M, Tondelli P, Schuppisser JP. How accurate is endorectal ultrasound in the preoperative staging of rectal cancer? Dis Colon Rectum 1993; 36:127–134.

49. Kruskal IB, Kane RA, Sentovich SM, Longmaid HE. Pitfalls and sources of error in staging rectal cancer with endorectal US. Radiographics 1997; 17:609–626.

50. Beynon J. An evaluation of the role of rectal endosonography in rectal cancer. Ann R Coll Surg Engl 1989; 71:131–139.

51. Rifkin MD, Ehrlich SM, Marks G. Staging of rectal carcinoma: prospective comparison of endorectal US and CT. Radiology 1989; 170:319–322.

52. Holdsworth PJ, Johnston D, Chalmers AG, et al. Endoluminal ultrasound and computed tomography in the staging of rectal cancer. Br J Surg 1988; 75:1019–1022.

53. Meyenberger C, Huch BRA, Bertschmger P, Zala GF, Klotz HP, Krestin GP. Endoscopic ultrasound and endorectal magnetic resonance imaging: a prospective, comparative study for preoperative staging and follow-up of rectal cancer. Endoscopy 1995; 27:469–479.

54. Kim NK, Kim MJ, Yun SH, Sohn SK, Min JS. Comparative study of transrectal ultrasonography, pelvic computerized tomography, and magnetic resonance imaging in preoperative staging of rectal cancer. Dis Colon Rectum 1999; 42:770–775.

55. Hunerbein M, Pegios W, Rau B, Vogl TJ, Felix R, Schlag PM. Prospective comparison of endorectal ultrasound, three-dimensional endorectal ultrasound, and endorectal MRI in che preoperative evaluation of rectal tumors. Preliminary results. Surg Endosc 2000; 14:1005–1009.

56. Hunerbein M, Totkas S, Moesta KT, Ulmer C, Handke T, Schlag PM. The role of transrectal ultrasound-guided biopsy in the postoperative follow-up of patients with rectal cancer. Surgery 2001; 129:164–169.

57. Rifkin MD, Wechsler RJ. A comparison of computed tomography and endorectal ultrasound in staging rectal cancer. Int J Colorectal Dis 1986; 1:219–223.

58. Waizer A, Zitron S, Ben-Baruch D, Baniel J, Wolloch Y, Dintsman M. Comparative study for preoperative staging of rectal cancer. Dis Colon Rectum 1989; 32:53–56.

59. Milsom JW, Graffner H. Intrarectal ultrasonography in rectal cancer staging and in the evaluation of pelvic disease. Clinical uses of intrarectal ultrasound. Ann Surg 1990; 212:602–606.

60. Beynon J, Mortensen NJ, Foy DM, Channer JL, Rigby H, Virjee J. Preoperative assessment of mesorectal lymph node involvement in rectal cancer. Br J Surg 1989; 76:276–279.

61. Detry RJ, Kartheuser AH, Lagneaux G, Rahier J. Preoperative lymph node staging in rectal cancer: a difficult challenge. Int J Colorectal Dis 1996; 11:217–221.

62. Thaler W, Watzka S, Martin F, et al. Preoperative staging of rectal cancer by endoluminal ultrasound vs. magnetic resonance imaging. Preliminary results of a prospective, comparative study. Dis Colon Rectum 1994; 37:1189–1119.

63. Romano G, Esercizio L, Santangelo M, Vallone G, Santangelo ML. Impact of computed tomography vs, intrarectal ultrasound on the diagnosis, resectability, and prognosis of locally recurrent rectal cancer. Dis Colon Rectum 1993; 36:261–265.

64. Spinelli P, Schiavo M, Meroni E, et al. Results of EUS in detecting perirectal lymph node metastases of rectal cancer: the pathologist makes the difference. Gastrointest Endosc 1999; 49:754–758.

65. Andreola S, Leo E, Belli F, et al. Manual dissection of adenocarcinoma of the lower third of the rectum specimens for detection of lymph node metastases smaller than 5 mm. Cancer 1996; 77:607–612.

66. Rodriguez-Bigas MA, Maamoun S, Weber TK, Penetrante RB, Blumenson LE, Petrelli NJ. Clinical significance of colorectal cancer: metastases in lymph nodes <5 mm in size. Ann Surg Oncol 1996; 3:124–130.

67. Orrom WJ, Wong WD, Rothenberger DA, Jensen LL, Goldberg SM. Endorectal ultrasound in the preoperative staging of rectal tumors. A learning experience. Dis Colon Rectum 1990; 33:654–659.

68. Burtin P, Rabot AF, Heresbach D, et al. Interobserver agreement in the staging of rectal cancer using endoscopic ultrasonography. Endoscopy 1997; 29:620–625.

69. Roubein LD, Lynch P, Glober G, Sinicrope FA. Interobserver variability in endoscopic ultrasonography: a prospective evaluation. Gastrointest Endosc 1996; 44:573–577.

70. Napoleon B, Pujol B, Berger F, Valette PJ, Gerard JP, Souquet JG. Accuracy of endosonography in the staging of rectal cancer treated by radiotherapy. Br J Surg 1991; 78:785–788.

71. Rau B, Hunerbein M, Barth C, et al. Accuracy of endorectal ultrasound after preoperative radiochemotherapy in locally advanced rectal cancer. Surg Endosc 1999; 13:980–984.

72. Dershaw DD, Enker WE, Cohen AM, Sigurdson ER. Transrectal ultrasonography of rectal carcinoma. Cancer 1990; 66:2336–2340.

73. Burtin P, Cellier P, Croue A, Arnaud JP, Carpentier S, Boyer J. Place of endorectal ultrasonography in the evaluation of staging of cancer of the rectum: before or after preoperative radiotherapy. Gastroenterol Clin Biol 1993; 17:287–291.

74. Williamson PR, Hellinger MD, Larach SW, Ferrara A. Endorectal ultrasound of T3 and T4 rectal cancers after preoperative chemoradiation. Dis Colon Rectum 1996; 39:45–49.

75. Gavioli M, Bagni A, Piccagli I, Fundaro S, Natalini G. Usefulness of endorectal ultrasound after preoperative radiotherapy in rectal cancer: comparison between sonographic and histopathologic changes. Dis Colon Rectum 2000; 43:1075–1083.

76. Sentovich SM, Blatchford GJ, Falk PM, Thorson AG, Christensen MA. Transrectal ultrasound of rectal tumors. Am J Surg 1993; 166:638–642.

77. Sailer M, Leppert R, Bussen D, Fuchs KH, Thiede A. Influence of tumor position on accuracy of endorectal ultrasound staging. Dis Colon Rectum 1997; 40:1180–1186.

78. Meijer S, Peretz T, Gaynor JJ, Tan C, Hajdu SI, Brennan MF. Primary colorectal sarcoma. A retrospective review and prognostic factor study of 50 consecutive patients. Arch Surg 1990; 125:1163–1168.

79. Hsieh JS, Huang CJ, Wang JY, Huang TJ. Benefits of endorectal ultrasound for management of smooth-muscle tumor of the rectum: report of three cases. Dis Colon Rectum 1999; 42:1085–10S8.

80. Van derBerg JC, Van Heesewijk JP, Van Es HW. Malignant stromal tumour of the rectum: findings at endorectal ultrasound and MM. Br J Radiol 20O0; 73:1010–1012.

81. Wolf O, Glaser F, Kuntz C, Lehnert T. Endorectal ultrasound and leiomyosarcoma of the rectum. Clin Investig 1994; 72:381–384.

82. Schroder J, Lohnert M, Doniec JM, Dohrmann P. Endoluminal ultrasound diagnosis and operative management of rectal endometriosis. Dis Colon Rectum 1997; 40:614–617.

83. Doniec JM, Luttges J, Lohnert M, Henne-Bruns D, Grimm H. Rectal ultrasound in the diagnosis of localized colitis cystica profunda (mucosal prolapse-rekted disease). Endoscopy 1999; 31:S55–S56.

84. Scullion DA, Zwirewich CV, McGregor G. Rerrorectal cystic hamartoma: diagnosis using endorectal ultrasound. Clin Radiol 1999; 54:338–339.

85. Oberwalder M, Tschmelitsch J, Conrad F, Offner F. Endosonographic image of a retrorectal bowel duplication: report of a case. Dis Colon Rectum 1998; 41:802–803.

86. Kassai M, Illenyi L, Horvath OP, Macdonald A. The hourglass appearance of the neurofibroma on rectal ultrasound. Surg Endosc 2002:79.

87. Gavioli M, Bagni A, Santacroce G, Piccagli I, Natalini G. Endorectal sonographic appearances of rectal MALT lymphoma, its response to therapy, and local recurrence. J Clin Ultrasound 2001; 29:401–405.

88. Sailer M, Bussen D, Fein M, et al. Endoscopic ultrasound-guided transrectal biopsies of pelvic tumors. J Gastrointest Surg 2002; 6:342–346.

89. Rosen M, Chan L, Beart RWJ, Vukasin P, Anthone G. Follow-up of colorectal cancer: a meta-analysis. Dis Colon Rectum 1998; 41:1116–1126.

90. Beynon J, Mortensen NJ, Foy DM, Charmer JL, Rigby H, Virjee J. The detection and evaluation of locally recurrent rectal cancer with rectal endosonography. Dis Colon Rectum 1989; 32:509–517.

91. Mascagni D, Corbellini L, Urciuoli P, Di MG. Endoluminal ultrasound for early detection of local recurrence of rectal cancer. Br J Surg 1989; 76:1176–1180.

92. Novell F, Pascual S, Viella P, Trias M. Endorectal ultrasonography in the follow-up of rectal cancer. Is it a better way to detect early local recurrence? Int J Colorectal Dis 1997; 12:78–81.

93. Ramirez JM, Mortensen NJ, Takeuchi N, Humphreys MM. Endoluminal ultrasonography in the follow-up of patients with rectal cancer. Br J Surg 1994; 81:692–694.

94. Rotondano G, Esposito P, Pellecchia L, Novi A, Romano G. Early detection of locally recurrent rectal cancer by endosonography. Br J Radiol 1997; 70:567–571.

95. Sailer M, Leppert R, Fuchs KH, Thiede A. Endorectal ultrasound for evaluating perirectal processes. Chirurgia 1995; 66:34–39.

96. Stergiou N, Riphaus A, Lange P, et al. Endoscopic snare resection of large colonic polyps: how far can we go. Int J Colorectal Dis 2003; 18:131–135.

97. Hurlstone DP, Sanders DS, Cross SS, et al. Colonoscopic resection of lateral spreading tumors: a prospective analysis of endoscopic mucosal resection. Gut 2004; 53:1334–1339.

98. Zhou PH, Yao LQ, Zhong YS, et al. Role of endoscopic miniprobe utaasonography in diagnosis of submucosal tumor of large intestine. World J Gastroenterol 2004; 10:2444–2446.

11 | Biofeedback for Pelvic Floor Disorders

Steve Heymen
UNC Center for Functional GI and Motility Disorders, University of North Carolina at Chapel Hill, Chapel Hill, North Carolina, U.S.A.

Han Kuijpers
Department of General Surgery, Ziekenhuis Gelderse Vallei Hospital, Ede, The Netherlands

INTRODUCTION

Biofeedback for pelvic floor muscle (PFM) disorders was first introduced in 1974 when Engel et al. (1) successfully treated patients with fecal incontinence (FI). In 1985, Bleijenberg and Kuijpers (2) published the first report of utilizing biofeedback for patients with constipation caused by paradoxical contractions of PFM during attempted. Reports describing biofeedback for treating patients with rectal pain have only been published in the last few years.

THEORY OF BIOFEEDBACK LEARNING

The type of learning on which biofeedback training is based is motor skills learning: the patient attempts to perform some action and uses feedback from the success or failure of his/her attempt to learn how to refine their performance (3). A good example is learning to shoot a basketball: the individual shoots repeatedly and learns from the successful shots how to shoot the ball more accurately. In the case of physiological responses such as sphincter contractions, however, feedback on the success or failure of attempts to control the PFMs may be difficult to perceive, especially if the muscle is initially quite weak. Consequently, biofeedback training involves detecting and transforming small changes in the muscle response to visual or auditory signals, which the patient can use to refine his/her motor skills. Biofeedback training sessions are usually supplemented by home practice (Kegel exercises), the purpose of which is to increase the strength or ability to relax PFMs and allow for weaning the patient from their dependence on the biofeedback instrumentation.

The purpose of biofeedback for treating FI is to improve the ability of the patient to voluntarily contract the external anal sphincter in response to rectal filling by improving the strength of the sphincter, by increasing the patient's ability to perceive weak distentions of the rectum, or by a combination of these two mechanisms. The purpose of biofeedback for treating constipation or rectal pain is to teach patients to retrain PFM relaxation during defecation. Biofeedback training for constipation is directed at coordinating PFM relaxation with a Valsalva maneuver (a downward intra-abdominal pressure to generate propulsive force).

TYPES OF BIOFEEDBACK TRAINING

Biofeedback training protocols for treating FI fall into three categories—pressure biofeedback, electromyography (EMG) biofeedback, and sensory discrimination training—and are described below.

Pressure Biofeedback

Biofeedback training to improve the strength of the external anal sphincter has most frequently been done by recording anal canal pressures and providing a visual or auditory signal, which is proportional to anal canal pressure. The patient is asked to squeeze as if preventing defecation, and is given visual feedback and verbal guidance on how to accomplish this. The patient may also be taught to inhibit inappropriate responses such as contraction of the abdominus rectus or gluteal muscles, which may accompany the contraction of the external anal sphincter. In most laboratories, patients have been asked to squeeze in response to distention of the rectum (accomplished by inflating a balloon in the rectum) (4,5), but in other laboratories, the patient is asked to squeeze without rectal distention (6).

Electromyography Biofeedback

Biofeedback training to strengthen PFMs may also be done by showing the patient a recording of the average electromyographic activity recorded from the striated muscles surrounding the anal canal (6). In electromyographic biofeedback training, the patient is usually asked to squeeze and relax repeatedly without the rectum being distended. Information on inappropriate abdominal wall contraction is often not provided with this type of biofeedback training. However, a second channel of abdominal electromyographic activity would improve discrimination of which muscle to tense (anal sphincter) and which muscle should remain relaxed (abdominal). Home exercises in which the patient is asked to repeatedly squeeze the PFMs (Kegel exercises) to further strengthen these muscles are usually requested whether the biofeedback training employs anal canal pressure or pelvic floor EMG.

Sensory Discrimination Training

Biofeedback training directed at increasing the patient's ability to perceive and respond to rectal distention (7,8) is based on sensory discrimination training: a catheter with a balloon attached to its tip is introduced into the rectum, and the balloon is distended with different volumes of air. The patient may be asked to report when the distention is felt, or may be asked to respond to the balloon distention by contracting the PFMs. In either case, large distention that the patient can easily perceive is presented first, and then the volume of rectal distention is gradually reduced until the patient has difficulty detecting when the balloon was distended. By repeatedly distending the balloon slightly above and then slightly below the patient's sensory threshold, and by providing feedback on accuracy of detection, the patient is taught to recognize weaker and weaker distention. In many laboratories, this type of sensory training is combined with sphincter-strengthening training by having the patient always contract in response to rectal distention and encouraging the patient to contract as strongly as possible while providing feedback on the strength of contraction as well as the accuracy of detection.

Biofeedback protocols for treating constipation or rectal pain primarily falls into two categories: EMG or the use of an anal canal pressure feedback device. Most studies in the last 10 years have employed pelvic floor EMG instead of anal canal pressure for biofeedback training.

FECAL INCONTINENCE
Epidemiology

FI is experienced by at least 2% to 4% of the population and 7% of people over 65 years of age (9–12); it is clearly not confined to the elderly. The true incidence is probably much higher due to the stigmata of the affliction leading to underreporting (13–16). Only approximately 30% of individuals with FI seek medical attention and despite significant associated morbidity, it is largely unrecognized by health-care professionals. Among women with symptoms of urinary incontinence, the prevalence of FI is about 20%, whereas 70% of individuals with FI have coexistent urinary incontinence (17,18). It accounts for costs of over US$400,000,000 per year for adult diapers in the United States (14); it is associated with poorer health status and limits the social activities of affected individuals.

Pathophysiology

Fecal continence is the ability to perceive, retain, and evacuate rectal contents at a suitable time and place.

The PFM are in a constant state of slight contraction resulting in an anorectal angle of 85° to 90°, so that they can immediately react with a contraction to increased rectal pressure. If the call to evacuate is voluntarily deferred, the subject consciously contracts the pelvic floor; the anorectal angle normally decreases (65–70°), and the anal canal closes.

Each phase of the mechanism of continence can be studied by specific functional tests, collectively termed "the colorectal laboratory" (19–21). These tests are performed both at rest and during maximal load or stimulation to assess maximal capacity of the areas studied. Anal manometry gives an objective, reliable, and reproducible assessment of anal sphincter function (22,23).

Many incontinent individuals have no feeling of urge and only realize that an uncontrolled loss of feces has occurred when they notice they have soiled themselves. Loss of small amounts of mucus that wets and stains underwear and clothing results in irritation of the perineal skin leading to itching, infection and ulceration. This can occur once per week or as often as several times daily. Several incontinence scores have been proposed in order to provide an objective tool to measure the severity of FI (24).

Incontinence is not a diagnosis but rather a symptom of various disorders and is generally considered a taboo subject. Many patients are depressed and embarrassed and have to continuously wear pads. For this reason, they do not seek medical advice and suffer social alienation and serious psychiatric isolation. They refrain from social activities and consequently become more and more isolated to the point where they are confined to their homes, afraid to visit neighbors, friends, and even family. These individuals are quite often told by friends, relatives, and their family doctors that there are very limited treatment options and that they should not complain. Finally, clinicians are beginning to realize that FI is common and presents an important problem in the care of the elderly where it is often combined with urinary incontinence.

Vaginal delivery plays an important role in the pathogenesis of FI. Causes of FI are neurogenic, obstetric, iatrogenic, traumatic, and congenital. The mechanisms involved are altered stool consistency, abnormal rectal compliance or capacity, decreased anorectal sensation, and impaired pelvic floor or anal sphincter function. Pudendal neuropathy is the most common cause of FI, particularly in older women. Intense and repeated straining leads to abnormal perineal descent and permanent distension and stretch-induced damage of the pudendal and perineal nerves, resulting in pelvic floor denervation. As a result, pelvic floor function diminishes. A decreased puborectalis function leads to an increased anorectal angle with loss of the feeling of urge and a high incidence of colorectal, gynecological, and urological prolapses (25). Decrease of external sphincter function leads to impaired squeeze pressures resulting in an inability to retain feces. Internal sphincter function is also impaired in neurogenic FI; however, this pathway is still unknown. Anal sensation is often absent, and childbirth is considered a causative factor. Multiparity, forceps delivery, increased duration of the second stage of labor, third-degree perineal tearing, and a high birth weight are important factors leading to pudendal nerve damage (26). Pudendal neuropathy may worsen with time. The impaired anal sphincter function is diagnosed by anal manometry. Similarly, pudendal nerve terminal motor latency (PNTML) demonstrates pudendal neuropathy, and endosonography may delineate unsuspected sphincter lesions. Function can be restored by relatively simple measures such as dietary alterations, use of constipating medications, and daily colonic irrigations. However, surgical options are limited. Results of postanal repair are moderate because the ability to retain feces and feel urge recurs in only 40% to 60% of individuals, and the quality of continence remains rather poor. Success does not appear to be related to reduction of the anorectal angle but more to restoration of anal sensation, while the effect on sphincter function remains in doubt. The procedure restores anatomy rather than function (27–29). Recent procedures such as the dynamic graciloplasty procedure (29) and artificial sphincter implantation (30) were promising, but are associated with high costs and complication rates. A colostomy is a last resort option, and preoperative counseling by a stoma therapist is of utmost importance.

Patients with obstetric sphincter rupture have the feeling of urge as the pelvic floor and puborectalis muscle are normal but cannot retain feces due to rupture of the sphincter complex. Anorectal manometric values are low, and the anterior defect can be demonstrated by digital examination, EMG, and endosonography. Dual pathology such as sphincter rupture and pudendal neuropathy occurs in approximately 20% and can be demonstrated by PNTML assessment. Surgery may be indicated, but is associated with poor outcome. Obstetric sphincter rupture can be treated by overlapping external sphincter repair. Good results are obtained in 85% to 90% of patients; poor results are due to preexisting pelvic floor denervation. The ability to retain feces is retained; however, residual minor incontinence to mucus and flatus may still persist as internal sphincter function cannot be restored despite adequate internal sphincter repair (31–33).

Denervation rather than sphincter transsection is frequently the cause of iatrogenic FI and is likely the result of distension of the sphincter complex by an overenthusiastic use of an anal retractor to obtain good exposure in treating fistulas, fissures, and hemorrhoids (25,34). Repair may be performed; however, results are only moderate; biofeedback treatment is becoming a suitable alternative.

Biofeedback for FI

The goal of biofeedback training for FI is to improve the ability of the patient to voluntarily contract the external anal sphincter and puborectalis muscles in response to rectal filling (Table 1). This is accomplished by (i) improving the strength of these PFMs, (ii) by increasing the patient's ability to perceive distensions of the rectum, or (iii) by a combination of these two mechanisms.

A comparison of treatment protocols is complicated by the use of different instrumentation that is necessitated by the various treatment strategies. While sensory training of the rectum utilizes an intrarectal pressure, balloon feedback device, coordination biofeedback training includes the addition of pressure transducers in the anal canal to measure PFM contractions to simultaneously feedback intrarectal and intra-anal pressures. Finally, strength training biofeedback may employ either anal canal pressure or intra-anal EMG feedback of PFM.

In a meta-analysis comparing the success rates of studies using coordination training (67%) to strength training (70%), Heymen et al. (63) found no significant difference between the two strategies (Table 1). Furthermore, the mean success rate for those strength training studies using EMG biofeedback was 74%, while the mean success rate for studies using anal canal pressure biofeedback strength training was 64%. Once again, this yielded no significant difference between "strength training strategies."

Research Design

The majority of the investigations of biofeedback for FI utilize uncontrolled experimental designs comparing pre- and post-treatment symptom frequency or severity. Only six studies of biofeedback for FI employed parallel designs (described below), and only three of these studies randomized subjects to treatment groups.

Loening-Baucke et al. (57) used a parallel design for treating children with myelomeningocele. They compared the use of a behavioral management strategy (toileting schedule) in four subjects to coordination biofeedback plus a toileting schedule in eight subjects, and found no difference in treatment outcomes. However, the sample size was small, and subjects were not randomly assigned to treatment. Guillemot et al. (43) also utilized a parallel group design comparing 16 subjects who received pressure biofeedback to eight subjects receiving medication. Again, subjects were not randomly assigned, but were allowed to select their preferred treatment. The investigators found significant improvements in the biofeedback group, but not the medication control group. Unfortunately, between-group comparisons are not interpretable due to the study design.

In a multiple baseline design, Latimer et al. (51) randomly assigned eight subjects to receive either strength or sensory training. Subjects were then crossed over to the alternate treatment. Finally, all eight subjects received coordination training. The positive findings in the first stage of treatment led the authors to conclude that coordination training was not necessary for the successful treatment of these subjects. However, the experimental design failed to account for the order effect of the treatments. Furthermore, this study also has inadequate sample size. Miner et al. (47) employed a more complicated crossover design. In this study, 25 adult patients were first randomized to receive three sessions of sensory biofeedback training or the same distensions of the rectum without feedback. The sensory training group showed significant reductions in frequency of incontinence, whereas the control group did not. Unfortunately, between-group differences were not significant. The control group subsequently received sensory biofeedback training and showed improved continence. All 25 patients were then randomized to receive either strength or coordination training, followed by another crossover to the other treatment. As a group, patients showed further improvements in

Table 1 Biofeedback for Fecal Incontinence Review of Literature 1974–1999

Author	Year	Sample	Design	Treatment	Sessions	Outcome	Measure
Heymen et al. (35)	1999	8/8/8/10	r,p	E/X/Y/Z	8	64/96/73/67%	R
Glia et al. (36)	1998	22	u	C	10	64%	—
Ko et al. (37)	1997	25	u	E	6.5	92%	—
Ho (38)	1997	6	u	P	?	100%	I by 90%
Rieger et al. (39)	1997	30	u	E	6	67%	I by 50%
Patankar et al. (6)	1997	77	u	Y	7	85%	—
van Tets et al. (40)	1996	12	u	E	5	0%	—
Rao et al. (41)	1996	19	u	P&S&C	7	100%	I by 50%
Sangwan et al. (42)	1995	28	u	P	3.75	75%	FI score
Guillemot et al. (43)	1995	16/8	p*	P or M	4	19%	—
Keck et al. (44)	1994	15	u	P	3	53%	I by 75%
Chiarioni (45)	1993	14	u	C	?	86%	—
McIntosh et al. (46)	1993	8	u	E	?	63%	I by 75%
Miner et al. (47)	1990	25	r,p,xx	S,P/C	3/3,3/3	76%	I by 75%
Riboli et al. (48)	1988	21	u	C	12	86%	—
Enck et al. (49)	1988	19	u	C	?	63%	—
Buser et al. (50)	1986	13	u	C	1 to 3	77%	I by 75%
Whitehead et al. (8)	1985	13	u	C	?	77%	—
Wald (7)	1984	11	u	C	?	73%	I by 75%
Latimer et al. (51)	1984	8	mbl	P/S,C	4/4/4	88%	I by 100%
MacLeod (52)	1983	50	u	E	?	74%	I by 90%
Wald (53)	1981	17	u	C	?	71%	I by 75%
Goldenberg et al. (54)	1980	12	u	C	?	83%	—
Cerulli et al. (55)	1979	50	u	C	?	72%	I by 90%
Engel et al. (1)	1974	7	u	C	4	100%	—
Iwai et al. (56)	1997	31	u	P	?	65%	—
Arhan et al. (57)	1994	47	u	C	3.7	50%	—
Loening-Baucke et al. (58)	1988	4/8	u,p	C/M	3	38%	—
Whitehead et al. (59)	1986	8	mbl	C,B	?	75%	I by 50%
Whitehead et al. (59)	1986	20	mbl	C/B	?	64%	I by 75%
Wald (60)	1983	15	u	C	2,3	47%	—
Whitehead et al. (61)	1981	6	u	C	?	75%	I by 75%
Wald (62)	1981	8	u	C	1 to 4	50%	—
Olness et al. (63)	1980	50	u	P	?	60%	—

Abbreviations: Treatment: E, electromyography strength training; P, pressure strength training; S, sensory training; C, coordination training; M, medical management; X, E&S; Y, E&H; Z, E&S&H; B, behavior modification. Designs: u, uncontrolled; r, randomized; p, parallel; p*, pt. chose Tx; mbl, multiple baseline; x, crossover. Measure: I, % of improved S's; R, % reduction in FI (group).

continence with this second phase of training; however, there were no significant differences between groups. The authors suggested that sensory training was the most important factor in the elimination of incontinence, although the results were not definitive due to limited statistical power of the small sample size and confounds from multiple crossovers. In addition, as with the Latimer et al. study, the results of this study lack external validity due to order effects of the treatment protocols. Whitehead et al. (59) compared coordination biofeedback combined with behavioral management to behavioral management alone in a select population of children with FI secondary to myelomeningocele. Subjects were assigned to one of two groups in an alternate assignment protocol. While both groups demonstrated significant improvement in the first month of behavioral treatment, there was no additional benefit reported with the addition of biofeedback in the second phase of treatment. The authors suggested that biofeedback was not superior to behavioral management for most children with myelomeningocele. However, a subgroup of patients with spinal cord lesions below L2 did demonstrate additional benefit from the biofeedback training. Heymen et al. (65) randomly assigned 40 adult subjects into one of four parallel treatment groups as follows: (i) EMG strength training; (ii) EMG strength training and sensory training; (iii) EMG strength training and the use of a home trainer; and (iv) a combination of EMG strength training, sensory and home trainer protocols. Although all four groups improved significantly, there were no statistically significant differences in outcome among the various treatment protocols. Unfortunately, due to the small sample size of each group, it is difficult to draw definitive conclusions in comparing the efficacy of the treatments in this study. While the outcomes of these studies are impressive, these results should be considered cautiously for one or more of the following reasons: (i) the lack of uniform criteria for inclusion or assessing outcome; (ii) diversity among treatment protocols, (iii) the lack of randomization of subjects, (iv) the lack of statistical power due to small sample size; and/or (v) order effects confounding attempts to compare treatment protocols.

CONSTIPATION
Epidemiology

Constipation is a common problem in the general population (66). This is not a disease, but merely a symptom and a heterogeneous condition encompassing different clinical subtypes. The prevalence of constipation in the United Kingdom and United States has been estimated as 0.9% and 1.2%, respectively, of physician visits yearly (9,67). One-third of young women and half of the middle-aged and older female population seek medical assistance for constipation. Furthermore, they have a significantly higher self-reported prevalence of constipation than do men. The prevalence of constipation increases with advancing age and may be a result of the aging process (9,68). This is a common complaint among geriatric patients and may result in significant morbidity, especially among nursing home residents, where it is only partly due to adverse drug effects (69,70).

The prevalence of irritable bowel syndrome (IBS) of which constipation is a symptom, ranges from 10% to 15%, constipation-predominant IBS occurring in approximately 5% of the population and more prevalent in females (71,72). When constipation is defined as the passage of two stools or less per week, the incidence is about 3%. The median frequency in a normal population is seven stools per week, 90% having between two motions per day, to one every two days. Approximately 3% have less than three bowel movements per week (9,10).

Pathophysiology

Patients with functional constipation suffer from a variety of symptoms such as abdominal pain, abdominal distension and cramps, nausea, and a feeling of the urge to defecate and rectal obstruction resulting in the need for straining, and is often associated with pain. The incidence of digital defecation is approximately 30% (21). The vast majority of patients can be successfully treated with laxatives, diet, and regular bowel habits. However, when conservative measures fail, a thorough evaluation of constipation is indicated to offer better management. As in FI, these tests are included in the colorectal laboratory (21–23).

Anal manometry is useful to demonstrate the presence of the internal sphincter inhibitory reflex, which excludes Hirschsprung's disease (19–22). Defecography is a suitable method to study the dynamics of rectal evacuation. During squeezing and straining, the mechanism of continence and defecation is suitably visualized, emphasizing the changes of the anorectal angle. Normal evacuation occurs when the anorectal angle increases by relaxation of the muscularis puborectalis and is therefore a reflection of the function of the pelvic floor (73). Pelvic floor EMG is another test to obtain information on pelvic floor function (74). Measurement of colonic transit time is an important tool in the evaluation of constipation. The technique with radio-opaque pellets is simple, safe, and reproducible, and allows the investigator to measure segmental colonic transit time (19,75). Approximately 30% of patients complaining of intractable constipation have normal colonic transit times in all three segments, whereas another 35% have delayed transit only in the rectosigmoidal segment. Most of these patients are unable to excrete barium during defecography. The anal canal remains closed, and the anorectal angle does not increase. Thus, a functional outlet is created. The pelvic floor contracts rather than relaxing, and feces cannot be excreted. Pelvic floor contraction during straining is confirmed by EMG, demonstrating electrical activity increase rather than decrease. This is caused by an abnormal use of a normal muscle. The terms "spastic pelvic floor syndrome," "puborectalis syndrome," "nonrelaxing pelvic floor," and "anismus" have all been proposed (76–78). These patients usually spend hours straining on a toilet in vain. Because the anal canal remains closed during straining due to external sphincter contraction, they cannot evacuate their bowels. This problem may also lead to incontinence due to pudendal nerve damage. Treatment options were based on weakening the muscle by impairing external sphincter function by partial sphincter division (78). However, with this technique, the results were either disappointing or were short term, lasting only a few weeks. Currently, injection of clostridium botulinum toxin seems to give good long-lasting results (79). Construction of a colostomy should be carried out with restraint. There is no indication for colonic resection because the colon itself is normal, as demonstrated by a normal transit time in most patients. Because this type of functional constipation is caused by abnormal function of a normal PFM, it should be classified as a behavioral disorder. Consequently, relearning normal muscle function during straining with biofeedback is indicated (2).

When transit time is delayed in all three segments and evacuation studies are normal, slow transit constipation is diagnosed and the presence of a neuromuscular disorder is suggested (80). Abnormal esophageal peristalsis, delayed gastric and gall bladder emptying, and delayed small-bowel transit are common in patients with slow-transit constipation (81,82). Several authors have reported favorable outcome of subtotal colectomy with ileorectal anastomosis. In fact, it only increases defecation frequency, but symptoms persist in 60% to 70% of patients (82–84). The liberal use of a colectomy should therefore be discouraged (82).

Biofeedback for Pelvic Floor Dyssynergia

Biofeedback training for constipation is directed at coordinating PFM relaxation with a Valsalva maneuver—a downward intra-abdominal pressure to generate propulsive force. Treatment instrumentation primarily falls into two categories: EMG or the use of an anal canal pressure feedback device. Most studies in the last 10 years have employed pelvic floor EMG instead of anal canal pressure for biofeedback training.

A meta-analysis comparing the success rates of studies utilizing these two protocols (Table 2) showed that the mean success rate for studies using pressure biofeedback (78%) was superior ($p < 0.05$) to the mean success rate for studies utilizing EMG biofeedback (70%) (115). However, the mean success rates comparing studies using intra-anal EMG sensors to studies using perianal EMG sensors were 69% and 72%, respectively, indicating no advantages for one type of EMG protocol over the other ($p = 0.43$). In the only study, which systematically compared the two types of biofeedback, Glia et al. (91) found EMG training to be superior to pressure biofeedback in a small sample (Table 2).

Research Design

As with the research for FI, the majority of the investigations of biofeedback for constipation utilize uncontrolled experimental designs comparing pre- and post-treatment symptom frequency or severity. There were only 10 (six pediatric and four adult) that have utilized some degree of experimental control. Of the 11 pediatric studies reviewed, 6 utilized parallel

Table 2 Biofeedback for Constipation Review of Literature 1980–2002

Author	Year	Sample size	Design	Treatment	Outcome	Sessions	Treatment success	Diagnosis
Dailianas et al. (85)	2000	11	u	P	64%	2	7 of 11	ob
McKee et al. (86)	1999	30	u	P,B	30%	3.5	9 of 30	ob
Rhee et al. (87)	1999	45	u	E	69%	8	31/45	an
Heymen et al. (35)	1999	36	r,p	E/X/Y/Z	?	?	No difference	pfd
Karlbom et al. (88)	1997	28	u	E	43%	8	12 of 28	pfd
Rao et al. (89)	1997	25	u	P	92%	6	23/25 by 50%	ob
Patankar et al. (6)	1997	86	u	E	73%	8	63/86	pfd
Rieger et al. (90)	1997	19	u	E	11%	6	2 of 19	const
Glia et al. (91)	1997	26	r,p	E*/P,B	90% and 60%	<11	9/10 and 6/10	pfd
Ko et al. (37)	1997	17	u	E	76%	4	13/17	pfd
Heah et al. (92)	1997	16	u	P	80%	4	4 of 5 by 90%	po
Ho et al. (93)	1996	62	u	P	90%	4	56/62	ob
Koutsomanis et al. (94)	1995	60	r,p	E*/B	69% and 64%	3 and 2	18/26 and 16/25	pfd
Hull (95)	1995	12	u	E*,S	82%	1–3	9 of 11	ob, po
Papachrysostomous (96)	1994	22	u	H,E,B	86%	HT 36 days	19/22	ob
Koutsomanis et al. (94)	1995	20	u	E	85%	4	17/20	pfd
Bleijenberg et al. (97)	1994	20	r,p	E/B	73% and 22%	8	8/11 and 2/9	pfd
Wexner et al. (98)	1992	18	u	E	89%	9	16/18	pfd
Turnbull and Ritvo PG (99)	1992	7	u	P,G	86%	4.5	6 of 7	const
Fleshman et al. (100)	1992	9	u	E,B	89%	12	8 of 9	pfd
Kawimbe et al. (101)	1991	15	u	E,H	Index	HT 3 wk	?/15	pfd
Lestar et al. (102)	1991	16	u	P,B	56%	1	9 of 16	pfd
Dahl et al. (103)	1991	14	u	E,S	93%	5	13/14	pfd
Emery et al. (104)	1988	65	u	E*	80%	?	52/65	pfd
Bleijenberg and Kuijpers (2)	1987	10	u	E,B	70%	10	7 of 10	pfd
Weber et al. (105)	1987	42	u	P	78% and 0%	4	20/26 and 0/16	rair, pfd
Nolan et al. (106)	1998	29	r,p	E*/M	43% and 53%	3.5	6/14 and 8/15	pfd
Ponticelli et al. (107)	1998	22	p	P,B/M	60% and 58%	Varied	6/10 and 7/12	sb
van der Plas et al. (108)	1996	71	r,p	E*,P/M	39% and 19%	5	15/39 and 6/32	enc
Cox et al. (109)	1994	26	p	E*/M	88% and 60%	2.5	11/13 and 8/13	pfd
Loening-Baucke (110)	1991	38	u	E*,P	37%	<7	14/38	pfd
Loening-Baucke (111)	1990	41	p	E*,P/M	55%/5%	<7	12/22 and 1/19	pfd
Keren et al. (112)	1988	12	u	P	100%	4	12 of 12	pfd
Veyrac et al. (113)	1987	12	u	P	83%	1	10 of 12	ob
Wald et al. (114)	1987	50	r,p	P/M	67% and 33%	3.5	6/9 and 3/9	pfd
Olness et al. (63)	1980	50	u	P	94%		47/50	enc

Abbreviations: Designs: u, uncontrolled; r, randomized; p, parallel. Treatment: E, electromyography; E*, electromyography, intra-anal; E*, electromyography, perianal; S, sensory; P, pressure; B, pass balloon; M, medical management; H, home trainers; G, general relaxation treatment; X, E&S; Y, E&H; Z, E&S&H. Diagnosis: ob, obstructed defecation; pfd, pelvic floor dyssynergia; const, constipated; rair, rectoanal inhibitory reflex; enc, encopresis; po, postoperative; sb, spina bifida; an, anismus.

research designs, but only three of these studies randomly assigned subjects to treatment. In all six of these pediatric studies, biofeedback was compared to traditional medical/behavior management such as laxative use and toileting schedules.

No significant difference between biofeedback and medical management was observed in the three pediatric studies utilizing a randomized, parallel design. Only one of these studies had a sample size that was sufficient to allow for meaningful statistical analysis. In this study, van der Plas et al. (108) compared biofeedback (a combination of anal canal pressure and perianal EMG) to medical management and found no significant difference between treatments in 71 subjects. Unfortunately, the method for determining outcome is not described. In addition, pelvic floor disorder (PFD) was identified in only 40% of subjects.

In another randomized study of subjects with mixed etiology, Wald et al. (114) found a trend for a subgroup of subjects, with PFD having a better outcome with pressure biofeedback than with mineral oil; however, there were no significant differences when evaluating the entire group. In the remaining pediatric study utilizing a randomized research design, Nolan et al. (106) found no advantages for perianal EMG biofeedback over medical management in a study where all subjects had PFD. Again, neither study had sufficient sample size to allow for meaningful analysis.

Three other pediatric studies utilized parallel design; however, these studies did not randomly assign subjects to treatment. In addition, these studies contained other research design flaws. While Cox et al. (109) matched subjects by age and gender, Loening-Baucke et al. (111) compared subjects in the biofeedback treatment group to subjects previously treated with medical management. Subjects were not matched, as in the Cox et al. (109) study. Furthermore, Ponticelli et al. (107) failed to identify how subjects were assigned to treatment or to identify the number of treatment sessions used. In addition, the criteria for determining outcome were confusing. However, unlike the randomized pediatric studies, these investigations had consistent subject selection. The etiology of constipation symptoms was consistent within each study, where children with PFD or children with a subtype of spina bifida were treated. Two of these studies found perianal EMG biofeedback to be superior to medical management or behavior management protocols; however, these studies also had insufficient sample size to provide reliable conclusions regarding outcome. The remainder of the pediatric investigations were uncontrolled.

Only four of the 27 adult (three included some pediatric subjects) studies utilized randomized parallel designs (91,94,97,116). Two of these studies compared EMG biofeedback to balloon defecation (94,97), and two studies compared different biofeedback techniques (91,116). As with the pediatric literature, only one well-controlled adult study had a sample size that was sufficient to provide meaningful statistical conclusions. In that study, Koutsomanis et al. (94) compared perianal EMG biofeedback and balloon defecation training to balloon defecation training alone and found no significant difference between treatments in 60 subjects. This study is one of a few (86,89,95), which address the question of adequate propulsive force during attempted defecation. In some cases, subjects may not be adequately pushing to generate propulsive force on the rectum, although the problem of excessive force is more often seen in these patients. The possible shortcomings of this study include a crossover to alternate treatment after only two unsuccessful sessions and that only 75% of subjects had PFD identified as the etiology for the constipation.

In a randomized study of 20 adult subjects with PFD, Bleijenberg et al. (97) found intra-anal EMG biofeedback to be superior to balloon defecation training. About 90% compared to 60% of subjects improved. In addition, the subjects who failed balloon defecation training were then given biofeedback, yielding an 80% success rate. Again the small sample size makes reliable conclusions regarding treatment outcome impossible.

Finally, two randomized studies directly compared different biofeedback protocols (91,116). All subjects in both studies were identified as having PFD. Heymen et al. (116) compared intra-anal EMG biofeedback to a combination of EMG and intrarectal balloon distension training, EMG and home trainers, or a combination of all three techniques. Although all groups showed significant improvement, no significant differences among treatment strategies were found. Glia et al. (91) found perianal EMG biofeedback to be superior to pressure biofeedback combined with balloon defecation training. However, as with most of the controlled studies reviewed, neither study had sufficient sample size to provide meaningful analysis. The remainder of the adult studies were not controlled.

RECTAL PAIN

The Rome II criteria for functional anorectal pain have identified two distinct anorectal pain disorders. They are levator ani syndrome and proctalgia fugax (117). While the two disorders may coexist, they differ based upon the duration, frequency, and characteristics of the pain.

Pathophysiology

Perineal pain syndromes are a great nuisance to clinicians as they are rare, and patients complain of severe, sometimes, intermittent perineal or anorectal pain or discomfort without any demonstrable abnormality (118–122). Furthermore, underlying psychiatric and emotional factors are often present. Most patients are referred by urologists, gynecologists, or orthopedic surgeons after thorough, negative investigation. Hysterectomy, hemorrhoidectomy, rectopexy, sphincterotomy, coccygectomy, pudendal nerve release, injection of botulinum A toxin, electro-galvanic stimulation (EGS), or anal stretch have all been advocated; however, the long-term results are disappointing (123–129). Patients with proctalgia fugax or levator syndrome complain of a sudden onset of severe rectal, anal, or perineal spastic pain, usually self-limiting and lasting for approximately 30 minutes; levator massage may be helpful. The pain in coccygodynia is a continuous burning sensation or dull ache and is localized around the sacrum and coccyx and is often made worse by sitting. In chronic idiopathic anal pain or descending perineum syndrome, pelvic, perineal, or anal pain is combined with a feeling of rectal obstruction or a bearing down discomfort (130). Thorough clinical and pelvic examination is necessary to exclude a colorectal, gynecological, urological, or orthopedic cause. However, these syndromes are difficult to manage. Specific operations such as coccygectomy and rectopexy have been tried but are often unsuccessful and often confound the problem (131). Therefore, they are not readily indicated. Although very often a cause is difficult to find, this does not mean that one does not exist. Tact, patience, and sympathy are important factors in treating these patients.

Biofeedback Treatment for Chronic Anorectal Pain

Although no controlled, parallel-group studies of treatment outcome are available, the following uncontrolled studies suggest that biofeedback training to teach pelvic floor relaxation may prove effective.

In 1991, Grimaud et al. (132) reported a prospective evaluation of 12 patients with chronic rectal pain; patients with proctalgia fugax and coccygodynia were excluded. Seventy-five percent of patients demonstrated pelvic floor dyssynergia when straining to defecate. Pressure biofeedback was provided on a weekly basis until all subjects reported being pain-free. All but one of the patients who had pelvic floor dyssynergia at pretreatment showed anal pressure relaxation at posttreatment. Only one patient reported a relapse of pain and was able to achieve alleviation of pain with one additional session.

Ger et al. (133) reported a retrospective evaluation of 60 consecutive patients diagnosed with chronic intractable rectal pain. Patients were allowed to choose among three treatment options: (i) EGS, (ii) biofeedback, or (iii) steroid caudal block (SCB). Biofeedback was conducted using an intra-anal EMG sensor. Of the 14 patients initially receiving biofeedback, 14.3% reported complete symptomatic relief (compared to 6.9% for EGS and 0% for SCB), and 28.6% reported acceptable improvement in the frequency and intensity of pain (compared to 31.0% for EGS and 18.2% for SCB). While biofeedback produced the highest success rate, it is considerably lower than the outcome of biofeedback for FI or constipation.

Gilliland at al. (134) retrospectively reviewed the medical records of 86 patients with rectal pain, who completed more than one session of intra-anal EMG biofeedback to assess the efficacy of biofeedback and to identify variables that may be predictive of success. Biofeedback was conducted using intra-anal EMG feedback. Thirty-four percent of patients reported symptomatic improvement. The only predictor of success was the completion of therapy versus premature termination of biofeedback training. Age, duration of symptoms, and the presence of paradoxical puborectalis contraction were not predictive of success.

Heah et al. (92) studied 16 patients with levator ani syndrome, who had an average duration of symptoms. Pain ratings decreased from a median of eight before treatment to a median of two after treatment; furthermore, patients reported a significant reduction in the use of nonsteroidal anti-inflammatory drugs (NSAIDs). However, pain reduction was not associated with significant reductions in anal canal pressures. Salzano et al. (135) treated 31 patients with chronic anal pain with pressure biofeedback, and all reported improvements in anal pain. In contrast to the previous study, these authors reported that symptom improvement was associated with significant reductions in anal canal pressures.

To date, no studies have included control groups with random assignment to treatment condition in order to control for placebo effects. Moreover, with the exceptions of the Heah et al. and the Grimaud et al. studies, investigators have not distinguished patients with proctalgia fugax from those with levator ani syndrome.

Given the different presentation of these disorders, it is reasonable to hypothesize that there may be different pathophysiological mechanisms underlying the disorders (e.g., smooth muscle spasm vs. spasm of striated PFMs). It is recommended that future research utilize the Rome II consensus criteria in selecting patient groups.

Presently, the findings of uncontrolled empirical studies suggest that biofeedback may be useful to some patients in managing chronic rectal pain. Biofeedback is not associated with side effects or adverse events that may occur as a result of medications or surgery nor has it been shown to worsen or exacerbate symptoms. Comparisons with other treatment alternatives such as surgery, EGS, sacral blockade, or analgesic medications suggest that biofeedback may be more effective. Given the significant disability associated with functional anorectal pain disorders, further development of biofeedback therapies and alternative treatment modalities is needed. However, future studies should focus on more restrictive and carefully characterized patient groups such as those with levator ani syndrome, who have elevated anal canal pressure or elevated pelvic floor EMG, and should consider the psychological symptoms, which have been associated with chronic rectal pain.

PSYCHOLOGICAL CONSIDERATIONS

While there is little available information regarding the incidence of psychopathology in fecal incontinent or rectal pain subjects, there is considerable evidence and interest in the role of psychopathology in constipation.

Fecal Incontinence

Several investigations have addressed the role of psychopathology in FI with mixed opinions. Among 33 adolescents with FI psychosocial impairment was significant on the Child Assessment Schedule, Child Behavior Checklist, and Youth Self-Report (136). Among community-dwelling adults, Huppe et al. (137) found that FI has a marked effect on a subject's sexuality and job function and may lead to nearly complete social isolation as a result of embarrassment. In a random sample of 704 residents of Olmsted County, Minnesota, who were 65 years or older, incontinent subjects showed impairment on the role functioning and current-health subscales of the SF-36 (a quality-of-life measure), even after statistical adjustment for the presence of chronic illness, number of medications taken, and impact on activities (138). Similarly, incontinent patients seen in an outpatient medical clinic in North Carolina had impairments on the SF-36 scales for bodily pain, role physical, mental health, and social functioning (139).

Conversely, Heymen et al. (140) reported that subjects with constipation and rectal pain showed significant elevations on somatization scales of the Minnesota Multiphasic Personality Inventory (MMPI), while scores for subjects with FI were within the normal range. Similarly, in another study comparing subjects with chronic constipation or FI to control subjects matched by age and gender, Fisher et al. (141) found constipation subjects to have significantly higher HAD depression subscale scores on the Hospital Anxiety and Depression (HAD) scale than controls, but subjects with FI were similar to controls on anxiety and depression scores on the HAD and General Health Questionnaire (GHQ). However, patients with FI, who had an unsuccessful surgical intervention, had significantly higher scores on these anxiety and depression scores than patients with FI in whom surgery was successful (138). This finding mirrors several investigations in which unsuccessfully treated subjects continued to show elevated psychological distress and those who were successfully treated for incontinence no longer demonstrated any elevations in psychopathology (142–144).

Constipation

Devroede et al. (145) and Kumar et al. (146) suggested that there may be a psychosomatic basis for chronic idiopathic constipation, including subjects with PFD. Nehra (147) reported that 65% of constipated subjects were diagnosed with various psychological disorders. Anxiety and/or psychological stress may contribute to the development of PFD by increasing the level of skeletal muscle tension. Using the MMPI assessment, Heymen et al. (140) found that subjects with PFD-type constipation and subjects with rectal pain showed a tendency to utilize somatization as a defense mechanism to manage psychological distress. This pattern was not seen in subjects with FI. Burnett et al. (139) reported significantly higher scores on the SCL-90R scales for anxiety, depression, hostility, interpersonal sensitivity, obsessive-compulsive traits, phobic anxiety, and somatization, for subjects with constipation. Similar studies reviewed by Whitehead (148) showed elevated levels of psychological distress in patients with symptoms of difficult defecation. Furthermore, inclusion of psychological treatment for subjects with constipation is frequently recommended in the literature (44,149–152).

Patients with symptoms of difficult defecation show significant impairments in the SF-36 scales for bodily pain, role physical (limitations in the ability to work or perform usual physical activities), and general health, even when the possible mediating effects of neuroticism (a personality trait associated with a generally pessimistic attitude) are statistically controlled (135).

While McKee et al. (153) hypothesized the possibility that constipation patients who benefit most from biofeedback have psychological difficulties as the predominant cause of their problem, some investigators (154) suggest psychopathology may be a consequence rather than a cause of constipation. Even in subjects whose constipation was attributed to slow colonic transit without PFD, Dykes et al. (155) found that 60% of subjects had an affective disorder, 66% had a previous affective disorder, and 33% had "distorted attitudes about food." This led these authors to recommend research comparing the effectiveness of biofeedback to psychotherapy for subjects with constipation.

Anxiety and/or psychological stress may also contribute to the development of pelvic floor dyssynergia by increasing the level of skeletal muscle tension. Heymen et al. (140) found clinically significant elevations on the MMPI scales for hypochondriasis and depression, and an elevation, which was nearly two standard deviations above normal for scale 3 (hysteria) in these patients. Burnett et al. (139) reported significantly higher scores on the SCL-90R scales for anxiety, depression, hostility, interpersonal sensitivity, obsessive-compulsive traits, phobic anxiety, and somatization. Similar studies showing elevated levels of psychological distress in patients with symptoms of difficult defecation were reviewed by Whitehead (148).

There are several studies reporting a history of a high incidence of sexual abuse for subjects with constipation. Leroi et al. (156) found a greater incidence of sexual abuse in women who had pelvic floor dyssynergia. These authors speculate that following the trauma of sexual abuse, any sensation of rectal fullness may trigger a memory of the original trauma and may lead to an involuntary contraction of the PFMs. Devroede (145) and Kumar et al. (146) also reported that many of their constipated subjects had a history of sexual or physical abuse. Lennard-Jones (152) recommends supportive psychotherapy, in addition to biofeedback, for those constipation subjects with a history of sexual abuse. Leroi et al. (155) found a greater incidence of sexual abuse in women with pelvic floor dyssynergia.

Children with Encopresis

Several investigators have reported the presence of psychosocial problems in encopretic children (112,157,158). However, other studies suggest that constipated children with pelvic floor dyssynergia have no more behavior problems than do children without pelvic floor dyssynergia (85,114,158,159).

Rectal Pain

Heymen et al. (140) reported that the MMPI profiles of patients with intractable rectal pain show a preoccupation with bodily symptoms and a fear of disease (shown by elevations on scales 1, 2, and 3 of the MMPI). Salzano et al. (135) also reported that these patients have psychological test scores showing elevated levels of anxiety. Given the significant disability associated with functional anorectal pain disorders, further developments of biofeedback therapies and alternative treatment modalities are needed. However, future studies should focus on more restrictive and more carefully characterized patient groups such as patients with levator ani syndrome, who have elevated anal canal pressure or elevated pelvic floor EMG and should take into account the psychological symptoms, which have been found to be associated with chronic rectal pain.

While comorbidity of psychological disorders with constipation and rectal pain appears to be quite high, it remains unclear whether psychopathology causes constipation or rectal pain, contributes to the maintenance of symptoms, or is simply a consequence of these very challenging disorders.

Many individuals with constipation show no elevations in psychological distress. However, the majority of the literature indicates that people with constipation do suffer from psychopathology more than the general public. Some investigations show resolution of psychological disorders after successfully treating constipation with biofeedback. This may indicate that the psychological distress was a result of suffering from constipation. However, this remains to be investigated.

Researchers asking similar questions regarding the role of psychopathology in subjects with IBS have discovered that these patients have higher levels of psychopathology than those with IBS, who have never sought treatment (72). Similar findings were reported in an extensive community-based investigation (72). This may reflect a higher incidence of psychopathology in individuals who seek versus those who do not seek treatment for functional disorders.

RECOMMENDATIONS

Biofeedback has advantages over surgical therapy in that it is a simple, rapid, and cost-effective procedure without any associated morbidity. Furthermore, it is a promising but inadequately tested therapy for FI, constipation, and perhaps, rectal pain.

The lack of controlled studies with long-term follow-up does not allow for definitive conclusions about its efficacy, but unexpectedly satisfying results, even in apparently desperate cases, warrant a trial with biofeedback in all motivated patients able to follow the instructions. Further work is needed to better define the population that is most likely to benefit from such therapy. In addition, well-controlled investigations comparing psychometric and quality-of-life measures pre- and post-treatment will continue to clarify the role of psychopathology in individuals with FI, constipation, and rectal pain.

REFERENCES

1. Engel BT, Nikoomanesh P, Schuster MM. Operant conditioning of rectosphincteric responses in the treatment of fecal incontinence. N Engl J Med 1974; 290:646–649.
2. Bleijenberg G, Kuijpers JHC. Treatment of the spastie pelvic floor syndrome with biofeedback. Dis Colon Rectum 1987; 30:108–111.
3. Whitehead WE, Thompson WG. Motility as a therapeutic modality: biofeedback. In: Schuster MM, ed. Atlas of Gastrointestinal Motility in Health and Disease. Baltimore: Williams & Wilkins, 1993:300–316.
4. Cerulli M, Nikoomanesh P, Schuster MM. Progress in biofeedback conditioning for fecal incontinence. Gastroenterology 1979; 76:742–746.
5. Glia A, Gylin M, Akerlund JE, et al. Biofeedback training in patients with fecal incontinence. Dis Colon Rectum 1998; 41:359–364.
6. Patankar SK, Ferrara A, Larach SW, et al. Electromyographic assessment of biofeedback training for fecal incontinence and chronic constipation. Dis Colon Rectum 1997; 40(8):907–911.
7. Wald A, Tunuguntla K. Anorectal sensorimotor dysfunction in fecal incontinence and diabetes mellitus. Modification with biofeedback therapy. N Engl J Med 1984; 310:1282–1287.
8. Whitehead WE, Burgio K, Engel BT. Biofeedback treatment of fecal incontinence in geriatric patients. J Am Geriatr Soc 1985; 33:320–324.
9. Walter S, Hallbook O, Gotthard R, Bergmark M, Sjodahl R. A population-based study on bowel habits in a Swedish community: prevalence of faecal incontinence and constipation. Scand J Gastroenterol 2002; 37:911–916.
10. Lynch AC, Dobbs BR, Keating J, Frizelle FA. The prevalence of faecal incontinence and constipation in a general New Zealand population; a postal survey. N Z Med J 2001; 114:474–476.

11. Francombe J, Carter PS, Hershman MJ. The aetiology and epidemiology of faecal incontinence. Hosp Med 2001; 62:529–532.
12. Perry S, Shaw C, McGrother C, et al. Prevalence of faecal incontinence in adults aged 40 years or more living in the community. Leicestershire MRC Incontinence Study Team. Gut 2002; 50: 480–484.
13. Hall W, McCracken K, Osterweil P, Guise JM. Frequency and predictors for postpartum fecal incontinence. Am J Obstet Gynecol 2003; 188:1205–1207.
14. Kalantar JS, Howell S, Talley NJ. Prevalence of faecal incontinence and associated risk factors; an underdiagnosed problem in the Australian community? Med J Aust 2002; 1762:54–57.
15. Faltin DL, Sangalli MR, Curtin F, Morabia A, Weil A. Prevalence of anal incontinence and other anorectal symptoms in women. Int Urogynecol J Pelvic Floor Dysfunct 2001; 12:117–120.
16. Edwards NI, Jones D. The prevalence of faecal incontinence in older people living at home. Age Ageing 2001; 30:503–507.
17. Eva UF, Gun W, Preben K. Prevalence of urinary and fecal incontinence and symptoms of genital prolapse in women. Acta Obstet Gynecol Scand 2003; 82:280–286.
18. Meschia M, Buonaguidi A, Pifarotti P, Somigliana E, Spennacchio M, Amicarelli F. Prevalence of anal incontinence in women with symptoms of urinary incontinence and genital prolapse. Obstet Gynecol 2002; 100:719–723.
19. Kuijpers JHC. Application of the colorectal laboratory in the diagnosis and treatment of functional constipation. Dis Colon Rectum 1990; 33:35–39.
20. Felt-Bersma RJF, Klinkenberg-Knol EC, Meuwissen SGM. Investigation of anorectal function. Br J Surg 1988; 75:53–55.
21. Smith LE. Practical Guide to Anorectal Testing. New York: Ikagu-Shoin, 1990.
22. Felt-Bersma RJF, Meuwissen SGM. Anal manometry. Int J Colorectal Dis 1990; 5:170–173.
23. Miller R, Bartolo DCC, Roe AM, Mortensen NJM. Assessment of microtransducers in anorectal manometry. Br J Surg 1988; 75:40–43.
24. Rockwood TH, Church JM, Fleshman JW, et al. Patient and surgeon ranking of the severity of symptoms associated with fecal incontinence: the fecal incontinence severity index. Dis Colon Rectum 1999; 42:1525–1532.
25. Kuijpers JHC, Scheuer M. Disorders of impaired fecal control: a clinical and manometric study. Dis Colon Rectum 1990; 33:207–211.
26. Snooks SJ, Swash M, Mathers SE, Henry MM. Effect of vaginal delivery on the pelvic floor: a 5-year follow-up. Br J Surg 1990; 77:1358–1360.
27. Womack NR, Morrisson JFB, Williams NS. Prospective study of the effects of postanal repair in neurogenic fecal incontinence. Br J Surg 1988; 75:48–52.
28. Scheuer M, Kuijpers HC, Jacobs PP. Postanal repair restores anatomy rather than function. Dis Colon Rectum 1989; 32:960–963.
29. Madoff RD, Rosen HR, Baeten CG, et al. Safety and efficacy of dynamic muscle plasty for anal incontinence: lessons from a prospective, multicenter trial. Gastroenterology 1999; 116:549–556.
30. Michot F, Costaglioli B, Leroi AM, Denis P. Artificial anal sphincter in severe fecal incontinence: outcome of prospective experience with 37 patients in one institution. Ann Surg 2003; 237:52–56.
31. Laurberg S, Swash M, Henry MM. Delayed external sphincter repair for obstetric tear. Br J Surg 1988; 75:786–788.
32. Jacobs PP, Scheuer M, Kuijpers JH, Vingerhoets MH. Obstetric fecal incontinenee. Role of pelvic floor denervation and results of delayed sphincter repair. Dis Colon Rectum 1990; 33:494–497.
33. Wexner SD, Marchetti F, Jagelman DG. The role of sphincteroplasty for fecal incontinence re-evaluated: a prospective physiologic and functional review. Dis Colon Rectum 1991; 34:22–30.
34. van Tets WF, Kuijpers JH, Tran K, Mollen R, van Goor H. Effects of Parks' anal retractor on anal sphincter pressures. Dis Colon Rectum 1997; 40:1042–1045.
35. Heymen S, Wexner SD, Vickers D, Nogueras JJ, Weiss EG, Pikarsky AJ. Prospective randomized trial comparing biofeedback techniques for patients with constipation. Dis Colon Rectum 1999; 42: 1388–1393.
36. Glia A, Gylin M, Akerlund JE, Lindfors U, Lindberg G. Biofeedback training in patients with fecal incontinence. Dis Colon Rectum 1988; 41:359–364.
37. Ko CY, Tong J, Lehman RE, Shelton AA, Schrock TR, Welton ML. Biofeedback is effective therapy for fecal incontinence and constipation. Arch Surg 1997; 132:829–833.
38. Yo YH, Tan M. Biofeedback therapy for bowel dysfunction following low anterior resection. Ann Acad Med Singapore 1997; 26:299–302.
39. Rieger NA, Watthow DA, Sarre RG, et al. Prospective trial of pelvic floor retraining in patients with fecal incontinence. Dis Colon Rectum 1997; 40:821–826.
40. van Tets WF, Kuijpers JH, Bleijenberg G. Biofeedback treatment is effective in neurologic fecal incontnience. Dis Colon Rectum 1996; 39:992–994.
41. Rao SS, Welcher KD, Happel J. Can biofeedback therapy improve anorectal function in fecal incontinence. Am J Gastroenterol 1996; 91:22,360–22,366.
42. Sangwan YP, Coller JA, Barrett RC, Roberts PL, Murray JJ, Schoetz DJ Jr. Can manometric parameters predict response to biofeedback therapy in fecal incontinence. Dis Colon Rectum 1995; 38:1021–1025.

43. Guillemot F, Bouche B, Gower-Rosseau C, et al. Biofeedback for the treatment of fecal incontinence: long-term clinical results. Dis Colon Rectum 1995; 38:393–397.

44. Keck JO, Staniunas RJ, Coller JA, et al. Biofeedback is useful in fecal incontinence but disappointing in constipation. Dis Colon Rectum 1994; 37:1271–1276.

45. Chiarioni G, Scattolini C, Bonfante F, Vantini I. Liquid stool incontinence with severe urgency: anorectal function and effective biofeedback treatment. Gut 1993; 34:1576–1580.

46. McIntosh LJ, Frahm JD, Mallett VT, Richardson DA. Pelvic floor rehabilitation in the treatment of incontinence. J Reprod Med 1993; 38:662–666.

47. Miner PB, Donnelly TC, Read NW. Investigation of mode of action of biofeedback in treatment of fecal incontinence. Dig Dis Sci 1990; 35:1291–1298.

48. Reboa G, Frascio M, Zanolla R, Pitto G, Riboli EB. Biofeedback training to obtain continence in permanent colostomy: experience of two centers. Dis Colon Rectum 1985; 28:419–421.

49. Enck P, Kranzle U, Schwiese J, et al. Biofeedback training in fecal incontinence. Dtsch Med Wochenschr 1988; 113:1789–1794.

50. Buser WD, Miner PB Jr. Delayed rectal sensation with fecal incontinence. Successful treatment using anorectal manometry. Gastroenterology 1986; 91:1186–1191.

51. Latimer PR, Campbell D, Kasperski J. A component analysis of biofeedback in the treatment of fecal incontinence. Biofeedback Self Regul 1984; 9:311–324.

52. MacLeod JH. Biofeedback in the management of partial anal incontinence. Dis Colon Rectum 1983; 26:244–246.

53. Wald A. Biofeedback therapy for fecal incontinence. Ann Intern Med 1981; 95:146–149.

54. Goldenberg DA, Hodges K, Hershe T, Jinich H. Biofeedback therapy for fecal incontinence. Am J Gastroenterol 1980; 74:342–345.

55. Cerulli MA, Nikoomanesh P, Schuster MM. Progress in biofeedback conditioning for fecal incontinence. Gastroenterology 1979; 76:742–746.

56. Iwai N, Iwata G, Kimura O, Yanagihara J. Is a new biofeedback therapy effective for fecal incontinence in patients who have anorectal malformations? J Pediatr Surg 1997; 32:1626–1629.

57. Arhan P, Faverdin C, Devroede G, et al. Biofeedback re-education of faecal incontinence in children. Int J Colorectal Dis 1994; 9:128–133.

58. Loening-Baucke V, Desch L, Wolraich M. Biofeedback training for patients with myelomeningocele and fecal incontinence. Dev Med Child Neurol 1988; 30:781–790.

59. Whitehead WE, Parker L, Bosmajian L, et al. Treatment of fecal incontinence in children with spina bifida: comparison of biofeedback and behavior modification. Arch Phys Med Rehab 1986; 67: 218–224.

60. Wald A. Biofeedback for neurologic fecal incontinence: rectal sensation is a determinant of outcome. J Pediatr Gastroenterol Nutr 1983; 2:302–306.

61. Whitehead WE, Parker LH, Masek BJ, Cataldo MF, Freeman JM. Biofeedback treatment of fecal incontinence in patients with myelomeningocele. Dev Med Child Neurol 1981; 23:313–322.

62. Wald A. Use of biofeedback in treatment of fecal incontinence in patients with meningomyelocele. Pediatrics 1981; 68:45–49.

63. Olness K, McParland FA, Piper J. Biofeedback: a new modality in the management of children with fecal soiling. J Pediatr 1980; 96:505–509.

64. Heymen S, Jones KR, Ringel Y, Scarlett Y, Whitehead WE. Biofeedback treatment of fecal incontinence: a critical review. Dis Colon Rectum 2001; 44:728–736.

65. Heymen S, Pikarsky AJ, Weiss EG, Vickers D, Nogueras JJ, Wexner SD. A prospective randomized trial comparing four biofeedback techniques for patients with fecal incontinence. Colorectal Dis 2000; 2:88–92.

66. Irvine EJ, Ferrazzi S, Pare P, Thompson WG, Rance L. Health-related quality of life in functional GI disorders: focus on constipation and resource utilization. Am J Gastroenterol 2002; 97:1986–1993.

67. Stewart WF, Liberman JN, Sandler RS, et al. Epidemiology of constipation (EPOC) study in the United States: relation of clinical subtypes to sociodemographic features. Am J Gastroenterol 1999; 94:3530–3540.

68. Chiarelli P, Brown W, McElduff P. Constipation in Australian women: prevalence and associated factors. Int Urogynecol J Pelvic Floor Dysfunct 2000; 11:71–78.

69. Robson KM, Kiely DK, Lembo T. Development of constipation in nursing home residents. Dis Colon Rectum 2000; 43:940–943.

70. van Dijk KN, de Vries CS, van den Berg PB, Dijkema AM, Brouwers JR, de Jong-van den Berg LT. Constipation as an adverse effect of drug use in nursing home patients: an overestimated risk. J Clin Pharmacol 1998; 46:255–261.

71. Saito YA, Schoenfeld P, Locke GR III. The epidemiology of irritable bowel syndrome in North America: a systematic review. Am J Gastroenterol 2002; 97:1910–1915.

72. Kuijpers JHC, Bleijenberg G. The spastic pelvic floor syndrome: a cause of constipation. Dis Colon Rectum 1985; 28:669–672.

73. Felt-Bersma RJF, Gort G, Meuwissen SGM. Normal values in anal manometry and rectal sensation; a problem of range. Hepatogastroenterol 1991; 38:444–449.

74. Bartolo DCC, Bartram CI, Ekberg O, et al. Symposium on proctography. Int J Colorectal Dis 1988; 3:67–89.

75. Metcalf AM, Phillips SF, Zinsheimer AR, Maccarthy RL, Beart RW, Wolff BG. Simplified assessment of segmental colonic transit. Gastroenterology 1987; 92:40–47.
76. Kuijpers JHC, Bleijenberg G. Assessment and treatment of obstructed defecation. Ann Med 1990; 22:405–411.
77. Preston DM, Lennard-Jones JE. Anismus in chronic constipation. Dig Dis Sci 1985; 30:413–418.
78. Kamm MA, Hawley PR, Lennard-Jones JE. Lateral division of the puborectalis muscle in the management of severe constipation. Br J Surg 1988; 75:661–663.
79. Hallaon RI, Melling J, Womack NR, Williams NS, Waldron DJ, Morrisson JFB. Treatment of anismus in intractable constipation with botulinum A toxin. Lancet 1988; 2:714–717.
80. Krishnamurthy S, Schuffler MD. Pathology of neuromuscular disorders of the small intestine and colon. Gastroenterology 1987; 93:630–639.
81. Mollen RM, Hopman WP, Oyen WJ, Kuijpers HH, Edelbroek MA, Jansen JB. Effect of subtotal colectomy on gastric emptying of a solid meal in slow-transit constipation. Dis Colon Rectum 2001; 44:1189–1195.
82. Mollen RM, Kuijpers HC, Claassen AT. Colectomy for slow-transit constipation: preoperative functional evaluation is important but not a guarantee for a successful outcome. Dis Colon Rectum 2001; 44:577–580.
83. Yoshioka K, Keighley MRB. Clinical results of colectomy for severe constipation. Br J Surg 1989; 76:600–604.
84. Pemberton JH, Rath DM, Ilstrup DM. Evaluation and surgical treatment of severe chronic constipation. Ann Surg 1991; 214:403–413.
85. Dailianas A, Skandalis N, Rimikis MN, Koutsoumanis D, Kardasi M, Archimadritis A. Pelvic floor study in patients with obstructive defecation influence of biofeedback. J Clini Gastroenterol 2000; 30:176–180.
86. McKee RF, McEnroe L, Anderson JH, Finlay IG. Identification of patients likely to benefit from biofeedback for outlet obstruction constipation. Br J Surg 1999; 86:355–359.
87. Rhee PL, Choi MS, Kim YH, et al. An increased rectal maximum tolerable volume and long anal canal are associated with poor short-term response to biofeedback therapy for patients with anismus with decreased bowel frequency and normal colonic transit time. Dis Colon Rectum 2000; 43:1405–1411.
88. Karlbom U, Hallden M, Eeg-Olofsson KE, Pahlman L, Graf W. Results of biofeedback in constipated patients: a prospective study. Dis Colon Rectum 1997; 40:1149–1155.
89. Rao SS, Welcher KD, Pelsing RE. Effects of biofeedback on anorectal function in obstructed defecation. Dig Dis Sci 1997; 42:2197–2205.
90. Rieger NA, Wattchow DA, Sarre RG, et al. Prospective study of biofeedback for treatment of constipation. Dis Colon Rectum 1997; 40:1143–1148.
91. Glia A, Glyin M, Gullberg K, Lindberg G. Biofeedback retraining in patients with functional constipation and paradoxical puborectalis contraction: comparison of anal manometry and sphincter electromyography for feedback. Dis Colon Rectum 1997; 40:889–895.
92. Heah SM, Ho YH, Tan M, Leong AF. Biofeedback is effective treatment for levator ani syndrome. Dis Colon Rectum 1997; 40:187–189.
93. Ho YH, Tan M, Goh HS. Clinical and physiologic effects of biofeedback in outlet obstruction constipation. Dis Colon Rectum 1996; 39:520–524.
94. Koutsomanis D, Lennard-Jones JE, Roy AJ, Kamm MA. Controlled randomized trial of visual biofeedback versus muscle training without a visual display for intractable constipation. Gut 1995; 37:95–99.
95. Hull TL, Fazio VW, Schroeder T. Paradoxical contraction in patients after pelvic pouch construction. Dis Colon Rectum 1995; 38(11):1144–1146.
96. Papachrysostomou M, Smith AN. Effects of biofeedback on obstructive defecation—reconditioning of the defecation reflex? Gut 1994; 35:252–256.
97. Bleijenberg G, Kuijpers HC. Biofeedback treatment of constipation: a comparison of two methods. Am J Gastroenterol 1994; 89:1021–1026.
98. Wexner SD, Cheape JD, Jorge JM, Heymen S, Jagelman DG. Prospective assessment of biofeedback for the treatment of paradoxical puborectalis contraction. Dis Colon Rectum 1992; 35:1193–1194.
99. Turnbull GK, Ritvo PG. Anal sphincter biofeedback relaxation treatment for women with intractable constipation symptoms. Dis Colon Rectum 1992; 35:530–536.
100. Fleshman JW, Dreznik Z, Meyer K, Fry RD, Carney R, Kodner IJ. Outpatient protocol for biofeedback therapy of pelvic floor outlet obstruction. Dis Colon Rectum 1992; 35:1–7.
101. Kawimbe BM, Papachrysostomou M, Binnie RN, Clare N, Smith AN. Outlet obstruction constipation (anismus) managed by biofeedback. Gut 1991; 32:1175–1179.
102. Lestar B, Pennickx F, Kerremans R. Biofeedback defaecation training for anismus. Int J Colorectal Dis 1991; 6:202–207.
103. Dahl J, Lindquist BL, Tysk C, Leissner P, Philipson L, Jarnerot G. Behavioral medicine treatment in chronic constipation with paradoxical puborectalis contraction. Dis Colon Rectum 1991; 34:769–776.
104. Emery Y, Descos L, Meunier P, Louis D, Valancogne G, Weil G. Terminal constipation caused by abdominopelvic asynchrony: analysis of etiological, clinical, manometric data and therapeutic results after rehabilitation by biofeedback. Gastroenterol Clin Biol 1988; 12:6–11.

105. Weber J, Ducrotte P, Touchais JY, Roussignol C, Denis P. Biofeedback training for constipation in adults and children. Dis Colon Rectum 1987; 30:844–846.

106. Nolan T, Catto-Smith T, Coffey C, Wells J. Randomized controlled trial of biofeedback training in persistent encopresis with anismus. Arch Dis Child 1998; 79:131–135.

107. Ponticelli A, Iacobelli BD, Silveri M, Broggi G, Rivosechi M, De Gennaro M. Colorectal dysfunction and faecal incontinence in children with spina bifida. Br J Urol 1998; 81(suppl 3):117–119.

108. Van der Plas RN, Benninga MA, Redekop WK, Taminiau JA, Buller HA. Randomized trial of biofeedback training for encopresis. Arch Dis Childhood 1996; 75:367–374.

109. Cox DJ, Sutphen J, Borowitz S, Dickens MN, Singles J, Whitehead WE. Simple electromyographic biofeedback treatment for chronic pediatric constipation/encopresis: preliminary report. Biofeedback Self Regul 1994; 19:41–50.

110. Loening-Baucke V. Persistence of chronic constipation in children after biofeedback treatment. Dig Dis Sci 1991; 36:153–160.

111. Loening-Baucke V. Modulation of abnormal defecation dynamics by biofeedback treatment in chronically constipated children with encopresis. J Pediatrics 1990; 116:214–222.

112. Keren S, Wagner Y, Heldenbert D, Golan M. Studies of manometric abnormalities of the rectoanal region during defecation in constipated and soiling children: modification through biofeedback therapy. Am J Gastroenterol 1988; 83:827–831.

113. Veyrac M, Granel D, Parelon G, Michel H. Idiopathic constipation in children. Value of treatment by biofeedback. Pediatrie 1987; 42:719–721.

114. Wald A, Chandra R, Gabel S, Chiponis D. Evaluation of biofeedback in childhood encopresis. J Pediatr Gastroenterol Nutr 1987; 6:554–558.

115. Heymen S, Jones KR, Scarlett Y, Whitehead WE. Biofeedback treatment of constipation: a critical review. Dis Colon Rectum. 2003; 46:1208–1217.

116. Heymen S, Wexner SD, Vickers D, Nogueras J, Weiss EG. A prospective randomized trial comparing four biofeedback techniques for patients with constipation [Abstr]. Gastroenterology 1996; 10:1678.

117. Whitehead WE, Wald A, Diamant N, Enck P, Pemberton J, Rao S. Functional disorders of the anus and rectum. In: Drossman DA, Corazziari E, Talley NJ, Thompson WG, Whitehead WE, eds. Rome II: The Functional Gastrointestinal Disorders. Falls Church, Virginia: Degnon Associates, 2000.

118. Wald A. Functional anorectal and pelvic pain. Gastroenterol Clin North Am 2001; 30:243–251.

119. Whitehead WE, Wald A, Diamant NE, Enck P, Pemberton JH, Rao SS. Functional disorders of the anus and rectum. Gut 1999; 45(suppl 2):II55– II59.

120. Wesselmann U, Burnett AL, Heinberg LJ. The urogenital and rectal pain syndromes. Pain 1997; 73:269–294.

121. Shafik A. Pudendal canal syndrome and proctalgia fugax. Dis Colon Rectum 1997; 40:504–506.

122. Hetrick DC, Ciol MA, Rothman I, Turner JA, Frest M, Berger RE. Musculoskeletal dysfunction in men with chronic pelvic pain syndrome type III: a case-control study. J Urol 2003; 170:828–831.

123. Ramsden CE, McDaniel MC, Harmon RL, Renney KM, Faure A. Nerve entrapment as source of intractable perineal pain. Am J Phys Med Rehabil 2003; 82:479–484.

124. Kamm MA, Hoyle CH, Burleigh DE, et al. Hereditary internal anal sphincter myopathy causing proctalgia fugax and constipation. A newly identified condition. Gastroenterology 1991; 100:805–810.

125. Morris L, Newton RA. Use of high voltage pulsed galvanic stimulation for patients with levator ani syndrome. Phys Ther 1987; 67:1522–1525.

126. Nicosia JF, Abcarian H. Levator syndrome. A treatment that works. Dis Colon Rectum 1985; 28: 406–408.

127. Katsinelos P, Kalomenopoulou M, Christodoulou K, et al. Treatment of proctalgia fugax with botulinum A toxin. Eur J Gastroenterol Hepatol 2001; 13:371–373.

128. Potter MA, Bartolo DC. Proctalgia fugax. Eur J Gastroenterol Hepatol 2001; 13:1289–1290.

129. Ramsey ML, Toohey JS, Neidre A, Stromberg LJ, Roberts DA. Coccygodynia: treatment. Orthopedics 2003; 26:403–405.

130. Henry MM, Parks AG, Swash M. The pelvic floor musculature in the descending perineum syndrome. Br J Surg 1982; 69:470–472.

131. van Tets W, Kuijpers JHC. Internal rectal intussusception—fact or fancy? Dis Colon Rectum 1995; 38:1080–1083.

132. Grimaud JC, Bouvier M, Naudy B, Guien C, Salducci J. Manometric and radiologic investigations and biofeedback treatment of chronic idiopathic anal pain. Dis Colon Rectum 1991; 34:690–695.

133. Ger GC, Wexner SD, Jorge JM, et al. Evaluation and treatment of chronic intractable rectal pain—a frustrating endeavor. Dis Colon Rectum 1993; 36:139–145.

134. Gilliland R, Heymen JS, Altomare DF, Vickers D, Wexner SD. Biofeedback for intractable rectal pain: outcome and predictors of success. Dis Colon Rectum 1997; 40:190–196.

135. Salzano A, Carbone M, Rossi E, et al. [Defecography and treatment of essential anal pain.] [Italian] Radiol Med 1999; 98:48–52.

136. Diseth TH, Emblem R. Somatic function, mental health, and psychological adjustment of adolescents with anorectal anomalies. J Pediatr Surg 1996; 31:638–643.

137. Huppe D, Enck P, Kruskemper G, May B. Psychosocial aspects of fecal incontinence [German]. Leber Magen Darm 1992; 22:138–142.

138. O'Keefe EA, Talley NJ, Zinsmeister AR, Jacobsen SJ. Bowel disorders impair functional status and quality of life in the elderly: a population-based study. J Gerontol A Biol Sci Med Sci 1995; 50:M184–M189.

139. Burnett C, Whitehead WE, Drossman D. Psychological distress and impaired quality of life in patients with functional anorectal disorders. Gastroenterology 1998; 114:A729.

140. Heymen S, Wexner SD, Gulledge AD. MMPI assessment of patients with functional bowel disorders. Dis Colon Rectum 1993; 36:593–596.

141. Fisher SE, Breckon K, Andrews H, Keighley M. Psychiatric screening for patients with faecal incontinence or chronic constipation referred for surgical treatment. Br J Surg 1989; 76:352–355.

142. Burgio KL, Locher J, Roth D, Goode P. Psychological improvements associated with behavioral and drug treatment of urge incontinence in older women. J Gerontol B Psychol Sci Soc Sci 2001; 56:P46–P51.

143. Millard RJ, Oldenburg B. The symptomatic, urodynamic and psychodynamic results of bladder re-education programs. J Urol 1983; 130:715–719.

144. Rosenzweig BA, Hischke D, Thomas S, Nelson A, Bhatia N. Stress incontinence in women: psychological status before and after treatment. J Reprod Med 1991; 36:835–838.

145. Devroede G, Girard G, Bouchoucha M, et al. Idiopathic constipation by colonic dysfunction. Relationship with personality and anxiety. Dig Dis Sci 1989; 34:1428–1433.

146. Kumar D, Bartolo DC, Devroede G, et al. Symposium on constipation. Int J Colorectal Dis 1992; 7: 47–67.

147. Nehra V, Bruce B, Rath-Harvey DM, Pemberton JH, Camilleri M. Psychological disorders in patients with evacuation disorders and constipation in a tertiary practice. Am J Gastroenterol 2000; 95:1755–1758.

148. Whitehead WE. Illness behaviour. In: Kamm NA, Lennard–Jones JE, eds. Constipation. Petersfield: Wrightson Biomedical Publishing, 1993:95–100.

149. Strickland M, Heymen S. Psychiatric treatment of constipation. In: Wexner SD, Bartolo DCC, eds. Constipation: Etiology, Evaluation and Management. London: Butterworth Heinemann, 1995: 251–261.

150. Heymen S, Wexner SD. Biofeedback for constipation. 2nd ed. In: Smith LE, ed. A Practical Guide to Anorectal Testing. New York: Igaku-Shoin, 1995:261–270.

151. Kuijpers HC. Application of the colorectal laboratory in diagnosis and treatment of functional constipation. Dis Colon Rectum 1990; 33:35–39.

152. Lennard-Jones JE. Clinical management of constipation. Pharmacology 1993; 47(suppl 1):216–223.

153. McKee RF, McEnroe L, Anderson JH, Finlay IG. Identification of patients likely to benefit from biofeedback for outlet obstruction constipation. Br J Surg 1999; 86:355–359.

154. Guerrero RA, Cavender CP. Constipation: physical and psychological sequelae. Pediatr Ann 1999; 28(5):312–316.

155. Dykes S, Smilgin-Humphreys S, Bass C. Chronic idiopathic constipation: a psychological enquiry. Eur J Gastroenterol Hepatol 2001; 1:39–44.

156. Leroi AM, Berkelmahs I, Denis P, Hemond M, Devroede G. Anismus as a marker of sexual abuse. Consequences of abuse on anorectal motility. Dig Dis Sci 1995; 40:1411–1416.

157. Loening-Baucke V. Factors determining outcome in children with chronic constipation and faecal soiling. Gut 1989; 30:999–1006.

158. Friman PC, Mathews JR, Finney JW, Christopherson ER, Leibowitz JM. Do encopretic children have clinically significant behavior problems? Pediatrics 1988; 82:407–409.

159. Loening-Baucke V, Cruikshank B, Savage C. Defecation dynamics and behavior profiles in encopretric children. Pediatrics 1987; 80(5):672–679.

12 ▌ Infectious Colitis

Derek Patel
Division of Gastroenterology, Department of Medicine, University of California–San Diego, San Diego, California, U.S.A.

John P. Cello
Department of Medicine and Surgery, University of California–San Francisco, San Francisco, California, U.S.A.

INTRODUCTION

The colon is a frequent target organ for enteric infections. Patients with infectious colitis may present with a broad spectrum of illnesses ranging from an essentially asymptomatic state of mild, self-limited diarrhea, to fulminant toxic colitis requiring aggressive resuscitation and surgical management. Early recognition of the signs and symptoms of infectious colitis and the expeditious identification of the pathogens allow for appropriate and prompt treatment. The focus of this chapter is on the clinical presentation, distinguishing features, and treatment of the commonly encountered etiologies of infectious colitis. Multiple organisms are associated with infectious colitis, and in this chapter they will be grouped into bacterial, parasitic, fungal, and viral agents. A summary of the presentations, endoscopic findings, diagnostic strategies, and therapies for the described infectious colitides can be found in Table 1.

BACTERIAL COLITIS
Nontyphoidal Salmonella

Salmonella infection is one of the most commonly reported causes of infectious colitis in the United States, and accounts for approximately one-third of the deaths resulting from food-borne illness in the United States (1). Fifty percent of cases of salmonella infection are linked to contaminated poultry, meats, eggs, and dairy products (2). The greatest risks occur in children under one year of age, although there is also a high attack rate and mortality in the elderly. Conditions that predispose to infection include hemolytic anemia, immunosuppression, and chronic schistosomiasis, the latter because salmonella multiply within the parasites, which then serve as a source for recurrent infection. Salmonella organisms are motile gram-negative bacilli. The most common serotypes in the United States are *Salmonella enteritides*, followed by *Salmonella typhimurium*, *Salmonella heidelberg*, *Salmonella newport*, and *Salmonella hadar*. Salmonella organisms most typically attack the small bowel, but the colon is often involved as well (3–5).

Patients with salmonellosis typically present with abdominal pain and symptoms of gastroenteritis, such as nausea, vomiting, and watery diarrhea. In those patients with colitis, diarrhea, occasionally bloody, may be present. Although the symptoms of gastroenteritis usually last only three to four days, the symptoms of colitis may continue for two to three weeks (2). On endoscopic examination of individuals with colitis, there may be diffuse involvement of the colon. However, as with most other causes of infectious colitis, the rectum is almost invariably involved. Common findings are mucosal edema, hyperemia, petechial hemorrhage, aphthous erosions, and small ulcerations (3,6). In more severe cases, deep ulcers with significant bleeding have been described (7,8). Although rare, there are reports of colitis complicated by toxic megacolon and spontaneous perforation (9,10). It is important to recognize that these features are not specific for Salmonella, and are common in other forms of colitis.

The diagnosis of salmonella infection is made by stool culture using routine media. Organisms at a count of 1×10^5 organisms per gram of feces result in the detection of greater

Table 1 Pathogens that Cause Colitis—Presentation, Endoscopic Findings, Diagnosis, and Therapy

Pathogen	Clinical presentation	Endoscopic findings	Diagnosis	Recommended therapy
Salmonella	Watery/bloody diarrhea, abdominal pain, nausea, vomiting	Diffuse edema, hyperemia, erosions/ shallow ulcers	Stool culture	Amoxicillin, TMP/SMX, quinolones[a]
Shigella, EIEC	Watery/bloody diarrhea, tenesmus, fever	Rectosigmoid edema, hyperemia, shallow ulcers; pancolitis rare	Stool culture	TMP/SMX, quinolones
Campylobacter	Watery/bloody diarrhea, abdominal pain, fever, headache	Segmental or diffuse edema, shallow ulceration	Stool culture	Erythromycin, quinolones[a]
EHEC (O157:H7)	Watery/bloody diarrhea, severe abdominal pain, occasionally hemolytic uremic syndrome	Edema, hyperemia, ulceration; proximal > distal, rectal sparing	Stool culture on sorbitol Mac-Conkey agar	Antibiotics not recommended
Tuberculosis	Abdominal pain, weight loss, nonbloody diarrhea, nausea, vomiting	Highly variable: deep linear or irregular ulcers, strictures, hypertrophic mass lesions; ileocecal area most common site	Endoscopic biopsy (acid-fast stain + PCR)	Three to four antituberculous drugs (Isoniazid, Rifampin, Pyrazinamide, Ethambutol)
Yersinia	Nonbloody diarrhea, fever, right lower quadrant abdominal pain; may be mistaken for appendicitis	Edema, hyperemia, shallow ulcerations of terminal ileum, cecum, and ascending colon	Stool culture on cold-enriched medium	Doxycycline, TMP/ SMX, Chloramphenicol, quinolones[a]
Chlamydia trachomatis	Proctalgia, tenesmus, blood/mucus in stool	Friability, ulceration in rectum	Culture, DFA of rectal swab	LGV immunotypes: Doxycycline, Tetracycline; NonLGV: Azithromycin, Doxycycline followed by Ofloxacin, Erythromycin
Neisseria gonorrhea	Often asymptomatic; may have pruritis ani, painful defecation	Mucous discharge, erythema, erosions, fissures in anal canal, rectum	Culture of rectal swab on Thayer–Martin agar	Ceftriaxone, Cefixime, Ciprofloxacin, Ofloxacin
Vibrio parahaemolyticus	Explosive watery diarrhea, abdominal pain, nausea, vomiting	Superficial ulcerations in distal colon	Stool culture on TCBS medium	Doxycycline, Tetracycline[a]
Aeromonas	Watery/bloody diarrhea, cramps, vomiting, fever	Edema, friability, erosions; may be left-sided or pancolitis	Stool culture	Quinolones, TMP/SMX[a]
Plesiomonas	Watery/bloody diarrhea, abdominal pain, vomiting, fever	Aphthous erosions in left colon	Stool culture	Quinolones, TMP/SMX[a]
Entamoeba histolytica	Variable: mild diarrhea and cramping to bloody diarrhea, tenesmus, abdominal pain, fever	Predominantly right-sided discrete shallow "punched out" ulcers with exudates; segmental masses of granulation tissue	Stool wet mount, stool culture, stool PCR, endoscopic biopsy (H&E, iron hematoxylin or immunohistochem-ical stain)	Metronidazole followed by Paromomycin, Iodoquinol
Trichuris trichiura	Often asymptomatic; may have mild	Coiled white 1 cm worms with heads	Stool wet mount, biopsy recovery of	Albendazole, Mebendazole

(Continued)

Table 1 Pathogens that Cause Colitis—Presentation, Endoscopic Findings, Diagnosis, and Therapy (*Continued*)

Pathogen	Clinical presentation	Endoscopic findings	Diagnosis	Recommended therapy
	diarrhea, bloody stool	embedded in mucosa; often found in cecum	worm	
Histoplasma	Watery/bloody diarrhea, weight loss, fever, abdominal pain	Erythema, ulcers, polyps/masses; most common in terminal ileum, cecum	Endoscopic biopsy (fungal stain, fungal culture)	Amphotericin B followed by Itraconazole
Cytomegalovirus	Watery/bloody diarrhea, abdominal pain, weight loss	Diffuse erythema with focal ulceration, subepithelial hemorrhage; pancolitis common	Endoscopic biopsy (H&E, PCR, immunostain, viral culture)	Ganciclovir, Foscarnet
Herpes simplex virus	Severe proctalgia, tenesmus, bloody stool	Small vesicles, shallow apthous ulcers in anus, distal rectum	Cell culture, DFA of anal/rectal swab	Acyclovir

[a]Antibiotics indicated in severe illness, young/elderly patients, immunosuppressed individuals, and pregnancy.
Abbreviations: TMP/SMX, trimethoprim-sulfamethoxazole; EIEC, enteroinvasive *E. coli*; EHEC, enterohemorrhagic *E. coli*; PCR, polymerase chain reaction; DFA, direct fluorescent antibody; LGV, lymphogranuloma venereum; H&E, hematoxylin and eosin; TCBS, thiosulfate-citrate-bile salts-sucrose agar.

than 90% of cases (11). In multiple studies, antibiotic treatment failed to alter the rate of clinical recovery from salmonella gastroenteritis (12–14). In fact, treatment may actually increase the duration of intestinal carriage, and thereby prolong fecal shedding (14–16). There are no prospective trials of antibiotic therapy in salmonella colitis. Thus, antibiotic treatment is not universally recommended. Antibiotics may be indicated; however, in the setting of particularly severe colitis or in patients at the extremes of age, immunosuppressed individuals, or pregnant women (17). The preferred antibiotics for the treatment of salmonella colitis include amoxicillin, trimethoprim-sulfamethoxazole (TMP/SMX), or quinolones.

Shigella and Enteroinvasive *Escherichia coli*

Shigella species infect over 200 million people annually, and are responsible for nearly 650,000 deaths worldwide each year (18). Infection is largely due to contaminated food and water, with most transmissions occurring person-to-person in a fecal-oral manner (2,19). *Shigella* can also be transmitted sexually, largely within the male homosexual population (20). *Shigella* is a nonlactose fermenting gram-negative rod of which humans are the only natural host. There are four species: *Shigella dysenteriae*, *Shigella flexneri*, *Shigella sonnei*, and *Shigella boydii*. The most common subgroup occurring in the United States is *Shigella sonnei* (21).

Shigellosis is characteristically a biphasic illness. Initially, constitutional symptoms such as fever, fatigue, and anorexia predominate. Nonbloody, watery diarrhea is also common. This is followed three to five days later by tenesmus and small volume bloody stool (21). Endoscopically, *Shigella* usually involves the rectosigmoid in a confluent manner, creating an appearance of hyperemic friable mucosa that is similar to idiopathic ulcerative colitis (22). The abnormalities can extend proximally, and rarely, pancolitis may result (22,23). Proximal disease has been found to be associated with a longer duration of diarrhea (22). Other nonspecific colonoscopic findings include edema with loss of vascular pattern, ulcers, and adherent mucopurulent membranes covering the mucosal surface (22,23). In the majority of patients, the aforementioned mucosal abnormalities are continuous and diffuse, but become patchy in distribution during clinical recovery. Pseudopolyps and strictures may also result from healing of *Shigella* colitis (24). While uncommon in the United States, obstruction, toxic megacolon, and perforation due to shigellosis occur regularly in developing countries (21,25,26).

The diagnosis of *Shigella* infection is made by stool culture on standard media. Although in the Western world, the disease course of *Shigella* colitis typically lasts less than one week, antibiotic therapy has been shown to shorten the duration of illness and reduce mortality (27,28). Given the ease of transmission and potential for causing life-threatening illness, antibiotic treatment is always indicated for documented shigellosis. Suggested antibiotics in adults include TMP/SMX and quinolones. Antimotility agents have been reported to worsen the symptoms, and may predispose to toxic megacolon, and therefore should be avoided (29).

Certain *Escherichia coli* (*E. coli*) strains known as enteroinvasive *E. coli* (EIEC) are closely related to *Shigella* and produce an identical clinical syndrome, although the infective dose for EIEC is at least at 1000-fold greater (2). Transmission of EIEC is usually food borne or waterborne, but person-to-person spread has been reported (30). This organism was responsible for a single widespread outbreak of dysentery associated with imported French Camembert cheese (31,32). Patients infected with EIEC typically present with watery diarrhea, but sometimes blood and mucus are found in the stool (30). Tenesmus and fever may also be present. The diagnosis of *E. coli* infection is made by culture of stool on routine media, but the possibility of EIEC must be mentioned in the request for culture. The disease course seems to be short, and antibiotics are often not needed. However, as in the case of *Shigella*, antibiotics would be expected to reduce the duration of illness. There are no clinical trials of antibiotics in the treatment of EIEC colitis to confirm this. Resistance to ampicillin and TMP/SMX is common; for this reason, quinolones are generally recommended (14).

Campylobacter

Campylobacter is the most frequently identified bacterial cause of diarrhea in the North America (33). The Centers for Disease Control estimates that 2.4 million *Campylobacter* infections occur annually in the United States, involving almost 1% of the entire population (34). Overall, *Campylobacter* infections are twice as common as *Salmonella*, and seven times more common than *Shigella* (35). Most *Campylobacter* infections in the developed countries are acquired during the preparation and eating of chicken (33). Person-to-person transmission is thought to play a minor role. *Campylobacter* is a motile gram-negative rod with a spiral shape. The most common *Campylobacter* species in humans is *Campylobacter jejuni*.

Patients with *Campylobacter colitis* present with fever, nausea, abdominal pain, and diarrhea (33). Prodromal symptoms such as coryza, headache, and malaise are common. More than half also have gross or occult fecal blood (36,37). Because of the frequency of bleeding, *Campylobacter* infection is sometimes mistaken for idiopathic inflammatory bowel disease. *Campylobacter colitis* is associated with the sequelae of reactive arthritis and Guillain-Barré syndrome (33,38). It is thought that approximately 30% of cases of Guillain-Barré syndrome are preceded by *Campylobacter* infection (39). Colonoscopic findings in patients with *Campylobacter colitis* range from segmental aphthous ulceration to a diffuse colitis with an edematous, exudative appearance, and spontaneous bleeding (40,41). Pseudomembranous colitis as well as toxic megacolon have been described (42–44).

Obtaining fecal culture for *Campylobacter* using standard media remains the best method of diagnosis. The clinical course of *Campylobacter colitis* is typically self-limited, but symptoms may last for more than one week in about 20% of the patients (42). Antibiotics benefit patients who have experienced more than seven days of symptoms, high fevers, or grossly bloody stool (33). Pregnant women and immunocompromised individuals likely should also receive antibiotics for the treatment of *Campylobacter colitis* (33). There is an alarming recent trend in the rapid emergence of antibiotic resistance (up to 84% in one study) due to the use of antibiotics in animals raised for food (45). Largely because of this, erythromycin has once again come to be considered the optimal drug for treatment of *Campylobacter* infection.

Escherichia coli O157:H7

Infection with *E. coli* O157:H7, also known as enterohemorrhagic *E. coli* (EHEC), was first recognized as a cause of human illness in 1982, when 47 individuals in Michigan and Oregon developed bloody diarrhea after eating contaminated hamburgers (46). Most cases of *E. coli* O157:H7 follow this pattern and are associated with outbreaks related to the consumption of undercooked mechanically processed ground beef contaminated with cattle feces during slaughter and processing (47). The low infectious dose required contributes to the person-to-person spread (48,49). Although it accounts overall for very few cases of diarrhea in North America, *E. coli* O157:H7 accounts for approximately 6% to 36% of the cases of bloody diarrhea (50–52). The high virulence of this organism is due to its production of large amounts of Shiga toxin.

Following ingestion, the incubation period for infection is three to five days. Patients typically experience the abrupt onset of nonbloody diarrhea that converts to frankly bloody stool after 24 to 48 hours (53). Often there is associated intense abdominal pain. Fatigue, headaches, and malaise are other commonly associated symptoms (54). Because of their often markedly bloody stool, patients with *E. coli* O157:H7 infection are frequently misdiagnosed with diverticular hemorrhage, ischemic colitis or idiopathic inflammatory bowel disease. Patients at the extremes of age are at increased risks for complications, such as hemolytic uremic syndrome (HUS), thrombotic thrombocytopenic purpura, and death (55). *E. coli* O157:H7 is associated with 75% to 90% of cases of HUS in North America, and overall, 8% of cases of *E. coli* O157:H7 infection result in HUS (50). Endoscopy in patients with *E. coli* O157:H7-associated hemorrhagic colitis usually reveals focal erythema, edema, superficial ulceration, and occasional pseudomembranes (56). The most serious abnormalities tend to be found in the cecum and ascending colon, with the disease taking on a less severe appearance distally (56). The rectum is typically spared, reminiscent of ischemic colitis (56).

The diagnosis of *E. coli* O157:H7 colitis is usually made on the basis of clinical findings, and is confirmed by serotyping sorbitol-negative *E. coli* isolates or by using tissue culture or gene probes to detect cytotoxin. Unless it is known that the microbiology laboratory routinely includes a sorbitol Mac-Conkey agar plate to screen all stool (many clinical microbiology labs do not), any physician considering this pathogen should specifically request this technique (57). The timing of stool collection is important, as virtually all stool specimens are positive within two days of symptoms, but only one-third are positive after seven days (58). Rapid nonculture-based tests are available for diagnosis, but these currently lack the sensitivity to replace the gold standard stool culture (59). Once the diagnosis of *E. coli* O157:H7 infection is made, a baseline complete blood count, electrolyte panel, and renal function tests should be checked to assist in monitoring for possible later complications such as HUS. Additionally, because of the possibility that an infected patient represents an index case in an outbreak, the treating physician should report a probable or definite *E. coli* O157:H7 infection to appropriate public health authorities urgently.

Despite dramatic hematochezia, most patients with *E. coli* O157:H7 colitis have a self-limited illness. It is generally recommended that antibiotics should be avoided in light of several published case series suggesting increased risks of HUS in patients receiving antibiotic treatment (60,61). This approach is somewhat controversial; however, a recent meta-analysis of nine published studies suggests no association between HUS and antibiotic use (62). Antimotility agents should also be avoided as they have been shown to prolong the duration of bloody diarrhea and increase the risk of HUS in children (48,63,64). Severe cases of *E. coli* O157:H7 colitis associated with renal failure and microangiopathic hemolytic anemia and thrombocytopenia may ultimately require treatment with steroids and/or hemodialysis.

Tuberculosis

Both *Mycobacterium tuberculosis* and *Mycobacterium bovis* can infect the intestinal tract. In the United States, tuberculosis occurs mainly in patients with AIDS, in prisoners, immigrants, the urban poor and the elderly, particularly those residing in nursing homes (65–68). Tuberculous enteritis occurs from swallowing infected sputum, ingesting contaminated milk, hematogenous spread or rarely, direct spread from adjacent infected organs (69). Only approximately 20% of patients with gastrointestinal (GI) involvement have concomitant pulmonary tuberculosis (69–71).

Patients with tuberculous colitis tend to have nonspecific symptoms including abdominal pain (in 90% of patients), weight loss, and diarrhea (69,72–74). Hematochezia is uncommon. Not infrequently, patients will have a palpable mass in the right lower quadrant (69). Endoscopically, disease may be primarily ulcerative, hypertrophic, or ulcero-hypertrophic, combining features of both. The ulcerative presentation, consisting of diffuse colitis with transverse ulcers and surrounding hypertrophic mucosa is most common (69,72,75,76). Hypertrophic disease is marked by inflammatory strictures and scarring as well as hypertrophic lesions resembling polyps and masses. These masses can be friable and necrotic, and are frequently mistaken for malignancy (69,70,72,75–78). The aforementioned abnormalities may be present diffusely, or may exist as skip lesions with normal intervening mucosa (75–77). While any region of the GI tract may be involved, the ileocecal area is the most common site (affected in 90% of patients with tuberculous enteritis) (69,75). Colonoscopy often reveals deformity of the cecum and ileocecal valve (Fig. 1) (72,77,79). Complications such as obstruction, free perforation, abscess, and massive hemorrhage have been described and are indications for surgical intervention (69,70).

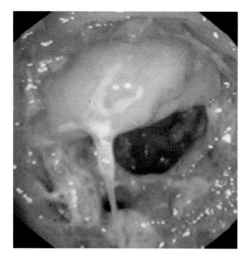

Figure 1 (*See color insert*) Tuberculous ileocolitis. There is marked ulceration and deformity of the ileocecal valve and cecum.

Stool culture has limited diagnostic utility in tuberculous colitis. The diagnostic procedure of choice is colonoscopy with biopsy, preferably from ulcer margins because granulomata are often submucosal (69,80,81). Even with optimal technique and an adequate number of biopsies, only 50% to 80% of cases can be diagnosed on the basis of histology and acid-fast staining (70). Polymerase chain reaction (PCR) of biopsy specimens results in a diagnostic sensitivity of 75% to 80% with a specificity of 85% to 95% (82,83). Overall, the total diagnostic yield of endoscopic biopsy has been reported at 81% (76). Serological methods for diagnosing tuberculosis using enzyme-linked immunosorbent assays and soluble antigen fluorescent antibody tests may assist in making the diagnosis (69). The treatment of tuberculous colitis is with three to four antituberculous drugs for a 6- to 12-month course. This typically results in a high cure rate of approximately 90% (69).

Yersinia enterocolitica

The first human isolates of this organism were described in 1939 (84). It was known by many names including *Pasteurella pseudotuberculosis* until 1964 when it was definitively named *Yersinia enterocolitica*. Yersinia is a non–lactose-fermenting, gram-negative coccobacillus found in stream and lake water, animals, and unprocessed milk.

Infection with *Yersinia enterocolitica* produces a spectrum of illness ranging from simple gastroenteritis to invasive ileitis and colitis mimicking Crohn's disease (85–87). Diarrhea and abdominal pain are the most common symptoms (85–88). Frankly, bloody diarrhea is uncommon. Approximately 40% of patients have symptoms suggestive of acute appendicitis (89). By endoscopy, terminal ileal involvement appears to be universal, and is distinguished by edema, hyperemia and irregularly shaped shallow ulcerations (89,90). In most patients there is contiguous inflammation of the ileocecal valve and cecum with edema and erythematous and friable mucosa (90). Small ulcerations resembling the typical aphthoid ulcers of Crohn's disease are frequently encountered (89,90). In up to 25% of cases, the ascending colon may be involved (90). Left-sided colonic disease appears to be rare, but has been described in infections of the 0:3 serotype (90). Uncommon, but reported, complications include toxic megacolon, perforation, and abscess formation (85,91).

Diagnosis is typically made on the basis of stool culture, but a special cold-enriched medium is required. Serology is a secondary alternative to culture, but low agglutinin titers may be difficult to interpret in immunosuppressed patients (85,92). Most illness due to Yersinia resolves without intervention. Antibiotics have not been shown to alter the course of uncomplicated disease, but have been recommended in patients with severe enteritis or the immunocompromised patient (14,85). Effective treatments include doxycycline, TMP/SMX, chloramphenicol, and quinolones.

Chlamydia trachomatis

Chlamydia trachomatis is an obligatory intracellular parasite closely related to gram-negative bacteria, and is best known as an etiology of nongonococcal urethritis. Anorectal infections with the lymphogranuloma venereum (LGV) immunotypes of *Chlamydia trachomatis* have been recognized for almost 70 years (93). More recently, it has been noted that both LGV and nonLGV immunotypes can cause proctitis and proctocolitis (94). In men, it is presumed that these infections result from passive anal intercourse (94,95). In women, the root of infection is either anal intercourse or direct extension of a genital tract infection into the rectum (94,95).

The typical symptoms of acute chlamydial proctocolitis are proctalgia and severe tenesmus with the passage of blood, mucus, and pus in the stool (96,97). Additional symptoms may include diarrhea, constipation, alternating constipation and diarrhea, and weight loss (95,96). LGV strains appear to cause more severe proctitis than nonLGV strains (94,95). The duration of symptoms in chlamydial proctocolitis can range from weeks to years (96). Endoscopy during the first few weeks after exposure may reveal nonspecific friable, hemorrhagic rectal mucosa with multiple discrete ulcerations (94). These changes may extend proximal to 25 cm from the anal verge (95,96). Chronic infection may result in a narrowing and distal stricture of the rectum known as proctitis obliterans (94,96). Severe stricturing may necessitate dilation, but this may be unsuccessful if scarring is significant. In such cases, surgery with or without preservation of the anal sphincter may be necessary (96). Other described complications include abscesses and fistula formation (94).

The diagnosis of chlamydial proctocolitis is made through culture or direct fluorescent antibody (DFA) testing of a rectal swab (98). Most other nonculture tests cannot be performed using rectal samples. Chlamydia serology may give false-positive results, because it may reflect other chlamydial infections. Treatment of chlamydial proctocolitis with antibiotics is recommended. For LGV immunotypes, doxycycline or tetracycline should be administered for three weeks. NonLGV chlamydial infections may be eradicated with a single dose of azithromycin or doxycycline followed by one week of ofloxacin or erythromycin.

Neisseria gonorrhea

Anorectal infection with the gram-negative intracellular diplococcus *Neisseria gonorrhea* has been observed since the end of the 19th century, and is common in both women and men who have sex with men (99). In these men, infection presumably results from direct anorectal inoculation; in women, penorectal contact or direct extension of a genital tract infection is postulated (99). Most patients with anorectal gonorrhea are asymptomatic (95,99). The most common complaints are pruritis ani, painful defecation, sensation of rectal fullness, mucoid discharge, and constipation (99,100). Hematochezia is very rare. Endoscopic findings are limited to the anal canal and rectum and include erythema, excessive rectal mucous, friability, superficial erosions, and fissures (95,99,100). Formation of fistulae and abscesses may occur on occasion (99). Rectal strictures, common in the past, are relatively rare in the antibiotic era (99).

The diagnosis of anorectal gonorrhea is typically made by culture of a rectal swab on Thayer-Martin agar. These swab specimens should be obtained by placing the swab approximately 1 in. into the anal canal and rotating it from side to side (99). The swab should not be used for culture if fecal material is obtained. Antibiotic treatment is recommended for cases of anorectal gonorrhea. Single doses of ceftriaxone, cefixime, ciprofloxacin, or ofloxacin are effective. Because chlamydial infections are often found in conjunction with gonorrhea, nonpregnant patients should also receive a single dose of azithromycin or a seven-day course of doxycycline or tetracycline (38,95). Follow-up posttreatment culture approximately 10 days after antibiotic therapy is completed is essential to document cure (100). Multiple sites in addition to the rectum should be cultured to verify eradication (100).

Other Bacterial Causes of Colitis: *Vibrio parahaemolyticus*, Aeromonas, and Plesiomonas

Vibrio parahaemolyticus is a halophilic (requiring sodium chloride for growth) organism found widely in marine environments, but seldom seen in fresh water or nonmarine locations. It was first identified as a cause of food-borne disease by Japanese investigators in 1950, and it is now recognized as the principal cause of food-borne outbreaks in Japan (101). Approximately 30 to 40 cases of *Vibrio parahaemolyticus* infection are reported annually in the Gulf Coast states of Alabama, Florida, Louisiana, and Texas (102). It is usually associated with the consumption of contaminated raw seafood. The clinical symptoms have their onset approximately 9 to 25 hours after ingestion (103). Infected individuals experience the sudden onset of profuse diarrhea with abdominal pain (103,104). Blood and mucus can be seen in the stool. Nausea, vomiting, headaches, and fevers are also often reported. Superficial mucosal ulcerations are found on flexible sigmoidoscopy (103). The diagnosis of *Vibrio parahaemolyticus* infection is made by stool culture by using special thiosulfate-citrate-bile salts-sucrose agar (TCBS) medium (105). The infection is typically self-limited, resolving in three to four days (106). The role of antibiotics is unknown, as no clinical trials have been performed. If treatment is required, due to the severity of symptoms, doxycycline or tetracycline appear to be the drugs of choice based on in vitro sensitivities (14).

Aeromonas are gram-negative flagellated bacilli widely distributed in fresh or brackish water, sewage and soil (107). There are various subspecies, but *Aeromonas hydrophila* and *Aeromonas sobria* are the strains most associated with human disease. *Aeromonas* was previously thought to be pathogenic only in immunocompromised hosts, but it is now known to be associated with GI infections in healthy individuals (107). The clinical symptoms of *Aeromonas* infection are due to an enterotoxin and occur after drinking untreated water or ingesting contaminated food, usually freshwater or marine-associated products (108,109). The typical symptoms include diarrhea, abdominal cramps, vomiting, and fever (107). Approximately one-quarter of patients have bloody stool (107). *Aeromonas colitis* is characterized on endoscopy by mucosal edema, loss of vascular markings, friability, superficial erosions, and overlying mucosa (107,110). Both segmental left-sided disease and pancolitis have been reported (107,110). *Aeromonas* infection is diagnosed by stool culture on routine media. The role of antibiotics in *Aeromonas* colitis is unclear, but treatment is indicated in prolonged illness (>1 week in duration). Oral quinolones and TMP/SMX are effective (14).

Plesiomonas is a gram-negative flagellated bacillus similar to *Aeromonas*, which is found in fresh water ecosystems and marine estuaries (109). Infection is strongly associated with consumption of uncooked shellfish, especially oysters (109,111). Patients with *Plesiomonas colitis* present with diarrhea, vomiting, fever, or bloody stool, typically 48 hours after eating contaminated food (111,112). Endoscopy may reveal aphthous lesions, sometimes bleeding, in the left colon (111,113). The diagnosis of *Plesiomonas* colitis is based on stool culture using routine media. Antibiotics have been recommended for severe infection (17). Oral quinolones and TMP/SMX are the most effective agents (114).

PARASITIC COLITIS
Entamoeba histolytica

Since Sir William Osler described the first North American case of amebiasis in 1890, *Entamoeba histolytica* has been recognized as a major source of illness worldwide (115). Infection is usually acquired by the ingestion of food or water contaminated with feces containing cysts (116). Venereal transmission through oral-fecal contact has also been described (117). No host other than humans is implicated in the life cycle of this parasite. Infection begins when the cyst is ingested, and the capsule is digested in the small bowel. The cyst then excysts and forms eight trophozoites. These colonize the colon and cause invasive disease or travel through the portal circulation to form liver abscesses. In the colon, infection is usually established in the cecum where there is stasis. Ten percent of the world's population is estimated to be infected with *Entamoeba histolytica* (118). The disease is most prevalent in the tropics and in areas with poor sanitation. The typical patient in the United States is young (age 20 to 40), an immigrant, Hispanic and male (9:1 male:female ratio) (117).

Following infection, there is an incubation period of one to three weeks. Typically, patients have a subacute presentation ranging from mild diarrhea to dysentery marked by abdominal pain, tenesmus, and bloody stool (115). Ten percent of patients may progress to fulminant colitis, which is associated with a high probability of mortality (115,119). The risks of fulminant amebic colitis may be increased in infected individuals with concomitant diabetes and chronic alcohol abuse (120). In invasive amebic colitis, endoscopy often demonstrates discrete shallow-based, flask-shaped ulcers covered with exudates (Fig. 2) (115,121). These ulcers may grow to over 2 cm in diameter. Most commonly, there is a right-sided predominance of these findings with skip lesions (115,121). The intervening mucosa is usually normal,

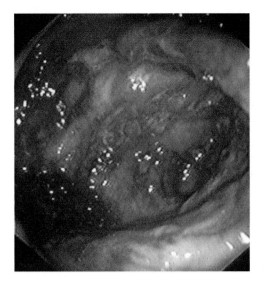

Figure 2 (*See color insert*) Amebic colitis. The colonic mucosa is erythematous and friable, with areas of discrete ulceration.

distinguishing this condition from ulcerative colitis. At times, however, amebic colitis may be indistinguishable from inflammatory bowel disease, with an endoscopic appearance of diffuse erythema, granularity, and friability. A study of patients with amebic colitis and concomitant amebic liver abscess found milder disease and exclusively right-sided endoscopic findings in these patients compared to those with amebic colitis alone (121). Localized infection may result in a segmental mass of granulation tissue known as an ameboma. This occurs in approximately 10% of patients with colonic disease, and is most common in the cecum, where it may be mistaken for carcinoma (115). Amebomas can result in obstruction or intussusception. Further complications of amebic colitis include appendicitis, strictures, and toxic megacolon (122). The latter has been associated with the use of steroids, which may be administered due to the misdiagnosis of amebic colitis as idiopathic inflammatory bowel disease (123,124).

The diagnosis of *Entamoeba histolytica* colitis is most frequently made during microscopic examination of fresh stool specimens, revealing erythrophagocytic trophozoites in over 90% of cases. Because organisms may be excreted in a noncyclic manner or may be unevenly distributed in the fecal specimen, at least three stool specimens should be examined to detect 85% to 95% of the infections (115). Stool culture is more sensitive than microscopy, but results may take up to one week (125). Stool antigen tests are now available, but are not as sensitive as culture. A PCR assay, which detects *Entamoeba histolytica*–specific DNA in fresh stool, is a rapid, sensitive, and specific manner of diagnosis, but is not yet widely available (126). The diagnostic yield from endoscopic biopsy is also high, as trophozoites are usually easily identified under light microscopy (115). Immunohistochemical staining may further increase yield. When obtaining sigmoidoscopic biopsy specimens with the intent of examining for *Entamoeba histolytica*, the procedure should be performed without bowel preparation to increase the chance of finding mobile trophozoites in the colonic mucus adherent to the biopsy specimen. Serologic testing may be helpful in confirmation of the diagnosis of amebic colitis, but because antiamebic antibodies may persist for months to years after the eradication of infection, a positive serology requires more rigid clinical and diagnostic correlation in endemic areas.

All patients with amebic colitis should be treated (127). The goals are to treat the invasive disease and to eradicate intestinal carriage of the parasite. Metronidazole is the drug of choice for invasive intestinal disease. Following a 5- to 10-day treatment course, a luminal agent is begun to eradicate intestinal carriage of the organism. The most commonly used drugs for this are paromomycin (7-day course) or iodoquinol (20-day course). Due to a 10% to 15% failure rate, patients should be tested for cure (115).

Trichuris trichiura

Trichuris trichiura is the third most common nematode, and is found only in humans (128). It is more commonly known as whipworm because of its whip-like appearance. *Trichuris* is found in the tropics and the southeastern United States, and infection is most frequent in areas without latrines, and in communities where untreated human fecal material is used as fertilizer (129). Infection begins with ingestion of embryonated ova. Digestive juices dissolve the shells of the ova, releasing larva that mature within the GI tract. Adult worms are 3–5 cm in length, and superficially invade and attach to the intestinal mucosa of the cecum where they may survive for several years.

Mild *Trichuris* infections are usually asymptomatic (129). Heavy infections are often associated with diarrhea, bloody stool, and anemia (130). Rectal prolapse, intussusception, colonic obstruction, and perforation have been described (131,132). The presence of this parasite is usually suspected on the basis of clinical symptoms, and the diagnosis is confirmed by finding the characteristic barrel-shaped ova in the feces (128). If endoscopy is performed in patients with severe infections, the worms may be seen as whitish coiled organisms about 1 cm in length, with their spiral heads embedded in the colonic mucosa (Fig. 3) (128,133,134). However, worms can be easily overlooked if colonic preparation is poor. Patients with *Trichuris* infections should be treated with a single dose of albendazole or three days of mebendazole.

FUNGAL COLITIS
Histoplasma capsulatum

Histoplasma capsulatum is a dimorphic fungus that exists as a mold in soil and as a yeast in tissues. In the United States, it is rarely encountered outside the rural valleys of Ohio, Mississippi, and Missouri, where it grows in soil contaminated with bird droppings. While infection is asymptomatic in most patients with normal immune function, immunosuppressed patients are at increased risk of disseminated histoplasmosis (135). GI involvement, including colitis, is found in up to 75% of patients with disseminated histoplasma infection (136).

Approximately one-half to two-thirds of patients with enteric histoplasmosis have symptoms of diarrhea, weight loss, fever, or abdominal pain (136,137). The terminal ileum and cecum are the most common sites of intestinal involvement in disseminated histoplasmosis, but virtually any area of the small or large bowel can be involved and pancolitis has been described (137,138). Endoscopic findings can be variable, but may include erythematous mucosa, ulcers with heaped-up margins, pseudopolyps, raised plaques, and fungating mass lesions having the appearance of a mucosal tumor (136–139). These mass lesions have been known to cause obstruction and result in perforation (137,140,141). Stricturing secondary to ulceration has also been described (142).

The diagnosis of histoplasma colitis is best made through identification of the characteristic intracellular oval budding yeast in colonic mucosa obtained by endoscopic biopsy (142). Fungal culture of biopsy specimens confirms the diagnosis. The treatment of enteric histoplasmosis requires intravenous amphotericin B as induction therapy (with a total dose of 1–2 g), followed by lifelong maintenance suppression using amphotericin B or oral intraconzole (143,144).

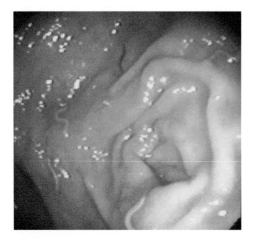

Figure 3   (*See color insert*) *Trichuris trichiura.* During colonoscopy, adult worms may be found attached to the cecal mucosa.

VIRAL COLITIS
Cytomegalovirus

Cytomegalovirus (CMV) is a double-stranded DNA virus in the human herpes virus family. It is present in a latent state in most adults, but replication and overt disease may occur in the setting of immune deficiency such as AIDS, posttransplantation immunosuppression, and chemotherapy. CMV infection can occur at any location along the GI tract. CMV is the most commonly identified pathogen in AIDS-related diarrhea when standard stool studies are negative (145). Approximately 10% of all AIDS patients suffer from CMV enteritis (146). This typically occurs in patients with CD4 counts below 150 cells/mm^3 (146,147). However, there are at least nine published reports of CMV colitis in immunocompetent patients (148).

Abdominal pain and diarrhea are the most common symptoms of CMV colitis, occurring in more than half of patients (146,149). Hematochezia is present in approximately 30% and weight loss is not uncommon (146,149,150). The colonoscopic appearance of CMV colitis is heterogeneous. Usually the entire colon is involved with the cecum and ascending colon most severely involved (148,149). Subepithelial hemorrhage, reminiscent of changes seen in ischemia, is a prominent endoscopic finding (Fig. 4) (149). Overall, the most common endoscopic presentation is diffuse colitis with focal ulceration (149). Ulcers may be well circumscribed with elevated margins, or aphthous in appearance. In almost three-quarters of patients, these abnormalities are pancolonic in distribution (149). Disease is limited to the right colon in 13% of patients (149). Additional endoscopic findings that have been encountered include plaque-like pseudomembranes and mass lesions known as viromas, which may resemble cancer (146,151–153). CMV colitis may be complicated by stricturing, perforation, bleeding, toxic megacolon, or fistula formation (146,154). One published review reported that one-quarter of patients required some manner of surgical intervention to treat these conditions (146).

Culture, antibody, antigen, or molecular studies of blood and stool cannot make the diagnosis of intestinal CMV disease. Rather, colonoscopy with biopsy is required to procure diagnostic specimens (147). At least six biopsy specimens using "jumbo" forceps should be taken from the ulcerating margins and base of the ulcers. These specimens should be stained with hematoxylin and eosin and examined for the cytomegalic changes of cytoplasmic or nuclear inclusions. The cytomegalic inclusion cells are to be found not only in the epithelial cells but also in the endothelial cells within the lamina propria and submucosa. Special antigenic and genomic stains and viral cultures of biopsy specimens may assist in the identification of CMV, but are not usually needed. While PCR assays hold the potential for rapid and accurate diagnosis, they remain a research tool at this point (155). When symptoms are present and CMV colitis is suspected, it is treated with a three-week course of intravenous ganciclovir or foscarnet (156). The results with this regimen are encouraging. In AIDS-associated CMV colitis, complete response was seen in 87% of patients (157). Relapse rates may approach 50%, but protease inhibitor therapy has been demonstrated to substantially reduce the risk of relapse and improve survival (157).

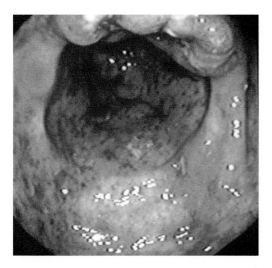

Figure 4 (*See color insert*) Cytomegalovirus colitis. Subepithelial hemorrhage and focal ulceration are common endoscopic findings.

Herpes Simplex Virus

Herpes simplex virus (HSV) is a double-stranded DNA virus. Humans are the only known natural reservoir for this infection. Clinical HSV disease may result from primary infection or secondary reactivation of latent disease. Secondary reactivation usually occurs in patients with CD4 counts less than 100 cells/mm^3 or in immunosuppressed transplant recipients (158–161). HSV is an uncommon cause of enteritis. Almost all occurrences are limited to the esophagus or rectum.

Acute proctitis is a classic manifestation of initial exposure to HSV (95). Patients present with low-grade fever, severe anorectal pain, tenesmus, and the passage of mucus or blood in their stool (95,162). Not infrequently, the patient experiences such pain that even a digital rectal examination is impossible without anesthesia. In many instances, an examination under general anesthesia is the only tolerable way to examine the anorectum in patients with herpetic proctocolitis. HSV frequently invades nerve ganglia, and urinary retention and constipation may be seen if the sacral nerve is involved (95,162). Endoscopic findings in HSV proctitis are prototypical in the distal 5 cm of the rectum. The typical lesions are small, sharply demarcated vesicles, or shallow ovoid ulcers with or without a vascular rim (162). These lesions often extend to the anal mucosa and perianal skin. A few cases of diffuse colonic disease, including one in an immunocompetent individual, have been described in the literature (159,163). In this aforementioned case, the endoscopic findings were aphthous ulcers and erosions with occasional pseudopolypoid lesions (163).

The diagnosis of HSV proctitis can often be made clinically, but should be confirmed through isolation of HSV using cell-culture techniques. A suitable sample may be obtained by swabbing an anal or biopsying a rectal lesion. The diagnosis can also be made by DFA testing of swab samples from herpetic lesions (95). Acute HSV proctitis should be treated with acyclovir five times a day for a 7- to 10-day course (164). Valacyclovir and famciclovir are presumably effective as well, but studies to confirm this are lacking. Intravenous acyclovir may rarely be necessary, if diarrhea precludes absorption of oral formulations.

GENERAL CONSIDERATIONS
Role of Colonoscopy in Diagnosis

Since its initial diagnostic application approximately 30 years ago, the role of colonoscopy in the evaluation and management of patients with suspected colitis has continued to evolve. Endoscopy has limited utility in the diagnosis of acute infectious diarrhea, which can be most effectively investigated using stool studies. However, it is cost-effective, and has a valuable role in the evaluation of chronic diarrhea, particularly in patients with a compromised immune system (145,165).

In the setting of infectious colitis, colonoscopy aids in determining the extent and pattern of disease. Most importantly, colonoscopic biopsy can help differentiate infectious colitis from inflammatory bowel disease (166). Due to the preservation of crypt architecture in infectious colitis, acute self-limited colitis can usually be distinguished from ulcerative colitis or Crohn's disease. Certain findings on biopsy might also suggest a specific diagnosis. For example, the presence of granulomata may suggest *Chlamydia trachomatis*, tuberculosis, histoplasmosis, or Yersinia infections. Typical viral inclusions can be seen in HSV and CMV infections, and parasites such as *Entamoeba histolytica* may be directly identified on biopsy specimens.

All patients with suspected infectious colitis need not undergo sigmoidoscopy or colonoscopy. Rather, endoscopic evaluation might be reasonably reserved for individuals with dysentery, persistent symptoms, or underlying immunocompromise. Such an approach has not been validated, but would be expected to yield diagnostic information that alters management in this group of patients. Although routine lower GI endoscopy is a safe procedure, it is contraindicated in acutely ill patients with fulminant colitis due to an increased risk of perforation. If colonoscopy or sigmoidoscopy is contemplated, gentle preparation of the bowel is needed, preferably with polyethylene glycol–based regimens or with saline cathartics. Irritant cathartics should be avoided. A limited examination, with judicious use of air insufflation to evaluate disease localization and obtain biopsies, is a reasonable approach.

Supportive Care

Similar to the patient with acute diarrhea, fluid and electrolyte replacement is the cornerstone of therapy for individuals suffering from infectious colitis (167). Patients with mild symptoms and with no or minimal clinical evidence of dehydration may take fluids orally. However, those with significant emesis or dehydration, or patients with fulminant colitis require intravenous fluid resuscitation and maintenance, as well as close monitoring of electrolytes and volume status.

During an episode of infectious colitis, the diet should probably be modified, as absorption of certain food items by the GI tract may be impaired. Except in cases of fulminant colitis, obstruction, or perforation, calories should be taken in to facilitate enterocyte renewal. The optimal foods in this setting include boiled starches and cereals such as potatoes, noodles, rice, wheat, or oats with some salt added. Yogurt, bananas, soup, and boiled vegetables are also appropriate. Once stools are formed, the diet may return to normal.

Role of Empiric Pharmacotherapy

When considering the institution of empiric antibiotic therapy in patients with infectious colitis, one must remember that the majority of cases are self-limited with symptoms resolving within one week of onset. Additional factors mitigating against routine use of antibiotics for all cases of infectious colitis include very limited evidence of treatment benefits, the costs of antibiotics, and the potential for the development of antibiotic resistance. Indiscriminate antibiotic use may exacerbate certain conditions, causing prolonged excretion of Salmonella (12,13), possible increased toxin production by *E. coli* O157:H7 (168,169), and worsening of *Clostridium difficile*–associated diarrhea.

The potential benefits of empiric treatment include more rapid symptom resolution, prevention of invasive disease, and decrease in the number of secondary cases through prevention of person-to-person spread. Those patients most susceptible to morbidity and mortality from infectious colitis, such as the elderly, diabetics, cirrhotics, pregnant women, immunocompromised individuals, and patients receiving chemotherapy, might be given consideration for empiric treatment with quinolone antibiotics. However, patients with symptoms of hemorrhagic colitis (suggestive of *E. coli* O157:H7 infection) or history of recent antibiotic use (at risk for *Clostridium difficile* infection) should not be treated empirically, and treatment should be based on documented etiology.

Antimotility agents and opioids are frequently used to improve the symptoms of diarrhea associated with infectious colitis. There is no evidence that these medications improve outcomes and in cases of *E. coli* O157:H7 and Shigella colitis, antimotility agents have been related to significant complications such as HUS and toxic megacolon (29,63). We do not recommend the routine use of these agents in the treatment of acute infectious colitis.

Role of Surgery

In the era of videoendoscopy, advanced imaging techniques, and potent antibiotics, surgery is rarely required for the diagnosis or treatment of infectious colitis. Today, the major role for surgery is in the management of the complications of infectious colitis. These include severe fulminant colitis refractory to antibiotic therapy, toxic megacolon, perforation, obstruction, refractory bleeding, and fistulae. Despite appropriate operative technique, mortality remains high in certain conditions such as fulminant amebic colitis and ulcerative tuberculous colitis (119,170). Surgical intervention tends to be more common in underdeveloped countries where infectious colitis is highly prevalent, antibiotics are less readily available, and patients are more likely to present in advanced stages of disease.

SUMMARY

Infectious colitis is caused by a variety of organisms, and may have an extremely varied presentation, course, and treatment response. While most diseases are self-limited and easily diagnosed through noninvasive means, endoscopy can aid in the evaluation of patients with prolonged symptoms or inconclusive stool studies. The majority of previously healthy adult patients will do well with supportive care alone. The empiric use of antibiotics is discouraged except in sick patients at high risk for complications. Antibiotics should be avoided in patients with hemorrhagic colitis caused by *E. coli* O157:H7 infection. Surgery is infrequently required in the diagnosis or treatment of infectious colitis, but retains an important role in the management of its complications.

REFERENCES

1. Mead PS, Slutsker L, Dietz V, et al. Food-related illness and death in the United States. Emerg Infect Dis 1999; 5:607–625.
2. Goldsweig CD, Pacheco PA. Infectious colitis excluding *E. coli* O157:H7 and *C. difficile*. Gastroenterol Clin North Am 2001; 30:709–733.
3. Mandal BK, Mani V. Colonic involvement in salmonellosis. Lancet 1976; 1:887–888.
4. Thomas M, Tillett HE. Letter: colonic involvement in salmonellosis. Lancet 1976; 1:1129–1130.
5. Boyd JF. Letter: colonic involvement in salmonellosis. Lancet 1976; 1:1415.
6. Dagash M, Hayek T, Gallimidi Z, Yassin K, Brook JG. Transient radiological and colonoscopic features of inflammatory bowel disease in a patient with severe Salmonella gastroenteritis. Am J Gastroenterol 1997; 92:349–351.
7. Maguire TM, Wensel RH, Malcolm N, Jewell L, Thomson AB. Massive gastrointestinal hemorrhage cecal ulcers and salmonella colitis. J Clin Gastroenterol 1985; 7:249–250.
8. Cariani G, Vandelli A. Salmonellosis-induced hemorrhage and ulcerations of the colon. Endoscopy 1993; 25:488.
9. Bellary SV, Isaacs P. Toxic megacolon (TM) due to Salmonella. J Clin Gastroenterol 1990; 12:605–607.
10. Tiao MM, Huang HC, Huang CB, Chuang JH, Shieh CS, Shen TL. Toxic megacolon in Salmonella colitis: report of two cases. Acta Paediatr Taiwan 2000; 41:43–46.
11. McCall CE, Martin WT, Boring JR. Efficiency of cultures of rectal swabs and faecal specimens in detecting salmonella carriers: correlation with numbers of salmonellas excreted. J Hyg (Lond) 1966; 64:261–269.
12. Sanchez C, Garcia-Restoy E, Garau J, et al. Ciprofloxacin and trimethoprim-sulfamethoxazole versus placebo in acute uncomplicated *Salmonella enteritis*: a double-blind trial. J Infect Dis 1993; 168: 1304–1307.
13. Kamath R. Antibiotic therapy for *Salmonella enteritis*. J Paediatr Child Health 1999; 35:338.
14. Oldfield EC III, Wallace MR. The role of antibiotics in the treatment of infectious diarrhea. Gastroenterol Clin North Am 2001; 30:817–836.
15. Aserkoff B, Bennett JV. Effect of antibiotic therapy in acute salmonellosis on the fecal excretion of salmonellae. N Engl J Med 1969; 281:636–640.
16. Neill MA, Opal SM, Heelan J, et al. Failure of ciprofloxacin to eradicate convalescent fecal excretion after acute salmonellosis: experience during an outbreak in health care workers. Ann Intern Med 1991; 114:195–199.
17. Wolf DC, Giannella RA. Antibiotic therapy for bacterial enterocolitis: a comprehensive review. Am J Gastroenterol 1993; 88:1667–1683.
18. Lindberg AA, Pal T. Strategies for development of potential candidate Shigella vaccines. Vaccine 1993; 11:168–179.
19. Mosley WH, Adams B, Lyman ED. Epidemiologic and sociologic features of a large urban outbreak of shigellosis. JAMA 1962; 182:1307–1311.
20. Dritz SK, Back AF. Letter: *Shigella enteritis* venereally transmitted. N Engl J Med 1974; 291:1194.
21. Acheson D, Keusch G. Shigella and enteroinvasive *Escherichia coli*. In: Blaser MJ, Smith PD, Ravdin JI, Greenberg HB, Guerrant RL, eds. Infections of the Gastrointestinal Tract. New York: Raven Press, 1995:763–784.
22. Speelman P, Kabir I, Islam M. Distribution and spread of colonic lesions in shigellosis: a colonoscopic study. J Infect Dis 1984; 150:899–903.
23. Khuroo MS, Mahajan R, Zargar SA, et al. The colon in shigellosis: serial colonoscopic appearances in *Shigella dysenteriae* I. Endoscopy 1990; 22:35–38.
24. Zalev AH, Warren RE. *Shigella colitis* with radiological and endoscopic correlation: case report. Can Assoc Radiol J 1989; 40:328–330.
25. Wilson AP, Ridgway GL, Sarner M, Boulos PB, Brook MG, Cook GC. Toxic dilatation of the colon in shigellosis. BMJ 1990; 301:1325–1326.
26. Upadhyay AK, Neely JA. Toxic megacolon and perforation caused by Shigella. Br J Surg 1989; 76:1217.
27. Keusch GT. Antimicrobial therapy for enteric infections and typhoid fever: state of the art. Rev Infect Dis 1988; 10(suppl 1):S199–S205.
28. Salam MA, Bennish ML. Antimicrobial therapy for shigellosis. Rev Infect Dis 1991; 13(suppl 4): S332–S341.
29. DuPont HL, Hornick RB. Adverse effect of lomotil therapy in shigellosis. JAMA 1973; 226: 1525–1528.
30. Nataro JP, Kaper JB. Diarrheagenic *Escherichia coli*. Clin Microbiol Rev 1998; 11:142–201.
31. Tulloch EF Jr., Ryan KJ, Formal SB, Franklin FA. Invasive enteropathic *Escherichia coli* dysentery. An outbreak in 28 adults. Ann Intern Med 1973; 79:13–17.
32. Marier R, Wells JG, Swanson RC, Callahan W, Mehlman IJ. An outbreak of enteropathogenic *Escherichia coli* foodborne disease traced to imported French cheese. Lancet 1973; 2:1376–1378.
33. Allos BM. *Campylobacter jejuni* infections: update on emerging issues and trends. Clin Infect Dis 2001; 32:1201–1206.

34. Friedman CR, Neimann J, Wegener HC, Tauxe RV. Epidemiology of *Campylobacter jejuni* infections in the United States and other industrialized nations. In: Nachamkin I, Blaser MJ, eds. Campylobacter. Washington, DC: ASM Press, 2000:121–138.

35. MacDonald KL, O'Leary MJ, Cohen ML, et al. *Escherichia coli* O157:H7, an emerging gastrointestinal pathogen. Results of a one-year, prospective, population-based study. JAMA 1988; 259: 3567–3570.

36. Blaser MJ, Berkowitz ID, LaForce FM, Cravens J, Reller LB, Wang WL. *Campylobacter enteritis*: clinical and epidemiologic features. Ann Intern Med 1979; 91:179–185.

37. Blaser MJ, Wells JG, Feldman RA, Pollard RA, Allen JR. *Campylobacter enteritis* in the United States. A multicenter study. Ann Intern Med 1983; 98:360–365.

38. Rautelin H, Koota K, von Essen R, Jahkola M, Siitonen A, Kosunen TU. Waterborne *Campylobacter jejuni* epidemic in a Finnish hospital for rheumatic diseases. Scand J Infect Dis 1990; 22:321–326.

39. Allos BM. Association between Campylobacter infection and Guillain-Barre syndrome. J Infect Dis 1997; 176(suppl 2):S125–S128.

40. Lambert ME, Schofield PF, Ironside AG, Mandal BK. *Campylobacter colitis*. Br Med J 1979; 1:857–859.

41. Loss RW Jr., Mangla JC, Pereira M. *Campylobacter colitis* present in as inflammatory bowel disease with segmental colonic ulcerations. Gastroenterology 1980; 79:138–140.

42. Allos BM, Blaser MJ. *Campylobacter jejuni* and the expanding spectrum of related infections. Clin Infect Dis 1995; 20:1092–1099.

43. Jackson TL Jr., Young RL, Thompson JS, McCashland TM. Toxic megacolon associated with *Campylobacter jejuni* colitis. Am J Gastroenterol 1999; 94:280–282.

44. Schneider A, Runzi M, Peitgen K, von Birgelen C, Gerken G. *Campylobacter jejuni*-induced severe colitis—a rare cause of toxic megacolon. Z Gastroenterol 2000; 38:307–309.

45. Hoge CW, Gambel JM, Srijan A, Pitarangsi C, Echeverria P. Trends in antibiotic resistance among diarrheal pathogens isolated in Thailand over 15 years. Clin Infect Dis 1998; 26:341–345.

46. Riley LW, Remis RS, Helgerson SD, et al. Hemorrhagic colitis associated with a rare *Escherichia coli* serotype. N Engl J Med 1983; 308:681–685.

47. Mead PS, Finelli L, Lambert-Fair MA, et al. Risk factors for sporadic infection with *Escherichia coli* O157:H7. Arch Intern Med 1997; 157:204–208.

48. Bell BP, Goldoft M, Griffin PM, et al. A multistate outbreak of *Escherichia coli* O157:H7-associated bloody diarrhea and hemolytic uremic syndrome from hamburgers. The Washington experience. JAMA 1994; 272:1349–1353.

49. Tuttle J, Gomez T, Doyle MP, et al. Lessons from a large outbreak of *Escherichia coli* O157:H7 infections: insights into the infectious dose and method of widespread contamination of hamburger patties. Epidemiol Infect 1999; 122:185–192.

50. Edelman R, Karmali MA, Fleming PA. From the National Institutes of Health. Summary of the International Symposium and Workshop on Infections due to Verocytotoxin (Shiga-like toxin)-producing *Escherichia coli*. J Infect Dis 1988; 157:1102–1104.

51. Pai CH, Ahmed N, Lior H, Johnson WM, Sims HV, Woods DE. Epidemiology of sporadic diarrhea due to verocytotoxin-producing *Escherichia coli*: a two-year prospective study. J Infect Dis 1988; 157:1054–1057.

52. Talan D, Moran GJ, Newdow M, et al. Etiology of bloody diarrhea among patients presenting to United States emergency departments: prevalence of *Escherichia coli* O157:H7 and other enteropathogens. Clin Infect Dis 2001; 32:573–580.

53. Ostroff SM, Kobayashi JM, Lewis JH. Infections with *Escherichia coli* O157:H7 in Washington State. The first year of statewide disease surveillance. JAMA 1989; 262:355–359.

54. Tarr PI, Neill MA. *Escherichia coli* O157:H7. Gastroenterol Clin North Am 2001; 30:735–751.

55. Griffin PM, Ostroff SM, Tauxe RV, et al. Illnesses associated with *Escherichia coli* O157:H7 infections. A broad clinical spectrum. Ann Intern Med 1988; 109:705–712.

56. Griffin PM, Olmstead LC, Petras RE. *Escherichia coli* O157:H7-associated colitis. A clinical and histological study of 11 cases. Gastroenterology 1990; 99:142–149.

57. Boyce TG, Pemberton AG, Wells JG, Griffin PM. Screening for *Escherichia coli* O157:H7—a nationwide survey of clinical laboratories. J Clin Microbiol 1995; 33:3275–3277.

58. Tarr PI, Neill MA, Clausen CR, Watkins SL, Christie DL, Hickman RO. *Escherichia coli* O157:H7 the hemolytic uremic syndrome—importance of early cultures in establishing the etiology. J Infect Dis 1990; 162:553–556.

59. Stapp JR, Jelacic S, Yea YL, et al. Comparison of *Escherichia coli* O157:H7 antigen detection in stool and broth cultures to that in sorbitol-MacConkey agar stool cultures. J Clin Microbiol 2000; 38:3404–3406.

60. Slutsker L, Ries AA, Maloney K, Wells JG, Greene KD, Griffin PM. A nationwide case-control study of *Escherichia coli* O157:H7 infection in the United States. J Infect Dis 1998; 177:962–966.

61. Wong CS, Jelacic S, Habeeb RL, Watkins SL, Tarr PI. The risk of the hemolytic-uremic syndrome after antibiotic treatment of *Escherichia coli* O157:H7 infections. N Engl J Med 2000; 342:1930–1936.

62. Safdar N, Said A, Gangnon RE, Maki DG. Risk of hemolytic uremic syndrome after antibiotic treatment of *Escherichia coli* O157:H7 enteritis: a meta-analysis. JAMA 2002; 288:996–1001.

63. Cimolai N, Carter JE, Morrison BJ, Anderson JD. Risk factors for the progression of *Escherichia coli* O157:H7 enteritis to hemolytic-uremic syndrome. J Pediatr 1990; 116:589–592.

64. Cimolai N, Basalyga S, Mah DG, Morrison BJ, Carter JE. A continuing assessment of risk factors for the development of *Escherichia coli* O157:H7-associated hemolytic uremic syndrome. Clin Nephrol 1994; 42:85–89.

65. Jereb JA, Kelly GD, Dooley SW Jr., Cauthen GM, Snider DE Jr. Tuberculosis morbidity in the United States: final data, 1990. MMWR CDC Surveill Summ 1991; 40:23–27.

66. Snider DE Jr., Roper WL. The new tuberculosis. N Engl J Med 1992; 326:703–705.

67. Rieder HL, Cauthen GM, Kelly GD, Bloch AB, Snider DE Jr. Tuberculosis in the United States. JAMA 1989; 262:385–389.

68. Mori MA, Leonardson G, Welty TK. The benefits of isoniazid chemoprophylaxis and risk factors for tuberculosis among Oglala Sioux Indians. Arch Intern Med 1992; 152:547–550.

69. Marshall JB. Tuberculosis of the gastrointestinal tract and peritoneum. Am J Gastroenterol 1993; 88:989–999.

70. Arnold C, Moradpour D, Blum HE. Tuberculous colitis mimicking Crohn's disease. Am J Gastroenterol 1998; 93:2294–2296.

71. al Karawi MA, Mohamed AE, Yasawy MI, et al. Protean manifestation of gastrointestinal tuberculosis: report on 130 patients. J Clin Gastroenterol 1995; 20:225–232.

72. Misra SP, Misra V, Dwivedi M, Gupta SC. Colonic tuberculosis: clinical features, endoscopic appearance and management. J Gastroenterol Hepatol 1999; 14:723–729.

73. Gilinsky NH, Marks IN, Kottler RE, Price SK. Abdominal tuberculosis. A 10-year review. S Afr Med J 1983; 64:849–857.

74. Klimach OE, Ormerod LP. Gastrointestinal tuberculosis: a retrospective review of 109 cases in a district general hospital. Q J Med 1985; 56:569–578.

75. Naga MI, Okasha HH, Ismail Z, El-Fatatry M, Hassan S, Monir BE. Endoscopic diagnosis of colonic tuberculosis. Gastrointest Endosc 2001; 53:789–793.

76. Kim KM, Lee A, Choi KY, Lee KY, Kwak JJ. Intestinal tuberculosis: clinicopathologic analysis and diagnosis by endoscopic biopsy. Am J Gastroenterol 1998; 93:606–609.

77. Pettengell KE, Pirie D, Simjee AE. Colonoscopic features of early intestinal tuberculosis. Report of 11 cases. S Afr Med J 1991; 79:279–280.

78. Park SJ, Han JK, Kim TK, et al. Tuberculous colitis: radiologic-colonoscopic correlation. Am J Roentgenol 2000; 175:121–128.

79. Han JK, Kim SH, Choi BI, Yeon KM, Han MC. Tuberculous colitis. Findings at double-contrast barium enema examination. Dis Colon Rectum 1996; 39:1204–1209.

80. Pulimood AB, Ramakrishna BS, Kurian G, et al. Endoscopic mucosal biopsies are useful in distinguishing granulomatous colitis due to Crohn's disease from tuberculosis. Gut 1999; 45:537–541.

81. Shah S, Thomas V, Mathan M, et al. Colonoscopic study of 50 patients with colonic tuberculosis. Gut 1992; 33:347–351.

82. Condos R, McClune A, Rom WN, Schluger NW. Peripheral-blood-based PCR assay to identify patients with active pulmonary tuberculosis. Lancet 1996; 347:1082–1085.

83. Tan MF, Ng WC, Chan SH, Tan WC. Comparative usefulness of PCR in the detection of *Mycobacterium tuberculosis* in different clinical specimens. J Med Microbiol 1997; 46:164–169.

84. Schleifstein JI, Coleman MB. An unidentified microorganism resembling B. Lignieri and Past. Pseudotuberculosis and pathogenic for man. NY State J Med 1939; 39:1749–1753.

85. Cover TL, Aber RC. *Yersinia enterocolitica*. N Engl J Med 1989; 321:16–24.

86. Gurgui Ferrer M, Prats Pastor G, Mirelis Otero B. *Yersinia enterocolitica*: intestinal features. Dig Dis 1990; 8:313–321.

87. Stolk-Engelaar VM, Hoogkamp-Korstanje JA. Clinical presentation and diagnosis of gastrointestinal infections by *Yersinia enterocolitica* in 261 Dutch patients. Scand J Infect Dis 1996; 28:571–575.

88. Simmonds SD, Noble MA, Freeman HJ. Gastrointestinal features of culture-positive *Yersinia enterocolitica* infection. Gastroenterology 1987; 92:112–117.

89. Vantrappen G, Ponette E, Geboes K, Bertrand P. Yersinia enteritis and enterocolitis: gastroenterological aspects. Gastroenterology 1977; 72:220–227.

90. Matsumoto T, Iida M, Matsui T, et al. Endoscopic findings in *Yersinia enterocolitica* enterocolitis. Gastrointest Endosc 1990; 36:583–587.

91. Sanford AH. *Yersinia enterocolitica* abscess of the transverse colon Report of a case. Dis Colon Rectum 1990; 33:985–986.

92. Bottone EJ, Sheehan DJ. *Yersinia enterocolitica*: guidelines for serologic diagnosis of human infections. Rev Infect Dis 1983; 5:898–906.

93. Bensaude R, Lambling A. Discussion of the aetiology and treatment of fibrous stricture of the rectum (including lymphogranuloma inguinale). Proc R Soc Med 1936; 29:1441–1460.

94. Quinn TC, Goodell SE, Mkrtichian E, et al. *Chlamydia trachomatis* proctitis. N Engl J Med 1981; 305:195–200.

95. Rompalo AM. Diagnosis and treatment of sexually acquired proctitis and proctocolitis: an update. Clin Infect Dis 1999; 28(suppl 1):S84–S90.

96. Annamunthodo H. Rectal lymphogranuloma venereum in Jamaica. Dis Colon Rectum 1961; 4:17–26.

97. Stamm WE, Quinn TC, Mkritichian EE, Wang SD, Schuffler MD, Holmes KK. *Chlamydia trachomatis* proctitis in homosexual men and heterosexual women. In: Marhd PA, Holmes KK, Oriel DJ, Piol P, Schacter J, eds. Chlamydia Infections. Amsterdam: Elsevier Biomedical, 1982:111–116.

98. Rompalo AM, Suchland RJ, Price CB, Stamm WE. Rapid diagnosis of *Chlamydia trachomatis* rectal infection by direct immunofluorescence staining. J Infect Dis 1987; 155:1075–1076.

99. Klein EJ, Fisher LS, Chow AW, Guze LB. Anorectal gonococcal infection. Ann Intern Med 1977; 86:340–346.

100. Quinn TC, Corey L, Chaffee RG, Schuffler MD, Brancato FP, Holmes KK. The etiology of anorectal infections in homosexual men. Am J Med 1981; 71:395–406.

101. Twedt RM. *Vibrio parahaemolyticus*. In: Doyle MP, ed. Foodborne Bacterial Pathogens. New York: Marcel Dekker, 1989:543–568.

102. Neill MA, Carpenter CCJ. Other pathogenic vibrios. In: Mandell GL, Bennett JE, Dolin R, eds. Principles & Practice of Infectious Disease. Vol. 2. New York: Churchill Livingstone, 2000:2272–2276.

103. Bolen JL, Zamiska SA, Greenough WB III. Clinical features in enteritis due to *Vibrio parahemolyticus*. Am J Med 1974; 57:638–641.

104. Barker WH Jr. *Vibrio parahaemolyticus* outbreaks in the United States. Lancet 1974; 1:551–554.

105. Feeley JC, Balows A. Vibrio. In: Lennette EH, Spaulding EH, Truant JP, eds. Manual of Clinical Microbiology. Washington, DC: American Society for Microbiology, 1974:238–245.

106. Agarwal RK, Kapoor KN, Kumar A. Virulence factors of aeromonads—an emerging food borne pathogen problem. J Commun Dis 1998; 30:71–78.

107. Deutsch SF, Wedzina W. Aeromonas sobria-associated left-sided segmental colitis. Am J Gastroenterol 1997; 92:2104–2106.

108. Holmberg SD, Schell WL, Fanning GR, et al. Aeromonas intestinal infections in the United States. Ann Intern Med 1986; 105:683–689.

109. Janda JM, Abbott SL. Unusual food-borne pathogens. Listeria monocytogenes, Aeromonas, Plesiomonas, and Edwardsiella species. Clin Lab Med 1999; 19:553–582.

110. Farraye FA, Peppercorn MA, Ciano PS, Kavesh WN. Segmental colitis associated with *Aeromonas hydrophila*. Am J Gastroenterol 1989; 84:436–438.

111. Holmberg SD, Wachsmuth IK, Hickman-Brenner FW, Blake PA, Farmer JJ III. Plesiomonas enteric infections in the United States. Ann Intern Med 1986; 105:690–694.

112. Kain KC, Kelly MT. Clinical features, epidemiology, and treatment of Plesiomonas shigelloides diarrhea. J Clin Microbiol 1989; 27:998–1001.

113. van Loon FP, Rahim Z, Chowdhury KA, Kay BA, Rahman SA. Case report of Plesiomonas shigelloides-associated persistent dysentery and pseudomembranous colitis. J Clin Microbiol 1989; 27:1913–1915.

114. Kain KC, Kelly MT. Antimicrobial susceptibility of Plesiomonas shigelloides from patients with diarrhea. Antimicrob Agents Chemother 1989; 33:1609–1610.

115. Li E, Stanley SL Jr. Protozoa. Amebiasis. Gastroenterol Clin North Am 1996; 25:471–492.

116. Katz DE, Taylor DN. Parasitic infections of the gastrointestinal tract. Gastroenterol Clin North Am 2001; 30:797–815.

117. Petri WA Jr., Upinder S, I RJ. Enteric amebiasis. In: Guerrant RL, Walker DH, Weller PF, eds. Tropical Infectious Diseases. Philadelphia: Churchill Livingstone, 1999:685–702.

118. The World Health Report 1995—bridging the gaps. World Health Forum 1995; 16:377–385.

119. Aristizabal H, Acevedo J, Botero M. Fulminant amebic colitis. World J Surg 1991; 15:216–221.

120. Takahashi T, Gamboa-Dominguez A, Gomez-Mendez TJ, et al. Fulminant amebic colitis: analysis of 55 cases. Dis Colon Rectum 1997; 40:1362–1367.

121. Sachdev GK, Dhol P. Colonic involvement in patients with amebic liver abscess: endoscopic findings. Gastrointest Endosc 1997; 46:37–39.

122. Gotohda N, Itano S, Okada Y, et al. Acute appendicitis caused by amebiasis. J Gastroenterol 2000; 35:861–863.

123. Stanley SL Jr. Amoebiasis. Lancet 2003; 361:1025–1034.

124. el-Hennawy M, Abd-Rabbo H. Hazards of cortisone therapy in hepatic amoebiasis. J Trop Med Hyg 1978; 81:71–73.

125. Parija SC, Rao RS. Stool culture as a diagnostic aid in the detection of Entamoeba histolytica in the faecal specimens. Indian J Pathol Microbiol 1995; 38:359–363.

126. Haque R, Ali IK, Akther S, Petri WA Jr. Comparison of PCR, isoenzyme analysis, and antigen detection for diagnosis of Entamoeba histolytica infection. J Clin Microbiol 1998; 36:449–452.

127. Ravdin JI. Amebiasis. Clin Infect Dis 1995; 20:1453–1464.

128. Yoshida M, Kutsumi H, Ogawa M, et al. A case of *Trichuris trichiura* infection diagnosed by colonoscopy. Am J Gastroenterol 1996; 91:161–162.

129. Grencis RK, Cooper ES. Enterobius, trichuris, capillaria, and hookworm including ancylostoma caninum. Gastroenterol Clin North Am 1996; 25:579–597.

130. MacDonald TT, Choy MY, Spencer J, et al. Histopathology and immunohistochemistry of the caecum in children with the Trichuris dysentery syndrome. J Clin Pathol 1991; 44:194–199.

131. Gilman RH, Chong YH, Davis C, Greenberg B, Virik HK, Dixon HB. The adverse consequences of heavy Trichuris infection. Trans R Soc Trop Med Hyg 1983; 77:432–438.

132. Fishman JA, Perrone TL. Colonic obstruction and perforation due to *Trichuris trichiura*. Am J Med 1984; 77:154–156.

133. Chandra B, Long JD. Diagnosis of *Trichuris trichiura* (whipworm) by colonoscopic extraction. J Clin Gastroenterol 1998; 27:152–153.

134. Joo JH, Ryu KH, Lee YH, et al. Colonoscopic diagnosis of whipworm infection. Hepatogastroenterology 1998; 45:2105–2109.

135. Goodwin RA, Loyd JE, Des Prez RM. Histoplasmosis in normal hosts. Medicine (Baltimore) 1981; 60:231–266.

136. Clarkston WK, Bonacini M, Peterson I. Colitis due to *Histoplasma capsulatum* in the acquired immune deficiency syndrome. Am J Gastroenterol 1991; 86:913–916.

137. Goodwin RA Jr., Shapiro JL, Thurman GH, Thurman SS, Des Prez RM. Disseminated histoplasmosis: clinical and pathologic correlations. Medicine (Baltimore) 1980; 59:1–33.

138. Reddy P, Gorelick DF, Brasher CA, Larsh H. Progressive disseminated histoplasmosis as seen in adults. Am J Med 1970; 48:629–636.

139. Cimponeriu D, LoPresti P, Lavelanet M, et al. Gastrointestinal histoplasmosis in HIV infection: two cases of colonic pseudocancer and review of the literature. Am J Gastroenterol 1994; 89:129–131.

140. Hung CC, Wong JM, Hsueh PR, Hsieh SM, Chen MY. Intestinal obstruction and peritonitis resulting from gastrointestinal histoplasmosis in an AIDS patient. J Formos Med Assoc 1998; 97:577–580.

141. Lee SH, Barnes WG, Hodges GR, Dixon A. Perforated granulomatous colitis caused by *Histoplasma capsulatum*. Dis Colon Rectum 1985; 28:171–176.

142. Fantry GT, Fantry LE, James SP. Histoplasmosis. In: Yamada T, Alpers DH, Laine L, Owyang C, Powell DW, eds. Textbook of Gastroenterology. Vol. 2. Philadelphia: Lippincott Williams & Wilkins, 1999:1653–1655.

143. McKinsey DS, Gupta MR, Riddler SA, Driks MR, Smith DL, Kurtin PJ. Long-term amphotericin B therapy for disseminated histoplasmosis in patients with the acquired immunodeficiency syndrome (AIDS). Ann Intern Med 1989; 111:655–659.

144. Wheat J, Hafner R, Wulfsohn M, et al. Prevention of relapse of histoplasmosis with itraconazole in patients with the acquired immunodeficiency syndrome. The National Institute of Allergy and Infectious Diseases Clinical Trials and Mycoses Study Group Collaborators. Ann Intern Med 1993; 118:610–616.

145. Bini EJ, Cohen J. Diagnostic yield and cost-effectiveness of endoscopy in chronic human immunodeficiency virus-related diarrhea. Gastrointest Endosc 1998; 48:354–361.

146. Karakozis S, Gongora E, Caceres M, Brun E, Cook JW. Life-threatening cytomegalovirus colitis in the immunocompetent patient: report of a case and review of the literature. Dis Colon Rectum 2001; 44:1716–1720.

147. Goodgame RW. Viral causes of diarrhea. Gastroenterol Clin North Am 2001; 30:779–795.

148. Sakamoto I, Shirai T, Kamide T, et al. Cytomegalovirus enterocolitis in an immunocompetent individual. J Clin Gastroenterol 2002; 34:243–246.

149. Wilcox CM, Chalasani N, Lazenby A, Schwartz DA. Cytomegalovirus colitis in acquired immunodeficiency syndrome: a clinical and endoscopic study. Gastrointest Endosc 1998; 48:39–43.

150. Chalasani N, Wilcox CM. Etiology and outcome of lower gastrointestinal bleeding in patients with AIDS. Am J Gastroenterol 1998; 93:175–178.

151. Falagas ME, Griffiths J, Prekezes J, Worthington M. Cytomegalovirus colitis mimicking colon carcinoma in an HIV-negative patient with chronic renal failure. Am J Gastroenterol 1996; 91:168–169.

152. Chow PK, Ho JM, Ling AE, Goh HS. CMV colitis masquerading as colon cancer—an unusual presentation of acquired immunodeficiency syndrome. Singapore Med J 1997; 38:32–34.

153. Olofinlade O, Chiang C. Cytomegalovirus infection as a cause of pseudomembrane colitis: a report of four cases. J Clin Gastroenterol 2001; 32:82–84.

154. Diaz-Gonzalez VM, Altemose GT, Ogorek C, Palazzo I, Pina IL. Cytomegalovirus infection presenting as an apple-core lesion of the colon. J Heart Lung Transplant 1997; 16:1171–1175.

155. Schafer P, Tenschert W, Cremaschi L, Gutensohn K, Laufs R. Utility of major leukocyte subpopulations for monitoring secondary cytomegalovirus infections in renal-allograft recipients by PCR. J Clin Microbiol 1998; 36:1008–1014.

156. Whitley RJ, Jacobson MA, Friedberg DN, et al. Guidelines for the treatment of cytomegalovirus diseases in patients with AIDS in the era of potent antiretroviral therapy: recommendations of an international panel. International AIDS Society-USA. Arch Intern Med 1998; 158:957–969.

157. Bini EJ, Gorelick SM, Weinshel EH. Outcome of AIDS-associated cytomegalovirus colitis in the era of potent antiretroviral therapy. J Clin Gastroenterol 2000; 30:414–419.

158. Bagdades EK, Pillay D, Squire SB, O'Neil C, Johnson MA, Griffiths PD. Relationship between herpes simplex virus ulceration and CD4+ cell counts in patients with HIV infection. AIDS 1992; 6: 1317–1320.

159. Adler M, Goldman M, Liesnard C, et al. Diffuse herpes simplex virus colitis in a kidney transplant recipient successfully treated with acyclovir. Transplantation 1987; 43:919–921.

160. Naik HR, Chandrasekar PH. Herpes simplex virus (HSV) colitis in a bone marrow transplant recipient. Bone Marrow Transplant 1996; 17:285–286.

161. Delis S, Kato T, Ruiz P, Mittal N, Babinski L, Tzakis A. Herpes simplex colitis in a child with combined liver and small bowel transplant. Pediatr Transplant 2001; 5:374–377.

162. Goodell SE, Quinn TC, Mkrtichian E, Schuffler MD, Holmes KK, Corey L. Herpes simplex virus proctitis in homosexual men. Clinical, sigmoidoscopic, and histopathological features. N Engl J Med 1983; 308:868–871.

163. Colemont LJ, Pen JH, Pelckmans PA, Degryse HR, Pattyn SR, Van Maercke YM. Herpes simplex virus type 1 colitis: an unusual cause of diarrhea. Am J Gastroenterol 1990; 85:1182–1185.
164. Rompalo AM, Mertz GJ, Davis LG, et al. Oral acyclovir for treatment of first-episode herpes simplex virus proctitis. JAMA 1988; 259:2879–2881.
165. Kearney DJ, Steuerwald M, Koch J, Cello JP. A prospective study of endoscopy in HIV-associated diarrhea. Am J Gastroenterol 1999; 94:596–602.
166. Surawicz CM. The role of rectal biopsy in infectious colitis. Am J Surg Pathol 1988; 12(suppl 1):82–88.
167. Duggan C, Santosham M, Glass RI. The management of acute diarrhea in children: oral rehydration, maintenance, and nutritional therapy. Centers for Disease Control and Prevention. MMWR Recomm Rep 1992; 41:1–20.
168. Walterspiel JN, Ashkenazi S, Morrow AL, Cleary TG. Effect of subinhibitory concentrations of antibiotics on extracellular Shiga-like toxin I. Infection 1992; 20:25–29.
169. Zhang X, McDaniel AD, Wolf LE, Keusch GT, Waldor MK, Acheson DW. Quinolone antibiotics induce Shiga toxin-encoding bacteriophages, toxin production, and death in mice. J Infect Dis 2000; 181:664–670.
170. Haddad FS, Ghossain A, Sawaya E, Nelson AR. Abdominal tuberculosis. Dis Colon Rectum 1987; 30:724–735.

13 | Pseudomembranous Colitis

Elizabeth Broussard and Christina M. Surawicz
Department of Medicine, University of Washington School of Medicine, Harborview Medical Center, Seattle, Washington, U.S.A.

Eileen Bulger
Department of Surgery, University of Washington School of Medicine, Seattle, Washington, U.S.A.

INTRODUCTION

Clostridium difficile is a gram-positive, anaerobic, spore-forming bacillus whose pathogenicity in the human gastrointestinal tract has paralleled advances in antimicrobial therapy. Prior to the age of antibiotics, *C. difficile* grew undisturbed in colonic mucosa, causing little damage or human disease. With the discovery of *C. difficile* as the causative agent for antibiotic-associated colitis, there has been a remarkable resurrection of this organism as pathogen, with intense scientific investigations examining epidemiology, pathophysiology, and effective clinical treatments that were developed within a few years of its rediscovery. Nosocomial outbreaks provided further opportunities for epidemiological study, and advances in molecular biology have resulted in cloning and sequencing of *C. difficile* toxins, prompting examination of cellular mechanisms of action. Despite the explosion of knowledge about the organism and associated disease, many questions remain. Areas for further study include effective methods of prevention, optimal treatment of recurrent disease, the role of host immune system factors, and possible prophylaxis with vaccine.

HISTORICAL PERSPECTIVE

The earliest report of *C difficile* was in 1893, when a patient of Dr. William Osler, a 22-year-old female, severely malnourished, presented with a history of nausea and vomiting for three months and had a dilated stomach with a palpable mass. She underwent surgical treatment of a cicatrizing ulcer in the pylorus and was treated postoperatively with enemas of whiskey and saline. At postoperative day 10, she experienced bloody diarrhea and tenesmus and died five days later. Autopsy was performed, which revealed "diptheritic" colitis and cecitis, and pseudomembranes in her colon (1). Since then, cases of cardiovascular insufficiency, colonic obstruction, heavy metal intoxication, sepsis, shock, spinal fracture, and uremia have all been sporadically associated with the finding of pseudomembranes. In 1935, Hall and O'Toole identified an organism in the normal colonic flora of healthy newborn infants, naming it *Bacillus difficilis*, because it was difficult to culture, and noted that it was fatal when injected into guinea pigs and rabbits (2). Because it was found in normal healthy infants, at that time, it was considered to be nonpathogenic in humans. In the 1950s, the introduction of broad-spectrum antibiotics chloramphenicol and tetracycline led to cases of antibiotic-associated diarrhea (AAD). The culprit was thought to be *Staphylococcus aureus* because it was frequently isolated in stools of affected patients and patients responded well to treatment with vancomycin (3). Pseudomembranous enterocolitis was a well-recognized clinical complication of surgical patients in the era prior to the introduction of antibiotics. Staphylococcal enterocolitis became much less frequent in the 1960s with the introduction of vancomycin and semisynthetic penicillinase-resistant β-lactam antimicrobials (4). Clindamycin was introduced in the 1960s as an agent to treat anaerobic infections, and with its increased use, more cases of pseudomembranous colitis were reported, without isolation of *S. aureus* in these cases.

In retrospect, 1974 was a banner year in terms of defining etiology and pathophysiology of disease associated with *C. difficile*. Tedesco reported that 200 patients treated with clindamycin developed serious diarrhea (21%) and pseudomembranous colitis (PMC) (10% of patients with diarrhea) and isolated a cytotoxic factor on tissue culture from their stools (5). The same year, Hafiz, described *C. difficile* as a bacterium that was widespread in nature, with most strains producing a toxin that was lethal in animals (6). Green showed cytotoxic changes in tissue culture monolayers inoculated with specimens from animals exposed to penicillins that died unexpectedly (7). Bartlett et al. and Larson et al. linked these findings together in 1977, when Bartlett demonstrated that cecal contents transferred from hamster to hamster could induce clindamycin-associated colitis, with only *C. difficile* being able to induce the same illness in other hamsters (8). The presence of toxin was suggested by the finding that a cell-free supernatant could produce the same illness. Larson described a cytotoxic factor in the stools of patients with PMC (9), thereby establishing the link between antibiotic-induced colitis in hamster models and presence of cytopathic toxin and disease in humans.

PATHOPHYSIOLOGY

The pathophysiology of PMC involves four main factors: (i) disturbance of normal colonic microflora, (ii) exposure to and colonization by *C. difficile*, (iii) production of toxin and toxin-mediated injury and inflammation, and (iv) host factors such as age, underlying disease, and immunologic status (10).

Disturbance of Normal Colonic Microflora

"Colonization resistance" is the term for the protective effect of the normal stable intestinal flora against overgrowth of pathogenic organisms. The specific organisms responsible have not yet been determined, although anaerobic bacteria such as *Lactobacillus* and group D enterococci were shown to be highly inhibitory toward *C. difficile* in vitro (11). In animal models, it has been shown that this flora barrier is disrupted by antibiotics, followed by infection with *C. difficile* (12–14). *C. difficile* can colonize the intestine of germ-free mice. Inoculation of these animals with fecal flora from normal mice led to the disappearance of *C. difficile* (13), confirming the importance of the normal flora in preventing colonization. In vitro, the growth of *C. difficile* is inhibited by emulsions of feces from healthy adults but not by sterile extracts (15). Healthy neonates and infants have poor colonization resistance because they have not yet developed stable and complex colonic microflora. Colonization resistance may rely upon the production of inhibitory fatty acids, toxin-degrading proteases, nutrient competition, the competition for attachment sites, or some combination of these factors (16). Antibiotics, other medications, or medical procedures eliminate or suppress normal flora to such an extent that colonization resistance is impaired, and *C. difficile* is free to grow and cause toxigenic diarrhea and inflammation.

Exposure to and Colonization by *Clostridium difficile*

The majority of exposures and infections are acquired while in the hospital setting, with ill patients on antibiotics, exposed to spores or vegetative *C. difficile* organisms, which are widespread and dormant in the hospital environment.

Most of our knowledge of the mode of transmission, routes of infection, and risk factors for *C. difficile* disease has been gained from sporadic outbreaks of *C. difficile* disease in hospitalized patients, starting in 1978. The sources of infection are not often identified. Savage and Alford reported a contaminated commode chair shared by two patients that transmitted *C. difficile* infection (17). Mogg et al. reported a contaminated sigmoidoscope as a source for an outbreak of pseudomembranous colitis (18).

Production of Toxin and Toxin-Mediated Injury and Inflammation

C. difficile diarrhea is toxin mediated. Pathogenic strains of *C. difficile* produce two large protein exotoxins, toxin A (308 kDa) and toxin B (275 kDa). Although toxin B was discovered earlier than toxin A, toxin A appeared first on the gas chromatography peaks and was thus named. The toxins are encoded by two distinct genes in proximity on the bacterial genome, similar in structure and sharing 49% homology at the level of amino acids (19–21). They bear no structural or functional relationship to other bacterial enterotoxins such as cholera toxin, *Escherichia coli* enterotoxin, or *Shiga* toxin (22). Toxin A is an inflammatory enterotoxin that causes fluid secretion, increased mucosal permeability, and enteritis and colitis after injection into animal

Table 1 Overview of Enterotoxicity for *Clostridium difficile* Toxins—Sequence of Events

Direct toxin effects on the enterocyte	Subsequent effects in lamina propria
Binding of toxin to receptors	Release of cytokines from enterocytes
Internalization	Activation of mast cells, afferent neurons
Inactivation of Rho	Activation of afferent neurons
Disaggregation of actin filaments	Release of mast cell products, substance P
Cell rounding	Regulation of adhesion molecules on vascular epithelium
Impairment of tight junctions	Recruitment of neutrophils
Diarrhea and inflammation	Diarrhea and inflammation

Source: From Ref. 33.

intestinal lumens (23) and weak cytotoxic activity against cultured cells (24,25). Toxin B is a potent cytotoxin but does not exhibit enterotoxic activity in animals in vivo (24,26–28). Initially, toxin B was thought not to be involved in the pathogenesis of *C. difficile* diarrhea and colitis in human beings because it did not have enterotoxic activity in animals. Recent evidence suggests that this is not the case. Both toxin A and B have been shown to cause injury and electrophysiologic changes in human colonic strips in vitro, with toxin B being 10 times more potent than toxin A in inducing these changes (29). Toxin A–negative/toxin B–positive strains of *C. difficile* from patients with AAD and colitis have been isolated, which suggests that toxin B alone may be pathogenic in human beings (30–34).

The cellular mechanisms of *C. difficile* toxins are targeted toward Rho family proteins, which are RhoGTPases–binding proteins that regulate actin filaments in all cells. Rho proteins are inactivated by *C. difficile* toxins; actin filaments disintegrate, causing cell dysfunction and cell rounding (29). This, in turn, increases tight junction permeability between the cells, causing leakage of fluids and soluble components into colonic lumen. Once enterotoxin binds to epithelial cell brush borders, inflammatory mediators such as leukotrienes, cytokines, and histamines attract inflammatory cells. Histologic examination may show focal ulceration of colonic mucosa associated with the eruption of purulent material including inflammatory cells, fibrin, and necrotic debris, which comprise the pseudomembrane. The adjacent mucosa may be intact, making the pseudomembrane appear as raised yellow or white plaques that are 2 to 4 mm in diameter. The patchy distribution of the pseudomembranes may be related to toxin dose response. When human colonic mucosal strips in vitro were exposed to toxin B in increasing concentrations, as toxin concentration increased, so did areas of tissue damage until the areas were nearly confluent (Table 1) (29,33).

Host Factors

It remains unknown why only some patients treated with a given antibiotic become colonized with *C. difficile*, and why only some patients who are colonized progress to symptoms. The ability of the host to mount an immune response may play a role. In a prospective study of nosocomial *C. difficile* infection, 51% of patients who acquired the organism remained asymptomatic. These asymptomatic carriers had serum levels of IgG antibody against toxin A, which were three times higher than in patients who developed *C. difficile* diarrhea. Patients were 48 times more likely to develop *C. difficile* diarrhea if they had a low serum level of IgG anti-toxin A rather than high antibody levels. IgG antitoxin B levels did not correlate with protection against *C. difficile* diarrhea, but did correlate with IgG anti-toxin A in asymptomatic carriers (34).

Almost all antibiotics have been associated with *C. difficile* diarrhea and colitis, including metronidazole and rarely vancomycin (35,36), but those most frequently associated include clindamycin, cephalosporins, ampicillin, and amoxicillin. Even after adjustment for other risk factors in multivariable analyses, these agents are associated with the highest risks of *C. difficile* diarrhea (37).

Age is an independent risk factor for developing *C. difficile* diarrhea (38,39). In England and Wales, 75% of all *C. difficile* reported to the Public Health Library Service Communicable Disease Surveillance Centre from 1992 to 1996 occurred in patients older than 62 years of age. Sicker patients with severe underlying disease at the time of admission to the hospital were eight times more likely to develop *C. difficile* infection compared with less ill patients (34).

The presence of a nasogastric tube, gastrointestinal procedures, acid antisecretory medications, intensive care unit stay, and duration of hospital stay have all been reported as risk factors for *C. difficile* infection, but degrees of association very from study to study, and these factors may serve as markers for severity of disease or older age or both; after controlling for confounding variables, their association with *C. difficile* loses significance (34,38,39).

EPIDEMIOLOGY
Prevalence

C. difficile is the leading cause of enteric nosocomial infection in U.S. hospitals, with an estimated three million new cases of diarrhea and colitis each year, affecting up to 10% of patients who are hospitalized for more than two days (40). Infection with *C. difficile* increases hospital length-of-stay in adults by an average of 8 days, and by an average of 36 additional days in elderly patients (41,42). In 1991, one study estimated the overall charges for an admitting diagnosis of *C. difficile*–associated disease (CDAD) averaged $5000 per admission and acquired cases resulted in additional hospital costs of $2000 (43). These costs include hospital microscopic laboratory assays, endoscopic examinations, antibiotic treatments, and per diem charges (43,44). Only 20,000 people acquire this infection annually as outpatients, with incidence as low as less than one case per 10,000 antibiotic prescriptions in one large outpatient setting (45). Colonization rates in asymptomatic individuals are surprisingly high. *C. difficile* can be isolated in 1% to 5% of healthy adults, 30% to 75% of healthy neonates, 9% to 14% of healthy infants under the age of one, and 10% to 30 % of inpatients without symptoms (39,46–49). Most asymptomatic colonized individuals will not progress to symptomatic disease.

A study determined that patients who developed infectious diarrhea after 48 hours of hospitalization were almost always infected with *C. difficile*, and that it was not cost effective to evaluate for any other enteric pathogen (50,51). *C. difficile* has also been frequently found in chronic-care facilities such as nursing homes. McFarland et al. reported a high percentage of patients (82%) with positive *C. difficile* cultures on discharge from the hospital, and these patients were more likely to be discharged to an extended care facility than those patients with negative *C. difficile* cultures (40). Among patients in two rehabilitation hospitals who were evaluated for diarrhea, 25% of them were positive for *C. difficile* (52). In the community, outbreaks in day-care centers have been reported, in which hands of teachers and children revealed the same strain of *C. difficile* (53).

Transmission

Routes of transmission are most often nosocomial, although sporadic cases of *C. difficile*-associated diarrhea occur in outpatient settings. One study showed that patients who were culture positive at time of hospital admission were most likely to have had prior exposure to that same hospital (54). The two major potential *C. difficile* reservoirs in hospitals are humans, symptomatic or asymptomatic, and inanimate objects (hospital surfaces) (55). Patient-to-patient transmission of *C. difficile* strains is the major mode of transmission, which has been confirmed by immunoblot typing (56). In one well-studied ward of medical and surgical patients, the rate of acquisition of *C. difficile* was shown to be linear at 8% per week (54).

Health-care workers may harbor intestinal infection but this has not shown to be a significant concern for transmission (50). Transient carriage on the health-care workers' hands, stethoscopes, and clothing is a far more likely culprit (41,57), as suggested by a reduction in *C. difficile* diarrhea associated with the use of gloves and careful hand washing after patient examination (47,55).

Contamination of environmental surfaces such as commodes, neonatal bathing tubs, telephones, and rectal thermometers have all been implicated as reservoirs of *C. difficile* (18,58,59). Measures that have been proposed to reduce cross-contamination and infection include use of disposable gloves, and disposable, single-use rectal thermometers (60), hand washing with chlorhexidine or other suitable disinfectant after patient contact, and disinfection of patient environment after discharge with agents that kill *C. difficile* spores, such as hypochlorous acid (61).

Newborns

Newborns acquire *C. difficile* from the hospital environment including the environmental surfaces of nurseries and neonatal intensive care units. A prospective study of three postnatal wards found colonization rates of infants as high as 52% as determined by daily stool cultures (58). Despite the fact that infants and children up to the age of two have reported colonization rates with *C. difficile*, of 25% to 80%, they rarely develop *C. difficile*-associated diarrhea (62,63). A possible mechanism for this phenomenon is the immaturity of the enterocytes with an absence of toxin receptor expression (64). Infants develop a serum and secretory antibody response during month 6 through month 12 when colonization with *C. difficile* peaks. After 12 to 24 months of age, about 50% to 60% of healthy children and adults have detectable serum and intestinal immunoglobulin levels to toxin A and toxin B, which persist throughout their lifetimes (65,66). Although infrequent, infants and children can get symptomatic CDAD and the diagnosis is often delayed.

Risk Factors

Major risk factors for *C. difficile* infection are advanced age, exposure to antibiotics, and hospitalization. In Sweden, a population-based study showed that the incidence of positive assays for *C. difficile* in individuals over the age of 60 was 20 to 100 times higher than those aged 10 to 20 (67). Nash et al. found that 62% of symptomatic patients were older than 60 (68). In an earlier Swedish survey, 63% of patients with *C. difficile* disease were older than 60, with all age groups represented (69). Older people get prescribed more antibiotics and have a higher incidence of intestinal neoplasms, intestinal surgery, and other factors that modify the immune system's ability to mount effective response, which can all contribute to their increased susceptibility to CDAD (70–72).

DIAGNOSTIC METHODS
Microbiologic Cultures

C. difficile is a fastidious anaerobic bacteria that must be inoculated in anaerobic cultures rapidly. Fresh stool, in a clean, watertight container should be processed within one to three hours or refrigerated if processing will be delayed (73). Cytotoxin titers will decrease over several days when held at 22°C to 27°C and *C. difficile* viability counts decrease when samples are frozen (74,75). No single assay meets ideal criteria for both high accuracy and rapid results. High sensitivity takes two to three days' processing time and usually requires specialized laboratory equipment. Fast results are not as specific and can lead to false diagnoses without confirmation by other assays. Combining selective plate or enrichment broth cultures and confirmatory identification tests may offer the most sensitive and specific means to isolate *C. difficile* (3).

Selective and Differential Media

C. difficile was initially named "difficult Clostridium" due to its resistance to isolation and growth on conventional media. It was not until 1979 that cefoxitin–cycloserine–fructose agar was developed, which selectively inhibited the growth of other enteric anaerobes, allowing differentiation of *C. difficile* from other clostridia (76). *C. difficile* colonies appear yellowish white, emit golden yellow fluorescence under UV light, distinctly smell like "an elephant house," and have a ground-glass appearance with magnification. These features are not unique to *C. difficile*; therefore, media selectivity has been improved with subsequent modifications including lowering cycloserine levels and adding sheep red blood cells and 0.1% sodium taurocholate (55,77).

Typing

An understanding of the epidemiology of CDAD depends on the development and application of new methods to allow typing or discrimination of different strains of *C. difficile*. Typing allows investigators to identify different strains in endemic disease as well as outbreaks, to examine modes of transmission and to address clinical issues such as whether diarrhea relapses are actually failure to eradicate specific strains or new infection with a new strain altogether.

A wide variety of methods have been utilized for typing. Methods are divided into phenotypic and genotypic characterizations. Phenotypic methods include susceptibility testing with antibiograms (78), susceptibility testing with bacteriocins and bacteriophages (79,80), polyacrylamide gel electrophoresis with radiolabeling (81) or with immunoblotting (82–84) based on cellular and surface protein patterns, and serotyping system using slide agglutination (85).

Genotypic methods do not depend on sample stability or culture conditions and have a theoretical advantage over phenotypic methods. These methods include examination of plasmid DNA as "plasmid fingerprints" or with restriction endonuclease analysis (86).

Latex Agglutination Assay

Latex agglutination assay (LAT) was first thought to be detecting *C. difficile* toxin A, or enterotoxin, but was later discovered to be detecting a glutamate dehydrogenase protein (87–90), which is found in nontoxigenic strains of *C. difficile*, other nonpathogenic clostridia and bacterial species such as *Clostridium sporogenes, Peptostreptococcus anaerobius, Bacteroides asaccharolyticus, Salmonella enteritidus, Shigella boydii*, and parasites such as *Blastocystis hominis* and *Giardia lamblia* (91,92). False-positive rates range from 1% to 32%, sensitivity ranges from 58% to 68%, and specificity ranges from 94% to 96% (59,93,94). Even though LAT is rapid, relatively inexpensive, and specific, it is not sufficiently sensitive to be used for routine laboratory detection of *C. difficile*.

Toxin Assay

Virtually all *C. difficile* strains produce both toxins A and B, which assures that cytotoxic activity is a reliable diagnostic test for CDAD (34,72,95,96). Recently, cases of CDAC have been attributed to strains producing only toxin B or undetectable toxin A. Some strains produce no toxin and presumably do not cause disease. The cytotoxin assay detects toxins capable of causing a cytopathic effect in tissue culture cell lines, usually fibroblasts, after 24 to 48 hours' incubation. A stool sample is collected and homogenized, centrifuged, and filtered. The cell-free supernatant is added to the tissue culture cell monolayer and incubated for 24 to 48 hours. A negative control using neutralizing *Clostridium sordellii* antitoxin, which cross-reacts with *C. difficile* cytotoxin, must be used to increase specificity. Stool must be diluted (1:10 to 1:100) because undiluted stool alone is cytopathic to most cell lines. Positive cytotoxin samples reveal the disintegration of the actin cytoskeleton, resulting in rounding of the cells and thinning of the cytoplasmic adherence projections. Negative cytotoxin samples and the negative control show normal cells. Cytotoxin is readily detected in diluted stool, with the limit of detection ranging from as little as 1 to 2 pg (10^{-12} g) to 3 to 5 ng/mL to cause cell rounding, depending on the cell lines (46,47,97). If performed correctly, the assay has both high sensitivity (67–100%) and high specificity (85–100%) (55). Sensitivity may be decreased by inactivation of toxins during transport and storage, by age and type of cell line utilized, and stool dilution titer (73,98–100).

Despite toxin assay being the current "gold standard" test for the diagnosis of CDAD, they still require refinement. The assays are not standardized, with different procedures, cell lines, fecal concentrations, inconsistent use of negative control, and added antibiotics and growth media that may affect the production of cytotoxin (101). In addition, there remain a significant number of cytotoxin-positive cultures in asymptomatic patients who carry *C. difficile*, and cytotoxin-negative findings in patients with *C. difficile* disease (97),(102). Furthermore, the assays require specialized facilities, cost about $30 to $40 each, and require 24 to 48 hours for results.

Enzyme-Linked Immunoassay

There are several commercially available enzyme-linked immunoassay (EIA) test kits that detect *C. difficile* toxins A and B, or toxin A by using a monoclonal antibody that reacts with an amino-terminal region epitope of the toxin A molecule (103–107). The kits that detect only toxin A will miss the 1% to 2% of *C. difficile* diarrhea that is due to variant strains that are toxin A negative/toxin B positive, and thus are less sensitive (33,105),(108). The EIA tests are, however,, easier to perform than cytotoxicity tests, relatively inexpensive, produce results in two to six hours, and exhibit high specificity (75–100%), but lower sensitivity (60–99%) than cytotoxicity tests (55).

Polymerase Chain Reaction

Using specific primers based on toxin A and toxin B genes, polymerase chain reaction (PCR) has been used to detect toxigenic *C. difficile* (42,109,110) with high sensitivity (100%) and high specificity (96.7–100%). Techniques to detect genes directly in feces have been developed, with

Table 2 Stool Tests for the Diagnosis of *Clostridium difficile* Infection

Diagnostic test	Detects	Advantages	Disadvantages
Cytotoxin assay	Toxin B	Gold standard, highly sensitive, highly specific	Requires tissue culture facility and takes 24–48 hrs
Enzyme immunoassay	Toxin A or B	Fast (2–6 hrs), easy to perform, high specificity	Not as sensitive as cytotoxin assay (80–85%)
Latex agglutination assay	Bacterial enzyme (glutamate dehydrogenase)	Fast, inexpensive, easy to perform	Low sensitivity and specificity
Culture	Toxigenic and nontoxigenic *C. difficile*	Sensitive; allows strain typing in epidemics	Requires aerobic culture, not specific for toxin-producing bacteria, and takes two to five days
Polymerase chain reaction	Toxin A or B genes in isolates or directly in feces	High sensitivity and high specificity	Requires expertise in molecular diagnostic techniques

Source: From Ref. 10.

reported 99% concordance with the cytotoxicity assay and high specificity (100%) and sensitivity (96.3%) (109). However, PCR assays are very labor intensive (Table 2).

Endoscopy and Histology

Endoscopic examination is generally not recommended in patients with clinical findings and positive stool toxin assay consistent with *C. difficile* diarrhea, except for special situations such as when the diagnosis remains in doubt or rapid diagnosis is necessary. Endoscopic examinations may reveal normal colon or may show nonspecific colitis in patients with mild to moderate diarrhea. The presence of pseudomembranes is virtually pathognomonic for *C. difficile* colitis in patients with AAD. Pseudomembranes appear as yellow or off-white raised plaques 0.2 to 2.0 cm in diameter interspersed with normal-appearing mucosa, with accompanying full-thickness bowel wall edema and hyperemia. (Fig. 1) The spectrum of PMC pathology has been divided into three distinct categories (111). Type 1 is the mildest form, with major inflammatory changes confined to superficial epithelium and subjacent lamina propria, and summit-like "volcano" lesions resulting from erupted polymorphonuclear cells and fibrin from the necrotic focus. Type 2 is characterized by more severe disruption of glands, marked secretion of mucin, and intense inflammation of the basal lamina. Type 3 is characterized by severe, intense necrosis of the full thickness of the mucosa with merging of plaques to form a confluent layer of pseudomembrane, which can mimic other forms of ischemic colitis and is not by itself diagnostic of PMC (Fig. 2).

The small focal plaques of type 1 PMC can be missed by sigmoidoscopy. In patients with suspected PMC, sigmoidoscopy detected 31% of plaques, while colonoscopy detected 85% of plaques in one study (112).

Most clinical laboratories currently test for toxin A or B or both, utilizing EIA. However, a negative test does not eliminate the possibility of disease, due to varying sensitivity and

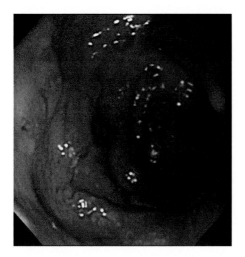

Figure 1 (*See color insert*) Typical endoscopic appearance of *Clostridium difficile* colitis with small white plaques.

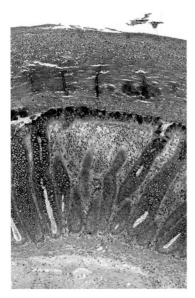

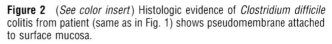

Figure 2 (*See color insert*) Histologic evidence of *Clostridium difficile* colitis from patient (same as in Fig. 1) shows pseudomembrane attached to surface mucosa.

specificity. If clinically indicated, the test should be repeated, or another test should be ordered and empiric therapy with antimicrobials should be initiated.

CLINICAL PRESENTATION AND COURSE

Diarrhea is the most common symptom of C. difficile disease. Diarrhea is generally defined as a change in bowel movement frequency with three or greater loose stools daily for at least two consecutive days. Diarrhea can consist of mucoid, greenish, foul-smelling, watery stools. Patients may complain of cramping abdominal pain, and have a low-grade fever and leukocytosis, and even a leukemoid reaction. Symptoms may present a few days after antibiotic therapy is initiated or up to eight weeks after discontinuation (4). The spectrum of disease conditions ranges from mild diarrhea that resolves with discontinuation of the offending antibiotic to severe, life-threatening, fulminant disease with toxic megacolon.

Antibiotic-Associated Diarrhea

Antibiotic diarrhea is diarrhea in the context of recent antibiotic use without evidence of colitis. The spectrum of severity of diarrhea can range from mild diarrhea that stops with discontinuation of antibiotic, to up to 20 to 30 diarrheal episodes daily for two to three months without treatment (5). The exact incubation period for symptomatic disease after colonization is not known but is likely less than seven days (early onset), with two days as median time of onset of symptoms (34,40,113,114), or longer, with symptoms starting two to six weeks after discontinuation of antibiotic (late onset) (3). The average duration of diarrhea is 8 to 10 days (115). Physical exam is usually normal except for minimal lower abdominal tenderness, without fever, leukocytosis, or dehydration. Stool cultures are positive for *C. difficile* in 11% to 33% patients (40,46).

The incidence of AAD varies from 3 to 30 in 100 hospital admissions, depending on antibiotics given, host factors, and underlying illnesses (40,116,117). About 10% to 20% of patients receiving clindamycin developed AAD, and 5% to 10% of patients receiving ampicillin developed AAD (118). In a study of 399 hospitalized patients, 90 developed AAD, with *C. difficile* attributed to approximately 25% of those AAD cases (40). Most AAD is unrelated to infection with *C. difficile* and may be due to osmotic diarrhea rather than infectious diarrhea. Osmotic diarrhea with antibiotic therapy occurs when antibiotics impair the ability of the intestinal microflora to break down unabsorbed carbohydrates (119). A small amount of dietary fiber and starch enters the colon intact, after passing through the small intestine without being digested. The microflora in the colon normally ferment the carbohydrates into short-chain fatty acids (SCFA) that are absorbed for fuel by colonic mucosa. With antibiotic therapy, bacterial fermentation of unabsorbed carbohydrates can change SCFA metabolism, resulting in osmotic diarrhea. Features that might help differentiate between osmotic (AAD) and infectious (*C. difficile*) diarrhea are as follows:

1. Approximately 50% of patients with *C. difficile* will have leukocytes in stool whereas those with osmotic diarrhea will have none
2. Fever and leukocytosis may be present in *C. difficile* infection but should be absent in osmotic diarrhea
3. Stopping oral intake will reduce stool frequency in osmotic diarrhea but will have no effect on *C. difficile* diarrhea (120).

Antibiotic-Associated Colitis

Antibiotic-associated colitis (AAC) includes patients taking antibiotics for six weeks or less, who experience diarrhea and who have colonic biopsy evidence of nonspecific inflammation without pseudomembranes. Patients experience a serious systemic illness with malaise, nausea, abdominal pain in right or left lower abdominal pain that is often relieved with defecation, anorexia, or rapid onset of mucous-containing or watery diarrhea, and may have 10 to 20 diarrheal episodes daily for over four weeks if untreated. Dehydration, low-grade fevers from 37°C to 38°C, and leukocytosis are commonly present (46). Erythema, friability, hyperemia, or frank hemorrhage can be seen endoscopically (47). The incidence of AAC ranges from 1 to 3/100,000 in outpatients to 1/100 to 1/1000 in inpatients (121). Stool cultures are positive for *C. difficile* or toxin in 65% to 70% of patients (118).

Pseudomembranous Colitis

This is the most severe form of *C. difficile* colitis. The prevalence ranges from 0.1% to 10.1% of inpatients who receive cephalosporins or penicillins (46). The incubation period can be as short as one to five days after antibiotic initiation, or up to one to five weeks after antibiotic completion. In PMC cases that receive no specific treatment, recovery usually occurs within seven days if antibiotics are stopped. If antibiotics are continued and diagnosis is delayed, PMC can last up to three weeks (3). Fulminant colitis and perforation have been associated with delayed diagnosis, with mortality up to 75% without treatment (5,18,122). Patients experience similar symptoms as with AAC, with 80% of PMC patients reporting watery diarrhea, abdominal cramps, leukocytosis, anorexia, and fevers (38–40°C). When performed, endoscopy usually shows pseudomembranes. In addition, upto 25% of PMC patients have hypoalbuminemia (46). Other complications include colonic perforations, toxic megacolon, severe fluid loss, and electrolyte imbalances. Nonspecific radiologic findings consistent with PMC include mucosal edema, thumbprinting, thickened colon, pancolitis, pericolonic inflammation with or without ascites, without involvement of small bowel (Fig. 3) (123).

Fulminant colitis occurs in 2% to 3% of patients and can lead to perforation, prolonged ileus, toxic megacolon, and death. Patients present with complaints of severe lower or diffuse abdominal pain and distention, diarrhea, high fever, chills, marked leukocytosis, and profuse diarrhea except in those patients with ileus and pooling of secretions in dilated, atonic colon. Metabolic acidosis is a sign of deterioration in status.

A severe complication of *C. difficile* colitis is toxic megacolon, which is a clinical diagnosis based upon massive dilatation of the colon plus fever and abdominal pain. Other X-ray findings include dilatation of the small intestine visible on plain abdominal radiographs, with air fluid levels that mimic intestinal obstruction or ischemia, and "thumb-printing" due to submucosal edema, or scalloping of the bowel wall due to edema or hemorrhage that occurs in intestinal ischemia, inflammation, or infection. This condition necessitates surgical intervention in 65% to 71% of cases, but still has high mortality rate of 35% (Fig. 4) (124).

Atypical Presentations

C. difficile can infect the small bowel (125) and in patients with prior proctocolectomy, ileitis with high ileostomy output has been described (126). Cellulitis, soft tissue infections and reactive arthritis, and osteomyelitis have all been described as well (125). While sterile arthritis can occur two to three weeks after onset of diarrhea caused by infection with *Shigella*,

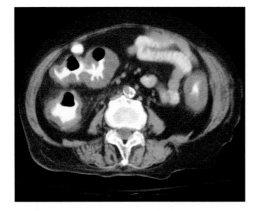

Figure 3 Abdominal computed tomography from a patient with *Clostridium difficile* colitis showing diffuse homogeneous transmural thickening of the colon from the rectum to the cecum. The wall measures up to 1 cm in maximal thickness. There is predominant fat stranding around the pericecal region and less fat stranding around the left periocolic gutter. *Source:* Courtesy of Dr. Ted Dubinsky, University of Washington, Seattle, Washington, U.S.A.

Salmonella, Yersinia, and *Campylobacter,* there have been 11 case reports of reactive oligoarthritis in patients after infection with *C. difficile.* After treatment with vancomycin for the *C. difficile,* the arthritis resolved (127). *C. difficile* cultured from pus, bone, and aspirated material has led to the association with osteomyelitis, with patient response to treatment with vancomycin (128,129). Pancreatic and splenic abscesses due to *C. difficile* infection have been reported in the absence of gastrointestinal disease. One case report documents primary infection of ascitic fluid with toxigenic *C. difficile,* without diarrhea, evidence of colitis, and growth of nontoxigenic *C. difficile* in stool, with successful treatment with two courses of metronidazole (130). *C. difficile* septicemia has been reported in fewer than 10 patients, with and without intestinal symptoms, with mortality rates as high as 83% (131). *C. difficile*-associated PMC may possibly activate or exacerbate hemolytic-uremic syndromes (HUS). Infection with typhoid, shigellosis, and verotoxin-producing *E. coli* can be complicated by HUS, which results in renal failure, microangiopathic hemolytic anemia, and thrombocytopenia. HUS has been infrequently associated with toxigenic *C. difficile.* Patients present with bloody diarrhea and rarely, pseudomembranes. Because most of the patients with *C. difficile*-associated HUS are children, *C. difficile* may play a causal role (132).

Protein-Losing Enteropathy

A subset of patients with indolent or subacute *C. difficile* infection develop hypoalbuminemia, ascites, and peripheral edema (133). These patients often relate a history of intermittent or low-grade diarrhea lasting one to four weeks, low-grade fever, abdominal pain, and anorexia.

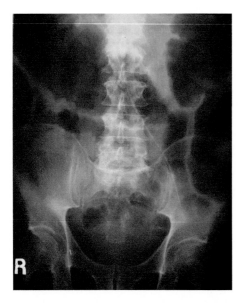

Figure 4 Abdominal X ray of a patient with *Clostridium difficile* colitis showing marked dilation of large bowel. *Source:* Courtesy of Dr. Ted Dubinsky, University of Washington, Seattle, Washington, U.S.A.

Pancolitis causes hypoalbuminemia as serum albumin leaks through damaged bowel wall, and that loss is not fully compensated for by increased hepatic synthesis, which results in rapid lowering of serum albumin to less than 2.0 g/dL. Protein-losing enteropathy has been associated with 12 of 12 patients with PMC, 6 of 14 (43%) with *C. difficile* diarrhea, and 50% of nursing home patients (133,134), in whom malnutrition should particularly be closely monitored and managed.

Possible Association with Inflammatory Bowel Disease

It was earlier thought that *C. difficile* could exacerbate inflammatory bowel disease (IBD), as some chronic IBD patients had *C. difficile* (135–137), but later studies of IBD patients who were not receiving antibiotics revealed no significant association with *C. difficile* (138). Infection with *C. difficile* may complicate the course of patients with IBD, by frequent prescription of antibiotics and hospitalizations, increasing the risk for acquiring *C. difficile* infection. Exacerbations of underlying IBD can mimic symptoms of *C. difficile* infection, including diarrhea, abdominal pain, and low-grade fever; so the diagnosis must be made promptly and the disease must be managed appropriately. Failure to diagnose *C. difficile* infection may lead to inappropriate treatment with corticosteroids or immunosuppressive therapy, and in one case report, resulted in death (139). Some patients develop *C. difficile* infection at the onset of the initial manifestation of IBD, which can lead to significant diagnostic confusion. Diarrhea from infection with *Shigella, Salmonella and Campylobacter* can also trigger an apparent flare of preexisting IBD or can trigger the initial attack of IBD (140).

Differential Diagnosis

The differential diagnosis of *C. difficile* diarrhea includes AAD, diarrhea caused by other enteric pathogens, diarrhea due to medications, ischemic colitis, IBD, and intra-abdominal sepsis (4).

Treatment
General Treatment Approaches
The treatment for CDAD should be determined by the severity of disease (55). No treatment is recommended for asymptomatic carriers, because most of these people will not progress to symptomatic disease (40,141). The first step in management is the discontinuation of the precipitating antibiotic (4,63). In one study of 20 patients with clindamycin-induced disease, published before the discovery of vancomycin as effective therapy, all patients recovered when clindamycin was discontinued (5). About 15% to 20% of cases of mild AAD will resolve in two to three days with nonspecific supportive measures such as oral or intravenous rehydration (44). Specific treatment against *C. difficile* incurs a risk of relapse following treatment completion (142). If discontinuation of the antibiotic is not feasible, then the regimen should be altered to agents that are less likely to exacerbate *C. difficile* diarrhea such as metronidazole, vancomycin, parenteral aminoglycoside, trimethoprim, rifampicin, or quinolones (63). Narcotic analgesics or antiperistaltic medications should be avoided because they may delay intestinal toxin clearance and perpetuate toxin-induced colonic damage or perpetuate ileus and toxic dilatation (143–146). Reducing diarrhea could theoretically lead to increased proximal absorption of metronidazole and cause failure of metronidazole treatment. Nearly all patients respond to oral metronidazole or vancomycin within two days of initiating specific therapy, even after relapses following specific treatment with the same drugs (44), with the mean time to resolution of diarrhea ranging from two to four days (147,148). However, patients with toxic megacolon or ileus may require treatment with oral agent and/or agents delivered by other routes (44). Patients should not be considered therapeutic failures until at least six days of treatment have been administered (55), and treatment is more likely to be successful if continued for 10 days (148). Testing for cure by sending cultures or toxin assays after treatment is not routinely recommended, because these do not accurately predict subsequent relapse (146).

Metronidazole and Vancomycin
Metronidazole (500 mg PO t.i.d.) (153) is the drug of choice for treatment of *C. difficile* disease. Vancomycin (125 mg PO q.i.d.) is a second-line agent, because while both drugs are equally effective in treating *C. difficile* infection (147), vancomycin usage can lead to the selection of vancomycin-resistant enterococci (154), and is far more expensive (121). At one northwest

tertiary care center each metronidazole 500 mg tablet costs $0.09, or $2.70 for 10-day course, compared to $203.60 for the same 10-day course with oral vancomycin.

Both drugs are highly active in vitro with an MIC_{90} of 0.4 for metronidazole and 1.6 µg/mL for vancomycin (148), with fecal drug concentrations of vancomycin, which is poorly absorbed, ranging from 2000 to 5000 µg/mL, which is several log_{10} higher than the MIC for *C. difficile* (155). There were some initial concerns about the therapeutic efficacy of metronidazole because it is well absorbed proximally, with fecal concentrations in healthy volunteers and *C. difficile* carriers being low or absent (156,157). However, bactericidal concentrations were found in all of the stool specimens from nine patients with CDAD, with metronidazole concentrations decreasing in feces as diarrhea improved, implying that either the drug is secreted directly through inflamed colonic mucosa or decreased transit time decreased drug absorption in diarrhea (158). Metronidazole is cytotoxic to facultative anaerobic bacteri and exerts its antimicrobial effects through the production of free radicals that are toxic to the microbe. Despite extensive worldwide use, acquired resistance to metronidazole among anaerobic bacteria is rare (159–161). There are occasional cases of *C. difficile* induced by metronidazole (36).

Metronidazole is well-proven effective treatment, with a clinical cure rate of 98% (148). In a randomized clinical trial comparing therapy of *C. difficile* diarrhea with either metronidazole or vancomycin, the only statistically significant difference between them was that vancomycin was more expensive. The duration of diarrhea, frequency of side effects, post-treatment relapse, and carriage of organism during recovery were not significantly different. Two of 42 patients (5%) treated with metronidazole and none of 52 patients treated with vancomycin failed to respond to therapy, which was not a statistically significant difference. Those two patients were cured when treatment was changed to vancomycin, leading some investigators to treat with vancomycin first in critically ill patients (4). Disadvantages of metronidazole are the adverse reactions associated with its use. In one institution, over a 10-year period, more than 600 patients received metronidazole for treatment of *C. difficile* diarrhea and only 1% experienced side effects (44). Adverse effects include nausea and vomiting, an unpleasant metallic taste, peripheral neuropathy with prolonged use, and a disulfiram-like reaction with alcohol. Metronidazole may potentiate the anticoagulant effects of warfarin, which can lead to prolonged prothrombin time. The use of metronidazole in pregnant and nursing women is somewhat controversial because it crosses the placenta and rapidly enters the fetal circulation. As a pregnancy category B drug, there are no adequate well-controlled studies showing safety in pregnant women and it should be avoided during the first trimester. Metronidazole has not been approved by the Food and Drug Administration specifically for the treatment of *C. difficile* diarrhea, but has been approved for the treatment of serious infections caused by susceptible anaerobic bacteria such as *C. difficile* (4). Oral doses of metronidazole are preferred but in patients who are severely ill and unable to take oral medications, intravenous metronidazole may be used although bactericidal concentrations may be decreased.

Vancomycin has been used successfully in the treatment of *C. difficile* colitis since 1978 (162). As the first agent shown to be effective for CDAD, it is the drug against which all subsequent therapies have been compared. When given orally, it is neither absorbed nor metabolized, excreted virtually unchanged in feces in high concentrations, making its pharmacokinetics ideal for the treatment of *C. difficile* diarrhea. Vancomycin may be administered by mouth, nasogastric tube, or enema (4,44) but should not be given intravenously because effective colonic concentrations in the lumen cannot be attained by this route (163,164). All patients treated with vancomycin 500 mg q.i.d. for 10 days in comparative trials have had resolution of diarrhea (147,165–168). This response rate decreased to 75% with lowering of dose from 500 mg q.i.d. to 125 mg q.i.d. and treatment for five days, but when treated at the lower dose for the full 10 days, all patients responded, with 15% relapse rate of patients treated (169). Within 72 hours of starting therapy, there was symptomatic improvement, and by the end of the 10-day treatment course, there was complete resolution of diarrhea and colitis in 96% of patients overall. An observational study at one institution of 122 patients treated with vancomycin revealed 99% response rate, 1% drug intolerance rate, and 10% relapse rate (Table 3) (44).

Vancomycin inhibits bacterial cell wall synthesis by blocking glycopeptide polymerization through tight binding with a portion of the cell wall precursor. Systemic side effects are rare, and adverse reactions with oral vancomycin include nausea, vomiting in 1 to 10%, and a bitter taste. It is a pregnancy category C drug. Despite its remarkable clinical efficacy,

Table 3 Antibiotic Therapy for *Clostridium difficile* Disease

Antibiotics	Dose	Cost for 10-day course	Patients studied	Cure	Relapse	Mean days to resolution	Reference
Metronidazole	250 mg q.i.d.	$2.70	42	40 (95%)	2 (5%)	2.4	(149)
Vancomycin	500 mg q.i.d.	$203.60	87	87 (100%)	13 (15%)	2.6–3.6	(149–151)
	125 mg q.i.d. 7 day		21	18 (86%)	6 (29%)	4.2	(152)
	125 mg q.i.d. 5 day		12	9 (75%)	?	<5	(124)
Bacitracin	25,000 units q.i.d.	$150	36	28 (78%)	10 (28%)	2.5–4.1	(151,152)
Teicoplanin	100 mg b.i.d.	N/A in United States	26	25 (96%)		3.4	(150)
Fusidic acid	0.5–1.5 g/day	N/A in United States					

Abbreviation: N/A, not available.
Source: From Refs. 55 and 153.

vancomycin is a currently considered a second-line agent for the treatment of *C. difficile*. As stated earlier, while it is as clinically effective as metronidazole, it may encourage the spread of vancomycin resistance among nosocomial bacteria, and it is expensive, with a 10-day course costing a hundred times more than metronidazole. The conditions under which oral vancomycin therapy should be initiated include (i) patient failure to respond to metronidazole, (ii) organism resistance to metronidazole, (iii) patient inability to tolerate metronidazole, allergy to metronidazole, concurrent treatment with ethanol-containing solution, (iv) patient is pregnant or a child under 10 years old, (v) critically ill patient with *C. difficile* diarrhea or colitis, and (vi) evidence that diarrhea is caused by *S. aureus* (4).

OTHER THERAPIES

Bacitracin (25,000 units q.i.d. for 7–10 days) has been studied in clinical trials for the treatment of *C. difficile* diarrhea, with overall response rate about 80%, relapse rate greater than 30%, and slower clinical response than vancomycin, possibly due to bacitracin resistance (4); overall it is less effective than metronidazole or vancomycin (148,149,166,167,170). Teicoplanin (100 mg b.i.d. for 10 days) was shown to be as effective as vancomycin for the treatment of *C. difficile* diarrhea, with a lower relapse rate of 7% (165,171). However, teicoplanin is expensive, has a propensity similar to that of vancomycin for encouraging the spread of vancomycin-resistant enterococci (4), and like bacitracin, is not readily available in oral formulation in the United States. Fusidic acid has been tested in a limited number of patients and has been found to be less effective than metronidazole or vancomycin, with a relapse rate of about 28% (171,172). Anion-binding resins such as cholestyramine or colestipol bind toxins A and B of *C. difficile*, but with limited and probably inadequate capacity in severe cases, and resultant low response rates (36%) (168). The resins may also bind vancomycin, diminishing its efficacy, and may cause severe constipation and intestinal obstruction with resolution of diarrhea. They are not recommended as primary therapy for *C. difficile* diarrhea (4,55). Because the disruption of normal colonic bowel flora leads to *C. difficile* disease, fecal enemas have been attempted as treatment (173), with marginal efficacy and low patient acceptance, as well as incurring the risk of transferring unapparent pathogens from donor to recipient (3).

SEVERE PSEUDOMEMBRANOUS COLITIS

Severe PMC occurs in 3% to 5% of patients with CDAD, with mortality rates as high as 65% (29,174,175). Many of the patients who develop severe PMC are often critically ill, with preexisting and substantial comorbidities (175,176). As with management of mild to moderate cases of *C. difficile* diarrhea, the first step is discontinuation of the inciting antibiotic if possible, followed by treatment with metronidazole or vancomycin. In the critically ill patient, vancomycin is recommended as first-line therapy (4), based on clinical observations that patients have responded more rapidly to vancomycin. Patients who cannot tolerate oral medications can be treated with intravenous metronidazole. In one series, six of eight patients with severe ileus were treated successfully with simultaneous intravenous metronidazole, vancomycin via nasogastric tube with intermittent clamping, and vancomycin retention enemas (500 mg every six hours) (44). Passive immunization with immunoglobulin products may be effective treatment for patients with severe PMC, who have low serum and fecal concentrations of antibody against *C. difficile* toxins (177–181). A few patients have been successfully treated with intravenous infusion of normal pooled human immunoglobulins, which increases serum IgG antitoxin levels (150,179). A vaccine has been developed and tested in human subjects based on formalin-inactivated *C. difficile* toxins (151,182). The *C. difficile* toxoid vaccine may be used to stimulate antitoxin antibody responses in healthy volunteers, producing a hyper-immune intravenous immunoglobulin against *C. difficile*, which can be used to treat patients with severe PMC (10).

Surgery

Patients with toxic megacolon, who have failed medical therapy and have impending or established bowel perforation, are candidates for surgical intervention (124,152), which in this setting is associated with a high mortality rate (32–50%) (124,152,183). In one hospital setting, 0.39% of patients with CDAD required surgical intervention, but among critically ill patients in an intensive care unit, 20.3% of patients with *C. difficile* colitis required surgical intervention. The operation of choice is subtotal colectomy and ileostomy (123,124,152). A literature review between 1976 and 1994 revealed that subtotal colectomy and ileostomy was associated with a failure rate of 24%, compared with nontherapeutic laparotomy, diverting stomas, and segmental resection, associated with failure rates of 77%, 75%, and 40%, respectively (184). One published nonrandomized experience reported a lower mortality rate (14%) for subtotal colectomy compared with left hemicolectomy (100%) (183). A recent review of 2334 patients with *C. difficile* colitis in one tertiary care center showed an increased incidence from 1998 to 2000, and an increase in the number of severe cases. Forty-four patients required a colectomy, with an overall death rate of 57%. Predisposing factors for *C. difficile* colitis were a recent surgical procedure and immunosuppression (185). Mortality after colectomy was associated with preoperative vasopressor requirements and age. These high mortality rates make the decision to operate difficult and reflect the severity of illness in this patient population.

RECURRENT *CLOSTRIDIUM DIFFICILE*

Despite initial treatment success, 15% to 20% of patients have recurrence of diarrhea in association with a positive stool test for *C. difficile* toxin (4,63). Recurrent symptoms appear most often within one to two weeks of discontinuing therapy, but can appear as late as one to two months. Symptomatic recurrence is rarely due to treatment failure or antimicrobial resistance to metronidazole or vancomycin, but presumably results from germination of *C. difficile* spores persisting in the colon despite treatment (186). One possible mechanism is the survival of spores in diverticula where they escape the normal cleansing action of diarrhea and avoid exposure to the high luminal concentrations of antibiotics. In addition, spores may be resistant to antibiotics. Colonic diverticula were present in 18 of 22 patients with relapse in one report (186). The mechanism of diarrhea relapse following therapy may be different for metronidazole and vancomycin. Because fecal concentrations of metronidazole decrease with resolution of diarrhea (187), remaining *C. difficile* spores in the colon can continue to germinate. Unlike metronidazole, vancomycin exerts a bacteriostatic effect on *C. difficile* at high concentrations achieved during therapy; so a large portion of organisms may remain viable during therapy (188). Recurrence results in most cases from reinfection with the same or different strain of *C. difficile* from the environment (189–191). One study using DNA fingerprinting showed that 56% of clinical recurrences were due to infection with a different strain of *C. difficile*, indicating the important role of impaired colonization resistance (191).

Approaches to management include conservative therapy, treatment with specific antibiotics against *C. difficile*, and probiotic therapy. The treatment of a first relapse does not differ from treatment of the initial episode (Table 4) (4). Diagnosis should be confirmed prior to reinstituting therapy. Patients with mild symptoms can be managed without antibiotic therapy, but if symptoms persist or are severe, a second 10- to 14-day course of metronidazole or vancomycin can be started. Most patients will respond again to the same specific therapy, and 92% will not experience further recurrences (44). Patients with a history of recurrence

Table 4 Practice Guidelines for Management of Relapses

Reconfirm the diagnosis

Discontinue medications that may be contributing to the diarrhea and treat the patient with nonspecific supportive therapy

If specific therapy is needed, treat the patient with a standard course of metronidazole given orally for 10 days or with vancomycin

When possible, avoid treating (minor) infections with antibiotics for the next two months after the treatment of a relapse

No treatment available in the United States has been proven to prevent recurrences. If the patient has suffered from multiple recurrences, consider using one of the following microbial regimens with or without one of the other therapeutic measures as an adjunct. (Not presented in order of preference)

Oral metronidazole (or vancomycin)

Specific therapy with vancomycin or metronidazole given orally for one to two months, either intermittently (such as every other day or week) or with gradual tapering

Oral vancomycin plus rifampin

Oral yogurt, *Lactobacillus* preparations, or *Lactobacillus* GG

Saccharomyces boulardii (500 mg orally b.i.d.), if available, may be given for one month, if the patient is not immunocompromised, beginning four days before a 10-day course of specific antibiotic therapy has been completed

Human immune globulin by intravenous infusion, for patients with documented deficiencies

Source: From Ref. 4.

have a higher risk of further episodes of *C. difficile* diarrhea after therapy is discontinued (192,193). Patients with at least one previous relapse had a subsequent relapse rate of 65% after standard therapy, without evidence to suggest that sequential episodes become progressively more severe or complicated.

Multiple recurrences of *C. difficile* diarrhea have been treated with a variety of treatment regimens. Confirmation of the diagnosis should always be the initial step. One approach is to give a prolonged course of vancomycin (or metronidazole) using a decreasing dosage schedule followed by pulse therapy. The rationale behind this is that pulse therapy allows *C. difficile* spores to vegetate on the off days and then be killed when the antibiotics are taken again. One report describes 22 patients with multiple relapses of *C. difficile* colitis, who were treated with pulse regimen of vancomycin with complete resolution of symptoms, with no relapses during the mean follow-up period of six months (186). A combination of vancomycin (125 mg PO q.i.d.) and rifampin (600 mg b.i.d. for seven days) was used successfully in a small, uncontrolled study of seven patients with relapsing disease (194), but there is no evidence that this combination of antibiotics has any unique activity against *C. difficile*. A recent study of 163 patients with recurrent *C. difficile* disease treated in the placebo arm of a study showed that pulsed and/or tapering vancomycin was more effective in preventing further recurrences than standard therapy (195).

An additional approach to multiple relapses of *C. difficile* diarrhea is to reconstitute the colonic flora with microorganisms. In one study, six patients with relapsing *C. difficile* colitis were treated with fresh feces enemas from a healthy relative or rectal infusions of a mixture of 10 different anaerobic and aerobic bacteria. The patients treated with the bacterial mix had *C. difficile* toxin lost from stools and bowel colonization by *Bacteroides* species, which had been absent from initial pretreatment stool samples and thus was thought to be one of the organisms that normally protects against pathogenic colonization with *C. difficile* (196). Uncontrolled trials suggest that oral administration of the probiotic *Lactobacillus* strain GG may also be beneficial (197). A more widely studied alternative is the administration of *Saccharomyces boulardii*, a nonpathogenic yeast used widely in Europe to prevent AAD (198). Animal studies suggest that *S. boulardii* also has therapeutic value by protecting against *C. difficile* toxin–induced colitis (199,200). A randomized, double-blinded, placebo-controlled trial involving 124 patients with *C. difficile* diarrhea looked at the efficacy of *S. boulardii* (500 mg b.i.d. for four weeks) in combination with metronidazole or vancomycin. *S. boulardii* significantly reduced recurrences compared with placebo in patients with multiple episodes (recurrence rate 35% vs. 65%), but not in those with an initial episode (recurrence rate 19% vs. 24%) (193). A later controlled trial confirmed the efficacy of *S. boulardii* in preventing further recurrences when combined with high-dose vancomycin (2 gm/day) but not low-dose vancomycin or metronidazole (201). The possible mechanisms for the action of *S. boulardii* on *C. difficile* infection include proteolysis of toxin A and its intestinal receptor by a yeast protease (200,202), a direct inhibition of *C. difficile* growth (199,203), and stimulation of intestinal disaccharidase activity possibly through *S. boulardii* release of polyamines (204,205).

Table 5 Practice Guidelines for Prevention of *Clostridium difficile* Diarrhea

1. Limit the use of antimicrobial drugs
2. Wash hands between contact with all patients
3. Use enteric (stool) isolation precautions for patients with *C. difficile* diarrhea
4. Wear gloves when contacting patients with *C. difficile* diarrhea/colitis or their environment
5. Disinfect objects contaminated with *C. difficile* with sodium hypochlorite, alkaline glutaraldehyde, or ethylene oxide
6. Educate the medical, nursing, and other appropriate staff members about the disease and its epidemiology

Source: From Ref. 4.

PREVENTION

C. difficile is a gastrointestinal tract pathogen that almost exclusively causes disease in the presence of antibiotic exposure. Despite the considerable knowledge that has resulted from the past three decades of scientific investigation, CDAD persists, and despite the best efforts at control and prevention, it is likely increasing in frequency (49,206,207). Incidence rates of nosocomial infection range from 0.1 to 30 per 1000 patients in nonepidemic settings (44,114,208–210), while in community settings, the prevalence ranges from 8 to 12 per 100,000 person-years (45,211). While it may be difficult to avoid antimicrobial therapy in order to decrease incidence of CDAD, the American College of Gastroenterology has published practice guidelines that are pragmatic and simple to implement (Table 5) (4). The most effective control measure directed at reduction in symptomatic *C. difficile* disease has been antimicrobial restriction. Clindamycin restriction first by voluntary educational modes, then by mandatory infectious disease approval restriction, resulted in a decline in CDAD rates from 22.5/1000 discharges to 7.4/1000 over 12 months, paralleling the decline in clindamycin usage (Table 6) (38,212). During the same time period, there were declines in the use of ampicillin, cephalosporin, and aminoglycosides. Early institution of enteric precautions and early empiric treatment of suspected CDAD were instituted as additional control measures. Effective restriction of clindamycin during a year-long hospital outbreak of CDAD resulted in a significant decrease in new cases of disease within three months (219). Other recommendations include handwashing with disinfectant soaps or chlorhexidine between contact with patients, wearing gloves when contacting patients with *C. difficile* diarrhea, and using enteric isolation precautions (4,55). A prospective controlled trial of vinyl glove use for handling body substances provides indirect evidence for the importance of personnel hand carriage of *C. difficile*; there was a significant decline in CDAD rates from 7.7 cases/1000 discharges before glove use to 1.5/1000 after glove use institution (48). Instruments and contaminated surfaces in rooms of patients with *C. difficile* diarrhea should be disinfected with sodium hypochlorite, alkaline glutaraldehyde, or ethylene oxide (4), because they are effective for killing the spores as well as the vegetative forms of *C. difficile* that persist on surfaces (40,41,220). The Society for Healthcare Epidemiology of America guidelines recommend that if rates of *C. difficile* diarrhea are high, electronic thermometers should be replaced with disposable thermometers, because this has been associated with a decreased incidence of *C. difficile* diarrhea (55,60,221).

Table 6 Intervention for the Control of Nosocomial Outbreaks of *Clostridium difficile*-Associated Disease

Patient population	Type of intervention	Frequency of positive cultures		Reference
		Before	**After**	
Environmental sites	Hypochlorite (500 ppm)	31%	16%	(213)
Adult inpatients	Education, vinyl glove	7.7/1000	1.5/1000	(35)
Environmental site	Environmental decontamination, handwashing, disposable equipment	21/150	0	(214)
Hospital staff	Bactericidal handwashing soap	88%	14%	(13)
Elderly patients	Increase infection control practice	13%	6.3%	(215)
Surgery patients	Enteric precautions, surveillance, terminal room, disinfection, cohorting, early treatment	1.5/1000	0.3/1000	(216)
Four wards	Infection control education	15/mo	5/mo	(217)
Inpatients	Single use disposable thermometers	2.7/1000	1.8/1000	(55)
Veterans hospital	Clindamycin restriction	7.7/mo	1.9/mo	(218)

Source: From Ref. 212.

The future of *C. difficile* disease research will be targeted toward effective treatment measures to control the disease, including passive and active immunization. There have been multiple approaches presented for the management of recurrent *C. difficile* diarrhea, but as yet there are no standard practice guidelines or treatment regimens supported by data. The pathophysiology, diagnosis, and treatment of AAD that is not due to *C. difficile* have yet to be fully explored and addressed. Improved standards of living have prolonged life in developed countries, and the growing elderly population is particularly vulnerable to endemic infection with and to outbreaks of *C. difficile*. Antibiotic resistance of *C. difficile* to metronidazole or vancomycin is rare but could be especially disastrous in this population. There has been tremendous progress in understanding this "difficult bacteria" since its first appearance in the stool of healthy newborns in the early 1900s. Continued advances in molecular biology, immunology, and epidemiology will further elucidate means to limit this pathogen and its ability to cause disease in adults.

ACKNOWLEDGMENT

The authors are grateful to Susan Sperline for expert manuscript preparation.

REFERENCES

1. Finney JM. Gast-enterostomy for cicatrizing ulcer of the pylorus. Johns Hopkins Bull 1893; 11:53–55.
2. Hall IC, O'Toole E. Intestinal flora in newborn infants with a description of a new pathogenic anaerobe *Bacillus difficilis*. Am J Dis Child 1935; 49:390.
3. McFarland LV. *Clostridium difficile*-associated disease. In: Surawicz CM, Owens RL, eds. Gastrointestinal and Hepatic Infections. Philadelphia: WB Saunders, 1995:153–175.
4. Fekety RF. Guidelines for the diagnosis and management of *Clostridium difficile*–associated diarrhea and colitis. Am J Gastroenterol 1997; 92:739–750.
5. Tedesco FJ, Barton RW, Alpers DH. Clindamycin–associated colitis. Ann Intern Med 1974; 81: 429–433.
6. Hafiz S. *Clostridium difficile* and its Toxins. Ph.D dissertation, University of Leeds, Leeds, UK, 1974.
7. Green RH. The association of viral activation with penicillin toxicity in guinea pigs and hamsters. Yale J Biol Med 1974; 47:166–181.
8. Bartlett JG, Chang TW, Gurwith M, et al. Antibiotic-associated pseudomembranous colitis due to toxin-producing clostridia. N Engl J Med 1978; 298:531–534.
9. Larson HE, Parry JV, Price AB, et al. Undescribed toxin in pseudomembranous colitis. Br Med J 1977; 1:1246–1248.
10. Kyne L, Farrell RJ, Kelly CP. *Clostridium difficile*. Gastroenterol Clin N Am 2001; 30:3.
11. Rolfe RD, Helebian S, Finegold SM. Bacterial interference between *Clostridium difficile* and normal fecal flora. J Infect Dis 1981; 143:470–475.
12. Onderdonk AB, Cisneros RL, Bartlett JG. *Clostridium difficile* in gnotobiotic mice. Infect Immun 1980; 28:277–282.
13. Wilson KH, Freter R. Interaction of *Clostridium difficile* and *Escherichia coli* with microflora in continuous–flow cultures and gnotobiotic mice. Infect Immun 1986; 54:354–358.
14. Wilson KH, Silva J, Fekety FR. Suppression of *Clostridium difficile* by normal hamster cecal flora and prevention of antibiotic-associated cecitis. Infect Immun 1981; 34:626–628.
15. Borriello SP, Barclay FE. An in-vitro model of colonization resistance to *Clostridium difficile* infection. J Med Microbiol 1986; 21:299–309.
16. Wilson KH, Perini F. Role of competition for nutrients in suppression of *Clostridium difficile* by the colonic microflora. Infect Immun 1988; 56:2610–2614.
17. Savage AM, Alford RH. Nosocomial spread of *C. difficile*. Infect Control 1983; 4:31–33.
18. Mogg GAG, Keighley MRB, Burdon DW, et al. Antibiotic-associated colitis: a review of 66 cases. Br J Surg. 1979; 66:738–742.
19. von-Eichel-Streiber C, Laufenberg-Feldmann R, Sartingen S, et al. Cloning of *Clostridium difficile* toxin B gene and demonstration of high N-terminal homology *between* toxin A and toxin B. Med Microbiol Immunol 1990; 179:271–279.
20. Sears CL, Kaper JB. Enteric bacterial toxins: mechanisms of action and linkage to intestinal secretion. Microbiol Rev 1996; 60:167.
21. Pothoulakis C. Pathogenesis of *Clostridium difficile*–associated diarrhea. Eur J Gastroenterol Hepatol 8:1041–1047.
22. Sullivan NM, Pellett S, Wilkins TD. Purification and characterization of toxins A and B of *Clostridium difficile*. Infect Immun 1982; 35:1032–1040.
23. Triadafilopoulos G, Pothoulakis C, O'Brien MJ, et al. Differential effects of *Clostridium difficile* toxins A and B on rabbit ileum. Gastroenterology 1987; 93:273–279.

24. Lyerly DM, Saum KE, MacDonald DK, et al. Effects of *Clostridium difficile* toxins given intragastrically to animals. Infect Immun 1985; 47:349–352.

25. Mitchell TJ, Ketley JM, Haslam SC, et al: Effect of toxin A and B of *Clostridium difficile* on rabbit ileum and colon. Gut 1986; 27:78–85.

26. Pothoulakis C, Barone LM, Ely R, et al. Purification and properties of *Clostridium difficile* cytotoxin B. J Biol Chem , 19; 261:1316–1386.

27. Riegler M, Sedivy R, Pothoulakis C, et al. *Clostridium difficile* toxin B is more potent than toxin A in damaging human colonic epithelium in vitro. J Clin Invest 1995; 95:2004–2011.

28. Brazier JS. The epidemiology and typing of *Clostridium difficile*. J Antimicrob Chemother 1998; 41(suppl C):47–57.

29. Kato H, Kato N, Katow S, et al. Deletions in the repeating sequences of the toxin A gene of toxin A-negative, toxin B-positive *Clostridium difficile* strains. FEMS Microbiol Lett 1999; 175:197–203.

30. Kato H, Kato N, Watanabe K, et al. Identification of toxin A-negative, toxin B-positive *Clostridium difficile* by PCR. J Clin Microbiol 1998; 36:2178–2182.

31. Limaye AP, Turgeon DK, Cookson BT, et al. Pseudomembranous colitis caused by toxin A(–) B (+) strain of *Clostridium difficile*. J Clin Microbiol 2000; 38:1696–1697.

32. Lyerly DM, Barroso LA, Wilkins TD, et al. Characterization of a toxin A-negative, toxin B-positive strain of *Clostridium difficile*. Infect Immun 1992; 60:4633–4639.

33. LaMont JT. Recent advances in the structure and function of *Clostridium difficile* toxins. In: Rambaud JC, LaMont JT, eds. Updates on *Clostridium difficile*. Paris: Springer-Verlag, 1996:73–82.

34. Kyne L, Warny M, Qamar A, Kelly CP. Asymptomatic carriage of *Clostridium difficile* and serum levels of IgG antibody against toxin A. N Engl J Med 2000; 342:390.

35. Hecht JR, Olinger EJ. *Clostridium difficile* colitis secondary to intravenous vancomycin. Dig Dis Sci 1989; 34:148–149.

36. Saginur R, Hawley CR, Bartlett JG. Colitis associated with metronidazole therapy. J Infect Dis 1980; 141:772–774.

37. Bignardi GE. Risk factors for *Clostridium difficile* infection. J Hosp Infect 1998; 40:1–15.

38. Brown B, Talbot GH, Axelrod R, et al. Risk Factors for *Clostridium difficile* toxin–associated diarrhea. Infect Control Hosp Epidemiol 1990; 11:283–290.

39. McFarland LV, Surawicz CM, Stamm WE. Risk factors for *Clostridium difficile* carriage and *c. difficile*-associated diarrhea in a cohort of hospitalized patients. J Infect Dis 1990; 162:678–684.

40. McFarland LV, Mulligan ME, Kwok RY, Stamm WE. Nosocomial acquisition of *Clostridium difficile* infection. N Engl J Med 1989; 320:204–210.

41. Kim KH, Fekety R, Batts DH, et al. Isolation of *c. difficile* from the environment and contacts of patients with antibiotic-induced colitis. J Infect Dis 1981; 143:42–44.

42. Wren B, Clayton C, Tabaqchali S. Rapid identification of toxigenic *Clostridium difficile* by polymerase chain reaction. Lancet 1990; 335:423.

43. Kofsky P, Rosen L, Reed J, et al. (1991) *Clostridium difficile*—a common and costly colitis. Dis Colon Rectum 34:244–248.

44. Olson MM, Shanholtzer CJ, Lee JT, Gerding DN. Ten years of prospective *Clostridium difficile*-associated disease surveillance and treatment at the Minneapolis VA medical center, 1982–1991. Infect Control Hosp Epdemiol 1994; 15:371–381.

45. Hirschorn LR, Trnka Y, Onderdonk A, et al. Epidemiology of community-acquired *Clostridium difficile*-associated diarrhea. J Infect Dis 1994; 169:127–133.

46. Bartlett JG. *Clostridium difficile*. Clinical considerations. Rev Infect Dis 1990; 12:S243–S251.

47. Trnka YM, LaMont JT. *Clostridium difficile* colitis. Adv Intern Med 1984; 29:85–107.

48. Johnson S, Gerding DN, Olson MM, et al. Prospective, controlled study of vinyl glove use to interrupt *Clostridium difficile* nosocomial transmission. Am J Med 1990; 88:137–140.

49. George RH. The carrier state: *Clostridium difficile*. J Antimicrob Chemother 1986; 18:47–58.

50. Siegel DL, Edelstein PH, Nachamkin I. Inappropriate testing for diarrheal diseases in the hospital. JAMA 1990; 263:979–982.

51. Yannelli B, Gurevich I, Schoch PE, et al. Yield of stool cultures, ova and parasite tests, and *Clostridium difficile* determinations in nosocomial diarrhea. Am J Infect Control 1988; 16:246–249.

52. Yablon SA, Krotenberg R, Fruhmann K. *Clostridium difficile*-related disease: evaluation prevalence among inpatients with diarrhea in two freestanding rehabilitation hospitals. Arch Phys Med Rehabil 1993; 74:913.

53. Kim K, Dupont HL, Pichering LK. Outbreaks of diarrhea associated with *c. difficile* and its toxin in daycare centers: evidence of person-to-person spread. J Pediatr 1983; 102:376–382.

54. Clabots CR, Johnson S, Olson MM, Peterson LR, Gerding DN. Acquisition of *Clostridium difficile* by hospitalized patients: evidence for colonized new admissions as a source of infection. J Infect Dis 1992; 166:561–567.

55. Gerding DN, Johnson S, Peterson LR, et al. *Clostridium difficile*-associated diarrhea and colitis. Infect Control Hosp Epidemiol 1995; 16:459–477.

56. Samore MH, Venkataraman L, DeGirolami PC, et al. Clinical and molecular epidemiology of sporadic and clustered cases of nosocomial *Clostridium difficile* diarrhea. Am J Med 1996; 100:32.

57. Fekety R, Kim KH, Brown D, et al. Epidemiology of AAC: isolation of *c. difficile* from the hospital environment. Am J Med 1981; 70:906–908.

58. Larson HE, Barclay FE, Honour P, et al. Epidemiology of *Clostridium difficile* in infants. J Infect Dis 1982; 146:727.
59. Shanholtzer CJ, Willard KE, Holter JJ, et al. Comparison of VIDAS C difficile toxin A immunoassay (CDA) with C difficile culture, cytotoxin, and latex test. J Clin Microbiol 1992; 30:1837–1840.
60. Brooks SE, Veal RO, Kramer M, Dore L, Schupf N, Adachi M. Reduction in the incidence of *Clostridium difficile*-associated diarrhea in an acute care hospital and a skilled nursing facility following replacement of electronic thermometers with single-use disposables. Infect Control Hosp Epidemiol 1992; 13:98–103.
61. Katz GW, Gitlin SD, Schaberg DR, et al. Acquisition of *Clostridium difficile* from the hospital environment. Am J Epidemiol 1988; 127:1289–1294.
62. Kelly CP, LaMont JT. *Clostridium difficile* infection. Ann Rev Med 1998; 49:375–390.
63. Kelly CP, Pothoulakis C, LaMont JT. *Clostridium difficile* colitis. N Engl J Med 1994; 330:257–262.
64. Eglow R, Pothoulakis C, Itzkowitz S, et al. Diminished *Clostridium difficile* toxin A sensitivity in newborn rabbit ileum is associated with decreased toxin A receptor. J Clin Invest 90:822–829, 1992.
65. Viscidi, R, Laughon, BE, Yolken R, et al. Serum antibody response to toxins A and B of *Clostridium difficile*. J Infect Dis 1983; 148:93.
66. Kelly CP, Pothoulakis C, Orellana J, et al. Human colonic aspirates containing immunoglobulin a antibody to *Clostridium difficile* toxin A inhibit toxin A receptor binding. Gastroenterology 1992; 102:35.
67. Karlstrom O, Fryklund B, Tullus K, Burman LG. A prospective nationwide study of *Clostridium difficile*–associated diarrhea in Sweden. Clin Infect Dis 1998; 26:141–145.
68. Nash JQ, Chattopadhyay B, Honeycombe J, et al. *C. difficile* and cytotoxin in routine faecal specimens. J Clin Pathol 1982; 35:561–565.
69. Aronsson B, Mollby R, Nord CE. Antimicrobial agents and *Clostridium difficile* in acute enteric disease: epidemiologic data from Sweden, 1980–82. J Infect Dis 1985; 151:476–481.
70. Cudmore MA, Silva J, Fekety R, et al. *C. difficile* colitis associated with cancer chemotherapy. Arch Intern Med 1982; 142:333–335.
71. Pierce PF, Wilson R, Silva J, et al. AAPMC: an epidemiologic investigation of a cluster of cases. J Infect Dis 1982; 145:269–274.
72. Morris G, Jarvis WR, Nunez-Montiel OL, et al. *C. difficile* colonization and toxin production in a cohort of patients with malignant hematologic disorders. Arch Intern Med 1984; 144:967–969.
73. Tichota-Lee J, Jaqua-Stewart MJ, Benfield D, et al. Effect of age on the sensitivity of cell cultures to *Clostridium difficile* toxin. Diag Microbiol Infect Dis 1987; 8:203–214.
74. Bowman RA, Riley TV. Laboratory diagnosis of *Clostridium difficile*-associated diarrhoea. Eur J Microbiol Infect Dis 1988; 7:476–484.
75. Chang TW, Laverman M, Bartlett JG. Cytotoxicity assay in antibiotic–associated colitis. J Infect Dis 1979; 140:765.
76. George WL, Sutter VL, Citron D, et al. Selective and differential medium for isolation of *Clostridium difficile*. J Clin Microbiol 1979; 9:217–219.
77. McFarland LV, Stamm WE. Review of *Clostridium difficile*-associated diseases. Am J Infect Control 1986; 14:99–109.
78. Burdon DW. *Clostridium difficile*: the epidemiology and prevention of hospital-acquired infection. Infection 1982; 10:203–204.
79. Sell TL, Schaberg DR, Fekety FR. Bacteriophage and bacteriocin typing scheme for *Clostridium difficile*. J Clin Microbiol 1983; 17:1147–1152.
80. Dei R. Observations on phage-typing of *Clostridium difficile*: preliminary evaluation of a phage panel. Eur J Epidemiol 1989; 5:351–354.
81. Tabaqchali S, Holland D, O'Farrell S, Silman R. Typing scheme for *Clostridium difficile*. Its application in clinical and epidemiological studies. Lancet 1984; 1:935–938.
82. Poxton IR, Aronsson B, Molby R, Nord CE, Collee JG. Immunochemical fingerprinting of *Clostridium difficile* strains isolated from an outbreak of antibiotic-associated colitis and diarrhea. J Med Microbiol 1984; 17:317–324.
83. Mulligan ME, Peterson LR, Kwok RY, Clabots CR, Gerding DN. Immunoblots and plasmid fingerprints compared with serotyping and polyacrylamide gel electrophoresis for typing *Clostridium difficile*. J Clin Microbiol 1988; 26:41–46.
84. Kato H, Cavallaro JJ, Kato N, et al. Typing of *Clostridium difficile* by western immunoblotting with 10 different antisera. J Clin Microbiol 1993; 31:413–415.
85. Nolan NPM, Kelly CP, Humphreys JFH, et al. An epidemic of pseudomembranous colitis: importance of person-to-person spread. Gut 1987; 28:1467–1473.
86. Clabots CR, Peterson LH, Gerding DN. Characterization of a nosocomial *Clostridium difficile* outbreak by using plasmid profile typing and clindamycin susceptibility testing. J Infect Dis 1988; 158:731–736.
87. Banno Y, Kobayashi T, Kono H, et al. Biochemical characterization and biologic actions of two toxins (D-1 and D-2) from *Clostridium difficile*. Rev Infect Dis 1984; 6:S11–S21.
88. Kamiya S, Nakamura S, Yamakawa K, et al. Evaluation of a commercially available latex immunoagglutination test kit for detection of *Clostridium difficile* D-1 toxin. Microbiol Immunol 1986; 30:177–181.

89. Lyerly DM, Wilkins TD. Commercial latex test for *Clostridium difficile* toxin A does not detect toxin A. J Clin Microbiol 1986; 23:622–623.

90. Lyerly DM, Barroso LA, Wilkins T. Identification of the latex test-reactive protein of *Clostridium difficile* as glutamate dehydrogenase. J Clin Microbiol 1991; 29:2639–2642.

91. Lyerly DM, Ball Dw, Toth J, Wilkins TD. Characterization of cross-reactive proteins detected by culturette brand rapid latex test for *Clostridium difficile*. J Clin Microbiol 1988; 26:397–400.

92. Qadri SM, Akhter J, Ostrawski S, et al. High incidence of false positives by a latex agglutination test for the diagnosis of *Clostridium difficile*-associated colitis in compromised patients. Diagn Microbiol Infect Dis 1989; 12:291–294.

93. Peterson LR, Olson MM, Shanholzter CJ, et al. Results of a prospective, 18-month clinical evaluation of culture, cytotoxin testing, and culturette brand (CDT) latex testing in the diagnosis of *Clostridium difficile*-associated diarrhea. Diagn Microbiol Infect Dis 1988; 10:85–91.

94. DiPersio JR, Varga FJ, Conwell DL, Kraft JA, Kozak KJ, Willis DH. Development of a rapid enzyme immunoassay for *Clostridium difficile* toxin A and its use in the diagnosis of c difficile-associated disease. J Clin Microbiol 1991; 29:2724–2730.

95. Boriello SP, Wren BW, Hyde S, et al. Molecular, immunological, and biological characterization of a toxin A–negative, toxin B–positive strain of *Clostridium difficile*. Infect Immun 1992; 60:4192–4199.

96. Torres JE. Purification and characterization of toxin B from a strain of *Clostridium difficile* that does not produce toxin A. J Med Microbiol 1991; 35:40–44.

97. McFarland LV, Elmer GW, Stamm WE, et al. Correlation of immunoblot type, enterotoxin production, and cytotoxin production with clinical manifestations of *Clostridium difficile* infection in a cohort of hospitalized patients. Infect Immun 1991; 59:2456–2462.

98. Brazier JS. The diagnosis of *Clostridium difficile*-associated disease. J Antimicrob Chemother 1998; 41(suppl C):29–40.

99. Peterson LR, Kelly PJ. The role of the clinical microbiology laboratory in the management of *Clostridium difficile*-associated diarrhea. Infect Dis Clin North Am 1993; 7:277–293.

100. Walker RC, Ruane PJ, Rosenblatt JE, et al. Comparison of culture, cytotoxicity assays, and enzyme–linked immunosorbent assay for toxin A and toxin B in the diagnosis of *Clostridium difficile*-related enteric disease. Diagn Microbiol Infect Dis 1986; 5:61–69.

101. Haslam SC, Ketley JM, Mitchell TJ, et al. Growth of *Clostridium difficile* and production of toxins A and B in complex and defined media. J Med Microbiol 1986; 21:293–297.

102. Lashner BA, Todorczuk J, Sahm DF, et al. *Clostridium difficile* culture-positive toxin-negative diarrhea. Am J Gastroenterol 1986; 81:940–943.

103. Barbut F, Kajzer C, Planas N, et al. Comparison of three enzyme immunoassays, a cytotoxicity assay, and toxigenic culture for the diagnosis of *Clostridium difficile*-associated diarrhea. J Clin Microbiol 1993; 31:963–967.

104. Doern GV, Coughlin RT, Wu L. Laboratory diagnosis of *Clostridium difficile*-associated gastrointestinal disease: comparison of monoclonal antibody enzyme immunoassay for toxins A and B with a monoclonal antibody enzyme immunoassay for toxin A only and two cytotoxicity assays. J Clin Microbiol 1992; 30:2042–2046.

105. Lyerly DM, Neville LM, Evans DT, et al. Multicenter evaluation of the *Clostridium difficile* TOX A/B TEST. J Clin Microbiol 1998; 36:184–190.

106. Merz CS, Kramer C, Forman M, et al. Comparison of four commercially available rapid enzyme immunoassays with cytotoxin assay for detection of *Clostridium difficile* toxins(s) from stool specimens. J Clin Microbiol 1994; 32:1142–1147.

107. Whittier S, Shapiro DS, Kelly WF, et al. Evaluation of four commercially available enzyme immunoassays for laboratory diagnosis of *Clostridium difficile*-associated diseases. J Clin Microbiol 1993; 31:2861–2865.

108. Bartlett JG. Antibiotic-associated diarrhea. N Engl J Med 2002; 346:334–339.

109. Alonso RMC, Pelaez T, Cercenado E, et al. Rapid detection of toxigenic *Clostridium difficile* strains by a nested PCR of the toxin B gene. Clin Microbiol Infect 1997; 3:145–147.

110. Kato N, Ou CY, Kato H, et al. Identification of toxigenic *Clostridium difficile* by the polymerase chain reaction. J Clin Microbiol 1991; 29:33–37.

111. Price AB, Davies DR. Pseudomembranous colitis. J Clin Pathol 1977; 30:1–12.

112. Seppala K, Hjelt L, Sipponen P. Colonoscopy in the diagnosis of AAC: a prospective study. Scand J Gastroenterol 1981; 16:465–468.

113. Johnson S, Clabots CR, Linn FV, et al. Nosocomial *Clostridium difficile* colonization and disease. Lancet 1990; 336:97–100.

114. Samore MH, DeGirolami PC, Tlucko A, et al. *Clostridium difficile* colonization and diarrhea at a tertiary care hospital. Clin Infect Dis 1994; 18:181–187.

115. Bartlett JG. AAPMC. Hosp Pract (Off Ed). 1981; 16:85–95.

116. Ramirez-Ronda CH. Incidence of clindamycin-associated colitis: comments and corrections. Ann Intern Med 1974; 81:860.

117. Brause BD, Romankiewicz JA, Gotz V, et al. Comparative study of diarrhea associated with clindamycin and ampicillin therapy. Am J Gastroenterol 1980; 73:244–248.

118. Bartlett JG. Antibiotic-associated colitis. J Clin Gastroenterol 1979; 8:783–801.

119. Rao SS, Edwards CA, Austen CJ, et al. Impaired colonic fermentation of carbohydrate after ampicillin. Gastroenterology 1988; 94:928.

120. LaMont JT. Clinical manifestations and diagnosis of *Clostridium difficile* infection. Uptodate December 2001.

121. Silva J. Update of pseudomembranous colitis. West J Med 1989; 151:644–648.

122. Parasakthi N, Puthucheary SD, Goh KL, et al. *Clostridium difficile* associated diarrhoea: a report of seven cases. Singapore Med J 1988; 29:504–507.

123. Cleary RK. *Clostridium difficile*-associated diarrhea colitis: clinical manifestations diagnosis treatment. Dis Colon Rectum 1998; 41:1435–1449.

124. Morris JB, Zollinger RM, Stellato TA. Role of surgery in antibiotic-induced pseudomembranous enterocolitis. Am J Surg 1990; 160:535–539.

125. Jacobs A, Barnard K, Fishel R, Gradon JD. Extracolonic manifestations of *Clostridium difficile* infections. Presentation of 2 cases and review of the literature. Medicine (Baltimore) 2001; 80:88.

126. Vesoulis Z, Williams G, Matthews B. Pseudomembranous enteritis after proctocolectomy: report of a case. Dis Colon Rectum 2000; 43:551.

127. Hannonen P, Hakola M, Mottonen T, et al. Reactive oligoarthritis associated with *Clostridium difficile* colitis. Scand J Rheumatol 1989; 18:57–60.

128. Riley TV, Karthigasu KT. Chronic osteomyelitis due to *Clostridium difficile*. Br Med J 1982; 284: 1217–1218.

129. Incave SJ, Muller DL, Krag MH, et al. Vertebral osteomyelitis caused by *Clostridium difficile*. A case report and review of the literature. Spine 1988; 13:111–113.

130. De Leeuw P, de Mot H, Dugernier T, et al. Primary infection of ascitic fluid with *Clostridium difficile*. J Infect 1990; 21:77–80.

131. Gerard M, Defresne N, Van der Auwera P, et al. Polymicrobial septicemia with *Clostridium difficile* in acute diverticulitis. Eur J Clin Microbiol Infect Dis 1989; 8:300–302.

132. Rooney N, Variend S, Taitz LS. Haemolytic uraemic syndrome and pseudomembranous colitis. Pediatr Nephrol 1988; 2:415–418.

133. Rybolt AH, Bennett RG, Laughon BE, et al. Protein-losing enteropathy associated with *Clostridium difficile* infection. Lancet 1989; 1:1353.

134. Bennett RG, Greenough WB III: *Clostridium difficile* diarrhea: a common—and overlooked—nursing home infection. Geriatrics 1990; 45:77–87.

135. Bennett JG. *Clostridium difficile* and IBD. Gastroenterology 1981; 80:863–865.

136. LaMont JT, Trnka YM. Therapeutic implications of *Clostridium difficile* toxin during relapse of chronic inflammatory bowel disease. Lancet 1980; 1:381.

137. Bolton RP, Sherriff RJ, Read AE. *Clostridium difficile* associated diarrhea: a role in IBD?. Lancet 1980; 1:383.

138. Meyers S, Mayer L, Bottone E, et al. Occurrence of *Clostridium difficile* toxin during the course of inflammatory bowel disease. Gastroenterology 1981; 80:697–700.

139. Johnson ST, Kent SA, O'Leary KJ, et al. Fatal pseudomembranous colitis associated with a variant *Clostridium difficile* strain not detected by toxin A immunoassay. Ann Intern Med 2001; 135:434–438.

140. Weber P, Koch M, Heizmann WR, et al. Microbic superinfection in relapse of inflammatory bowel disease. J Clin Gastroenterol 1992; 14:302.

141. Johnson S et al. Treatment of asymptomatic *Clostridium difficile* carriers (fecal excretors) with vancomycin or metronidazole. A randomized, placebo-controlled trial. Ann Intern Med 1992; 117:297–302.

142. Bartlett JG. The 10 most common questions about *Clostridium difficile*-associated diarrhea/colitis. Infect Dis Clin Pract 1992; 1:254–259.

143. Novak E, Lee JG, Seckman CE, Phillips JP, DiSanto AR. Unfavorable effect of atropine-diphenoxylate (Lomotil) therapy in lincomycin-caused diarrhea. JAMA 1976; 235:1451–1454.

144. Walley T, Milson D. Loperamide related toxic megacolon in *Clostridium difficile* colitis. Postgrad Med J 1990; 66:582.

145. George WL, Rolfe RD, Finegold SM. Treatment and prevention of antimicrobial agent-induced colitis and diarrhea. Gastroenterology 1980; 79:366–372.

146. Cone JB, Wetzel W. Toxic megacolon secondary to pseudomembranous colitis. Dis Colon Rectum 1982; 25:478–482.

147. Teasley DG, Gerding DN, Olson MM, et al. Prospective randomized trial of metronidazole versus vancomycin for *Clostridium difficile*-associated diarrhea and colitis. Lancet 1983; ii:1043–1046.

148. Peterson LR, Gerding DN. Antimicrobial agents in *Clostridium difficile*-associated intestinal disease. In: Rambaud J-C, Ducluzeau R, eds. *Clostridium difficile*-Associated Intestinal Diseases. Paris, France: Springer-Verlag, 1990:115–127.

149. Tedesco FJ. Bacitracin therapy in antibiotic-associated pseudomembranous colitis. Dig Dis Sci 1980; 25:783–784.

150. Salcedo J, Keates S, Pothoulakis C, et al. Intravenous immunoglobulin therapy for severe *Clostridium difficile* colitis. Gut 1997; 41:366–370.

151. Kohoff KL, Wasserman SS, Genevieve A, et al. Safety and immunogenicity of increasing doses of a *Clostridium difficile* toxoid vaccine administered to healthy adults. Infect Immun 2001; 69:988–995.

152. Bradbury AW, Barrett S. Surgical aspects of *Clostridium difficile* colitis. Br J Surg 1997; 84:150–159.

153. Surawicz CM. Rambaud JC, LaMont JT, eds. Updates on *Clostridium difficile*. Paris: Springer-Verlag, 1996:105–115.
154. Recommendations for preventing the spread of vancomycin resistance: recommendations of the hospital infection control practices advisory committee (HICPAC). Am J Infect Control 1995; 23:87–94.
155. Silva J Jr., Batts DH, Fekety R, Plouffe JF, Rifkin GD, Baird I. Treatment of *Clostridium difficile* colitis and diarrhea with vancomycin. Am J Med 1981; 71:815–822.
156. Hoverstad T, Carlstedt-Duke B, Lingaas E, et al. Influence of ampicillin, clindamycin, and metronidazole on faecal excretion of short-chain fatty acids in healthy subjects. Scand J Gastroenterol 1986; 21:621–628.
157. Arabi Y, Dimock F, Burdon DW, Alexander-Williams J, Keighly MRB. Influence of neomycin and metronidazole on colonic microflora of volunteers. J Antimicrob Chemother 1979; 5:531–537.
158. Ings RM, McFadzean JA, Ormerod WE. The fate of metronidazole and its implications in chemotherapy. Xenobiotica 1975; 5:223–235.
159. Cuchural GJ, Tally FP, Jacobus NV, et al. Antimicrobial susceptibilities of 1,292 isolates of the bacteroides fragilis group in the United States: comparison of 1981 with 1982. Antimicrob Agents Chemother 1984; 26:145.
160. Musial CE, Rosenblatt JE. Antimicrobial susceptibilities of anaerobic bacteria isolated at the mayo clinic during 1982 through 1987: comparison with results from 1977 through 1981. Mayo Clin Proc 1989; 64:392.
161. Barbut F, Decre D, Burghoffer B, et al. Antimicrobial susceptibilities and serogroups of clinical strains of *Clostridium difficile* isolated in France in 1991 and 1997. Antimicrob Agents Chemother 1999; 43:2607.
162. Keighly MR, Burdon DW, Arabi Y, et al. Randomized controlled trial of vancomycin for pseudomembranous colitis and postoperative diarrhoea. BMJ 1978; 2:1667–1669.
163. Kleinfeld DI, Sharpe RJ, Donta ST. Parenteral therapy for antibiotic-associated pseudomembranous colitis. J Infect Dis 1988; 157:389.
164. Oliva SL, Guglielmo BJ, Jacobs R, et al. Failure of intravenous vancomycin and intravenous metronidazole to prevent or treat antibiotic-associated pseudomembranous colitis [letter]. J Infect Dis 1989; 159:1154–1155.
165. deLalla F, Nicolin R, Rinaldi E, et al. Prospective study of oral teicoplanin versus oral vancomycin for therapy of pseudomembranous colitis and *Clostridium difficile*-associated diarrhea. Antimicrob Agents Chemother 1992; 36:2192–2196.
166. Dudley MN, McLaughlin JC, Carrington G, Frick J, Nightingale CH, Quintiliani R. Oral bacitracin versus vancomycin therapy for *Clostridium difficile*-induced diarrhea: a randomized double blind trial. Arch Intern Med 1986; 146:1101–1104.
167. Young GP, Ward PB, Bayley N, et al. Antibiotic-associated colitis due to *Clostridium difficile*: double-blind comparison of vancomycin with bacitracin. Gastroenterology 1985; 89:1038–1045.
168. Mogg GAG, Arabi Y, Youngs D, et al. Therapeutic trials of antibiotic associated colitis. Scand J Infect Dis 1980; (suppl 22):41–45.
169. Fekety R, Silva J, Kauffman C, Buggy B, Deery G. Treatment of antibiotic-associated *Clostridium difficile* colitis with oral vancomycin: comparison of two dosage regimens. Am J Med 1989; 86:15–19.
170. Chang TW, Gorbach SL, Bartlett JG, et al. Bacitracin treatment of antibiotic-associated colitis and diarrhea caused by *Clostridium difficile* toxin. Gastroenterology 1980; 78:1584–1586.
171. Wenisch C, Parschalk B, Hasenhundl M, et al. Comparison of vancomycin, teicoplanin, metronidazole, and fusidic acid for the treatment of *Clostridium difficile*-associated diarrhea. Clin Infect Dis 1996; 22:813–818.
172. Cronberg S, Castor B, Thoren A. Fusidic acid for the treatment of antibiotic-associated colitis induced by *Clostridium difficile*. Infection 1984; 12:276–279.
173. Bowden TA, Mansberger AR, Lykins LE. Pseudomembranous enterocolitis: mechanism for restoring flora homeostasis. Am Surg 1981; 47:178–183.
174. Jobe BA, Grasley A, Deveney KE, et al. *Clostridium difficile* colitis: an increasing hospital-acquired illness. Am J Surg 1995; 169:480–483.
175. Kyne L, Merry C, O'Connell B, et al. Factors associated with prolonged symptoms and severe disease due to *Clostridium difficile*. Age Ageing 1999; 28:107–113.
176. Anand A, Bashey B, Mir T, et al. Epidemiology, clinical manifestations and outcome of *Clostridium difficile*-associated diarrhea. Am J Gastroenterol 1994; 89:519–523.
177. Aronsson B, Granstrom M, Mollby R, et al. Serum antibody response to *Clostridium difficile* toxins in patients with *Clostridium difficile* diarrhoea. Infection 1985; 13:97–101.
178. Johnson S, Gerding DN, Janoff EN. Systemic and mucosal antibody responses to toxin A in patients infected with *Clostridium difficile*. J Infect Dis 1992; 166:1287–1294.
179. Leung DY, Kelly CP, Boguniewicz M, et al. Treatment with intravenously administered gamma globulin of chronic relapsing colitis induced by *Clostridium difficile* toxin. J Pediatr 1991; 118:633–637.
180. Mulligan ME, Miller SD, McFarland LV, et al. Elevated levels of serum immunoglobulins in asymptomatic carriers of *Clostridium difficile*. Clin Infect Dis 1993; 16(suppl 4):S239–S244.
181. Warny M, Vaerman JP, Avesani V, et al. Human antibody response to *Clostridium difficile* toxin A in relation to clinical course of infection. Infect Immun 1994; 62:384–389.
182. Gorbach SL. Antibiotics and *Clostridium difficile*. N Engl J Med 1999; 341:1690–1691.

183. Lipsett PA, Samantaray DK, tam ML, et al. Pseudomembranous colitis: a surgical disease. Surgery 1994; 116:491–496.
184. Grundfest-Broniatowski S, Quader M, Alexander F, et al. *Clostridium difficile* colitis in the critically ill. Dis Colon Rectum 1996; 39:619–623.
185. Synnott K, Mealy K, Merry C, et al. Timing of surgery for fulminating pseudomembranous colitis. Br J Surg 1998; 85:229–231.
186. Tedesco FJ, Gordon D, Fortson WC. Approach to the patient with multiple relapses of antibiotic-associated pseudomembranous colitis. Am J Gastroenterol 1985; 80:867–868.
187. Bolton RP, Culshaw MA. Fecal metronidazole concentrations during oral and intravenous therapy for antibiotic-associated colitis due to *Clostridium difficile*. Gut 1986; 27:1169–1172.
188. Levett PN. Time-dependent killing of *Clostridium difficile* by metronidazole and vancomycin. J Antimicrob Chemother 1991; 27:55–62.
189. Walters BA, Roberts R, Stafford R, Seneviratne E. Relapse of antibiotic associated colitis: endogenous persistence of *Clostridium difficile* during vancomycin therapy. Gut 1983; 24:206.
190. Young G, McDonald M. Antibiotic-associated colitis: why do patients relapse? Gastroenterology 1986; 90:1098.
191. Wilcox MH, Fawley WN, Settle CD, Davidson A. Recurrence of symptoms in *Clostridium difficile* infection—relapse or reinfection? J Hosp Infect 1998; 38:93.
192. Fekety R, McFarland LV, Surawicz CM, et al. Recurrent *Clostridium difficile* diarrhea: characteristics of and risk factors for patients enrolled in a prospective, randomized, double-blinded trial. Clin Infect Dis 1997; 24:324–333.
193. McFarland LV, Surawicz CM, Greenberg RN, et al. A randomized placebo-controlled trial of *Saccharomyces boulardii* in combination with standard antibiotics for *Clostridium difficile*. JAMA 1994; 271:1913–1918. [published erratum appears in JAMA 1994; 272(7):518].
194. Buggy BP, Fekety R, Silva Jr J. Therapy of relapsing *Clostridium difficile*-associated diarrhea and colitis with the combination of vancomycin and rifampin. J Clin Gastroenterol 1987; 9:155–159.
195. McFarland LV, Elmer GW, Surawicz CM. Breaking the cycle: treatment strategies for 163 cases of recurrent *C. difficile* disease. Am J Gastroenterol 2002; 971:1769–1775.
196. Tvede M, Rask-Madsen J. Bacteriotherapy for chronic relapsing *Clostridium difficile* diarrhoea in six patients. Lancet 1989; 1:1156.
197. Gorbach SL, Chang TW, Goldin B. Successful treatment of relapsing *Clostridium difficile* colitis with *lactobacillus* GG. Lancet 1987; 2:1519.
198. Elmer GW, Surawicz CM, McFarland LV. Biotherapeutic agents. A neglected modality for the treatment and prevention of selected intestinal and vaginal infections. JAMA 1996; 275:870.
199. Elmer GW, McFarland LV. Suppression by *Saccharomyces boulardii* of toxigenic *Clostridium difficile* overgrowth after vancomycin treatment in hamsters. Antimicrob Agents Chemother 1987; 31:129.
200. Pothoulakis C, Kelly CP, Joshi MA, et al. *Saccharomyces boulardii* inhibits *Clostridium difficile* toxin A binding and enterotoxicity in rat ileum. Gastroenterology 1993; 104:1108.
201. Surawicz CM, McFarland LV, Greenberg RN, Rubin M, Fekety R, Mulligan ME, et al. The search for a better treatment for recurrent *Clostridium difficile* disease: use of high-dose vancomycin combined with *Saccharomyces boulardii*. Clin Infect Dis 2000; 31:1012–1017.
202. Castagliuolo I, LaMont JT, Baker C, et al. Purified *Saccharomyces boulardii* protease inhibits C. difficile toxin A effects in rat ileum [abstr]. Gastroenterology 1995; 108:A792.
203. Massot J, Sanchez O, Astoin R, et al. Bacterio-pharmacological activity of *Saccharomyces boulardii* in clindamycin-induced colitis in the hamster. ArzneimForch/Drug Res 1984; 34:794–797.
204. Buts JP, Bernasconi P, Van Craynest M, Maldague P, DeMeyer R. Response of human and rat intestinal mucosa to oral administration of *Saccharomyces boulardii*. Pediatr Res 1986; 20:192–196.
205. Buts JP, Keyser ND, Raedemaeker LD. *Saccharomyces boulardii* for *Clostridium difficile*-associated enteropathies in infants. J Pediatr Gastroenterol Nutr 1994; 16:419–425.
206. Nath SK, Thornley JH, Kelly M, et al. A sustained outbreak of *Clostridium difficile* in a general hospital: persistence of a toxigenic clone in four units. Infect Control Hosp Epidemiol 1994; 15:382–389.
207. Silva J Jr. *Clostridium difficile* nosocomial infections-still lethal and persistent. Infect Control Hosp Epidemiol 1994; 15:382–389.
208. Struelens MJ, Maas A, Nonhoff C, et al. Control of nosocomial transmission of *Clostridium difficile* based on sporadic case surveillance. Am J Med 1991; 91(suppl 3B):S138–S144.
209. Alfa MJ, Du T, Beda G. Survey of incidence of *Clostridium difficile* infection in Canadian hospitals and diagnostic approaches. J Clin Microbiol 1998; 36:2076–2080.
210. Samore MH. Epidemiology of nosocomial *Clostridium difficile* diarrhoea. J Hosp Infect 1999; 43(suppl):S183–S190.
211. Levy DG, Stergachis A, McFarland LV, et al. Antibiotics and *Clostridium difficile* diarrhea in the ambulatory care setting. Clin Ther 2000; 22:91–102.
212. McFarland LV. Nosocomial acquisition and risk factors for *Clostridium difficile* disease. In: Rambaud JC, LaMont JT, eds. Updates on *Clostridium difficile*. Paris: Springer-Verlag, 1996:37–50.
213. Kaatz GW, Gitlin SD, Schaberg Dr, et al. Acquisition of clostridium difficile from the hospital environment. Am J Epidemiol 1988; 127:1289–94.
214. Testore GP, Pantosti A, Cerquetti M. et al. Evidence for cross-infection in an outbreak of clostridium difficile-associated diarrhoea in a surgical unit. J Med Microbiol 1988; 26:125–128.

215. Cartmill TD, Panigrahi H, Worsley MA, McCann DC, Nice CN, Keith E. Management and control of a large outbreak of diarrhoea due to clostridium difficile. J Hosp Infect. 1994; 27(1):1–15.

216. Struelens MJ, Mass A, Nonhoff C, et al. Control of nosocomial transmission of clostridium difficile based on sporadic case surveillance. Am J Med 1991; 91:1385–1445.

217. Zafer AB, Gaydos LA, Furlong WB, Nguyen MH, Mennonna PA. Effectiveness of infection control program in controlling nosocimial clostridium difficile. Am J Infect Control. 1998; 26(6):588–93.

218. Pear SM, Williamson TH, Bettin Km, et al. Derease in nosocomial clostridium difficile-associated diarrhea by restricting clindamycin use. Ann Intern Med 1994; 120:272–277.

219. Pear SM, Williamson TH, Bettin KM, et al. Decrease in nosocomial *Clostridium difficile*-associated diarrhea by restricting clindamycin use. Ann Intern Med 1994; 120:272–277.

220. Fekety R. Antibiotic-associated colitis. In: Mandell G, Bennett JE, Dolin R, eds. Principles Practice of Infectious Diseases. 4th ed. New York: Churchill Livingstone, 1996:978–806.

221. Jernigan JA, Siegman-Igra Y, Guerrant RC, et al. A randomized crossover study of disposable thermometers for prevention of *Clostridium difficile* and other nosocomial infections. Infect Control Hosp Epidemiol 1998; 19:494–499.

222. McFarland LV, Coyle MB, Kremer WH, Stamm WE. Rectal swab cultures for *Clostridium difficile* surveillance studies. J Clin Microbiol 1987; 25:2241–2242.

223. Dove CH, Wang SZ, Price SB, et al. Molecular characterization of the *Clostridium difficile* toxin A gene. Infect Immun 1990; 58:480–488.

224. Eriksson S, Aronsson B (1989). Medical implications of nosocomial infection with *Clostridium difficile*. Scand J Infect Dis 21:733–734.

225. Barroso LA, Wang SZ, Phelps CJ, et al. Nucleotide sequence of *Clostridium difficile* toxin B gene. Nucl Acids Res 1990; 18:4004.

226. Gerding DN, Olson MM, Peterson LR, et al. C. *difficile*-associated diarrhea and colitis in adults. Arch Intern Med 1986; 146:95–100.

14 | Colon Ischemia

Lawrence J. Brandt
Divsion of Gastroenterology, Departments of Medicine and Surgery, Albert Einstein College of Medicine, Montefiore Medical Center, Bronx, New York, U.S.A.

Scott J. Boley
Department of Surgery, Albert Einstein College of Medicine, Montefiore Medical Center, Bronx, New York, U.S.A.

INTRODUCTION

Colon ischemia is a frequent disorder of the large bowel and is the most common form of intestinal ischemic injury. There have been several changes in our concepts of this disease, from its early descriptions. In the 1950s, colon ischemia was considered synonymous with colon infarction or gangrene. Now we recognize that colon ischemia describes a pathophysiologic process that leads to a spectrum of clinical disorders including reversible colopathy (mucosal or intramural hemorrhage), transient colitis, chronic colitis, stricture, gangrene, and fulminant universal colitis. Previously, colon ischemia was thought of as a disease affecting older individuals, in whom an etiology was rarely discovered. Today, an increasing number of young people are being diagnosed with colon ischemia, mainly those who have an underlying thrombophylic condition, patients on a wide variety of medications, or those who use illicit drugs such as cocaine. Finally, we are learning that whereas the majority of patients with colon ischemia do well, there are some in whom prognosis is more guarded. This is especially true when only the right side of the colon is affected [within the distribution of the superior mesenteric artery (SMA)], as is seen in dialysis patients, patients recovering from cardiac surgery, patients who have had shock or sepsis, and when the SMA flow is compromised.

COLONIC CIRCULATION

The SMA and inferior mesenteric arteries (IMA) supply blood to the colon, although review of hundreds of vascular dissections and countless mesenteric angiograms has revealed incredible variation in vascular anatomy (1). In general, the SMA supplies the ascending colon and most of the transverse colon, while the IMA supplies the descending colon, sigmoid, and upper rectum. Major branches of the SMA are the ileocolic, right colic, and middle colic arteries; the IMA usually gives off the left colic artery, which divides into an ascending and descending branch; other branches are the sigmoid vessels before the IMA ends as the superior hemorrhoidal artery (Fig. 1).

Numerous communications between the celiac axis, SMA, IMA, and iliac artery beds provide the colon with abundant collateral circulation. Collateral flow around small arterial branches is made possible by multiple arcades within the colonic mesentery, and SMA or IMA occlusions may be bypassed by one or more of a series of connections between these two vessels, including the marginal artery of Drummond, the central anastomotic artery, and the arc of Riolan. Within the bowel wall, there also is a network of communicating submucosal vessels that can maintain viability of short segments of the colon if the extramural arterial blood supply has been compromised. Despite this vast collateral circulation, however, there still remains a weak link in the anastomoses between the middle colic and left colic arteries in the region of the splenic flexure. Hall et al. showed, by measurements of tissue

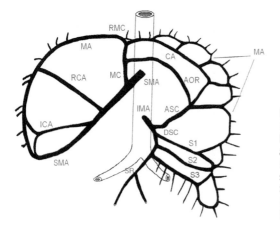

Figure 1   Schematic diagram of colon blood flow. *Abbreviations*: AOR, arc of Riolan; CA, central artery; ICA, ileocolic artery; IMA, inferior mesenteric artery; MA, marginal artery; MC, middle colic artery; RCA, right colic artery; RMC, right middle colic artery; SA, sigmoid artery; SMA, superior mesenteric artery; SR, superior rectal artery; S1, S2, S3, sigmoid arteries; ASC, ascending branch of IMA; DSC, descending branch of IMA. *Source*: From Ref. 1a.

oxygen tension, that after ligation of the IMA at its origin, the marginal artery system remains able to supply adequate flow to the transverse colon and descending colon, but not the sigmoid colon (2). Furthermore, using laser Doppler flowmetry, Dworkin and Allen-Mersh demonstrated that there is a 50% reduction in perfusion of the sigmoid colon after ligation of the IMA (3). The splenic flexure and sigmoid are thus "watershed" areas of the colon and are most often affected by ischemia. Conversely, the rectum, because of its dual blood supply from the splanchnic and systemic colon circulations, is the least affected.

DEMOGRAPHICS

The incidence of colon ischemia is underestimated and not precisely known for several reasons. First, the diagnosis is usually made after the period of ischemia has passed and blood flow to the affected segment has returned to normal. Many cases of transient or reversible ischemia are probably missed because the condition resolves before medical attention is sought or because diagnostic studies are not performed early enough in the course of illness. Second, because the colon, like other organs in the body, reacts to a wide variety of insults in only a limited number of ways, colon damaged by ischemia resembles colon damaged by infectious or toxic agents and inflammatory processes. Therefore, colon ischemia is often misdiagnosed and confused with other disorders, notably inflammatory bowel disease (IBD). In two retrospective studies of 154 patients in whom new-onset colitis was identified after the age of 50, approximately 75% had definite or probable colon ischemia, half of whom had been diagnosed erroneously with IBD (4,5).

In our tertiary care hospital, colon ischemia accounts for approximately 1 in 2000 hospital admissions and is seen in approximately 1 in 100 flexible sigmoidoscopies and colonoscopies. A study of medical claims data from a large health care organization calculated a crude incidence rate of 7.2 cases per 100,000 person · years of observation in the general population and in contrast to 42.8 cases per 100,000 person · years for a population with irritable bowel syndrome (5a). Colon ischemia has no gender predilection and more than 90% of patients with colon ischemia are older than 60 years. Colon ischemia affecting young persons has been documented in case reports or series of relatively few patients in whom causes have been identified in up to 46% of subjects.

PATHOPHYSIOLOGY AND ETIOLOGY

The colon has an inherently lower blood flow than the small intestine, and is therefore, more sensitive to ischemic injury during acute reductions in blood flow. Moreover, experimental studies have shown that functional motor activity of the colon is accompanied by diminished blood flow, in contrast to blood flow to the small intestine, which increases markedly during digestion and periods of increased peristalsis. In addition, the pronounced effects of "straining" on systemic arterial and venous pressure in constipated, compared with nonconstipated subjects, provides indirect evidence that constipation may accentuate the adverse circulatory effects of defecation. Geber (6) postulated "the combination of normally low blood flow and decreased blood flow during functional activity would seem to make the colon rather unique among all areas of the body where increased motor activity is usually accompanied by an increased blood flow and more susceptible to pathology." Other factors that decrease colon blood flow are changes in the environment and emotionally stressful situations. Experiments evaluating the hypothalamic influence on gastrointestinal (GI) blood flow in the awake cat model suggest that of the entire GI tract, the colon blood flow is most affected by autonomic stimulation (7). What ultimately triggers an episode of colon ischemia, however, remains conjectural in most instances. Whether it is an increased demand by colonic tissues superimposed on an already marginal blood flow or whether the flow itself is acutely diminished has yet to be determined. Colon ischemia is a disease mainly occurring in the elderly; therefore, an association with degenerative changes of the mesenteric vasculature has been postulated. Autopsy studies have shown abnormal musculature in the wall of the superior rectal artery in the elderly population (8), and postmortem angiographic studies have revealed an age-related tortuosity of the longer colonic arteries, which may cause increased resistance to colonic blood flow, thus predisposing the colon to ischemia (9). Despite such suggestive evidence for a vascular or autonomic cause of colon ischemia, most cases have no identifiable cause. These "spontaneous" episodes are thought to be the result of local nonocclusive ischemia in association with small vessel disease. Colonic blood flow can be further compromised by reductions in systemic perfusion, as is seen in patients with congestive heart failure or shock or those on hemodialysis. Colon ischemia resulting from such hemodynamic insults is usually within the distribution of the SMA and hence affects the ascending colon.

Many causes of colon ischemia have been identified in recent years, mainly related to acquired or hereditary prothrombotic conditions, drug and medication use, infectious agents, and autoimmune disorders with a vasculitic component (Table 1). Potential causes are found more often in younger rather than older subjects; however, even in the small number of younger individuals who have been reported, at least 50% of the causes remain unexplained (10). A report by Koutroubakis et al. (11) identified one or more predisposing prothrombotic abnormalities in 72% of 36 patients with colon ischemia. Such disorders included activated protein C resistance (28%), C677T methyl tetrahydrofolate reductase (23%), factor V Leiden (23%), antiphospholipid antibody (19%), protein S deficiency (14%), antithrombin deficiency (11%), protein C deficiency (6%), and prothrombin 20210A (3%). While there may be some question regarding the accuracy of the assays in this report, there is no doubt that thrombophilic states are being increasingly identified in a wide variety of inflammatory disorders and conditions with venous thromboses. A prothrombotic cause for a venous occlusion with subsequent ischemic injury of the colon is contrary to the prevailing view that colon ischemia results from localized areas of nonocclusive ischemia in small arteries. Classic work in the early and mid-1960s by Allen and Boley, however, did show a variety of venous and arterial lesions in various colitides, including ischemic enterocolitis (12,13). The possibility that colonic ischemia may be associated with prothrombotic disorders raises the question of whether patients with colonic ischemia should have screening for these underlying conditions or whether these coagulation disorders are merely epiphenomena and of little significance (14). Conceivably, patients with underlying coagulation or immune disorders are also at increased risk for the irreversible types of colon ischemia such as chronic ischemic colitis and stricture formation. In a group of 36 patients with colon ischemia, so-called "IBD-specific pANCA" was positive in seven, all of whom had chronic disease; only two patients with reversible colon ischemia had a positive test and both results were in low titer only (15).

Three infectious agents may produce colon ischemia (Fig. 2): one bacteria (*Escherichia coli* O157:H7), and two viruses [cytomegalovirus (CMV) and hepatitis B]. Thus, a thorough stool analysis should be done to exclude a potential cause of infection in all cases of suspected colon ischemia and segmental colitis. *E. coli* O157:H7 most commonly manifests as hemorrhagic colitis and may be accompanied by hemolytic uremic syndrome or thrombotic thrombocytopenic purpura (16). It usually is transmitted in food-borne outbreaks and most often affects the young and the elderly. *E. coli* O157:H7 produces colon ischemia by its Shiga-like toxins that damage vascular endothelium, diminish prostacyclin synthesis, aggregate platelets, and cause platelet-fibrin thrombi. The most common method to diagnose infection with this bacterium is by culturing the stool on MacConkey-sorbitol agar; the organism ferments sorbitol slowly or does not ferment it at all. We demonstrated the presence of *E. coli* O157:H7 in archival paraffin-embedded tissue sections from 3 of 11 patients with ischemic colitis (17).

Table 1 Causes of Colon Ischemia

Noniatrogenic causes	Iatrogenic causes
Nonocclusive ischemia	Surgical
Cardiac failure or arrhythmias	Aneurysmectomy
Shock	Aortoiliac reconstruction
Obstructing colon carcinoma	Gynecologic operations
Volvulus	Exchange transfusion
Strangulated hernia	Colon bypass
Arterial embolus	Lumbar aortography
IMA thrombosis	Colectomy with IMA ligation
Cholesterol emboli	Laparoscopy
Phlebosclerosis	Colonoscopy
Pancreatitis	Barium enema
Amyloid	Medications[a]
Idiopathic dysautonomia	Digitalis
Allergy	Estrogens
Trauma	Danazol
Ruptured ectopic pregnancy	Progestins
Long-distance running	Gold compounds
Hematologic disorders	Psychotropic drugs
Sickle cell disease	Sumatriptan
Polycythemia vera	Cocaine
Paroxysmal nocturnal hemoglobinuria	NSAIDs
Protein C and S deficiencies	Imipramine
Antithrombin III deficiency	Golytely
Factor V Leiden	Penicillin
Activated protein C resistance	Methamphetamines
Prothrombin 20210A mutations	Vasopressin
Vasculitis	Ergot
Systemic lupus erythematosus	Oral saline laxatives
Rheumatoid arthritis	Interferon alpha
Thromboangiitis obliterans	Kayexalate
Takaysu arteritis	Glycerin enema
Periarteritis nodosa (idiopathic and hepatitis B-related)	Flutamide
Kawasaki disease	Pit viper toxin
Infections	Phenylephrine
Bacteria (E. coli O157:H7)	Alosetron
Viral (cytomegalovirus, hepatitis B)	Immunosuppressive agents
Parasitic (*Angiostrongylus costaricensis*)	

[a]Any medication that has constipation as an adverse effect can potentially cause colon ischemia.
Abbreviations: IMA, inferior mesenteric artery; NSAIDs, nonsteroidal anti-inflammatory drugs.

CMV infection occurs almost exclusively in the presence of immunocompromise, as in persons with AIDS or those taking medications (especially corticosteroids and cyclosporine) after transplantation or as therapy for IBD. CMV has a predilection for endothelial cells and can cause an obliterative arteritis. Erythema and submucosal hemorrhage may be seen in approximately 20% of cases, ulceration is typical, and pseudomembranes are occasionally present; hepatitis B virus with polyarteritis is another cause of colon ischemia.

A complete medication history is important in evaluating the possible causes of a bout of colon ischemia. Medications may have a direct effect on the local or systemic vasculature or they may cause severe constipation and secondary colon ischemia; an obstructing stool mass may give rise to increased intraluminal pressure, similar to overdistention of the colon by insufflation of air during colonoscopy or barium during barium enema examination. Commonly used medications that have been associated with colon ischemia include nonsteroidal anti-inflammatory agents, digitalis, imipramine, danazol, sumatriptan, and pseudoephedrine. Cases of colon ischemia attributed to alosetron, a 5-HT$_3$ receptor inhibitor used to treat diarrhea-predominant irritable bowel syndrome in women, resulted in the temporary removal of the drug from the market. The mechanism for ischemia from this drug is not well understood because the serotonin receptors it is antagonistic for are not found on the colonic vasculature. Postulated mechanisms include potentially severe constipation or an excess of 5-HT$_3$ which may "cross-talk" with other serotonin neurotransmitter receptors and stimulate vasoconstriction; this process may be exaggerated by atherosclerosis. Interestingly, one patient with colon

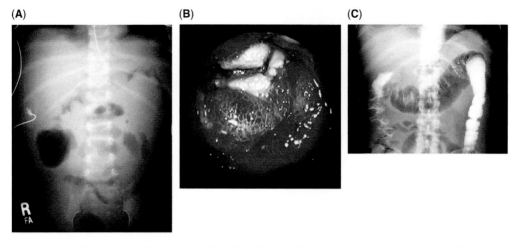

(A) **(B)** **(C)**

Figure 2 Infectious causes of ischemic colitis. (**A**) Plain film of the abdomen showing ischemic colitis in a young boy. There is thumbprinting of the transverse colon and narrowing of the descending colon and sigmoid. The abnormal colon had to be resected after which full recovery was made. (**B**) (*See color insert*) Colonoscopic view of the rectum of a patient with AIDS and cytomegatovirus-induced ischemic proctocolitis. There is significant mucosal and submucosal hemorrhage and edema. (**C**) Barium enema revealing dramatic thumbprinting of the ascending colon in a man with polyarteritis-associated hepatitis B.

ischemia attributed to alosetron had positive immunoperoxidase staining for *E. coli* O157:H7 on the colon resection specimen.

Cocaine and amphetamines are well-known causes of colon ischemia; a history of illicit drug use should always be sought in any young patient who develops colon ischemia. Oral contraceptives also convey an increased risk of colon ischemia, especially in women who carry the mutation for Factor V Leiden.

PATHOLOGY

Morphologic changes after colon ischemia vary with the duration and severity of the injury (18). The mildest changes consist of mucosal and submucosal hemorrhage and edema, with or without partial necrosis, and ulceration of the mucosa. These hemorrhages are either resorbed (reversible colopathy) or the overlying mucosa ulcerates (transient colitis) and perhaps sloughs. More severe injury results in more extensive damage, resulting in granulation tissue replacing the mucosa and submucosa. Eventually, the mucosa may regenerate over the submucosa, which is widened and edematous and contains abundant granulation and fibrous tissue. These changes in the submucosa and the presence of iron-laden macrophages are characteristic of ischemic injury. With moderate-to-severe injury, chronic ulcerations, crypt abscesses, and even pseudopolyps develop, which can mimic IBD or infectious colitis (Fig. 3); pseudomembranes can also be seen and the differential diagnosis between ischemic colitis with pseudomembranes and pseudomembranous colitis with ischemia may be difficult. Occasionally, the inflammatory response and granulation tissue are extremely abundant and can cause a heaping up of the mucosa and submucosa, resembling a stricturing or polypoid neoplasm (Figs. 4A and B) (19). With more severe and prolonged ischemia, the muscularis propria may be damaged and replaced by fibrous tissue and subsequent stricture formation (Fig. 5). Patients with this type of ischemic injury usually present with increasing constipation or even colonic obstruction; the latter may be the initial manifestation of a previous silent ischemic injury. In the most severe form of ischemic damage, there is transmural infarction of all colon layers, with gangrene and perforation.

CLINICAL MANIFESTATIONS AND DIAGNOSIS
Presentation

Colon ischemia typically presents with the sudden onset of mild, cramping abdominal pain, usually localized to the left lower quadrant. Less commonly, the pain is severe, or conversely,

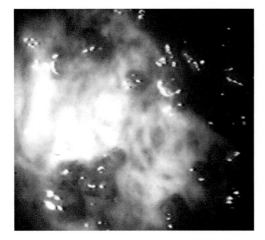

Figure 3 (*See color insert*) Colonoscopic image showing extensive pseudopolyp formation and ulceration in a patient with ischemic colitis.

in some patients, the description of the pain can only be elicited retrospectively, if at all. An urgent desire to defecate frequently accompanies or follows the pain and is followed within 24 hours by the passage of either bright red or maroon blood in the stool. The bleeding is neither vigorous nor hemodynamically significant, and blood loss requiring transfusion is sufficiently rare that its occurrence suggests an alternative explanation. Physical examination is limited to mild-to-severe abdominal tenderness in the location of the involved segment of colon. Depending on the severity and duration of the ischemic insult, the patient may develop fever, leukocytosis, or both. Generally, there is no hypotension, signs of sepsis, peritonitis, or acidemia, unless gangrene and/or perforation is present.

Distribution

Any portion of the colon may be affected, but the splenic flexure and descending and sigmoid colon are the most common sites (Fig. 6). Certain specific causes tend to affect certain areas of the colon more than others, but no prognostic implications can be derived from the distribution of disease, except in the case of colon ischemia involving only the ascending colon, which has a poorer prognosis than colon ischemia involving any other segment (19a). Nonocclusive ischemic injuries tend to involve the "watershed" areas of the colon—the splenic flexure and sigmoid-descending colon junction; ligation of the IMA produces changes in the sigmoid. Ischemic proctitis may be a manifestation of systemic lupus erythematosus especially when accompanied by the antiphospholipid (anticardiolipin) antibody syndrome. Isolated right colon ischemia is seen in patients with SMA disease, in systemic low-flow states such as cardiogenic shock, and in patients with chronic renal failure that requires hemodialysis and in

(A)   **(B)**

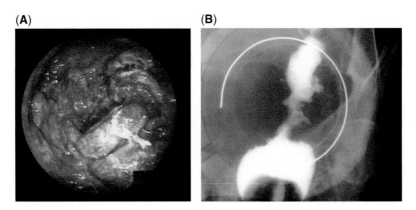

Figure 4 Two examples of colon ischemia mimicking a neoplasm. (**A**) (*See color insert*) Colonoscopic view of a polypoid heaped-up mass, which, on biopsy, revealed changes compatible with ischemia. The mass resolved within two to three weeks. (**B**) Spot film from a barium enema showing rectosigmoid ischemia mimicking an apple-core lesion.

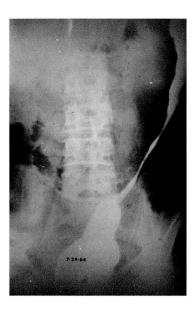

Figure 5 Barium enema showing a long, smooth ischemic stricture of the descending colon.

whom repeated episodes of hypotension and major fluid shifts occur. The length of affected bowel also varies with the cause of the ischemic injury. For example, atheromatous emboli result in short segment changes, and nonocclusive injuries usually involve much longer segments of colon.

Natural History

Despite similarities in the initial presentation of most episodes of colon ischemia, outcome cannot be predicted at its onset unless the initial physical findings indicate an unequivocal intra-abdominal catastrophe (Table 2). The ultimate course of an ischemic insult (i) depends on many factors, including the cause; (ii) the caliber of the occluded vessel; (iii) the duration and degree of ischemia; (iv) the rapidity of onset of ischemia; (v) the condition of the collateral circulation; (vi) the metabolic requirements of the affected bowel; (vii) the quantity, type, and virulence of the bowel flora; and (viii) the presence of associated conditions, such as colonic distention.

Most commonly, symptoms subside within 24 to 48 hours, and clinical, roentgenographic, and endoscopic evidence of healing is seen within two weeks. More severe, but still reversible, ischemic damage may take one to six months to resolve; however during this time, the patient is usually asymptomatic. The vast majority of patients with colon ischemia have reversible disease. Approximately 60% to 70% of patients with reversible disease exhibit only colonic hemorrhage or edema (reversible colopathy), whereas the others develop

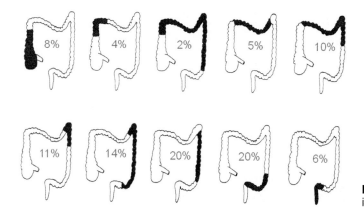

Figure 6 Distribution of colon ischemia in 250 cases.

Table 2 Types and Approximate Incidences of Colon Ischemia

Type	Incidence (%)
Reversible colopathy	>30–40
Transient colitis	>15–20
Chronic ulcerating colitis	<20–25
Stricture	<10–15
Gangrene	<15–20
Fulminant universal colitis	<5

transient colitis. In approximately 20% to 30% of cases, irreversible disease ultimately develops. In approximately two-third of these patients, colon ischemia follows a more protracted course, developing into either chronic ulcerating segmental colitis or ischemic stricture. The remaining one-third develop signs and symptoms of an intra-abdominal catastrophe, such as gangrene with or without perforation, which becomes obvious within hours of the initial presentation.

Before the onset of symptoms, most patients with colon ischemia are well or in their usual states of chronic ill health. Patients who develop colon ischemia after a major cardiac event, such as congestive heart failure, myocardial infarction, or new-onset arrhythmia, or during hemodialysis have a particularly poor prognosis. These are typically elderly individuals taking digitalis preparations, which may act as potent splanchnic vasoconstrictors, exacerbating the already compromised colonic perfusion. In some reports (20,21), approximately 30% of colon ischemia cases requiring hospitalization occurred immediately following episodes of systemic hypotension. In one series, (21) 12 of 13 patients with colon ischemia who presented in shock died.

Diagnosis

If colon ischemia is suspected and the patient has no signs of peritonitis, colonoscopy or the less attractive combination of sigmoidoscopy and a gentle barium enema should be performed on the unprepared bowel within 48 hours of the onset of symptoms. Computed tomography is frequently used to evaluate patients with abdominal pain and can certainly demonstrate the presence and location of a colitic process; it is, however, a nondiagnostic test and doesn't differentiate among the various causes of colitis. During colonoscopy and barium enema examination, care should be taken not to overdistend the colon because high intraluminal pressure may aggravate ischemic damage, particularly in patients with vasculitis (22). At intraluminal pressures greater than 30 mmHg (pressures that can be achieved during colonoscopy and barium enema examinations), colon blood flow decreases, blood is shunted from the mucosa to the serosa, and there is a drop in the arteriovenous oxygen difference (23). This occurrence is rare, but can be minimized by the use of CO_2 rather than air for the insufflating agent; CO_2 is a vasodilator and is rapidly absorbed from the intestinal lumen, thereby minimizing distention (24).

Colonoscopy is preferable to radiologic studies for diagnosis because it is more sensitive in diagnosing mucosal abnormalities and because biopsy specimens may be obtained (25). It is also preferable to flexible sigmoidoscopy because many episodes of colon ischemia are beyond the level reached by the sigmoidoscope. Hemorrhagic nodules seen at colonoscopy represent bleeding into the submucosa and are equivalent to so-called "thumbprinting" on barium enema studies. Segmental distribution of these findings, with or without ulceration, is highly suggestive of colon ischemia, but the diagnosis cannot be made conclusively on a single colonoscopic study unless gangrene is seen.

The initial diagnostic study should be performed within 48 hours of the onset of symptoms, because thumbprinting disappears within days as the submucosal hemorrhages are resorbed or the overlying mucosa ulcerates or sloughs (Fig. 7). Studies performed one week after the initial study-should reflect evolution of the injury—either normalization or replacement of the thumbprints with a segmental colitis pattern. Universal colonic involvement favors true ulcerative colitis, whereas fistula formation suggests Crohn's disease. Occasionally, an abundant inflammatory response can produce heaping up of the mucosa and submucosa, which resembles a stricture or a neoplasm (Fig. 4).

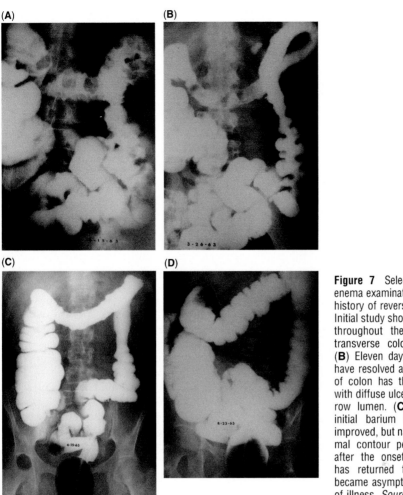

Figure 7 Selected films from barium enema examinations showing the natural history of reversible colon ischemia. (**A**) Initial study shows dramatic thumbprints throughout the involved area of the transverse colon and splenic flexure. (**B**) Eleven days later, the thumbprints have resolved and the involved segment of colon has the appearance of colitis with diffuse ulceration and a tubular narrow lumen. (**C**) One month after the initial barium enema, the colon has improved, but narrowing and loss of normal contour persist. (**D**) Five months after the onset of disease, the colon has returned to normal. The patient became asymptomatic after three weeks of illness. *Source*: From Ref. 25a.

Biopsies of nodules identified early in the course of disease reveal submucosal hemorrhage, while biopsies of adjacent normal-appearing mucosa usually show only nonspecific inflammatory changes (26). Histologic evidence of mucosal infarction or ghost cells, although rare, is pathognomonic for ischemia; more common changes are vascular congestion and acute and chronic inflammation.

At the time of onset of symptoms, colon blood flow typically has returned to normal, and, therefore, mesenteric angiography usually is not indicated. An exception to this rule is when the clinical presentation does not allow a clear distinction to be made between colon ischemia and acute mesenteric ischemia; then administration of air during flexible sigmoidoscopy can be used to reveal thumbprinting not otherwise visible on abdominal plain films. No thumbprinting or thumbprinting isolated to the ascending colon suggests SMA disease and the need for angiography. Similarly, thumbprinting that affects the ascending colon as part of more extensive involvement can be viewed as reflecting colon ischemia. Because untreated acute mesenteric ischemia progresses rapidly to an irreversible outcome and optimal diagnosis and treatment of this condition require angiography, the diagnosis of acute mesenteric ischemia must be established or excluded prior to any contrast studies; residual contrast will obscure the mesenteric vessels and, therefore, preclude an adequate angiographic examination and intervention.

A few suggestions regarding colonoscopy in patients with proven or suspected colon ischemia: Colonoscopy should not be performed in patients who have peritonitis and in whom colon perforation is suspected. If mucosal gangrene is found during colonoscopy, it is prudent to cease the examination. In patients at high risk for colon ischemia, e.g., after aortic aneurysm repair, who develop symptoms typical of colon ischemia and in whom computed tomography scan shows segmental colon thickening, a judgment must be made as to whether the small risk of colonoscopy with biopsy is worth the benefit of observing endoscopic findings compatible with colon ischemia and obtaining supporting histopathology. It is sometimes more prudent to accept the diagnosis of colon ischemia as probably correct and to begin the patient on broad-spectrum antibiotics, reserving colonoscopy for the patient whose course is complicated or casts doubt on the diagnosis.

MANAGEMENT

Guidelines for the management of patients with colon ischemia have been published by the American Gastroenterological Association (Fig. 8) (27,28).

General Principles

Once the diagnosis of colon ischemia has been established and the physical examination does not suggest gangrene or perforation, the patient is treated expectantly. Most patients do not require hospital admission. Those whose bleeding or abdominal pain is severe enough to warrant admission are given parenteral fluids and the bowel is placed at rest. Broad-spectrum antibiotics that provide coverage for *Enterococcus* and anaerobic organisms are administered, although the data supporting this recommendation are limited. Antibiotic therapy will not prevent colonic infarction, but has been shown to reduce the length of the bowel damaged by an episode of ischemia and to increase the time before irreversible ischemic changes occur. Cardiac function is optimized to ensure adequate systemic perfusion. In patients with colon ischemia associated with major cardiovascular incidents, medications that cause mesenteric vasoconstriction (e.g., digitalis and vasoconstrictors) should be withdrawn if possible. The urine output is monitored and maintained with parenteral isotonic fluids. If the colon appears distended, either clinically or radiologically, it can be decompressed with a rectal tube, with or without gentle saline irrigations. Contrary to their efficacy in ulcerative colitis, parenteral corticosteroids are contraindicated because they may increase the possibility of perforation and secondary infection.

Although rarely needed, blood products should be administered according to the patient's requirements. Serum potassium and magnesium levels must be monitored because the levels of these electrolytes may be disturbed by the associated diarrhea and tissue necrosis.

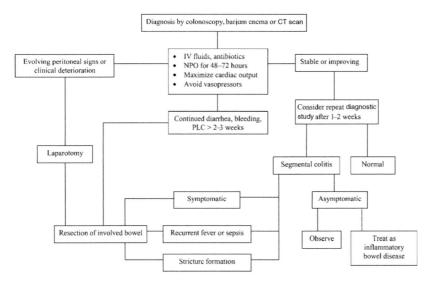

Figure 8 Management of colon ischemia. Solid lines indicate accepted management plan; dashed line indicates alternative management plan. *Abbreviations*: CT, computed tomography; IV, intravenous; NPO, nil per os; PLC, protein-losing colopathy. *Source*: Modified from Ref. 27.

Patients with significant diarrhea are begun on parenteral nutrition early. As with other potential surgical conditions, narcotics should be withheld until it is clear that an intra-abdominal catastrophe is not present. Stimulatory cathartics are contraindicated. No attempt should be made to prepare the bowel for surgery in the acute phase because this may precipitate a perforation. Increasing abdominal tenderness, guarding, rebound tenderness, rising temperature, and paralytic ileus during the period of observation suggest colonic infarction. These signs, although not distinct indicators of transmural ischemia or infarction, dictate the need for expedient laparotomy and resection of the abnormal segment of colon. At laparotomy, the serosal appearance of infarcted colon ranges from that of wet tissue paper to that of mottled, thickened, aperistaltic bowel. The resected specimen should be opened in the operating suite and examined for mucosal injury; if the margins are involved, additional colon should be removed until they appear grossly normal.

Reversible Lesions

In the mildest cases of colon ischemia, in which signs and symptoms of illness disappear within 24 to 48 hours, submucosal and intramural hemorrhages are resorbed, and there is complete clinical and radiologic resolution within one to two weeks. In such cases, no further therapy is indicated. More severe ischemic insults result in necrosis of the overlying mucosa, with ulceration and inflammation and subsequent development of a segmental colitis. Varying amounts of mucosa may slough, but healing occurs within several months. Patients with such protracted healing usually are clinically asymptomatic even in the presence of persistent radiologic or endoscopic evidence of disease. These asymptomatic patients are placed on a high-residue diet to, hopefully, avoid stricture formation. Follow-up evaluations are performed to confirm complete healing or the development of a stricture or persistent colitis. Recurrent episodes of sepsis in asymptomatic patients with unhealed areas of segmental ischemic colitis are usually caused by bacterial translocation through the diseased segment of bowel and are an indication for elective resection.

Irreversible Lesions

Patients with persistent diarrhea, rectal bleeding, sepsis, or protein-losing colopathy for more than 10 to 14 days frequently develop perforation. Hence, early resection is indicated to prevent this complication. In those instances in which the patient has had a concurrent or recent myocardial infarction or if the patient has major medical contraindications to the surgery, a six- to eight-week trial of prolonged parenteral nutrition with concomitant intravenous antibiotic therapy may be considered as an alternative, albeit less optimal, method of management.

When surgery is undertaken, standard bowel prep with a large-volume colon lavage solution and intravenous and oral antibiotics are used; enemas should not be used to prepare the bowel. Despite a normal serosal appearance, there may be extensive mucosal injury, and the extent of resection should be guided by the distribution of disease as seen on the preoperative studies rather than the appearance of the serosal surface of the colon at the time of surgery. As in all resections for colon ischemia, the specimen must be opened at the time of surgery to ensure normal mucosa at the margins. If at the time of surgery, the rectum is involved, a mucous fistula or Hartmann's procedure with an end colostomy should be performed. The mucous fistula can be fashioned through the diseased bowel and in some cases this segment will heal sufficiently to allow subsequent restoration of bowel continuity; local steroid enemas may be helpful in this setting, although parenteral steroids are contraindicated. A simultaneous, proctocolectomy rarely is indicated except in the case of colon ischemia after abdominal aortic replacements.

Patients with chronic segmental ulcerating ischemic colitis are frequently misdiagnosed as having IBD, especially if not seen during the acute episode. The de novo occurrence of a segmental area of colitis (or stricture) in an elderly patient should be considered most likely ischemic and treated accordingly (Figs. 9A and B). Patients with chronic segmental ischemic colitis, initially, are managed symptomatically. Local corticosteroid enemas may be helpful, but parenteral steroids should be avoided. Medications conventionally used to treat IBD are usually without benefit in patients with chronic ischemic colitis. In patients whose symptoms cannot be controlled by medication, segmental resection of the diseased bowel should be performed to avoid disease recurrence.

(A)   **(B)**

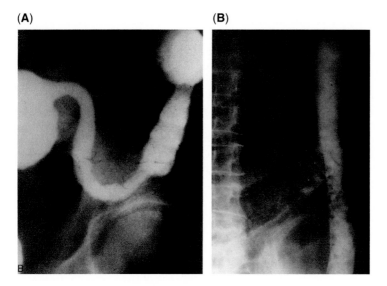

Figure 9 Barium enema appearance of chronic segmental ischemic colitis that mimics Crohn's disease. (**A**) Narrowed, tubular, ahaustral sigmoid flanked by normal colon on both sides. (**B**) Narrow ahaustral descending colon with pseudopolyps. *Source*: From Ref. 26.

Ischemic Stricture

Approximately 10% of patients will develop a stricture after a bout of severe colon ischemia as a consequence of damage to the muscularis propria and its replacement with fibrous tissue (Fig. 10) (10). These patients may not present during the acute episode of ischemia, but rather with what may appear as a sudden new-onset constipation or colon obstruction, weeks to months later. Patients with ischemic strictures may be observed if they are asymptomatic, because some strictures will regress with no specific therapy. Symptoms from strictures, however, such as worsening constipation, warrant more aggressive management. While gentle use of bulk laxatives may dilate strictures, it is hazardous and may produce total obstruction if they are used in a zealous fashion. Endoscopic dilation may be attempted if the stricture is short, although there are no data on the efficacy of this approach. Most symptomatic strictures can be surgically resected, with good results.

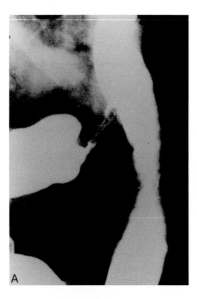

Figure 10 Barium enema revealing a short ischemic stricture with characteristics of a carcinoma. *Source*: From Ref. 26.

Colon Ischemia Complicating Aortic Aneurysm Surgery

Although mesenteric vascular reconstruction is not indicated in the vast majority of cases of colon ischemia, it may be required to prevent colon ischemia during and after aortic reconstruction surgery. In retrospective studies, the reported incidence of colon ischemia complicating aortic surgery is 1% to 2%, while in prospective and endoscopic studies, this complication is reported in 3% to 7% of elective cases (29,30). The incidence of colon ischemia after the repair of ruptured aortic aneurysms has been reported to be as high as 60% (31). Although clinical evidence of this complication occurs in only 1% to 2% of patients, when it does occur, it is responsible for approximately 10% of the deaths that occur after aortic replacement (32). Factors that contribute to postoperative colon ischemia include rupture of the aneurysm, hypotension, operative trauma to the colon, hypoxemia, dysrhythmias, long cross-clamp time, and improper management of the IMA during aneurysmectomy.

The most important aspect of the management of colon ischemia after aortic surgery is its prevention. Collateral blood flow to the left colon after occlusion of the IMA comes from the SMA via the arc of Riolan (also known as "the meandering artery"), the central anastomotic artery, or the marginal artery of Drummond, and from the internal iliac arteries via the middle and inferior rectal arteries. If these collateral pathways are intact, the risk of postoperative colon ischemia can be minimized by intraoperative preservation. Aortography and a full mechanical and antibiotic bowel preparation are recommended before aortic reconstruction. Aortography is advised to determine the patency of the celiac axis, SMA, IMA, and internal iliac arteries.

The presence of a meandering artery does not in and of itself allow safe ligation of the IMA, because the blood flow in the meandering artery frequently originates from the IMA and reconstitutes an obstructed SMA (Fig. 11). Ligation of the IMA in the latter colon circumstance can be catastrophic, with resultant infarction of the small and large bowel. Ligation of the IMA is safe only when it has been confirmed angiographically that the blood flow in the meandering artery is from the SMA to the IMA (Fig. 12) (33). Reimplantation of the IMA and revascularization of the SMA are required, therefore, in those instances when the SMA is occluded or tightly stenosed and the IMA provides inflow to the meandering artery. Occlusion of both internal iliac arteries on the preoperative arteriogram indicates that the rectal blood flow is dependent on collateral flow from the IMA or from the SMA via the meandering artery. In this circumstance, reconstitution of flow to one or both hypogastric arteries is desirable at the time of aneurysmectomy (Fig. 13). At surgery, cross-clamp time should be minimized, and hypotension must be avoided. If a meandering artery is identified,

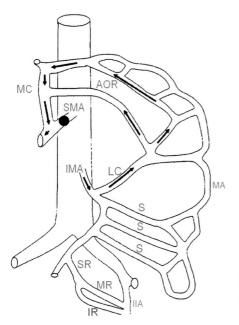

Figure 11 Collateral blood flow from the IMA via the MA and AOR to an occluded SMA. *Abbreviations*: AOR, arc of Riolan; IIA, internal iliac artery; IMA, inferior mesenteric artery; IR, inferior rectal artery; LC, left colic artery; MA, marginal artery; MC, middle colic artery; MR, middle rectal artery; S, sigmoid arteries; SMA, superior mesenteric artery; SR, superior rectal artery. *Source:* From Ref. 33.

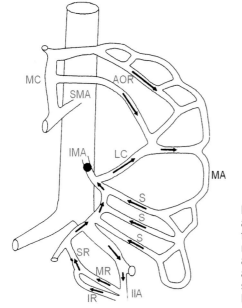

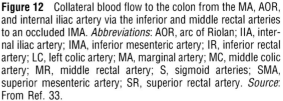

Figure 12 Collateral blood flow to the colon from the MA, AOR, and internal iliac artery via the inferior and middle rectal arteries to an occluded IMA. *Abbreviations*: AOR, arc of Riolan; IIA, internal iliac artery; IMA, inferior mesenteric artery; IR, inferior rectal artery; LC, left colic artery; MA, marginal artery; MC, middle colic artery; MR, middle rectal artery; S, sigmoid arteries; SMA, superior mesenteric artery; SR, superior rectal artery. *Source*: From Ref. 33.

it should be carefully preserved. Because the serosal appearance of the colon is not a reliable indicator of collateral blood flow, several methods have been suggested to determine the need for IMA reimplantation. Stump pressure in the transected IMA of greater than 40 mmHg, or a mean IMA stump pressure–to–mean systemic blood pressure ratio of greater than 0.40 indicates adequate collateral circulation and can be used reliably to avoid IMA reimplantation. Doppler ultrasound flow signals at the base of the mesentery and at the serosal surface of the colon with temporary IMA inflow occlusion suggest that the IMA can be ligated safely without reimplantation.

Tonometric determination of intramural pH of the sigmoid colon has been used to infer that colonic blood flow during aneurysmectomy is inadequate and to predict postoperative colon ischemia (34). A tonometric balloon is passed through the anus into the sigmoid colon before cross-clamping of the aorta, thereby enabling the evaluation of colonic intramural pH

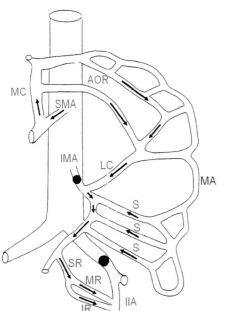

Figure 13 The entire rectal blood flow is dependent on collateral flow after occlusion of both internal iliac arteries. In this figure, the IMA is also occluded, leaving rectal blood flow dependent on collateral flow from the SMA via the AOR and the MA and then via the superior rectal vessel to the middle and inferior rectal arteries. *Abbreviations*: AOR, arc of Riolan; IIA, internal iliac artery; IMA, inferior mesenteric artery; LC, left colic artery; MA, marginal artery; MC, middle colic artery; MR, middle rectal artery; S, sigmoid arteries; SMA, superior mesenteric artery; SR, superior rectal artery. *Source*: From Ref. 33.

before and after occlusion and restoration of aortic flow. Intramural pH is a metabolic marker of tissue acidosis, and intramural acidosis reflects clinically significant ischemia and indicates the need for revascularization while the abdomen is open. An abnormal tonometric study of the sigmoid colon, loss of arterial pulsation, diminished stump pressures, and decreased transcolonic oxygen saturation after aortic surgery are indications for reimplantation of the IMA. When IMA reimplantation is deemed necessary, the IMA should be excised with a patch of the aortic wall (Carrell patch), and this patch should be sutured into the side of the aortic prosthesis.

If the SMA is occluded, it can be revascularized by reimplantation into the graft wall or, alternatively, by creating a lateral extension of the prosthesis and performing an end-to-side anastomosis with the SMA. Use of these adjunctive procedures has both substantially reduced the incidence of colon ischemia and eliminated it as a cause of death after aortic surgery.

The difficulty in accurately assessing colon ischemia after surgery and the significant mortality rates associated with occurrence mandate that postoperative colonoscopy be performed in high-risk patients. Patients at high risk for the development of postoperative colon ischemia after aortic reconstruction are those with ruptured abdominal aortic aneurysms, prolonged cross-clamping time, a patent IMA on preoperative aortography, nonpulsatile flow in the internal iliac arteries at surgery, and postoperative diarrhea. In such patients, colonoscopy is routinely performed within two to three days of the operation, and if colon ischemia is identified, therapy (nothing by mouth, adequate hydration, and antibiotics) is begun before major complications develop. Clinical deterioration, indicating progression of the ischemic insult to transmural necrosis necessitates reoperation. These patients should undergo resection of the abnormal segment of colon and colostomy. Primary anastomosis is contraindicated due to the potential contamination of the aortic prosthesis in the event of an anastomotic leak. If the rectum is involved, it must also be resected. Every effort should be made to protect the aortic graft from contamination; therefore, the retroperitoneum overlying the graft should be closed using local tissues or the omentum.

Colitis Associated with Colon Carcinoma

Acute colitis in patients with colon carcinoma of the colon has been recognized for many years. The colitis is usually, but not always, proximal to the tumor and occurs with and without clinical obstruction. It is of ischemic origin and has the typical radiologic and endoscopic appearance of ischemic colitis (Figs. 14A and B). Clinically, patients may present with symptoms of colon ischemia or with symptoms related to the primary cancer. In most cases, however, the predominant complaints are related to the ischemic episode—sudden onset of mild-to-moderate abdominal pain, fever, bloody diarrhea, and abdominal tenderness.

It is imperative for the gastroenterologist and radiologist, as well as the surgeon to be aware of this association. The gastroenterologist doing the colonoscopy and the radiologist doing the barium enema or computed tomographic scan must be careful to exclude cancer

(A)

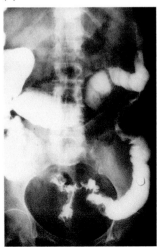

(B)

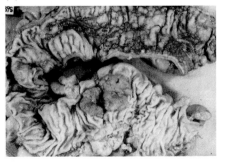

Figure 14 (**A**) Barium enema showing a segment of ischemic colitis in the descending colon and a non obstructing carcinoma in the sigmoid colon. (**B**) Gross specimen from the same patient demonstrating typical segmental ischemic colitis with normal colon between the neoplasm and the colitis. *Source*: From Ref. 26.

in every case of colon ischemia; for the surgeon, it is vital to examine any colon resected for cancer to exclude the presence of an ischemic process in the area of the anastomosis, because such involvement may lead to stricture or leak.

Colon Ischemia as a Manifestation of Acute Mesenteric Ischemia

Colon ischemia isolated to the right side of the colon occurs in about 25% of patients hospitalized with colon ischemia and may be a manifestation of SMA occlusion (19a). Any such evidence of colon ischemia isolated to the right colon is an indication for vascular imaging (CT angiography or conventional mesenteric angiography) before discharge to evaluate the status of the SMA. Patients with isolated right colon ischemia have a worse prognosis than do patients with colon ischemia involving other segments of the colon or when the right side of the colon is involved along with other segments (19a). The demonstration of a partially or completely obstructed SMA is an indication for revascularization of this artery.

REFERENCES

1. Michels NA. Blood Supply and Anatomy of the Upper Abdominal Organs with a Descriptive Atlas. Philadelphia, PA: JB Lippincott, 1955.
1a. Kornblith PL Boley SJ whitehouse BS. Anatomy of the splanchnic circulation. Surg Clin North Am 1992; 72:31–43.
2. Hall NR, Finan PJ, Stephenson BM, et al. High tie of the inferior mesenteric artery in distal colorectal resections-a safe vascular procedure. Int J Colrectal Dis 1995; 10: 29–32.
3. Dworkin MJ, Allen-Mersh TC. Effect of inferior mesenteric artery ligation on blood flow in the marginal artery-dependent sigmoid colon. J Am Coll Surg 1996; 183:357–360.
4. Brandt LJ, Boley SJ, Goldberg L, et al. Colitis in the elderly: a reappraisal. Am J Gastroenterol 1981; 76:239–245.
5. Wright HG. Ulcerating colitis in the elderly. Epidemiological and clinical study of an in-patient hospital population submitted as thesis for M.D. degree. Yale University, 1970.
5a. Cole JA, Cook SF, Sands BE, et al. Occurrence of colon ischemia in relation to irritable bowel syndrome. Am J Gastroenterol 2004; 99:486–491.
6. Geber WF. Quantitative measurements of blood flow in various areas of the small and large bowel. Am J Physiol 1960; 198:985–986.
7. Delaney JP, Leonard AS. Hypothalamic influence on gastrointestinal blood flow in the awake cat. Fed Proc 1970; 29:A80.
8. Quirke P, Campbell I, Talbot IC. Ischaemic proctitis and adventitial fibromuscular dysplasia of the superior rectal artery. Br J Surg 1984; 71:33–38.
9. Binns JC, Issacson P. Age related changes in the colonic blood supply: their relevance to ischemic colitis. Gut 1978; 19:384–390.
10. Preventza OA, Lazaridis KN, Sawyer MD. Ischemic colitis in young adults: a single institution experience. Gastroenterol 1999; 116:S0207.
11. Koutroubakis IE, Sfiridaki A, Theodoropoulou E, et al. Role of acquired and hereditary thrombotic risk factors in colon ischemia of ambulatory patients. Gastroenterol 2001; 121:561–565.
12. Allen AC. A unified concept of the vascular pathogenesis of enterocolitis of varied etiology: a pathophysiologic analysis. Am J Gastroenterol 1971; 55:347–378.
13. Boley SJ, Schwartz S, Krieger H, et al. Further observations on reversible vascular occlusion of the colon. Am J Gastroenterol 1965; 44:260–268.
14. Brandt LJ. Thrombophilia and colon ischemia: *aura popularis*? Gastroenterol 2001; 121:724–729.
15. Persky S, Tobak J, Brandt LJ. Perinuclear anti-neutrophil cytoplasmic antibodies (p-ANCA) are present in some patients with colon ischemia. Gastroenterol 2001; 120:A281.
16. Su C, Brandt LJ. *Escherichia coli* 0157:H7 infection in humans. Ann Int Med 1995; 123:698–714.
17. Su C, Brandt LJ, Sigal S, et al. The immunohistological diagnosis of *E. coli* 0157:H7 colitis: possible association with colonic ischemia. Am J Gastroenterol 1998; 93:1055–1059.
18. Mitsudo S, Brandt LJ. Pathology of intestinal ischemia. Surg Clin NA 1992; 72:43–63.
19. Brandt LJ, Katz HJ, Wolf EL. Simulation of colonic carcinoma by ischemia. Gastroenterol 1985; 88: 1137–1142.
19a. Sotiriadis J, Khorshidi I, Brandt LJ. Does colon ischemia have a worse prognosis when isolated to the right side? Gastroenterology 2006; 130:T1037 (A460).
20. Arnott ID, Ghosh S, Ferguson A. The spectrum of ischaemic colitis. Euro J Gastroenterol Hepatol 1999; 11:295–303.
21. Guttormson NL, Bubrick MP. Mortality from ischemic colitis. Dis Colon Rectum 1989; 26:469–472.
22. Church JM. Ischemic colitis complicating flexible endoscopy in a patient with connective tissue disease. Gastrointest Endosc 1995; 41:181–182.

23. Boley SJ, Agrawal GP, Warren AR, et al. Pathophysiologic effects of bowel distention on intestinal blood flow. Am J Surg 1969; 117:228–234.
24. Brandt LJ, Boley SJ, Sammartano RJ. Carbon dioxide and room air insufflation of the colon. Gastrointest Endosc 1986; 32:324–329.
25. Scowcroft CW, Sanowski RA, Kozarek RA. Colonoscopy in ischemic colitis. Gastrointest Endosc 1981; 27:156–161.
25a. Boley SJ, Schwartz SS. Colon ischemia: reversible ischemia reasons. In: Boley SJ, Schwartz SS, William LF, eds. Vascular Disorders of the Intestines. New York: Appleton, Century-Cropts, 1971.
26. Boley SJ, Brandt LJ, Veith FJ. Ischemic disorders of the intestine. Curr Prob Surg 1978; 15:1–85.
27. Brandt LJ, Boley SJ. AGA technical review on intestinal ischemia. Gastroenterol 2000; 118:954–968.
28. American Gastroenterological Association Medical Position Statement: Guidelines on Intestinal Ischemia. Gastroenterol 2000; 118:951–953.
29. Ernst CB, Hagihara PE, Daugherty ME, et al. Ischemic colitis incidence following abdominal aortic reconstruction: a prospective study. Surgery 1976; 80: 417–421.
30. Zelenock GB, Strodel WE, Knol JA, et al. A prospective study of clinically and endoscopically documented colonic ischemia in 100 patients undergoing aortic reconstructive surgery with aggressive and direct revascularization: comparison with historic controls. Surgery 1989; 106:771–780.
31. Hagihara PE, Ernst CB, Griffen WB. Incidence of ischemic colitis following abdominal aortic reconstruction. Surg Gynecolog Obstet 1979; 149:571–573.
32. Kim MW, Hundahl SA, Dang CR, et al. Ischemic colitis following aortic aneurysmectomy. Am J Surg 1983; 145:392–394.
33. Kaley R, Boley SJ. Colonic bleeding and ischemia. In: Zuidema GP, Yeo C, eds. Shackelfords Surgery of Alimentary Tract. 5th ed. Philadelphia: WB Saunders.
34. Schiedler MG, Cutler BS, Fiddian-Green RG. Sigmoid intramural pH for prediction of ischemic colitis during aortic surgery: a comparison with risk factors and inferior mesenteric artery stump pressures. Arch Surg 1987; 122:881–886.

15 | Radiation Injury to the Colon: Colopathy and Proctopathy

Joseph Ahn
Department of Medicine, Hepatology Division, Rush University Medical Center, Chicago, Illinois, U.S.A.

Roger Hurst
Department of Surgery, University of Chicago Medical Center, Chicago, Ilinois, U.S.A.

Eli D. Ehrenpreis
Section of Gastroenterology, Department of Medicine, University of Chicago Hospitals, University of Chicago Medical Center, Chicago, Illinois, U.S.A.

INTRODUCTION

Radiation injury to the gastrointestinal tract was first described in 1897, two years after the discovery of X-rays by Wilhelm Roentgen (1). Subsequently, although ionizing radiation was found to be an effective treatment of breast, skin, and other detectable malignancies it was limited by the complications of skin burns and hyperemia. Supervoltage radiation techniques allow the utilization of high radiation doses for the treatment of neoplasms without skin complications; unfortunately, radiation-induced deep tissue damage has become a significant problem with its use. Radiation injury to the colon may be concomitant with small bowel injury. It is seen most often with irradiation of pelvic malignancies: prostate, cervix, uterus, bladder, colon, rectum, and ovaries. During the last 25 years, in spite of improved knowledge and technical advancements in computer-aided dosimetric analysis, brachytherapy, megavoltage equipment, radioprotective techniques and compounds, the prevalence of radiation-induced gastrointestinal injury is estimated to be between 2% and 20% (2–7). However, these estimates are based on retrospective studies comprised of small groups of heterogeneous patients with a wide variety of primary malignancies treated, radiotherapy techniques used, radiation injury locations and severity, and duration of follow-up. The use of radiation in up to 50% of cancer treatment (1), and the increased availability of chemotherapy agents that may sensitize the colon to radiation has made colonic injury from radiation a significant and persistent problem. Moreover, the rectum's proximity to the organs that are common targets for radiation therapy, as well as its susceptibility to significant chronic radiation injury in the setting of few proven therapeutic options has made radiation proctopathy a difficult clinical entity for managing physicians. This chapter discusses the epidemiology, pathology, pathogenesis, clinical features and treatment options along with the prognosis and future direction of radiation-induced colorectal injury. In this chapter, data on rectal injury (proctopathy) will be separated from injury to other parts of the colon (colopathy) to reflect the two main bodies of literature on colonic radiation injury.

GENERAL RADIATION PHYSIOLOGY

An understanding of the pathophysiology of radiation injury to the colon requires an explanation of some basic terminology of radiation therapy (8,9). Radiation is classified into two categories: ionizing and nonionizing. Radiation is said to be ionizing if it involves the transfer of energy that causes the displacement of negatively charged electrons from their orbit, leading to molecular bond rupture and the production of charged particles and ions. Nonionizing radiation comprises the ubiquitous forms present in our environment (Fig. 1) (8). Examples of nonionizing radiation include microwaves, radio waves, ultraviolet waves, infrared and visible light such as the sun and laser light. Ionizing radiation is the most common vehicle for

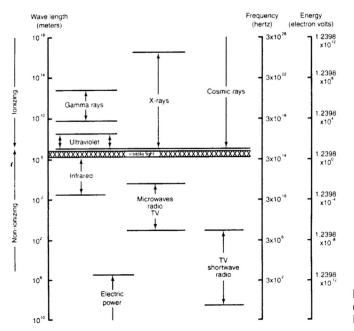

Figure 1 The characteristics of the electromagnetic waves. *Source*: From Ref. 8.

radiation therapy, specifically X-rays and gamma rays (8). Ionizing radiation can further be classified as electromagnetic and particulate. Electromagnetic radiation waves have no mass or charge and their energy is determined by their wavelength and frequency.

Particulate radiation is composed of electrons, alpha particles, beta particles, protons, neutrons, and other charged particles with variable masses.

X-rays and gamma rays are the primary modalities of radiotherapy practice, but particulate forms of radiation such as proton beams and neutron beams are being increasingly utilized. X-rays and gamma rays have low to moderate energy and relatively deep penetration of tissue (9). X-rays are produced via X-ray machines such as the linear accelerator, while gamma rays are emitted spontaneously by radioactive substances such as ^{60}Co (8). X-rays and gamma rays cause damage by the photoelectric and the Compton process in which the displaced electron ejected by the X-ray photons interacts with nearby water molecules to form free radicals (10). The free radicals go on to cause single and double strand breakage in the DNA, in addition to disrupting cellular structures leading ultimately to injury or death of the affected cell.

$$H_2O + e^- \rightarrow H_2O^+ + H_2O \rightarrow H_3O^+ + OH^- \rightarrow \text{Cellular and DNA damage}$$

In addition to the cytotoxic aspects of radiation, there is a humoral inflammatory tissue response leading to changes in the tissue levels of prostaglandins, prostacyclins, and other vasoactive substances. It is thought that these substances lead to vascular changes, increased permeability, and chemotaxis that contribute to chronic radiation pathology.

Radiation Units

The Roentgen (R) is the generic unit of exposure such that 1 R is the dose of radiation that causes ionization of 1 cm^3 of air at standard temperature and pressure such that the ions will carry one electrostatic unit of electrical charge. The measurement of clinical radiation effects has classically been done via the rad, which is the dose of radiation that results in the absorption of energy of 100 ergs per gram of tissue. The rad has been supplanted by the Gray (Gy), the SI term, which is equal to 100 rad; 1 rad equals 1 cGy (Table 1) (11).

The concept of "minimal and maximal tolerance" to radiation dose in various tissue types is defined by the term "total dose" (TD). The TD 5/5 and TD 50/5 are the doses at which 5% and 50% of exposed patients will have clinically evident radiation injury in five years

Table 1 Definitions and Units

Unit	Abbreviation	Quantity measured	Definition
Roentgen	R	Exposure	Dose of radiation that produces ionization of a standard volume of so that the ions will carry one electrostatic unit of electric charge
Rad	Rad	Dose	Dose of radiation that results in the absorption of 100 ergs per gram of tissue
Gray	Gy	Dose	SI unit of absorption corresponding to 100 rad. $1\,Gy = 1\,Joule/kg = 10^7\,ergs$
Rem	Rem	Dose equivalence	Used mainly to compare types of radiation. Reflects biologic response to radiation

Source: From Ref. 11.

(Table 2) (12). These values help guide the intensity of radiotherapy to maximize therapeutic killing of tumor cells while minimizing normal tissue injury. The TD 5/5 and TD 50/5 doses were proposed to be 45 to 60 Gy for the large intestine and 55 to 80 Gy for the rectum (13). However, these doses are not clearly established and are dependent on the assumption of a standard fractionation regimen using standard doses and exact dose delivery to the target tissue.

The response of cells to various doses and types of radiation exposure can be plotted with "Survival" on the y-axis and "Dose" on the x-axis (Figure 2). For particulate radiation, the curve reflects an exponential relationship of decreasing survival with increased dose. For electromagnetic radiation, specifically X-rays, the curve is initially linear followed by a shoulder region where cell survival decreases in proportion to the square of the dose. With increasing dose, this shoulder region returns to a linear relationship. The shoulder region is thought to represent sublethal damage such as single strand DNA breaks that can be repaired over time. This is the rationale for fractionation of the total dose of radiation over a period of time such that the sublethal damage to healthy tissue can have a chance of repair. In contrast, particulate radiation has no shoulder region because its direct ionizing effects causes double stranded DNA breaks and other cellular damage that are beyond the cell's ability for repair (Fig. 2) (14).

Tissue Effects of Radiation

Factors that influence tissue effects of radiation can be divided into several categories: physical, chemical, and biological (8). From these factors that influence radiation injury to the colon, the four important concepts of repair, reoxygenation, redistribution, and repopulation provide the rationale for modern fractionated radiotherapy.

The physical factors affecting the severity of tissue injury are the total radiation dose, the dose rate, the volume or size of exposure, and the techniques of radiation delivery and protective maneuvers used to minimize damage. Table 3 lists the typical radiation dose schemes for sites associated with bowel injury. The response to radiation insult is proportional to the total dose, but also on the dose rate. Because of this, prolongation of the course of radiation treatment and increasing the time between fractions of radiation reduces tissue damage by allowing time for

Table 2 Minimal and Maximal Tolerance Doses

Organ	Pathology	TD 5/5	TD 50/5	Whole vs. partial organ
Fetus	Death	200	400	Whole
Bone marrow	Pancytopenia, aplasia	250, 3000	450, 4000	Whole, segmental
Kidney	Nephrosclerosis	1500, 2000	2000, 2500	Partial, whole
Liver	Hepatitis	1500, 2500	2000, 4000	Partial, whole
Lung	Pneumonitis	1500, 3000	2500, 3500	Partial, whole
Stomach	Perforation, ulcer, hemorrhage	4500	5500	100 cm
Intestine	Perforation, ulcer, hemorrhage	4500, 5000	5500, 6500	400 cm, 100 cm
Heart	Pericarditis, pancarditis	4500, 7000	5500, 8000	60%, 25%
Spinal cord	Infarction, necrosis	4500	5500	10 cm
Brain	Infarction, necrosis	5000	6000	Whole

Abbreviation: TD, total dose.
Source: From Ref. 12.

(A)   **(B)**

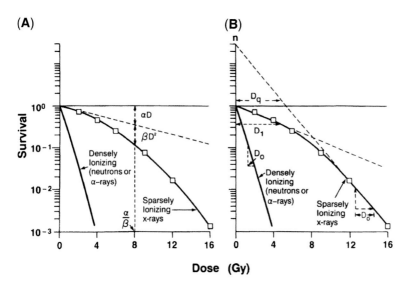

Figure 2   Cell survival curve. The fraction of cells surviving (logarithmic *Y* axis) is plotted against the dose (linear *X* axis). For sparsely ionizing radiation, there is an initial (*shallow slope*, described by D_1) linear relationship, followed by a shoulder (representing the cell's ability to repair sublethal damage, described by the parameters *n* and D_q), followed by a final (*steep slope*, described by D_0) linear relationship. For densely ionizing radiation, the cell survival curve is a straight line (described by D_0), as repair of double-stranded breaks is minimal. There are two components to cell killing by radiation, one that is proportional to the dose (mediated by the term α), and the other that is proportional to the square of the dose (mediated by the term β). The dose at which these linear and quadratic components are equal is α/β, in this case 8 Gy. *Abbreviation:* Gy, Gray. *Source:* From Ref. 14.

cells to repair sublethal injury. Repair is the first important factor in determining radio-sensitivity of cells.

The response of the tumor and the normal colonic tissue is also dependent on the volume of exposure. Radiation delivery can be done by X-ray beams using external sources such as linear accelerators or by gamma rays using radioactive substances such as ^{60}Co. Radiation can also be delivered by brachytherapy: the insertion of radioactive isotopes such as cesium into body cavities (endocavitary therapy) or directly into tissues (interstitial therapy). These various techniques differ in the energy levels of radiation delivered, the field size of exposure, the precision of delivery, and the penetration of the radiation into tissues. For example, rectal injury from external beam radiotherapy for prostate cancer is influenced by the movement of the rectum into and out of the field during the therapy over the radiation course. Work is being done to minimize rectal exposure and reduce rectal toxicity during external beam therapy by using different beam arrangements and computer aided three-dimensional (3-D) treatment planning (15–19). There have been some efforts for prevention of gastrointestinal injuries by minimizing bowel presence in the treatment field by bowel exclusion and shielding procedures. Surgical partitioning of the abdominal and pelvic cavities

Table 3   Typical Radiation Dose Schemes for Sites Associated with Bowel Injury

Site of cancer	Total dose (cGy)	Fraction size (cGy)
Prostate	6600–8000	180–200
Bladder	6000–7000	180–200
Seminoma	2500–4000	150–175
Rectum	4500–5400	180–200
Colon	4500–5000	180–200
Ovary	2500–5000	150–200
Uterus, intact	4500–8500[a]	180–200
Uterus, post-op	4500–6500[a]	180–200
Cervix, intact	4500–8500[a]	180–200
Cervix, post-op	4500–6500[a]	180–200
Vagina	4500–8500[a]	150–200

[a]Includes brachytherapy dose.

have been studied using omentum as well as synthetic materials. However, these methods appear to be more effective in reducing small bowel sequelae than in preventing proctopathy or colopathy (20,21). They also carry a significant risk of complications such as herniation, small bowel obstruction, ileus, wound dehiscence, and wound infection (22,23). Calculations of radiation dose delivery can also be done with brachytherapy and implants can be positioned to minimize rectal and colonic damage.

The degree of radiation-induced injury is also influenced by the coadministration of radioprotective and radiosensitizing chemical factors. Oxygen interacts with radiation-induced free radicals to produce compounds such as peroxide, which goes on to cause permanent change in the irradiated target tissue (8). In vitro studies have shown that oxygen potentiates cell killing by radiation, and that oxygen reduction has a protective effect. Therefore, tumors with hypoxia due to decreased vascularity are less sensitive to radiation damage than the surrounding normal tissue with normal oxygen tension. Thus, oxygen tension needs to be increased in these tumor cells before they can be effectively treated with radiotherapy. It has been found that the proportion of hypoxic cells in a tumor is roughly equivalent at the beginning and end of a fraction of radiotherapy. Spacing apart the fractions of radiation treatment allows the hypoxic, radioresistant cells that survive the initial radiation fraction to shift to an oxygenated state and become more radiosensitive for the next fraction of radiation. This phenomenon, called reoxygenation, is another rationale for fractionated radiotherapy (8).

Amifostine (WR-2721) is an organic thiophosphate compound whose active metabolite acts as a radioprotector. This metabolite (WR-1065) is radioprotective by its action as a free radical scavenger, by inducing cellular anoxia and possibly by upregulating DNA repair and apoptosis. Amifostine has been used intravenously and subcutaneously to reduce the severity of radiation toxicity (24). It has also been shown to reduce acute and late gastrointestinal toxicity in pelvic radiation for advanced rectal cancer (25). However, a phase I/II placebo controlled study in which increasing doses of WR-2721 enemas were given 45 minutes before each radiation treatment to 24 patients failed to demonstrate protection of the rectosigmoid mucosa. A more recent phase I study has shown encouraging data that rectal amifostine given 30 minutes before radiation may safely reduce rectal radiation damage in prostate radiotherapy (26).

Chemotherapy is often given in conjunction or in series with radiotherapy for pelvic and abdominal malignancies for synergistic or additive tumor control. Many of these chemotherapy agents are also radiosensitizers (27). Chemotherapy agents alone can injure intestinal epithelial cells and impair their function in addition to interfering with stem cell proliferation. When combined with radiotherapy, they enhance the frequency and severity of epithelial cell dysfunction and compromise the repair process (28). These include agents such as adriamycin, actionmycin D, methotrexate, 5-fluorouracil, and bleomycin (4). Five-fluorouracil is an important element in the treatment of gastrointestinal malignancies, and has been shown to increase acute complications without significantly increasing chronic intestinal complications (29,30).

Biological factors that influence tissue response to radiation exposure are the tissue repair rate and the timing of the radiation relative to the cell cycle. The cell cycle for mammalian cells is divided into four phases: mitosis (M), followed by G_1, followed by the DNA synthesis (S), then by G_2 and back to mitosis. In general, cells are most sensitive to radiation in the M and G_2 phases and most resistant in the S phase (31). Rapidly dividing cells such as those found in malignant and intestinal tissue are more radiosensitive because they redistribute the cells faster throughout the cell cycle back into M and G_2 in time for the next fraction of radiation. This phenomenon, called redistribution, explains why acute radiation toxicity is seen more in the rapidly dividing mucosal cells of the intestines than in the slowly dividing cells of the endothelium. Another biological factor is repopulation, or the ability of the cell population to undergo successful mitosis and division to replace the lost cells following radiation. Like redistribution, it is cell-type specific and requires sufficient time between radiation doses to allow for growth.

Radiation damage to the gastrointestinal system may be increased by patient-specific risk factors such as previous abdominal surgery, adhesions, or colitis by causing fixation of the intestines in the radiation field. Damage could theoretically also be exacerbated by factors that predispose to secondary vascular changes: diabetes mellitus, peripheral vascular disease, atherosclerosis, and collagen vascular disease (32,33). However, there is no evidence that there is any significant correlation of radiation injury to the above-mentioned risk factors (2,6,34,35).

Effects of Radiation on Colon and Rectal Cells

The large intestine mucosa is composed of a single layer of epithelial cells, the majority of which are goblet cells with fewer absorptive glandular cells. These glandular cells perform the duties of fluid and electrolyte absorption and lubrication of the feces. Epithelial cells of the colon originate from undifferentiated stem cells in the base of the crypts of Lieberkuhn, which divide to maintain the complete cell turnover rate of four to eight days. The stem cells divide at the germinal centers in the crypts and move up to the mucosa as transitional cells and mature before arriving to replace the dying or sloughed epithelium. The mucosa rests on the more slowly dividing endothelium comprised of interstitial connective tissue and vasculature.

Acute Response

Acute effects of radiation are seen most dramatically in the rapidly proliferating epithelium with immediate cell death, apoptosis, or cessation of mitosis. Within 12 to 24 hours of exposure, epithelial cell death leads to focal denudation or even erosion of the mucosa. This is compounded by stem cell death and dysfunction so that there is an inadequate replacement of dead and dying epithelial cells. The rate of repair, regeneration, and repopulation of the epithelial stem cells determines whether the mucosal injury becomes significant. If radiation damage is too great, the loss of a functional mucosal epithelium will lead to the disruption of the colon's secretory, absorptive, and barrier functions. Microulcerations will expand to form erosions with subsequent bleeding. Translocation of gut bacteria into the vasculature may result in bacteremia and sepsis. Recovery will occur in spite of the severe acuity of the damage if the radiation insult is not overwhelming. However, some epithelial abnormalities may persist (35,36).

Chronic Response

Endothelial or vascular cells are less sensitive to early radiation injury but do sustain acute injury that is rarely evident in the immediate setting. Acute vascular changes may occur with a resultant decrease in mucosal blood flow, which can potentiate epithelial cell damage. Acute vascular damage leads to capillary swelling, increased vascular permeability and interstitial edema. Because these are slowly dividing cells, delayed effects are seen usually more than six months to years from the time of radiation damage. Chronic injury may result in progressive ischemia caused by fibrosis of the endothelium and connective tissue. This insidious ischemia most often leads to mucosal injury rather than ulceration and necrosis. Radiation may induce abnormal fibroblast function causing fibrosis. At times, fibrosis may result in stricture formation as well as fistulas between irradiated organs. The result of this chronic process is a thickened, ulcerated, fibrotic bowel and rectum.

Acute injury poses less of a significant clinical problem because it is usually self-limited and responds to modification of the radiation regimen or symptom-directed therapy. On the other hand, chronic injury to the colon and rectum presents a more daunting clinical problem due to the underlying pathology that is often refractory to current therapeutic options.

PATHOLOGY

The temporal occurrence of radiation pathology can be divided into immediate (less than 24 hours), early (24 hours to six months), and delayed (greater than six months) damage. The rectum and sigmoid colon are the most common sites of injury due to their reduced mobility from being fixed as well as their proximity to radiation targets such as the cervix and the prostate.

Acute

Acute changes are mainly inflammatory, and are most obvious in the mucosa. Within hours of radiation exposure, epithelial cell death can be seen with the surviving cells often exhibiting atypical features: enlargement, loss of nuclear polarity, reduced mitoses, and decreasing proliferation rates. The undifferentiated stem cells at the base of the crypts of Lieberkuhn are also affected so that with escalating exposure, the rate of repopulation, regeneration, and maturation cannot keep up with the epithelial cell death. This leads to focal and diffuse ulcer formation and erosions (9,37,38).

Inflammatory changes are seen with infiltration of neutrophils and plasma cells and loss of lymphocytes from the lamina propria. An increase in permeability causes hyperemia and edema with swelling of the mucosa and submucosa as seen on microscopy (4,39–41). There may also be variable amount of fibrin deposition in the submucosa (11). An increase in eosinophils along with other inflammatory cells and sloughed, dead epithelial cells contribute to crypt abscess formation (37,42). The submucosa may have sustained damage and have fibrinous deposition but may not show evidence of damage early on in radiation exposure (11).

Chronic

Delayed or chronic lesions can be seen from six months to 30 years after therapy, but usually manifest within one to five years. They are mainly due to delayed submucosal damage to the blood vessels and connective tissue that causes a progressive ischemia. Histologically, there are little or no inflammatory changes. Nevertheless, the epithelium demonstrates atrophy with occasional atypical nuclei present. There may be delayed necrosis with ulcerations and thickening with fibrosis (11). Fibrosis is seen in a heterogeneous pattern throughout the stroma and is thought to be a delayed expression of radiation injury due to ischemia and fibroblast dysfunction. Fibrinous exudate deposition is thought to be due to secondary damage of the vasculature with basement membrane disruption, activation of the coagulation system, and depletion of plasminogen activator with reduction in ability to break down and resorb fibrin deposition (43). Atypical, large fibroblasts with multiple cytoplasmic projections, irregular and hyperchromatic nuclei are found with the extensive fibrosis (44).

Vascular damage that leads to vascular insufficiency and ischemic changes is most evident in the capillary system because the capillary endothelium is very radiosensitive. Endothelial cells degenerate, detach from the basement membrane, or have swelling of their cytoplasm such that the capillary lumen becomes obstructed (43). The luminal obstruction is perpetuated by thrombosis due to fibrin and platelet aggregation as well as endothelial cell rupture. These endothelial cells with irregular walls and luminal thrombosis contribute to the formation of telangiectasias. Moreover, there is not only capillary damage but also a significant loss of capillaries relative to larger vessels, as the capillaries do not have the supportive scaffolding of smooth muscle, and connective tissue of large vessels. Thus, less damage is seen with increasing arterial size. The obliterative damage, luminal obstruction, and overall loss of capillaries is progressive and a significant cause of ischemia. Smaller arterioles also have subendothelial and adventitial fibrosis with hyalinization of the media with lipid laden macrophages or foam cells often residing in the intima. Although capillary and small arteriole changes are most common, venous lesions are also seen (45).

Vascular complications lead to the formation of visible telangiectatic vessels that are often friable and prone to bleeding (46). Progressive ischemia causes necrosis and fibrosis. The necrosis occasionally leads to ulcer formation. Complications of radiation-induced ulceration include perforation, abscess formation, and fistula formation between irradiated organs. The ischemic and atypical fibroblast-induced fibrosis over time forms strictures and adhesions. The strictures are due to submucosal and serosal fibrosis (43). These late complications contribute to the clinical presentation of chronic radiation colopathy and proctopathy.

Over the years, there have been approximately 60 cases of secondary malignancy found in sites of radiation treatment. Secondary cancers cannot be attributed to radiation sequelae unless they arise in an irradiated segment of bowel, are flanked by tissue on either side with chronic radiation changes, and occur at least 5 to 10 years after the treatment (47). There have been data that suggest a relative risk of 2 to 3.6 of secondary cancer following radiation therapy to the bowel (48). In spite of this, it is unclear whether the increase in secondary cancers may be due to mutations in oncogenes or radiation-induced immunosuppression and tumor promotion (46,49).

CLINICAL MANIFESTATIONS

Patients with primary malignancies of the prostate, testes, uterus, cervix, bladder, and colon who undergo radiation therapy may present with acute or chronic radiation damage to the rectum and colon. Up to 30% to 50% of patients may develop acute gastrointestinal side effects from radiation to the colon and rectum (4,50). In one study, 50% of patients undergoing radiation therapy to the prostate, reported acute gastrointestinal side effects that had a moderate to severe impact on their daily living (51). The field of literature on this topic is best divided into information on injury to the colon (colopathy) and rectal damage (proctopathy).

Radiation Colopathy

Published data on the acute and chronic symptoms of radiation colopathy alone have been limited. This is because the radiation treatment fields often include both the small and large intestine as well as the rectum. Symptoms of radiation colopathy are often nonspecific or difficult to localize. Acute symptoms of radiation colopathy include nausea, vomiting, diarrhea, pain, and occasionally bleeding. The pain is often nonspecific but may be cramping and diffuse. Nausea and vomiting may be due to the systemic effects of radiation, which are mediated by neurotransmitters and endogenous splanchnic chemicals on the central and enteric nervous system (52). Diarrhea, characterized by six or more stools per day, develops within two to four weeks and is usually self-limited. It can be due to small intestinal injury but primarily is caused by decreased colonic water reabsorption and altered motility. The symptoms of nausea, pain, diarrhea, and tenesmus usually halt within four to six weeks after completion of the radiation therapy (6,51,53).

Late symptoms of radiation colopathy are most often the result from strictures, fistulas, ulcerations, perforation, and abscess formation (2,7). Chronic colopathy can present with diarrhea, but this is usually seen in conjunction with proctopathy. Crampy abdominal pain with associated tenesmus is experienced by a minority of patients. Strictures and adhesions can cause colonic obstruction that present with symptoms such as cramps, abdominal pain, nausea, vomiting, and narrowing of the stool caliber (54). Ulcerations and abscesses present with localized abdominal pain, fevers, and peritoneal signs if perforation has occurred (50). Fistulas cause symptoms unique to the anatomical location and pathway of the fistula (6). Among the fistulas, connections from the large intestine to the bladder, vagina, or small intestine are the most common.

Radiation Proctopathy

Because the rectum is the most common site of injury following pelvic irradiation and is easily accessible for evaluation, most published literature on gastrointestinal injury from radiation is on proctopathy. Acute radiation proctopathy occurs in up to 30% of patients undergoing pelvic irradiation. This is characterized by diarrhea, mucoid rectal discharge, pain with defecation, and urgency (55,56). Rectal bleeding may be present, but not of the severity as seen with chronic radiation proctopathy. There is some suggestion that the severity of acute symptoms may predict the likelihood and severity of late symptoms (57–59).

The most common sign of chronic radiation proctopathy is bleeding. This bleeding arises from fragile telangiectasias and friable mucosa that easily bleed in response to minor trauma such as stool passage (6,33,50,60). On occasion, bleeding may be severe enough to cause transfusion-dependent anemia. Impaired rectal compliance and anal sphincter dysfunction may cause other symptoms such as evacuation difficulty, frequent elimination, incontinence, and urgency (61). Direct nerve damage, internal and external sphincter muscle damage, and chronic fibrosis have been implicated in anal sphincter dysfunction (47,62,63).

DIAGNOSIS
Acute

Physical findings in acute proctocolopathy are nonspecific. Patients with acute radiation proctocolopathy with nausea and vomiting may have plain films that show ileus and altered motility. Barium studies of the rectum and colon reveal mucosal edema and occasional ulcerations. There may be colonic spasms, and thumbprinting may be seen at sites of focal edema (64). Endoscopic investigation shows rectal and colonic mucosa that is edematous and congested with granular textures, friability, and ulcerations (65,66). These diagnostic findings of radiation injury may be nonspecific or not present. The endoscopic findings may be mimicked by inflammatory bowel disease, ischemic colitis, and other infectious colitis. Moreover, the severity and extent of radiation injury may not correlate with the severity and nature of the clinical manifestations.

Chronic

Barium studies may reveal absent haustra, and thickening of the affected segments with narrowing due to fibrosis (67). Strictures, fistulas, and ulcerations can also be seen and must be differentiated from recurrent tumor (68). Computed tomography scans can help to detect recurrence of the primary malignancy, locate abscesses, fistulas, and thickening of the colon and rectum (69). Endoscopic findings include mucosal pallor and telangiectasias (Fig. 3). Ulcerations and stricture formation are less common (66). Endoscopic ultrasound may show segmental thickening of the rectal wall and loss of normal haustra (70).

Anorectal manometry in patients with established symptoms of chronic radiation proctopathy have provided some explanation for the fecal urgency, incontinence, and pain. A reduction in rectal compliance and capacitance has been noted. Anal sphincter effects have included decreased basal resting pressures and voluntary maximal pressures. Increased rectal sensitivity to distention has also been demonstrated (62,63,71–75). Iwamoto et al. studied 31 patients receiving radiation therapy for cervical cancer. All patients underwent anorectal manometry at baseline, during therapy, and at six months after therapy. This study demonstrated that one-third of patients had an acute and chronic reduction in rectal compliance and capacitance following radiation therapy (76). Two other prospective studies compared rectal manometry before and after radiation therapy for pelvic malignancy (61,77). The first study of 35 patients found a reduction in rectal compliance, an increase in rectal sensitivity, and a decrease in minimal basal and maximal anal squeeze pressures. This suggested that radiation caused rectal wall injury and internal and external anal sphincter dysfunction (61). Further analysis showed that this acute dysfunction and a decrease in rectal volumes for perception and desire to defecate had predictive significance on chronic anorectal dysfunction and symptoms (74). Further studies to determine the mechanisms of radiation-induced symptoms of proctopathy are awaited (78,79).

Classification Systems

Diagnostic classification systems have also been proposed by several groups. They include the LENT system: late effects of radiation on normal tissue, and the SOMA parameters: subjective, objective, management criteria, analytical laboratory, and imaging procedures (12,29,80). This system was proposed to replace many existing late-effects assessment scales including the Radiation therapy oncology group (RTOG)/European organization for research and treatment of cancer (EORTC), which was most widely used (81). A valid diagnostic system is necessary for comparison and sharing of data and research on radiation injury as well as to optimize radiation therapy techniques for maximum tumor killing with minimal normal tissue damage. The Late effects of normal tissue (LENT)/Subjective, objective management and analytic scales (SOMA) system is an improvement on the RTOG/EORTC scale, but needs further validation and adjustments based on prospective randomized studies (82–84).

In our current pharmacotherapeutic trials for functional symptoms of radiation proctopathy, we propose the use of a modified Likert scale to quantify the severity and frequency of symptoms. Frequency and severity of symptoms are scored using the following scales and combined to give a total score (Table 4). Pre- and posttreatment total scores are compared to assess the effectiveness of therapy. Endoscopic grading of injury severity also suffers from a lack of a universally accepted scale. However visualization of a confluence or patches of telangiectasias appears to correlate with increased risk for bleeding (85).

(A)   **(B)**   **(C)**

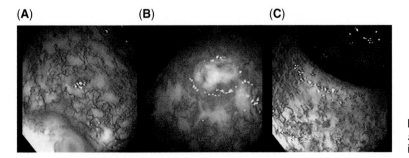

Figure 3 (*See color insert*) Endoscopic findings in radiation proctopathy.

Table 4   Modified Likert Scale

Symptoms	Severity	Frequency
Diarrhea		
Urgency		
Rectal pain		
Tenesmus		
Rectal bleeding		
Fecal incontinence		
Other symptoms		
Total score		

Frequency	Score
Monthly	1
Weekly	2
Several times a week	3
Daily	4
Throughout the day	5

Severity	Score	Explanation
No problem	1	
Mild problem	2	Can be ignored when you do not think about it
Moderate problem	3	Cannot be ignored; no effect on daily activities
Severe problem	4	Influences your concentration on daily activities
Very severe problem	5	Markedly influences your daily activities and/or requires rest

MEDICAL AND ENDOSCOPIC THERAPY

An analysis of the published literature on management of radiation colopathy and proctopathy reveals that the overwhelming majority of articles are case reports. Fewer than 10 randomized trials have been performed (86). These studies are all essentially focused on proctopathy. The data often reflects retrospective analysis of a small number of heterogeneous patients with inconsistent symptomatic and endoscopic grading of the baseline disease state. Without a universally accepted or utilized grading system, consistent comparison of baseline and endpoint has not been possible. Thus, the therapeutic value or efficacy of a treatment is often equivocal and studies cannot be directly compared. What is more, the natural history of radiation colopathy and proctopathy has not been fully elucidated. Moreover, the patients in the medical literature may not be representative of routine patients with these diseases due to selection bias. Given these limitations, management of patients with symptomatic radiation colopathy and proctopathy has often been empirical based upon individual and institutional experience (Table 5). Nevertheless, some basic concepts stand out:

1. Acute radiation symptoms are usually self-limited and treated symptomatically.
2. Rectal bleeding secondary to telangiectasias is treated topically, generally with cautery or sclerosis.
3. Virtually no pharmacotherapeutic studies have addressed functional symptoms of radiation proctopathy as a separate entity.

Radiation Colopathy

As mentioned, the therapy of acute and chronic colopathy has lacked controlled trials. Treatment is generally targeted at symptoms. Severe, acute symptoms are generally managed by the radiation oncologist by adjustments to the radiation course via a small reduction of the dose fraction or splitting of the therapy into twice daily treatments (87).

Methods for prevention of radiation colopathy are under study. Performance of radiation therapy aims to minimize complications by accurate radiation planning and dosing techniques such as 3-D conformal radiotherapy, and by adjustments of dosage and fractionation scheduling if early symptoms develop. Proposed prevention options have included the use of prophylactic antibiotics, aspirin, elemental diets, and radioprotective drugs. Elemental diets are thought to be radioprotective by reducing pancreatobiliary secretions and improving nutrient absorption (88).

Table 5 Medical and Endoscopic Therapy for Radiation Colopathy and Proctopathy

Medical	Endoscopic
Antiemetics (PO)	Heater probe
Antidiarrheals (PO)	Bipolar electrocoagulator
Anticholinergics (PO)	Nd:YAG laser
Amifostine (WR-2721) (IV, SC)	Argon laser
Sucralfate (PO)	KTP laser
Short chain fatty acids (butyric acid) (PO)	Argon plasma coagulator
5-Aminosalicyclic acid (PO, PR)	
Corticosteroids (PO, PR)	
Pentosan polysulfate (PO)	
Retinol palmitate (PO)	
Antioxidants (vitamin C, E) (PO)	
Formalin (PR)	
Hyperbaric oxygen	
Metronidazole (PO)	
Hormone therapy (estrogen, progestin) (PO)	
Misoprostol (PO)	
Total parenteral nutrition	

Note: PO, oral; PR, enema; Nd:YAG, neodymium:yttrium aluminum garnet; KTP, potassium titanyl phosphate.

The radioprotective drug WR-2721 has shown promise as a free radical scavenger in preventing radiation damage.

Pharmacotherapy

Conservative treatment using antidiarrheals such as loperamide or diphenoxylate with dietary avoidance of lactose and other osmotic agents are effective for diarrhea. Abdominal or rectal pain and cramping can be treated with antispasmodics, anticholinergics, and mild analgesics, or narcotics. Nausea and vomiting at this stage responds to 5-hydroxytryptamine type-3 receptor blockers such as ondansetron as well as to general antiemetics such as metoclopropamide and prochlorperazine. Supplemental oral nutrition and even total parenteral nutrition may be an important arsenal in complete patient care, but there is little evidence that it impacts the outcome or severity of radiation colopathy (89). Sigmoid disease may benefit from treatment directed at proctopathy due to its close proximity.

Endoscopy

Endoscopic treatment of colopathy is limited mainly to cautery or sclerosing of sigmoid telangiectasias that are often contiguous with rectal lesions. This will be covered in more detail below.

PROCTOPATHY

Therapy for radiation proctopathy has benefited from evidence from a few randomized controlled trials. However, most drug trials have failed to show therapeutic benefit or have had conflicting results. Nevertheless, several show promise but require confirmation in larger, randomized trials.

Pharmacotherapy

Patients with tenesmus and rectal discharge from acute proctopathy can be treated with Sitz baths, analgesic or narcotics, steroid enemas, and dietary adjustments to increase stool bulk. Symptomatic treatments including antidiarrheals and anticholinergics for diarrhea and rectal pain have also been used with success. Preventive studies are under way and are currently focused on WR-2721 and sucralfate (26).

5-Aminosalicyclic Acid

5-aminosalicyclic acid (5-ASA) is the active component of sulfasalazine, which is used to treat ulcerative colitis (90). Its effective use in ulcerative colitis led to studies using oral and rectal preparations that showed disappointing results (91–93). A randomized trial of prophylactic 5-ASA during radiotherapy for prostate cancer was ended early when the 5-ASA group had a sixfold greater acute proctopathy symptom development when compared to placebo (94). Because 5-ASA may work by decreasing prostaglandins, and a recent trial of prostaglandin E1 (misoprostol) showed improvement of acute radiation proctopathy, 5-ASA may actually worsen radiation injury to the colon and rectum (95).

Steroids

Anti-inflammatory agents such as corticosteroids have been recommended as treatment for radiation injury despite a lack of clinical trial data. It would be anticipated that the anti-inflammatory effects of corticosteroids have little effect on the telangiectasias, anorectal compliance, or fibrostenosis of chronic radiation proctopathy. Several small trials, however, appeared to show some benefit but most showed little evidence for efficacy (91,93,96). Conversely, corticosteroid enemas may exacerbate hemorrhoids and bleeding from rectal telangiectasias (70).

Sucralfate

Sucralfate is a highly sulfated polyanionic disaccharide used for treatment of gastric and duodenal ulcers. Its mechanism of action for mucosal protection is postulated to be due to formation of a protective barrier to fecal toxins by adherence to positively charged proteins on ulcer bases (97). Sucralfate may also induce angiogenesis, encourage epithelial regeneration by binding basic fibroblastic growth factor, and increase cytoprotection by inducing prostaglandin secretion (98–101). One study demonstrated no benefit of rectal sucralfate during radiotherapy of the prostate in the reduction of symptoms of acute radiation proctopathy (51). Two randomized, placebo-controlled trials reported reduction of acute and chronic bowel discomfort in patients given prophylactic oral sucralfate during radiotherapy for localized malignancies of the pelvis (102,103). In more recent randomized controlled trials, oral sucralfate given during pelvic radiation therapy did not reduce the symptoms of acute radiation toxicity (104,105). In one of these studies, an increase in fecal incontinence and nausea were more common in patients taking sucralfate compared to the placebo group (104). The other study demonstrated that patients receiving sucralfate had increased risk of acute bleeding compared to placebo (105). The cause of these toxicities in the sucralfate group was unclear.

Several retrospective reports have suggested that oral or rectal sucralfate may improve symptoms in chronic radiation proctosigmoidopathy (106–109). A prospective, open-label study of 26 patients followed for an average of 45 months found that topical sucralfate induced lasting remission in the majority of patients with moderate to severe bleeding from radiation proctosigmoidopathy (110). A randomized controlled trial of 37 patients comparing rectal sucralfate versus rectal steroids and oral 5-ASA found that both treatments were effective, but that sucralfate enemas had a better clinical response and were tolerated better by patients. These differences were not statistically significant. No changes in the severity of findings on endoscopy were seen with either treatment (96).

Pentosan Polysulfate

Pentosan polysulfate is a heparin-like macromolecule with anticoagulant and fibrinolytic effects that is used for interstitial cystitis and chronic radiation cystitis. Grigsby et al. performed a phase I/II trial of 13 patients with chronic radiation proctopathy. This group found that 9 out of the 13 patients obtained a complete response defined as a complete disappearance of symptoms. This was based on a graded scale of symptoms and lifestyle modifications or disruptions scored from one to five (111). However, four patients out of the nine responders had relapsed at one year, and one patient developed a maculopapular rash that was attributed to the pentosan polysulfate.

Short Chain Fatty Acids

Short chain fatty acids (SCFA) are an important source of energy for colonic mucosa with butyric acid being the most important (112). They are produced by bacterial fermentation of nonabsorbed carbohydrates. They were effective in treating diversion colitis, and this success led to studies in radiation colopathy. SCFA may increase mucosal blood flow and exert a trophic effect on colonic mucosa by promoting proliferation and cell differentiation (113,114).

A randomized, double-blind, crossover trial of topical butyric acid on 20 patients with acute radiation proctopathy found that butyric acid led to remission in their symptoms (115). An initial case report of seven patients with chronic radiation proctopathy showed promise of clinical, endoscopic, and histologic improvement (116). Another report of six patients with chronic radiation proctopathy suggested clinical improvement that was not statistically significant (117). Talley et al. performed a randomized, double-blind, controlled, crossover trial in 15 patients with chronic radiation proctopathy. This trial showed a statistically insignificant improvement in the total symptom score and histology in patients on SCFA. Endoscopic appearances were largely unchanged by the SCFA treatment (118). A more recent randomized, double-blind, controlled trial of 19 patients with chronic radiation proctopathy showed a tendency of diminished rectal bleeding in the treated group. However, there was no statistically significant endoscopic or histologic improvement or sustained long-term benefit compared to placebo (112).

Antioxidants

Chronic radiation proctopathy characterized by fibrosis and vascular insufficiency due to collagen proliferation and chronic ischemia are postulated to be a result of reactive oxygen metabolites. Antioxidants such as vitamins E and C were studied in chronic radiation proctopathy based on the hypothesis that counteracting reactive oxygen metabolites may slow or stop the vicious cycle of fibrosis and ischemia. One open-label trial enrolled 20 patients taking daily vitamin E (400 IU, three times a day) and vitamin C (500 mg, three times a day), and found that it was associated with an improvement in their symptoms of bleeding, diarrhea, and urgency as well as their lifestyle. The patients graded the severity and frequency of rectal bleeding, rectal pain, diarrhea, and fecal urgency as assessed by a telephone questionnaire. They also filled out a questionnaire at baseline and one year after treatment, regarding the impact of these symptoms on their lifestyle. However, the study had a high drop-out rate, no control group, and may have been prone to recall bias (119).

Hyperbaric Oxygen

Hyperbaric oxygen therapy acts by increasing tissue oxygenation, increasing capillary angiogenesis, reducing edema, and inhibiting bacterial growth and toxin production (120). A number of case studies with less than 50 patients have reported improvement or cessation of rectal bleeding with hyperbaric oxygen therapy in chronic radiation proctopathy (86,121–130). However, these reports could not be compared directly because of variations in the hyperbaric oxygen pressures and duration used as well as heterogeneous patient populations enrolled. Most studies also did not have statistical measurement or analysis of the stated improvement. Hyperbaric oxygen has potential side effects of middle ear and sinus barotrauma, pulmonary oxygen toxicity, chest tightness, and central nervous system toxicity including ocular damage (86,121–130). The average number of treatment sessions was 24, with the range of 12 to 40 sessions (126). The expense for these hyperbaric oxygen treatments is significant, and the equipment is only available at specialized centers.

Formalin

Topical formalin is a solution of formaldehyde gas that is used for refractory radiation-induced cystitis (131). It has also been used commercially for embalming, fireproofing, glues, adhesives, and tanning (132). Topical formalin solution had been reported as early as 1986 to be successful in controlling bleeding from radiation-induced proctopathy (133). Its purported mechanism of action is local chemical cauterization by sealing in fragile telangiectasias on contact. The formalin seals oozing from neovascularized telangiectasias that develops from chronic radiation injury. More than 10 reports comprising more than 150 patients have differed on the technique of administration and on the duration of therapy. The formalin may be applied by direct contact to the visualized telangiectasias using sponges or gauze or may be irrigated into the rectum using anoscopes (134,135). Often, general anesthesia was utilized. The formalin was kept in contact for a fixed total time or until the bleeding ceased. These studies reported success in these heterogeneous patients who had often failed medical or surgical therapy (136–141). The overall outcome was excellent for controlling rectal bleeding with a median follow-up period of close to one year. Relapses usually responded to repeat applications of formalin. Unfortunately, severe anal pain, anal ulcerations, anal fissures, and worsening of strictures have been reported (134,135,140,141). Therefore, care must be taken to protect the perianal area with draping and lubrication to avoid direct formalin contact injury.

Miscellaneous

Other medical therapies that have been studied include metronidazole, hormonal therapy, and transexamic acid. There has been one study on metronidazole with and without corticosteroid and 5-ASA enemas for 60 chronic radiation proctopathy patients. It showed favorable outcomes for the metronidazole group by a lower bleeding, ulceration, diarrhea, and edema rate up to 12 months after treatment (142). Hormonal therapy using estrogen progestin has been limited to case studies that report bleeding cessation but also worsening cardiovascular disease (143–146). Our group has promising data on the use of oral retinol palmitate for treatment (147). As mentioned above, functional symptoms of radiation proctopathy have yet to be studied in pharmacological trials.

Endoscopy

Chronic, recurrent hematochezia after radiation therapy may be more likely from discrete telangiectasias rather than diffuse proctopathy or colopathy (148). Endoscopic therapy is an important mainstay for patients with rectal bleeding because it can treat discrete problem areas by the obliteration of the telangiectasias and bleeding sites. Because minor bleeding is self-limited and is amenable to iron supplementation, only those patients with persistent or severe bleeding are likely to benefit from endoscopic cauterization. Patients who benefit from endoscopic treatment are those who have chronic rectal bleeding from endoscopically proven radiation telangiectasias and mucosal abnormalities (148,149). They are also those who have been refractory to conservative medical therapy and have become transfusion dependent (150). It is also important to rule out tumor recurrence and nonrectal causes of bleeding.

Endoscopic cauterization of bleeding can be done by contact or noncontact methods. Contact endoscopic probes include the bipolar eletrocoagulation and heater probes. Noncontact endoscopic photocoagulation has been done using the neodymium:yttrium:aluminum:garnet (Nd:YAG) laser or argon plasma coagulation. Most patients require multiple endoscopic treatment sessions before bleeding ceases.

The bipolar electrocoagulation and the heater probes cause direct contact coagulation of focal bleeding telangiectasias. Scarring of the tissue and reepithelialization with normal tissues occur over time until the bleeding telangiectasias are obliterated. A randomized, prospective trial using bipolar electrocoagulation and heater probe for chronic rectal bleeding found that severe bleeding episodes decreased and patient-reported symptoms improved (148). Another preliminary study reported that contact coagulation was superior to Nd:YAG laser in safety and efficacy (151). However, the contact method may itself induce bleeding by direct trauma and require significantly longer treatment sessions (150,152).

Laser therapy using Nd:YAG and argon lasers have been studied and found to be effective in the short term for radiation-induced rectal bleeding. The Nd:YAG trials enrolled between 4 and 59 patients, and used variable power settings and had different follow-up times. All of the studies found that the majority of patients with bleeding responded within two to three treatment sessions (153–159). The Nd:YAG laser has a wavelength of $1.06\,\mu m$ and is invisible with a depth of penetration up to 5 mm (153). It is able to coagulate large vessels up to 5 mm in diameter and induces a homogeneous tissue coagulation (160). In comparison, the argon laser has a depth of penetration of 2 mm, and is able to coagulate vessels up to 1 to 2 mm in diameter. Both lasers are preferentially absorbed more efficiently by the darker ectatic blood vessels as opposed to the lighter radiation injured mucosa (150). The Nd:YAG laser's deeper penetration and wider coagulation diameter allows greater possibility of controlling bleeding from larger vessels with an increased risk of transmural necrosis with perforation and ulcerations. The deeper penetration may coagulate submucosal vessels and aggravate the ischemic irradiated tissue to stricture and fistula formation (159). Complication rates have varied between 5% and 15% including ileus, perforation, pain, fistula, and ulcerations (158). The argon beam laser appears to be safer with less fibrosis, stricture formation, and transmural inflammation (161).

The development of the argon plasma coagulation has decreased the use of Nd:YAG and argon lasers for management of radiation-induced gastrointestinal bleeding. Argon plasma coagulation is the application of an ionized stream of argon gas toward the target tissue. It is not a laser, but uses a high-voltage spark at the tip of the probe to ionize a stream of gas that is sprayed toward the target tissue. With the usual setting of 50 W, the depth of penetration is 2 to 3 mm and can coagulate linearly and tangentially. It has been used to control superficial bleeding during hepatic surgery. In the setting of radiation proctopathy, argon coagulation may be advantageous compared to the laser therapy because of its ease of application, lower risk of damage with a reduced and more predictable depth of penetration, and lower cost. Argon plasma coagulation has been found to be safe and effective with an average of two to four sessions for complete symptom relief (162–166). It may be easier if the coagulation is done in the retroflexed position. To this end, we recommend use of the smaller upper endoscopes rather than sigmoidoscopes or colonoscopes to facilitate the ease of treatment.

Endoscopic therapies along with formalin have become mainstays in the treatment of persistent bleeding from chronic radiation proctosigmoidopathy because of their safety profile and efficacy. Although there have been no direct comparisons to medical therapies, given the relative ineffectiveness of pharmacologic therapy, it is generally reasonable to utilize endoscopic cauterization. The choice of vehicle for cauterization will depend on local availability and experience, although argon plasma coagulation seems to have the greatest ease and safety.

SURGICAL THERAPY

A majority of colorectal radiation injuries can be managed without the need for surgery. Surgical intervention, however, is required for cases of intractable bleeding, intestinal obstruction, perforation, fistula formation, or fecal incontinence. Because surgical treatment of radiation injuries, particularly surgical resection of the radiated rectum, is associated with a high risk for perioperative morbidity and even mortality, careful assessment of the relative virtues of operative versus nonoperative management must be undertaken. Additionally, a realistic appreciation of what surgery can accomplish in these difficult cases must be acknowledged.

Most cases of severe radiation proctopathy can be successfully palliated with a simple diverting stoma without resection of the affected rectum (167). Diversion of the fecal stream from the rectum is effective for cases complicated by severe diarrhea, incontinence, strictures, and fistula formation. It is also an effective treatment for intractable bleeding or pain. Intestinal stoma formation affords effective palliation of colovaginal fistulas, but healing of these fistulas with simple diversion is unlikely to occur. In most cases, an end colostomy with a Hartmann's closure of the distal segment is preferred. In cases of radiation-induced stricture, a Hartmann's closure is to be avoided and either a double-barreled colostomy or an end stoma with a mucus fistula should be performed. This approach prevents the accumulation of mucus and distention in the segment proximal to the obstruction that would otherwise occur if the rectal stump proximal to the stricture were closed. Complications associated with colostomy formation for the treatment of radiation proctitis include peristomal fistula, stomal retraction, and necrosis (168). Utilization of healthy proximal bowel that is well mobilized to prevent tension on the stoma site can minimize these problems. When a diverting stoma is utilized for the treatment of radiation proctopathy, the stoma will often be permanent as healing of a diverted rectum sufficient to allow reestablishment of the intestinal continuity without resection or reconstruction, is uncommon.

Resection with anastomosis may be considered for patients if diversion does not satisfactorily control symptoms or if the stoma itself is otherwise poorly tolerated. Resection of the rectum with successful low colorectal or coloanal anastomosis (preferably with construction of a colonic J-pouch) can allow for reestablishment of the intestinal continuity and continence (169–172). These procedures, however, have been associated with high-complication rates and poor long-term functional results for many patients (173–175). In fact, for patients with radiation injury extending to the sphincter muscles, the functional results after resection and anastomosis may be worse than the inconveniences associated with an ileostomy or colostomy. If such a reconstructive procedure is performed, it should be accompanied by a temporary fecal diversion.

Due to the differences in radiation techniques and the considerable variability in individual response to radiation therapy, the perioperative course is difficult to predict on an individual basis and absolute guidelines for the safety of surgical resection and anastomosis are limited. In general, however, it has been recommended that resection and reconstructive procedures not be performed when the prognosis for long-term survival is poor, when the radiation injury extends to below the midrectum, or when the total pelvic radiation has exceeded 6000 cGy (175). These guidelines may have to be violated in extreme cases, but as a rule, surgical management of complications related to radiation proctopathy should be based on as simple a procedure as possible to ameliorate symptoms and extend life (173,175,176).

CONCLUSION

Radiation proctocolopathy is an unfortunate sequelae of radiation therapy. Although elucidation of its natural history will continue to be a challenge, accurate measurement of its incidence and prevalence will aid in developing universally accepted diagnostic criteria. Diagnostic criteria need to be developed to encompass the functional symptoms of radiation proctopathy. Finally, the review of treatment options reveals a great need for randomized control studies. Further studies to compare medical therapy to endoscopic or surgical therapies remain to be carried out. Finally, focusing future research on prevention of radiation injury by developing improved radiotherapy protocols and techniques may be the best option to reduce the impact of this challenging disease.

ACKNOWLEDGMENTS

The authors thank Ashesh Jani, M.D., Department of Radiation Oncology at the University of Chicago, for his assistance in reviewing the radiation oncology aspects of this chapter.

REFERENCES

1. Walsh D. Deep tissue traumatism from Roentgen ray exposure. BMJ 1897; 2:272.
2. Decosse JJ, Rhodes RS, Entz WB, Reagan JW, et al. The natural history and management of radiation induced injury of the gastrointestinal tract. Ann Surg 1969; 170:369–384.
3. Buchi K. Radiation proctopathy: therapy and prognosis. J Am Med Assoc 1991; 265:1180.
4. Kinsella TJ, Bloomer WD. Tolerance of the intestine to radiation therapy. Surg Gynecol Obstet 1980; 151:273–284.
5. Cho KH, Lee CK, Levitt SH. Proctitis after conventional external radiation therapy for prostate cancer: importance of minimizing posterior rectal dose. Radiology 1995; 195:699–703.
6. Gilinsky NH, Burns DG, Barbezat GO, et al. The natural history of radiation-induced proctosigmoiditis: an analysis of 88 patients. Q J Med 1983; 52:40–53.
7. Fischer L, Kimose HH, Spjeldnaes N, Wara P. Late progress of radiation-induced proctitis. Acta Chir Scand 1990; 156:801–805.
8. Fajardo LF, Berthrong M, Anderson R. Basic radiation, physics, chemistry and biology B.M. In: Fajardo LF, Anderson RE, eds. Radiation Pathology. New York: Oxford University Press, 2001:3–17.
9. Ming S, Goldman H. Disorders common to the gastrointestinal tract. In: Ming GHS, ed. Pathology of the Gastrointestinal Tract. Williams and Wilkins: Baltimore, 1998:210–217.
10. Hall EJ. The physics and chemistry of radiation absorption. In: Hall EJ, ed. Radiobiology for the Radiologist. Philadelphia: J.B. : Lippincott, 1994:1–13.
11. Berthrong M, Fajardo LF. Radiation injury in surgical pathology. Part II. Alimentary tract. Am J Surg Pathol 1981; 5(2):153–178.
12. Rubin P, Constine LS, Fajardo LF, et al. Overview: late effects of normal tissues (LENT) scoring system. Int J Radiat Oncol Biol Phys 1995; 31(5):1041–1042.
13. Rubin P, Casarett GW. A direction for clinical radiation pathology. In: Frontiers of Radiation Therapy and Oncology. University Park Press: Baltimore, 1972:1–16.
14. Hall EJ. Cell survival curves. In: Hall EJ, ed. Radiobiology for the Radiologist. Philadelphia: J.B. Lippincott, 1994:29–44.
15. Hanks GE, Schultheiss TE, Hanlon AL, Hunt M, et al. Optimization of conformal radiation treatment of prostate cancer: report of a dose escalation study. Int J Radiat Oncol Biol Phys 1997; 37(3):543–550.
16. Ling CC, Burman C, Chui CS, et al. Conformal radiation treatment of prostate cancer using inversely-planned intensity-modulated photon beams produced with dynamic multileaf collimation. Int J Radiat Oncol Biol Phys 1996; 35:721.
17. Fraass BA, Kessler ML, McShan DL, et al. Optimization and clinical use of multisegment intensity-modulated radiation therapy for high-dose conformal therapy. Semin Radiat Oncol 1999; 9:60.
18. Zelefsky MJ, Cowen D, Fuks Z, et al. Long term tolerance of high dose three-dimensional conformal radiotherapy in patients with localized prostate carcinoma. Cancer 1999; 85:2460–2468.

19. Dearnaley DP, Khoo VS, Norman AR, et al. Comparison of radiation side-effects of conformal and conventional radiotherapy in prostate cancer: a randomised trial. Lancet 1999; 353:267–272.
20. Lechner P, Cesnik H. Abdominopelvic omentopexy: Preparatory procedure for radiotherapy in rectal cancer. Dis Colon Rectum 1992; 35:1157–1160.
21. Hoffman JP, Lanciano R, Carp NZ, et al. Morbidity after intraperitoneal insertion of saline-filled tissue expanders for small bowel exclusion from radiotherapy treatment fields: a prospective four-year experience with 34 patients. Am Surg 1994; 60:473–482.
22. Trimbos JB, Snijders-Keilholz T, Peters AA. Feasibility of the application of a resorbable polyglycolic-acid mesh (Dexon mesh) to prevent complications of radiotherapy following gynecological surgery. Eur J Surg 1991; 157:281–284.
23. Van Kasteren YM, Burger CW, Meijer OW, et al. Efficacy of a synthetic mesh sling in keeping the small bowel in the upper abdomen to prevent radiation enteropathy in gynecologic malignancies. Eur J Obstet Gynecol Reprod Biol 1993; 50:211–218.
24. Koukourakis MI, Kyrias G, Kakolyris S, Kouroussis C, et al. Subcutaneous administration of amifostine during fractionated radiotherapy: a randomized phase II study. J Clin Oncol 2000; 18(11):2226–2233.
25. Liu T, Liu Y, He S, et al. Use of radiation with or without WR-2721 in advanced rectal cancer. Cancer 1992; 69:2820–2825.
26. Ben-Josef E, Han S, Tobi M, et al. Intrarectal application of amifostine for the prevention of radiation-induced rectal injury. Semin Radiat Oncol 2002; 12(1):81–85.
27. Sokol GH, Maickel RP. Radiation Drug Interactions in the Treatment of Cancer. Wiley and Sons: New York, 1980.
28. Hall EJ. Radiobiology for the Radiologist. Philadelphia: J.B. Lippincott, 1994.
29. Coia LR, Myerson RJ, Tepper JE. Late effects of radiation therapy on the gastrointestinal tract. Int J Radiat Oncol Biol Phys 1995; 31(5):1213–1236.
30. Krook JE. Effective surgical adjuvant therapy for high risk rectal carcinoma. NEJM 1991; 324:709–715.
31. Hall EJ. Radiosensitivity and cell age in the mitotic cycle. In: Hall EJ, ed. Radiobiology for the Radiologist. Philadelphia: JB Lippincott, 1994:91–105.
32. Potish RA. Importance of predisposing factors in the development of enteric damage. Am J Clin Oncol 1982; 5:189–194.
33. Cox JD, Byhardt RW, Wilson JF, Haas JS, et al. Complications of radiation therapy and factors in their prevention. World J Surg 1986; 10:171–188.
34. Potish RA, Jones TK, Levitt SH. Factors predisposing to radiation-related small-bowel damage. Radiology 1979; 132:479–482.
35. Lanciano RM, Martz K, Montana GS, Hanks GE. Influence of age, prior abdominal surgery, fraction size, and dose on complications after radiation therapy for squamous cell cancer of the uterine cervix. Cancer 1992; 69:2124–2130.
36. Hageemann RF, Sigdestad CP, Lesher S. Intestinal cryp survival and total crypt levels of proliferating cellularity following irradiation: fractionated X-ray exposure. Radiation Res 1981; 47:149.
37. Gelfand MD, Tepper M, Katz LA, et al. Acute irradiation proctitis in man. Development of eosinophilic crypt abscesses. Gastroenterology 1968; 54:401–411.
38. Sedgwick DM, Howard GCW, Ferguson A. Pathogenesis of acute radiation injury to the rectum: a prospective study in patients. Int J Colorectal Dis 1994; 9:23–30.
39. Haboubi NY, Schofield PF, Rowland PL. The light and electron microscopic features of early and late phase radiation-induced proctitis. Am J Gastroenterol 1988; 83(10):1140–1144.
40. Carr KE, Hume SP, Ettarh R, et al. Radiation-induced changes to epithelial and non-epithelial tissue. In: Dubois A, Livengood D, eds. Radiation and the Gastrointestinal Tract. CRC Press: Boca Raton, 1994:113.
41. Berthrong M. Pathologic changes secondary to radiation. World J Surg 1986; 10(2):155–170.
42. Weisbrot IM, lieber AF, Gordon BS. The effects of therapeutic radiation on colon mucosa. Cancer 1975; 36:931–940.
43. Fajardo LF, Berthrong M, Anderson RE. Overview of radiation injury in organs and tissues. In: Fajardo LF, Anderson RE, eds. Radiation Pathology. New York: Oxford University Press, 2001:155–163.
44. Sher ME, Bauer J. Radiation induced enteropathy. Am J Gastroenterol 1990; 85(2):121–128.
45. Hasleton PS, Carr N, Schofield PF. Vascular changes in radiation bowel disease. Histopathology 1985; 9:517–534.
46. Fajardo LF, Berthrong M. Radiation injury in surgical pathology. Am J Surg Pathol 1981; 5:153–279.
47. Fajardo LF, Berthrong M, Anderson RE. Large intestine and anal canal. In: Fajardo LF, Anderson RE, eds. Radiation Pathology. New York: Oxford University Press, 2001:239–247.
48. Sandler RS, Sandler DP. Radiation-induced cancers of the colon and rectum: assessing the risk. Gastroenterology 1983; 84:51–57.
49. Little JB. Cellular effects of ionizing radiation I and II. NEJM 1968; 278:308.
50. Galland RB, Spencer J. The natural history of clinically established radiation enteritis. Lancet 1985; 1:1257–1258.
51. O'Brien PC, Franklin CI, Dear KB, et al. A phase III double-blind randomised study of rectal sucralfate suspension in the prevention of acute radiation proctitis. Radiother Oncol 1997; 45(2):117–123.

52. Young RW. Mechanisms and treatment of radiation-induced nausea and vomiting. In: Davis CJ, Grahame-Smith DG, eds. Nausea and Vomiting: Mechanisms and Treatment. Springer-Verlag: Berlin, 1986:94–109.
53. Pilepich MV, Krall J, George FW, et al. Treatment related morbidity in phas III RTOG studies of extended field irradiation for carcinoma of the prostate. Int J Radiat Oncol Biol Phys 1984; 10: 1861–1867.
54. Roswit B. Complications of radiation therapy: the alimentary tract. Semin Roentgenol 1974; 9(1): 51–63.
55. Schultheiss TE, Lee WR, Hunt MA, et al. Late GI and GU complications in the treatment of prostate cancer. Int J Radiat Oncol Biol Phys 1997; (1):3–11.
56. Babb RR. Radiation proctopathy: a review. Am J Gastroenterol 1996; 91(7):1309–1311.
57. Bourne RG, Kearsley JH, Grove WD, et al. The relationship between early and late gastrointestinal complications of radiation therapy for carcinoma of the cervix. Int J Radiat Oncol Biol Phys 1983; 9:1445–1450.
58. Denham JW, O'Brien PC, Dunstan RH, et al. Is there more than one late radiation proctitis syndrome? Radiother Oncol 1999; 51:43–53.
59. Wang CJ, Leung SW, Chen HC, et al. The correlation of acute toxicity and late rectal injury in radiotherapy for cervical carcinoma: evidence suggestive of consequential late effect (CQLE). Int J Radiat Oncol Biol Phys 1998; 40(1):85–91.
60. Lucarotti ME, Mountford RA, Bartolo DC. Surgical management of intestinal radiation injury. Dis Colon Rectum 1991; 34(10):865–869.
61. Yeoh EK, Russo A, Botten R, et al. Acute effects of therapeutic irradiation for prostatic carcinoma on anorectal function. Gut 1998; 43(1):123–127.
62. Varma JS, Smith AN, Busuttil A. Function of the anal sphincters after chronic radiation injury. Gut 1986; 27:528–533.
63. Varma JS, Smith AN. Internal anal sphincter damage in radiation proctitis. Gut 1984; 25:564.
64. Novak JM, Collins JT, Donowitz M, et al. Effects of radiation on the human gastrointestinal tract. J Clin Gastroenterol 1979; 1:9–39.
65. Den Hartog Jager FC, van Haastert M, Battermann JJ, et al. The endoscopic spectrum of late radiation damage of the rectosigmoid colon. Endoscopy 1985; 17:214–216.
66. Reichelderfer M, Morrisey JF. Colonoscopy in radiation colitis. Gastrointest Endosc 1980; 26:41–43.
67. Den Hartog Jager FC, Cohen P, van Haastert M. Late radiation injury of the rectum and sigmoid colon: barium enema findings in 92 patients. Br J Radiol 1989; 62:807.
68. Gajraj H, Daries DR, Jackson BT. Synchronous small and large bowel cancer developing after pelvic irradiation. Gut 1988; 29:126.
69. Doubleday LC, Bernardino ME. CT findings in the perirectal area following radiation therapy. J Comput Assist Tomogr 1980; 4:634.
70. Earnest DL. Treatment of radiation enterocolitis. In: In: Therapy of Digestive Disorders. WB Saunders: Philadelphia, 2000:541–555.
71. Varma JS, Smith AN, Busuttil A. Correlation of clinical and manometric abnormalities of rectal function following chronic radiation injury. Br J Surg 1985; 72:875–878.
72. Broens P, Van Limbergen E, Penninckx F, Kerremans R. Clinical and manometric effects of combined external beam irradiation and brachytherapy for anal cancer. Int J Colorectal Dis 1998; 13:68–72.
73. Yeoh EK, Sun WM, Russo A, et al. A retrospective study of the effects of pelvic irradiation for gynecological cancer on anorectal function. Int J Radiat Oncol Biol Phys 1996; 35(5):1003–1010.
74. Yeoh EK, Botten R, Russo A, et al. Chronic effects of therapeutic irration for localized prostatic carcinoma on anorectal function. Int J Radiat Oncol Biol Phys 2000; 47(4):915–924.
75. Kim GE, Lim JJ, Park W, et al. Sensory and motor dysfunction assessed by anorectal manometry in uterine cervical carcinoma patients with radiation-induced late rectal complications. Int J Radiat Oncol Biol Phys 1998; 41(4):835–841.
76. Iwamoto T, Nakahara S, Mibu R, et al. Effect of radiotherapy on anorectal function in patients with cervical cancer. Dis Colon Rectum 1997; 40(6):693–697.
77. Meerwaldt JH, Luijsterburg HW. Rectal compliance following pelvic irradiation: a prospective study. Radiother Oncol 1996; 40(suppl 1):S33.
78. Vordermark D. Is there more than one radiation-induced fecal incontinence syndrome? Int J Radiat Oncol Biol Phy 2001; 49(1):280.
79. O'Brien PC. Radiation injury of the rectum. Radiother Oncol 2001; 60:1–14.
80. Pavy JJ, Denekamp J, Letscher J, et al. Late effects toxicity scoring: the SOMA scale. Radiother Oncol 1995:11–15.
81. Late effects consensus conference. RTOG/EORTC. Radiother Oncol 1995; 35:5–7.
82. LENT SOMA tables. Int J Radiat Oncol Biol Phys 1995; 31:1048–1092.
83. LENT SOMA tables. Radiother Oncol 1995; 35:17–60.
84. Anacak Y, Yalman D, Ozsaran Z, et al. Late radiation effects to the rectum and bladder in gynecologic cancer patients: the comparison of LENT/SOMA and RTOG/EORTC late-effects scoring systems. Int J Radiat Oncol Biol Phys 2001; 50(5):1107–1112.
85. Wachter S, Gerstner N, Goldner G, et al. Endoscopic scoring of late rectal mucosal damage after conformal radiotherapy for prostate carcinoma. Radiother Oncol 2000; 54:11–19.

86. Denton AS, Andreyev JH, Forbes A, Maher EJ. Systematic review for non-surgical interventions for the management of late radiation proctitis. Br J Cancer 2002; 87(2):134–143.

87. Perez CA, Brady LW. Principles and Practice of Radiation Oncology. 3rd ed. Philadelphia: Lippincott-Rave, 1998.

88. McArdle AH, Reid EC, Laplante MP, et al. Prophylaxis against radiation injury: the use of elemental diet prior to and during radiotherapy for invasive bladder cancer and in early postoperative feeding following radical cystectomy and ileal conduit. Arch Surg 1986; 121:879.

89. Brown MS, Buchanan RB, Karran SJ. Clinical observations on the effects of elemental diet supplementation during irradiation. Clin Radiol 1980; 31:19.

90. Asad Khan Ak, Piris J, Truelove SC. An experiment to determine the active therapeutic moiety of sulphasalazine. Lancet 1979; 2:1894–1898.

91. Goldstein F, Khoury J, Thornton JJ. Treatment of chronic radiation enteritis and colitis with salicylazosulfapyridine and systemic corticosteroids. A pilot study. Am J Gastroenterol 1976; 65(3):201–208.

92. Baum CA, Biddle WL, Miner PB Jr. Failure of 5-aminosalicyclic acid enemas to improve chronic radiation proctopathy. Dig Dis Sci 1989; 34(5):758–760.

93. Triantafillidis JK, Dadioti P, Nicholakis D, et al. High doses of 5-aminosalicyclic acid enemas in chronic radiation proctitis: Comparison with betamethasone enemas. Am J Gastroenterol 1989; 84:1587–1588.

94. Freund U, Scholmerich J, Siems H, Kluge F, Schafer HE, Wannemacher M. Severe side-effects with the application of mesalazine (5-aminosalicyclic acid) during radiotherapy. Strahlenther Onkol 1987; 163(10):678–680.

95. Khan AM, Birk JW, Anderson JC, et al. A prospective randomized placebo-controlled doubleblinded pilot study of misoprostol rectal suppositories in the prevention of acute and chronic radiation proctopathy symptoms in prostate cancer patients. Am J Gastroenterol 2000; 95(8): 1961–1966.

96. Kochhar R, Patel F, Dhar A, et al. Radiation induced proctosigmoiditis: prospective, randomized, double-blind controlled trial of oral sulfasalazine plus rectal steroids versus rectal sucralfate. Dig Dis Sci 1991; 36(1):103–107.

97. McCarthy DM. Sucralfate. NEJM 1991; 325:1017–1025.

98. Szabo S, Hollander D. Pathways of gastrointestinal protection and repair: mechanism of action of sucralfate. Am J Med 1989; 86:23–31.

99. Szabo S, Vatay P, Scarbrough E, et al. Role of vascular factors including angiogenesis in the mechanism of ation of sucralfate. Am J Med 1991; 91:158–160.

100. Tarnawski A, Hollander D, Krause WJ, et al. Does sucralfate affect the normal gastric mucosa? Histologic, ultrastructural, and functional assessment in the rat. Gastroenterology 1986; 90:893–905.

101. Burch RM, McMillan BA. Sucralfate induces proliferation of dermal fibroblasts and keratinocytes in culture and granulation tissue formation in full thickness skin wounds. Agents Actions 1991; 34: 229–231.

102. Valls A, Algara M, Domenech M, et al. Efficacy of sucralfate in the prophylaxis of diarrhoea secondary to acute radiation-induced enteritis. Preliminary results of a double blind randomised trial. Med Clin (Barc) 1991; 96:449–452.

103. Henriksson R, Franzen L, Littbrand B. Prevention and therapy for radiation-induced bowel discomfort. Scand J Gastroenterol 1992; 27(suppl 191):7–11.

104. Martenson JA, Bollinger JW, Sloan JA, et al. Sucralfate in the prevention of treatment-induced diarrhea in patients receiving pelvic radiation therapy: a north central cancer treatment group phase III double-blind placebo-controlled trial. J Clin Oncol 2000; 18(6):1239–1245.

105. Kneebone A, Mameghan H, Bolin T, et al. The effect of oral sucralfate on the acute proctitis associated with prostate radiotherapy: a double-blind, randomized trial. Int J Radiat Oncol Biol Phys 2001; 51(3):628–635.

106. Stockdale AD, Biswas A. Case report: long-term control of radiation proctitis following treatment with sucralfate enemas. Br J Surg 1997; 84(3):379.

107. Oliveira L. Management of radiation proctopathy with sucralfate suspension enema: preliminary results. Dis Colon Rectum 1998; 41(4):A36–37.

108. Kochhar R, Sharma SC, Gupta BB, Mehta SK. Rectal sucralfate in radiation proctitis. Lancet 1988; 2:400.

109. Sasai T, Hiraishi H, Suzuki Y, Masuyama H, et al. Treatment of chronic post-radiation proctitis with oral administration of sucralfate. Am J Gastroenterol 1998; 93(9):1593–1595.

110. Kochhar R, Sriram PVJ, Sharma SC, et al. Natural history of late radiation proctosigmoiditis treated with topical sucralfate suspension. Dig Dis Sci 1999; 44(5):973–978.

111. Grigsby PW, Pilepick MV, Parsons CL. Preliminary results of a phase I/II study of sodium pentosanpolysulfate in the treatment of chronic radiation-induced proctitis. Am J Clin Oncol 1990; 13(1):28–31.

112. Pinto A, Fidalgo P, Cravo M, et al. Short chain fatty acids are effective in short-term treatment of chronic radiation proctopathy: randomized, double-blind, controlled trial. Dis Colon Rectum 1999; 42(6):788–795.

113. Mortensen FV, Nielsen H, Mulvany MJ, et al. Short chain fatty acids dilate isolated human colonic resistance arteries. Gut 1990; 31:1391–1394.

114. Frankel WL, Zhang W, Singh A, et al. Mediation of the trophic effects of short chain fatty acids on the rat jejunum and colon. Gastroenterolgy 1994; 106:375–380.

115. Vernia P, Fracasso PL, Casale V, et al. Topical butyrate for acute radiation proctitis: randomised cross-over trial. Lancet 2000; 356:1232–1235.

116. Al-Sabbagh R, Sinicrope FA, Sellin JH, et al. Evaluation of short-chain fatty acid enemas: treatment of radiation proctitis. Am J Gastroenterol 1996; 91(9):1814–1816.

117. Mamel JJ, Chen M, Combs W, et al. Short-chain fatty acid (SCFA) enemas are useful for the treatment of chronic radiation proctitis. Gastroenterology 1995; 108:A305.

118. Talley NA, Chen F, King D, et al. Short-chain fatty acids in the treatment of radiation proctitis: a randomized, double-blind, placebo-controlled, cross-over pilot trials. Dis Colon Rectum 1997; 40:1046–1050.

119. Kennedy M, Bruninga K, Mutlu EA, et al. Successful and sustained treatment of chronic radiation proctitis with antioxidant vitamins E and C. Am J Gastroenterol 2001; 96(4):1080–1084.

120. Zel G. Hyperbaric oxygen therapy in urology. AUA Update Ser 1990; 9:114.

121. Charenau J, Bouachour G, Person B, et al. Severe hemorrhagic radiation proctitis advancing to gradual cessation with hyperbaric oxygen. Dig Dis Sci 1991; 36(3):373–375.

122. Williams JA, Clarke D, Denis EJ, et al. The treatment of pelvic soft tissue radiation necrosis with hyperbaric oxygen. Undersea Hyper Med 1992; 24(3):181–184.

123. Nakada T, Kubota Y, Sasagawa I, et al. Therapeutic experience of hyperbaric oxygenation in radiation colitis. Dis Colon Rectum 1993; 36:962–965.

124. Warren DC, Freehan P, Slade JB, Cianci PE. Chronic radiation proctopathy treated with hyperbaric oxygen. Undersea Hyper Med 1997; 24(3):181–184.

125. Feldmeier JJ, Heimach RD, Davolt DA, Court WS, Stegmann BJ, Sheffield PJ. Hyperbaric oxygen as an adjunctive treatment for delayed radiation injuries of the abdomen and pelvis. Undersea Hyper Med 1996; 23:205–213.

126. Woo TCS, Joseph D, Oxer H. Hyperbaric oxygen treatment for radiation proctopathy. Int J Radiat Oncol Biol Phys 1997; 38(3):619–622.

127. Gouello JP, Bouachour G, Person B, et al. Contribution of hyperbaric oxygen in irradiation-induced digestive disorders: 36 observations. La Presse Medicale 1999; 28:1053–1057.

128. Kitta T, Shinohara N, Shirato H, Otsuka H, Koyanagi T. The treatment of chronic radiation proctopathy with hyperbaric oxygen in patients with prostate cancer. BJU Int 2000; 85(3):372–374.

129. Bem J, Bem S, Singh A. Use of hyperbaric oxygen chamber in the management of radiation-related complications of the anorectal region: report of two cases and review of the literature. Dis Colon Rectum 2000; 43(10):1435–1438.

130. Mayer R, Klemen H, Quehenberger F, Sankin O, Mayer E, Hackl A, et al. Hyperbaric oxygen–an effective tool to treat radiation morbidity in prostate cancer. Radiother Oncol 2001; 61(2):151–156.

131. Shrom SH, Donaldson MH, Duckett JW, Wein AJ. Formalin treatment of intractable hemorrhagic cystitis: a review of the literature with 16 additional cases. Cancer 1976; 38:785–789.

132. Hong JJ, Park W, Ehrenpreis ED. Review article: current therapeutic options for radiation proctopathy. Aliment Pharmacol Ther 2001; 15:1253–1262.

133. Rubinstein E, Ibsen T, Rasmussen RB, et al. Formalin treatment of radiation-induced hemorrhagic proctitis. Am J Gastroenterol 1986; 81(1):44–45.

134. Seow-Chen F, Goh H-S, Eu K-W, et al. A simple and effective treatment for hemorrhagic radiation proctopathy using formalin. Dis Colon Rectum 1993; 36:135–138.

135. Saclarides TJ, King DG, Franklin JL, et al. Formalin instillation for refractory radiation-induced hemorrhagic proctopathy. Report of 16 patients. Dis Colon Rectum 1996; 39(2):196–199.

136. Biswal BM, Lal P, Rath GK, et al. Intrarectal formalin application, an effective treatment for grade III haemorrhagic radiation proctitis. Radiother Onco 1995; 35:212–215.

137. Mathai V, Seow-Choen F. Endoluminal formalin therapy for haemorrhagic radiation proctitis. Br J Surg 1995; 82:190.

138. Counter SF, Froese DP, Hart MJ. Prospective evaluation of formalin therapy for radiation proctopathy. Am J Surg 1999; 177(5):396–398.

139. Pikarsky AJ, Belin B, Efron J, et al. Complications following formalin instillation in the treatment of radiation induced proctitis. Int J Colorectal Dis 2000; 15(2):96–99.

140. Ouwendijk R, Tetteroo GW, Bode W, de Graaf EJR. Local formalin instillation: an effective treatment for uncontrolled radiation-induced hemorrhagic proctitis. Dig Surg 2002; 19(1):52–55.

141. Luna-Perez P, Rodriguez-Ramirez SE. Formalin instillation for refractory radiation-induced hemorrhagic proctitis. J Surg Oncol 2002; 80(1):41–44.

142. Cavcic J, Turcic J, Martinac P, et al. Metronidazole in the treatment of chronic radiation proctitis: clinical trial. Croat Med J 2000; 41(3).

143. Wurzer H, Schfhalter-Zoppoth I, Brandstatter G. Hormonal therapy in chronic radiation colitis. Am J Gastroenterol 1998; 93(12):2536–2538.

144. Niv Y, Henkin Y. Estrogen-progestin therapy and coronary heart disease in radiation-induced rectal telangiectases. J Clin Gastroenterol 1995; 21(4):295–297.

145. Van Cutsem E, Rutgeerts P, Vantrappen G. Treatment of bleeding gastrointestinal vascular malformations with oestrogen-progesterone. Lancet 1990; 335:953–955.

146. Van Cutsem E, Rutgeerts P, Vantrappen G. Long-term effects of hormonal therapy for bleeding gastrointestinal vascular malformations. Eur J Gastroenterol Hepatol 1993; 5:439–443.
147. Levitsky J, Hong JJ, Jani AB, Ehrenpreis ED. Oral vitamin A therapy for a patient with a severely symptomatic post radiation anal ulceration: report of a case. Dis Colon Rectum. In press.
148. Jensen DM, Machicado GA, Cheng S, et al. A randomized prospective study of endoscopic bipolar electrocoagulation and heater probe treatment of chronic rectal bleeding from radiation telangiectasia. Gastrointest Endosc 1997; 45(1):20–25.
149. Ahlquist DA, Gostout CJ, Viggiano TR, et al. Laser therapy for severe radiation-induced rectal bleeding. Mayo Clin Proc 1986; 61:927–931.
150. Swaroop VS, Gostout CJ. Endoscopic treatment of chronic radiation proctopathy. J Clin Gastroenterol 1998; 27(1):36–40.
151. Michispoulos S, Isibouris P, Balta A, et al. Study comparing Nd-YAG laser and heater probe efficacy on chronic rectal bleeding of radiation colitis. Gastroenterology 1998; 114:29.
152. Viggiano TR, Zighelboim J, Ahlquist DA, et al. Endoscopic Nd:YAG laser coagulation of bleeding from radiation proctopathy. Gastrointest Endosc 1993; 39(4):513–517.
153. Leuchter RS, Petrilli ES, Dwyer RM, et al. Nd:YAG laser therapy of rectosigmoid bleeding due to radiation injury. Obstet Gynecol 1982; 59(6):S65–S67.
154. Berken CA. Nd:YAG laser therapy for gastrointestinal bleeding due to radiation colitis. Am J Gastroenterol 1985; 80(9):730–731.
155. Rutgeerts P, Van Gompel F, Geboes K, et al. Long term results of treatment of vascular malformations of the gastrointestinal tract by Neodymium-YAG laser photocoagulation. Gut 1985; 26:586–593.
156. Alexander TJ, Dwyer RM. Endoscopic Nd:YAG laser treatment of severe radiation injury of the lower gastrointestinal tract: long-term follow-up. Gastrointest Endosc 1988; 34(5):407–411.
157. O'Connor JJ. Argon laser treatment of radiation proctitis. Arch Surg 1989; 124(6):749.
158. Taylor JG, DiSario JA, Buchi KN. Argon laser therapy for hemorrhagic radiation proctopathy: long-term results. Gastrointest Endosc 1993; 39(5):641–644.
159. Buchi KN, Dixon JA. Argon laser treatment of hemorrhagic radiation proctitis. Gastrointest Endosc 1987; 33(1):27–30.
160. Carbatzas C, Spencer GM, Thorpe SM, Sargeant LR, Bown SG. Nd:YAG laser treatment for bleeding from radiation proctitis. Endoscopy 1996; 28:497–500.
161. Hunter JG, Burt RW, Becker JM, et al. Colonic mucosal lesions: evaluation of monopolar electrocautery, argon laser, and neodymium:YAG laser. Curr Surg 1984; 41:373–375.
162. Silva RA, Correia AJ, Dias LM, et al. Argon plasma coagulation therapy for hemorrhagic radiation proctosigmoiditis. Gastrointest Endosc 1999; 50(2):221–224.
163. Fantin AC, Binek J, Suter WR, et al. Argon beam coagulation for treatment of symptomatic radiation-induced proctitis. Gastrointest Endosc 1999; 49(4):515–518.
164. Tam W, Moore J, Schoeman M. Treatment of radiation proctitis with argon plasma coagulation. Endoscopy 2000; 32(9):667–672.
165. Kaassis M, Oberti E, Burtin P, Boyer J. Argon plasma coagulation for the treatment of hemorrhagic radiation proctitis. Endoscopy 2000; 32(9):673–676.
166. Chutkan R, Lipp A, Waye J. Argon plasma coagulator: a new and effective modality for treatment of radiation proctits. Gastrointest Endosc 1997; 45:AB27.
167. Jao SW, Beart RW, Gunderson LL. Surgical treatment of radiation injuries of the colon and rectum. Am J Surg 1986; 151:272–277.
168. Marks G, Mohiudden M. The surgical management of the radiation-induced intestine. Surg Clin North Am 1983; 63(1):81–95.
169. Allen-Mersh TG, Wilson EJ, Hope-Stone HF, et al. The management of late radiation-induced rectal injury after treatment of carcinoma of the uterus. Surg Gynecol Obstet 1987; 164:521–524.
170. Cross MJ, Frazee RC. Surgical treatment of radiation enteritis. Am Surg 1992; 58:132–135.
171. Gazet JC. Parks' coloanal pull-through anastomosis for severe, complicated radiation proctitis. Dis Colon Rectum 1985; 28(2):110–114.
172. Nowacki MP, Szawlowski AW, Borrowski A. Parks' coloanal sleeve anastomosis for treatment of postirradiation rectovaginal fistula. Dis Colon Rectum 1986; 29:817–820.
173. Anseline PF, Lavery IC, Fazio VW, et al. Radiation injury of the rectum. Evaluation of surgical treatment. Ann Surg 1981; 194(6):716–724.
174. Browning GG. Late results of mucosal proctectomy and colo-anal sleeve anastomosis for chronic irradiation rectal injury. Br J Surg 1987; 74:31–34.
175. Corman ML. Colon and Rectal Surgery. Lippincott-Raven: Philadelphia, 1998:1064–1066.
176. Miholic J, Schwarz C, Moeschl P. Surgical therapy of radiation-induced lesions of the colon and rectum. Am J Surg 1988; 155:761–764.

16 | Acute Lower Gastrointestinal Tract Bleeding

Lawrence R. Schiller
Department of Gastroenterology, Baylor University Medical Center, Dallas, Texas, U.S.A.

Warren Lichliter
Department of Colon and Rectal Surgery, Baylor University Medical Center, Dallas, Texas, U.S.A.

INTRODUCTION
Definition

Acute lower gastrointestinal tract bleeding is defined as the recent onset of gross gastrointestinal bleeding from a site distal to the ligament of Treitz. Severe acute lower gastrointestinal tract bleeding is associated with unstable vital signs, rapidly developing anemia, and/or a need for transfusion. Operationally, this definition is equivalent to voluminous hematochezia (gross red rectal bleeding), although it does not exclude melena (black stools due to gastrointestinal bleeding). The source is not usually apparent on clinical grounds, making for an overlap with acute upper gastrointestinal tract bleeding until endoscopic or radiographic studies define the site of blood loss with more precision (1–6). Approximately 10% to 15% of patients presenting with voluminous hematochezia have a source in the upper gastrointestinal tract. Relatively few disorders typically present with severe acute lower gastrointestinal tract bleeding. Many more lesions in the lower gastrointestinal tract produce lesser degrees of bleeding, although most occasionally can produce voluminous hemorrhage. This chapter focuses on the diagnosis and management of severe acute lower gastrointestinal tract bleeding.

Some authorities distinguish between lower tract bleeding and small bowel bleeding, limiting "lower" gastrointestinal tract bleeding to bleeding due to lesions within the reach of the colonoscope (terminal ileum, colon and rectum). This has not been accepted universally and the more inclusive definition will be used in this chapter.

The severity criterion (unstable vital signs, anemia, and need for transfusion) are included to differentiate more severe acute lower gastrointestinal tract bleeding from chronic blood loss characterized by a positive fecal occult blood test and "terminal" hematochezia due to lesions in the rectal outlet (e.g., hemorrhoids and fissures). Thus, by definition, patients with severe acute lower gastrointestinal tract bleeding have a potentially life-threatening problem. Severity varies widely, however. Published mortality rates vary from 3% to 5% per episode, but death is usually due to complications of shock or comorbid illness rather than blood loss itself (1–7). Spontaneous cessation of bleeding is common in most cases, but bleeding often recurs.

Epidemiology

The incidence of acute lower gastrointestinal tract bleeding is approximately 25 cases per 100,000 adults per year (3). This represents 15% to 30% of the incidence of acute upper gastrointestinal tract hemorrhage. Bleeding is more frequent in men than in women, and the incidence increases with age. The average age of patients presenting with acute lower gastrointestinal tract bleeding is 71 years (5).

Costs

Costs associated with lower gastrointestinal tract bleeding have been evaluated in a recent survey from Canada. Adjusting for currency differences but not international differences in medical costs, direct costs per episode averaged $3580 (8). Given an annual incidence of 45,000 cases in the United States each year, this would amount to an aggregate expense of $161 million annually. It is likely that the actual costs in the United States are at least twice as high.

CLINICAL CLASSIFICATION AND DIFFERENTIAL DIAGNOSIS
Clinical Classification

The ultimate classification of lower gastrointestinal bleeding is by etiology, but clinical classification by presentation and severity is the most useful way to direct patient care. Under this clinical classification, patients are divided into those with hematochezia of either low volume or high volume, those with melena due to chemical changes in the hemoglobin molecule, and those with occult gastrointestinal bleeding. Such a classification scheme allows for appropriate evaluation and speedier detection of the underlying cause (Table 1).

Low-Volume Hematochezia

The causes of low-volume hematochezia are usually located within the distal colon, rectum, or anal canal and include hemorrhoids, fissures, low-lying polyps or tumors, proctitis of any sort, diversion colitis, rectal ulcer, and endometriosis. These lesions are within easy reach of a sigmoidoscope and ordinarily do not pose an immediate threat to life. Bleeding from hemorrhoids is occasionally quite copious and is often bright red because of the arterialized blood supply to the anal cushions. Other sources of "terminal" hematochezia typically produce darker crimson bleeding and almost never produce voluminous bleeding.

High-Volume Hematochezia

High-volume hematochezia is a different matter. While some of the same lesions that cause low-volume hematochezia sometimes can produce severe bleeding, a different, and more extensive differential diagnosis must be considered when red rectal bleeding is voluminous. Lesions from as high as the esophagus must be considered; therefore, a regional differential diagnosis must be considered. Upper gastrointestinal tract lesions that can produce hematochezia include esophageal varices, Mallory-Weiss tears, peptic ulcers, Dieulafoy lesions, and aortoenteric fistulas. Small bowel sources include jejunal diverticulosis, Meckel's diverticulum, small bowel ulceration (especially those due to nonsteroidal anti-inflammatory drugs), and intussusception.

Table 1 Differential Diagnosis of Rectal Bleeding by Presentation[a]

	Hematochezia			
Diagnosis	High volume	Low volume	Melena	Occult bleeding
Colonic sources				
Diverticulosis	++	+	+/−	−
Angioectasia	++	++	+/−	−
Colonic varices	++	+	+/−	−
Neoplasia	+/−	+	+	++
Colitis/ulceration	+/−	+	+/−	++
Dieulafoy lesion	++	+	+/−	−
Endometriosis	+/−	+	+/−	−
Rectoanal sources				
Hemorrhoids	+	++	−	+
Fissure	−	++	−	+
Small bowel sources				
Angioectasia	+	+	++	+
Jejunal diverticulosis	+/−	+	++	−
Meckel's diverticulum	+	++	++	−
Enteritis/ulceration	−	+	+	++
Neoplasia	−	−	+	++
Aortoenteric fistula	++	+	+	−
Dieulafoy lesion	+	++	+	−
Upper tract lesions				
Esophageal varices	+	+	++	−
Mallory-Weiss tear	+	+	++	−
Peptic ulcer	+	+	++	+
Dieulafoy lesion	+	+	++	−

[a]Key to symbols: ++, likely presentation; +, possible presentation; +/−, unlikely presentation; −, rare presentation/never seen.

Colonic sources include diverticulosis, angiodysplasia, and other vascular lesions such as colonic varices, and colitis of any cause. In general, upper tract lesions and small intestinal lesions must be bleeding briskly to cause hematochezia. Approximately 11% of patients with hematochezia have bleeding upper gastrointestinal tract lesions, and 9% have small bowel lesions as a cause of bleeding.

Melena

When bleeding is slower, chemical reactions in the gut lumen digest the blood and produce melena instead of hematochezia. The most effective melena-producing reaction occurs when gastric acid acts on blood leaking into the upper gastrointestinal tract, but melena can occur with bleeding as distal as the right colon due to other denaturing reactions by both luminal enzymes and bacteria. Thus, the differential diagnosis of hematochezia and melena is similar, although the frequency with which specific bleeding lesions present with different stool colors varies (Table 1).

Occult Gastrointestinal Bleeding

When bleeding is slow and of low volume, there may be no visible blood or blood products in the stool, and bleeding is said to be occult. Such bleeding is usually detected by chemical (guaiac-based pseudoperoxidase reaction) or immunological methods. Any lesion that bleeds might produce a positive fecal occult blood test as its sole manifestation, but this is very unlikely for some lesions which almost always bleed voluminously (Table 1).

Pseudobleeding

Another situation to consider is pseudobleeding. Ingestion of food dyes or intensely colored vegetables such as beets can impart a red color to stools that could be mistaken for hematochezia. Likewise, melena may be simulated by ingestion of bismuth (e.g., PeptoBismol) or charcoal. It is important to confirm the presence of blood in the stool with a fecal occult blood test before launching into an extensive evaluation of a patient reporting red or black stools.

SPECIFIC CAUSES OF LOWER GASTROINTESTINAL TRACT BLEEDING
Diverticulosis

Massive lower gastrointestinal tract bleeding is most often due to diverticular disease of the colon (see Chapter 19) (1–7). Bleeding is due to rupture of vasa recta, arteries that are located at the apex or neck of the diverticulum, and rarely it is associated with acute diverticulitis. Bleeding therefore can be quite voluminous, and is unheralded by abdominal pain or fever. Although most previous experience suggests that bleeding is most often due to diverticula in the right colon, a recent study suggests that most diverticular hemorrhage originates in the left colon where most of the diverticula are located (1). Bleeding diverticulosis typically occurs in older patients who often have comorbidities, such as cardiovascular disease, that make resuscitation more difficult and lead to excess morbidity and mortality. Accurate diagnosis may be impeded by the frequent occurrence of asymptomatic diverticulosis in older individuals, and the propensity of blood from any source to fill existing diverticula. Surgery is rarely needed acutely because more than 80% of patients with diverticular hemorrhage spontaneously stop bleeding, and nonoperative therapy usually can control bleeding (see below). However, recurrent episodes of diverticular bleeding, seen in 25% of patients with diverticular hemorrhage, may require operative management (2).

Angiodysplasia and Vascular Ectasia

Angiodysplasia and other vascular ectasias (e.g., angiomas, and arteriovenous malformations) are commonly found in the right colon, but can occur anywhere in the colon and small intestine, especially in older patients (9,10). They are dilatations of submucosal capillaries or veins that are uncommon in asymptomatic individuals. Bleeding from these lesions tends to be less severe than diverticular hemorrhage and often is intermittent. It is not clear what causes these lesions. Occasionally, they are seen as part of Osler–Weber–Rendu disease, but most are thought to be acquired lesions. An association with calcific aortic stenosis has been proposed, but the pathogenesis of mucosal ectasias in aortic stenosis remains speculative. Studies show that incidentally discovered angiodysplasias rarely bleed over a three-year period, and therefore endoscopic treatment of nonbleeding lesions is not advisable (11).

Dieulafoy Lesions

Dieulafoy lesions are pathologically different than angioectasias, and consist of large mucosal arterioles that are placed anomalously close to the lumen. These have a propensity to rupture, causing brisk pinpoint bleeding from what otherwise seems like normal mucosa. Because there are no ulcers or other evidence of their presence, these lesions are difficult to detect endoscopically when they are not bleeding. Most symptomatic Dieulafoy lesions are found in the stomach, but up to one-third are extragastric (12,13). Clinically Dieulafoy lesions behave more like bleeding diverticula than angiodysplasias, producing voluminous hemorrhage that sometimes recurs. If the lesion is identified, endoscopic therapy is usually successful in stopping bleeding.

Colonic Varices

Patients with portal hypertension develop spontaneous portasystemic shunts in several areas including the colon and rectum. It has been estimated that about 10% of patients with portal hypertension and 60% of patients who have had bleeding esophageal varices develop rectal varices (14,15). Fortunately, bleeding from colorectal varices is uncommon, affecting perhaps one-third of those patients who develop colorectal varices. Treatment analogous to that for bleeding esophageal varices can be useful.

Meckel's Diverticulum

Meckel's diverticulum occurs in 1% to 2% of the population and is often asymptomatic (16). It has been estimated that the lifetime risk of any diverticulum-related symptoms developing in people with Meckel's diverticula is only 4.2% (17). Hemorrhage occurs as a complication, most often in children between the ages of 10 and 15, but can occur in adults, usually before the age of 40. In many individuals, bleeding is associated with peptic ulceration adjacent to heterotopic gastric mucosa in the diverticulum, but this is not universally the case. Patients presenting with a bleeding Meckel's diverticulum usually have maroon stools and behave clinically like patients with upper gastrointestinal tract bleeding due to peptic ulcer (large initial bleed with recurrent, substantial bleeding episodes). Resection of the diverticulum is curative.

Postpolypectomy Bleeding

Clinically significant bleeding complicates polypectomy in approximately 0.2% to 6% of patients (18). It may occur up to two weeks after the procedure, but usually occurs within 72 hours. Removal of large polyps (greater than 2 cm) or sessile lesions and concurrent use of anticoagulation or antiplatelet therapy with aspirin or other drugs may lead to hemorrhage, but the data supporting this is only observational (18). Repeat colonoscopy and identification of the bleeding site coupled with appropriate endoscopic therapy is usually adequate to control bleeding.

Colitis and Ulcers

Colitis of any etiology may cause rectal bleeding, but rarely produces severe acute lower gastrointestinal tract hemorrhage. Infections with organisms that invade the mucosa or cause ulcers, such as *Shigella*, *Campylobacter*, some strains of *E. coli*, and *cytomegalovirus*, can cause significant hemorrhage occasionally. Inflammatory bowel disease (i.e., Crohn's disease and ulcerative colitis) rarely causes severe acute bleeding, but may require surgery to control bleeding because endoscopically treatable lesions are seldom found in this setting (19). Ischemic colitis typically produces acute low-volume hematochezia that spontaneously resolves. In contrast, radiation colitis typically causes chronic low-volume hematochezia. Ulcers in the lower gastrointestinal tract of any cause (e.g., due to nonsteroidal anti-inflammatory drugs or stercoral ulcers) may produce voluminous bleeding.

Neoplasia

Carcinomas, lymphomas, and benign polyps in the small bowel and colon characteristically produce occult gastrointestinal bleeding and chronic anemia, not voluminous acute hemorrhage. Occasionally, brisk bleeding is encountered with these lesions, especially if present in the rectum or anus.

Endometriosis

Ectopic endometrial tissue may involve the wall of the colon and produce cyclic bleeding in synchrony with the menstrual cycle. The bleeding is usually a low-volume hematochezia and may be overshadowed by other symptoms of endometriosis, such as abdominal pain or obstruction (20).

Aortoenteric Fistula

An unusual but potentially fatal complication of treatment of an aortic aneurysm by surgical placement of a prosthetic graft is development of an aortoenteric fistula (21). These typically form between the proximal anastomosis and the duodenum, but can occur elsewhere in the gut. Rarely they can occur without any preceding surgical intervention (22). Clinically, a "herald" bleed of minor significance often presages an exsanguinating hemorrhage. Thus, any patient presenting with rectal bleeding who has had an aortic aneurysm repair should have this condition excluded. Diagnostic testing with endoscopy, computerized tomography, and even angiography can be misleading, and so any patient after aortic aneurysm repair with undiagnosed gastrointestinal bleeding may need surgical exploration to exclude aortoenteric fistula.

MANAGEMENT OF ACUTE LOWER GASTROINTESTINAL TRACT BLEEDING
Initial Assessment

Because severe acute lower gastrointestinal tract bleeding is associated with some degree of hemodynamic instability, prompt assessment of the patient's circulatory status and adequate volume resuscitation is essential (1–6,23,24).

The initial evaluation should include a focused clinical history. This should include the patient's report of the color of the stool (use of a color chart can facilitate the identification of the color), and an estimate of the duration and severity of rectal bleeding. Any previous history of lower gastrointestinal tract bleeding should be recorded. Use of nonsteroidal anti-inflammatory drugs (associated with ulceration in the small bowel and colon) or digoxin (associated with colonic ischemia) and any antecedent hypotension should be noted. Other important historical points include previous surgery or radiation therapy, recent polypectomy, and constipation or dyschezia.

The initial physical examination includes assessment of volume status by checking for postural changes in blood pressure and pulse. Of course, if the bleeding patient is already hypotensive and tachycardic while supine, demonstration of orthostasis may be fraught with hazard and should be deferred. The abdomen should be examined carefully with particular attention to the presence or absence of peritoneal signs, signs of chronic liver disease, and evidence of aortic aneurysm. A digital rectal examination should be done to assess stool color and consistency personally and to test for occult blood.

Resuscitation

Simultaneously with this rapid preliminary evaluation, blood samples should be sent to the laboratory for a complete blood count including platelet count, coagulation tests (prothrombin time and partial thromboplastin time), serum chemistries, and blood typing in anticipation of the need for transfusion. At least one large bore intravenous line should be started; patients who are hypotensive should have two lines inserted, including a central venous catheter. Saline or lactated Ringer's solution should be infused at a rapid rate pending the return of the laboratory tests. In patients, in shock, consideration should be given to placement of an arterial catheter to facilitate hemodynamic monitoring, an indwelling urinary catheter to monitor urinary output, and a nasogastric tube to look for evidence of upper gastrointestinal tract hemorrhage.

Table 2 Indicators of Increased Severity of Lower Gastrointestinal Tract Bleeding

Abnormal vital signs
Tachycardia
Hypotension
Severe anemia (<8 g/dL)
Large transfusion requirement (>3–4 units/24 hr)
Continued or recurrent bleeding
Comorbid conditions
Previous aortic surgery
Abnormal endoscopic findings
Diverticulum or colon ulcer with stigmata of recent hemorrhage
Ischemic colitis
Cancer

Source: Adapted from Refs. 7, 25, and 26.

Packed red blood cells should be infused when available if the patient is presented in shock. In those with lesser degrees of blood loss in whom intravenous fluid is sufficient to restore vital signs to normal, transfusion can be elective. Most patients without comorbid conditions can tolerate hematocrits of 25% to 30% and need not be transfused unless bleeding has not stopped. Patients with cardiopulmonary diseases should be transfused to maintain their hematocrits greater than 30%. The initial hematocrit may not reflect blood loss accurately, and the need for transfusion should be reevaluated by sequential measurement of vital signs, rechecking the hematocrit at intervals, and monitoring the response to resuscitation. Continued bleeding and its effect on the circulatory system and other organs is the leading cause of morbidity and mortality in these patients.

Blood platelets should be infused in patients with severe thrombocytopenia (platelet count $<20{,}000/\text{mm}^3$) or documented platelet dysfunction. Coagulopathy should be assessed and treated. In patients taking warfarin, fresh frozen plasma may be needed to reverse the drug effect. Vitamin K should only be administered to those in whom reanticoagulation is not anticipated, because reestablishment of a therapeutic prothrombin time may be very difficult after giving vitamin K. If heparin therapy is needed, it should be monitored closely and partial thromboplastin times should be kept at the minimum therapeutic level (usually twice normal).

During this initial phase of resuscitation, the severity of the bleeding can be assessed according to criteria displayed in Table 2. This classification allows some insight into the likelihood that serious interventions will be needed: interventions are more likely in patients with shock or who experience severe or continuing bleeding. Additional predictors of severity include syncope, lack of abdominal tenderness, and aspirin use (25). Patients with severe bleeding and patients with moderately severe bleeding who have significant comorbidities should be managed in an intensive care unit or close observation area. Those with lesser problems can be managed on a regular hospital floor.

Diagnostic Testing

As the patient stabilizes, diagnostic testing can start. The goal is to identify the source of bleeding so that definitive treatment can be undertaken. Initially, simple tests can provide a diagnosis. For patients with hematochezia, anoscopy, proctoscopy, or bedside sigmoidoscopy may lead to a diagnosis. A limited examination may also be useful in patients who have physical findings of a rectal mass, a history of surgery that may have compromised the inferior mesenteric artery (e.g., aortic aneurysm resection), or recent distal polypectomy. These examinations may be difficult due to incomplete bowel preparation. Unless there is unequivocal evidence of a bleeding source, the evaluation of more proximal sites still is necessary. Passage of a nasogastric tube and inspection of an aspirate of gastric contents for blood might identify a proximal source. The absence of blood in a nasogastric aspirate does not exclude the possibility of an upper gastrointestinal tract source; therefore, upper gastrointestinal tract endoscopy may still be necessary.

For patients who stabilize quickly and seem to have stopped bleeding, prompt gastrointestinal lavage with a poorly absorbable polyethylene glycol–electrolyte solution and urgent colonoscopy has become the standard diagnostic approach (6,24). This technique can identify most colonic sources and may permit the application of endoscopic therapy to oozing lesions. Quick preparation followed immediately by colonoscopy is preferred to emergency colonoscopy without preparation, because lesions may be difficult to identify when blood and stool fill the colon. If possible, the ileum should be intubated or at least the ileocecal valve should be observed for a short time to see if blood is coming from above. If no source is identified by colonoscopy, upper gastrointestinal endoscopy should be performed to exclude an upper tract source.

The diagnostic yield of urgent colonoscopy in acute lower gastrointestinal bleeding is greater than 80% (27). Features that improve diagnostic yield are adequate preparation and prompt performance as the preparation is completed. This allows the preparation solution to wash through the colon as the examination is done and facilitates identification of active bleeding. Active bleeding coming from a point in otherwise normal mucosa is characteristic of a Dieulafoy lesion. Active bleeding may also be seen coming from a diverticulum or vascular malformation. Stigmata of recent hemorrhage may also be seen, such as a protruding artery, pigmented protuberance, or adherent clot. If a discrete bleeding lesion or stigmata of recent hemorrhage cannot be identified, colonoscopy may allow identification of the level of bleeding and lesions that may or may not be related to the bleeding source, such as polyps, diverticula, and angiodysplasia.

In patients who have continuing bleeding or rebleeding and in those in whom a diagnosis is not made after colonoscopy and endoscopy, a radionucleide bleeding scan may identify a possible location of bleeding (28). In order for the scan to be most effective, dynamic imaging after infusion of technetium-labeled red blood cells is essential. Static imaging often fails to accurately identify the site of bleeding and use of unbound technetium may lead to nonspecific activity in the gut lumen as this isotope can be excreted into the gut. Bleeding rates as low as 0.1 mL/min can be detected by a careful study. The positive predictive value of a properly done scan is approximately 90%, but false positives and false negatives continue to be problematic for patient management (29). It is important to recognize that—at best—a bleeding scan only identifies a site of bleeding and not a specific lesion causing the bleeding.

Better delineation of a bleeding site can be obtained by angiography. This technique is best applied to patients with continuing, undiagnosed bleeding. Bleeding has to be fairly brisk (greater than 0.5 mL/min) in order to be detected angiographically, but is very accurately localized if it is demonstrated. Thus, as compared with radionucleide scintigraphy, angiography is less sensitive, but more specific. Some radiologists will not perform angiography, unless a patient can be shown to have active bleeding by a technetium-tagged red blood cell scan. Vascular lesions are readily demonstrated, and therapy can be applied (see below).

Other diagnostic tests that can be applied include a radioisotope Meckel's scan (using unbound technetium that can be secreted by heterotopic gastric mucosa in the diverticulum), push enteroscopy, capsule enteroscopy, and small bowel radiography. These techniques are designed to explore small bowel sources of bleeding. In general, they are used in patients who have stopped bleeding and who are still undiagnosed. In particular, small bowel radiography in which barium is introduced into the gastrointestinal tract should be reserved for stable patients in whom bleeding has stopped, because it precludes other radiographic and angiographic techniques until the barium has cleared. Recently, triphasic helical computed tomography scanning has been proposed as a valuable diagnostic test for acute lower gastrointestinal tract bleeding (30). Its ultimate role in these patients still needs to be defined.

Treatment
Endoscopic Therapies
Several endoscopic treatments have been used to treat actively bleeding lesions encountered during colonoscopy. In general, these are adapted from endoscopic treatments employed in the upper gastrointestinal tract, but have somewhat greater risk because the colon wall is thinner than that of the upper gastrointestinal tract. Injection of epinephrine into the area of the bleeding vessel, thermal coagulation with heater probes, bipolar electrodes or argon plasma coagulation, and mechanical occlusion with hemoclips have been described (1,27,31).

Injection of bleeding sites with 1 to 2 mL of 1:10,000 epinephrine solution can slow or arrest bleeding in many cases (1). Injection should start on the side of a lesion furthest from the tip of the colonoscope (to allow an unobstructed view of the bleeding site, and a wheal should be built up with blanching of the surrounding mucosa. Additional injections can be made more distally. Injection should be continued until there is some resistance to further injection, because the main mechanism by which injection controls bleeding is tamponade of the bleeding vessel and not just vasospasm. Injection can be used alone or in combination with other modalities to control bleeding. Injection of sclerosing solutions should be avoided in the colon because of a risk of perforation. If used, the volume injected should be kept less than 0.5 mL per injection.

Thermal coagulation is another technique that can be applied to bleeding lesions in the colon. Direct coaptive coagulation, in which a probe is used to apply pressure to "seal" the leaking blood vessel, has been favored by most investigative endoscopists when a discrete bleeding source is identified (actively bleeding Dieulafoy lesion and visible vessels). Circumferential application of the probe can be used when more diffuse lesions such as angiodysplasia are encountered. The optimal power settings are not well defined for bleeding lesions in the colon. In general, lower settings should be used to avoid perforation. Combination of epinephrine injection and thermal coagulation is probably more effective than either modality alone. Laser and argon beam coagulation are best reserved for more diffuse lesions, such as angiodysplasia and radiation colitis.

Mechanical occlusion of bleeding vessels with clips, loops and bands has been used by some endoscopists, but has not been studied extensively. These devices are most attractive for small bleeding lesions, such as polyp stalks or visible vessels. Suction ligators must be used with great caution in the colon because of the possibility that the full thickness of the colon will be ligated, producing necrosis and perforation.

Angiographic Therapies

Angiographic therapies include intra-arterial vasopressin infusion and embolization (32–34). Vasopressin infused at a rate of 0.2 to 0.4 U/min can control 80% to 90% of bleeding in patients with diverticulosis. Vasopressin administration can be complicated by coronary artery spasm, and nitroglycerin may have to be administered. Vasopressin infusion may stop bleeding long enough to restore hemodynamic stability, but bleeding may recur when the infusion is turned off. For this reason, angiographic embolization of the arterial branch supplying a bleeding lesion has been applied. Embolization should be considered only when a bleeding source has been identified and is designed to reduce perfusion pressure of the bleeding vessel. The risk is that thrombosis may occur, carrying with it the danger of producing colonic ischemia. With more modern techniques of superselective catheterization, this risk may be acceptably low (32,35).

Surgery

Despite major advances in endoscopic and angiographic therapies for the management of acute lower gastrointestinal bleeding, most surveys still report a 10% to 20% requirement for emergency surgical intervention (36,37). In addition, surgery may be required to localize the site of bleeding in up to 50% of cases (blind look laparotomy). Moreover, up to 15% of patients rebleed in the early postoperative period, and require a second operation with an attendant increase in mortality (38–40).

Surgery is indicated when a lesion has been identified but bleeding cannot be controlled, or when no specific lesion is identified but continued bleeding becomes life-threatening. Indeed, instability of the patient may limit the ability to perform any diagnostic procedures other than nasogastric tube insertion and lavage. Recurrent hemorrhage is another indication for surgery.

Some experts set an arbitrary limit of blood transfusions as an indication for surgery, but the overall condition of the patient and the progress made in controlling hemorrhage is probably a better basis for the decision to operate. Most quantitative guidelines suggest that transfusion of more than six units of packed red blood cells in less than 24 hours or 8 to 10 units per bleeding episode warrant operative intervention. Patients with continued bleeding who require more than 10 units of packed red blood cells to maintain hemodynamic stability have an increased mortality (39).

Whenever possible, surgery should be done electively, after other diagnostic and therapeutic modalities have been tried and the patient's condition has been stabilized. This permits the best outcomes, and is associated with lower rebleeding rates than "blind" resections (40).

Conversely, delay of surgery in an unstable patient to obtain diagnostic tests may lead to higher morbidity and mortality.

Once a decision has been made to operate, individual considerations can help in planning the surgical procedure. For example, preexisting chronic diarrhea or fecal incontinence may limit the extent of resection that is considered or may even mandate that an ostomy should be created. Patients with symptomatic diverticular disease in the left colon who have localized bleeding in the right colon might benefit more from a subtotal colectomy and ileorectal anastomosis than from a more limited right colectomy. Patients at high risk for surgery may require a quick operation that might preclude more time-consuming procedures such as subtotal colectomy or intraoperative endoscopy. Such patients might not tolerate the risks of anastomosis, especially if ischemia is a consideration, and this may dictate creation of an ostomy with Hartmann's pouch or mucous fistula.

Prior to any surgery, the patient should be volume resuscitated including transfused and appropriately hemodynamically monitored. Consideration should be given to central venous access and arterial monitoring as well as obviously an indwelling bladder catheter and nasogastric tube. All surgery should be performed in the modified lithotomy position, so that transanal access can be obtained for any necessary colonoscopy and similarly the anesthesiologist should be aware that the gastroenterologist may be performing upper endoscopy and/or small bowel enteroscopy. Due to the timing of surgery, mechanical bowel preparation may not have been possible, but in general can be used even through a nasogastric tube in the preoperative phase. Fortunately, blood is a good cathartic and the colon is usually relatively clean in these cases. However, intraoperative lavage, fecal diversion, and subtotal colectomy all remain potential options none of which mandate a preoperative bowel preparation. If possible, oral neomycin and erythromycin or neomycin and metronidazole may be given the day prior to surgery, but in general, in cases of acute gastrointestinal hemorrhage, only intravenous antibiotics are possible. Broad-spectrum parenteral antibiotics should be given "on-call" to the operating room, and sequential compression stockings and possibly either heparin or fragmented heparin may be used for thrombosis prophylaxis. Once the patient has been anesthetized and positioned, transrectal irrigation with normal saline until clear may be useful. The catheter may be left in place to help prevent blood accumulation.

Operative procedures can be broadly classified into two clinical scenarios: those done in patients in whom localization studies could not be done because of the severity of bleeding or in whom localization studies were uninformative; and those done in patients in whom a presumed source of bleeding has been identified. In the first group, a "blind-look laparotomy" is done. In the second group, a "directed laparotomy" is done. It should be pointed out that—in the first group—there may have been diagnostic procedures, such as endoscopy or colonoscopy, that limit the differential diagnosis before laparotomy is done. It should also be noted that sometimes the presumed source of bleeding in the second group is incorrect, and so the surgeon must keep an open mind when exploring the patient's abdomen.

An additional point to be considered is the role of laparoscopy in the approach to patients with acute lower gastrointestinal tract bleeding. Because of the need to manually palpate the bowel for lesions and to direct passage of an endoscope for intraoperative enteroscopy, open laparotomy is preferable to laparoscopy. Also, emergent operative intervention in unstable patients requires as expeditious a procedure as possible, arguing against laparoscopy.

"Blind-look laparotomy" requires the surgeon to be ready for anything. If possible, preoperative mechanical bowel preparation should be done, even using the nasogastric tube to infuse lavage solution. Oral neomycin and erythromycin or neomycin and metronidazole should be given ahead of the surgery. If time does not allow mechanical and antibiotic preparation, intraoperative lavage, fecal diversion, and subtotal colectomy remain as potential operative options, none of which mandate a preoperative bowel preparation. Patients should be given systemic antibiotics prior to incision, and patients should be placed in a modified lithotomy position to facilitate anastomosis or endoscopy.

The initial goal of the surgeon is to rule out bleeding proximal to the ileocecal valve. The stomach and duodenum should be inspected and a careful, systematic examination of the small intestine should be performed. Particular attention should be paid to the mesenteric attachment of the bowel, where jejunal diverticula are located, but sometimes difficult to visualize. Mass lesions, induration of the bowel with associated ulcer, mesenteric inflammation or thickening (sometimes seen with carcinoid tumors) should be sought. Two situations may be confusing.

First, the presence of large amounts of bile in the bowel can look like blood when observed transmurally; aspiration or enterotomy may be needed to distinguish bile from blood. Second, an incompetent ileocecal valve may allow blood from the colon to reflux into the ileum, making the source seem like it is in the small intestine.

In unstable patients, inability to exclude the small bowel as a source of bleeding may necessitate creation of an ileostomy with a mucous fistula or colectomy with ileostomy and Hartmann's pouch. This approach allows more rapid identification of continued small bowel bleeding and facilitates ileoscopy postoperatively.

In stable patients, the inability to exclude the small bowel as a source of bleeding dictates the need for endoscopic enteroscopy either transorally or transanally. During oral enteroscopy, the gastroenterologist advances an enteroscope or pediatric colonoscope past the ligament of Treitz and into the jejunum and ileum. The room lights are turned off and the bowel is telescoped over the scope while the gastroenterologist looks at the mucosa and the surgeon looks at the transilluminated wall of the intestine looking for arteriovenous malformations. If such lesions are identified, they can be ligated or the involved segment can be resected. Operative enteroscopy can be quite challenging due to overinflation of the gut and operative injury to the bowel may be misinterpreted as a bleeding site. Nevertheless, its usefulness has been confirmed in several studies. Intraoperative colonoscopy may also be helpful.

If the small bowel is identified as the source of bleeding, operative findings dictate the appropriate management: for example, a local resection for Meckel's diverticulum, or a more extensive resection for jejunal diverticulosis or small bowel neoplasm. If exploration identifies the colon as the source of bleeding, operative management can proceed with the same considerations as when preoperative evaluation has identified colonic bleeding.

"Directed laparotomy" for suspected colonic bleeding involves a difficult choice for the surgeon: whether to perform a limited resection or more extensive resection of the colon. If a particular portion of the colon is implicated as the source of bleeding by radionucleide scintigraphy, angiography or other techniques, it can be removed selectively. This carries the risk that the wrong section will be removed, and that bleeding will recur. Historically, "blind" segmental resections for colonic bleeding were associated with rebleeding rates of up to 40% with associated mortality of 5% to 30%. With modern localization techniques, the rebleeding rate after limited colonic resection is much lower, approximately 5% to 20% (40). An alternative approach is subtotal colectomy with ileorectal anastomosis (41,42). This procedure has reduced rebleeding rates to as low as 2% with mortality rates of 10% to 15%. As mentioned earlier, the presence of comorbid lesions elsewhere in the colon also may mandate a more extensive resection.

The decision about the extent of colonic resection depends on the balance between rebleeding rates, acute morbidity and mortality, and long-term bowel function. Because rebleeding rates, morbidity and mortality are comparable in modern series of limited and extensive resections, concerns about intractable diarrhea and fecal incontinence have dominated decision making in the operating room. Recent series suggest that the rates of these complications are similar with limited and extensive resections, and is only a clinically important problem in 5% of patients of age 65 years and older (43).

OUTCOMES

Overall mortality in acute lower gastrointestinal bleeding increases with age, transfusion requirements, comorbid conditions, and the frequency of rebleeding. Operative morbidity and mortality rates can be quite high in patients with lower gastrointestinal tract bleeding due to comorbid conditions, such as congestive heart failure or chronic pulmonary disease, that are more common in an elderly population (44). Endoscopic stigmata of recent hemorrhage may be another risk factor for recurrent bleeding (26). In-hospital rebleeding rates range from 10% to 15%. In general, observation for 48 to 72 hours is acceptable once bleeding has subsided. During this time, vital signs and hematocrit should continue to be closely monitored.

Patients who survive their first episode of diverticular hemorrhage have a 10% risk of rebleeding in the first year and a 25% risk over four years (7). Patients who survive a second diverticular bleed have a 50% chance of developing further bleeding episodes, raising the issue of elective colectomy (3).

REFERENCES

1. Gostout CJ. Acute Lower Gastrointestinal Bleeding. In: Brandt LJ, ed. Clinical Practice of Gastroenterology. Philadelphia: Current Medicine, 1999:651–662.
2. Stollman NH, Raskin JB. Diagnosis and management of diverticular disease of the colon in adults. Ad Hoc Practice Parameters Committee of the American College of Gastroenterology. Am J Gastroenterol 1999; 94:3110–3121.
3. Longstreth GF. Epidemiology and outcome of patients hospitalized with acute lower gastrointestinal hemorrhage: a population-based study. Am J Gastroenterol 1997; 92:419–424.
4. Zuckerman GR, Prakash C. Acute lower intestinal bleeding: part I: clinical presentation and diagnosis. Gastrointest Endosc 1999; 48:606–617.
5. Zuckerman GR, Prakash C. Acute lower intestinal bleeding: part II: etiology, therapy, and outcomes. Gastrointest Endosc 1999; 49:228–238.
6. Zuccaro G Jr. Management of the adult patient with acute lower gastrointestinal bleeding. American College of Gastroenterology Practice Parameters Committee. Am J Gastroenterol 1998; 93:1202–1208.
7. Terdiman JP. Colonoscopic management of lower gastrointestinal hemorrhage. Curr Gastroenterol Rep 2001; 3:425–432.
8. Comay D, Marshall JK. Resource utilization for acute lower gastrointestinal hemorrhage: the Ontario GI bleed study. Can J Gastroenterol 2002; 16:677–682.
9. Reinus JF, Brandt LJ. Vascular ectasias and diverticulosis. Common causes of lower intestinal bleeding. Gastroenterol Clin North Am 1994; 23:1–20.
10. Foutch PG. Angiodysplasia of the gastrointestinal tract. Am J Gastroenterol 1993; 88:807–818.
11. Foutch PG, Rex DK, Lieberman DA. Prevalence and natural history of colonic angiodysplasia among healthy asymptomatic people. Am J Gastroenterol 1995; 90:564–567.
12. Norton ID, Petersen BT, Sorbi D, Balm RK, Alexander GL, Gostout CJ. Management and long-term prognosis of Dieulafoy lesion. Gastrointest Endosc 1999; 50:762–767.
13. Schmulewitz N, Baillie J. Dieulafoy lesions: a review of 6 years of experience at a tertiary referral center. Am J Gastroenterol 2001; 96:1688–1694.
14. Shudo R, Yazaki Y, Sakurai S, Uenishi H, Yamada H, Sugawara K. Clinical study comparing bleeding and nonbleeding rectal varices. Endoscopy 2002; 34:189–194.
15. Hosking SW, Smart HL, Johnson AG, Triger DR. Anorectal varices, haemorrhoids, and portal hypertension. Lancet 1989; 1:349–352.
16. Mackey WC, Dineen P. A fifty year experience with Meckel's diverticulum. Surg Gynecol Obstet 1983; 156:56–64.
17. Soltero MJ, Bill AH. The natural history of Meckel's diverticulum and its relation to incidental removal. A study of 202 cases of diseased Meckel's diverticulum found in King County, Washington over a fifteen year period. Am J Surg 1976; 132:168–173.
18. Sorbi D, Norton I, Conio M, Balm R, Zinsmeister A, Gostout CJ. Postpolypectomy lower GI bleeding: descriptive analysis. Gastrointest Endosc 2000; 51:690–696.
19. Pardi DS, Loftus EV Jr., Tremaine WJ, et al. Acute major gastrointestinal hemorrhage in inflammatory bowel disease. Gastrointest Endosc 1999; 49:153–157.
20. Yantiss RK, Clement PB, Young RH. Endometriosis of the intestinal tract: a study of 44 cases of a disease that may cause diverse challenges in clinical and pathologic evaluation. Am J Surg Pathol 2001; 25:445–454.
21. Antinori CH, Andrew CT, Santaspirt JS, et al. The many faces of aortoenteric fistulas. Am Surg 1996; 62:344–349.
22. Lemos DW, Raffetto JD, Moore TC, Menzoian JO. Primary aortoduodenal fistula: a case report and review of the literature. J Vasc Surg 2003; 37:686–689.
23. Lingenfelser T, Ell C. Lower intestinal bleeding. Best Pract Res Clin Gastroenterol 2001; 15: 135–153.
24. Eisen GM, Dominitz JA, Faigel DO, et al. American Society for Gastrointestinal Endoscopy Standards of Practice Committee. An annotated algorithmic approach to acute lower gastrointestinal bleeding. Gastrointest Endosc 2001; 53:859–863.
25. Strate LL, Orav EJ, Syngal S. Early predictors of severity in acute lower intestinal tract bleeding. Arch Intern Med 2003; 163:838–843.
26. Kanwal F, Dulai G, Jensen DM, et al. Major stigmata of recent hemorrhage on rectal ulcers in patients with severe hematochezia: endoscopic diagnosis, treatment, and outcomes. Gastrointest Endosc 2003; 57:462–468.
27. Jensen DM, Machicado GA. Colonoscopy for diagnosis and treatment of severe lower gastrointestinal tract bleeding: routine outcomes and cost analysis. Gastrointest Endosc Clin N Am 1997; 7:477–498.
28. O'Neill BB, Gosnell JE, Lull RJ, et al. Cinematic nuclear scintigraphy reliably directs surgical intervention for patients with gastrointestinal bleeding. Arch Surg 2000; 135:1076–1081.
29. Levy R, Barto W, Gani J. Retrospective study of the utility of nuclear scintigraphic-labelled red cell scanning for lower gastrointestinal bleeding. ANZ J Surg 2003; 73:205–209.
30. Ernst O, Bulois P, Saint-Drenant S, Leroy C, Paris JC, Sergent G. Helical CT in acute lower gastrointestinal bleeding. Eur Radiol 2003; 13:114–117.

31. Jensen DM, Machicado GA, Jutabha R, Kovacs TO. Urgent colonoscopy for the diagnosis and treatment of severe diverticular hemorrhage. N Engl J Med 2000; 342:78–82.
32. Luchtefeld MA, Senagore AJ, Szomstein M, Fedeson B, Van Erp J, Rupp S. Evaluation of transarterial embolization for lower gastrointestinal bleeding. Dis Colon Rectum 2000; 43:532–534.
33. Funaki B. Endovascular intervention for the treatment of acute arterial gastrointestinal hemorrhage. Gastroenterol Clin North Am 2002; 31:701–713.
34. Darcy M. Treatment of lower gastrointestinal bleeding: vasopressin infusion versus embolization. J Vasc Interv Radiol 2003; 14:535–543.
35. Horiguchi J, Naito A, Fukuda H, et al. Morphologic and histopathologic changes in the bowel after super-selective transcatheter embolization for focal lower gastrointestinal hemorrhage. Acta Radiol 2003; 44:334–339.
36. Breen E, Murray JJ. Pathophysiology and natural history of lower gastrointestinal bleeding. Semin Colon Rectal Surg 1997; 8:128–137.
37. Klas JV, Madoff RD. Surgical options in lower gastrointestinal bleeding. Semin Colon Rectal Surg 1997; 8:172–177.
38. Darby CR, Berry AR, Mortensen N. Management variability in surgery for colorectal emergencies. Br J Surg 1992; 79:206–210.
39. Bender JS, Wiencek RG, Bouwman DL. Morbidity and mortality following total abdominal colectomy for massive lower gastrointestinal bleeding. Am Surg 1991; 57:536–540.
40. Parkes BM, Obeid FN, Sorensen VJ, Horst HM, Fath JJ. The management of massive lower gastrointestinal bleeding. Am Surg 1993; 59:676–678.
41. Field RJ Sr, Field RJ Jr., Shackleford S. Total abdominal colectomy for control of massive lower gastrointestinal bleeding. J Miss State Med Assoc 1994; 35:29–33.
42. Baker R, Senagore A. Abdominal colectomy offers safe management for massive lower GI bleed. A Surg 1994; 60:578–581.
43. Farner R, Lichliter W, Kuhn J, Fisher T. Total colectomy versus limited colonic resection for acute lower gastrointestinal bleeding. Am J Surg 1999; 178:587–591.
44. Brackman MR, Gushchin VV, Smith L, Demory M, Kirkpatrick JR, Stahl T. Acute lower gastroenteric bleeding retrospective analysis (the ALGEBRA study): an analysis of the triage, management and outcomes of patients with acute lower gastrointestinal bleeding. Am Surg 2003; 69:145–149.

17 | Vascular Disorders of the Colon

Omar S. Nehme
Division of Gastroenterology, Indiana University School of Medicine, Indianapolis, Indiana, U.S.A.

Jeffrey B. Raskin
Division of Gastroenterology, Miami Miller School of Medicine, University of Miami/Jackson Memorial Medical Center, Miami, Florida, U.S.A.

INTRODUCTION

Abnormalities of gastrointestinal (GI) vasculature are diverse, and are often incidentally discovered during imaging, angiographic, and endoscopic studies performed for various reasons. Patients with such abnormalities are often asymptomatic; however, chronic blood loss resulting in anemia, and severe acute GI bleeding can also be modes of presentation (1). Recognition of such abnormalities and familiarity with diagnostic modalities and therapeutic options are essential in caring for such patients. In this chapter, we will review the vascular abnormalities that involve the colon (Table 1).

VASCULAR ECTASIAS (ARTERIOVENOUS MALFORMATIONS)

This class of lesions encompasses the most common vascular abnormalities of the lower GI tract and with diverticulosis representing one of the two most common causes of lower GI bleeding. The reported incidence of colonic arteriovenous malformations (AVMs) in different series of patients presenting with a lower GI bleed has been largely variable, with 20% being a rough estimate of this incidence. Some series reported AVMs as the most common cause of lower GI bleeding in patients above the age of 65 (2,3). Colonic AVMs are most commonly described in the cecum, but may be present throughout the colon. They can be variable in size, single or multiple. Multiple AVMs can be associated with disease entities such as hereditary telangiectasia, Osler–Weber–Rendu (OWR) disease, and the Calcinosis, Raynaud's, Esophageal dysmotility, Sclerodactyly, and Telangiectasia (CREST) syndrome in association with scleroderma.

Vascular ectasias represent a dilated complex of arterioles, venules and communicating capillaries. Development of such dilation is commonly thought to be related to increased pressure within the colonic lumen. Luminal pressure changes and increased predisposition to ischemia associated with aging may explain the predominance of such lesions in the middle-aged and the elderly (3,4). In addition, the greater tension in the cecal wall may explain the preponderance of these lesions in the right colon.

AVMs are usually less than 10 mm in diameter, and can be diagnosed by means of colonoscopy and/or angiography. Such lesions are felt to be acquired and should be differentiated from congenital vascular malformations (e.g., OWR disease).

Bleeding from AVMs is a well-described entity that represents a common source of GI bleeding in the elderly (Fig. 1). Such bleeding is most often felt to be intermittent and subacute often leading to significant anemia. As a result of the nature of the bleeding, stool fecal occult blood tests are not always positive. More brisk bleeding is associated with the passage of maroon colored or tarry stools. Although the incidence of subacute versus acute bleeding from AVMs is not well documented, the incidence of recurrent bleeding from untreated AVMs has been reported to be as high as 80% (5). Several reports have suggested a higher incidence of AVMs in patient's with aortic stenosis (Heyde's syndrome), chronic renal insufficiency, and von Willebrand's disease. Such observations have not been well validated by means of controlled studies. Many authors have questioned whether the increased incidence noted in the latter two conditions is a result of increased bleeding from AVMs secondary to the coagulopathy that is often noted in these patients. In addition, there are some reports of an increased

Table 1 Colonic Vascular Lesions

Arteriovenous malformations
Osler–Weber–Rendu disease
Hemangioma
Dieulafoy lesion
Rectal varices
Portal hypertensive colopathy

incidence of aortic stenosis in patients with GI AVMs. Other reports have also attributed the bleeding from AVMs in patients with aortic stenosis to acquired von Willebrand factor (6–8).

DIAGNOSIS

AVMs are most typically seen at the time of the colonoscopy. Differentiating AVMs from vascular abnormalities associated with inflammatory bowel disease, radiation, ischemia, and other disorders can be a difficult process. In addition, the endoscopic appearance of vascular ectasia can be influenced by the patient's blood pressure and volume status. Meperidine (Demerol), which is often used for sedation during colonoscopy, is believed to make AVMs less visible (possibly due to blood pressure and flow changes). Some experts advocate the use of reversal agents such as naloxone, once the cecum is intubated when such findings are expected to improve the visualization of AVMs (9). In our experience, it is important to look for AVMs at the time of scope insertion and prior to obtaining any mucosal biopsies. This technique helps avoid confusing AVMs with mucosal trauma induced by the colonoscopy and/or biopsy forceps. A relatively new technique in diagnosing colonic AVMs is helical computed tomographic angiography (CTA). Junquera et al. compared this technique to colonoscopy combined with visceral angiography. They reported the sensitivity and specificity of CTA in detecting colonic AVMs to be 70% and 100%, respectively (10). Should the results of further studies confirm this estimate, then CTA promises to be an effective and minimally invasive tool for diagnosing colonic AVMs. Although there have been case reports of right colonic AVMs diagnosed by capsule endoscopy, this technique is primarily utilized for visualizing the small intestine, and there are no published studies specifically regarding its use to visualize the cecum and right colon. Several systems have been proposed for the classification of colonic angiodysplasia. One system considers three main factors which are the location of the lesions (gastric, duodenal, jejunal, and colonic); size of the lesions (less than 2 mm in diameter, 2–5 mm, and greater than 5 mm); and number of lesions (unique, 2–10, and greater than 10). Such systems are useful mainly for research purposes and their clinical significance remains unknown (11).

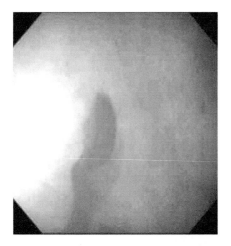

Figure 1 (*See color insert*) Colonic arteriovenous malformation with active bleeding. *Source*: Courtesy of Emad Y. Rahmani, Department of Surgery, Indiana University School of Medicine, Indianapolis, Indiana, U.S.A.

MANAGEMENT

In view of the low risk of bleeding from colonic AVMs incidentally found at the time of colonoscopy, no specific endoscopic therapy is generally recommended. In patients presenting with bleeding or anemia associated with heme positive stools, endoscopic and angiographic techniques can be utilized for diagnostic and therapeutic purposes. Most GI bleeds resulting from AVMs can be controlled without surgery. Resuscitation with fluids and blood products, optimizing the patient's coagulation status and early diagnostic and therapeutic intervention often result in a good clinical outcome (12). On angiography, AVMs often appear as dilated, slow filling, and early emptying veins. When seen by colonoscopy, they appear as flat or slightly raised red lesions, which often have a spider-like appearance. Larger polypoid vascular lesions have been described but are less frequent (13).

Angiography can be utilized to identify and treat active bleeding but the rate of bleeding has to exceed 0.5 cc/min for angiography to be diagnostic (14,15). Active bleeding appears as contrast extravasation. Infusion of vasoconstrictor agents (such as vasopressin) at the time of angiography, and embolization of the bleeding vessel have been described as modalities of controlling bleeding secondary to angiodysplasia (2,16–18). Although a high success rate of both modalities has been reported in some series, such interventions have the potential for inducing colonic ischemia/infarction. It has been suggested that slower infusion rates of vasoconstrictors in smaller arteries may help avoid such complications.

Other complications described with the use of angiographic techniques include the formation of hematomas, pseudoaneurysms, and arterial thrombosis. Superselective catheter placement has been described, and is associated with a decreased risk of bowel infarction; however, this risk remains considerable especially if vasopressin infusion is used (19,20).

Since the 1970s, endoscopic interventions to control bleeding from AVMs have been described. Different techniques aimed at ablating the vascular lesions have included sclerotherapy, electrocoagulation, neodymium:yttrium aluminum garnet (Nd:YAG) laser, and most recently argon plasma coagulation (APC) (21–24).

Other forms of therapeutic endoscopic interventions such as the use of hemoclips and banding may prove to be of benefit in treating bleeding AVMs (25). Whether using APC or electrocoagulation to treat bleeding AVMs, the mucosa should be cauterized until it is white with obliteration of the visualized lesion (Fig. 2). The use of APC is preferred over Nd:YAG laser therapy because the light wave of the former penetrates more superficially, thus decreasing the risk of perforation. Rebleeding occurs in 10% to 30% of treated patients, and most cases of rebleeding are due to missed lesions or incompletely cauterized lesions (24,26).

In a series of 100 patients with bleeding AVMs who were medically treated (with iron, blood transfusions, and hormonal therapy) for two years prior to endoscopic therapy, the mean hematocrit was noted to be 37.3 after endoscopic intervention (vs. 26.8) and the number of units blood transfused per year was 1.3 in the same group (vs. 4.3) (26).

Another form of nonsurgical intervention in patients with AVMs involves the use of hormonal therapy. This controversial therapy with estrogen derivatives has been mostly

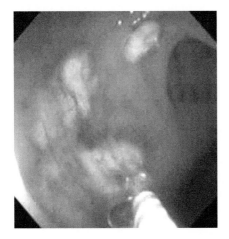

Figure 2 (*See color insert*) Colonic arteriovenous malformation posttreatment with BICAP cautery. *Source*: Courtesy of Emad Y. Rahmani, Department of Surgery, Indiana University School of Medicine, Indianapolis, Indiana, U.S.A.

investigated in patients with OWR disease, in patients with AVMs and renal failure. Results of hormonal therapy have been contradictory. Earlier studies suggested a beneficial effect associated with the use of hormonal therapy in patients with AVM-related blood loss (27,28). However, a recent multicenter placebo-controlled trial from Spain showed no benefit from using hormonal therapy in cases of bleeding AVMs (29). Although the type and dosage of hormonal therapy could potentially alter the outcome, the results of such studies raise important questions regarding the routine use of hormonal therapy in managing patients with chronic bleeding from AVMs.

Observational studies and case reports have also suggested a beneficial effect associated with the use of somatostatin analogues (Octreotide). This medication may help control bleeding by causing a reduction in splanchnic blood flow. Larger controlled studies are needed before a broader use of this class of medications can be recommended (30,31).

In patients whose bleeding cannot be controlled with the above methods, or in whom recurrent bleeding occurs, surgical intervention is indicated. Since the majority of colonic AVMs are localized in the cecum and ascending colon, a right hemicolectomy is often the procedure of choice. Following surgery, cases of obscure recurrent bleeding are occasionally managed by means of a subtotal colectomy. In a study by Jensen and Machicado, in which patients were followed post endoscopic intervention for AVM bleeding, 18% of the patients required surgery for recurrent bleeding (23). If the localization of the bleeding point is not possible prior to surgical intervention, then the use of intraoperative enteroscopy and colonoscopy may be of benefit in identifying the source of blood loss. If expert intraoperative endoscopic evaluation reveals no specific bleeding point, and if the presentation and data are suggestive of a colonic bleed, a subtotal colectomy may be cautiously considered. The performance of either an ileorectal anastomosis or an ileostomy depends upon the preoperative and intraoperative hemodynamic, nutritional, and other systemic factors.

OSLER–WEBER–RENDU DISEASE

Although GI lesions of OWR are primarily localized in the proximal GI tract, colonic lesions have been well described. This entity has an autosomal dominant form of inheritance, and is characterized by recurrent epistaxis and the presence of AVMs in different organ systems. Its prevalence in the United States is one to two patients per 100,000 population. Equal incidence in males and females has been reported. Diagnostic and therapeutic interventions in patients with OWR and colonic bleeding are identical to the ones used in patients with sporadic AVMs. A better response to hormonal therapy has been reported in this subgroup of patients. It is important to recognize the coexistence of telangiectasia in the stomach and small intestine of these patients (32). While these concomitant lesions are rare in patients with acquired AVMs, the involvement of the mucous membranes in patients with OWR, explains the epistaxis, which is often a presenting sign. Additionally, the vascular lesions of OWR often involve all layers of the bowel wall contrary to acquired AVMs, which are confined to the mucosal and submucosal layers.

Another systemic disease causing colonic vascular malformations is the CREST variant of scleroderma. This entity is more common in females. The prevalence of scleroderma in the United States is 240 cases per million; however, the true incidence and prevalence of CREST is not known (33). The telangiectasia in these patients often involve the skin and the upper GI tract; however, bleeding secondary to small intestinal and colonic telangiectasia has been reported (34).

HEMANGIOMA

Hemangiomas represent a congenital anomaly in which a proliferation of vascular endothelium leads to a mass that resembles neoplastic tissue (hamartoma). Colonic hemangiomas are variable in size, and can be localized or present in other organ systems.

Although most colonic hemangiomas produce blood loss at a slow rate, large rectal hemangiomas may lead to massive lower GI bleeding. Small lesions maybe amenable to endoscopic intervention; however, larger lesions require surgical resection (35). GI hemangiomas have been associated with the blue rubber bleb nevus syndrome. Patients with this syndrome

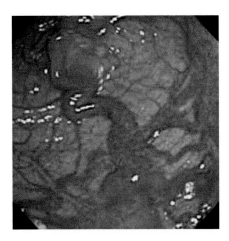

Figure 3 (*See color insert*) Rectal varices. *Source*: Courtesy of Emad Y. Rahmani, Department of Surgery, Indiana University School of Medicine, Indianapolis, Indiana, U.S.A.

are reported to have bluish raised lesions (hemangioma) that may be diffuse, but tend to spare the mucous membranes. Small bowel and colonic hemangioma have been described in association with this syndrome. Patients with anemia are best managed with iron supplementation. In the rare cases where patients present with acute lower GI bleeding, surgical resection of the involved segment is indicated. Such cases may be well suited to preoperative endoscopic ink marking to facilitate laparoscopic or laparoscopic-assisted resection. Endoscopic interventions have proven to be effective in select cases (36,37). Rectal hemangiomas have also been associated with Klippel–Trenaunay syndrome, which consists of vascular nevi and osseous hypertrophy of the lower limbs. Lower GI bleeding can be secondary to blood loss from the hemangiomas, or to bleeding from rectal varices, which have been reported in this patient population (38). The presence of phleboliths on imaging studies may help in differentiating large rectosigmoid hemangiomas from other lesions such as carcinoma and radiation stricture (39).

DIEULAFOY LESION

Dieulafoy lesion (Exulceratio Simplex) is a well-recognized cause of GI bleeding. This lesion which is caused by a large caliber artery that protrudes through a mucosal defect was described by Georges Dieulafoy in the late 19th century. These lesions are most frequently located in the proximal stomach in the proximity of the gastroesophageal junction. Dieulafoy lesions of the small intestine and colon have been reported, and 3% of patients with these lesions present with rectal bleeding only (40,41). Endoscopic management of these lesions is associated with a relatively low risk of rebleeding (10–20%). Reported modalities of endoscopic therapy include injection with a sclerosant, electrocoagulation (42,43), as well as the use of mechanical

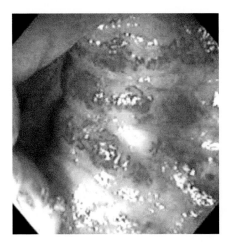

Figure 4 (*See color insert*) Portal hypertensive colopathy. *Source*: Courtesy of Emad Y. Rahmani, Department of Surgery, Indiana University School of Medicine, Indianapolis, Indiana, U.S.A.

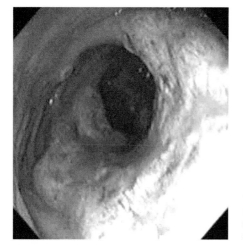

Figure 5 (*See color insert*) Portal hypertensive colopathy posttreatment with argon plasma coagulation. *Source*: Courtesy of Emad Y. Rahmani, Department of Surgery, Indiana University School of Medicine, Indianapolis, Indiana, U.S.A.

devices such as endoloop and endoscopic clipping (44). In cases with severe bleeding, which prevents adequate endoscopic visualization, the diagnosis can be accomplished by means of visceral angiography. In patients who are known to be at high risk for undergoing surgery, an attempt at embolizing the bleeding vessel should be made (45).

RECTAL VARICES AND PORTAL COLOPATHY

In patients with portal hypertension, varices can form between the hemorrhoidal veins of the portal and systemic circulation. In this patient population, the incidence of rectal varices is reported to be greater than 50% (Fig. 3). In patients with rectal variceal bleeding, endoscopic therapeutic techniques include sclerotherapy (46), and banding (47). Such techniques may result in rectal ulcerations that may result in delayed rectal bleeding. In addition to endoscopic intervention (Figs. 4 and 5), the use of somatostatin infusion may help to control bleeding secondary to portal hypertensive colopathy (48,49).

Refractory bleeding may be controlled by means of angiographic embolization (50). Placement of intrahepatic portosystemic shunt has been reported to be effective in controlling bleeding from rectal varices. In addition to varices, patients with portal hypertension are reported to have an increased incidence of telangiectasia, and loss of the normal colon vascular pattern. These findings have been labeled as portal hypertensive colopathy, and may mimic the changes seen with inflammatory bowel disease.

Endoscopic findings range from mild erythema to angiodysplasia with subepithelial hemorrhage (Fig. 4). When compared with colonoscopy, the use of rectal ultrasonography has been reported to provide earlier detection of distal colonic mucosal changes secondary to portal hypertension (51). Attempts have been made to classify colopathy based on the degree of involvement (52). No correlation has been noted between the severity of portal hypertensive gastropathy, and the presence of portal hypertensive colopathy. Some studies, however, have reported a predominance of severe portal colopathy in patients with large esophageal varices (53). Surgery can be exceptionally perilous and should be avoided whenever possible.

CONCLUSION

Vascular malformations and aberrant blood vessels can occur throughout the GI tract. Although a small percentage of these lesions are present at birth, the majority are acquired and detected during adulthood. In the colon, angiodysplasia is primarily found proximal to the splenic flexure. Although a large number of these lesions remain asymptomatic throughout life, up to 30% of cases of lower GI bleeding could be explained by this entity. Recent advances in endoscopy and radiology have made the detection of most of these lesions easier. Pharmacologic interventions to control blood loss from these lesions are limited at best.

Contrary to small bowel vascular malformations, which are often distal and outside the reach of enteroscopes (including push enteroscopy), colonic lesions are accessible and amenable to endoscopic therapy. The main difficulty arises in identifying all present lesions at the time of colonoscopy. The ease of detection can be affected by the patient's preparation, anatomy, type of sedation, etc. For refractory lesions, angiography with embolization is an attractive diagnostic and therapeutic option; however, colonic ischemia as a result of such interventions remains a significant risk. For these refractory cases, surgical intervention also remains an option. The extent of colonic resection largely depends on the adequacy of pre- and intraoperative localization using endoscopic and angiographic techniques. Total colectomy is very cautiously reserved for patients with refractory bleeding and poor localization. Capsule video endoscopy and enteroscopy are valuable tests, prior to colonic surgery, to rule out the possibility of small bowel malformations that could be contributing to the patient's symptoms.

REFERENCES

1. Elta G. Urgent colonoscopy for acute lower-GI bleeding. Gastrointest Endosc 2004; 59(3):402–408.
2. Browder W, Cerise EJ, Litwin MS. Impact of emergency angiography in massive lower gastrointestinal bleeding. Ann Surg 1986; 204:530–536.
3. Boley SJ, DiBiase A, Brandt LJ, Sammartano RJ. Lower intestinal bleeding in the elderly. Am J Surg 1979; 137:57–64.
4. Rogers BH. Endoscopic diagnosis and therapy of mucosal vascular abnormalities of the gastrointestinal tract occurring in elderly patients and associated with cardiac, vascular, and pulmonary disease. Gastrointest Endosc 1980; 26:134–138.
5. Gupta N, Longo WE, Vernava AM III. Angiodysplasia of the lower gastrointestinal tract: an entity readily diagnosed by colonoscopy and primarily managed nonoperatively. Dis Colon Rectum 1995; 38:979–982.
6. Imperiale TF, Ransohoff DF. Aortic stenosis, idiopathic gastrointestinal bleeding, and angiodysplasia: is there an association? A methodologic critique of the literature. Gastroenterology 1988; 95:1670–1676.
7. Veyradier A, Balian A, Wolf M, et al. Abnormal von Willebrand factor in bleeding angiodysplasias of the digestive tract. Gastroenterology 2001; 120:346–353.
8. Oneglia C, Sabatini T, Rusconi C, et al. Prevalence of aortic valve stenosis in patients affected by gastrointestinal angiodysplasia. Eur J Med 1993; 2:75–78.
9. Brandt LJ, Spinnell MK. Ability of Naloxone to enhance the colonoscopic appearance of normal colon vasculature and colon vascular ectasias. Gastrointest Endosc 1999; 49:79–83.
10. Junquera F, Quiroga S, Saperas E, et al. Accuracy of helical computed tomographic angiography for the diagnosis of colonic angiodysplasia. Gastroenterology 2000; 119:293–299.
11. Schmit A, van Gossum A. Proposal for an endoscopic classification of digestive angiodysplasias for therapeutic trials. Gastrointest Endosc 1998; 48:659.
12. Trudel JL, Fazio VW, Sivak MV. Colonoscopic diagnosis and treatment of arteriovenous malformations in chronic lower gastrointestinal bleeding: clinical accuracy and efficacy. Dis Colon Rectum 1988; 31:107–110.
13. Koziara FJ, Brodmerkel GJ, Boylan JJ, Ciambotti GF, Agrawal RM. Bleeding from polypoid colonic arteriovenous malformations. Am J Gastroenterol 1996; 91(3):584–586.
14. Emanuel RB, Weiser MM, Shenoy SS, Satchidanand SK, Asirwatham J. Arteriovenous malformations as a cause of gastrointestinal bleeding; the importance of triple vessel angiographic studies in diagnosis and prevention of rebleeding. J Clin Gastroenterol 1985; 7:237–246.
15. Boley SJ, Sprayregen S, Sammartano RJ, Adams A, Kleinhaus S. The pathophysiologic basis for the angiographic signs of vascular ectasias of the colon. Radiology 1977; 125:615–621.
16. Uflacker R. Transcatheter embolization for treatment of acute lower gastrointestinal bleeding. Acta Radiol 1987; 28:425–430.
17. Sniderman KW, Franklin J, Sos TA. Successful transcatheter gelfoam embolization of bleeding cecal vascular ectasia. Am J Roentgenol 1978; 131:157–159.
18. Sherman LM, Shenoy SS, Cerra FB. Selective intra-arterial vasopressin: clinical efficacy and complications. Ann Surg 1979; 189:298–302.
19. DeBarros J, Rosas L, Cohen J, Vignati P, Sardella W, Hallisey M. The changing paradigm for the treatment of colonic hemorrhage: superselective angiographic embolization. Dis Colon Rectum 2002; 45:802–808.
20. Gordon RL, Ahl KL, Kerlan RK, et al. Selective arterial embolization for the control of lower gastrointestinal bleeding. Am J Surg 1997; 174:24–28.
21. Cello JP, Grendell JH. Endoscopic laser treatment for gastrointestinal vascular ectasias. Ann Intern Med 1986; 104:352–354.
22. Naveau S, Aubert A, Poynard AT, Chaput J. Long term results of treatment of vascular malformations of the gastrointestinal tract by Neodymium YAG laser photocoagulation. Dig Dis Sci 1990; 35:821–826.
23. Jensen DM, Machicado GA. Bleeding colonic angioma: endoscopic coagulation and follow-up. Gastroenterology 1985; 88:1433.

24. Grund K, Straub T, Farin G. Argon plasma coagulation (APC) in flexible endoscopy. Experience with 2193 applications in 1062 patients. Gastrointest Endosc 1999; 49(4):1999.
25. Ohta S, Yukioka T, Ohta S, Miyagatani Y, Matsuda H, Shimazaki S. Hemostasis with endoscopic hemoclipping for severe gastrointestinal bleeding in critically ill patients. Am J Gastroenterol 1996; 91:701–704.
26. Jensen D, Machiado G. Control of bleeding. In: Raskin JB, Nord SJ, eds. Colonoscopy Principles and Techniques. New York: Igaku-Shoin, 1995:323–325.
27. Barkin JS, Ross BS. Medical therapy for chronic gastrointestinal bleeding of obscure origin. Am J Gastroenterol 1998; 93:1250–1254.
28. Bronner MH, Pate MB, Cunningham JT, Marsh WH. Estrogen-progesterone therapy for bleeding telangiectasias in chronic renal failure: an uncontrolled trial. Ann Intern Med 1986; 105:371–374.
29. Junquera F, Feu F, Papo M. A multicenter, randomized, clinical trial of hormonal therapy in the prevention of rebleeding from gastrointestinal angiodysplasia. Gastroenterology 2001; 121:1073–1079.
30. Andersen MR, Aaseby J. Somatostatin in the treatment of gastrointestinal bleeding caused by angiodysplasia. Scand J Gastroenterol 1996; 31:1037–1039.
31. Nardone G, Rocco A, Balzano T, Budillon G. The efficacy of octreotide therapy in chronic bleeding due to vascular abnormalities of the gastrointestinal tract. Aliment Pharmacol Ther 1999; 13:1429–1436.
32. Longacre AV, Gross CP, Gallitelli M, Henderson KJ, White RI Jr, Proctor DD. Diagnosis and management of gastrointestinal bleeding in patients with hereditary hemorrhagic telangiectasia. Am J Gastroenterol 2003; 98(1):59–65.
33. Mayes M. Scleroderma epidemiology. Rheumatic Dis Clin North Am 2003; 29(2):239–254.
34. Duchini A, Sessoms SL. Gastrointestinal hemorrhage in patients with systemic sclerosis and CREST syndrome. Am J Gastroenterol 1998; 93(9):1453–1456.
35. Fishman SJ, Smithers CJ, Folkman J. Blue rubber bleb nevus syndrome: Surgical eradication of gastrointestinal bleeding. Annals Surg 2005; 241(3):523–528.
36. Nijhawan S, Kumar D, Joshi A, et al. Endoscopic band ligation for non variceal bleed. Ind J Gastroenterol 2004; 23(5):186–187.
37. Ng WT, Kong CK. Argon plasma coagulation for blue rubber bleb nevus syndrome in a female patient. Eur J Pediatr Surg 2003; 13(2):137–139.
38. Mussack T, Siveke JT, Pfeifer KJ, Folwaczny C. Klippel-Trenaunay syndrome with involvement of coecum and rectum: a rare cause of lower gastrointestinal bleeding. Eur J Med Res 2004; 9(11):515–517.
39. Levy AD, Abbott RM, Rohrmann CA Jr., Frazier AA, Kende A. Gastrointestinal hemangiomas. Am J Roentgenol 2001; 177:1073–1081.
40. Barlow TF, Bentley FH. Arteries, veins, and arteriovenous anastomosis in the stomach. Surg Gynecol Obstet 1951; 93:657.
41. Fockers P, Tytgat G. Dieulafoy's disease. Gastrointest Endosc Clin North Am 1996; 6:739–752.
42. Schmulewitz N, Baillie J. Dieulafoy lesions: a review of 6 years of experience at a tertiary referral center. Am J Gastroenterol 2001; 96(6):1688–1694.
43. Abdulian JD, Santoro MJ, Chen YK, Collen MJ. Dieulafoy-like lesion of the rectum presenting with exanguinating hemorrhage: successful endoscopic sclerotherapy. Am J Gastroenterol 1993; 88(11): 1939–1941.
44. Gimeno-Garcia AZ, Parra-Blanco A, Nicolas-Perez D, Ortega Sanchez JA, Medina C, Quintero E. Management of colonic Dieulafoy lesions with endoscopic mechanical techniques: report of two cases. Dis Colon Rectum 2004; 47(9):1539–1043.
45. Ashour MA, Millward SF, Hadziomerovic A. Embolotherapy of a Dieulafoy lesion in the cecum: case report and review of the literature. J Vasc Intervent Radiol 2000; 11(8):1059–1062.
46. Yamanaka T, Shiraki K, Ito T. Endoscopic sclerotherapy for acute rectal varices bleeding in a patient with liver cirrhosis. Hepato-Gastroenterology 2002; 49(46):941–943.
47. Firoozi B, Gamagaris Z, Weinshel EH, Bini EJ. Endoscopic band ligation of bleeding rectal varices. Dig Dis Sci 2002; 47(7):1502–1505.
48. Rana SS, Dutta U, Sinha SK, Kochhar R, Nagi B, Bhasin DK. Severe acute bleeding from portal colopathy controlled by somatostatin: a case report. Trop Gastroenterol 2004; 25(3):144–145.
49. Yoshie K, Fujita Y, Moriya A, Kawana I, Miyamoto K, Umemura S. Octreotide for severe acute bleeding from portal hypertensive colopathy: a case report. Eur J Gastroenterol Hepatol 2001; 13(9):1111–1113.
50. Hidajat N, Stobbe H, Hosten N, et al. Transjugular intrahepatic portosystemic shunt and transjugular embolization of bleeding rectal varices in portal hypertension. Am J Roentgenol 2002; 178(2):362–363.
51. Dhiman RK, Saraswat VA, Choudhuri G, Sharma BC, Pandey R, Naik SR. Endosonographic, endoscopic, and histologic evaluation of alterations in the rectal venous system in patients with portal hypertension. Gastrointest Endosc 1999; 49(2):218–227.
52. Miranda M, Domingues A. Hypertensive portal colopathy in Schistosomiasis mansoni-proposal for a classification. Memorias do Insituto Oswaldo Cruz 1999; 99(suppl 11):1999.
53. Naveau S, Bedossa P, Poynard T, Mory B, Chaput JC. Portal hypertensive colopathy. A new entity. Dig Dis Sci 1991; 36(12):1774–1781.

18 ▎ Irritable Bowel Syndrome

Kevin W. Olden
Division of Gastroenterology, Mayo Clinic Scottsdale, Scottsdale, Arizona, U.S.A.

Adriane Budavari
Department of Medicine, Mayo Clinic Scottsdale, Scottsdale, Arizona, U.S.A.

INTRODUCTION

No reference work covering disorders of the colon would be complete without a chapter covering irritable bowel syndrome (IBS). IBS is the most common disorder seen in gastrointestinal practice. Despite tremendous advances, which have occurred in the care of colonic disorders in the last 30 years, IBS remains a significant challenge for physicians, for a number of reasons. The first is that IBS has no pathognomonic structural, biochemical, or physiologic markers to identify it. Secondly, the symptoms of IBS, i.e., pain, constipation, and/or diarrhea and bloating can be seen in an extremely wide spectrum of gastrointestinal disorders. This presents at first glance a significant diagnostic and therapeutic challenge. However significant advances in our understanding of IBS have occurred in the last 10 years. This is particularly true in the areas of IBS diagnosis and treatment. It will be the purpose of this chapter to review the epidemiology, clinical presentation, and psychosocial correlates of IBS. A rational approach to diagnosis will be proposed, and recommendations for treatment emphasizing new and emerging agents will be discussed in detail. Although the treatment of IBS has been a somewhat nihilistic area of medical practice, an emerging realization of the importance of this somewhat perplexing disorder has produced a body of new knowledge to help us effectively treat these often long-suffering patients.

EPIDEMIOLOGY

The prevalence of IBS has been shown to be between 10% and 25% worldwide. One large community-based epidemiologic survey reported an 11.2% prevalence of IBS in the United States (1). Similar prevalence rates have been shown in other countries (1–3). These and other studies have not demonstrated any strong cultural differences; in fact, the prevalence of IBS worldwide seems to remain amazingly stable. However, it is clear that only a certain percentage of people with IBS ultimately seek treatment. One community-based sample in England found the prevalence of IBS to be 13% in women and 5% in men (1). However, only half of the subjects ultimately sought medical care. The dichotomy between patients who meet the diagnostic criteria for IBS in the community and those who actually seek medical care for their IBS was further studied by Drossman (4). In this landmark study, subjects were recruited from three populations: (i) patients from a university-based gastrointestinal (GI) clinic specializing in the treatment of IBS, consisting of individuals who chose to seek medical care for IBS, designated "IBS patients." (ii) Subjects recruited from the same university's undergraduate student population who met the diagnostic criteria for IBS but who chose not to seek care, the "IBS nonpatient" group. (iii) The final group consisted of undergraduate students from the same university who had no symptoms of IBS, serving as normal controls. All subjects were administered the McGill pain questionnaire as well as other psychological instruments to measure levels of pain, psychological distress, and coping abilities. The findings were dramatic in that subjects with IBS who chose to seek medical care (IBS patients) were significantly more likely to be psychologically impaired as compared to both the positive control group

(IBS nonpatients) and subjects who had no symptoms of IBS. This study suggested that IBS care seekers represent a unique subset of individuals who are more emotionally distressed than people who have identical symptoms and who chose not to seek care (4).

These findings were replicated by Whitehead and colleagues who studied a group of urban churchgoers who met the diagnostic criteria for IBS (study population) as well as subjects with documented lactose intolerance (positive controls) and individuals with no bowel symptoms (negative controls). In this study the IBS patients, although having symptoms quite similar to individuals with lactose intolerance, were more likely to seek health care and also more likely to be emotionally distressed and to have more pain than either the lactose-intolerant individuals or the normal controls (5). These studies emphasize that patients who seek care for IBS are a unique subgroup of the universe of individuals with IBS, a point worth remembering as clinicians treat patients with IBS.

PATHOPHYSIOLOGY

The pathophysiology of IBS remains in many ways a mystery. Multiple mechanisms have been proposed to explain the genesis of IBS symptoms, including altered motility, inflammatory factors, psychological factors, visceral hypersensitivity, and alterations in brain function. However, no single pathophysiologic mechanism has been shown to explain the multiple symptoms of IBS. These competing theses will be discussed individually, but may obviously overlap or be synergistically important.

Motility Abnormalities

In the years from the late 1940s to the early 1990s, the majority of research within the field of IBS was focused on disturbances of gastrointestinal motility. At first glance this approach would seem to be reasonable. The symptoms of IBS such as diarrhea, constipation, and bloating are all suggestive of abnormal GI motility. Nonetheless, although altered motor function has been identified in patients with IBS (6), the correlation between symptoms and motility abnormalities has been poor. A number of studies have demonstrated that patients with IBS can experience significant symptoms while showing little or no abnormalities in GI motility. Likewise, patients found to have significant motility abnormalities of the colon or small bowel often have no symptoms of IBS. This would suggest that factors other than abnormal motility play a role in the generation of IBS symptoms.

Visceral Hypersensitivity

Pain is a prominent symptom in many patients with IBS. In an attempt to better define the mechanism of IBS related pain, more recent studies have evaluated abnormalities in visceral sensation in patients with IBS. These studies have most often used balloon distention in the rectum, sigmoid, and/or ileum, or have used electrical stimulation of the rectum to demonstrate abnormalities in pain perception in IBS patients. These studies have fairly consistently demonstrated lower pain thresholds in patients with IBS when compared with non-IBS controls (7). Other studies have demonstrated abnormal somatic pain thresholds in patients with IBS suggesting that the hyperalgesia in IBS patients is not localized to the viscera. Abnormal central nervous system (CNS) processing of pain may also play a role in symptom generation in IBS patients. Studies have demonstrated abnormal activation of the anterior cingulate gyrus and the prefrontal cortex in the brains of IBS patients compared to non-IBS controls (8).

Inflammatory Factors in Irritable Bowel Syndrome

Approximately one third of patients with IBS report the initial onset of their IBS symptoms following an episode of acute gastrointestinal infection (9). This finding has led to speculation that there may be an infectious and/or inflammatory etiology for IBS (10), an exciting hypothesis worthy of further investigation. Complicating the issue is the fact that one study showed that the presence of psychosocial difficulties was a more powerful predictor of which patients with these physiological abnormalities would go on to develop symptoms of IBS (11).

THE ROLE OF STRESS

Research has shown that severe life stress frequently occurs immediately prior to the onset of IBS symptoms (12). Life stressors can also play a role in symptom exacerbation, health care behavior, and outcomes (13). In regard to IBS, the term "stress" is used to signify environmental events (stressors) as well as any incongruity between the stressors and one's adaptation such as coping and calling on social support. Numerous studies of IBS and other functional GI disorders (FGID) have used the Life Events and Difficulty Scale (LEDS) (12,14,15) to show an association between stress and IBS and other GI disorders. Creed et al. used the LEDS to demonstrate that stressful life events were more common in individuals with FGID (60–66% of FGID patients had experienced severe life events compared to 25% of healthy controls). Interestingly, although the frequency of life events was similar in patients with FGID and organic GI diseases, severe negative life events (bereavement, marital separation, court appearance with threat of imprisonment) were more common in the FGID group, and these events almost always preceded the onset of symptoms. In this study, the magnitude of the level of stress in FGID was similar to that occurring in patients who had taken a deliberate overdose of psychiatric medications (12).

Evidence suggests that the presence of life stressors is also an important predictor of symptom exacerbation, treatment-seeking behavior (16), and outcome (17). The precise mechanisms by which stressful life events ultimately translate into disturbed gut function or symptoms in FGID remain unclear. In general, compared to healthy controls, patients with IBS have increased motor reactivity to various stressors including balloon distension (7), and changes in various neuropeptides (7,18,19), as well as physical and psychological stressors (20,21). This being said, it is clear that the relationship between physiological responses and symptom generation needs to be further studied.

THE ROLE OF PSYCHIATRIC DISORDERS

The relationship between FGID and psychiatric disorders has been noted for many years (22), although early reports relied mainly on clinical impressions and were thus prone to bias. Since the advent of formal diagnostic criteria for both psychiatric and FGID (the American Psychiatric Diagnostic and Statistical Manual of Mental Disorders, currently in its fourth edition, DSM-IV, and the ROME II criteria, respectively) investigators have been able to systematically study this relationship.

Among patients with IBS studied at tertiary centers, the most frequent psychiatric diagnostic categories are (i) anxiety disorders (panic and generalized anxiety disorder); (ii) mood disorders (major depression and dysthymic disorder); and (iii) somatoform disorders (pain disorder and somatization disorder) (23). These psychiatric diagnoses often antedate the onset of the bowel disorder. While there are no data to definitively confirm a causative role for psychiatric disorders in the generation of IBS, it is generally accepted that the presence of psychiatric disturbance can have a significant impact on symptom severity, health care–seeking and other illness behavior, and the therapeutic approach and clinical outcome.

Psychiatric disorders are more common in patients with IBS seen in referral centers as opposed to those patients seen in community clinics or those who do not seek medical care. When evaluating for the presence of psychiatric disorders in patients with IBS who are seen at referral centers, most investigators have found a prevalence of between 42% and 61% in their IBS patients. The psychiatric diagnoses most commonly seen are anxiety and/or mood disorders. This is significantly greater than that seen in the control groups (24). Generally, when patients from tertiary care centers have been studied, and lifetime psychiatric diagnoses considered, even higher rates (up to 94%) of psychological disturbance have been reported (25).

Psychiatric comorbidity in IBS patients has been shown to influence disease severity. Recent data suggest that altered perception of visceral stimuli in CNS may be at least partially responsible. Blomhoff et al. compared IBS patients with and without phobic anxiety to see if this comorbid psychiatric disorder influenced brain information processing of auditory stimuli, and tried to detect possible consequences with respect to visceral sensitivity thresholds and IBS disease severity. This study used event-related potentials, auditory-presented words with emotional content, barostat-assessed visceral sensitivity thresholds, and symptom levels in 11 female IBS patients with comorbid phobic anxiety disorder and 22 age-matched female IBS patients without comorbidity. They found that the IBS patients with comorbid anxiety disorders showed differences in central processing of emotional stimuli (26). The presence of phobic anxiety in these patients seemed to interfere with the processing of visceral information in the frontal cerebral cortex of the brain and in turn tended to affect visceral sensitivity, and increased IBS symptomatology. This link may provide a clue as to the mechanistic link regarding the contribution of psychiatric comorbidity to the severity and duration of intestinal disorders.

The presence of a concomitant psychiatric diagnosis with IBS tends to be associated with poorer clinical outcomes. Conversely, treatment of a comorbid psychiatric disturbance in a patient with IBS can result in improvement in the patient's IBS symptoms (27). For instance, panic disorder has been frequently linked to IBS (28,29). When patients with both IBS and panic disorder are treated for their panic disorder the patient's IBS symptoms almost always also improve (13,28). This highlights the importance of recognizing and treating comorbid psychiatric disorders in IBS patients.

THE ROLE OF ABUSE

Research suggests a strong epidemiological relationship between self-reported sexual and physical abuse and FGID (30,31). In a landmark study, Drossman et al. interviewed 206 women attending a university-based GI clinic and found that patients with FGID reported a significantly higher rate of early sexual and physical abuse compared to female patients with organic GI diseases (53% vs. 37%) (32). These findings have been replicated by other investigations (30,33–35). These studies consistently reported rates of abuse in the 30% to 56% range for IBS patients seen at referral centers in the United States and in Europe.

The high frequencies of abuse are not unique to IBS. High prevalences of abuse have been reported by patients with chronic or recurrent painful nongastrointestinal functional conditions such as chronic pelvic pain, chronic headaches, and fibromyalgia (36,37), as well as patients with certain behavioral disorders such as bulimia, morbid obesity, and substance abuse (38). Furthermore, there is some evidence to suggest that the association of abuse with IBS or any other chronic painful condition also depends on the clinical setting in which the patient is seen (39,40). In fact, it could be argued that the high prevalence of abuse histories among patients with IBS seen at referral centers is a product of selection bias—that is, it is more closely associated with the clinical setting than with IBS per se. It has been noted that the frequency of abuse in patients with IBS in primary care settings is lower. In one study, the rate was one-half of that seen in tertiary care centers (39). Leroi and colleagues attempted to address this issue by investigating a cohort of 144 patients seen in a tertiary care, university-based GI clinic, and a community GI practice. They found that 40% of the patients ultimately diagnosed with a lower GI tract FGID had been sexually abused compared with only 10% of patients who ultimately received an organic diagnosis ($p < 0.0003$), a finding that held true in both the referral center and community settings (41).

Abuse history has important implications for the evaluation and management of patients. It increases the likelihood of consulting a physician (42), of having more severe GI symptoms (43), more non-GI symptoms (39), and of having associated psychiatric disturbances (44), all of which lead to greater disability and overall poorer outcome. For instance, Drossman et al found that GI patients with abuse histories reported 70% more severe pain ($p < 0.0001$); 40% greater psychological distress ($p < 0.0001$); spent over two-and-a-half times more days in bed in the previous three months (11.9 days vs. 4.5 days, $p < 0.0007$); had almost twice as poor daily function ($p < 0.0001$); saw physicians more often (8.7 visits vs. 6.7 visits over six months, $p < 0.03$); and even underwent more surgical procedures (4.9 vs. 3.8, $p < 0.04$) than women who had no abuse history (40).

The definition of physical and sexual abuse in these studies varies, and it is important to determine which types of abuse tend to be associated with poorer outcomes. Leserman and coworkers found that among GI patients, rape (penetration), multiple abuse experiences, and abuse perceived as life threatening were associated with poorer health status (40). This has led to the development of an abuse severity scale to try to quantify abuse severity with the hope that this in turn can predict adverse health outcome (43). To address this issue Leserman and colleagues interviewed 239 women presenting for treatment of FGID at a university-based gastroenterology clinic and found that 55.2% experienced some type of sexual abuse and 48.5% had some history of physical abuse. When severity of abuse was measured by structured interview, patients with sexual abuse were more likely to have increased levels of pain, non-GI somatic complaints, in-bed disability days, lifetime surgeries, and psychological distress, as well as poor overall functional status (45).

The reason why abuse, particularly in childhood, would lead to increased levels of functional bowel complaints and psychiatric disturbance remains incompletely understood. Some authors (31) have suggested that abuse history is not etiologic for IBS, but is associated with a tendency to communicate psychological distress through physical symptoms. The presence of an abuse history and associated difficulties may produce a chronic state of symptom amplification originating either at the CNS level (hypervigilance to body sensations) or gut level (visceral hypersensitivity and conditioned hypermotility). It may influence the individual's appraisal of those symptoms (causing increased health-care seeking and health anxiety), and perhaps even lead to unwarranted feelings of guilt and responsibility, making spontaneous disclosure unlikely (46). Eventually, a vicious cycle of health-care seeking and repeated referrals develops if the health-care system provides only symptomatic treatments and does not address the abuse issues (45).

In conclusion, patients with IBS attending referral centers commonly suffer from high frequencies of sexual and physical abuse (31). Alarmingly, physicians are often unaware of this abuse history. In Drossman's study, the physicians knew about the abuse history in only 17% of cases, and 30% of the victims had never previously disclosed this history to anyone (32). Abusive experiences negatively impact health status (45). Recording an abuse history should be routinely included with other aspects of history taking in patients who present to gastroenterology practices with symptoms suggestive of FGID.

SYMPTOM-BASED DIAGNOSTIC CRITERIA

One of the most basic challenges in effectively making a diagnosis of IBS is the fact that the disorder has no anatomic, physiologic, or biochemical markers. The traditional approach to GI diagnosis such as physical examination, endoscopy, and biochemical testing and imaging studies will yield no abnormalities in an IBS patient. This makes these studies of limited usefulness in terms of *establishing* an affirmative diagnosis of IBS (as opposed to excluding organic pathology). To meet this challenge, symptom-based criteria have been established for the diagnosis of IBS.

The concept of symptom-based diagnostic criteria is not unique to gastroenterology. Psychiatry has effectively used symptom-based criteria in the diagnosis of psychiatric disorders for the last 20 years. The DSM-IV has provided a meaningful tool for the symptom-based diagnosis of psychiatric disorders (47). In addition, other nongastrointestinal functional disorders have been characterized using symptom-based criteria. The American College of Rheumatology Diagnostic Criteria for fibromyalgia is an excellent example (48). There are multiple advantages for having standardized criteria for IBS. First, they provide a common language for diagnosis in clinical practice. Secondly, they provide a universal "yardstick" for outcome measures in treatment trials. Finally, standardized criteria provide a common starting point for epidemiologic studies to better define the incidence and prevalence of IBS. However, it is important to distinguish between standardized diagnostic criteria that have been designed mainly for clinical care and those for use in clinical research. Often the inclusion criteria for coding in epidemiologic studies do not efficiently lend itself to the use of standardized diagnostic criteria. The use of symptom clusters for inclusion criteria in epidemiologic surveys, while less specific than standardized diagnostic criteria, is a reasonable and efficient way to survey for the prevalence of IBS in populations.

DEVELOPMENT OF STANDARDIZED DIAGNOSTIC CRITERIA

The process of developing symptom-based criteria for IBS has become increasingly sophisticated over the last 25 years. A key event in this process was the development of the Manning criteria in 1978, which have proven to be a reasonable tool for diagnosis of IBS (Table 1) (49). Further, the Manning criteria have been found to be equally applicable to African-American populations, as well as Caucasians (50).

Table 1   Comparison of Diagnostic Criteria for Irritable Bowel Syndrome

Manning criteria	Rome criteria	Revised Rome criteria (65)

Abdominal pain that is relieved with a bowel movement
Pain associated with more frequent stools
Sensation of incomplete evacuation
Passage of mucus
Abdominal distention
	Continuous or recurrent symptoms of:
	  Abdominal pain, relieved with defecation, or associated with change in frequency or consistency of stool;
	  and/or
	  Disturbed defecation (two or more of):
	    Altered stool frequency
	    Altered stool form (hard or loose/watery)
	    Altered stool passage (straining or urgency, feeling of incomplete evacuation)
	    Passage of mucus
	  Usually with
	  Bloating or feeling of abdominal distension
		At least 12 weeks or more, which need not be consecutive, in the preceding 12 months of abdominal discomfort or pain that has two out of three features:
		  Relieved with defecation;
		  and/or
		  Onset associated with a change in frequency of stool;
		  and/or
		  Onset associated with a change in form (appearance) of stool.
		Symptoms that cumulatively support the diagnosis of irritable bowel syndrome:
		  Abnormal stool frequency (for research purposes "abnormal" may be defined as greater than 3 bowel movements per day and less than 3 bowel movements per week;
		  Abnormal stool form (lumpy/hard or loose/watery stool);
		  Abnormal stool passage (straining, urgency, or feeling of incomplete evacuation);
		  Passage of mucus;
		  Bloating or feeling of abdominal distension.

However, the ability of the Manning criteria to be equally applicable to men and women has been the subject of some debate. In a study of 97 subjects (61 women and 36 men), Smith and colleagues found that the Manning criteria correlated significantly with a diagnosis of IBS in women ($p < 0.01$), but did not discriminate IBS definitively in men. The authors concluded that significant gender differences exist when using the Manning criteria for the diagnosis of IBS and that these criteria may not be an ideal instrument for the diagnosis of IBS in men (51). However, the Smith study suffered from a small sample size relative to other studies on this topic. Also, in this study the clinicians evaluating the subjects had some difficulty in distinguishing between a diagnosis of IBS and organic disorders based on their low confidence ratings. This is in contrast to a study by Taub where the same symptom criteria used to identify IBS was applied to both males and females in the same study (50). These findings were similar to those of Talley et al. who found that the Manning criteria had a higher predictive value in younger patients and in women as opposed to men (52). An attempt to improve on the Manning criteria using expert panels was first attempted in 1988. The goal of the so-called Rome working teams was (and remains) to refine and develop symptom-based diagnostic criteria for IBS and other FGID that would be accepted by the majority of experts in the field. The resulting Rome I diagnostic criteria for IBS were published in 1990. The Rome criteria (Rome II) were subsequently revised in 1999. The Manning, Rome I, and Rome II diagnostic criteria are listed in Table 1.

Saito and colleagues compared the Manning criteria to the Rome I criteria as well as the revised Rome II criteria for the diagnosis of IBS. They found that the prevalence of IBS in a population-based cross-sectional survey was 20.4% using two symptoms of the Manning criteria, and 8.5% using the three defecation disorder criteria of Rome I. Agreement between the original Rome criteria and the "revised" Rome II criteria was greater than 90% in their sample (53). Further evaluation of the sensitivity and specificity of the Rome II criteria compared to the previous Rome I and Manning criteria was undertaken by Boyce and colleagues who surveyed 4500 individuals from Australia. The sample included both male and female adults over

18 years old. They found a 13.6% prevalence of IBS according to the Manning criteria compared to 4.4% using the Rome I criteria, and 6.9% using the Rome II criteria. Thus, patients who met the Rome I criteria for the diagnosis of IBS also met the Rome II diagnostic criteria. However, patients who met the Manning criteria for the diagnosis of IBS were less likely to be diagnosed with IBS by the Rome II criteria. The authors concluded that the new Rome II criteria might be unnecessarily restrictive for use in generalized clinical practice (54).

The use of the Rome II criteria can be extremely helpful in terms of establishing a clinical picture, which is consistent with IBS, and their sensitivity and specificity seem to be quite good. The important practical question that remains, however, is whether these diagnostic criteria can actually help us eliminate unnecessary diagnostic studies in clinically evaluating the IBS patient.

THE ROLE OF DIAGNOSTIC TESTING

The symptoms of IBS are often quite vague. Patients who complain of bloating and/or abdominal pain may present an endless list of diagnostic possibilities. Likewise, common IBS symptoms such as diarrhea or constipation have an extensive differential diagnosis. Pursuing all diagnostic possibilities via an extensive workup can lead to much unnecessary and costly testing. This futility, in turn, can subject the patient to unneeded expense, inconvenience, and suffering. The key to planning a diagnostic work up for patients with vague abdominal symptoms, which may or may not represent IBS, is astute history taking and judicious use of the Rome criteria for the diagnosis of IBS. The first key step in taking a history of patients with vague GI symptoms is to search for "alarm symptoms." These symptoms, when present, should rapidly shift the physician's differential diagnosis toward structural or inflammatory conditions of the GI tract. The patient who reports fevers, weight loss, skin rashes, arthritis, or who have positive occult blood in the stool or a mass palpable in the abdomen on physical examination clearly requires a workup to further explain those findings, in contrast to the patient with no "alarm" symptoms at all. Hamm and colleagues studied 1452 patients who met the Rome I criteria for IBS for at least a period of six months prior to entry into a clinical trial. Colonoscopy was performed in patients who were 50 years or older, and flexible sigmoidoscopy was performed in patients younger than 50 years. Thyroid stimulating hormone (TSH), hydrogen breath (H_2) testing for lactose malabsorption, and stool studies for ova and parasites were also performed. The investigators found that evaluation of the colonic mucosa endoscopically yielded abnormalities only 2% of the time. Of the seven patients found to have a colonic endoscopic abnormality, only three had colitis and one patient had a colonic obstruction that may have been contributing to symptoms of abdominal pain or altered bowel habits. Abnormal TSH was found in 6% of the patients (50% hypothyroid and the other half hyperthyroid). Examination of the stool for ova and parasites was positive only 2% of the time, with organisms of low pathogenicity found exclusively. Interestingly, lactose malabsorption was diagnosed in 23% of the patients using H_2 breath testing. The authors noted that these latter three findings compared favorably to the incidence of thyroid dysfunction, parasitic infection, and lactose malabsorption in the general population in the United States. They concluded that the low detection rates, additional cost, and inconvenience to patients generated by these studies made them of minimal usefulness and that their routine utilization in patients who met the Rome I criteria for IBS be reconsidered (55).

At this point, it seems reasonable to recommend the use of basic screening laboratory studies to further search for an anatomic, inflammatory, or infectious source of the patient's symptoms. Obtaining a complete blood count (CBC) and a chemistry panel would be reasonable, as these studies are often a routine part of an office visit for any GI complaint. Further, these studies have been recommended by expert reviews put forth to help clarify the physician's approach to IBS (56).

However, it is not uncommon for patients presenting with symptoms that are ultimately diagnosed as IBS to undergo more extensive diagnostic testing. The literature supporting the utility of various diagnostic studies for the treatment of IBS is difficult to interpret. Many of the studies are retrospective. Others drew patients from tertiary referral settings and may not accurately represent patients seen in the wider spectrum of gastroenterology practice. In an attempt to clarify the situation, Tolliver and colleagues studied 196 patients who met the Rome I criteria for IBS who were prospectively evaluated using CBC, erythrocyte sedimentation rate

(ESR), stool for ova and parasites, TSH, and structural evaluation of the colon either by barium enema, flexible sigmoidoscopy, or colonoscopy (57). The authors found that the ESR and examination of the stool for ova and parasites had no diagnostic yield in their sample. Likewise, none of their 196 patients had abnormalities in the white blood cell count or hemoglobin. Less than 1% had abnormalities in liver enzymes or in their thyroid profiles. Interestingly, 34 of the 196 patients (21.9%) had structural abnormalities of the colon. However, closer examination of these data reveals that the majority of the lesions were colonic polyps (4.5%), asymptomatic diverticulosis (8.6%), or hemorrhoids (5.6%). Colon cancer, colitis, and colonic lipoma were all identified in only one patient each. With the exception of the two patients with colon cancer and colitis, respectively, it is unlikely that any of the structural abnormalities found could explain the patients' symptoms. The patients in this study also underwent H_2 breath testing to diagnose lactose malabsorption. Forty-eight patients (25.8%) showed evidence of lactose malabsorption, with 52% of those with lactose malabsorption unaware of this association with their symptoms. However, the investigators did not specify the ethnic background of the patients studied; so this sample may have overly represented ethnic groups at higher risk for lactose malabsorption. Tolliver and colleagues recommended omitting ESR and thyroid testing as part of the routine workup for IBS. Likewise, they recommended testing for ova and parasites only when patients have been in an area known to be endemic for parasites. A further recommendation was that structural evaluation of the colon should be guided by established colon cancer screening guidelines.

The usefulness of sigmoidoscopy, particularly sigmoidoscopy with rectal biopsy, has also been the subject of some controversy in the diagnosis of IBS. Although recommended by some experts, the use of routine sigmoidoscopy for the diagnosis of IBS has also been subject to some criticism (58). To evaluate the usefulness of sigmoidoscopy and, specifically, the role of rectal biopsy in patients who meet the diagnostic criteria for IBS, MacIntosh and colleagues evaluated 89 patients who met either the Rome I or Manning criteria for IBS and compared them to 59 controls. All patients underwent sigmoidoscopy with rectal biopsy. Biopsy specimens were read by two pathologists blinded to the patients' IBS status. None of the IBS subjects had evidence of melanosis coli or met the diagnostic criteria for microscopic or collagenous colitis. The authors concluded that patients who meet symptom-based criteria for IBS and who have an endoscopically normal distal colon on flexible sigmoidoscopy are unlikely to have histologic abnormalities in the rectum. They felt that routine rectal biopsies were a costly and unnecessary undertaking in the evaluation of patients with presumed IBS (59). One weakness of this study, however, is that patients with the constipation-predominant as well as the alternating (constipation/diarrhea) patterns of IBS symptoms along with patients who had diarrhea-predominant IBS were all included in the study. This might have led to an underestimation of the usefulness of rectal biopsy in a diarrhea-predominant IBS population.

The usefulness of imaging studies has also been a subject of some controversy in the diagnosis of IBS. The role of abdominal ultrasound in IBS was evaluated by Francis and colleagues who studied 125 patients (100 women and 25 men) who met the diagnostic criteria for IBS using the Rome I criteria. In this study, 20% of the females and 8% of the males had an ultrasound abnormality. However, none of those abnormalities led to additional therapeutic measures. Likewise, none of the findings on ultrasound could be considered by the investigators to entirely account for the patient's presenting symptoms. Eight percent of the female IBS subjects had a pelvic abnormality, and again, it was not considered to be of any clinical consequence in any of the subjects. The authors concluded that using the Rome criteria to achieve a "positive diagnosis of IBS" was a safe practice and that routine use of ultrasound of the abdomen in patients suspected of having IBS was unnecessary. They further concluded that routine use of ultrasound in the evaluation of patients with IBS could be counterproductive by detecting minor abnormalities that could further obfuscate the clinical picture. Another interesting aspect of this study was that sigmoidoscopy was also performed on all patients, and additionally, in patients older than 45 years, a barium enema or colonoscopy was also undertaken. The authors found all of the imaging studies of the colon to be normal except for a few cases of uncomplicated diverticular disease (60). These latter findings are consistent with the findings of Tolliver et al. (57,59) further supporting the concept that routine use of colonic imaging in patients who meet Rome diagnostic criteria for IBS, and who have no alarm symptoms, is probably not useful. This conclusion is further supported in the findings of Hamm and colleagues discussed above. In their study, all patients underwent colonic imaging either via colonoscopy or radiography within two years of entering the study. Colonic abnormalities were detected in only 2% of the patients. These abnormalities may have contributed to symptoms of abdominal pain or altered bowel habits in only four of the seven patients. Because 98% of their patients had normal colonic evaluations despite the fact that the mean age of the patient population was 45, the investigators concluded that colonic imaging added little to the differential diagnosis of IBS (55).

DIFFERENTIAL DIAGNOSIS

The differential diagnosis of IBS can at first seem daunting. Symptoms of chronic constipation and/or diarrhea, abdominal pain, and bloating have an almost unlimited list of diagnostic possibilities. A key point needs to be established in effectively approaching the differential diagnosis of IBS. That is, almost without exception, the disorders listed in Table 2 have unique symptoms that can help differentiate them from IBS on the basis of history taking and physical examination. These so-called "alarm features" are a key component to directing a physician toward or away from a diagnosis of IBS. Indeed the Rome II criteria demand the absence of other inflammatory, structural, or biochemical abnormalities, which could possibly be causing the patient's symptoms as a requirement for meeting the diagnostic criteria for IBS. A list of these alarm symptoms and their potentially associated diseases is outlined in Table 2. While appropriate diagnostic testing in the suggestive setting is encouraged, the authors recommend judicious and selective use rather than "all-patients, all-tests" approach. A suggested diagnostic approach to the patient with suspected IBS is provided in Figure 1.

TREATMENT
The Physician–Patient Relationship

An effective physician–patient relationship is an integral aspect of the treatment of IBS. This is supported by the fact that patients with IBS have up to a 90% placebo response rate. It is important to obtain a thorough history, including a psychosocial and abuse history using a nonjudgmental, patient-centered approach. The physician should provide a thorough explanation of the diagnosis and reassure the patient using terminology the patient can understand. The physician should give the patient realistic expectations regarding prognosis. It is important for patients with IBS to have an ongoing relationship with their physician. While this is an oft-quoted general platitude, there is evidence to support that allowing patients to ask questions and offering reassurance improves prognosis in IBS (61). Together, these measures can have a significant impact upon patient anxiety and can help patients participate fully in their care. An effective physician–patient relationship can also decrease the need for additional testing in patients concerned about a "missed" diagnosis.

Stratification of Treatment

Treatment recommendations for patients with IBS have been categorized into subgroups based upon symptom severity. Although these subgroups were originally created to assist with

Table 2 Alarm Symptoms and Their Potentially Associated Diseases

Symptom	Possible cause
Weight loss	Cancer, IBD, malabsorption
Anemia	IBD, celiac disease, cancer
Fevers	Infections, lymphoma, IBD, rheumatoid disorders
Skin rashes	IBD, celiac disease, rheumatoid disorders
Stool occult blood	Cancer, IBD
Nighttime diarrhea	IBD, neuroendocrine tumors, microscopic cavity carcinoid
Flushing	Carcinoid or pheochromocytoma tumors
New onset >50 yrs of age	Cancers, IBD, mesenteric insufficiency

Abbreviation: IBD, inflammatory bowel disease.

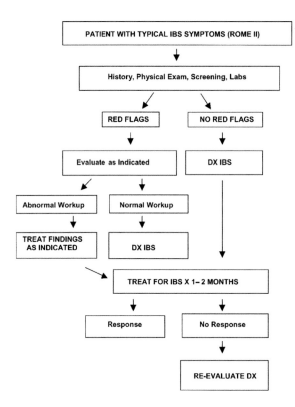

Figure 1 Algorithm depicting potential diagnostic approach.

stratification of patients enrolled in clinical trials, categorization of patients based upon symptom severity is also useful in clinical practice.

The Patient with Mild Symptoms

Approximately 70% of patients with IBS have "mild" symptoms that can be managed with measures such as patient education, reassurance, and lifestyle modification. Dietary modification to reduce the intake of lactose and other nonabsorbable sugars such as sorbitol and fructose, as well as fat alcohol, and caffeine may be recommended in these patients. Patients in this subgroup with constipation-predominant symptoms may benefit from a high-fiber diet or fiber supplementation. One key element of the treatment of IBS patients is education. It has been shown that patients with IBS report a need for more and better information regarding their illness (62).

The Patient with Moderate Symptoms

Approximately 25% of patients with IBS have "moderate" symptoms. Although these patients may have increased levels of psychological distress, they do not tend to have severe psychosocial or psychiatric disturbances. Pharmacotherapy in these patients should be symptom focused. In addition to bowel-directed medical treatment such as fiber supplementation, intermittent laxatives or antidiarrheals, anticholinergics, and smooth muscle relaxants, the use of antidepressants may also be helpful in these patients (discussed further below). It has been suggested that these patients may benefit from a multidimensional approach to treatment including medications as well as behavioral treatments, such as hypnosis and relaxation training (62). Patient education obviously also plays a key role in helping these patients fully understand and cope with their illness.

The Patient with Severe Symptoms

Five percent of patients with IBS are classified as having "severe" symptoms. These patients describe constant pain and have high levels of disability. These patients often have significant functional impairment and lower overall quality of life. These patients are quite likely to have comorbid psychiatric diagnoses including anxiety disorders, major depressive disorder, and somatoform disorders as a part of their clinical picture. These patients also have high rates of major social trauma in their lives such as the death of a parent or spouse. Finally, these patients are much more likely to have high rates of physical and/or sexual abuse. Multimodal treatments combining medical management with education seems to be particularly promising approaches to the patient with moderate-to-severe IBS (62). Likewise, psychotherapeutic approaches have also been demonstrated to be particularly helpful in patients with severe refractory IBS. Creed and colleagues studied 255 patients referred for treatment of severe IBS. They randomized this sample to one of three treatment arms. The first was a psychotherapy arm consisting of approximately eight hours of psychotherapy delivered over a three-month period. The second arm consisted of patients randomized to paroxetine 20 mg/day for three months. The third group continued with usual medical treatment with no psychiatric or psychopharmacologic intervention. Eighty-five patients were randomized in each group. They calculated quality of life on entry and exit to the study, IBS symptom etiology, psychological distress as measured by the symptom check list-90 symptom check list-90 (SCL-90). A measure of a subject overall emotional state and hospital costs during the study and in follow-up. Patients were followed up at three months and 15 months after cessation of the intervention. Both psychotherapy and paroxetine were superior to standard treatment for improving the physical aspects of health-related quality of life as measured on the short form-36 (SF-36). A vacinated generic quality of life measure. On the physical component score ($p < 0.001$). However, there were no significant differences in the psychological components of the SF-36. In the one-year follow-up to the study, the subjects randomized to psychotherapy had a significant reduction in health care costs compared to treatment as usual. This did not occur in the paroxetine group. Investigators concluded that in subjects with severe IBS both psychotherapy and paroxetine improved health-related quality of life without increasing the cost of treatment. In addition, psychotherapy was specifically associated with reduction of overall health care costs. This study demonstrates the utility of multimodality treatment combining standard medical treatment, psychopharmacologic intervention, and behavioral strategies. It can be anticipated that additional studies designed along this line will be appearing in the future and allow us to refine our approach to patients with IBS, particularly refractory patients (63).

Drug Treatment of Irritable Bowel Syndrome

The selection of medications for use in patients with IBS is based upon the predominant symptom pattern and the severity of the patient's symptoms.

Irritable Bowel Syndrome with Constipation

Fiber may be useful in patients with constipation-predominant IBS, although the literature on the efficacy of fiber is equivocal. Fiber supplementation certainly can reduce constipation associated with IBS. However, it can also be associated with bloating and abdominal cramping, which makes its use for the treatment of IBS less than optimal. The recommended fiber intake for these patients is 20 to 30 g/day. In addition to fiber, polyethylene glycol solution has been shown to be useful in alleviating the constipation associated with IBS (64).

Irritable Bowel Syndrome with Diarrhea

Loperamide, a nonabsorbable opioid, has been shown to slow intestinal transit, increase water and ion absorption, and increase rectal sphincter tone leading to improvement of diarrhea and rectal urgency in patients with diarrhea-predominant IBS. Because loperamide does not cross the blood brain barrier, it is preferred over other narcotic medications. Cholestyramine has also demonstrated benefit in diarrhea-predominant IBS. It has been suggested that the mechanism of action may relate to bile acid sequestration in patients with idiopathic bile acid malabsorption contributing to symptoms of IBS. However, patients may have difficulty in tolerating cholestyramine.

Antidepressants

Antidepressants have been used for many years in the treatment of IBS. The initial rationale for using these medications was their proven efficacy for the treatment of peripheral

Table 3 Antidepressant Dosing Guidelines

Antidepressant	GI dosage (mg)	Range (mg/day)
Amitriptyline	10–200	50–300
Imipramine	10–200	75–300
Clomipramine	25–250	25–250
Doxepin	10–200	75–300
Fluoxetine	10–20	20–80
Paroxetine	10–20	20–50
Sertraline	25–50	50–200
Trazodone	25–300	150–600

neuropathy and other neuropathic pain syndromes (65). However, the rationale for the use of antidepressants in IBS is more complex. Tricyclic antidepressants have been shown in numerous studies to relieve diarrhea, constipation, abdominal pain, and bloating in patients with IBS (66). This effect is independent of their antidepressant effect. Likewise, tricyclic antidepressants seem to have their effect independent of their anticholinergic effect (67). They seem to be helpful in treating both the constipation- and diarrhea-predominant forms of IBS. However, their usefulness is limited by the fact that many patients find the side effects associated with antidepressant use intolerable.

In addition, antidepressants have been shown to be useful in IBS patients with concomitant psychiatric disorders as well as in IBS patients with no signs of psychiatric disturbance (68). Psychiatric disorders that are most commonly associated with IBS are panic disorder, major depressive disorder, and phobias. All of these conditions have been shown to be responsive both to tricyclic antidepressants and to the selective serotonin reuptake inhibitors. The importance of screening for psychiatric disorders in patients with IBS, particularly those who are refractory to standard medical management, can help identify individuals who will benefit particularly well from the addition of antidepressant agents to their regimen. For patients who do not have a concomitant psychiatric disorder, tricyclic antidepressants in doses far lower than are usually used for the treatment of depression and anxiety can be employed. In patients who have a concomitant psychiatric disorder, standard antidepressant doses are usually needed (Table 3).

Serotonergic Agents

It has been known for many years that 90% of the serotonin receptors present in the body are located in the gut. Research over the last 10 years has demonstrated multiple roles for various serotonin receptor subtypes in both visceral perception and motor function of the gut. There has been extensive research to develop serotonergically active agents that could influence the disturbances of bowel sensation and function seen in IBS. This line of investigation has led to the development of a number of new agents, some of which are currently available and others still in development. A list of newly available and emerging agents is outlined in Table 4. The first of these was alosetron, a serotoneric type 3 (5-HT$_3$) antagonist. Alosetron has been shown to decrease visceral sensation, thereby reducing pain and rectal urgency in IBS associated with constipation. Alosetron has been associated with high degrees of patient satisfaction and significant improvement in the patient's overall well being (69). The major issue confronting alosetron is the fact that it has been associated, for reasons, which remain unclear, with ischemic colitis (70) that led to the drug being transiently withdrawn from the market. However, because of its high efficacy and high degree of patient satisfaction, regulatory authorities in the United States have reapproved the drug under controlled prescribing circumstances. Alosetron is currently approved for the treatment of severe IBS in women. Another new agent is tegaserod, which is a 5-HT$_4$ partial agonist. Tegaserod is currently available in the United States for the treatment of IBS with associated constipation in women. To date, no significant safety issues have been seen with this drug, although early trials suggested a potential increased risk of gall bladder surgery. Likewise, patient satisfaction, improvements in global well-being, and improvement in the specific IBS symptoms of pain, bloating, and constipation have all been documented with this drug (71).

In addition to the two agents discussed above, there are additional serotonergically active agents that are in development. One is prucalopride, which is a 5-HT$_4$ *full* antagonist.

Table 4 New and Emerging Drugs for Irritable Bowel Syndrome

Name	Action	Indication	Status
Alosetron	5-HT$_3$ antagonist	Women IBS-C	Available
Tegaserod	5-HT$_4$ partial agonist	Women IBS-C	Available
Lubiprostone	ClC$_3$ Activation	IBS-C	In trials

Abbreviations: IBS, irritable bowel syndrome.

This drug currently remains in development and has not yet entered clinical trials; so no clinical data is available. Cilansetron is a 5-HT$_3$ antagonist that has also been designed to treat IBS with associated diarrhea. It is currently in the final stages of Phase III of the clinical trials. Data regarding its efficacy and safety should be available within the next year.

Novel Agents and Approaches

In addition to antidepressants and the gut-specific serotonergic agents, a number of new compounds aimed at other receptor sites in the gut are being investigated for the treatment of IBS. For some time, the kappa opiate antagonist fedotozine has been studied for the treatment of IBS, specifically for the treatment of pain and bloating. Kappa opiate receptors are found only in the gut. The theoretical advantage of fedotozine is that it does not interact with the opiate receptor that is responsible for the euphoria and extraintestinal pain relief seen with traditional narcotic analgesics. To date, clinical trials using fedotozine have been inconclusive, and it remains unclear whether this agent offers significant therapeutic benefit to patients with IBS (72). However other kappa opiate agonists as well as chloride channel type 2 activation such as lubiprostone are being studied in IBS.

In addition to the kappa opiate agonists, antagonists to the inflammatory mediator neurokinin (NK antagonists) are currently being investigated to treat a presumed inflammatory response in IBS. It has been postulated that this inflammatory response may lead to stimulation of visceral afferent nerve endings causing pain, discomfort, and altered motility.

Behavioral Treatment of Irritable Bowel Syndrome

The biopsychosocial nature of IBS would suggest that its effective treatment does not depend only on medical management. An emerging body of literature is appearing to support the efficacy of a variety of behavioral interventions for the treatment of IBS. Psychotherapy, particularly cognitive behavioral therapy, hypnosis, and psychodynamic psychotherapy have all been used with great effectiveness in the treatment of patients with IBS (73). A number of studies have now demonstrated that the use of psychotherapy can decrease gastrointestinal symptoms and health-care utilization, as well as increase the patient's overall sense of well being.

SUMMARY

IBS is a common, chronic gastrointestinal disorder that is commonly seen both in primary care and in GI specialty practice. It is a disorder of gastrointestinal motility, which is influenced by, but not caused by, stress and psychosocial dysfunction. The evaluation of the patient with IBS-like symptoms needs to be prudent. The use of symptom-based criteria as typified by the Rome II diagnostic criteria to make a "positive" as opposed to an exclusionary approach to diagnosis has been shown to be a safe and rational approach. When evaluating the patient with suspected IBS, it is important to evaluate the psychosocial dimensions of the patient's life, specifically inquiring about the presence of physical or sexual abuse and the presence of social losses such as the death of a parent while in childhood. In addition, screening for *selected* psychiatric disorders is also of great importance. It is only by exploring all of these dimensions, physical, social, and psychological, that an appropriate treatment plan for patients with IBS can be formulated. Further, diagnostic testing should be selective and judicious.

The treatment of patients with IBS depends not only on effective medical management, such as dietary manipulation and use of medications directed at gut function, but also may include the judicious use of antidepressants and newer agents acting on the various neurotransmitter systems in the gut (74). Behavioral interventions such as hypnotherapy and psychotherapy increasingly play an important role in the treatment of IBS. Adopting a multi-modal approach to the treatment of IBS seems to be the most effective approach for these patients. It allows the physician to bring a perspective that is both reassuring and empowering for the patient. Most importantly, it provides the foundation for an effective physician–patient partnership to maximize the combined energy of both parties to ameliorate the patient's IBS symptoms.

REFERENCES

1. Heaton KW, O'Donnell LJD, Braddon FEM, et al. Symptoms of irritable bowel syndrome in a British urban community: consulters and nonconsulters. Gastroenterology 1992; 102:1962–1967.
2. Schlemper RJ, Van Der Werf SDJ, Vandenbroucke JP, et al. Peptic ulcer, non-ulcer dyspepsia and irritable bowel syndrome in the Netherlands and Japan. Scand J Gastroenterol 1993; 28(200):33–41.
3. Kang JY, Yap I, Gwee KA. The pattern of functional and organic disorders in an Asian gastroentero-logical clinic. J Gastroenterol Hepatol 1994; 9:124–127.
4. Drossman DA, McKee D, Sandler R, et al. Psychosocial factors in the irritable bowel syndrome. A multivariate study of patients and nonpatients with irritable bowel syndrome. Gastroenterology 1988; 95:701–708.
5. Whitehead WE, Bosmajian L, Zonderman AB, et al. Symptoms of psychologic distress associated with irritable bowel syndrome: comparison of community and medical clinic samples. Gastroenterology 1988; 95:709–714.
6. McKee DP, Quigley EMM. Intestinal motility in irritable bowel syndrome: is IBS a motility disorder? Part 2. Motility of the small bowel, esophagus, stomach and gall-bladder. Dig Dis Sci 1993; 38(10): 1773–1782.
7. Whitehead WE, Holtkotter B, Enck P, et al. Tolerance for rectosigmoid distention in irritable bowel syndrome. Gastroenterology 1990; 98:1187–1192.
8. Silverman DHS, Munakata J, Ennes H, et al. Regional cerebral activity in normal and pathological perception of visceral pain. Gastroenterology 1997; 112:64–72.
9. Rodriguez LAG, Ruigomez A. Increased risk of irritable bowel syndrome after bacterial gastroent-eritis: cohort study. Br Med J 1999; 318:565–566.
10. Neal KR, Hebdon J, Spiller R. Prevalence of gastrointestinal symptoms six months after bacterial gastroenteritis and risk factors for development of the irritable bowel syndrome. Br Med J 1997; 314:779–782.
11. Gwee KA, Leong YL, Graham C, et al. The role of psychological and biological factors in postinfective gut dysfunction. Gut 1999; 44:400–406.
12. Creed FH, Craig T, Farmer RG. Functional abdominal pain, psychiatric illness and life events. Gut 1988; 29:235–242.
13. Olden KW, Brotman AW. Irritable bowel/irritable mood: the mind/gut connection. Harv Rev Psychiatr 1998; 6:149–154.
14. Gilligan I, Fung L, Piper DW, et al. Life event stress and chronic difficulties in duodenal ulcer: a case control study. J Psychosom Res 1987; 31:117–123.
15. Ellard K, Beaurepaire J, Jones M, et al. Acute and chronic stress in duodenal ulcer disease. Gastroen-terology 1990; 99:1628–32.
16. Whitehead WE, Crowell MD, Robinson JC, et al. Effects of stressful life events on bowel symptoms: subjects with irritable bowel syndrome compared to subjects without bowel dysfunction. Gut 1992; 33:825–830.
17. Bennett EJ, Tennant CC, Piesse C, et al. Level of chronic life stress predicts clinical outcome in irritable bowel syndrome. Gut 1998; 43:256–262.
18. Preston DM, Adrian TE, Christofides ND, et al. Positive correlation between symptoms and circulat-ing motilin, pancreatic polypeptide and gastrin concentrations in functional bowel disorders. Gut 1986; 26:1059–1064.
19. Sjölund K, Ekman R, Lindgren S, et al. Disturbed motilin and cholecystokinin release in the irritable bowel syndrome. Scand J Gastroenterol 1996; 31:1110–1114.
20. Welgan P, Meshkinpour H, Beeler M, et al. Effect of anger on colon motor and myoelectric activity in irritable bowel syndrome. Gastroenterology 1988; 94:1150–1156.
21. Whorwell PJ, Houghton LA, Taylor EE, et al. Physiological effects of emotion: assessment via hypnosis. Lancet 1992; 340:69–72.
22. Bockus HL, Bank J, Wilkinson SA. Neurogenic mucous colitis. Am J Med Sci 1928; 176:813–829.
23. Drossman DA, Creed FH, Olden KW, et al. Psychosocial aspects of the functional gastrointestinal dis-orders. In: Drossman DA, Corazziari E, Talley NJ, et al., eds. Rome II: The Functional Gastrointestinal Disorders: Diagnosis, Pathophysiology and Treatment: A Multinational Consensus. McLean, VA: Degnon and Associates, 2000:157–245.
24. Toner BB, Garfinkel PE, Jeejeebhoy KN. Psychological factors in irritable bowel syndrome. Can J Psychiatr 1990; 35:158–161.

25. Walker EA, Katon WJ, Roy-Byrne PP, et al. Histories of sexual victimization in patients with irritable bowel syndrome or inflammatory bowel disease. Am J Psychiatr 1993; 150:1502–1506.
26. Blomhoff S, Spetalen S, Jacobsen MB, et al. Phobic anxiety changes the function of brain–gut axis in irritable bowel syndrome. Psychosom Med 2001; 63:959–965.
27. Noyes RJ, Cook C, Garvey M, et al. Reduction of gastrointestinal symptoms following treatment for panic disorder. Psychosomatics 1990; 31:75–79.
28. Lydiard RB, Greenwald S, Weissman MM, et al. Panic disorder and gastrointestinal symptoms: findings from the NIMH Epidemiologic Catchment Area project. Am J Psychiatr 1994; 151:64–70.
29. Zaubler TS, Katon W. Panic disorder and medical comorbidity: a review of the medical and psychiatric literature. Bull Menninger Clin 1996; 60(suppl A):A12–A38.
30. Delvaux M, Denis P, Allemand H. French club of digestive motility: sexual and physical abuses are more frequently reported by IBS patients than by patients with organic digestive diseases or controls: results of a multicenter inquiry. Eur J Gastroenterol Hepat 1997; 9:3345–3352.
31. Drossman DA, Talley NJ, Olden KW, et al. Sexual and physical abuse and gastrointestinal illness: review and recommendations. Ann Intern Med 1995; 123:782–794.
32. Drossman DA, Leserman J, Nachman G, et al. Sexual and physical abuse in women with functional or organic gastrointestinal disorders. Ann Intern Med 1990; 113:828–833.
33. McCauley J, Kern DE, Kolodner K, et al. Clinical characteristics of women with a history of childhood abuse. JAMA 1997; 277:1362–1368.
34. Scarinci IC, McDonald-Haile JM, Bradley LA, et al. Altered pain perception and psychosocial features among women with gastrointestinal disorders and history of abuse: a preliminary model. Am J Med 1994; 97:108–118.
35. Talley NJ, Fett SL, Zinsmeister AR. Self-reported abuse and gastrointestinal disease in outpatients: association with irritable bowel-type symptoms. Am J Gastroenterol 1995; 90:366–371.
36. Laws A. Sexual abuse history and women's medical problems. J Gen Intern Med 1993; 8:441–443.
37. Katon W, Sullivan M, Walker E. Medical symptoms without identified pathology: relationship to psychiatric disorders, childhood and adult trauma, and personality traits. Ann Intern Med 2001; 134:917–925.
38. Leserman J, Drossman DA. The reliability and validity of a sexual and physical abuse history questionnaire in female patients with gastrointestinal disorders. Behav Med 1995; 21:141–150.
39. Longstreth GF, Wolde-Tsadik G. Irritable bowel-type symptoms in HMO examinees: prevalence, demographics, and clinical correlates. Dig Dis Sci 1993; 38:1581–1589.
40. Drossman DA, Li Z, Leserman J, et al. Health status by gastrointestinal diagnosis and abuse history. Gastroenterology 1996; 110:999–1007.
41. Leroi AM, Bernier C, Watier A, et al. Prevalence of sexual abuse among patients with functional disorders of the lower gastrointestinal tract. Int J Colorect Dis 1995; 10:200–206.
42. Talley NJ, Fett SL, Zinsmeister AR. Gastrointestinal tract symptoms and self-reported abuse: a population-based study. Gastroenterology 1994; 107:1040–1049.
43. Leserman J, Li Z, Drossman DA, et al. Impact of sexual and physical abuse dimensions on health status: development of an abuse severity measure. Psychosom Med 1997; 59:152–160.
44. Blanchard EB, Keefer L, Payne A, et al. Early abuse, psychiatric diagnoses and irritable bowel syndrome. Behav Res Ther 2002; 40:289–298.
45. Leserman J, Drossman DA, Li Z, et al. Sexual and physical abuse in gastroenterology practice: how types of abuse impact health status. Psychosom Med 1996; 58:4–15.
46. Drossman DA. Irritable bowel syndrome and sexual/physical abuse history. Eur J Gastroenterol Hepat 1997; 9:327–330.
47. American Psychiatric Association. Diagnostic and Statistical Manual of Mental Disorders. Washington, DC: American Psychiatric Association, 1994.
48. Wolfe F, Smythe HA, Yunus MB, et al. The American College of Rheumatology 1990 criteria for the classification of fibromyalgia: report of the multicenter criteria committee. Arthritis Rheum 1990; 33(2):160–172.
49. Manning AP, Thompson WG, Heaton KW. Towards positive diagnosis of the irritable bowel. Br Med J 1978; 2(653):654.
50. Taub E, Cuevas JL, Cook EW, et al. Irritable bowel syndrome defined by factor analysis: gender and race comparisons. Dig Dis Sci 1995; 40(12):2647–2655.
51. Smith RC, Greenbaum DS, Vancouver JB, et al. Gender differences in Manning criteria in irritable bowel syndrome. Gastroenterology 1991; 100:591–595.
52. Talley NJ, Phillips SF, Melton J III, et al. Diagnostic value of the Manning criteria in irritable bowel syndrome. Gut 1990; 31:77–81.
53. Saito YA, Locke GR, Talley NJ, et al. A comparison of the Rome and Manning criteria for case identification in epidemiological investigations of irritable bowel syndrome. Am J Gastroenterol 2000; 95:2816–2824.
54. Boyce PM, Koloski NA, Talley NJ. Irritable bowel syndrome according to varying diagnostic criteria: are the new Rome II criteria unnecessarily restrictive for research and practice? Am J Gastroenterol 2000; 95:3176–3183.
55. Hamm LR, Sorrells SC, Harding JP, et al. Additional investigations fail to alter the diagnosis of irritable bowel syndrome in subjects fulfilling the Rome criteria. Am J Gastroenterol 1999; 94:1279–1282.

56. Olden KW. Diagnosis of irritable bowel syndrome. Gastroenterol 2002; 122:1701–1714.

57. Tolliver BA, Herrera JL, DiPalma JA. Evaluation of patients who meet clinical criteria for irritable bowel syndrome. Am J Gastroenterol 1994; 89(2):176–178.

58. Smith RC. Diagnosing the irritable bowel syndrome. Ann Intern Med 1992; 117(12):1056–1057.

59. MacIntosh DG, Thompson WG, Patel DG, Barr R, Guindi M. Is rectal biopsy necessary in irritable bowel syndrome? Am J Gastroenterol 1992; 87(10):1407–1409.

60. Francis CY, Duffy JN, Whorwell PJ, et al. Does routine abdominal ultrasound enhance diagnostic accuracy in irritable bowel syndrome? Am J Gastroenterol 1996; 91:1348–1350.

61. Dancey CP, Backhouse S. Towards a better understanding of patients with irritable bowel syndrome. J Adv Nurs 1993; 18:1443–1450.

62. Heymann-Monnikes I, Arnold R, Florin I, et al. The combination of medical treatment plus multicomponent behavioral therapy is superior to medical treatment alone in the therapy of irritable bowel syndrome. Am J Gastroenterol 2000; 95:981–994.

63. Creed F, Fernandes L, Guthrie E, Palmer S, et al. The cost-effectiveness of psychotherapy and paroxetine for severe irritable bowel syndrome. Gastroenterology 2003; 124:303–317.

64. Schiller LR. The therapy of constipation. Aliment Pharmacol Ther 2001; 15:749–763.

65. Onghena P, Van Houdenhove B. Antidepressant-induced analgesia in chronic non-malignant pain: a meta-analysis of 39 placebo-controlled studies. Pain 1992; 49(2):205–219.

66. Jackson JL, O'Malley PG, Tomkins G, et al. Treatment of functional gastrointestinal disorders with antidepressant medications: a meta-analysis. Am J Med 2000; 108:65–72.

67. Greenbaum DS, Mayle JE, Vanegeren LE, et al. Effects of desipramine on irritable bowel syndrome compared with atropine and placebo. Dig Dis Sci 1987; 32(3):257–265.

68. Budavari AI, Olden KW. The use of antidepressants in irritable bowel syndrome. Pract Gastroenterol 2002; 42(3):13–27.

69. Camilleri M, Mayer EA, Drossman DA, et al. Improvement in pain and bowel function in female irritable bowel patients with alosetron, a 5HT 3-receptor antagonist. Aliment Pharmacol Ther 1999; 13:1149–1159.

70. Anonymous. Alosetron (Lotronex) for treatment of irritable bowel syndrome. Med Lett 2000; 42:53.

71. Novick J, Miner P, Krause R, et al. A randomized, double-blind, placebo-controlled trial of tegaserod in female patients suffering from irritable bowel syndrome with constipation. Aliment Pharmacol Ther 2002; 16:1877–1888.

72. Dapoigny M, Abitbol JL, Fraitag B. Efficacy of peripheral kappa agonist fedotozine versus placebo in treatment of irritable bowel syndrome: a multicenter dose-response study. Dig Dis Sci 1995; 40(10):2244–2248.

73. Camilleri M. Management of the irritable bowel syndrome. Gastroenterology 2001; 120:652–668.

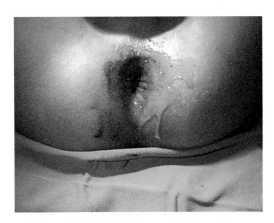

Figure 3.1 Young patient with rectal fecaloma producing hypotonic anus and soiling. (*See p. 38*)

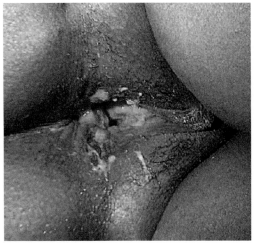

Figure 3.2 Patulous anus. (*See p. 43*)

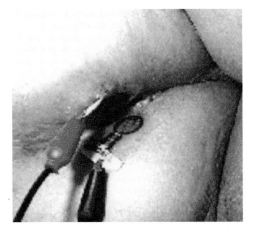

Figure 3.13 Electrical stimulation. (*See p. 50*)

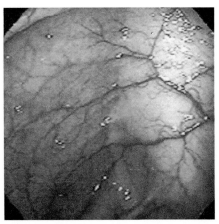

Figure 6.4 The hepatic flexure is frequently identified by the bluish hue resulting from its close proximity to the liver. (*See p. 140*)

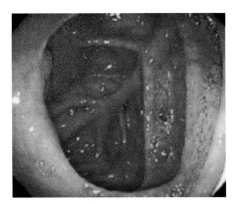

Figure 6.5 The characteristic notch of the superior lip of the ileocecal valve is demonstrated. The opening to the ileum lies on the inferior aspect of the fold. (*See p. 140*)

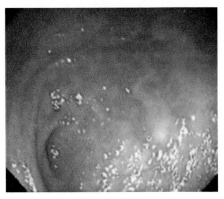

Figure 6.6 The appendiceal orifice is typically seen as a crescent-shaped slit as shown here but may have other appearances. Multiple, small erythematous halos are commonly seen near the appendiceal orifice. (*See p. 141*)

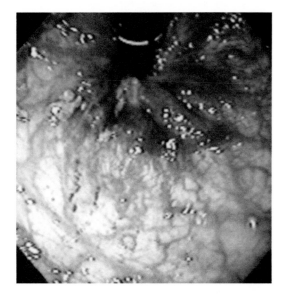

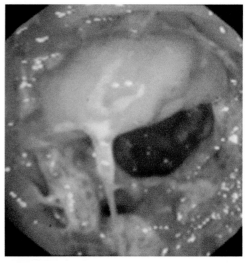

Figure 6.7 Prior to the removal of the colonoscope from the rectum, a retroflexion of the instrument tip should be performed to inspect the distal rectum, an area that may easily be missed on the forward view. (*See p. 150*)

Figure 12.1 Tuberculous ileocolitis. There is marked ulceration and deformity of the ileocecal valve and cecum. (*See p. 284*)

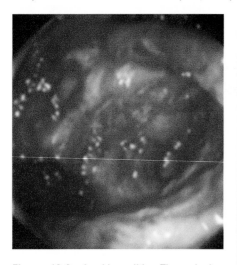

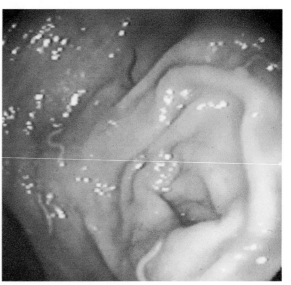

Figure 12.2 Amebic colitis. The colonic mucosa is erythematous and friable, with areas of discrete ulceration. (*See p. 287*)

Figure 12.3 *Trichuris trichiura.* During colonoscopy, adult worms may be found attached to the cecal mucosa. (*See p. 288*)

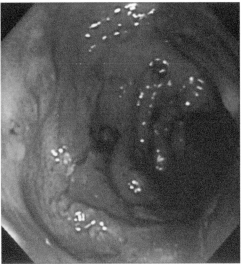

Figure 12.4 Cytomegalovirus colitis. Subepithelial hemorrhage and focal ulceration are common endoscopic findings. (*See p. 289*)

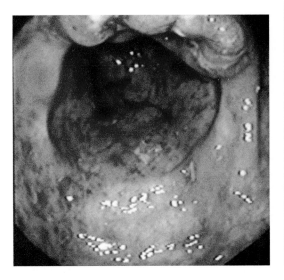

Figure 13.1 Typical endoscopic appearance of *Clostridium difficile* colitis with small white plaques. (*See p. 305*)

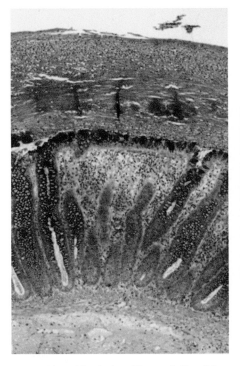

Figure 13.2 Histologic evidence of *Clostridium difficile* colitis from patient (same as in Fig. 13.1) shows pseudomembrane attached to surface mucosa. (*See p. 306*)

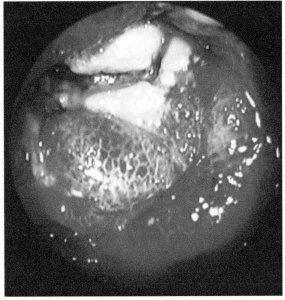

Figure 14.2 Infectious causes of ischemic colitis. (**B**) Colonoscopic view of the rectum of a patient with AIDS and cytomegatovirus-induced ischemic proctocolitis. (*See p. 327*)

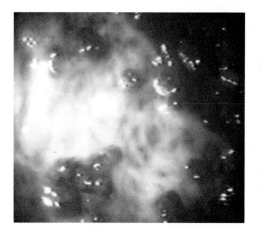

Figure 14.3 Colonoscopic image showing extensive pseudopolyp formation and ulceration in a patient with ischemic colitis. (*See p. 328*)

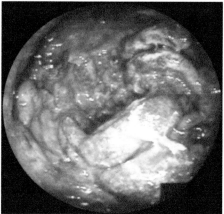

Figure 14.4 (**A**) Colonoscopic view of a polypoid heaped-up mass, which, on biopsy, revealed changes compatible with ischemia. (*See p. 328*)

(A) **(B)** **(C)**

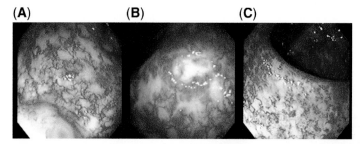

Figure 15.3 Endoscopic findings in radiation proctopathy. (*See p. 349*)

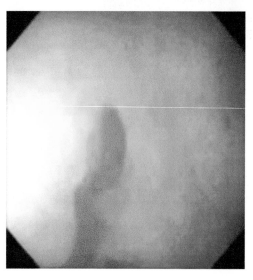

Figure 17.1 Colonic arteriovenous malformation with active bleeding. (*See p. 376*)

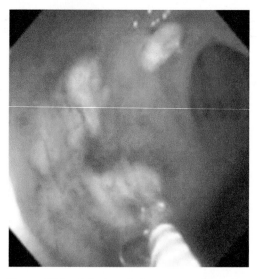

Figure 17.2 Colonic arteriovenous malformation posttreatment with BICAP cautery. (*See p. 377*)

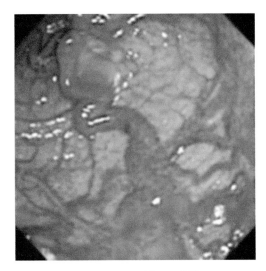

Figure 17.3   Rectal varices. (*See p. 379*)

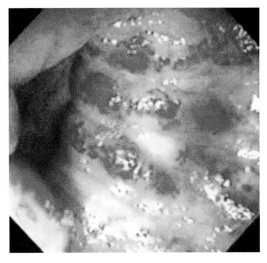

Figure 17.4   Portal hypertensive colopathy. (*See p. 380*)

(A)

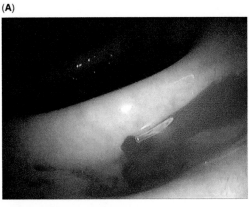

(B)

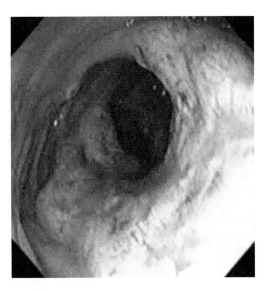

Figure 17.5   Portal hypertensive colopathy posttreatment with argon plasma coagulation. (*See p. 380*)

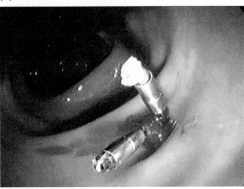

Figure 19.11   (**A**) Endoscopic view of actively bleeding diverticulum. (**B**) Hemostasis after endoclip placement. (*See p. 426*)

(A)

(B)

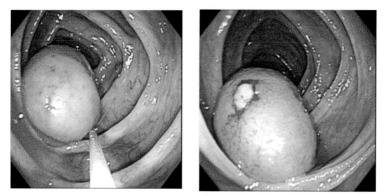

Figure 24.1 **(A)** Large submucosal lesion of the colon. **(B)** The naked fat sign. Diagnosis of lipoma is conclusive when fat extrudes from the biopsy-on-biopsy site of a submucosal colonic lesion. (*See p. 518*)

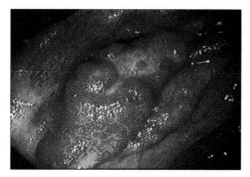

Figure 24.2 An example of primary colorectal lymphoma that presented as an ulcerated submucosal lesion. (*See p. 521*)

(A)

(B)

(C)

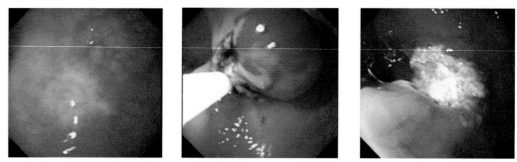

Figure 24.3 An example of a rectal carcinoid lesion. **(A)** The lesion was submucosal; previous biopsy of the site showed carcinoid. **(B)** Rubber band placement at the lesion base to protrude the submucosa. A snare loop has been positioned below the rubber band. **(C)** Lesion following complete resection. (*See p. 533*)

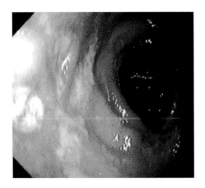

Figure 26.2 Macroscopic features of moderate to severe ulcerative colitis. (*See p. 587*)

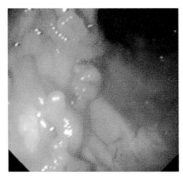

Figure 26.3 Macroscopic appearance of long-standing ulcerative colitis. (*See p. 587*)

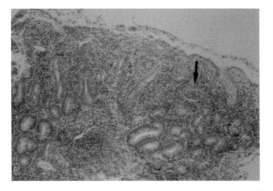

Figure 26.6 Microscopic findings showing active chronic ulcerative colitis including superficial ulcerations, crypt distortion, marked mononuclear inflammation within the lamina propria, and crypt abscess (*arrow*). (*See p. 589*)

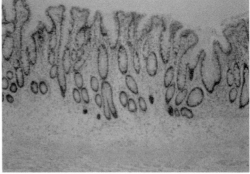

Figure 26.7 Microscopic findings showing inactive (quiescent) ulcerative colitis including crypt distortion and atrophy and paucity of inflammatory cells. (*See p. 589*)

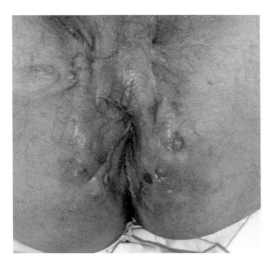

Figure 32.2 Chronic case of perianal abscess. (*See p. 708*)

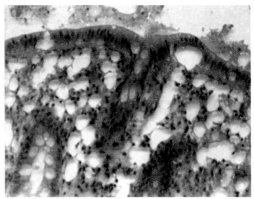

Figure 34.3 Microscopic picture of pneumatosis cystoides intestinalis. (*See p. 743*)

(A)

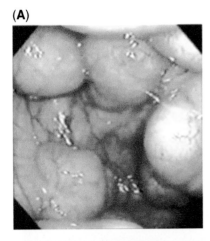

Figure 34.5 Pneumatosis cystoides intestinalis. (**A**) Endoscopic appearance of normal mucosa overlying gas-filled pockets. (*See p. 744*)

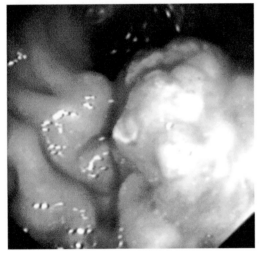

Figure 34.6 Colitis cystica profunda. Endoscopic view of sigmoid involvement demonstrating edematous mucosa overlying a mass. (*See p. 744*)

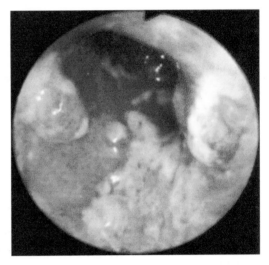

Figure 34.9 Malakoplakia. Endoscopic view of colonic involvement revealing yellowish mucosal discoloration with ulceration and irregularity. (*See p. 748*)

(A)   **(B)**

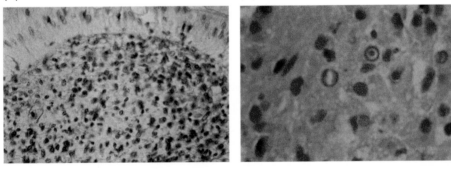

Figure 34.10 Malakoplakia. Photomicrograph at low (**A**) and high (**B**) power demonstrating characteristic Von Hansemann cells with Michaelis–Gutmann bodies. (*See p. 749*)

19 | Diverticular Disease

Jeffrey M. Fox
Department of Internal Medicine and Gastroenterology, The Pernaneate Medical Group, Inc., San Rafael, California, U.S.A.

William Schecter
Department of Clinical Surgery, University of California–San Francisco, and Department of Surgery, San Francisco General Hospital, San Francisco, California, U.S.A.

Neil Stollman
Division of Gastroenterology, University of California–San Francisco, San Francisco, and East Bay Endosurgery, Oakland, California, U.S.A.

INTRODUCTION

Diverticular disease of the colon is extremely common in developed countries and results in a significant health burden. Two decades ago, diverticulosis affected 30 million people in the United States, resulted in 200,000 hospitalizations, and cost over $30 million annually (1). Because the prevalence of diverticulosis increases with age, we will likely see a continued rise in societal impact from this condition as the population ages. Despite the morbidity observed in patients with symptomatic diverticular disease, the majority (80%) of patients with diverticulosis will remain entirely asymptomatic. This fact makes the pathogenesis and natural history of diverticular disease somewhat difficult to study. Some authors even question whether asymptomatic diverticulosis is, in fact, a "disease" at all. Nevertheless, important advances have been made in our understanding of diverticular disease and in the approach to treatment in the last few decades. In this chapter, we review the incidence, pathophysiology, clinical presentation, and treatment of diverticular disease of the colon. Particular emphasis will be placed on the role of colonoscopy in the diagnosis and management of diverticular disease and on the emerging role of minimally invasive surgical management of diverticular complications.

HISTORICAL ASPECTS

Diverticular disease of the colon is often characterized as a "20th century" disorder. In reality, diverticular disease has been described for centuries. The initial description of diverticular disease of the colon was made by the French surgeon Alexis Littre in 1700 (2). In 1849, the French pathologist Jean Cruveilhier described herniations of the colonic mucosa through gaps in the muscular layer in necropsy specimens (3). Ernst Graser used the term "peridiverticulitis" in 1899 to describe inflammation in sigmoid diverticula, while also observing that the sites of penetration of vasa recta through the colon muscle wall were also the sites of diverticular formation (4). William Mayo in 1907 reported on the surgical treatment of severe diverticulitis, recognizing then that most cases were mild and resolved with conservative therapy (5). In 1908, Telling described a series of 80 cases of sigmoid diverticulitis and suggested that the condition may be more common than previously thought (6). The first demonstration of diverticula on contrast radiographs of the colon was reported in 1914 (7). Medical textbooks began to include discussions of diverticular disease in the 1920s, but it was not until the 1960s that extensive epidemiological research demonstrated its prevalence and associated complications.

EPIDEMIOLOGY

The prevalence of diverticulosis in the general population is difficult to measure, mainly because the majority of patients are asymptomatic. Furthermore, the findings of population-based studies of diverticular disease incidence are somewhat difficult to interpret. Autopsy series may underestimate its prevalence if small diverticula are missed at autopsy, whereas barium enema (BE) series may represent overestimates, because examinations are generally performed on patients with gastrointestinal (GI) symptoms and may select for patients with diverticulosis (8,9). The initial studies performed earlier in the 20th century reported prevalence rates of 2% to 10% (8); however, studies in recent decades estimate a much higher prevalence of colonic diverticulosis. The incidence of diverticular disease clearly increases with age, varying from less than 10% in those under 40 years to an estimated 50% to 66% of patients over age 80 (8,10,11). Diverticulosis appears to be equally prevalent in men and women, although men predominate in young "precocious" cases (discussed later).

Diverticulosis has been termed a "disease of Western civilization," because of its striking geographic variability. The disorder is extraordinarily rare in rural Africa and Asia; conversely, the highest incidence rates are seen in the United States, Europe, and Australia (8). Within a given country, the prevalence of colonic diverticula may also vary among ethnic groups. For example, the incidence of diverticulitis in Chinese inhabitants of Singapore was found to be 0.14 cases per 1 million population per year versus 5.41 cases in European inhabitants (12). An autopsy study of Japanese-born individuals who migrated to Hawaii revealed a prevalence of diverticulosis of 52%, significantly greater than that of native-born Japanese remaining in mainland Japan (13). Urbanization within a country also seems to lead to an increase in diverticulosis. While the earlier data in Singapore showed the disease to be quite rare, a more recent follow-up autopsy series revealed diverticulosis in 19% of colons examined, a marked increase, attributed mainly to dietary changes (14). Arabs residing in Israel, a country that has undergone a marked Westernization in the past 40 to 50 years, have shown sharply increasing rates of diverticulosis on barium studies over a 10-year span (15). In the same study, Ashkenazi Jews residing in Israel, with genetic roots in Westernized countries in the United States and Europe, started this surveillance period with an already high prevalence of diverticulosis and remained high at the 10-year follow-up.

Aside from geography and ethnicity, other inherited and acquired risk factors have been statistically associated with diverticular disease, although causality is unclear (Table 1). The role of dietary fiber in the pathogenesis of this disorder will be detailed later in the chapter.

NATURAL HISTORY

Much of the sentinel data on the natural history of this disease was reported by Parks in Belfast in the 1960s and 1970s (11,16). It must be recognized, however, that much of these data are derived from "symptomatic" index patients, while it is known that the large majority, perhaps 80%, of patients with diverticulosis will remain entirely "asymptomatic" throughout their lives. Parks' observation that patients with many diverticula were on average older than those with few diverticula suggests that the disease is, to some extent, progressive (16). In contrast, patients with total colonic involvement were on average somewhat "younger" than those with segmental disease, suggesting that disease pattern may be determined early on and then remain more or less constant, rather than increasing over time in number and extent of disease. Similarly, Horner

Table 1 Risk Factors for Diverticulosis

Associated with increased risk
  Increasing age
  Dietary meat intake
  Living in Western countries (e.g., United States,
    Western Europe, and Australia)
  Connective tissue diseases
Associated with decreased risk
  Dietary fiber intake
  Living in predominantly rural Asian or African countries
    (e.g., Kenya, Jordan, and Thailand)
Equivocal or no association
  Gender
  Alcohol
  Smoking
  Colorectal cancer
  Polycystic kidney disease

reviewed BE studies in 183 patients with diverticulosis, who had repeat examinations an average of 4.4 years apart (17). He noted no apparent progression of disease in 70% of patients.

The fact that diverticulosis and colorectal cancer are both "Westernized" diseases (unusual in developing countries) has suggested to some a causal relationship between the two entities (18). Both diseases are very common in the elderly, but their co-occurrence may be entirely coincidental. Moreover, two studies addressing this issue met with conflicting results, and both used "symptomatic" diverticular patients as controls (19,20); thus, a significant selection and/or detection bias may exist. It seems more likely, as Painter and Burkitt suggested (8), that the Western diet, low in fiber and high in carbohydrates and fat, is an important etiology for both conditions.

PATHOLOGIC ANATOMY

The colon is lined by mucosa, submucosa, and muscularis mucosa surrounded by a complete circular layer of smooth muscle. External to this layer are three incomplete rows of linear smooth muscle, the taenia coli. One band (the mesenteric taenia) lies immediately adjacent to the mesentery; the other two (the antimesenteric taenia) are equally spaced 120° apart. The colon is enclosed in a serosal lining, which is continuous with the visceral peritoneum. Slack reported in 1962 the typical locations of four parallel rows of diverticula in a series of autopsy- or surgically removed colons (21). He noted "four rows, which arise between the mesenteric and antimesenteric taenia...in close association with the mesenteric border of the two antimesenteric taenia and the two borders of the mesenteric taenia." The propensity for diverticula to form at these sites has been amply confirmed. The relative weakness of the muscle wall at these areas that permits herniation is felt to be secondary to the vascular anatomy of the colon. The major colonic vessels reach the bowel via the mesentery, giving rise to the vasa recta. These small arteries penetrate the circular smooth muscle at specific sites between smooth muscle fascicles to anastomose with the submucosal plexus and supply the mucosa. These sites of penetration correspond to the sites where diverticula are found (i.e., on both sides of the mesenteric taenia and the mesenteric sides of the antimesenteric taenia). Thus, weakness of the muscular wall where vessels penetrate appears to allow the mucosa and submucosa to herniate, leading to diverticular formation. A consequence of this anatomic sequence is that diverticula are surrounded by a rich arterial plexus of the vasa recta, with branches typically coursing over the "dome" of the sac. This is relevant to the nature of bleeding from diverticula, which is generally arterial, and often clinically significant (see section "Hemorrhage").

Colonic diverticula are thus, strictly speaking, "pseudodiverticula," in that they are herniations of the mucosa and submucosa through a weakness in the muscle lining but do not themselves include the muscle layers surrounding the colon (Fig. 1). "True" diverticula, in which all layers herniate, uncommonly occur as isolated findings throughout the intestines and may be congenital in origin. Diverticula can vary in number from one to literally hundreds. They typically measure 5 to 10 mm in diameter but can exceed 2 cm. An entity of giant colonic diverticula has been described, with sizes up to 25 cm. Most giant diverticula are single, located in the sigmoid colon, and arise from the antimesenteric border of the colon.

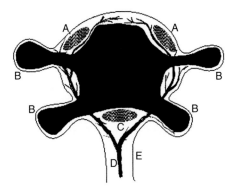

Figure 1 Cross-sectional schematic diagram of diverticulosis of the colon. *A*, antimesenteric taenia; *B*, diverticula; *C*, mesenteric taenial; *D*, arterial branch; *E*, mesentery.

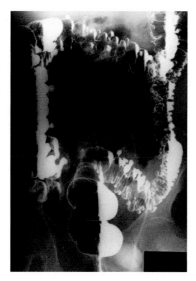

Figure 2 Double-contrast barium enema demonstrating right- and left-sided diverticulosis.

They may be asymptomatic, detected incidentally as a round air density or air-fluid level on abdominal radiographs, or may present with infection, obstruction, or perforation (22).

A fascinating epidemiological finding is the differential clustering of diverticula in the right or left sides of the colon of people in different parts of the world. In Western societies, diverticula occur mainly in the distal or left-sided colon, with up to 90% of patients having involvement of the sigmoid colon and only 15% having right-sided involvement (with or without left colon involved) (2,11,21,23). This is in contrast to Asian countries, in which right-sided involvement seems more prominent, with ascending colon involvement reported in 74% of 1014 consecutive autopsy colons from Singapore, compared with 23% for the sigmoid colon (14). A barium enema (BE) study in Singapore also revealed right-sided involvement in 70% (24). A more recent study in Japan showed that the prevalence of right-sided diverticulosis found on BE doubled (rose from 10% of the population to 20%) in the time period from the early 1980s to the late 1990s, while diverticulosis in the left colon remained the same during that same time (about 4%) (25). An autopsy study of Hawaiian Japanese revealed right colonic diverticula in 50% of cases, compared with sigmoid involvement in 18% (13). While these Asian patients may be somewhat younger than their Western, sigmoid-predominant counterparts, the structural morphology of these pseudodiverticula appears identical on the right and left sides of the colon. Thus, it appears that while environmental factors (e.g., diet) dramatically affect the prevalence of this disorder, genetic and/or racial factors seem to define its anatomic location. Additionally, a blending of different genetic and cultural lineages could explain why many people in the United States develop diverticulosis on both sides of the colon (Fig. 2).

ETIOLOGY AND PATHOGENESIS

Research pertaining to the etiology of colonic diverticulosis has focused mainly in three areas: (i) defects in the colonic wall structure and resistance, (ii) abnormal motility producing increased intraluminal pressures, and (iii) the role of dietary fiber. Undoubtedly, these mechanisms act synergistically to produce herniation of the colonic mucosa, and their distinction may be artificial. Each is summarized briefly below.

Colonic Wall Resistance

As previously mentioned, the sites at which the vasa recta vessels penetrate the muscle wall are the same areas in which diverticula form. Despite suggestions that venous distention or atherosclerotic changes in older people might further weaken this defect, there is no evidence to support that the vessels themselves play an active role in diverticular formation. Painter and Burkitt eloquently summarized that the vasa recta's "passage through the colonic wall charts a course for the mucosal herniation to follow ... but they are not responsible for their appearance" (10). Early anatomic descriptions of diverticular colons reported thickening of the muscle wall and shortening of the taenia, with a resulting accordion- or concertina-like bunching of the folds. Routine histology, however, did not generally reveal muscle hypertrophy. Electron microscopic studies have confirmed that diverticular colonic walls have structurally normal muscle cells, but contain a greater than 200% increase in elastin deposition between the muscle cells in the taenia, compared with those without diverticula (26). The elastin is laid down in a contracted form, resulting in shortening of the taenia and bunching of the circular muscle. It is possible that age-related changes in collagen composition may also play an etiologic role in weakening colonic wall resistance, for example, an increase in Type III collagen synthesis has been described (27). The importance of gut wall connective tissue is also underscored by the increased development of diverticula in patients with connective tissue disorders such as Ehlers–Danlos syndrome, Marfan's syndrome, or scleroderma (1).

Disordered Motility

The possibility of an altered colonic motility playing an etiologic role in diverticular disease began to be explored in earnest in the 1960s. Arfwidsson et al. in 1964 performed manometry on patients with or without sigmoid diverticula (28). Higher resting, postprandial, and neostigmine-stimulated luminal pressures were found in the diverticular patients compared with controls. Painter was unable to replicate the finding of increased resting pressures (intraluminal hypertension) but did confirm elevated pressures in response to neostigmine or morphine in patients with sigmoid diverticula (29). Painter additionally performed simultaneous manometry and cineradiography in these patients (29,30), and postulated a theory of segmentation in which contraction of the colon at haustral folds causes the colon to act not as a continuous tube, but as a series of discrete "little bladders." He proposed that this segmentation not only had a physiologic role in delaying transport and augmenting water reabsorption, but also could generate excessively high pressures within each segment or "bladder," forcing the mucosa to herniate. He further suggested that the Western diet may alter colonic motility in some way as to cause hypersegmentation and an increased propensity for diverticula formation. These earlier manometry studies involved placing catheters 20 cm from the anus (recording over a 10 cm span) through rigid sigmoidoscopes. These recordings thus consequently evaluated the rectum more than the sigmoid colon. A more recent study, using a colonoscopically placed catheter at 55 cm from the anus (recording over a 30 cm span), replicated Arfwidsson's findings of increased resting and postprandial pressures in patients with diverticulosis (31). Another study compared sigmoid motility in patients with or without symptomatic diverticular disease (32) and found that patients with symptomatic disease (complicated or uncomplicated) had higher motility indices than either asymptomatic patients or normals, implying that this finding might have utility in identifying patients at risk for symptomatic or complicated disease. In addition to increased resting and postprandial contraction amplitude, one study found retropropagation of contractile waves in diverticular segments of colon, indicating that motility may be abnormal not only in magnitude but in direction as well (33). The predominance of right-sided diverticula in Asia led Sugihara to compare motility patterns in the right colon of patients with such diverticula (34). Using a colonoscopically placed-microtransducer, higher basal and neostigmine-induced right-sided pressures were documented in the patients with right-sided diverticulosis compared with controls. This finding suggests that abnormal motility also may play a role in the pathogenesis of proximal colonic diverticula.

The molecular basis for the abnormal motility is not yet clear. An increase in the activity of excitatory cholinergic nerves has been demonstrated in diverticular colons compared to controls, as well as diminished activity of nonadrenergic, noncholinergic inhibitory nerves by nitric oxide (35). This suggests, perhaps, an imbalance in the normal excitatory/inhibitory influences favoring excitation and, hence, increased tonicity. Interestingly, a recent study of the tachykinin neurotransmitter system showed a decreased contractility of circular muscle induced by substance P in diverticular colons than normal ones (36). Motility abnormalities appear to exist in diverticular disease at both a gross and a molecular level, and more data are needed to characterize the complex role of different molecular influences on motility in this disease.

Wynne-Jones agreed that high intraluminal pressures predispose to diverticular disease but suggested an alternative hypothesis to increased intrinsic motor tone (37). He postulated that the Westernized, urbanized lifestyle is impermissive of flatus, thus forcing the continuously descending air to return to the upper rectum and sigmoid, causing circular muscle shortening and hypersegmentation. Rigorous confirmation of this hypothesis is still elusive.

Dietary Fiber

The wide geographic variability of diverticular disease and its correlation with a Westernized diet have long suggested a dietary factor in its pathogenesis. Further support for such a factor was the observation that clinical diverticular disease began to emerge in the decades following the introduction of steel rolling mills, which greatly reduce the fiber content of milled grains. Humans, whose diet is remarkably low in vegetable fiber, are the only nondomesticated animals to develop colonic diverticula. Burkitt and Painter were among the most eloquent and early proponents of this theory, in fact, labeling diverticulosis a "deficiency disease" that, like scurvy, should be avoidable with dietary changes (10). In a landmark study, they recorded transit times and stool weights from more than 1200 individuals in the U.K. and rural Uganda (38). The United Kingdom patients, eating a refined Western diet low in fiber, had transit times of approximately 80 hours and mean stool weights of 110 g/day. In marked contrast, the rural Ugandans, eating very high fiber diets, had transit times of 34 hours and stool weights of more than 450 g/day. The long intestinal transit time and smaller volume stools were felt to increase intraluminal pressure, predisposing to diverticular herniation, whereas bulkier stools require less colonic contraction and lower wall pressures. As reasonable as this postulate seems, studies in Western populations comparing transit times and stool volumes in patients with and without diverticular disease have failed to show significant differences. Nonetheless, corroborative animal data do exist; most notably a study of 1800 Wistar rats fed diets of varying fiber contents throughout their natural life span (39). Forty-five percent of the rats on the lowest fiber diet developed diverticula, compared with only 9% of those fed the highest fiber diet. Interestingly, the diverticula formed were mainly right sided, but histologically occurred at points of blood vessel penetration of the muscular wall, as do human diverticula. In humans, other indirect and direct evidence exist with respect to the etiological role of fiber in diverticulosis. In the United States, fiber intake decreased by 28% during the period from 1909 to 1975 (1), a period of dramatic "growth" for the prevalence of diverticular disease. In a British study, a group of vegetarians, with a higher level of fiber intake than nonvegetarians, had a lower prevalence of diverticulosis (12% vs. 33%) (40). Dietary influences for diverticulosis may also be different on the right and left sides of the colon. Right-sided diverticular disease was shown in an Asian study to have no association with fruit and vegetable intake or supplemental fiber intake, though prior meat consumption was strongly associated with right-sided disease (41). Whether these associations apply to Westerners with right-sided diverticulosis is not known. A discussion of the potential role of fiber in the "treatment" of diverticular disease is addressed later in this chapter.

UNCOMPLICATED DIVERTICULOSIS
Clinical Features

As noted, the large majority of patients with diverticulosis will remain entirely asymptomatic. Others will have symptoms attributed to their disease but will lack serious or life-threatening features, so-called symptomatic uncomplicated diverticular disease (SUDD); these patients are discussed in this section. Patients with diverticulitis, bleeding, and other associated complications such as obstruction, stricture, or fistulization are described in a following section on symptomatic *complicated* diverticular disease.

The Asymptomatic Patient
Asymptomatic diverticular disease (ADD) is usually an incidental finding in patients undergoing evaluation for other indications such as occult blood loss or colon cancer screening. With a larger number of people undergoing endoscopic screening for colon cancer, more asymptomatic people with diverticular disease are likely to be identified. There is no clear indication for any therapy or follow-up in these patients, because the majority will remain asymptomatic throughout their lifetime. One study, however, has suggested a possible "prophylactic" benefit of a high-fiber diet. In a prospective study of 51,529 U.S. male health professionals followed over four years, 385 (0.75%) new cases of symptomatic diverticular disease were identified (42). Prior dietary habits were assessed from a food questionnaire administered at study entry.

A significant inverse association was found between dietary fiber intake and the risk of subsequently developing clinically evident diverticular disease. Other findings included that the most "protective" fiber was that from fruits or vegetables, as compared with the more frequently taken cereal fibers, and that a high intake of total fat and red meat was also associated with an increased risk of developing symptomatic disease. Further analysis of this cohort supported the protective effect of the insoluble component of fiber, particularly cellulose (43). These findings suggest that patients with ADD may benefit from increasing their fruit and vegetable fiber intake while decreasing their fat and red meat consumption.

The Symptomatic Uncomplicated Patient

Other patients come to clinical attention because of nonspecific abdominal complaints and may then be found to have diverticulosis coli. A causative relationship between the diverticulosis and the abdominal symptoms is often difficult to establish. Most such patients present with left-sided lower abdominal pain. By definition, such patients do not have findings suggestive of intra-abdominal infection such as fever, leukocytosis, or peritoneal signs. The pain is often exacerbated by eating and diminished with defecation or the passage of flatus, presumably due to lowered intracolonic pressure. Patients may also report other symptoms of colonic dysfunction, including bloating, constipation, diarrhea, or the passage of mucus. Physical examination may reveal fullness or mild tenderness in the left-lower quadrant, but frank rebound or guarding is absent. Occult blood in the stool should never be attributed to diverticulosis without a complete colonic evaluation; in fact, rates of occult bleeding in patients with diverticulosis are similar to that of healthy controls (44). Laboratory studies should be normal.

Diagnostic Modalities: The Role of Colonoscopy

For many years, the BE examination had been the standard investigation in SUDD patients. Barium studies can provide information on the number and location of colonic diverticula but cannot discern their clinical significance. Despite its time-honored tradition, caution has been expressed about a significant diagnostic error rate for BE examinations in patients with colonic diverticulosis. Boulos et al. reported on 65 symptomatic patients who had double-contrast BE studies revealing sigmoid diverticulosis (45). All of these patients underwent subsequent colonoscopy. About 19 neoplastic lesions (17 polyps and 2 carcinomas) were reported on BE. Colonoscopy revealed no polyps in 9 of these 17 (53%) and confirmed only one of the two carcinoma readings. In 46 BEs showing only diverticulosis and no neoplasia, colonoscopy revealed (unreported) polyps in eight and carcinomas in three, with a false-negative error rate of 24%. Overall, the BE interpretation was wrong in 32%. The authors recommend routine colonoscopy in all patients with symptomatic diverticular disease (Fig. 3), particularly to exclude neoplasia. A number of other aspects of colonoscopy in patients with SUDD bear mention. In the early 1970s, the presence of diverticulosis was felt by some to be a relative contraindication to colonoscopy for fear of an increased likelihood of perforation

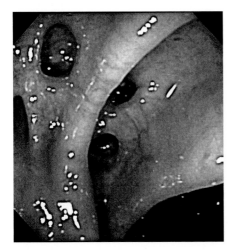

Figure 3 Endoscopic view of sigmoid diverticulosis, demonstrating the in-line orientation of the diverticula.

(46,47). Further data, however, have not supported this fear. Brayko et al. insufflated air into fresh cadaveric sigmoid colons with diverticula and recorded manometric burst pressures (48). All of the colons developed serosal lacerations followed by mucosal rupture at the antimesenteric border, and all of the ruptures occurred at least 2 cm from the nearest diverticula. No diverticular "blowout" occurred. The mean pressure causing rupture was 226 mmHg. This pressure is much higher than that encountered during routine colonoscopy, even with the tip of the instrument against the colon wall or during a cough or Valsalva maneuver. These data and many years of clinical experience have demonstrated the relative safety of colonoscopy in patients with SUDD. One must remain cautious, however, in the face of undiagnosed or subclinical diverticulitis with undetected microperforation and always be judicious with air insufflation. This is particularly true if the head of the colonoscope might be in the neck of a diverticula, because very high local pressures can develop within the diverticula itself.

The diverticular colon can be difficult to examine colonoscopically because of spasm, luminal narrowing from prominent enlarged folds, fixation from prior inflammation and pericolic fibrosis, or confusion between luminal and diverticular openings. Force should never be applied in these circumstances, because an instrumental perforation can occur. The use of a smaller diameter colonoscope may be necessary in examining the difficult colon. Bat and Williams reported a success rate of over 90% with a pediatric colonoscope in cases in which an adult colonoscope could not be passed through the sigmoid due to varying nonstricture-related causes (e.g., looping, fixation, etc.) (49). While specific data are not given regarding success in patients in whom diverticulosis was the sole reason for failure with the adult scope, 44% of these patients had diverticular disease. Kozarek reported the use of the small-caliber upper endoscope in 31 patients who had unsuccessful left colon examinations, 17 (55%) of whom had severe diverticulosis (50). The right colon was reached in 73% of these examinations, allowing therapeutic maneuvers in five patients. The shorter scope length, however, required frequent patient position changes and hook-and-pull maneuvers to telescope the colon over the short shaft. A novel technique, termed the "sigmoid flotation maneuver," has been reported to have facilitated colonoscopy in six technically difficult cases of severe diverticular disease (51). The technique involves distending the colonic lumen with 100 to 300 mL of water, which reportedly opens and straightens the lumen, thus allowing easier passage of the colonoscope. Another entity with which a colonoscopist should be familiar is the inverted diverticulum, where the diverticular pouch bulges into the lumen instead of outside of it. An inverted diverticulum resembles a polyp and can confuse the endoscopist who is not familiar with this phenomenon. The radiographic manifestations of inverted diverticula on BE have been described in six cases, manifested as broad-based sessile polyps with characteristic central umbilication (52). An inverted diverticulum is suggested endoscopically by the gross appearance of normal overlying mucosa, surrounding diverticula, a broad fleshy stalk, the "pillow" sign, and a "replaceable" lesion. Removal is best avoided when these features are encountered. Inadvertent colonoscopic diverticulectomy has been reported in three patients, as well as one surgical sigmoidectomy for a 3 cm "polyp" that was in fact an inverted diverticulum (53–55). Interestingly, all three colonoscopic diverticulectomy patients had uneventful recoveries with conservative therapy.

Differential Diagnosis: Relationship to Irritable Bowel Syndrome

In a patient with nonspecific symptoms of colonic dysfunction, the demonstration of diverticula radiographically or colonoscopically adds little to the diagnostic probabilities or management because of the high prevalence of this finding in the general population. One must be careful to consider alternative diagnoses before attributing the symptoms solely to diverticulosis. These nonspecific presenting symptoms of diverticulosis overlap considerably with those of the irritable bowel syndrome (IBS). Some have postulated that diverticula are, in fact, a late consequence of IBS. In Denmark, Otte et al. reviewed 69 patients with IBS, 24 (35%) of whom had diverticula (56). Over a five- to seven-year follow-up period, they could detect no difference in symptoms or prognosis between those with or without diverticula. This finding led them to conclude that there is no basis to consider symptomatic diverticular disease as a separate entity from IBS. Ritchie reported on the similarity of pain sensation from rectal balloon distention in patients with IBS and those with diverticulosis (57). Whether these two disorders are distinct entities is unknown and probably not clinically important, because both are treated in a similar fashion with equally good prognoses.

Treatment
Dietary Fiber
The possible protective effect of fiber in asymptomatic patients has already been mentioned. There have been multiple uncontrolled studies demonstrating the salutary effect of fiber supplements in patients with nonspecific symptoms and diverticulosis, but the high placebo response rate in these patients and lack of a control group make this data suspect. Brodribb in Oxford, England, published the first randomized, double-blind trial of a high-fiber diet in 18 patients with symptomatic diverticular disease (58). While a significant placebo effect was observed at one month; by three months, there was a statistically significant decrease in bowel symptoms in patients on the high-fiber diet. An important clinical lesson from this trial is that patients should gradually increase their dietary fiber over a few weeks. They should also be cautioned that their symptoms might initially worsen before improving and that such improvement may take months. In a larger study of fiber supplementation in patients with diverticular disease, patients took bran or placebo in a four-month, double-blind, crossover study (59). Unlike Brodribb's data, there was no improvement in symptom end points, despite documenting decreased bowel transit times and significant increases in stool weight and frequency. Despite the conflicting data and the certainty that diverticula do not "regress" with an increased fiber intake, some amelioration of symptoms in patients with uncomplicated disease can be expected with a high-fiber diet.

Medications
The hypermotility of the colon in diverticulosis suggests that anticholinergic or antispasmodic agents such as dicyclomine or hyoscyamine might improve symptoms by diminishing muscular contraction. Nonetheless, there are no adequately controlled therapeutic trials documenting such a benefit. Intravenous glucagon has been reported to offer short-term relief of pain, presumably as a result of smooth muscle relaxation (59). There is no rationale for the use of antibiotics or narcotic analgesics in uncomplicated diverticular disease.

Surgery
Surgical intervention is generally not considered for patients with true uncomplicated diverticulosis, because the risks of surgery would outweigh the benefits in most cases. However, some patients may have an unclear disease presentation; for example, patients with atypical or "smoldering" diverticulitis may demonstrate pain in a characteristic pattern but show no signs of systemic inflammation such as fever or leukocytosis. A cohort of 47 such patients at the Mayo clinic, who underwent sigmoid resection with primary anastomosis for their symptoms, were retrospectively examined (60). Although all the patients lacked systemic signs of inflammation, 76% of the resected specimens had evidence of acute or chronic diverticular inflammation. Additionally, complete resolution of symptoms occurred in 76.5% of patients after resection and 88% of them being pain-free at a minimum of 12 months of follow-up. Hence, it appears that there is a group of patients with "uncomplicated" diverticulosis in whom surgery is appropriate, though most of these individuals probably have low-grade or uncomplicated "diverticulitis," for whom chronic symptoms are a clearer indication for surgery. This finding underscores the importance of clinical follow-up and an open mind regarding those patients with apparent uncomplicated disease but whose symptoms do not follow the expected benign course with conservative treatment. Given cost conscious out-patient treatment, many patients are repeatedly treated with oral antibiotics and have chronic diverticulitis but are never hospitalized. These patients may benefit from a colectomy despite never having been hospitalized. Conversely, patients who have been hospitalized once or even twice may permanently avoid surgery.

COMPLICATED DIVERTICULAR DISEASE

Diverticulitis, defined as inflammation and/or infection associated with diverticula, is probably the most common clinical manifestation of this disorder, affecting an estimated 10% to 25% of patients with diverticula (11). It is generally the result of perforation of a single diverticulum (61). When this results in a localized phlegmon, the term "uncomplicated diverticulitis" is used. "Complicated" diverticulitis refers to cases associated with obstruction, free perforation with peritonitis, fistula, or abscess formation (62). Besides diverticulitis, the other major form of complicated diverticular disease is bleeding, which will be discussed later in the chapter.

Just as diverticular disease, in general, appears to be increasingly common, its complications appear to be increasing in incidence as well. In the period from 1986 to 2000, a university hospital in northern Finland showed an increase of 50% in annual cases of perforated diverticulitis (63). Over about the same period in a university hospital in Texas, the rate of diverticular perforation nearly quadrupled (64).

Uncomplicated Diverticulitis
Pathophysiology
The process through which a diverticulum becomes inflamed has been likened to that causing appendicitis, in that it becomes obstructed by inspissated stool in its neck. This fecolith abrades the mucosa of the sac, causing low-grade inflammation and further blocking drainage. Pathologically, this is evident as lymphoid tissue hyperplasia and aggregation at the apex of the sac (65). The obstruction may then cause an expansion of the normal bacterial flora, diminished venous outflow with localized ischemia, and altered mucosal defense mechanisms. One such alteration is a defective CD2 pathway-induced apoptosis, which has been found in lamina propria lymphocytes in patients with diverticulitis, possibly leading to an upregulation of the local immune response in these patients similar to Crohn's and ulcerative colitis patients (66). The cascade of events initiated by obstruction allows bacteria to breach the mucosa and extend the process through the full wall thickness, ultimately leading to perforation (67). Perforation can involve diverticula both along the mesenteric and along the antimesenteric taenia (68). The extent and localization of the perforation will determine its clinical behavior. Microperforations may remain very well localized, contained by the pericolic fat and mesentery, and cause small pericolic abscesses. Larger macroperforations can result in a more extensive abscess formation, which may track longitudinally around the bowel wall. This process can form a large inflammatory mass, with possible later fibrosis, extension to other organs, and/or fistulous disease. Free perforation into the peritoneum causing frank bacterial peritonitis can be life threatening, but is fortunately very uncommon, with a population incidence of 4 cases per 100,000 population per year (63,69). Hinchey et al. reported a staged grading system reflecting the degree of perforation (Table 2) (70). That staging system was subsequently modified by Sher and co-workers (Table 2) (71).

Clinical Features
Patients with acute diverticulitis classically present with left lower quadrant abdominal pain, reflecting the marked propensity for this disorder to occur in the sigmoid colon in Western countries. Patients with a redundant sigmoid colon may well manifest suprapubic or right-sided pain. Asian patients have predominantly right-sided diverticula. In one series from Hong Kong, 96% of patients with diverticulitis had right lower quadrant pain as their initial complaint (72). The pain may be intermittent or constant and is frequently associated with a change in bowel habits, either diarrhea or constipation (73). Hematochezia is rare. Anorexia,

Table 2 Staging and Classifications

Hinchey Classification of Diverticular Perforation
Stage I: confined pericolic abscess
Stage II: distant abscess (retroperitoneal or pelvic)
Stage III: generalized peritonitis due to rupture of a pericolic or pelvic abscess (noncommunicating with bowel lumen because of obliteration of diverticular neck by inflammation)
Stage IV: fecal peritonitis due to free perforation of a diverticulum (communicating)
Modified Hinchey Classification System
Stage I: pericolic abscess
Stage IIA: distant abscess amenable to percutaneous drainage
Stage IIB: complex abscess associated with fistula
Stage III: generalized purulent peritonitis
Stage IV: fecal peritonitis

Source: From Refs. 70 and 71.

nausea, and vomiting may occur. Dysuria and urinary frequency may be reported by patients, reflecting a sympathetic cystitis induced by bladder irritation from the nearby inflamed sigmoid colon.

Physical examination usually discloses localized tenderness, generally in the left lower quadrant, although, as noted, right-sided signs do not preclude diverticulitis. Guarding and rebound tenderness may be present, as may a tender, cylindrical, and palpable mass. Bowel sounds are typically depressed but may be normal in mild cases or increased in the presence of obstruction. Rectal examination may disclose tenderness or a mass, particularly, with a low-lying pelvic abscess. Fever is present in the majority of patients, while hypotension and shock are unusual. The white blood corpuscles (WBC) count is frequently elevated, although one study reported a normal WBC count ($<11,000/um^3$), with no left shift in 46% of patients (73). No other laboratory abnormalities are routinely helpful.

Differential Diagnosis
Acute Appendicitis
Acute appendicitis is the misdiagnosis most frequently made in patients with acute diverticulitis. Patients with a redundant sigmoid colon or with right-sided diverticula may present with right-sided symptoms. In Hong Kong, where awareness of right predominant diverticulosis is presumably high, 34 of 35 patients with right-sided diverticulitis were initially felt to have acute appendicitis (72). While appendicitis is, on average, a disease of much younger patients than is acute diverticulitis, there is a wide range of ages for both, and clinical suspicion must remain high when diagnosing one or the other on clinical grounds. In fact, one study reported that patients with right-sided diverticulitis were actually younger than left-sided patients and were operated on earlier, more frequently for mistaken diagnoses (74).

Inflammatory Bowel Disease
Ulcerative colitis, with its typical features of bloody diarrhea and mucus, should be fairly easy to distinguish from diverticulitis. Crohn's disease, however, may mimic diverticulitis. With its transmural involvement, Crohn's colitis may present with abdominal pain, fever, and leukocytosis. Fistulas can complicate both diseases. Aphthous ulcers, anorectal involvement, and chronic diarrhea should suggest a possible diagnosis of Crohn's colitis. The coexistence of both diseases in the same patient has been well described. A series of patients from London's St. Mark's Hospital with both Crohn's colitis and diverticulosis has been reported (75). Only one of 26 patients had a normal anorectal region, suggesting a useful point of discrimination. Six patients with localized Crohn's disease of the colon in association with diverticulosis, all without perianal disease or systemic manifestations, have also been reported (76). All underwent localized resection for presumed diverticulitis with no reported recurrences. A segmental colitis has been described associated with diverticula, with sparing of the remaining colon and no specific alternative diagnosis (such as infectious or ischemic colitis) (77). These patients presented mainly with hematochezia and diarrhea, without overt diverticulitis. The majority had endoscopic and clinical remission at 12 months. In a separate study, a group of patients undergoing sigmoid resection with findings of both diverticulitis and Crohn's disease–like changes were studied (78). Only patients with prior Crohn's in other parts of the bowel had evidence of active Crohn's postoperatively. About 23 or 25 patients without preexisting Crohn's had no recurrences of disease, which is not the typical natural history for Crohn's. This study suggests that the majority of patients with coexisting diverticulitis and Crohn's may actually have diverticulitis alone with an idiosyncratic inflammatory response that is histologically similar to, but prognostically different from, Crohn's disease.

Colon Cancer
Colon carcinoma and diverticulosis both affect mainly the distal colon of aging patients, particularly in developed Western countries. Speculation as to a causative relationship has been previously discussed. Most likely, both are consequences of the same environmental effects, mainly dietary. Nonetheless, both can present with perforation, obstruction, or fistula formation. Differentiation obviously has critical prognostic importance. Chronic symptoms of weight loss or bleeding should raise suspicion for carcinoma. Although usually difficult to distinguish by imaging, findings on abdominal contrast tomography that favor colon cancer as the diagnosis include enlarged pelvic lymph nodes or liver metastases, while pericolonic

inflammation or segmental involvement of greater than 10 cm favors diverticulitis (79). Because both cancer and diverticulitis can present with obstruction or perforation, surgical exploration and resection may be necessary to make a precise diagnosis. In uncomplicated cases, elective colonoscopy and/or BE after the acute inflammation has resolved will allow for exclusion of luminal malignancy.

Ischemic Colitis
The elderly with diverticulosis may have diffuse atherosclerotic vascular disease and thus are also at risk for ischemic colitis. Features helpful in differentiating the two include the presence of thumbprinting on abdominal X rays and hematochezia, both suggesting ischemia as a more likely cause of the patients' abdominal pain. In difficult cases, a limited flexible sigmoidoscopy with minimal air insufflation may be helpful in identifying ischemic mucosal changes.

Peptic Ulcer Disease
Free air in the abdomen or peritonitis may be present in perforated ulcers or diverticula. A careful history for preexistent ulcer disease, dyspepsia, or nonsteroidal anti-inflammatory drug (NSAID) use may help in the differentiation.

Others
Gynecologic disorders, such as ruptured ovarian cysts, ovarian torsion, ectopic pregnancy, or pelvic inflammatory disease, can resemble acute diverticulitis in female patients. Pelvic or transvaginal sonography may be helpful in obtaining an accurate diagnosis. Meckel's diverticulitis and other forms of colitis such as pseudomembranous or amebic can also mimic diverticulitis.

Diagnostic Modalities
Most patients with acute diverticulitis present with signs and symptoms sufficient to justify the clinical diagnosis and institute empiric therapy. However, the diagnosis of diverticulitis based solely on clinical criteria can be inaccurate. Emergency surgery for presumed diverticulitis, without the benefit of radiological confirmation, carries a misdiagnosis rate as high as 34% to 67% (80). Therefore, radiological studies to confirm the diagnosis of diverticulitis are often employed. Plain radiography should generally be performed in most patients as part of their initial evaluation. Further studies should be reserved for those patients in whom the diagnosis remains uncertain, response to empiric treatment is suboptimal, or a complication is suspected.

Plain Radiography
An erect chest radiograph, together with erect and supine abdominal radiographs, should generally be performed on patients with clinically significant abdominal pain. The erect chest film has the dual purpose of detecting a pneumoperitoneum, which has been reported to be present in up to 11% of patients with acute diverticulitis (81) and to assess cardiopulmonary status in a generally elderly population with frequent comorbid illness. Abdominal X rays have been reported to be abnormal in 30% to 50% of patients with acute diverticulitis (81,82). Findings include small- or large-bowel dilation or ileus, bowel obstruction, or soft-tissue densities, suggesting abscesses.

Contrast Enema Examinations
Since the demonstration by Case in 1914 of diverticula on BE examination (7), contrast enemas became the diagnostic standard for many years. The choice of contrast material to be used remains somewhat controversial. While barium is less expensive than water-soluble contrast media and provides better mucosal detail, the possibility of a perforation is a relatively strong contraindication to its use, for fear of fecal/barium peritonitis with its attendant management difficulties. Hence, only water-soluble contrast enema should be used in the setting of acute diverticulitis (83). A gentle, single-contrast study should be performed and terminated, once significant findings have been discovered. An attempt to visualize the entire colon should be deferred to a later date when the acute attack has resolved. Air (double)-contrast studies are not indicated. Findings considered "diagnostic" of diverticulitis include demonstration of extravasated contrast material outlining an abscess cavity, an intramural sinus tract, or fistula (2,84). Extensive diverticulosis, spasm, mucosal thickening or spiking, or deformed sacs

are suggestive but are nonspecific signs. An extraluminal mass compressing or displacing the bowel is said to be the most common finding in severe diverticulitis (85), although this finding is clearly not specific for this diagnosis. Obviously, the absence of any diverticula or associated findings should invoke a reconsideration of the diagnosis. In retrospective analysis, contrast enema has been shown to have a sensitivity of 62% to 94% (62,86) in detecting acute diverticulitis, with false-negative results in 2% to 15% (62).

Computerized Tomography
Because diverticulitis is mainly an extraluminal disease, luminal contrast studies may be inaccurate. In recent years, computerized tomography (CT) scanning has been assuming an increasing role. Most now consider CT the procedure of choice, replacing contrast enemas. CT has the ability to image transmural or extraluminal disease and adjacent structures and has therapeutic potential in the percutaneous drainage of abscesses. Abdominal and pelvic scanning is generally performed with water-soluble contrast, both orally to opacify the small bowel and rectally to better evaluate the rectosigmoid. If not contraindicated, intravenous contrast is generally used as well. CT criteria suggestive of diverticulitis include the presence of diverticula with pericolic infiltration of fatty tissue (often appearing as fat "stranding" or "streaking"), thickening of the colonic wall, and abscess formation. In the earliest large retrospective series of CT findings in diverticulitis, Hulnick et al. (87) reported the finding of pericolic fat inflammation in 98%, diverticula in 84%, a colonic wall thickness greater than 4 mm in 70%, and an abscess in 35%. Contrast enema examinations in the same patients underestimated the extent of disease in 15 of 37 cases (41%), leading the authors to conclude that CT should be the initial examination of choice in patients with diverticulitis. Numerous subsequent trials have been performed comparing these two modalities in patients with suspected diverticulitis, the largest of which comprised over 400 patients, and have consistently reported a sensitivity of 93% to 98% and a specificity of 75% to 100%, significantly more accurate than contrast enemas (84,88,89). Recent data have also found CT to be highly sensitive and specific for right-sided diverticulitis and in helping to differentiate diverticulitis from colorectal cancer of the ascending colon and cecum (90,91). While some reports show a lower sensitivity of CT for diverticulitis (92,93), and respecting issues of cost, availability, and local expertise, we believe that in cases in which the diagnosis is in doubt or clinical deterioration occurs, CT has become the more suitable primary radiological modality. Conversely, in patients with mild disease and in whom the diagnosis is straightforward, CT scan is usually unnecessary.

Ultrasonography
Based on its relatively low cost, convenience, and noninvasive nature, ultrasonography has been advocated as a potentially useful modality in diverticulitis. Characteristic findings implying active inflammation have included bowel-wall thickening, presence of diverticula or abscesses, and hyperechogenicity of the bowel wall. Prospective series have reported a sensitivity of 84% to 98% and specificity of 80% to 93% (94,95). One study of 71 patients with suspected diverticulitis reported a negative predictive value of 100% with ultrasound (96). The addition of a graded compression technique to identify focal tenderness and displace obscuring bowel gas may improve accuracy (97). A recent trial comparing ultrasonography with CT revealed equally good accuracy (98). Sonography may also be useful in female patients, to exclude pelvic/gynecologic pathology. Despite these data, the examination remains very operator dependent, especially for the detection of interloop abscesses, air-filled abscesses, or disease complications posterior in the abdomen that may not be well visualized. Ultrasound therefore remains a second-line diagnostic tool to be used in selected circumstances or for research.

Magnetic Resonance Imaging
With limited resolution secondary to motion artifact introduced by peristalsis and respiration, the potential role of magnetic resonance imaging remains to be demonstrated. Whether decreased scan times and intraluminal contrast agents will overcome these limitations remains to be seen.

Endoscopy
Due to the risk of perforation, either from the instrument itself or insufflation of air, endoscopy is generally avoided in the initial evaluation of the patient with acute diverticulitis. Its use

should be limited to situations in which the diagnosis of diverticulitis is unclear. In such cases, a limited rigid or flexible sigmoidoscopy with minimal air insufflation may be helpful to exclude other diagnoses such as inflammatory bowel disease, carcinoma, or ischemic colitis. Once the acute setting has passed, however, a colonoscopy should be routinely performed to confirm the diagnosis and to "clear" the colon of competing diagnoses, particularly neoplasia.

Treatment
One of the initial decisions in uncomplicated diverticulitis involves a determination of the need for hospitalization. This ultimately depends on the impression of the physician, based on an individual patient's initial clinical presentation. Although no hard generalizations can be made about treatment, guidelines can be applied to the majority of patients. Factors to be considered include the patient's ability to tolerate oral intake, severity of illness, comorbid diseases, and available outpatient support systems (e.g., a reliable family).

An appropriate candidate for outpatient management would be one with mild symptoms, no peritoneal signs, the ability to take oral fluids, and a supporting home network. These patients should be treated with a clear liquid diet and antibiotics. When cultured, the majority of diverticular abscesses grow mixed aerobic and anaerobic infections, with the most common single organisms being *Escherichia coli, Streptococcal spp.*, and *Bacteroides fragilis* (99). Hence, oral antibiotics with broad-spectrum coverage, such as amoxicillin/clavulanate, sulfamethoxazole/trimethoprim with metronidazole, or a fluoroquinolone with metronidazole have been recommended as reasonable choices (100). Patients treated as an outpatient should have close follow-up. They should be instructed to call the physician for increasing pain, fever, or inability to tolerate oral fluids, all of which could indicate the development of complications and may necessitate hospitalization. Symptomatic improvement should generally be evident within two to three days, at which time the diet may be slowly advanced. Antibiotic treatment should be continued for 7 to 10 days.

Elderly patients, immunosuppressed patients, those with severe comorbid disease, and those with high fevers or significant leukocytosis with acute diverticulitis should be hospitalized. These patients should have their bowels rested with either clear liquids or nothing by mouth. Intravenous fluid therapy to maintain or restore intravascular volume, balance electrolytes, and ensure adequate urinary output should be initiated. Broad-spectrum intravenous antibiotics should be started. Recommended combination regimens include anaerobic coverage with metronidazole or clindamycin and gram-negative coverage with an aminoglycoside (e.g., gentamycin and tobramycin), monobactam (e.g., aztreonam), or a third-generation cephalosporin (e.g., ceftazidime, cefotaxime, and ceftriaxone) (100). Single-agent coverage with intravenous second-generation cephalosporins such as cefoxitin or cefotetan or beta-lactamase inhibitor combinations such as ampicillin/sulbactam or ticarcillin/clavulanate are reasonable alternative therapies. Symptomatic improvement with decreasing fever and leukocytosis should be observed within two to three days, at which point the diet may be advanced. If improvement continues, patients may be discharged but should complete a 7- to 10-day oral antibiotic course. Failure to improve with conservative medical therapy warrants a diligent search for complications, consideration of alternative diagnoses, and surgical consultation. The majority of patients hospitalized with acute diverticulitis will respond to conservative medical therapy, but it has been estimated that 15% to 30% will require surgery during that admission (1,2,16,62). Surgical treatment of complications such as perforation, abscess, fistula, or obstruction is discussed in the section on complicated diverticulitis, later in this chapter.

For the majority of patients who respond well to conservative therapy, another important clinical question involves the likelihood of recurrence and the role of elective or prophylactic surgical resection. The risk of recurrent symptoms following an attack of acute diverticulitis has been variously reported to range from as low as 7% to as high as 45%. Many authors report the risk of recurrence to be about 33% (1,2,16,62). A second attack requiring readmission has been reported in 25% and a third attack in 6% (16). Half of these second attacks occurred within one year and 90% within five years of the initial attack. Recurrent attacks are less likely to respond to medical therapy and have a higher mortality rate (16,62); thus, most authorities would agree that elective resection is indicated after two attacks of uncomplicated diverticulitis (101–103). Most patients after elective resection for recurrent diverticulitis report having a good functional outcome and low rates of recurrent disease (104). Not surprisingly, the patients with significant IBS symptoms prior to elective resection have less successful symptom resolution after elective resection. The risk–benefit analysis of any given approach to uncomplicated diverticulitis must be individualized for a specific patient. Consideration must be given to the severity and responsiveness of the attack, the general health of the patient, and the risk to the patient of a subsequent attack. The risk of the resection itself is a factor as well, and this area is evolving. Increasingly favorable experiences with laparoscopic resections for diverticular disease are being reported (discussed later in this chapter), which should lower the threshold for resection in some patients by lowering the operative morbidity. An elective sigmoid resection is a reasonable approach after even a single attack in selected cases.

Diverticulitis: Special Issues

The Young Patient

Diverticulitis is relatively uncommon in patients less than 40 years old, representing 2% to 5% of all diverticulitis patients (2,16). Because it is uncommon in these age groups, the diagnosis of acute diverticulitis is often missed (40–80% of the time) or mistaken for other diagnoses, such as appendicitis or inflammatory bowel disease. Like diverticulitis in older patients, the disease is mainly sigmoid in location, although one report has described a right-sided predominance in younger Israeli patients (74). However, unlike the older patients, there seems to be a significant male predominance in these patients (2,105,106). The disease is thought to be more virulent in younger patients, with 66% to 88% of patients reportedly requiring urgent surgery during their initial attack, and to have a higher risk of recurrence or complication compared with older patients (2,106,107). When patients with acute diverticulitis are managed nonoperatively, youth and radiographic severity of the initial episode appear to be independent variables associated with poor outcome in their subsequent course (108). The younger patients may do worse in large part due to delay in diagnosis. Many authors conclude that an elective segmental colectomy in a healthy young person is indicated after one well-documented episode of uncomplicated diverticulitis, because of the low risk of surgery and the high risk of recurrence and complication after nonoperative treatment of diverticulitis in young patients (62,102,108). Others, however, have recently questioned this assertion, based on some investigations that do not support a more aggressive course in younger patients (74,101,109).

The Immunocompromised Patient

Physicians are seeing an increasing number of immunosuppressed patients, from causes including AIDS, iatrogenic immunosuppression with chemotherapy, post–organ transplant, steroid use, renal failure, or cirrhosis. Such patients with diverticulitis may present with much more subtle signs and symptoms than immunocompetent patients and represent a more difficult diagnostic challenge. Although diverticulitis in such patients does not appear to be more common, it appears to have graver consequences. Perkins et al. (110), in comparing the clinical course of acute diverticulitis in 10 immunosuppressed patients with 76 nonimmunosuppressed ones, found that 24% of nonsuppressed patients failed medical therapy, whereas 100% of immunosuppressed patients required surgery. Another series compared the outcome of acute diverticulitis in 40 immunocompromised patients with that in 169 immunocompetent patients (111). The immunocompromised patients had a higher rate of free perforation (43% vs. 14%), need for surgery (58% vs. 33%), and postoperative mortality (39% vs. 2%) than the noncompromised patients. In solid organ transplant populations, such as heart, lung, and kidney, mortality from diverticulitis has been found to be extremely high, ranging from 25% to 100% (112–114). Due to this high risk, many advocate elective resection after one attack in an immunosuppressed patient (9,102).

Recurrent Diverticulitis After Resection

Operative management of recurrent disease is often technically challenging due to inflammation and adhesions. Up to 10% of patients will have symptomatic recurrent diverticulitis after surgical resection, and reoperation may be required in 2% to 3% (101,104,115,116). One study showed the mean length of time from elective resection to recurrence in these patients to be 25 months (104). In a series of 501 patients from the Mayo Clinic, who had resection and reanastomosis for diverticular disease, a higher recurrence rate was found when the sigmoid colon was used for the distal resection margin, compared with the rectum (116). The authors thus suggested that the entire distal colon be removed during resection with anastomosis to the proximal rectum. This would theoretically decrease the risk of recurrence in remaining sigmoid diverticula. The proximal anastomosis should be made at a noninflamed area of normal colon but need not include all diverticular disease present (62,101). This finding has been confirmed by Thaler et al. from the Cleveland Clinic, Florida, U.S.A. (117).

Specialization and Quality of Care

Because diverticulitis is so common, it is diagnosed in diverse practice settings, from the primary care office visit to the hospital emergency room. People affected with diverticulitis may be managed by a primary physician, such as a family practitioner or internist, a general surgeon, or a subspecialist such as a gastroenterologist or a colorectal surgeon. The demands of a changing physician work force have necessitated management of increasingly complex medical problems by nonspecialists. In most cases, it may be appropriate for a generalist to manage patients with diverticulitis without consulting a specialist. However, a study considering retrospectively an Illinois registry of patients hospitalized for diverticulitis showed that patients with a gastroenterologist as the attending physician, compared to a family practitioner or internist, had shorter length-of-stay, lower readmission rates, and a trend toward lower complication rate and mortality (118). The cost of the hospitalization, however, was not significantly impacted by the person primarily directing care. The decreased length of stay for the gastroenterologist-managed patients probably was offset by increased (and earlier) use of diagnostic modalities. Similarly, in managing diverticulitis complicated by fistulas, colorectal surgeons have been shown to have better surgical outcomes, including lower complication rates and shorter hospital stays, than general surgeons (119). These data imply that early consultation with a subspecialist, though not always necessary or available at every institution, might improve quality of care in the inpatient management of diverticulitis.

Complicated Diverticulitis
Abscess

When perforation of a colonic diverticulum occurs, the ability of the pericolic tissues to control the spread of the inflammatory process will determine subsequent clinical behavior and treatment. A localized phlegmon initially develops with a limited spread. Further spread can lead to the formation of larger local or distant abscesses. The Hinchey and Modified Hinchey grading systems discussed earlier classifies Stage I disease as a localized pericolic abscess and Stage II as a distant retroperitoneal or pelvic abscess. Stages III and IV refer to generalized purulent or fecal peritonitis and require urgent surgical intervention. Clinical signs suggesting abscess formation include a tender mass on physical examination or persistent fever and/or leukocytosis despite an adequate trial of appropriate intravenous antibiotics. Once an abscess is suspected, radiographic evaluation with a CT scan is the best modality for making the definite diagnosis and following its course over time. CT scan is also valuable as a guide for percutaneous drainage.

Small pericolic abscesses (Stage I) can often be treated conservatively with antibiotics and bowel rest (101). In one series of 140 consecutive patients with acute diverticulitis, 10 were found to have pericolic abscesses, seven of whom (70%) responded successfully to conservative treatment (120). The authors reasonably postulated that this favorable prognosis may be due to a persistent fistula between the abscess and the colon, thus permitting spontaneous internal drainage. Conservative, noninterventional management of abscesses should be considered only in stable patients who demonstrate unequivocal improvement in pain, fever, tenderness, and leukocytosis over the first few days of therapy.

Increasingly, radiological drainage is an option that is employed as an adjunct to, and sometimes in place of, surgical drainage (Fig. 4). First touted in the early 1980s (121), CT scan–guided percutaneous drainage of abdominal abscesses has assumed a prominent complementary role with surgery. The immediate advantage of percutaneous catheter drainage is rapid control of sepsis and patient stabilization without the need for and risk of general anesthesia. It will often eliminate the need for a multiple-stage procedure with colostomy (122), instead allowing for temporary palliative drainage and subsequent single-stage resection in three to four weeks. Two retrospective series have reported success rates of 74% and 80% in stabilizing patients and safely allowing for subsequent single-stage procedures (123,124). A surgical procedure is required in the acute setting in the 20% to 25% of patients in whom

(A) **(B)**

(C)

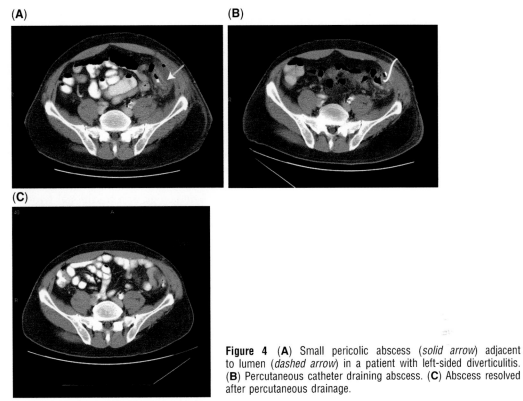

Figure 4 (**A**) Small pericolic abscess (*solid arrow*) adjacent to lumen (*dashed arrow*) in a patient with left-sided diverticulitis. (**B**) Percutaneous catheter draining abscess. (**C**) Abscess resolved after percutaneous drainage.

the abscess is multiloculated, anatomically inaccessible for drainage or not resolving with drainage. Again, a single-stage procedure is preferable for complicated diverticulitis if appropriate conditions are met; these conditions appear to be made increasingly possible with the assistance of percutaneous drainage.

When the patient with a localized abscess is unstable or not improving with medical and/or percutaneous management, exploratory surgery is usually needed. In cases where surgical intervention is deemed necessary, the approach has evolved over the last half-century. Historically, a three-stage management was preferred for complicated diverticulitis of all severity. The first procedure involves a proximal colostomy, drainage of the intra-abdominal abscess, and oversewing or patching with the omentum, the site of perforation, if found. The second procedure is devoted to resecting the diseased bowel, with the anastomosis still protected by the proximal postoperative colostomy. Unfortunately, the third procedure is for restoration of bowel continuity. Although the multiple-stage surgical approach to diverticular disease was generally effective for management of abscess formation, it is generally desirable to limit the number of laparotomies to minimize morbidity and time of hospitalization. In the last few decades, two-stage management (Hartmann procedure, described below under "free perforation") and, increasingly, management with a single operation (resection with primary anastomosis) have become the preferred surgical approaches. The switch to fewer operations has been made without a discernable compromise in overall outcomes relative to three-stage approaches. In a series of 140 patients treated for complicated diverticulitis, primary resection with anastomosis was performed in 61% of patients with a mortality rate of 1%, whereas those who underwent a three-stage approach had a mortality of 14% (125). Such studies can be biased, however, by the fact that patients with more advanced disease and at higher risk for mortality usually require more extensive intervention and are often not candidates for resection with primary anastomosis. Nevertheless, single-stage management of complicated diverticulitis is possible and is being increasingly utilized in appropriate patients.

A recent task force by the American Society of Colon and Rectal Surgeons specifically addressed the ideal extent of bowel resection (101). In elective cases, attempts should be made to remove all of the diseased colon. It is not critical, however, to remove all diverticular colon in portions that are not hypertrophied or inflammatory. The entire "sigmoid" colon should be removed, however, because this is the most common location for initial disease and recurrence (see section "Recurrent diverticulitis after resection" above). When primary anastomosis is chosen, it should be made to normal rectum and should be free of tension to optimize results.

Restoring bowel continuity after multiple-stage operations can be technically challenging and carries a risk of anastomotic leakage and mortality. Because of this risk, only about half of patients undergoing a proximal-end colostomy will ultimately have an additional procedure performed for colostomy let down (126); the remainder end with a permanent colostomy long term. For this reason, it may be desirable, when appropriate, to perform a primary anastomosis at the time of surgery for complicated diverticulitis. In order to do so, bowel preparation is thought to be necessary, though some investigators have challenged this concept (127). For elective resection, when perforation is not a concern, bowel preparation is performed prior to the operation, usually as an outpatient. This can be done with either a one-day sodium phosphate or polyethylene glycol-electrolyte lavage or a traditional two- or three-day mechanical preparation; both types have been shown to have similar outcomes in a randomized trial (128). In the setting of urgent or emergent surgery when free perforation is suspected, bowel lavage is being performed increasingly in an "on-table" fashion, thereby allowing a primary anastomosis to be performed in a single stage (129–131).

Free Perforation

Severe peritonitis (Hinchey Stage III or IV) is a surgical emergency and requires urgent operative intervention. Although uncommon in the antibiotic era, mortality from generalized peritonitis has been reported in the 12% to 26% range (132). Early identification of free perforation is critical. Although CT scan can confirm the diagnosis in ambiguous cases, an abdominal series showing free intraperitoneal air combined with high clinical suspicion is ground alone for exploration. Broad-spectrum intravenous antibiotics such as a second-or third-generation cephalosporin and metronidazole should be immediately instituted.

The desired method of surgical management for generalized peritonitis, as for localized abscesses, is controversial. The common options are as follows: (i) "primary resection" of the diseased sigmoid colon with either proximal end colostomy and oversewing of the rectal stump (the Hartmann procedure) or primary colorectal anastomosis and (ii) secondary resection with the initial operation to form a diverting colostomy and suture the perforation, if possible, and subsequent procedures to resect the diseased colon and restore bowel continuity. In most cases of free perforation, unlike cases of diverticulitis with lower severity, at least two separate operations are necessary, regardless of whether primary or secondary resection is performed. As previously noted, in many cases, restoration of the anastomosis is not possible, and the colostomy becomes permanent. The descending colon selected for anastomosis may have scattered diverticular outpouchings but should not have muscle hypertrophy.

It seems more pathophysiologically attractive to resect the diseased bowel at the initial operation. However, there is no clear consensus over whether primary or secondary resection is more beneficial for peritonitis from diverticulitis. The sigmoid colon is the most common location for diverticulitis and its complications in Western nations, and therefore most studies addressing surgical outcomes refer to sigmoid disease. Retrospective studies suggest an advantage for primary over secondary resection with respect to morbidity and mortality (132–134). To date, two prospective randomized trials have been performed comparing primary versus secondary sigmoid resection for generalized purulent or fecal peritonitis. The conclusions about the optimal approach were conflicting. The first (135) involved 62 patients at a single center with peritonitis and macroscopic evidence of sigmoid diverticulitis at laparotomy. Patients were randomized to transverse colostomy with suture of visible perforation and coverage with an omental flap, followed by later elective resection and a third procedure for colostomy closure, if possible (secondary resection, three-stage) versus immediate resection with proximal end colostomy, mucus fistula, or the Hartmann procedure for the distal bowel, and delayed second procedure for elective anastomosis and colostomy closure (primary resection, two-stage). No patients underwent primary resection with primary anastomosis, meaning all patients required at least two operations. The patients who underwent primary resection for purulent peritonitis had significantly more deaths than the secondary resection group ($6/25$ vs. $0/21$, $p = 0.024$). No significant difference was found between groups for death from fecal peritonitis. The primary resection group were found to have significantly fewer days in hospital during the first year after the initial operation. Overall, the authors concluded that secondary resection was superior to primary resection for purulent peritonitis, though there was no difference for fecal peritonitis or overall. The main limitation of this study was that baseline characteristics differed between groups with respect to gender and proportion with fecal and purulent peritonitis. Also, the sample size calculations were not described a priori, and the study was probably underpowered to detect overall mortality differences. The second trial (136) corrected for these limitations by performing a multicenter trial that enrolled 105 patients, meeting their expected sample size requirement. The groups were similar on all major baseline variables. Similar surgical approaches were employed on the primary and secondary resection groups as in the above study. However, this study showed that postoperative peritonitis and early reoperation occurred less frequently after primary than secondary resection. Additionally, the primary resection group had shorter hospital stays after the first procedure. No difference in mortality between groups was found. Overall, with respect to mortality, neither primary nor secondary sigmoid resection has been proven to be superior. Patients who undergo primary resection clearly spend less time hospitalized, while secondary resection may be slightly more desirable for purulent peritonitis, though this needs to be proven in other groups. Practically, the decision of primary or secondary resection is made intraoperatively based on the extent of disease, the difficulty of bowel mobilization, and the degree of peritoneal contamination. With the current evidence, it is justifiable to perform either type of procedure for sigmoid diverticulitis complicated by generalized peritonitis, as specific situations and local expertise dictate.

Regardless of approach, surgery for complicated diverticulitis has evolved over the decades into a relatively safe procedure with one of the highest success rates of any of the common GI procedures (137). The safety can be optimized by a tension-free anastomosis constructed in nondiverticular bowel. High ligation of the inferior mesenteric vessels, splenic flexure mobilization, and eve-extended resection may all be necessary to help achieve this goal. Due to the heterogeneity of underlying disease, it is difficult to estimate exact rates of specific procedure-related complications. One such complication is accidental ureteral injury. In patients with an extensive inflammatory process from diverticulitis extending to the retroperitoneum, ureter injury can be a difficult complication to avoid. Although uncommon, it can result in serious morbidity such as renal failure (138). A technique, which is gaining acceptance, is the placement of prophylactic ureteral stents preoperatively to prevent ureteral injury during surgery, both with open and with laparoscopic approaches (137–140). Particularly in patients with a large inflammatory mass or phlegmon, ureteral stents theoretically allow quicker and safer dissection through easier identification of the ureters. Although published evidence is sparse regarding the effectiveness of this approach, it is logical to attempt to protect the ureters because the incidence of this injury is not insignificant (about 2% of laparotomies for diverticulitis), and there is some evidence that stenting can be performed safely at minimal additional cost or operative time (139).

Right-Sided Diverticulitis

In Western countries, diverticulitis of the ascending colon or cecum is uncommon, due to the relatively low incidence of diverticula in these portions of the colon. In Asia, right-sided diverticulitis is the predominant form. Especially in younger patients, however, the diagnosis of right-sided diverticulitis is more difficult to make than in left-sided disease, and is very difficult to distinguish clinically from acute appendicitis. To distinguish the two, patients with diverticulitis tend to be older, and have a lower frequency of nausea and vomiting than patients with appendicitis (141). Radiologically, right-sided diverticulitis and appendicitis are also easily confused, especially with the presence of a local abscess (Fig. 5). There is an estimated preoperative misdiagnosis rate in right-colon inflammatory conditions of 40% to 92% (141–143). Even with excellent imaging, the diagnosis of right-sided diverticulitis is frequently made at laparotomy. The general principles of surgical management are the same in right- and left-sided disease: resection of diseased bowel, often with diversion stoma created (i.e., ileostomy) and a second stage for forming anastomosis if bowel preparation is not possible in the primary operation. As in left-sided diverticulitis, the exact operative approach depends on the extent of colon that is involved. With diverticulitis confined to the ascending colon, a right hemicolectomy with ileocolonic anastomosis may suffice. With isolated cecal involvement, a cecectomy and ileocolonic anastomosis is usually performed. Although right-sided diverticulitis occurs infrequently,

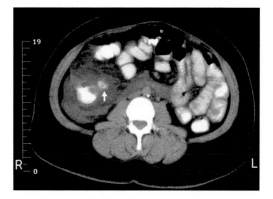

Figure 5 Contrast-filled cecum with extravasated contrast filling an abscess cavity (*arrow*) in a patient with right-sided diverticulitis.

it should be part of the differential diagnosis for any patient with right-lower quadrant symptoms. The much more common complication associated with right-colonic diverticula is hemorrhage, which will be discussed later in the chapter.

Fistulas

When a diverticular phlegmon or abscess extends or ruptures into an adjacent organ, fistulas can occur. Fistulas are thought to develop in less than 5% of patients with diverticulitis, but are present in about 20% of those who require surgical management (144). In a Cleveland Clinic review of 84 patients seen over 26 years with internal fistulas caused by diverticular disease, 65% were colovesical (145). There was a 2:1 male predominance, attributed to the protection given the bladder by the uterus, which is supported by the 50% incidence of previous hysterectomy in female patients with colovesical fistulas. In another review of 76 patients with enterovesical fistulas, the majority of which were diverticular, pneumaturia was present in 57% and fecaluria in 42% (146). Although pneumaturia may also be caused by emphysematous cystitis, fecaluria is pathognomonic for enterovesical fistula. Cystoscopy, cystography, and BE are useful diagnostically (Fig. 6), though demonstration of the fistula itself is often difficult. In both of the above series, single-stage operative resection with fistula closure and primary anastomosis could be performed in 75% of patients. Presumably, single-stage management is possible so frequently in the presence of fistulas to extracolonic organs because the fistula has effectively "decompressed" the inflammatory process. Colovaginal fistulas are the next most common internal fistula, representing approximately 25% of all cases (145). The passage of stool or flatus per vagina is pathognomonic. Frequent vaginal infections or copious discharge should prompt consideration of the diagnosis. Many patients with colovaginal fistula have undergone a previous hysterectomy. Treatment is the surgical resection of the diseased segment of colon, with repair of the contiguous organ, again which can generally

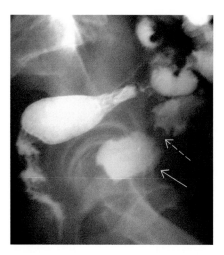

Figure 6 Water-soluble contrast enema demonstrating contrast within bladder (*solid arrow*) due to colovesical fistula (*dashed arrow*).

be performed as a single-stage procedure (101). Coloenteric, colouterine, and colouretral fistulas occur but much less commonly. Spontaneous colocutaneous fistulas are very rare and more frequently follow prior surgical repair. Other rare fistula types which have been reported as a presumed or documented complication of diverticulitis include colocholecystal, coloappendiceal, and colosalpingal. Although diverticular disease is a common cause of fistulization from the colon to adjacent organs, other conditions such as inflammatory bowel disease, pancreatitis, radiation enteritis and colitis, and malignancy can also cause fistulas, and these diagnoses must be entertained when a fistula involving the colon is discovered.

Obstruction

Obstruction may accompany diverticular disease either acutely or chronically. During an attack of acute diverticulitis, partial colonic obstruction can occur due to relative luminal narrowing from the pericolic inflammation (Fig. 7) and/or compression from abscess formation. Obstruction can be confirmed with a gentle water-soluble contrast enema in a patient not suspected to have free perforation (144) while simultaneously excluding a sigmoid cancer. Complete obstruction is unusual. Colonic ileus or pseudo-obstruction can also occur. These conditions usually improve with effective medical therapy including antibiotics, bowel rest, and nasogastric suction. Should they fail to resolve with medical management, prompt surgical consultation is indicated. Acute diverticulitis can cause small-bowel obstruction mechanically if a loop of small intestine becomes incorporated into the inflammatory mass by localized irritation or by the development of an ileus. The obstruction should improve as the inflammation subsides. Surgical intervention may be required for persistent obstruction not responding to medical therapy. Ideally, a modified bowel preparation with gentle irrigation enemas and/or low-dose oral laxatives can be given over a period of a few days preoperatively (144), thereby allowing the possibility of primary anastomosis in some cases. In cases when bowel preparation is not possible, the Hartmann procedure is usually performed.

The Role of Colonoscopy in Chronic Obstruction

Recurrent attacks of diverticulitis, which may be subclinical, can initiate progressive fibrosis and stricturing of the colonic wall in the absence of ongoing inflammation. In such cases, high-grade or complete obstruction can occur, requiring surgical therapy. A more insidious presentation with nonspecific symptoms is not uncommon. Frequently, a stricture of uncertain etiology is demonstrated on BE. The critical issue is to distinguish between a diverticular stricture and a stenosing neoplasm. An accurate diagnosis will help guide the correct surgical procedure. Colonoscopy plays an important role in such patients. Forde and Treat reported on the utility of colonoscopy in 181 patients with strictures of unclear etiology found on barium studies (147). About 70% of these strictures were in the sigmoid colon. The stricture could be

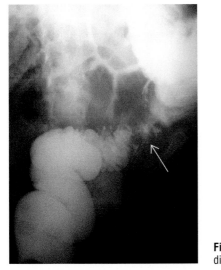

Figure 7 Partial colonic obstruction (*arrow*) due to sigmoid diverticulitis.

traversed and its etiology diagnosed with colonoscopy in 97 (54%). Of the 84 (46%) patients in whom they could not traverse the stricture, biopsy and cytology revealed a diagnosis of carcinoma in 24 (29%). Overall, colonoscopy was informative in 67% of patients. Strictures in which malignancy cannot be excluded despite colonoscopic and radiographic examinations should undergo surgical resection. A trial of endoscopic therapy can reasonably be attempted in patients in whom neoplasm is felt to be sufficiently excluded. A 1986 American Society for Gastrointestinal Endoscopy survey reported on 64 patients who underwent hydrostatic balloon dilation of colonic strictures (148). There was a 79% technical success rate, and 56% of the patients had immediate symptomatic improvement. Three perforations occurred (two at anastomotic strictures), and significant hemorrhage developed in two patients (one a diverticular stricture and the other neoplastic). Only 5 of these 64 balloon dilations were performed for diverticular strictures. In these patients, technical success was accomplished in all five patients (100%), and greater than three-month symptomatic relief occurred in two of three reported patients. Forde reported their experience in 14 patients with strictures of varying etiologies, utilizing various techniques, including bouginage, balloon, laser, electrocautery, and a blunt-dilating endoscope (149). Multiple treatments were required in most cases, and there were no perforations or bleeding complications. The authors concluded that, based on their experience, dilations with a balloon, bougie, or a dilating endoscope are most useful in strictures resulting from inflammatory disease. They felt that laser and electrocautery therapies were most useful for strictures caused by carcinoma and anastomotic webs. Another series reported on 27 patients with recurrent Crohn's disease, who underwent transendoscopic hydrostatic balloon dilations for anastomotic strictures (150). About 18 of 27 patients (67%) were successfully dilated, without recurrent obstructive symptoms developing during a mean follow-up of 19 months. One patient sustained a perforation during balloon dilation, which was treated successfully by bowel resection. While no equivalent series has been reported specifically for diverticular strictures, this technique may be a reasonable therapeutic option in patients who are unwilling to undergo or who are at significant risk for surgery. It has been suggested that an upper endoscope may be preferable for balloon dilation of colonic strictures due to its shorter length and greater tip deflection (151). Some feel that balloon dilation may be accomplished safely without fluoroscopy (151). Early and preliminary experience with colonic metal stents suggests that they may have a role in colonic obstruction due to diverticular disease, particularly in providing temporary decompression, allowing for bowel preparation and a subsequent single-stage resection without diversion (152,153).

Laparoscopic Surgery for Complicated Diverticular Disease

With the increasing ability to manage surgical problems in other parts of the digestive system laparoscopically, there has been a growing worldwide interest in applying laparoscopic techniques to colorectal disease. However, there are a number of technical limitations that make the role of laparoscopy less clear for diseases of the colon than for other conditions (154). Nevertheless, laparoscopic approaches have some distinct advantages over open techniques (Table 3). If outcomes between laparoscopic and open operations were found to be similar, laparoscopic may be more desirable.

Table 3 Laparoscopic vs. Open Sigmoidectomy

Advantages
   Less intraoperative trauma
   Less postoperative pain
   Shorter hospitalization
   Reduced disability
   Improved cosmesis
   Fewer postoperative adhesions
Disadvantages
   Multiple intra-abdominal locations, requiring repositioning of instruments, ports, and personnel
   Highly vascularized mesentery, vascular control long and arduous
   Anastomosis more difficult to perform laparoscopically than open
   Loss of tactile evaluation of bowel
   Longer operative time

The laparoscopic sigmoidectomy technique is detailed elsewhere (154). Briefly, the procedure begins with creation of three trocar sites (or more in selected cases): an optic trocar superior to the umbilicus and two trocars in the right lower quadrant (103). Pneumoperitoneum is created, and dissection is begun, beginning with either lateral mobilization or vessel ligation on the mesosigmoid. The mesenteric attachments are freed, and parietal peritoneum divided into the splenic flexure, which is then mobilized. The rectosigmoid junction is then divided by an endoscopic linear cutting stapler. An incision is made, usually in one of the lower quadrants, for extracting the bowel, completing the proximal resection, and placing the anvil of the stapling device. This minilap is sometimes being made at the start of the procedure to allow the entry of a hand to assist the laparoscopic resection (155). A stapling device is then transanally placed, and the anastomosis is completed. The anastomosis integrity is confirmed either endoscopically, with air, or with methylene blue. Routine use of a 33-mm circular stapler for the anastomosis helps insure adequate lumenal diameter and, therefore, conversely, absence of significant muscular hypertrophy in the descending colon.

No randomized trials currently exist comparing laparoscopic management of diverticular complications to open, so the current data are based on experience with other diseases, case–control studies, and anecdotal reports. However, there have been a number of case series published in the last 10 years, a few of which now describe experience with over 100 patients having undergone laparoscopic sigmoid or total colectomy for diverticular disease (156–161). In these descriptive studies, time to dietary intake ranged two to four days, hospital stay ranged four to eight days, and operative time ranged 160 to 240 minutes. In those studies that compared open to laparoscopic procedures, the laparoscopic approach was superior with respect to time to oral intake and length-of-stay, while open procedures had a shorter operative time. The morbidity for laparoscopic resection ranged from 5% to 25%, with the most common complications being hematoma, abscess, bleeding, transit disorders, and urinary tract infection. Not surprisingly, the highest complication rates were noted when laparoscopic sigmoid resection was performed in the setting of more advanced disease (i.e., Hinchey Stage II–IV) (71). There did not seem to be a significant difference between overall morbidity and costs between open and laparoscopic methods when cases of similar severity were compared. There is also a laparoscopic-to-open conversion rate of 4% to 15%. One group identified three factors as predictive of cases that would require open conversion: diagnosis of malignancy, obesity, and surgeon inexperience (162). As with all types of procedures, there is a learning curve with a threshold above which an operator becomes "up to speed." With laparoscopic colorectal surgery, this threshold is probably in the range of 30 to 50 cases (157,163).

In a consensus development conference, the role of laparoscopic management of complicated diverticular disease was addressed (103). It was determined by this group that laparoscopic sigmoid colectomy was only appropriate for elective cases of uncomplicated diverticulitis, restricted to surgeons who are experienced in laparoscopic management of colorectal disease. The group also stated that the management of complicated diverticulitis (up to Hinchey Stage II), after percutaneous drainage of abscess, may be justified. Finally, it was underscored that randomized trials comparing open to laparoscopic techniques in appropriate cases need to be performed before any conclusions about the relative benefits of laparoscopy versus open surgery for diverticulitis can be made. Until that time, open methods should remain the standard-of-care for surgical management of complicated diverticular disease. Most recently, in a complete paradigm shift and almost a reversion to three-staged procedures, laparoscopy with lavage with or without fibrin glue or omental patching of a perforation in diverticulitis has been safely employed (156,164). These patients who initially presented with peritonitis or even perforation were spared an emergent resection and a stoma. Adoption of this methodology has been very limited.

HEMORRHAGE

Bleeding from diverticula, vascular ectasias, colitis, and neoplasms is responsible for the majority of lower GI bleeding (23,165–167). Two recent reports describe diverticula as the most common bleeding source identified in patients with lower GI bleeding, accounting for 30% to 40% of cases where such a source was found (168,169). Nonetheless, a precise determination of each of these lesions' respective responsibility is limited by a number of factors, including the extent of investigation undertaken in different studies (e.g., angiography, colonoscopy, and resection), the fact that these are relatively common lesions in the elderly population with bleeding, and that their presence alone does not unequivocally define their significance. The best evidence that a specific lesion is the bleeding source is direct visualization of an actively bleeding lesion endoscopically or by extravasation from a specific lesion at angiography. Unfortunately, such confirmation with colonic bleeding is only available in a minority of cases (165,166). Quinn proposed five clinical criteria for the diagnosis of colonic diverticular hemorrhage (170): (i) passage of bright red or maroon blood per rectum, (ii) radiographic evidence of diverticula, (iii) no other demonstrable cause of hemorrhage on BE or sigmoidoscopy, (iv) no blood in a gastric aspirate and/or no abnormality found on an upper GI series, and (v) normal blood coagulation parameters. In a series of 43 patients over age 65 with severe hemorrhage and a discharge diagnosis of diverticulosis, no patient fulfilled all five criteria and 19 (44%) fulfilled four of five (165).

Epidemiology

Severe hemorrhage has been reported to occur in 3% to 5% of patients with diverticulosis (23,171,172). Despite the fact that most diverticula are in the left colon in Western individuals, the site of bleeding diverticula is often in the proximal colon (23,171,173). In two early series of patients with diverticular bleeding, 12/13 (92%) and 9/18 (50%) were localized to the right colon (174,175). A recent large series of 180 Asian patients admitted to the hospital with diverticular disease supported this trend, with both a higher bleeding rate and greater need for surgery with right-sided compared to left-sided disease (176).

Pathophysiology

The pathogenesis of diverticular bleeding has been elucidated in part by Meyers et al., using sophisticated microangiographic techniques on resected colonic specimens from patients with arteriographically documented bleeding diverticula (173). Three-dimensional histologic reconstructions were created to evaluate blood vessel–diverticular relationships. These studies demonstrated a consistent finding of intimal thickening and medial thinning of the vasa recta as it coursed over the dome of the diverticulum. These changes, occurring eccentrically toward the lumen of the diverticulum, led to a segmental weakening of the artery, thus predisposing to its rupture. This arterial lesion was not seen in nonbleeding diverticula from the same patients. The factor(s) that initiates this isolated, asymmetric arterial change or the precipitating event leading to its rupture is unknown. Inflammation does not appear to be a contributing factor, because it is absent histologically in resected bleeding diverticula. This is in concordance with the general clinical impression that bleeding rarely, if ever, complicates diverticulitis.

The association of NSAID use with peptic ulcer disease and upper GI bleeding is well documented. More recent data have also implicated these agents in lower GI and specifically diverticular bleeding. A large prospective series of over 100 patients with lower GI bleeding (in which 50% were diverticular) reported a bleeding risk with NSAIDs equal to that of duodenal ulcer (177). Further support for this association is provided by the Health Professionals Follow-up Study of over 35,000 male health professionals aged 40 to 75 years at baseline and free of diverticular disease at entry (178). Over four years of follow-up, regular NSAID use was associated with an overall increased risk of diverticular bleeding. In addition to an increased bleeding risk, NSAIDs have also been shown to confer a three-fold increased risk of diverticular perforation (179). Other studies have confirmed a higher overall complication rate and more severe complications in patients with diverticular disease, who take NSAIDs (180,181). Hence, it is logical that those who have an episode of diverticular bleeding and are concurrently taking NSAIDs should be told to discontinue them, if possible, to decrease their risk of complications, particularly bleeding. Whether patients with diverticulosis without prior bleeding episode should be counseled as well to avoid NSAIDs, as is done for ulcer patients, or utilize COX-2 selective agents is still unclear. A multicenter trial comparing peptic ulcer complications in rheumatoid arthritis patients randomized to naproxen (conventional NSAID) or rofecoxib (COX-2 selective agent) was reanalyzed for lower GI bleeding complication rates (182). The relative risk of lower GI bleeding from all causes was 0.46 in patients taking rofecoxib compared to those taking naproxen, a significant difference. The number of patients who were confirmed to have diverticular bleeding in the rofecoxib group was also lower than the naproxen group, though this difference was not significant due to a low number of confirmed cases in both groups. More research in this area will be necessary before firm recommendations on NSAID use in patients with diverticular disease can be made, but clearly, patients with complicated diverticular disease should be queried about NSAID use, and if present, counseled to discontinue, or minimize use, if possible.

Clinical Features

The clinical presentation of patients with diverticular hemorrhage is usually one of an abrupt, painless onset. The patient may have mild lower abdominal cramps followed by the urge to defecate. The arterial nature of the bleeding is manifested by the passage of voluminous red or maroon blood or clots. While melena can occasionally occur with slowly bleeding right colon lesions, the arterial nature of diverticular bleeding makes this presentation uncommon. The presence of colonic diverticula should not be considered an adequate explanation for a positive fecal occult blood test or as an etiology of iron-deficiency anemia. The natural history of diverticular hemorrhage has been well reported. Bleeding ceases spontaneously in 70% to 80% of patients, and rebleeding rates range from 22% to 38% in reported series (171,172,175). The chance of a third bleeding episode can be as high as 50% (171), leading many to recommend surgical resection after a second bleeding episode, similar to the recommendations made for recurrent diverticulitis (102).

Diagnosis and Management

The diagnosis and treatment of patients with lower GI bleeding, in general, is beyond the scope of this chapter and has been reviewed comprehensively elsewhere (172,183). A treatment algorithm summarizing the important decisions to be made in someone who is actively bleeding from diverticula is included (Fig. 8). Fluid and blood product resuscitation requires immediate attention. Excluding an upper GI source by nasogastric lavage or upper endoscopy is warranted, inasmuch as 10% to 15% of patients with hematochezia will have an upper GI-tract etiology. Flexible sigmoidoscopy is an appropriate initial approach to rule out an obvious rectosigmoid lesion, and can be performed unprepped or after enema administration. If no etiology is found with flexible sigmoidoscopy, further evaluation with noninvasive (nuclear scintigraphy) or invasive techniques (angiography, colonoscopy) can be undertaken in an attempt to localize and/or treat the bleeding source.

Nuclear Scintigraphy

Nuclear scintigraphy, also referred to as tagged red blood cell scan, has a number of theoretical advantages in the evaluation of lower GI bleeding. It is noninvasive, technically simple, relatively inexpensive, and quite sensitive to bleeding rates as low as 0.1 mL/min. Furthermore, once labeled, red cells remain active for up to 24 hours, permitting repetitive imaging in the patient with intermittent bleeding (Fig. 9) (184). At best, however, nuclear scans provide information only about the site of the bleeding, not its etiology, and they have no therapeutic potential. Even their accuracy at predicting the correct bleeding site has been questioned. One study reported a surgical error rate of at least 42% when localization was guided solely by red-cell scintigraphy (185). Given its very high sensitivity and relative simplicity, however, many centers use scintigraphy as a screening test prior to angiography. This is done primarily to minimize the number of negative angiograms performed and to allow for the rapid selection of a specific artery for injection (184).

Angiography

Angiography has a theoretical sensitivity for lower GI bleeding at a rate of 0.5 mL/min. This figure has been derived from animal studies, and some have questioned its equivalent sensitivity in humans (166). One theoretical utility of diagnostic angiography is to identify the site of bleeding with enough accuracy to direct segmental surgical resection (see below). An additional utility for angiography, however, is its therapeutic potential. Intra-arterial vasopressin has been demonstrated to control lower GI hemorrhage in up to 91% of patients (186). This therapy is usually only temporary, however, and up to half of the patients will rebleed with cessation of the infusion. Nonetheless, in a surgical candidate, temporary control of

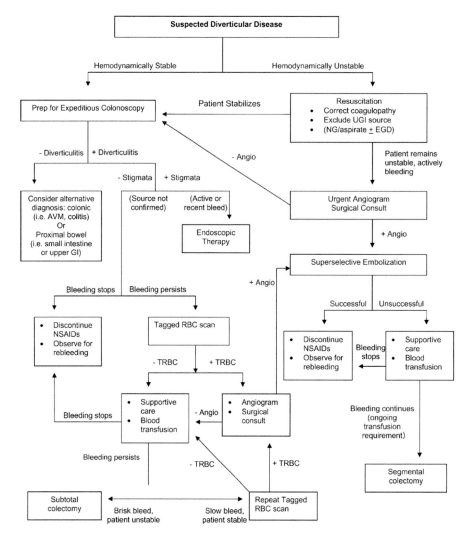

Figure 8 Algorithm for managing suspected diverticular hemorrhage. *Abbreviations*: NSAIDs, nonsteroidal anti-inflammatory drugs; TRBC, tagged red blood cell; EGD, esophagogastroduodenoscopy.

bleeding is quite helpful because it will allow for a semielective surgical procedure in a well-prepared patient, rather than an emergency resection, with a concomitant reduction in surgical morbidity (186). While transcatheter arterial embolization had previously been felt to carry a high risk of bowel infarction, embolization of a very distal bleeding branch, the so-called subselective embolization, has been demonstrated to be feasible, effective, and safe (Fig. 10) (187,188).

Colonoscopy

For the majority of patients, diverticular bleeding is self-limited. Subsequent colonoscopy should be performed to elucidate the bleeding source, if possible, but more importantly to exclude neoplasia. In a review of over 2000 colonoscopies for overt or occult rectal bleeding, neoplastic polyps were found in 32% and carcinoma in 19% (189). Another retrospective study focused at the yield of colonoscopy in 258 patients with rectal bleeding, who had negative sigmoidoscopies and single-contrast BEs that were normal or showed only diverticulosis (190). The overall incidence of significant findings was 41%, including carcinoma in 29 patients (11%) and telangiectasias in 17 (7%). A more recent prospective study from Ontario found colonoscopy more sensitive than the combination of sigmoidoscopy and barium examination for the diagnosis of adenoma, carcinoma, and angiodysplasia (191). The increased ability to

(A)   **(B)**

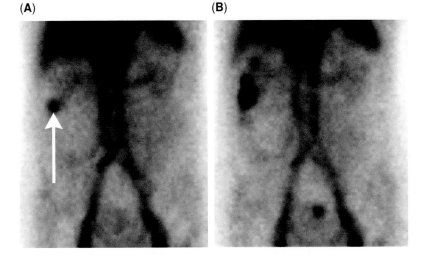

Figure 9 Nuclear scintigram of active colonic bleeding from diverticulosis. (**A**) Early image showing site of bleeding at hepatic flexure (*arrow*). (**B**) Later image showing accumulation of radionuclide at site of bleeding and spread to distal portions of colon.

diagnose vascular ectasias and diverticula (which cause the majority of bleeding), the ability to exclude neoplasia, and the therapeutic potential of colonoscopy (Fig. 11) support its utility as a primary investigation in patients with lower GI bleeding.

The role of colonoscopy during an episode of "acute" lower GI bleeding is being redefined. A 1974 report cited the utility of colonoscopy in the diagnosis and management of 17 of 18 cases of acute hemorrhage (192). Forde reported in 1981 on the value of emergent colonoscopy in 25 patients with acute bleeding (193). The only preparation was via enema, and a WaterPik was used with a double-channel instrument to lavage clots. The bleeding site was localized in eight patients (32%), with four operations averted. Diverticulosis was found in five patients and carcinoma in three. One perforation was reported of an actively bleeding diverticulum. While the diagnostic role of colonoscopy was becoming increasingly appreciated, its therapeutic role remained unclear. Indeed, a 1984 editorial opined that "colonoscopy offers no possibility of staunching blood arising from a diverticulum . . . " (194). The use of the rapid oral purge, initially with saline and now with electrolyte solutions, in preparing the colon for emergent colonoscopy was first reported in abstract form in 1983 (195). Subsequent publications by the same group and others (196,197) have expanded the experience with this technique, demonstrating that it was safe and effective in patients with acute GI bleeding. Patients are given the solution orally or via nasogastric tube until the rectal effluent is clear, which usually requires approximately three to four hours. Actively bleeding diverticula were seen in 17% and 22% of patients in these two early studies. Endoscopic interventions were effective in 39% and 50%

(A)   **(B)**   **(C)**

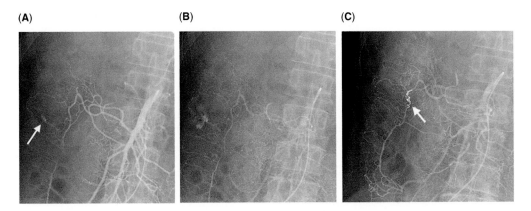

Figure 10 (**A**) Superior mesenteric angiogram showing extravasation (*arrow*) from distal arterial branch within a diverticulum in the ascending colon. (**B**) Later image shows pooling of contrast at site of extravasation. (**C**) Hemostasis achieved after placement of embolization coils (*arrow*).

(A)   **(B)**

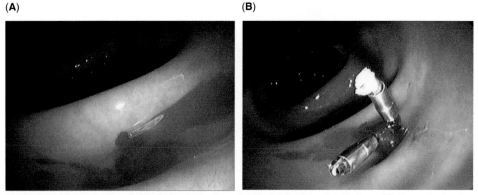

Figure 11 (*See color insert*) (**A**) Endoscopic view of actively bleeding diverticulum. (**B**) Hemostasis after endoclip placement. *Source*: Courtesy of Janak Shah, MD.

of patients, although none for bleeding diverticula. A case report in 1985 described cessation of hemorrhage from an actively bleeding diverticulum with local irrigation of 4 mL of 1:1000 epinephrine (198). Although this technique has not seemed to gain wide acceptance, it likely represents the first report of therapeutic colonoscopy directed at diverticular bleeding. In 1986 Johnston and Sones reported three patients with actively bleeding diverticula, who were successfully treated with heater probe coagulation (199). Their technique involved placing the probe in the diverticulum with "modest" appositional force and delivering a mean energy of 173 J. They noted immediate cessation of bleeding in all three patients, no recurrence, and no complications. Savides and Jensen reported their experience with three patients with recurrent diverticular bleeding (200). All three were found to have a visible vessel at the edge of the diverticulum. Endoscopic coagulation was accomplished with six to seven one-second pulses with a Gold probe (Microvasive-Boston Scientific Inc., Watertown, Massachusetts, U.S.A.) set at 4 on a 50-W bipolar generator. No bleeding occurred during or after the procedure, and no patient had further bleeding. Fouch described successful endoscopic therapy in three of four patients with diverticular bleeding from a pigmented protuberance using bipolar cautery (201). Injection hemostasis for diverticular bleeding was first reported in a case report from Italy in 1990 (202), with a subsequent case reported in 1993 (203). Control of bleeding was achieved in both cases by using 1:10,000 epinephrine injected into the neck of the diverticulum with a standard sclerotherapy needle. A total of 16-mL was used in one case, with the amount not reported in the other. Neither patient had recurrent bleeding, and no complications were reported. The injection of a fibrin sealant has also been described in a case report (204), as has the use of a modified banding device (205) and an endoscopic clipping device (206).

Most recently, Jensen has described his group's experience evaluating the role of colonoscopy in diverticular hemorrhage (207). In a cohort of 48 patients, 10 patients had definite signs of diverticular hemorrhage and were treated endoscopically with injection of 1 to 2 mL of 1:20,000 epinephrine in four quadrants, followed by bipolar coagulation with 10 to 15 w of power, moderate appositional pressure directly on the vessel, and one second pulses until coagulation, and flattening of the vessel was achieved. None of these endoscopically treated patients had recurrent bleeding or required surgery. They were compared to 17 patients in a prior cohort, who were not treated colonoscopically, of whom nine had additional bleeding and six required surgery. The authors concluded that such therapy may prevent recurrent bleeding and decrease the need for surgery. While this is compelling data, the study design was suboptimal, utilizing a historical cohort design rather than a true, randomized trial. Further, such therapy may well be applicable to only a small subset of patients with lower intestinal bleeding. If, for example, only 25% to 40% of all patients with lower intestinal bleeding are bleeding from a diverticulum, and if only 20% of such patients have identifiable lesions amenable to endoscopic treatment, then only 5% to 8% of all lower GI bleeding patients will be candidates for such therapy. Nonetheless, we are clearly beginning to characterize and define the role of colonoscopy in this arena and anticipate its playing an increasing role in years to come.

Prognosticating outcomes and predicting rebleeding based on endoscopic findings has not been as well validated in lower GI bleeding as it clearly is in upper GI bleeding.

Table 4 Indications for Operative Management of Bleeding Diverticula

Large transfusion requirement (e.g., >6 units packed red blood cells)
Recurrent hemorrhage
Hemodynamic instability not resolving with resuscitation

Nonetheless, Foutch reported on 13 patients with acute lower GI bleeding in which a specific diverticulum was unequivocally identified as the cause of bleeding (208). He defined stigmata of significant and insignificant hemorrhage, analogous to the endoscopic stigmata widely used in upper GI bleeding. The four patients (31%) with "significant" stigmata (three with a visible vessel inside the diverticula and one with an adherent clot with active bleeding) had a statistically significant increase in rebleeding, transfusion requirements, and need for surgical or endoscopic treatment relative to the nine patients (69%) with ulcerations that were judged insignificant. An additional report has histopathologically demonstrated that a "pigmented protuberance" in a diverticulum was a sentinel clot rather than a visible vessel (195). Whether the colonoscopic appearance of bleeding diverticula will have as significant a prognostic utility as such stigmata do with peptic ulcers will require prospective trials with larger numbers of patients.

Surgery

Surgery in lower GI bleeding is usually avoided until medical, endoscopic, or angiographic therapies fail. Because diverticular bleeding spontaneously stops in the majority of patients, surgical management is infrequently required. The primary indications for operative management of diverticular hemorrhage are listed in Table 4.

When surgery is necessary, a partial colectomy is preferred to a subtotal colectomy whenever possible. Segmental resection is most commonly performed if the bleeding site is clearly identified from a therapeutically unsuccessful angiographic or endoscopic procedure. The rebleeding rate compiled from seven series was 6% in 167 patients who underwent segmental resections for angiographically documented bleeding sites (186). Although endoscopic, nuclear and angiographic methods should theoretically make segmental resection possible in all actively bleeding patients, exact localization of a bleeding site is often difficult. A recent large, single-center series reported that of 65 patients undergoing selective angiography, only 12% underwent directed resection without further bleeding, while a nearly equivalent number (11%) had complications from the procedure (209).

In patients with persistent bleeding and no identification of a likely bleeding site, a subtotal colectomy may be required. Those who require subtotal colectomy as a "last resort," though they usually stop bleeding, have extremely high morbidity and mortality rates (210). This fact may be in part due to the number of invasive tests required and delay in definitive management in attempting to localize the bleeding source, hence selecting for sicker patients. Additionally, a "blind" segmental colectomy carries with it a risk of not resecting the bleeding lesion when the source is more proximal (small bowel arteriovenous malformation). In a series of 10 blind subtotal colectomies for presumed diverticular hemorrhage, four patients were subsequently found to have a small bowel source (211). Finally, with an anastomosis to the proximal rectum in an emergency (unprepped) situation, the risk of anastomotic failure was high. In one series, over half of the patients who underwent emergency blind colectomy experienced anastomotic leak and/or peritonitis (175). For these reasons, subtotal colectomy without bleeding localization should generally be avoided until all other possibilities have been exhausted.

SUMMARY

Diverticulosis is an increasingly common disorder in developed countries. Although up to two-thirds of those individuals over age 80 are affected, most people will never develop symptoms in their lifetime. The etiology of colonic diverticula remains elusive, though altered colonic wall resistance, colonic dysmotility, and fiber deficiency appear to contribute. Dietary fiber may also play a preventive role and should be recommended to those with asymptomatic or mild disease. The symptoms of SUDD disease can be nonspecific and may overlap with those of a number of other conditions, particularly IBS. However, more severe or complicated diverticulitis is much more clinically distinctive and requires appropriate diagnosis and treatment. Medical management of diverticulitis involves a combination of antibiotics and, where appropriate, percutaneous drainage. Surgical management is indicated electively after multiple attacks of diverticulitis, depending on age and severity, and more urgently for complications such as abscess, free perforation, fistula, or obstruction. Although open surgical methods are still most commonly used to treat diverticulitis, laparoscopic sigmoidectomy is the preferred alternative for elective cases. With further technical refinements and expertise, laparscopy may be the chosen approach in the emergent setting as well, possibly to facilitate drainage, irrigation, and primary closure of any perforation. Hemorrhage is the other main complication of diverticular disease. Bleeding, unlike diverticulitis, often involves right-sided diverticulosis and is associated with NSAID use. Although bleeding usually spontaneously stops, nuclear, endoscopic, angiographic, and/or surgical methods are often needed to achieve hemostasis. Colonoscopy can be useful across the full spectrum of diverticular disease, both diagnostically, to document diverticula and exclude alternative diagnoses, and therapeutically, to dilate strictures or locate and stop hemorrhage.

REFERENCES

1. Almy TP, Howell DA. Medical progress. Diverticular disease of the colon. N Engl J Med 1980; 302(6):324–331.
2. Roberts PL, Veidenheimer MC. Current management of diverticulitis. Adv Surg 1994; 27:189–208.
3. Cruveilhier S. Traite de Anatomie Pathologique. Paris: Balliere et Cie 1849; 1(1):592–593.
4. Graser E. Uber multiple falsche darmdivertikel in der fleura sigmoidea. Muench Med Wochenschr 1899; 46:74.
5. Mayo W, Wilson LB, Giffin HZ. Acquired diverticulitis of the large intestine. Surg Gynecol Obstet 1907; 5:8–15.
6. Schoetz DJ Jr. Diverticular disease of the colon: a century-old problem. Dis Colon Rectum 1999; 42(6):703–709.
7. Case J. The roentgen demonstration of multiple diverticula of the colon. Am J Roentol 1914; 2: 654–658.
8. Painter NS, Burkitt DP. Diverticular disease of the colon: a deficiency disease of Western civilization. Br Med J 1971; 2(759):450–454.
9. Schoetz DJ Jr. Uncomplicated diverticulitis. Indications for surgery and surgical management. Surg Clin North Am 1993; 73(5):965–974.
10. Painter NS, Burkitt DP. Diverticular disease of the colon: a 20th century problem. Clin Gastroenterol 1975; 4(1):3–21.
11. Parks TG. Natural history of diverticular disease of the colon. Clin Gastroenterol 1975; 4(1):53–69.
12. Kyle J, Adesola AD, Tinckler LF, deBeaux J. Incidence of diverticulitis. Scand J Gastroenterol 1967; 2:77–80.
13. Stemmermann GN, Yatani R. Diverticulosis and polyps of the large intestine. A necropsy study of Hawaii Japanese. Cancer 1973; 31(5):1260–1270.
14. Lee YS. Diverticular disease of the large bowel in Singapore. An autopsy survey. Dis Colon Rectum 1986; 29(5):330–335.
15. Levy N, Stermer E, Simon J. The changing epidemiology of diverticular disease in israel. Dis Colon Rectum 1985; 28(6):416–418.
16. Parks TG. Natural history of diverticular disease of the colon. A review of 521 cases. Br Med J 1969; 4(684):639–642.
17. Horner JL. Natural history of diverticulosis of the colon. Am J Dig Dis 1958; 3(5):343–350.
18. Burkitt DP. Related disease—related cause? Lancet 1969; 2(7632):1229–1231.
19. Morini S, De Angelis P, Manurita L, Colavolpe V. Association of colonic diverticula with adenomas and carcinomas. A colonoscopic experience. Dis Colon Rectum 1988; 31(10):793–796.
20. Stefansson T, Ekbom A, Sparen P, Pahlman L. Increased risk of left sided colon cancer in patients with diverticular disease. Gut 1993; 34(4):499–502.
21. Slack WW. The anatomy, pathology, and some clinical features of divericulitis of the colon. Br J Surg 1962; 50:185–190.
22. Levi DM, Levi JU, Rogers AI, Bergau DK, Wenger J. Giant colonic diverticulum: an unusual manifestation of a common disease. Am J Gastroenterol 1993; 88(1):139–142.
23. Reinus JF, Brandt LJ. Vascular ectasias and diverticulosis. Common causes of lower intestinal bleeding. Gastroenterol Clin North Am 1994; 23(1):1–20.
24. Chia JG, Wilde CC, Ngoi SS, Goh PM, Ong CL. Trends of diverticular disease of the large bowel in a newly developed country. Dis Colon Rectum 1991; 34(6):498–501.
25. Miura S, Kodaira S, Shatari T, Nishioka M, Hosoda Y, Hisa TK. Recent trends in diverticulosis of the right colon in Japan: retrospective review in a regional hospital. Dis Colon Rectum 2000; 43(10): 1383–1389.

26. Whiteway J, Morson BC. Elastosis in diverticular disease of the sigmoid colon. Gut 1985; 26(3):258–266.

27. Bode MK, Karttunen TJ, Makela J, Risteli L, Risteli J. Type I and III collagens in human colon cancer and diverticulosis. Scand J Gastroenterol, 2000; 35(7):747–752.

28. Arfwidsson S, Knock NG, Lehmann L, Winberg T. Pathogenesis of multiple diverticula of the sigmoid colon in diverticular disease. Acta Chir Scand 1964; 63(Suppl):1–68.

29. Painter NS. The aetiology of diverticulosis of the colon with special reference to the action of certain drugs on the behaviour of the colon. Ann R Coll Surg Engl 1964; 34:98–119.

30. Painter NS, Truelove SC, Ardran GM, Tuckey M. Segmentation and the localization of intraluminal pressures in the human colon with special reference to the pathogenesis of colonic diverticula. Gastroenterology 1965; 49:169–177.

31. Trotman IF, Misiewicz JJ. Sigmoid motility in diverticular disease and the irritable bowel syndrome. Gut 1988; 29(2):218–222.

32. Cortesini C, Pantalone D. Usefulness of colonic motility study in identifying patients at risk for complicated diverticular disease. Dis Colon Rectum 1991; 34(4):339–342.

33. Bassotti G, Battaglia E, Spinozzi F, Pelli MA, Tonini M. Twenty-four hour recordings of colonic motility in patients with diverticular disease: evidence for abnormal motility and propulsive activity. Dis Colon Rectum 2001; 44(12):1814–1820.

34. Sugihara K, Muto T, Morioka Y. Motility study in right sided diverticular disease of the colon. Gut 1983; 24(12):1130–1134.

35. Tomita R, Fujisaki S, Tanjoh K, Fukuzawa M. Role of nitric oxide in the left-sided colon of patients with diverticular disease. Hepatogastroenterology 2000; 47(33):692–696.

36. Liu L, Shang F, Markus I, Burcher E. Roles of substance P receptors in human colon circular muscle: alterations in diverticular disease. J Pharmacol Exp Ther 2002; 302(2):627–635.

37. Wynne-Jones G. Flatus retention is the major factor in diverticular disease. Lancet 1975; 2(7927): 211–212.

38. Burkitt DP, Walker AR, Painter NS. Effect of dietary fibre on stools and the transit-times and its role in the causation of disease. Lancet 1972; 2(7792):1408–1412.

39. Fisher N, Berry CS, Fearn T, Gregory JA, Hardy J. Cereal dietary fiber consumption and diverticular disease: a lifespan study in rats. Am J Clin Nutr 1985; 42(5):788–804.

40. Gear JS, Ware A, Fursdon P, et al. Symptomless diverticular disease and intake of dietary fibre. Lancet 1979; 1(8115):511–514.

41. Lin OS, Soon MS, Wu SS, Chen YY, Hwang KL, Triadafilopoulos G. Dietary habits and right-sided colonic diverticulosis. Dis Colon Rectum 2000; 43(10):1412–1418.

42. Aldoori WH, Giovannucci EL, Rimm EB, Wing AL, Trichopoulos DV, Willett WC. A prospective study of diet and the risk of symptomatic diverticular disease in men. Am J Clin Nutr 1994; 60(5):757–764.

43. Aldoori WH, Giovannucci EL, Rockett HR, Sampson L, Rimm EB, Willett WC. A prospective study of dietary fiber types and symptomatic diverticular disease in men. J Nutr 1998; 128(4):714–719.

44. Nakama H, Fattah AS, Zhang B, Kamijo N, Uehara Y. Association of diverticulosis coli and vascular ectasias and the results of fecal occult blood test. Hepatogastroenterology 2000; 47(35):1277–1279.

45. Boulos PB, Karamanolis DG, Salmon PR, Clark CG. Is colonoscopy necessary in diverticular disease? Lancet 1984; 1(8368):95–96.

46. Williams CB, Lane RH, Sakai Y. Colonoscopy: an air-pressure hazard. Lancet 1973; 2(7831):729.

47. Wolff WI, Shinya H. Polypectomy via the fiberoptic colonoscope. Removal of neoplasms beyond reach of the sigmoidoscope. N Engl J Med 1973; 288(7):329–332.

48. Brayko CM, Kozarek RA, Sanowski RA, Howells T. Diverticular rupture during colonoscopy. Fact or fancy? Dig Dis Sci 1984; 29(5):427–431.

49. Bat L, Williams CB. Usefulness of pediatric colonoscopes in adult colonoscopy. Gastrointest Endosc 1989; 35(4):329–332.

50. Kozarek RA, Botoman VA, Patterson DJ. Prospective evaluation of a small caliber upper endoscope for colonoscopy after unsuccessful standard examination. Gastrointest Endosc 1989; 35(4):333–335.

51. Falchuk ZM, Griffin PH. A technique to facilitate colonoscopy in areas of severe diverticular disease. N Engl J Med 1984; 310(9):598.

52. Glick SN. Inverted colonic diverticulum: air contrast barium enema findings in six cases. AJR Am J Roentgenol 1991; 156(5):961–964.

53. Ladas SD, Prigouris SP, Pantelidaki C, Raptis A. Endoscopic removal of inverted sigmoid diverticulum— is it a dangerous procedure?. Endoscopy 1989; 21(5):243–244.

54. Dumas O, Jouffre C, Desportes R, Etaix JP, Barthelemy C, Audigier JC. Inverted sigmoid diverticulum: a misleading polyp. Gastrointest Endosc 1991; 37(5):587–588.

55. Schuman BM. Endoscopic diverticulectomy in the sigmoid colon. Gastrointest Endosc 1982; 28(3):189–190.

56. Otte JJ, Larsen L, Andersen JR. Irritable bowel syndrome and symptomatic diverticular disease— different diseases?. Am J Gastroenterol 1986; 81(7):529–531.

57. Ritchie J. Similarity of bowel distension characteristics in the irritable colon syndrome and diverticulosis. Gut 1977; 18:A990.

58. Brodribb AJ. Treatment of symptomatic diverticular disease with a high-fibre diet. Lancet 1977; 1(8013):664–666.

59. Ornstein MH, Littlewood ER, Baird IM, Fowler J, Cox AG. Are fibre supplements really necessary in diverticular disease of the colon? A controlled clinical trial. Br Med J (Clin Res Ed), 1981; 282(6273):1353–1356.

60. Horgan AF, McConnell EJ, Wolff BG, The S, Paterson C. Atypical diverticular disease: surgical results. Dis Colon Rectum 2001; 44(9):1315–1318.

61. Berman LG, Burdick D, Heitzman ER, Prior JT. A critical reappraisal of sigmoid peridiverticulitis. Surg Gynecol Obstet 1968; 127(3):481–491.

62. Roberts P, Abel M, Rosen L, et al. Practice parameters for sigmoid diverticulitis: supporting documentation. Dis Colon Rectum 1995; 38:125–132.

63. Makela J, Kiviniemi H, Laitinen S. Prevalence of perforated sigmoid diverticulitis is increasing. Dis Colon Rectum 2002; 45(7):955–961.

64. Schwesinger WH, Page CP, Gaskill HV III, et al. Operative management of diverticular emergencies: strategies and outcomes. Arch Surg 2000; 135(5):558–562; discussion 562–563.

65. Morson BC. Pathology of diverticular disease of the colon. Clin Gastroenterol 1975; 4(1):37–52.

66. Boirivant M, Marini M, Di Felice G, et al. Lamina propria T cells in Crohn's disease and other gastrointestinal inflammation show defective CD2 pathway-induced apoptosis. Gastroenterology 1999; 116(3):557–565.

67. Williams RA, Davis IP. Diverticular disease of the colon. In: Haubrick WS, Schaffner F, eds. Bockus Gastroenterology. Philadelphia: Saunders WB, 1995:1637–1656.

68. Tagliacozzo S, Tocchi A. Antimesenteric perforations of the colon during diverticular disease: possible pathogenetic role of ischemia. Dis Colon Rectum 1997; 40(11):1358–1361.

69. Hart AR, Kennedy HJ, Stebbings WS, Day NE. How frequently do large bowel diverticula perforate? An incidence and cross-sectional study. Eur J Gastro Hepatol 2000; 12(6):661–665.

70. Hinchey EJ, Schaal PG, Richards GK. Treatment of perforated diverticular disease of the colon. Adv Surg 1978; 12:85–109.

71. Sher ME, Agachan A, Bortul M, Nogueras JJ, Weiss EG, Wexner SD. Laparoscopic surgery for diverticulitis. Surg Endosc 1997; 11:264–277.

72. Markham NI, Li AK. Diverticulitis of the right colon—experience from Hong Kong. Gut 1992; 33(4):547–549.

73. Ambrosetti P, Robert JH, Witzig JA, et al. Acute left colonic diverticulitis: a prospective analysis of 226 consecutive cases. Surgery 1994; 115(5):546–550.

74. Reisman Y, Ziv Y, Kravrovitc D, Negri M, Wolloch Y, Halevy A. Diverticulitis: the effect of age and location on the course of disease. Int J Colorectal Dis 1999; 14(4–5):250–254.

75. Schmidt GT, Lennard-Jones JE, Morson BC, Young AC. Crohn's disease of the colon and its distinction from diverticulitis. Gut 1968; 9(1):7–16.

76. McCue J, Coppen MJ, Rasbridge SA, Lock MR. Coexistent Crohn's disease and sigmoid diverticulosis. Postgrad Med J 1989; 65(767):636–639.

77. Imperiali G, Meucci G, Alvisi C, et al. Segmental colitis associated with diverticula: a prospective study. Gruppo di Studio per le Malattie Infiammatorie Intestinali (GSMII). Am J Gastroenterol 2000; 95(4):1014–1016.

78. Goldstein NS, Leon-Armin C, Mani A. Crohn's colitis-like changes in sigmoid diverticulitis specimens is usually an idiosyncratic inflammatory response to the diverticulosis rather than Crohn's colitis. Am J Surg Pathol 2000; 24(5):668–675.

79. O'Malley ME, Wilson SR. Ultrasonography and computed tomography of appendicitis and diverticulitis. Semin Roentgenol 2001; 36(2):138–147.

80. Wexner SD, Dailey TH. The initial management of left lower quadrant peritonitis. Dis Colon Rectum 1986; 29(10):635–638.

81. Kourtesis GJ, Williams RA, Wilson SE. Surgical options in acute diverticulitis: value of sigmoid resection in dealing with the septic focus. Aust N Z J Surg 1988; 58(12):955–959.

82. Morris J, Stellato TA, Lieberman J, Haaga JR. The utility of computed tomography in colonic diverticulitis. Ann Surg 1986; 204(2):128–132.

83. Gottesman L, Zevon SJ, Brabbee GW, Dailey T, Wichern WR Jr. The use of water soluble contrast enema in the diagnosis of acute left quadrant peritonitis. Dis Colon Rectum 1984; 27(2):84–88.

84. Doringer E. Computerized tomography of colonic diverticulitis. Crit Rev Diagn Imaging 1992; 33(5):421–435.

85. McKee RF, Deignan RW, Krukowski ZH. Radiological investigation in acute diverticulitis. Br J Surg 1993; 80(5):560–565.

86. Shrier D, Skucas J, Weiss S. Diverticulitis: an evaluation by computed tomography and contrast enema. Am J Gastroenterol 1991; 86(10):1466–1471.

87. Hulnick DH, Megibow AJ, Balthazar EJ, Naidich DP, Bosniak MA. Computed tomography in the evaluation of diverticulitis. Radiology 1984; 152(2):491–495.

88. Cho KC, Morehouse HT, Alterman DD, Thornhill BA. Sigmoid diverticulitis: diagnostic role of CT—comparison with barium enema studies. Radiology 1990; 176(1):111–115.

89. Ambrosetti P, Jenny A, Becker C, Terrier TF, Morel P. Acute left colonic diverticulitis—compared performance of computed tomography and water-soluble contrast enema: prospective evaluation of 420 patients. Dis Colon Rectum 2000; 43(10):1363–1367.

90. Jang HJ, Lim HK, Lee SJ, Lee WJ, Kim EY, Kim SH. Acute diverticulitis of the cecum and ascending colon: the value of thin-section helical CT findings in excluding colonic carcinoma. AJR Am J Roentgenol 2000; 174(5):1397–1402.

91. Jang HJ, Lim HK, Lee SJ, Choi SH, Lee MH, Choi MH. Acute diverticulitis of the cecum and ascending colon: thin-section helical CT findings. AJR Am J Roentgenol 1999; 172(3):601–604.

92. Johnson CD, Baker ME, Rice RP, Silverman P, Thompson WM. Diagnosis of acute colonic diverticulitis: comparison of barium enema and CT. AJR Am J Roentgenol 1987; 148(3):541–546.

93. Stefansson T, Nyman R, Nilsson S, Ekbom A, Pahlman L. Diverticulitis of the sigmoid colon. A comparison of CT, colonic enema and laparoscopy. Acta Radiol 1997; 38(2):313–319.

94. Verbanck J, Lambrecht S, Rutgeerts L, et al. Can sonography diagnose acute colonic diverticulitis in patients with acute intestinal inflammation? A prospective study. J Clin Ultrasound 1989; 17(9):661–666.

95. Zielke A, Hasse C, Nies C, et al. Prospective evaluation of ultrasonography in acute colonic diverticulitis. Br J Surg 1997; 84(3):385–388.

96. Wilson SR, Toi A. The value of sonography in the diagnosis of acute diverticulitis of the colon. AJR Am J Roentgenol 1990; 154(6):1199–1202.

97. Schwerk WB, Schwarz S, Rothmund M. Sonography in acute colonic diverticulitis. A prospective study. Dis Colon Rectum 1992; 35(11):1077–1084.

98. Pradel JA, Adell JF, Taourel P, Djafari M, Monnin-Delhom E, Bruel JM. Acute colonic diverticulitis: prospective comparative evaluation with US and CT. Radiology 1997; 205(2):503–512.

99. Brook I, Frazier EH. Aerobic and anaerobic microbiology in intra-abdominal infections associated with diverticulitis. J Med Microbiol 2000; 49(9):827–830.

100. Chow AW. Appendicitis and diverticulitis. In: Hoeprich PD, Jordan MC, Ronald AR, eds. Infectious Diseases: A Treatise of Infectious Processes. Philadelphia: Lippincott, 1994:878–881.

101. Wong WD, Wexner SD, Lowry A, et al. Practice parameters for the treatment of sigmoid diverticulitis—supporting documentation. The Standards Task Force. The American Society of Colon and Rectal Surgeons. Dis Colon Rectum 2000; 43(3):290–297.

102. Stollman NH, Raskin JB. Diagnosis and management of diverticular disease of the colon in adults. Ad Hoc Practice Parameters Committee of the American College of Gastroenterology. Am J Gastroenterol 1999; 94(11):3110–3121.

103. Kohler L, Sauerland S, Neugebauer E. Diagnosis and treatment of diverticular disease: results of a consensus development conference. The Scientific Committee of the European Association for Endoscopic Surgery. Surg Endosc 1999; 13(4):430–436.

104. Thorn M, Graf W, Stefansson T, Pahlman L. Clinical and functional results after elective colonic resection in 75 consecutive patients with diverticular disease. Am J Surg 2002; 183(1):7–11.

105. Acosta JA, Grebenc ML, Doberneck RC, McCarthy JD, Fry DE. Colonic diverticular disease in patients 40 years old or younger. Am Surg 1992; 58(10):605–607.

106. Konvolinka CW. Acute diverticulitis under age forty. Am J Surg 1994; 167(6):562–565.

107. Freischlag J, Bennion RS, Thompson JE Jr. Complications of diverticular disease of the colon in young people. Dis Colon Rectum 1986; 29(10):639–643.

108. Chautems RC, Ambrosetti P, Ludwig A, Mermillod B, Morel P, Soravia C. Long-term follow-up after first acute episode of sigmoid diverticulitis: is surgery mandatory? a prospective study of 118 patients. Dis Colon Rectum 2002; 45(7):962–966.

109. Spivak H, Weinrauch S, Harvey JC, Surick B, Ferstenberg H, Friedman I. Acute colonic diverticulitis in the young. Dis Colon Rectum 1997; 40(5):570–574.

110. Perkins JD, Shield CF III, Chang FC, Farha GJ. Acute diverticulitis. Comparison of treatment in immunocompromised and nonimmunocompromised patients. Am J Surg 1984; 148(6):745–748.

111. Tyau ES, Prystowsky JB, Joehl RJ, Nahrwold DL. Acute diverticulitis. A complicated problem in the immunocompromised patient. Arch Surg 1991; 126(7):855–858; discussion 858–859.

112. Lederman ED, Conti DJ, Lempert N, Singh TP, Lee EC. Complicated diverticulitis following renal transplantation. Dis Colon Rectum 1998; 41(5):613–618.

113. Maurer JR. The spectrum of colonic complications in a lung transplant population. Ann Transplant 2000; 5(3):54–57.

114. Khan S, Eppstein AC, Anderson GK, et al. Acute diverticulitis in heart-and lung transplant patients. Transpl Int 2001; 14(1):12–15.

115. Frizelle FA, Dominguez JM, Santoro GM. Management of post-operative recurrent diverticulitis: a review of the literature. J R Coll Surg Edinb 1997; 42(3):186–188.

116. Benn PL, Wolff BG, Ilstrup DM. Level of anastomosis and recurrent colonic diverticulitis. Am J Surg 1986; 151(2):269–271.

117. Thaler K, Weiss EG, Nogueras JJ, Arnaud JP, Wexner SD, Bergamaschi R. Recurrence rates at a minimum 5 year follow up: laparoscopic versus open sigmoid resection for uncomplicated diverticulitis. Surg Laparosc Endosc Percut Tech 2003; 13:325–327.

118. Zarling EJ, Piontek F, Klemka-Walden L, Inczauskis D. The effect of gastroenterology training on the efficiency and cost of care provided to patients with diverticulitis. Gastroenterology 1997; 112(6):1859–1862.

119. Di Carlo A, Andtbacka RH, Shrier I, et al. The value of specialization—is there an outcome difference in the management of fistulas complicating diverticulitis. Dis Colon Rectum 2001; 44(10):1456–1463.

120. Ambrosetti P, Robert J, Witzig JA, et al. Incidence, outcome, and proposed management of isolated abscesses complicating acute left-sided colonic diverticulitis. A prospective study of 140 patients. Dis Colon Rectum 1992; 35(11):1072–1076.

121. Gerzof SG, Robbins AH, Johnson WC, Birkett DH, Nabseth DC. Percutaneous catheter drainage of abdominal abscesses: a five-year experience. N Engl J Med 1981; 305(12):653–657.

122. Saini S, Mueller PR, Wittenberg J, Butch RJ, Rodkey GV, Welch CE. Percutaneous drainage of diverticular abscess. An adjunct to surgical therapy. Arch Surg 1986; 121(4):475–458.

123. Stabile BE, Puccio E, vanSonnenberg E, Neff CC. Preoperative percutaneous drainage of diverticular abscesses. Am J Surg 1990; 159(1):99–104; discussion.

124. Schechter S, Eisenstat TE, Oliver GC, Rubin RJ, Salvati EP. Computerized tomographic scan-guided drainage of intra-abdominal abscesses. Preoperative and postoperative modalities in colon and rectal surgery. Dis Colon Rectum 1994; 37(10):984–988.

125. Hackford AW, Schoetz DJ Jr., Coller JA, Veidenheimer MC. Surgical management of complicated diverticulitis. The Lahey Clinic experience, 1967 to 1982. Dis Colon Rectum 1985; 28(5):317–321.

126. Desai DC, Brennan EJ Jr., Reilly JF, Smink RD Jr. The utility of the Hartmann procedure. Am J Surg 1998; 175(2):152–154.

127. Trillo C, Paris MF, Brennan JT. Primary anastomosis in the treatment of acute disease of the unprepared left colon. Am Surg 1998; 64(9):821–824; discussion 824–825.

128. Fleites RA, Marshall JB, Eckhauser ML, Mansour EG, Imbembo AL, McCullough AJ. The efficacy of polyethylene glycol-electrolyte lavage solution versus traditional mechanical bowel preparation for elective colonic surgery: a randomized, prospective, blinded clinical trial. Surgery 1985; 98(4):708–717.

129. Lee EC, Murray JJ, Coller JA, Roberts PL, Schoetz DJ Jr. Intraoperative colonic lavage in nonelective surgery for diverticular disease. Dis Colon Rectum 1997; 40(6):669–674.

130. Wedell J, Banzhaf G, Chaoui R, Fischer R, Reichmann J. Surgical management of complicated colonic diverticulitis. Br J Surg 1997; 84(3):380–383.

131. Dudley HA, Racliffe AG, McGeehan D. Intraoperative irrigation of the colon to permit primary anastomosis. Br J Surg 1980; 67(2):80–81.

132. Krukowski ZH, Matheson NA. Emergency surgery for diverticular disease complicated by generalized and faecal peritonitis: a review. Br J Surg 1984; 71(12):921–927.

133. Nagorney DM, Adson MA, Pemberton JH. Sigmoid diverticulitis with perforation and generalized peritonitis. Dis Colon Rectum 1985; 28(2):71–75.

134. Rodkey GV, Welch CE. Changing patterns in the surgical treatment of diverticular disease. Ann Surg 1984; 200(4):466–478.

135. Kronborg O. Treatment of perforated sigmoid diverticulitis: a prospective randomized trial. Br J Surg 1993; 80(4):505–507.

136. Zeitoun G, Laurent A, Rouffet F, et al. Multicentre, randomized clinical trial of primary versus secondary sigmoid resection in generalized peritonitis complicating sigmoid diverticulitis. Br J Surg 2000; 87(10):1366–1374.

137. Wolff BG, Devine RM. Surgical management of diverticulitis. Am Surg 2000; 66(2):153–156.

138. Beahrs JR, Beahrs OH, Beahrs MM, Leary FJ. Urinary tract complications with rectal surgery. Ann Surg 1978; 187(5):542–548.

139. Chahin F, Dwivedi AJ, Paramesh A, et al. The implications of lighted ureteral stenting in laparoscopic colectomy. JSLS 2002; 6(1):49–52.

140. Dwivedi A, Chahin F, Agrawal S, et al. Laparoscopic colectomy vs open colectomy for sigmoid diverticular disease. Dis Colon Rectum 2002; 45(10):1309–1314; discussion 1314–1315.

141. Nirula R, Greaney G. Right-sided diverticulitis: a difficult diagnosis. Am Surg 1997; 63(10):871–873.

142. Sarkar R, Bennion RS, Schmit PJ, Thompson JE. Emergent ileocecectomy for infection and inflammation. Am Surg 1997; 63(10):874–877.

143. Violi V, Roncoroni L, Boselli AS, Trivelli M, Peracchia A. Diverticulitis of the caecum and ascending colon: an unavoidable diagnostic pitfall? Int Surg 2000; 85(1):39–47.

144. Rothenberger DA, Wiltz O. Surgery for complicated diverticulitis. Surg Clin North Am 1993; 73(5):975–992.

145. Woods RJ, Lavery IC, Fazio VW, Jagelman DG, Weakley FL. Internal fistulas in diverticular disease. Dis Colon Rectum 1988; 31(8):591–596.

146. McBeath RB, Schiff M Jr., Allen V, Bottaccini MR, Miller JI, Ehreth JT. A 12-year experience with enterovesical fistulas. Urology 1994; 44(5):661–665.

147. Forde KA, Treat MR. Colonoscopy in the evaluation of strictures. Dis Colon Rectum 1985; 28(10):699–701.

148. Kozarek RA. Hydrostatic balloon dilation of gastrointestinal stenoses: a national survey. Gastrointest Endosc 1986; 32(1):15–19.

149. Oz MC, Forde KA. Endoscopic alternatives in the management of colonic strictures. Surgery 1990; 108(3):513–519.

150. Blomberg B, Rolny P, Jarnerot G. Endoscopic treatment of anastomotic strictures in Crohn's disease. Endoscopy 1991; 23(4):195–198.

151. Lewis BS. Obstruction. In: Raskin JB, Nord JH, eds. Colonoscopy: Prinicples and Techniques. New York: IgakuShoin, 1995:333–334.

152. Davidson R, Sweeney WB. Endoluminal stenting for benign colonic obstruction. Surg Endosc 1998; 12(4):353–354.

153. Tamim WZ, Ghellai A, Counihan TC, Swanson RS, Colby JM, Sweeney WB. Experience with endoluminal colonic wall stents for the management of large bowel obstruction for benign and malignant disease. Arch Surg 2000; 135(4):434–438.

154. Wexner SD, Moscovitz ID. Laparoscopic colectomy in diverticular and Crohn's disease. Surg Clin North Am 2000; 80(4):1299–1319.

155. Mooney MJ, Elliott PL, Galapon DB, James LK, Lilac LJ, O'Reilly MJ. Hand-assisted laparoscopic sigmoidectomy for diverticulitis. Dis Colon Rectum 1998; 41(5):630–635.

156. Franklin ME Jr, Dorman JP, Jacobs M, Plasencia G. Is laparoscopic surgery applicable to complicated colonic diverticular disease?. Surg Endosc 1997; 11(10):1021–1025.

157. Stevenson AR, Stitz RW, Lumley JW, Fielding GA. Laparoscopically assisted anterior resection for diverticular disease: follow-up of 100 consecutive patients. Ann Surg 1998; 227(3):335–342.

158. Kockerling F, Schneider C, Reymond MA, et al. Laparoscopic resection of sigmoid diverticulitis. Results of a multicenter study. Laparoscopic Colorectal Surgery Study Group. Surg Endosc 1999; 13(6):567–571.

159. Schlachta CM, Mamazza J, Poulin EC. Laparoscopic sigmoid resection for acute and chronic diverticulitis. An outcomes comparison with laparoscopic resection for nondiverticular disease. Surg Endosc 1999; 13(7):649–653.

160. Bouillot JL, Berthou JC, Champault G, et al. Elective laparoscopic colonic resection for diverticular disease: results of a multicenter study in 179 patients. Surg Endosc 2002; 16(9):1320–1323.

161. Trebuchet G, Lechaux D, Lecalve JL. Laparoscopic left colon resection for diverticular disease. Surg Endosc 2002; 16(1):18–21.

162. Schlachta CM, Mamazza J, Seshadri PA, Cadeddu MO, Poulin EC. Determinants of outcomes in laparoscopic colorectal surgery: a multiple regression analysis of 416 resections. Surg Endosc 2000; 14(3):258–263.

163. Schlachta CM, Mamazza J, Seshadri PA, Cadeddu M, Gregoire R, Poulin EC. Defining a learning curve for laparoscopic colorectal resections. Dis Colon Rectum 2001; 44(2):217–222.

164. Regenet N, Tuech JJ, Pessaux P, Ziani M. Intraoperative colonic lavage of primary anastomosis versus Hartmann's procedure for complex diverticular disease of the colon. Hepatogastroenterology 2002; 49:664–667.

165. Boley SJ, DiBiase A, Brandt LJ, Sammartano RJ. Lower intestinal bleeding in the elderly. Am J Surg 1979; 137(1):57–64.

166. Potter GD, Sellin JH. Lower gastrointestinal bleeding. Gastroenterol Clin North Am 1988; 17(2): 341–356.

167. Gostout CJ, Wang KK, Ahlquist DA, et al. Acute gastrointestinal bleeding. Experience of a specialized management team. J Clin Gastroenterol 1992; 14(3):260–267.

168. Longstreth GF. Epidemiology and outcome of patients hospitalized with acute lower gastrointestinal hemorrhage: a population-based study. Am J Gastroenterol 1997; 92(3):419–424.

169. Peura DA, Lanza FL, Gostout CJ, Foutch PG. The American College of Gastroenterology Bleeding Registry: preliminary findings. Am J Gastroenterol 1997; 92(6):924–928.

170. Quinn WC. Diverticular disease of the colon with hemorrhage: a study of 78 cases. Am Surg 1960; 26:171–174.

171. McGuire HH Jr., Haynes BW Jr. Massive hemorrhage for diverticulosis of the colon: guidelines for therapy based on bleeding patterns observed in fifty cases. Ann Surg 1972; 175(6):847–855.

172. Zuckerman GR, Prakash C. Acute lower intestinal bleeding. Part II: etiology, therapy, and outcomes. Gastrointest Endosc 1999; 49(2):228–238.

173. Meyers MA, Alonso DR, Gray GF, Baer JW. Pathogenesis of bleeding colonic diverticulosis. Gastroenterology 1976; 71(4):577–583.

174. Casarella WJ, Kanter IE, Seaman WB. Right-sided colonic diverticula as a cause of acute rectal hemorrhage. N Engl J Med 1972; 286(9):450–453.

175. McGuire HH Jr. Bleeding colonic diverticula. A reappraisal of natural history and management. Ann Surg 1994; 220(5):653–656.

176. Wong SK, Ho YH, Leong AP, Seow-Choen F. Clinical behavior of complicated right-sided and left-sided diverticulosis. Dis Colon Rectum 1997; 40(3):344–348.

177. Wilcox CM, Alexander LN, Cotsonis GA, Clark WS. Nonsteroidal antiinflammatory drugs are associated with both upper and lower gastrointestinal bleeding. Dig Dis Sci 1997; 42(5):990–997.

178. Aldoori WH, Giovannucci EL, Rimm EB, Wing AL, Willett WC. Use of acetaminophen and nonsteroidal anti-inflammatory drugs: a prospective study and the risk of symptomatic diverticular disease in men. Arch Fam Med 1998; 7(3):255–260.

179. Goh H, Bourne R. Non-steroidal anti-inflammatory drugs and perforated diverticular disease: a case-control study. Ann R Coll Surg Engl 2002; 84(2):93–96.

180. Wilson RG, Smith AN, Macintyre IM. Complications of diverticular disease and non-steroidal anti-inflammatory drugs: a prospective study. Br J Surg 1990; 77(10):1103–1104.

181. Campbell K, Steele RJ. Non-steroidal anti-inflammatory drugs and complicated diverticular disease: a case-control study. Br J Surg 1991; 78(2):190–191.

182. Laine L, Connors LG, Reicin A, et al. Serious lower gastrointestinal clinical events with nonselective NSAID or coxib use. Gastroenterology 2003; 124(2):288–292.

183. Zuccaro G Jr. Management of the adult patient with acute lower gastrointestinal bleeding. American College of Gastroenterology. Practice Parameters Committee. Am J Gastroenterol 1998; 93(8): 1202–1208.

184. Alavi A, Ring EJ. Localization of gastrointestinal bleeding: superiority of 99mTc sulfur colloid compared with angiography. AJR Am J Roentgenol 1981; 137(4):741–748.

185. Hunter JM, Pezim ME. Limited value of technetium 99m-labeled red cell scintigraphy in localization of lower gastrointestinal bleeding. Am J Surg 1990; 159(5):504–506.

186. Browder W, Cerise EJ, Litwin MS. Impact of emergency angiography in massive lower gastrointestinal bleeding. Ann Surg 1986; 204(5):530–536.

187. Luchtefeld MA, Senagore AJ, Szomstein M, Fedeson B, Van Erp J, Rupp S. Evaluation of transarterial embolization for lower gastrointestinal bleeding. Dis Colon Rectum 2000; 43(4):532–534.

188. Gordon RL, Ahl KL, Kerlan RK, et al. Selective arterial embolization for the control of lower gastrointestinal bleeding. Am J Surg 1997; 174(1):24–28.

189. Shinya H, Cwern M, Wolf G. Colonoscopic diagnosis and management of rectal bleeding. Surg Clin North Am 1982; 62(5):897–903.

190. Tedesco FJ, Waye JD, Raskin JB, Morris SJ, Greenwald RA. Colonoscopic evaluation of rectal bleeding: a study of 304 patients. Ann Intern Med 1978; 89(6):907–909.

191. Irvine EJ, O'Connor J, Frost RA, et al. Prospective comparison of double contrast barium enema plus flexible sigmoidoscopy v colonoscopy in rectal bleeding: barium enema v colonoscopy in rectal bleeding. Gut 1988; 29(9):1188–1193.

192. Deyhle P, Blum AL, Nuesch HJ. Emergency coloscopy (sic) in the management of perianal hemorrhage. Endoscopy 1974; 6:229–232.

193. Forde KA. Colonoscopy in acute rectal bleeding. Gastrointest Endosc 1981; 27(4):219–220.

194. Schuman BM. When should colonoscopy be the first study for active lower intestinal hemorrhage? Gastrointest Endosc 1984; 30(6):372–373.

195. Jensen DM, Machicado GA. Emergent colonoscopy in patients with severe hematochezia. Gastrointest Endosc 1983; 9:177.

196. Caos A, Benner KG, Manier J, et al. Colonoscopy after Golytely preparation in acute rectal bleeding. J Clin Gastroenterol 1986; 8(1):46–49.

197. Jensen DM, Machicado GA. Diagnosis and treatment of severe hematochezia. The role of urgent colonoscopy after purge. Gastroenterology 1988; 95(6):1569–1574.

198. Mauldin JL. Therapeutic use of colonoscopy in active diverticular bleeding. Gastrointest Endosc 1985; 31(4):290–291.

199. Johnston J, Sones J. Endoscopic heater probe coagulation of the bleeding colonic diverticulum. Gastrointest Endosc 1986; 32:160.

200. Savides TJ, Jensen DM. Colonoscopic hemostasis for recurrent diverticular hemorrhage associated with a visible vessel: a report of three cases. Gastrointest Endosc 1994; 40(1):70–73.

201. Foutch PG, Zimmerman K. Diverticular bleeding and the pigmented protuberance (sentinel clot): clinical implications, histopathological correlation, and results of endoscopic intervention. Am J Gastroenterol 1996; 91(12):2589–2593.

202. Bertoni G, Conigliaro R, Ricci E, Mortilla MG, Bedogni G, Fornaciari G. Endoscopic injection hemostasis of colonic diverticular bleeding: a case report. Endoscopy 1990; 22(3):154–155.

203. Kim YI, Marcon NE. Injection therapy for colonic diverticular bleeding. A case study. J Clin Gastroenterol 1993; 17(1):46–48.

204. Andress HJ, Mewes A, Lange V. Endoscopic hemostasis of a bleeding diverticulum of the sigma with fibrin sealant. Endoscopy 1993; 25(2):193.

205. Witte JT. Band ligation for colonic bleeding: modification of multiband ligating devices for use with a colonoscope. Gastrointest Endosc 2000; 52(6):762–765.

206. Hokama A, Uehara T, Nakayoshi T, et al. Utility of endoscopic hemoclipping for colonic diverticular bleeding. Am J Gastroenterol 1997; 92(3):543–546.

207. Jensen DM, Machicado GA, Jutabha R, Kovacs TO. Urgent colonoscopy for the diagnosis and treatment of severe diverticular hemorrhage. N Engl J Med 2000; 342(2):78–82.

208. Foutch PG, Rex DK, Lieberman DA. Diverticular bleeding: are nonsteroidal anti-inflammatory drugs risk factors for hemorrhage and can colonoscopy predict outcome for patients? Prevalence and natural history of colonic angiodysplasia among healthy asymptomatic people. Am J Gastroenterol 1995; 90(10):1779–1784.

209. Cohn SM, Moller BA, Zieg PM, Milner KA, Angood PB. Angiography for preoperative evaluation in patients with lower gastrointestinal bleeding: are the benefits worth the risks?. Arch Surg 1998; 133(1):50–55.

210. Setya V, Singer JA, Minken SL. Subtotal colectomy as a last resort for unrelenting, unlocalized, lower gastrointestinal hemorrhage: experience with 12 cases. Am Surg 1992; 58(5):295–299.

211. Gianfrancisco JA, Abcarian H. Pitfalls in the treatment of massive lower gastrointestinal bleeding with "blind" subtotal colectomy. Dis Colon Rectum 1982; 25(5):441–445.

20 | Megacolon

Hélio Moreira, Jr.
Colorectal Service, Department of Surgery, Medical School of the Federal University of Goiás, Goiânia, Goiás, Brazil

Joffre Marcondes Rezende
Gastroenterology Service, Department of Internal Medicine, Medical School of the Federal University of Goiás, Goiânia, Goiás, Brazil

INTRODUCTION

Megacolon may result from a variety of clinical conditions and can be classified as two major categories—acute or chronic. Acute megacolon may be due to distal obstruction, metabolic disturbances, or inflammatory disorders of the bowel. This chapter will only discuss chronic causes of megacolon (Table 1).

CHAGASIC MEGACOLON

Chagas disease remains a medical challenge in South American countries, especially in Brazil. It has an estimated incidence of over 16 to 18 million people, approximately 2 million of whom are in Brazil (1). The disease is caused by *Trypanosoma cruzi*, a protozoan that uses some mammals, including humans, as its host and is transmitted by insects (reservatory) that carry *T. cruzi* in their digestive tracts. When the infected insect bites the skin, its feces may come into contact with the wound surface, thereby contaminating the person or animal. The incidence of Chagas' disease is endemic in impoverished areas of Brazil. While this disease was originally confined to South America, recent estimates indicate that 350,000 people in the United States are seropositive, a third of whom are thought to have chronic Chagas' disease (2).

Pathogenesis

In addition to insect bites, Chagas' disease may be transmitted by blood transfusion in humans (3). This may represent a future health problem in developed countries in which Latin American population immigration has increased and serology for Chagas' disease is not routinely undertaken for blood donors.

As *T. cruzi* reaches the blood vessels in infected individuals, it is systemically spread, resulting in tissue lesions to various organs. The three important clinical stages for Chagas' disease are discussed in the following sections.

Acute Stage

The acute stage presents with nonspecific symptoms, varying from mild to severe general malaise, thereby making early diagnosis of Chagas' disease difficult. Infected individuals will present with fever, hepatosplenomegaly, generalized edema, and lymphadenopathy. At later stages, diffuse skin exanthema, diarrhea, and vomiting may also be present. Acute myocardiopathy may be detected in approximately 30% of patients; however symptoms spontaneously subside within four to eight weeks without any permanent sequelae. The acute stage is usually recognized in children younger than 15 years of age. Severe clinical manifestations, including myocarditis and meningoencephalitis, are usually seen in younger children, and may even be fatal in children under two years of age.

There are specific clinical signs that are indicative of Chagas' disease. The portal of entry of *T. cruzi* in the skin surface becomes inflamed, the so-called chagoma. Because the insect usually bites at night when the face is often the only uncovered area, the face is the most common portal of entry for the *T. cruzi* infection. Unilateral or bilateral reddish painless

Table 1   Classification of Megacolon

Acute megacolon	Acquired
Obstructive cause (mechanical)	Infection
Adhesion	Chagasic megacolon
Neoplasia	Drug induced
Volvulus	Cathartics
Stricture	Anticholinergics
Toxic megacolon	Ganglionic blocking agents
Inflammatory bowel disease	Anti-Parkinsonian
Ulcerative colitis	Narcotics
Crohn's disease	Functional disorders
Infectious colitis	Colonic inertia
Pseudomembranous colitis (*Clostridium difficile*)	Outlet obstruction
Amebic colitis	Idiopathic megacolon
Intestinal pseudo-obstruction (colon dysmotility) or Ogilvie's syndrome	Neurological and muscular diseases
Ileus	Parkinson's disease
Postoperative ileus	Spinal cord injury
Inflammatory disease	Myotonia dystrophica
Electrolyte disturbances	Neurofibromatosis
Cardiac failure	Miscellaneous
Vascular insufficiency	Lead poisoning
Atonic colon	Porphyria
Chronic megacolon	Psychogenic megacolon
Congenital	
Hischsprung's disease	

periophthalmic cellulitic areas, the so-called Romana sign, are typical manifestations of acute Chagas' disease (Fig. 1).

Indeterminate Stage

The asymptomatic indeterminate stage usually commences 8 to 10 weeks after the acute stage and may last indefinitely. Despite normal chest X-ray, electrocardiogram, and absence of all clinical manifestations, serological tests for Chagas' disease remain positive; parasitemia may be recognized in 20% to 60% of patients. These patients are generally asymptomatic for a prolonged period of time and, subsequently, become the reservoir that sustains the disease cycle, especially if they are potential blood donors.

Chronic Stage

Only 30% of patients will progress from an indeterminate Chagas' disease to a chronic cardiac, digestive, or, rarely, neurological stage; this usually occurs 10 to 20 years after infection (4).

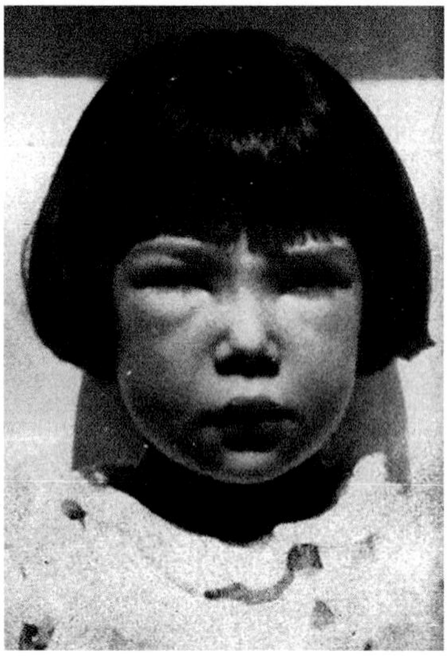

Figure 1   "Romana" sign, suspicion of acute chagasic infection.

Chagasic Cardiopathy

The most common ventricular conduction defects seen in patients with Chagas' disease include right bundle block and left anterior hemiblock. Clinical manifestations include heart failure and arrhythmias; therefore these patients commonly require pacemakers. Severe complications include both peripheral and pulmonary embolism and even sudden death. A variety of arrhythmias may occur, including bradycardia, sinoatrial block, sustained ventricular tachycardia, and ventricular fibrillation. Primary T-wave changes and Q waves are also detected in these patients although, interestingly, coronary vessels are preserved.

Digestive Form

There are two clinical manifestations of digestive Chagas' disease: megacolon and mega-esophagus. Both clinical conditions deteriorate over time and frequently coexist in the same patient.

Chagasic Mega-esophagus.   Patients with megaesophagus will initially present with dysphagia for solid dry foods; this progressively deteriorates, becoming symptomatic for liquids as well.

Chagasic Megacolon.   Patients with chagasic megacolon usually become symptomatic in their fourth or fifth decade of life. Chronic constipation that progressively deteriorates associated with a history of contact with disease carriers is the key aspect to suspecting chagasic colopathy.

   Koeberle (5) histologically demonstrated why these patients become constipated. The protozoa in the bowel wall cause an inflammatory response, which ultimately causes damage to the Meissner and Auerbach neural plexus. Colonic physiology is a complex multifactorial event that is regulated by a wide variety of neurotransmitters. The result of various colonic stimuli, osmolarity of the feces, and the intestinal flora determines the intestinal transit time. In physiological conditions, it results in an atonic propulsive contraction of the colon. The consequence of neural damage to the bowel is increased colonic transit time (6). Moreover, chagasic colopathy includes the presence of internal sphincter achalasia, further exacerbating the constipation (7).

   It may take years or even decades before the development of any clinical manifestation. Chronic constipation, which progressively deteriorates, is the main complaint. It is usually associated with abdominal cramping, flatulence, abdominal distention, and cathartic dependency. Severe cases are usually associated with generally poor health and malnutrition, especially when associated with mega-esophagus. It is quite common for patients to have one bowel movement every 10 days (Table 2), while more severely afflicted individuals may have a bowel movement only once every four months. Complications may occur in 50% of patients, including fecaloma and volvulus. These situations may be life threatening, especially if the general condition of the patient is very poor.

   A patient presenting with a fecaloma usually complains of rectal pain and a sensation of incomplete evacuation. In addition, they may present with paradoxical diarrhea and fecal incontinence, depending on the size and location of the fecaloma. High fecalomas may be identified on physical examination of the abdomen as an abdominal mass, can be palpated in the sigmoid area, and the "Gersuny" sign is quite common.

Table 2   Severity of Constipation in Patients with Chagasic Megacolon

Number of days without bowel movement	Number of patients	%
1–5	54	11.5
6–10	106	22.6
11–15	39	8.3
16–20	83	17.7
21–25	06	1.2
26–30	107	22.9
>30	74	15.8
Total	469	100

Patients with chagasic megacolon may present with sigmoid volvulus in 25% of cases (8). Clinical manifestations include severe abdominal cramping, bowel obstruction, and, in cases of vascular ischemia of the sigmoid, toxemia and peritonitis; volvulus is rarely associated with a fecaloma.

Chagasic megacolon is associated with chagasic mega-esophagus or chagasic cardiopathy in approximately 60% of patients (4). Therefore, patients commonly complain of dysphagia, heartburn, regurgitation, palpitation, dyspnea, and arrhythmia. The association of different types of Chagas' diseases increases the morbidity and mortality.

Diagnosis

Clinical manifestations of progressive chronic constipation, especially when associated with dysphagia or cardiac symptoms, are suspects for chagasic megacolon. Patients are generally from areas endemic for Chagas' disease and relate a history of contact with a disease carrier; they may also have relatives with Chagas' disease.

Complementary tests are necessary to establish an accurate diagnosis. Serological tests may confirm Chagas' disease; Guerreiro–Machado is a complement-fixation test and is most commonly available. However, the 90% sensitivity associated with this test may determine the necessity of other serological tests, including enzyme linked immunosorbent assay, indirect hemagglutination, or indirect immunofluorescence (9). A barium enema is also important to help confirm chagasic megacolon when a large megacolon is present. However, unlike megaesophagus, chagasic colopathy will initially become a dolichocolon and then dilate. Therefore, a normal barium enema will not exclude the diagnosis of chagasic megacolon (Fig. 2).

On occasion, a patient may present with chronic constipation with positive epidemiology, positive serological tests for Chagas' disease, and a normal barium enema. Considering that, in endemic areas, the incidence of positive serology for Chagas' disease is approximately 8% of the district population and that only 30% of these patients will ultimately become symptomatic, it is reasonable to question whether the patient is actually constipated due to a chagasic colopathy. In these situations, anorectal manometry plays an important role in determining the diagnosis of chagasic colopathy, as the absence of the inhibitory rectoanal reflex is expected (Fig. 3) (10).

Treatment
Clinical Management

Clinical management for patients with chagasic megacolon is controversial. Highly selected patients with significant comorbidity and associated severe cardiopathy may be treated with

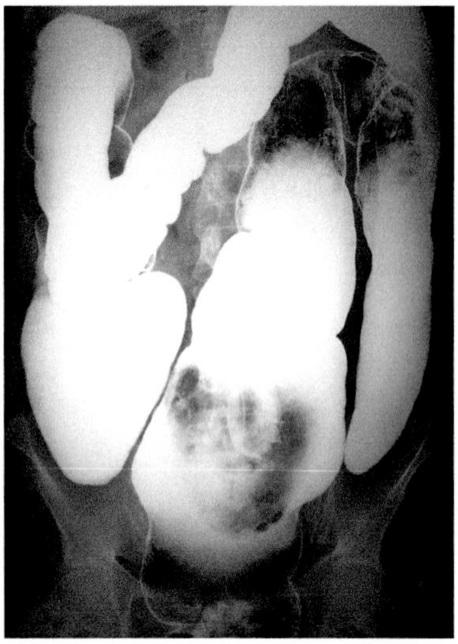

Figure 2   Barium enema of a patient with chagasic megacolon.

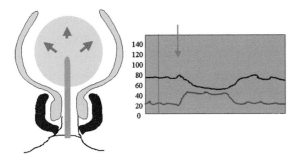

Figure 3 Anorectal manometry shows achalasia of the internal sphincter in a chagasic patient.

cathartic drugs and retrograde lavage. However, even after successful management, the risk of volvulus in this group remains as high as 30%. Therefore, the indication for this clinical management schema should be restricted to a very select group of patients. Although some authors advocate conservative nonoperative management for asymptomatic patients, considering the natural history of the disease where constipation progressively worsens, it is wise to consider a definitive surgical treatment while these patients are younger, with better nutritional status, and a lower morbidity and mortality rate.

Surgical Treatment

Several surgical techniques have been described for the treatment of chagasic megacolon. Some have been abandoned due to associated high morbidity and recurrence rates. Currently, there are two major surgical procedures for chagasic megacolon, the Duhamel–Haddad technique and its modifications (Fig. 4) (11) and low anterior resection (12). In our department, we have been performing the Duhamel–Haddad procedure for chagasic megacolon since 1970. According to our experience, the Duhamel–Haddad technique when performed by an experienced surgical team, is associated with the following:

Low recurrence rates: Symptomatic recurrence after the Duhamel–Haddad surgery is expected in less than 3% of patients. Moreover, even if symptoms do recur, they are usually less severe than prior to surgery. Recurrence after a Duhamel–Haddad procedure usually results from an inadequate initial surgical technique, including a long rectal stump, low colorectal septum, and reoperations.

Low morbidity and mortality rates: The advantage of the Duhamel–Haddad surgery is that it may be performed in two stages, seven days apart. The first stage includes transection of the rectal stump at the promontory level and pull-through of the colon in the presacral and submucosal space (Fig. 5), avoiding a colonic anastomosis. The anastomosis is subsequently performed in a second stage, seven days after the initial procedure. At that time, anastomoses may be postponed if septic complications are observed, including retrorectal and rectal stump abscess. With an experienced surgical team, morbidity and mortality rates are reportedly quite low at 15% and 1%, respectively. As a result, over the last decade, some

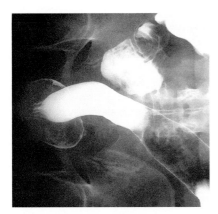

Figure 4 Postoperative barium enema in a chagasic patient submitted to a Duhamel–Haddad surgery.

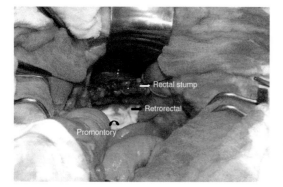

Figure 5 Duhamel–Haddad surgery: first stage, transection of the rectal stump at the promontory level and pull-through of the colon in the presacral and submucosal space.

authors have advocated immediate stapled colorectal anastomosis, thereby reducing hospitalization (13). The main potential surgical complication after the Duhamel–Haddad surgery is necrosis of the pulled-through colon. This life-threatening complication demands emergent surgery with resection of the necrosed colon and construction of an end colostomy. Therefore, for inexperienced surgeons, immediate colorectal anastomoses after Duhamel–Haddad surgery should be avoided.

Good long-term results: Long-term follow-up remains a challenge in this subset of patients because they usually come from rural areas where contact is extremely difficult. Moreover, because these patients are usually impoverished, frequent follow-up is unaffordable. Nevertheless, because recurrent symptoms are rarely seen in our institution, we can only assume that the treatment of chagasic megacolon using the Duhamel–Haddad technique is associated with low recurrence rates.

CONGENITAL MEGACOLON

The congenital absence of the Auerbach's and Meissner's autonomic plexuses in the colonic wall can extend proximally for a variable distance from the rectum, involving the entire colon and a portion of the terminal ileum, as described by Hirschsprung in 1887 (14). However, the disease is usually restricted to the rectum or rectosigmoid area in approximately 77% of cases. Symptoms are often present at birth and include abdominal distension and failure of the meconium to pass. Other symptoms also include repeated vomiting, chronic constipation, and delayed growth due to malnutrition. In addition, there is usually a zone of hypoganglionosis between the normal and the aganglionic bowel. When the diseased segment reaches or includes the small intestine, the disease is referred to as "long-segment disease." Conversely, when the diseased segment includes only a portion of the large intestine, it is called "short-segment disease."

Incidence

The incidence of Hirschsprung's disease (HD) is 1:5000 live births with a male preponderance of 3:1 in short-segment but equal gender distribution in long-segment disease (15). In addition, there is a recognized increased incidence in patients with Down syndrome.

Etiology and Pathology

Most cases of HD are due to sporadic genetic mutations. Individuals with a family history of HD are at an increased risk (16) and are strongly urged to undergo genetic counseling and analysis. The anatomic-pathological basis for HD is the absence of ganglionic cells in the distal or "narrowed"colonic segment, with hyperplasia and hypertrophy of the nonmyelinic neural bundles of the myenteric plexus of Auerbach, Meissner (superficial submucosa), and Henle (deep submucosa). This defect may be related to the cephalad–caudal mismigration of the vagus neural crist, as a consequence of deletion of the long arm of chromosome 10. Histochemistry shows increased acetylcholinesterase activity in the enlarged nerve fibers (17).

Classification and Clinical Manifestation

Symptoms may be present in earlier stages according to the extent of the aganglionic segment. Newborns with HD have a delayed first bowel movement and may also present with bilious vomiting and abdominal distention. Furthermore, chronic constipation is present from birth. Digital examination may be followed by an explosive elimination of liquid feces and gas. Symptoms may alternate between constipation and diarrhea. Cecal perforation may be the first clinical manifestation, although enterocolitis may develop before or after surgical treatment. Enterocolitis is associated with a poor prognosis (18); worrisome signs may include fever, abdominal distention, vomiting, diarrhea, and rectal bleeding.

Diagnosis may be established in older children as obstructive symptoms become more rare over time and constipation becomes the major symptom. Paradoxical diarrhea and fecal incontinence may also be expected due to rectal fecal impaction. A significant growth delay is commonly seen in these individuals. As with younger children, teenagers and adults with HD have usually experienced lifelong severe constipation. The extent of the respective aganglionic segment will determine the severity of the constipation.

Diagnosis

Clinical manifestations raise the possibility of HD. Initially, evaluation should include a physical examination, which reveals abdominal distention and, occasionally, the presence of a fecaloma. Further tests may include barium enema, rectal biopsy, and anal manometry.

Barium Enema

The typical plain abdominal radiograph features colonic distention with less small bowel distension and occasional air fluid levels; alternatively, the radiograph may be normal or show obstruction or generalized distension. A barium enema with the catheter situated just inside the anal margin shows a narrow nondistended rectum with a transition to dilated colon. These telltale signs may be subtle if the infant is examined at an early age and fecal impaction is not significant. However, most infants are diagnosed as neonates. An irregular "saw tooth" appearance of the rectum is a valuable sign. In total colonic HD, the colon may be either normal or decreased in caliber as the clinical presentation raises suspicion. The rare delayed presentation of HD is severe chronic constipation. The narrow aganglionic distal segment is easily demonstrated on barium enema (Figure 6A and B).

Anorectal Manometry

Anorectal manometry plays an important role in the diagnosis of HD. Callaghan and Nixon (19) demonstrated achalasia of the internal anal sphincter in patients with HD.

Rectal Biopsy

Rectal biopsy provides a definitive diagnosis of HD. It is usually performed by resecting a 3 to 5 cm full-thickness flap of the posterior rectal wall, starting at 2 cm above the dentate line.

(A)   **(B)**

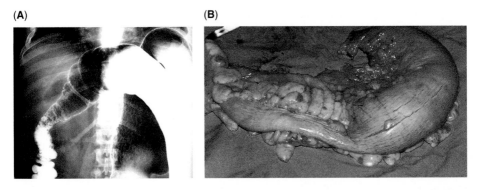

Figure 6   Barium enema of a narrowed aganglionic segment of rectosigmoid colon in an adult patient with Hirschsprung's disease (HD) (**A**). Rectosigmoid surgical specimen of a patient with HD (**B**). Note that the diseased segment is not dilated.

Histology shows increased neural amyelinic bundles in the aganglionic segment. Some authors include a segment of the internal sphincter in the specimen in the hopes of symptomatic improvement, especially for short-segment congenital megacolon. Thus, the procedure can be diagnostic and therapeutic in patients with ultrashort-segment disease.

Surgical Treatment

Surgical management may be a primary curative procedure or a diverting colostomy with subsequent definitive surgical treatment. Definitive surgery includes one of four pull-through surgical procedures: the Swenson (20), the Soave (21), the Martin (22), and the Duhamel (23) procedures.

Colostomy

There are specific situations where a colostomy is an excellent option, including the following:

- Malnourished patients with a high operative risk
- Premature infants
- Stenosis or fistulas followed by unsuccessful surgery
- Colonic perforation.

A colostomy has gradually become a rare indication. Currently, it is generally preferable to perform a definitive surgery as an initial approach, even in neonates. The colostomy should be performed as close as possible to the transitional aganglionic segment. A Hartmann's operation is usually preferred in order to prevent distal fecalomas. The colostomy will be subsequently closed during the definitive surgery without an additional surgical stage.

Swenson Procedure

Swenson et al. proposed this surgical technique in 1948. It was the first surgical technique based on the pathophysiology of HD (20). The affected aganglionic segment is resected and the proximal ganglionic colon is mobilized to reach the perineum. The rectum is fully mobilized to the levator ani muscles and everted through the anal canal. The colon is then pulled through the rectal lumen and exteriorized in the perineum. The diseased rectum is resected approximately 1 cm above the dentate line. A colorectal anastomosis is performed and the colon is placed back into the pelvis. This surgery is associated with several major functional disorders, particularly sexual impotence and fecal incontinence, due to neural stretching. Consequently, this procedure has been abandoned as an option for the treatment of HD.

Soave Procedure

Soave's technique was first described in 1964, consisting of both an abdominal and perineal surgery phase (21). The aim of this surgery was to prevent complications associated with the Swenson's procedure; therefore the rectum was left in situ and resected at the level of the sacral promontory. A circular mucosectomy of the rectum is performed, leaving 1 cm of mucosa above the dentate line. The proximal innervated colon is pulled through the rectal muscular tunica and exteriorized in the perineum, leaving a 5 cm colonic segment in the perineum; this segment is resected between the 10th and 15th postoperative days. The main postoperative complication is anal stenosis that necessitates frequent anal dilatation.

Martin Procedure

This surgical technique was proposed for selected HD patients with total colonic aganglionosis (22). A subtotal colectomy is performed, which includes the right and transverse colon. The ganglionic distal ileum is pulled through the retrorectal space, as with the Duhamel procedure. A long laterolateral anastomosis is performed between the ileal segment and left colon. The aim of this surgery is to combine the ability of peristaltic ileum (nonaffected portion) with the ability of the left aganglionic colon to absorb liquid.

Duhamel Procedure

The Duhamel procedure was proposed in 1956 as a surgical option for the treatment of HD and is currently the most commonly employed surgical technique. This technique can be performed using a laparoscopic approach, with good cosmetic results and similar clinical outcomes when compared to laparotomy. Long-term follow-up will demonstrate if laparoscopy will ultimately be associated with a lower incidence of bowel obstruction due to less adhesion formation.

IDIOPATHIC MEGARECTUM AND MEGACOLON

The definition of megacolon varies in the literature. Most researchers use the criterion of a cecum greater than 12 cm. However, it does not include measurement of the left colon that is more commonly seen as a dilated segment. Many factors influence the result of a bowel measurement, including individual anatomy, solution used for the contrast enema, air pressure applied after instillation of the rectal contrast, ability of the patient to retain the contrast (patient's continence status), and the distance of the X-ray machine from the patient.

While the megacolon itself should not always be considered as an abnormal finding, the associated clinical presentation does make it a relevant finding. Chronic constipation, radiologic megacolon, or megarectum with normal myenteric ganglia and no organic etiology are the default definitions for patients with idiopathic megacolon (IMC).

Incidence

Megabowel is more equally distributed between genders when compared with the predominantly male distribution of HD. However, like HD, megabowel is usually seen in younger individuals.

Pathophysiology

The pathophysiology of this condition remains poorly elucidated. The associated feature is that fatty acids appear to reduce the volume of the proximal large bowel (24). Opiate narcotics reduce the propensity of colonic constriction (25).

The control of colonic contractility is a complex interaction of intrinsic colonic nerves, splanchnic nerve control, and central nervous system input. The final common pathway of intrinsic nerve control of colonic motility is via postganglionic nerves: stimulatory cholinergic nerves and inhibitory nitric oxide–releasing nerves. Evidence suggests that excessive production of nitric oxide may be the mechanism responsible for acute megacolon (26); however, there is no evidence for a potential role of nitric oxide in chronic megacolon.

Animal studies have shown that the splanchnic nerves can dramatically affect colonic motility by either contracting or, conversely, relaxing the colon (27). Extrinsic adrenergic nerves mainly seem to act by reducing acetylcholine release from intrinsic postganglionic nerves, although a direct action on smooth muscle cells cannot be excluded. At this time, the respective roles of the intrinsic and splanchnic nerves in inducing megacolon must be clarified.

Some authors (28–30) have revealed silver-staining anatomical abnormalities of the myenteric plexus. They have also observed abnormal neurons with small dark nuclei without nucleoli or visible chromatin structure. However, this plexus damage may be due to chronic laxative abuse. IMC may also be acquired as a psychologic consequence of refusal during toilet training, resulting in a chronic outlet obstruction, which ultimately results in colorectal dilatation.

Clinical Features

Dilatation of the rectum and/or colon, in the absence of demonstrable organic disease, is an uncommon and poorly characterized condition; IMC may be associated with sigmoid volvulus. Patients with idiopathic megarectum (IMR), present with soiling and fecal impaction compared to patients with IMC, whose symptoms are variable and include constipation or increased bowel frequency with persistence of rectal fullness, abdominal pain, and a variable need for laxatives. Patients with IMR are generally younger than patients with IMC, becoming symptomatic in childhood, while half of the patients with IMC develop symptoms as adults. Patients with IMR may present with a maximum anal resting pressure below normal, indicating sphincter damage or inhibition. Gatuso et al. (31) demonstrated that both IMR and IMC patients had altered rectal sensitivity to distension, suggesting that despite the lack of rectal dilatation, IMC has altered viscoelasticity, tone, or sensory function.

Physical Examination

Physical examination generally reveals a distended abdomen, which may or may not be tense, and tympany is invariably present. Most patients present with painless constipation, although colicky pain may occur. Constipation is the predominant symptom of megacolon. Frequent and severe abdominal pain, which is relieved by evacuation, is more likely to be attributed to irritable bowel syndrome. A sensation of incomplete evacuation is usually associated with an outlet obstruction (rectocele, anismus, perineal descent, and sigmoidocele). If megacolon is secondary to any or several of these mechanisms, treatment should initially be focused on the primary disorder. Digital rectal examination may demonstrate a hard mass of stool immediately cephalad to the anorectal ring. Megarectum, with a chronically distended rectum, tends to cause the anus to gape open secondary to internal anal sphincter dysfunction. These patients may present with factitious diarrhea secondary to overflow incontinence.

Investigation

Laboratory studies are important to exclude other etiologies, including electrolyte abnormalities; in addition, thyroid function tests should also be performed. After plain films reveal the megacolon, a barium contrast enema may be helpful to assess the size and length of the colon, determine the presence of megacolon, megarectum, or both, and exclude other causes of bowel obstruction. Colonoscopy or flexible sigmoidoscopy may be used to exclude an obstructive/mechanical cause of colonic dilatation.

Colonic Transit Study

Distinguishing a colonic inertia etiology from that of a functional outlet obstruction is probably best accomplished by colonic marker transit studies. There are numerous ways to perform this test. One method is to instruct the patient to consume 30 g of daily dietary fiber and to discontinue all laxatives, enemas, and constipating medications for at least two days prior to, as well as during, the test. The patient ingests the markers and abdominal plain films are obtained on the fifth postingestion day. Patients with colonic inertia will have markers distributed throughout the large bowel, while patients with outlet obstruction exhibit markers normally distributed throughout the colon, but accumulating in the rectum (Fig. 7A and B).

Anorectal Manometry

Anorectal manometry may help to distinguish congenital megacolon from acquired megacolon. The presence of a rectoanal inhibitory response means that there are intact ganglia, and the patient does not have HD. However, conversely, if the inhibitory response is absent, a rectal biopsy is required to confirm the diagnosis of HD.

(A)   **(B)**

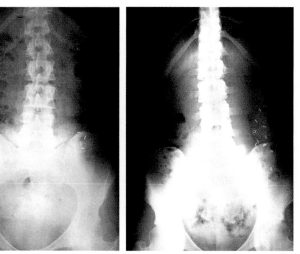

Figure 7 Colonic transit study shows a delayed transit time five days after taking the sitz markers, suggesting colonic inertia (**A**) and an outlet obstruction (**B**).

Cinedefecography

Outlet obstruction may be a cause of constipation. Paradoxical contraction of the puborectalis muscle, rectocele, sigmoidocele, and rectoanal intussusception are all common causes of difficult rectal emptying, which may in turn result in colon and rectal dilation. These entities are well documented using cinedefecography or dynamic proctography (32). The patient's rectum is filled using a contrast with a consistency similar to that of fecal material. The patient is then placed on a commode and a lateral view of the pelvis is obtained using fluoroscopy. Next, the patient is asked to contract the anal canal, followed by evacuation of the contrast. This entire event is recorded and radiographs are taken during "rest," "squeeze," and "push" maneuvers.

Once a definitive causative diagnosis is obtained, specific medical or surgical treatment may be considered, as discussed elsewhere in this textbook. However, this can be summarized as follows:

Rectocele: Surgical repair is recommended for patients who have significant constipation including a sensation of incomplete evacuation, digital evacuation, and protrusion of the posterior vaginal wall during evacuation. These rectoceles are usually radiologically larger than 3 cm and do not completely empty during evacuation.

Paradoxical contraction of the puborectalis muscle: Surgery is usually associated with a high incidence of fecal incontinence as division of the puborectlis muscle is performed (33). A new medical approach has been recently proposed with injection of botulinum toxin into the puborectalis muscle, prompting temporary relaxation (34). However, long-term follow-up is necessary to clarify the efficacy of this method. Biofeedback therapy (35,36) includes six to eight sessions of a retraining program in which the patient learns (or relearns) to contract and relax the pelvic floor muscles under audiovisual assistance. The technique of biofeedback as well as its results, is described in greater detail elsewhere in this textbook.

Treatment

Chronic constipation with megacolon usually requires a multidisciplinary approach, including a gastroenterologist, nutritionist/dietitian, psychiatrist, and possibly a surgeon.

A recommended regimen for chronic megacolon in a stable patient is as follows.

Consume bulking agents/bowel agents (30–35 gm daily of insoluble fiber): Patients with acquired, nonacute megacolon should follow a high-fiber diet, which usually helps to improve symptoms of constipation. A wide variety of over-the-counter agents are available for this purpose and typically contain psyllium husk or cellulose; each patient may respond differently to each agent. Some patients with severe constipation state that a high-fiber diet produces greater difficulty with constipation or worsening of abdominal bloating. Exacerbation of constipation usually occurs in patients who, despite a high-fiber diet, still have a low fluid intake, which is also an essential measure. A minimum of 2 L to 3 L of nonalcoholic or noncaffeinated beverages per day is recommended. Laxatives may be considered and continued if deemed helpful. The best laxatives for this purpose are osmotic agents such as magnesium salts, sorbitol, or lactulose (the latter two agents may increase flatulence). Patients should be encouraged to ingest sufficient amounts to produce a result. Physical activity is also important; besides increasing the strength of the accessory muscles of evacuation—the abdominal wall muscles—exercise can have a great psychosocial effect on these patients. Stimulant laxatives are best left as a last resort because they may induce difficult colonic evacuation. Typical stimulant laxatives are senna- and bisacodyl-containing medications. Many patients use "natural herbal" laxatives; these agents typically contain cascara sagrada (Table 3). Chronic catharctic laxative abuse is associated with a high incidence of melanosi coli, drug dependence, and megacolon.

Progressively alter and/or individualize the fiber and fluid intake regimen: A drastic and sudden change in dietary habits is usually an unsuccessful measure because patient adherence to this regimen is very low. Multifactorial abnormalities, such as psychological disorders, past history of sexual abuse, depression, a stressful lifestyle, and food intake disorders are commonly associated with constipation.

Surgical Treatment

Surgery is usually recommended if dilatation is persistent or worsened despite employment of all of the above medical measures (37–45). Segmental colectomy has been recommended as a

Table 3 Classification of Laxative Drugs

Mechanism	Agent
Bulk agents	Methylcellulose, carboxymethylcellulose plantago psyllium, *Plantago ovata*, agar, wheat flour
Emollients or surfactants	Sodium docusate
Lubricants	Mineral oil, glycerine, liquid paraffin
Saline solutions	Magnesium hydroxate, magnesium sulphate, sodium sulphate
Contact stimulant agents	Cascara sagrada, senna, aloes, fenolftalein, bisacodil, sodium picosulphate, castor oil, monobasic sodium phosphate
Osmotic agents	Lactulose, polyethyleneglycol, mannitol 10–20%, macrogol 3350
Prokinetics	Cisapride, prostigmine, physiostigmine, tegaserode

surgical treatment for patients with segmental delayed transit time. However, highly disappointing outcomes have been reported (46).

Total abdominal colectomy with ileorectal anastomosis is the operation of choice for megacolon with a normal-sized rectum (38), while total proctocolectomy with ileostomy and total proctocolectomy with ileoanal anastomosis may be recommended for those patients with associated megarectum (47).

Functional disorders of the digestive tract are very common. Associated functional disorders in the same patient, with similar clinical features, make precise diagnosis challenging for the specialist. IBS with symptoms of constipation may be confused with colonic inertia, or even with functional constipation. More importantly, they are eventually associated with IMC as a consequence of chronic constipation. An accurate definition of the initial cause of symptoms is essential to achieve good therapeutical results. For instance, IMC associated with IBS is usually associated with a poor surgical result; despite normalization of bowel habits, chronic debilitating abdominal pain remains in the majority of the patients, while others may present with diarrhea (48).

Complications

Fortunately, free perforation rarely occurs. Perforation is generally due to overdistension of the bowel or stercoral ulcers. If the etiology is overdistension, cecal perforation typically occurs. Stercoral ulcers typically occur in the sigmoid/rectosigmoid region.

Prognosis

Prognosis is related to the severity of the megacolon and to the severity of the patient's comorbid diseases. While some patients cannot be managed on any type of bowel program and require immediate surgery, other patients may be successfully maintained on a strict bowel regimen. However, no detailed longitudinal studies have been performed to assess strict prognostic associations or indicators. Patient education with regard to a strict bowel program is essential to management. Maintaining effective management requires extensive effort and discipline on the part of both the health-care provider and the patient. To this end, educating the patient about the entire process is crucial.

REFERENCES

1. Status of Chagas' disease in the region of the Américas. Epidemiol Bull 1984; 5(2):5–9.
2. WHO. Control of Chagas' disease. Report of a WHO expert committee, Geneva WHO technical report series 1991; 811:95.
3. Schmunis GA. Chagas' disease and blood transfusion. In: Dodd RY, Barker LE, ed. Infection Immunity and Blood Transfusion. New York: Alan R. Liss Inc., 1985:127–145.
4. de Rezende JM de, Moreira H. Chagasic megaesophagus and megacolon. Historical review and present concepts. Arq Gastroenterolog São Paulo 1988; 25(special issue)32:43.
5. Koeberle F. Patologia y anatomia patológica de la enfermedad de Chagas. Bol Sanit Panam 1988; 51:404.
6. Habr-Gama A. Motilidade do colon sigmoide e reto (contribuição a fisiopatologia do megacolo chagásico). Thesis, Faculty of Medicine, University of São Paulo, 1996.
7. Moreira H. Estudo eletromanométrico da atividade motora do coto retal e do colo descendente em pacientes chagásicos submetidos as operações de Hartmann e de Duhamel. Revista Goiana Méd 1974; 20:125.

8. Moreira H. Tratamento cirúrgico do volvulo de sigmóide no megacolo chagásico. Revista Goiana Méd 1979; 778:73–76.
9. de Freitas JLP. Contribuição para o estudo do diagnóstico da moléstia de Chagas por processos de laboratório. Thesis, Faculty of medicine, University of São Paulo, 1947.
10. Habr-Gama A, Costa Curta L, Raia A. Anatomia e fisiologia do esfíncter interno do ânus. Ver Bras Coloproctologia 1970; 3:21.
11. Haddad J. Tratamento do megacolo adquirido pelo abaixamento retro-retal do colo com colostomia perineal (operação de Duhamel modificada). Revista Hosp Clin Fac Méd São Paulo 1968; 23(5):235–253.
12. Cardoso AA. A retossigmoidectomia no tratamento do megacolon chagásico. Revista Goiana Méd 1959; 5:103.
13. Lins Neto MAF. Operação de Duhamel modificada com anastomose colorretal imediata para o tratamento do megacolon chagásico. Thesis, Faculty of Medicine, University of São Paulo, 1997.
14. Hirschsprung H. Stuhltragheit neugeborener in folge von dilatation und hypertrophie des colons. Jahrb Kinderh 1887; 27:1.
15. Kleinhaus S, Baley SJ, Sheran M, Sieber WK. Hirschsprung's disease—a survey of members of the Surgical Section of the American Academy of Pedeatrics. J Pediatr Surg 1979; 14:588–597.
16. Gabriel SB, Salomon R, Pelet A, et al. Segregation at three loci explains familial and population risk in Hirschsprung's disease. Nat Genet 2002; 31:89–93.
17. Briner J, Oswald HW, Hirsig J. Neuronal intestinal displasia – clinical and histochemical findings and its association with Hirschsprung's disease. Z Kinderchir 1986; 41:282.
18. Lanna Sobrinho JMD, Tatsuo ES, Lanna JCBD. Anomalias congênitas dos intestinos. In: Dani R, Castro LP, eds. Gastroenterologia Clínica Vol. 1. 3rd ed. Rio de Janeiro: Guanabara Koogan 1993:663–673.
19. Callaghan RP, Nixon HH. Megarectum: physiological observations. Arch Dis Child 1964; 39:153–157.
20. Swenson O, Neuhauser EBD, Pickett LK. New consepts of etiology, diagnosis and treatment of congenital megacolon. Pediatrics 1949; 4:201.
21. Soave F. Hirschsprung's disease: a new surgical technique. Arch Dis Child 1964; 39:116.
22. Matin LW. Surgical treatment of total colonic aganglionosis. Ann Surg 1972; 176:343.
23. Duhamel B. Une nouvelle operation pour le megacolon congenital: rabaissement retro-rectal et trananal du colon te son application possible au traitement de quelques autres malformations. Presse Med 1956; 64:2249–2250.
24. Sellin J, Shelat H. Short-chain fatty acid (SCFA) volume regulation in proximal and distal rabbit colon is different. J Membr Biol 1996; 150:83–88.
25. Holzer P. Opioids and opioids receptors in the enteric nervous system: from a problem in opioid analgesia to a possible new prokinetic therapy in humans. Neurosci Lett 2004; 361(1–3):192–195.
26. Shet SG, La Mont JT. Toxic megacolon. Lancet 1998; 351:509.
27. Bagnol D, Herbrecht F, Jule Y, Jarry T, Cupo A. Changes in enkephalin immunoreactivity of sympathetic ganglia and digestive tract of the cat after splanchnic nerve ligation. Regul Pept 1993; 47(3):259–273.
28. Dyer NH, Dawson AM, Smith BF, Tood IP. Obstruction of bowel due to lesion in the myenteric plexus. Br Med J 1969; 1:686–689.
29. Smith B, Grace RH, Tood IP. Organic constipation in adults. Br J Surg 1977; 64:313–314.
30. Schuffler MD, Jonak Z. Chronic idiopathic pseudo-obstruction caused by a degenerative disorder of the myenteric plexus: the use of Smith's method to define the neuropathology. Gastroenterology 1982; 82:476–486.
31. Gatuso JM, Kamm MA, Abassi M, Talbot IC. First description of the pathology of idiopathic megarectum and megacolon. Gut 1993; 34:S49.
32. Farouk R, Duthie GS, Bartolo DCC. Functional anorectal disorders and physiological evaluation. In: Beck DE, Wexner SD, eds. Fundamentals of Anorectal Surgery. New York: McGraw-Hill, Inc., 1992.
33. Pinho M, Yoshioka K, Keighley MRB. Long-term resultscof anorectal myectomy for chronic constipation. Br J Surg 1989; 76:1163–1164.
34. Hallan RI, Williams NS, Melling J, Waldron DJ, Womack NR, Morison JF. Treatment of anismus intractable constipation with botulinum A toxin. Lancet 1988; 2:714–717.
35. Wexner SD, Cheape JD, Jorge JM, et al. Prospective assessment of biofeedback for the treatment of paradoxical puborectalis contraction. Dis Colon Rectum 1992; 35:145–150.
36. Glliland R, Heymen S, Altomare DF, Park UC, Vickers D, Wexner SD. Outcome and predictors of success of biofeedback for constipation. Br J Surg 1997; 84:1123–1126.
37. Correa Neto A. Tratamento cirúrgico do megacolon pela ressecção dos esfíncteres funcionais do colon. Revista de Cir de SP 1934; 1:249.
38. Correa Neto A. Megacolon. Revista Assoc Méd Bras 1955; 1(4):353.
39. Celso NM. Tratamento do megacolon adquirido pela anorretomiectomia. Revista Assoc Méd Minas Gerais 1962; 13:139–146.
40. Vasconcelos E. Nova técnica de abaixamento do colon sem sutura no megacolo. Revista do Hosp das Clinicas Fac Méd S Paulo 1961; 16:355.
41. Almeida AD. Sigmoidectomia abdominal no tratamento do megacolon. Revista Paul Méd 1963; 62:349.
42. Vasconcelos E. Colectomia subtotal e anastomose ceco-retal no tratamento do megacolo do adulto. Revista Hosp Clin Fac Méd S Paulo 1964; 19:321.

43. Cutait DE, Figlioni FJ. Megacolon adquirido: nova técnica de anastomose colorretal na retossigmoi-dectomia abdomino-perineal. Revista Paulista de Méd 1962; 60:447.
44. Haddad J, Raia A, Correa Neto A. Abaixamento retro-retal do colon com colostomia perineal no tra-tamento do megacolon adquirido. Operação de Duhamel modificada. Revista da Ass Méd Bras 1965; 11:83–88.
45. Moreira H, Rezende JM, Sebba F, Azevedo IF, Leite ACA, Soares EP. Chagasic Megacolon. Coloproc-tology 1985; 5:260–266.
46. Wexner SD, Moreira H Jr. Surgical management of constipation. In: Cameron JL, ed. Current Surgical Therapy. St Louis: Mosby, 1998.
47. Stabile G, Kamm MA, Hawley PR. Colectomy for idiopathic megarectum and megacolon. Gut 1991; 32(12):1538–1540.
48. Nicholls RJ, Kamm MA. Proctocolectomy with restorative ileoanal reservoir for severe idiopathic con-stipation. Report of two cases. Dis Colon Rectum 1988; 31(12):968–969.
49. Verne GN, Hocking MP, Davis RH, et al. Long-term response to sub-total colectomy in colonic inertia. J Gastrointest Surg 2002; 6(5):738–744.

21 | Pseudo-Obstruction (Ogilvie's), Cathartic Colon–Laxative Abuse, and Melanosis

Laura Gladstone
Division of Colon and Rectal Surgery, Swedish Medical Center, Seattle, Washington, U.S.A.

Mitchell Bernstein
Division of Colon and Rectal Surgery, College of Physicians and Surgeons, Columbia University, and Anorectal Physiology Laboratory and The Continence Center, St. Luke's/Roosevelt Hospital Center, New York, New York, U.S.A.

Alex Teixeira
Department of Gastroenterology, Brockton Hospital, Brockton, Massachusetts, U.S.A.

Arthur Harris
Division of Gastroenterology and Hepatology, Weill Medical College at Cornell University, New York, New York, U.S.A.

ACUTE COLONIC PSEUDO-OBSTRUCTION

Pseudo-obstruction of the colon, characterized by colonic ileus with extreme dilatation of the right colon and cecum in the absence of mechanical obstruction, was first recognized as a clinical entity in 1948. The English surgeon Sir W. Heneage Ogilvie reported two such cases and proposed a pathophysiologic mechanism of the disorder. Previously, the medical literature had only made note of a similar functional occlusion of the small intestine, first described in 1896 as "spastic ileus" (1). In a paper entitled "Large-Intestine Colic Due to Sympathetic Deprivation," Ogilvie described two patients with colicky abdominal pain, distention, and constipation who, despite normal barium enemas, had symptoms of colonic obstruction, which were so convincing that both were taken to surgery. In the operating room, both patients were found to have normal colons with malignant infiltration of the subdiaphragmatic sympathetic plexus. From this finding, he surmised that interruption of the sympathetic supply to the colon left parasympathetic innervation from sacral nerves unopposed (2). The term "intestinal pseudo-obstruction" was first used to describe this condition in 1958 (3). Current consensus is that colonic ileus caused by malignant infiltration of the celiac plexus as reported by Ogilvie, along with various syndromes described throughout the medical literature including "idiopathic large-bowel obstruction," "false colonic obstruction," "pseudo-obstruction of the colon," "colonic ileus," "idiopathic nontoxic megacolon," and "nonobstructive colonic dilatation" are all examples of the broader disorder now referred to as "acute colonic pseudo-obstruction" (ACPO) (1,4–6).

PRESENTATION AND ETIOLOGY

The true incidence of ACPO is not known, most likely because it can go unnoticed and spontaneously resolve. Most attempts to quantify the incidence of ACPO have been retrospective reviews and, because the vast majority of cases of colonic pseudo-obstruction are considered a complication of the primary diagnosis, it may be underreported or missed in a retrospective chart review. Often ACPO is not clinically recognized until massive abdominal distention occurs (7). A study of patients in a New Zealand hospital over a nine-year period revealed that 10.6% of patients treated for colonic obstruction fit the criteria of ACPO (8). In addition, mild cases can be mistaken for simple constipation and treated with enemas, often with resolution as an outpatient.

The hallmark feature of colonic pseudo-obstruction is a nontender yet markedly distended, tympanic abdomen. This distention can be accompanied by a myriad of signs and symptoms including crampy abdominal pain, nausea, vomiting, constipation or decreased stool and flatus, and diarrhea (1,3,8–11). On physical examination, bowel sounds can be normal, increased or decreased, but rarely absent. Rectal examination usually reveals absence of stool. Tenderness is typically absent and should be a cause of concern because it develops in up to 87% of patients with ischemic or perforated bowel. Tenderness in the right iliac fossa is most concerning for incipient cecal perforation, with diffuse tenderness suspicious for perforation and peritonitis. Fever occurs in 37% of patients, more commonly when ischemia or perforation is present. Leukocytosis is present in 27% of those without as opposed to up to 100% of patients with ischemia or perforation (3,11). The diagnosis of ACPO is usually confirmed by plain abdominal radiograph showing a markedly dilated colon, with a cecal diameter greater than 9 cm.

The patient population prone to developing ACPO is diverse, and demographic data vary widely depending on the population studied. The first cases described by Ogilvie were older male patients with retroperitoneal tumors. Many of the cases subsequently described in the literature were those of young women who were postpartum from either normal vaginal or cesarian delivery. Since those early reports, ACPO has been linked to a wide variety of medical conditions, surgical procedures, and medications (Table 1). About 56% to 65% of ACPO patients have sustained trauma or undergone a surgical procedure, notably orthopedic surgery, pelvic surgery, renal transplants, and cardiac surgery (10,12–14). Medical conditions such as chronic obstructive pulmonary disease (COPD), sepsis, renal failure, metabolic and electrolyte derangements, chronic bed rest, or a generally debilitated condition have also been associated with ACPO (Table 1). Greater than three-quarters of patients will have more than one identifiable risk factor, but on rare occasions, no identifiable cause can be found, and the ACPO is considered idiopathic (1,3,4,6,10–12) ACPO occurs more frequently in males, with an incidence of 1.5 to 3 times higher in males than that in females (7,8,10,11,13,15). ACPO occurs over a broad age range with an overall average age in the sixth to seventh decade; however, the average age of women with ACPO is slightly less than that of men due to the development of ACPO after obstetrical procedures (5,6,10–13,15,16).

PATHOPHYSIOLOGY

Colonic motility depends on a delicate balance between sympathetic and parasympathetic activity. Parasympathetic stimulation is excitatory and results in increased colonic contractility and motility, whereas sympathetic stimulation results in inhibition of muscle contraction with contraction of sphincters. The parasympathetic nerve supply to the colon

Table 1 Medical Conditions, Surgical Procedures, and Medications Associated with Acute Colonic Pseudo-Obstruction

Medical conditions	Surgical Procedures	Medications
Normal vaginal delivery	Abdominal surgery	Tricyclic antidepressants
Burns/trauma	Pelvic surgery:	Calcium channel blockers
Retroperitoneal disease	Urologic	Clonidine
MI/CHF	Gynecologic	Theophylline
Sepsis	Caesarian section	Chemotherapy
Neurologic disease/stroke	Renal transplant	Narcotics
Uremia/renal failure	Cardiac surgery	Benzodiazepines
Liver failure	Spinal surgery	Digoxin
Electrolyte imbalance	Joint surgery	Phenothiazines
Pneumonia	Neurosurgery	
COPD/respiratory failure	Peripheral vascular surgery	
Malignancy		
Herpes Zoster virus		
Alcohol abuse		
Diabetes		

Abbreviations: COPD, chronic obstructive pulmonary disease; MI, myocardial infarction; CHF, congestive heart failure.

is mostly from the vagus nerve, with the distal colon supplied by nerves from sacral segments S2 to S4. Parasympathetic fibers synapse with nerve cells in the enteric plexus to increase or decrease activity but do not directly initiate muscular activity themselves. Sympathetic stimulation to the proximal large bowel comes from the superior mesenteric plexus, and the distal colon receives input from fibers of the upper and lower divisions of the hypogastric plexus (1).

In his original 1948 paper, Ogilvie suggested that sympathetic deprivation caused unopposed parasympathetic stimulation leading to excessive and uncoordinated contraction resulting in functional obstruction (2). This theory is no longer popular. While it is still theorized that ACPO is caused by a disruption between sympathetic and parasympathetic stimulation, it is more commonly believed that the deprivation is in the parasympathetic supply to the colon, by excessive sympathetic stimulation, impairment of sacral parasympathetic outflow, or imbalance between proximal and distal parasympathetic signals (1,10). Currently, the most widely accepted theory is that ACPO is caused by a derangement of sacral parasympathetic pathways with impairment of distal colon motility. With increased tone of the distal colon, a functional obstruction could clinically mimic a mechanical obstruction. This is well illustrated by the classic abdominal radiograph showing a markedly distended right colon with a "cutoff" at the splenic flexure, the transition zone between vagal and sacral parasympathetic supplies (1,10,17). Strong support for the suppression of parasympathetic input to the colon as the central event underlying ACPO also comes from the success of neostigmine therapy in the treatment of the disorder (18). Animal studies have identified mechano-receptors in the colonic wall, which, when stimulated, activate a reflex arc involving colonic afferent pathways and efferent nerves from the sympathetic prevertebral ganglia resulting in the inhibition of motor activity in the large bowel. If such a colocolonic reflex were present in the human colon, this would explain the cycle of progressive and maintained colonic distension, which characterizes pseudo-obstruction (3,17). Histological studies of autopsy and surgical specimens of colon in patients diagnosed with ACPO have revealed no structural abnormality in the nerves or smooth muscle (5,17).

Colonic dilatation is accompanied by an increased risk of perforation. While the entire colon can be dilated with pseudo-obstruction, the cecum has the highest risk of rupture based on the Law of LaPlace, $T = \pi dP$ (T = tension, d = diameter, P = intraluminal pressure). This law predicts that at a fixed pressure in a cylinder, wall tension is highest where the diameter is greatest (19,20). At larger diameters, progressively smaller increases in volume markedly increase wall tension primarily affecting the serosa. This increase in wall tension also causes gradual cessation of lymphatic, venous, and finally arterial circulation, resulting in early mucosal ischemia most often involving the antimesenteric side (20,21). Thus, perforation occurs from both "outside-in" and "inside-out." The pathophysiology of colonic perforation was demonstrated in one study in which the intraluminal pressures required to damage human cadaver colons was investigated. The authors observed cecal rupture at pressures that were half of those tolerated by the sigmoid, thereby validating the Law of LaPlace. Air insufflation under high pressure caused serosal and superficial muscle tears followed by mucosal disruption. Serosal tears were usually linear, often beginning in and following the course of the teniae coli, located on the antimesenteric side of the colon. Areas of pneumatosis with air blebs dissecting into the mesentery usually developed after serosal splitting, but before tearing of the outer and inner muscular layers and actual mucosal rupture (22).

DIAGNOSIS

Once the diagnosis of ACPO is suggested by the history and physical examination, plain abdominal radiographs are the most useful initial test. Marked dilatation of the proximal colon with distal collapse is seen. The classic X ray of a patient with ACPO shows an air-filled cecum measuring nine or more centimeters, often with a clear cutoff at the splenic flexure or along the descending colon (Figs. 1 and 2). About 9 cm is generally accepted as the upper limit of normal cecal size based on a 1956 study of barium enemas in which 97% of normal patients had a cecal diameter of less than 9 cm (1,19). Upright or decubitus films must be obtained to evaluate for free air due to perforation, although pneumoperitoneum may not be visible if a pinhole

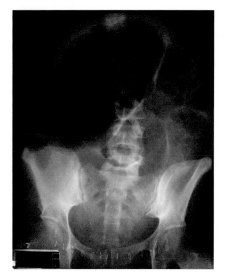

Figure 1 Supine view of a 37-year-old woman five days after cesarian section with a disproportionately large cecum and air-fluid levels.

perforation has rapidly sealed. Distended loops of small bowel are sometimes seen, and the colon is predominantly filled with air and minimal fluid; thus air–fluid levels are rare. The haustral and mucosal pattern of the colon is maintained with well-defined septa and a smooth inner colonic contour (Figs. 3 and 4) (3,11). In one large series, the mean initial cecal diameter at the time of diagnosis was 13.1 cm. Patients with viable bowel had an average cecal diameter of 12.9 cm, and those who were subsequently diagnosed with ischemia or perforation presented with a cecal diameter of 15.9 cm. Patients with pneumoperitoneum on their initial film had an average cecal diameter of 10.3 cm, suggesting spontaneous sealing of micro-perforations precluding complete decompression (11).

The diagnosis of ACPO is necessarily one of exclusion. Once the diagnosis is suggested by plain radiographs without evidence of peritonitis, mechanical bowel obstruction must be ruled out. Malignancy, colonic volvulus, and fecal impaction are high in the differential diagnosis. A contrast enema is the study of choice in this setting. This can either confirm the diagnosis of ACPO or reveal the site of a mechanical obstruction. Water-soluble contrast is recommended over barium in case a perforation is present or occurs during administration. The study can be preceded by proctosigmoidoscopy to exclude an obstructing rectal cancer (3). While primarily diagnostic, contrast enema can also be therapeutic as the hyperosmolality of

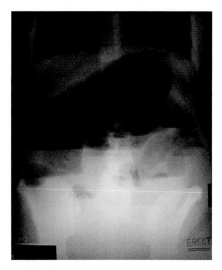

Figure 2 Upright view of a 37-year-old woman five days after cesarian section with a disproportionately large cecum and air-fluid levels.

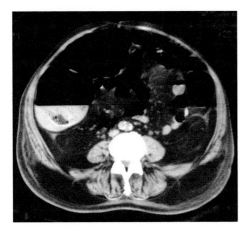

Figure 3 Computed tomography scan of an 87-year-old man who developed acute colonic pseudo-obstruction after repair of a broken hip.

water-soluble contrast increases water content and bulk volume of stool, which decreases intestinal transit time by promoting bulk flow. Reflex peristalsis can occur after distention of the colon with contrast, and rectal contraction can be stimulated by its hyperosmotic and irritant properties, treating the condition as it is diagnosed (23). The risk of perforation from contrast enema is approximately 1% (11). If the results of contrast enema are equivocal, colonoscopy should be performed in order to satisfactorily rule out mechanical obstruction. Contrast enema has traditionally been performed preferentially over colonoscopy, as it is often easier to obtain acutely, is less costly, and is simpler and safer to perform in patients with unprepped colons.

TREATMENT AND OUTCOMES
Conservative Management

Historically, ACPO was treated expectantly, with surgery reserved for patients who failed conservative management. More recently, however, invasive treatment has moved away from operative intervention as other modalities of therapy have been developed. Most patients have an initial period of conservative or expectant management subsequent to diagnosis. This consists of restriction of oral intake, gentle enemas, treatment of metabolic derangements or other inciting factors, a decrease in or cessation of narcotic administration, and, occasionally, a nasogastric and/or rectal tube (Fig. 5) (3,9,11,13). Frequent serial abdominal exams are required to evaluate for change in abdominal pain, tenderness, or distention, and plain

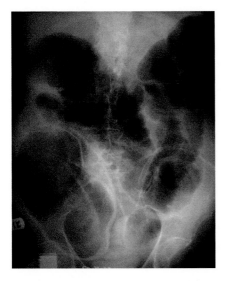

Figure 4 An 82-year-old woman admitted with abdominal distention found to have gynecologic cancer. The radiograph shows cecal dilation and an air-filled colon with a maintained haustral pattern and smooth inner contour along with distended small bowel.

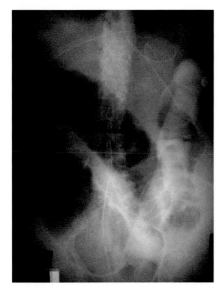

Figure 5   Patient in Figure 4 with nasogastric and rectal tubes with small amount of improvement in cecal dilation.

abdominal radiographs are recommended every 12 to 24 hours to evaluate for further increase in cecal diameter (11). Patients often improve with simple observation and restriction of oral intake, usually within two to six days (8,9,11). However, patients with ACPO will often relapse after an initial period of improvement, with an overall success rate of 53% with conservative therapy alone (12).

Cecal perforation is the main complication in patients with ACPO (Fig. 6). Studies done prior to the advent of aggressive endoscopic and pharmacologic management found cecal perforation rates with observation alone to range from 14% to 40% (3,11,12,24). It is unclear whether the primary predictor of cecal perforation is the size or duration of the cecal distention. In a large review, 13% of patients with ACPO developed perforations or ischemia, none of whom had a cecal diameter less than 12 cm. However, 7% of patients with a cecal diameter of 12 to 14 cm developed compromised bowel, as did 23% of those with a cecum measuring greater than 14 cm (11). There is also evidence to support a relationship between perforation and duration of colonic distention in a retrospective study showing that patients with perforations had an average of five days of cecal distention as opposed to two days in those who did not, with cecal diameters of 15 and 14 cm, respectively (25). While most deaths in patients with ACPO are due to underlying illness in generally debilitated patients, perforation of

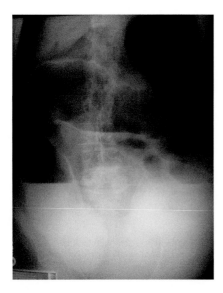

Figure 6   Patient in Figures 4 and 5 after perforation with massive amount of free air.

the cecum causes mortality rates to sharply increase from 10% to 15% to 40% to 50%, correlating with patient age as well as cecal diameter and delay of decompression (3,4,11,20,24). Patients over 60 years of age with ACPO are four times more likely to die than patients under age 40. Mortality in patients with a cecal diameter of greater than 14 cm is double that of patients with a cecum that measures 14 cm or less; patients who undergo decompression at sooner than four days have a mortality almost half that of those who remain distended for four to seven days, and five times less than those with a delay in decompression of greater than seven days (11). Therefore, if a patient demonstrates no significant improvement after 48 to 72 hours, conservative treatment should be abandoned for mechanical or pharmacologic decompression.

Endoscopic Management

Prior to 1977, operative decompression by surgical cecostomy was routinely performed when the patient's cecal diameter reached 12 cm because the risk of perforation and subsequent mortality rate were high. In 1977, Kukora and Dent reported the first series of ACPO patients successfully treated with endoscopic decompression (26). Their work was based on the first report of a successful reduction of a sigmoid volvulus using a fiberoptic scope one year prior.

Colonoscopy in patients with ACPO is often difficult to perform due to retained stool and the possibility of worsening distension caused by insufflation and irrigation. Gentle saline enemas can be administered to improve visibility, and carbon dioxide is often used as the insufflating agent as its rapid absorption minimizes additional distention and acts as a vasodilator to increase mucosal blood flow (3,10). Colonoscopic complications, mainly perforation, occur on average in 3% of patients, with a mortality rate of 1% (5,10,11,13,15,19). These rates reflect the complexity of performing therapeutic colonoscopy in a patient with pseudo-obstruction compared to diagnostic colonoscopy with accepted complication and mortality rates of 0.2% and 0.06%, respectively (27).

While endoscopic decompression is often successful initially, colonic distention frequently recurs, sometimes acutely. Rates of success following initial colonoscopy range from 61% to 100% (average 83%) with recurrence in up to 65% (average 23%). The average time for recurrent significant distention after colonoscopy is two to four days. Serial decompressions are performed in up to one-third of patients. There are no identified clinical predictors for failure of endoscopy and no correlation between initial and sustained success. It is clear, however, that success rates decrease and recurrence rates increase with each subsequent endoscopic procedure. Ultimate success rates with endoscopic decompression range from 73% to 90%. Surgical intervention is required in 10% to 20% of patients due to repeated failure to decompress or identification of ischemia during endoscopy (3,5,9–13,15). Ischemia is observed in 7% to 14% of patients undergoing colonoscopy for ACPO (13,19,20).

Successful endoscopic decompression is defined as a decrease in or resolution of abdominal distention and related symptoms, as well as a decrease in cecal diameter on follow-up abdominal film; both are related to achieving proximity to the cecum during colonoscopy. Endoscopy is almost twice as likely to be successful if the cecum or ascending colon is reached than if the hepatic flexure is not passed (10). There is an average decrease of 37% in cecal diameter when the cecum is reached with the endoscope as opposed to a 23% decrease when the colonoscope only reaches the transverse colon. A decrease in cecal diameter of just 15% occurs when only the splenic flexure is reached (15). Initial cecal size may be a predictor of successful decompression. One study found that of the patients who were successfully decompressed, recurrence occurred in those with a larger cecal diameter at the onset (10). Often, a markedly improved physical exam and resolution of symptoms are typically accompanied by a small change in cecal diameter on X ray of 2 to 4 cm, still potentially leaving the cecum in excess of 9 cm. LaPlace's Law accounts for the fact that a significant clinical improvement accompanies a small radiological change; a small decrease in diameter provides a significant decrease in intraluminal pressure (5,13,28).

The placement of a long intestinal tube during colonoscopy can provide prolonged decompression. Techniques for employing these tubes include passage over a guide wire or piggybacking a tube to the colonoscope with a snare. Placement and position of the tube can be confirmed with a supine abdominal X ray. The tube should be maintained on low intermittent suction and flushed with saline to maintain patency (13,29). Results with decompression tubes are varied, with some studies showing no difference with or without tube placement while others demonstrate improved rates of successful decompression. In a small group of patients undergoing multiple decompression procedures, 90% of patients were successfully decompressed when the tube was placed in the cecum or ascending colon. Eighty-three percent of patients were successfully decompressed when the decompression tube was placed in the transverse colon. Success rates dropped to only 60% with tubes left in the splenic flexure and descending colon. This suggests that colonoscopy could be terminated in the transverse colon if a decompression tube is placed, decreasing the risk of a prolonged and difficult colonoscopic procedure (13).

Pharmacological Management

Neostigmine is among the latest in the pharmacologic armamentarium for the treatment of ACPO. Neostigmine is a parasympathomimetic that competes with acetylcholine for attachment to acetylcholinesterase at sites of cholinergic transmission. This increases the availability of acetylcholine by inhibiting its hydrolysis, thereby theoretically restoring peristalsis. Neostigmine undergoes hydrolysis by cholinesterase and is also metabolized by microsomal enzymes in the liver (7,17,24). The successful treatment of ACPO with neostigmine lends support to the hypothesis that ACPO is related to deficient parasympathetic transmission. In addition, the use of neostigmine reflects a shift in the therapeutic treatment of ACPO. Endoscopic decompression "passively" treats the symptom (colonic distention) by removing the air from within the colon that is often a temporizing measure. Conversely, neostigmine is believed to have a direct therapeutic effect on the bowel itself, which results in resolution of symptoms.

The first work with parasympathomimetic anticholinesterases is often credited to Bernard Catchpole and Julian Neely in 1969 and 1971, respectively. They wrote extensively on the pathophysiology of ileus and described case reports in which they administered physiostigmine, first used for ileus in 1904, and neostigmine, which was introduced in 1931 with successful resolution of ileus (30). The success of these early experiments was duplicated in 1992 by Hutchinson and Griffiths (31). They treated a series of patients with colonic pseudo-obstruction with a regimen of 20 mg of intravenous (IV) guanethidine, an adrenergic blocker, followed by 2.5 mg of neostigmine over one minute with insertion of a rectal tube. Their initial results were favorable, with 8 of 11 patients showing clinical improvement with passage of flatus and decreased distention within 10 minutes. Passage of flatus and decreased abdominal distention were noted to occur only after the administration of neostigmine, with no significant response during guanethidine infusion. Similar success was seen in a subsequent study using neostigmine alone (32,33). This supports the theory of parasympathetic suppression rather than overactive sympathetic activity as the mechanism of ACPO.

Numerous studies performed since then have confirmed the effectiveness of neostigmine therapy in the treatment of ACPO. The doses administered range from 2 to 2.5 mg given in either concentrated or diluted form over 1 to 60 minutes. Some studies included the placement of rectal tubes, and cardiac monitoring is always recommended (7,14,18,24,34). Results have been very favorable, with better results in patients who receive a concentrated dose IV push. When 2.5 mg of neostigmine diluted in 100 mL is administered over one hour, initial success averages 75% with an overall success of 82% after repeated administrations. Patients first begin passing flatus within 20 minutes to three to four hours with this regimen (7,14). In patients who receive the 2.5 mg of neostigmine pushed over 1 to 3 minutes, time to pass flatus ranges from 30 seconds to 20 minutes, with immediate relief in 86% to 94% of patients and sustained response in up to 100% of patients (16,18,24,33,34). Use of neostigmine is contraindicated in patients taking beta blockers, those with acidosis, or those with recent myocardial infarction due to an increased risk of dysrhythmias. Adverse reactions to neostigmine therapy include transient bradycardia (atropine should be readily available), abdominal pain, nausea, lightheadedness, and sweating; no deaths have been attributed to the use of neostigmine (7,14,17,18,24,33,34). The incidence of significant bradycardia may be decreased or eliminated with the slow bolus technique of infusion, but may diminish its effectiveness. A second dose of neostigmine can be administered within one hour if no immediate response occurs (16,17). The change in cecal diameter after neostigmine therapy has been shown to be greater than that seen with endoscopic decompression, with a mean decrease of 4.8 cm (16). After decompression, patients require continued serial exams and radiographs to observe for recurrence. As patients continue to pass flatus and stool, they can be cautiously returned to a diet.

Neostigmine is the only pharmacologic agent indicated for the primary treatment of ACPO. Cisapride, a 5-Hydroxytryptamine-4 (5-HT$_4$) receptor agonist that can induce colonic contraction by enhancing the release of acetylcholine in the myenteric plexus of the gut wall, erythromycin, a macrolide antibiotic that binds to motilin receptors with prokinetic properties in the upper gut, and octreotide, a somatostatin analogue that promotes the migrating motor complex, as well as Reglan, naloxone, beta blockers, and epidural anesthesia have not reliably shown to be effective (3,13,17,23,24). Oral neostigmine or pyridostigmine is being investigated for maintenance therapy after successful pharmacologic decompression; however, early reports have been largely anecdotal.

Surgical Management

Prior to the regular use of endoscopic decompression in the management of ACPO, surgical intervention was the standard therapy in patients who failed conservative management. Currently, with routine use of colonoscopy and the use of neostigmine therapy gaining wider acceptance, the number of surgeries performed for ACPO has markedly dropped. The goal of therapy in patients with ACPO is often to avoid any surgical intervention due to the high postoperative morbidity and mortality associated with this patient population.

Nonetheless, there are some indications for surgical intervention in patients with ACPO other than failure of medical and endoscopic management. The development of right lower quadrant tenderness with localized or generalized peritonitis, ischemia or necrosis seen during endoscopic evaluation, or development of free air on plain film during serial radiographic evaluations are all indications for surgery (3,11). In the absence of ischemic or perforated bowel, a tube cecostomy is recommended. This is the simplest procedure to perform and it usually does not require a second surgical procedure for closure. It can be performed through a limited right lower quadrant incision, often using only local anesthesia. If ischemia or perforation is present, a laparotomy should be performed via a vertical midline incision, with the operation dictated by the condition of the bowel. A well-localized area of ischemia or a small perforation in the cecum can be excised and exteriorized, or intubated with a Foley catheter as a formal cecostomy. Extensive necrosis or large perforation requires a right colectomy. The remaining bowel, especially the ascending and transverse colon, should be inspected for signs of ischemia with appropriate management (3,11,20). Immediate anastomosis following right colectomy can be performed on rare occasions; however, fecal contamination or areas of questionable bowel viability often dictate the need for an ileostomy (3,11).

The mortality rate of patients undergoing operative decompression and resection ranges from 30% to 60% (3,11,12,24), which is higher than in conservatively treated patients, and reflects that surgery is often performed because of ischemic or perforated bowel. Mortality directly correlates with bowel viability; there is a 26% mortality rate in patients with viable bowel as opposed to a 44% rate with ischemic bowel. Additionally, morbidity and mortality vary based on the procedure performed. Tube cecostomy has the lowest mortality rate (15%) but highest complication rate (9%), while resection with ileostomy or colostomy reportedly has the highest mortality rate (40%) but the lowest morbidity rate (3%) (11).

In an attempt to minimize the morbidity and mortality of surgical intervention, minimally invasive procedures are being applied to patients with ACPO. Laparoscopic cecostomy has the advantage over an open cecostomy performed through a right lower quadrant incision in that the entire colon can be assessed for viability. Laparoscopic cecostomy is achieved through percutaneous placement of a Foley catheter into the cecum and then anchoring the cecum to the anterior abdominal wall with T-fasteners. Alternatively, if the cecum is reached during colonoscopy, a percutaneous endoscopic cecostomy or can be performed (35). Computed tomography (CT)–guided percutaneous decompression of the cecum has also been described via posterior puncture of the retroperitoneal ascending colon (36).

SUMMARY

ACPO has numerous etiologies, all with the presumed pathophysiology of an imbalance between parasympathetic and sympathetic innervation of the colon. Patients require either medical or surgical intervention, vary in age, and often have multiple comorbidities. A suggestive history and physical exam, a dilated right colon or cecum that exceeds 9 cm on plain

Table 2 Treatment of Acute Colonic Pseudo-Obstruction

Conservative	Endoscopic	Pharmacologic	Surgical

NPO
Correct electrolytes
Limit narcotics
Enemas +/− NG or
  rectal tube
Serial exams and X rays
Patient repositioning
Further intervention if no
  improvement in 48–72 hrs
	CO_2 insufflation
	May require serial
	  decompression
	Decompression tube
	  insertion
		2.5 mg neostigmine over
		  1–3 min with cardiac
		  monitoring, atropine
		Can be repeated
		  if needed
			Indications include:
			  Failure of medical and
			    endoscopic
			    management
			  Development of
			    localized or
			    generalized peritonitis
			  Ischemia or necrosis
			    seen during
			    endoscopy
			  Free air on X ray

Abbreviation: NG, nasogastric; NPO, nil per os.

abdominal radiograph, and the absence of mechanical obstruction are sufficient to make a diagnosis of ACPO. Laboratory tests are generally nondiagnostic and nonspecific. If no evidence of ischemia or perforation are present, and distention does not exceed 12 cm, early management entails observation with restriction of oral intake, nasogastric tube decompression, correction of metabolic derangements, withdrawal of inciting medications, serial exams, and at least one set of abdominal X rays per day. If after 48 to 72 hours, no improvement is noted, the patient develops evidence of peritonitis, or if cecal distention progresses, immediate decompression is indicated (Table 2).

While colonoscopy is well established as an effective intervention, it is often merely a temporizing measure. Colonoscopy works by reducing cecal pressure and wall tension through the removal of gas and stool, thereby reducing the likelihood of perforation; however, colonoscopy does not address the underlying etiology of ACPO or offer therapeutic benefit to the colon itself. Serial procedures carry higher failure and recurrence and complication rates. In addition, perforation due to colonoscopy is associated with significant mortality. As well, endoscopic decompression requires sedation and access to appropriate staff and equipment, and can be a source of discomfort to the patient.

Neostigmine therapy has become an accepted, safe means of decompression and is believed to enhance parasympathetic transmission and augment peristaltic activity in the colon. It requires fewer repeat procedures than colonoscopy and carries a lower complication and mortality rate. Basic cardiac monitoring is all that is required. Initial decompression is generally more successful with neostigmine than with endoscopic decompression and is associated with a higher long-term success rate.

With the regular use of neostigmine, the number of patients who have required surgical intervention has decreased, thereby lowering the incidence of morbidity and mortality. Prior to the use of neostigmine, the rate of patients requiring surgery for refractory critical colonic distention was 16%, which has dropped dramatically to 4% in studies where neostigmine was used. With this reduction in operative intervention comes a corresponding decrease in mortality from 24% in the preneostigmine time to just 2% postneostigmine (5–7,10–16,18,24,33,34). Most deaths are attributed to the generally debilitated condition of the typical patient with ACPO and not to colonic pathology, unless ischemia or perforation occurs. Mortality is higher in older patients and those who develop ischemia or perforation, and who experience a delay in decompression. Therefore, if ACPO is recognized early, the patient's physical and X-ray examinations followed closely, and decompression attempted pharmacologically, using neostigmine, colonic distention can be successfully treated in most cases.

CATHARTIC COLON—LAXATIVE ABUSE AND MELANOSIS

Laxatives are widely used in clinical practice and are generally viewed in Western society as harmless or "benign" drugs. In the United States, laxatives are freely available for self-medication (primarily over-the-counter) and it is estimated that 20% to 25% of otherwise healthy Americans spend more than $400 million per year on laxatives (37). If taken on an occasional basis, they usually produce few unwanted or serious side effects. Many factors contribute to the use of these medications, including aging of the population, misconception as to what is normal bowel movement frequency, and fear of the consequences of constipation.

The laxative abuse syndrome can be considered as a type of Munchausen syndrome characterized by frequent or surreptitious abuse of these agents. It is often confused with irritable bowel syndrome, inflammatory bowel disease, or malabsorption syndromes, because symptoms may include diarrhea (sometimes alternating with constipation), vague abdominal pain, nausea, vomiting, and weight loss. Psychiatric disturbances also commonly coexist, particularly eating disorders such as anorexia nervosa and bulimia. Quite often, chronic laxative abuse accompanies severe physical, psychological, social, or even financial problems. Because of the low profile and general social acceptability of these drugs, laxative abuse is often unsuspected and can be extremely difficult to detect.

Patients who abuse laxatives can be classified into two major categories:

Habitual laxative abusers: They are generally middle-aged to elderly people who initially began using laxatives for a variety of reasons including distorted perceptions about normal bowel habits, chronic constipation associated with poor dietary habits, and decreased mobility, or side effects from concomitant drug therapy. These patients are unaware of the harmful effects of laxative abuse and are coaxed into admission only when thoroughly questioned.

Surreptitious laxative abusers: These individuals may be further subdivided into three groups: (i) patients (usually women) with eating disorders due to excessive weight; (ii) young-to-middle-age individuals who often work in medically related fields; and (iii) children who are given laxatives as a form of abuse.

Laxatives fall into five categories according to their mode of action as bulking agents, lubricants, osmotics, stimulant laxatives, and rectal enemas (Table 3).

Side effects related to laxative abuse are numerous and although often related to a specific laxative group, occur across a range of socioeconomic classes. The most frequent gastrointestinal side effects are diarrhea, often alternating with constipation, nausea and vomiting, weight loss, steatorrhea, malabsorption, protein-losing enteropathy, melanosis coli, and cathartic colon. Diarrhea may be profound with up to 20 bowel movements per day. In severe cases, white and red blood cells may be identified in the stool, further complicating the diagnostic process.

Melanosis coli is actually a misnomer that refers to the presence of brown pigment, identified as lipofuscin rather than melanin in the phagosomes (lysosomes) of macrophages in the lamina propia of the large-bowel mucosa. Although initially described by Cruveihier in 1829, Virchow first coined the term "melanosis coli" in 1857 (39). For many years, the

Table 3 Five Categories of Laxatives According to Their Mode of Action

Bulking agents: These include agents of dietary or processed natural fibers (bran and psyllium) and chemically modified cellulose (methylcellulose) and synthetic polymers. They work by increasing intraluminal volume (from water retention), thus stimulating motility and increasing the transit time of luminal contents through the colon, the end result being softer, more bulky stools. Additionally, once in the colon, these agents are subject to bacterial fermentation that produces short-chain fatty acids that also increase water retention, luminal osmolarity, and overall fecal mass.

Lubricants: Liquid paraffin (mineral oil) is the major lubricant laxative. When given orally or rectally, it decreases water absorption and softens the stool helping to promote evacuation. Although no longer commonly prescribed because of the risk of adverse effects (e.g., aspiration and anal seepage), it remains readily available over-the-counter.

Osmotic: These drugs include salts of poorly absorbable cations (magnesium) or anions (phosphate and sulfate), in addition to lactulose and sorbitol. The latter two are sugars that are poorly absorbed in the small bowel and subsequently broken down by bacteria in the colon. This group also includes the polyethylene glycol compounds, which stimulate colonic water retention, although stool osmolarity remains near normal.

Stimulant laxatives: Medications in this class stimulate intestinal motility and/or affect epithelial transport of water and electrolytes. Agents belonging to this group include the diphenylmethane derivatives (phenolphthalein, bisacodyl, and sodium picosulfate), anthraquinones [casanthrol (aloe), senna, and cascara], ricinoleic acid (castor oil) and surface-acting agents (docusates). Phenolphthalein has been removed from the market in the United States, because animal studies have suggested it might be carcinogenic (38), prompting at least one European country to investigate the safety of other anthraquinone agents.

Rectally Instilled Enemas: These usually administer either sodium phosphate or tap water. Although usually safe when used intermittently, if taken regularly these can result in significant metabolic disturbances such as water intoxication, hyponatremia, hypokalemia, hypocalcemia, hyperphosphatemia, and even seizures.

Source: From Ref. 38.

medical literature evidenced a strong association between melanosis coli and laxative abuse, specifically the anthraquinone laxative. However, most recent studies have suggested that melanosis coli is the result of phagocytosis of epithelial cells, which have undergone apoptosis. This recognition has led many to theorize that melanosis coli is, instead, a nonspecific marker of increased apoptosis in the colon, which may result from laxative abuse or many possible etiologies (40). Recently, melanosis coli was reported in a patient receiving topical anthralin for psoriasis (41). Nonsteroidal anti-inflammatory drugs have also been proposed as playing a role in the development of melanosis (42,43).

Experiments have demonstrated melanosis coli within one year of continued anthraquinone laxative use and its disappearance 6 to 11 months after drug cessation (43). Although most commonly seen in the rectum and cecum, it may affect the entire length of the colon, including the appendix, but rarely involves the small bowel. The incidence at autopsy varies from 0.25% to 5.3% when detected macroscopically, and up to 59.9% on light microscopy (40,44).

Some studies have suggested an increased incidence of colon cancer in patients with melanosis coli. A recent study by Nusko et al. (45), however, found no increase in the incidence of colon carcinoma in cases of melanosis coli, although adenomas were more commonly identified. The reasoning behind this finding is that melanosis coli facilitates detection of diminutive polyps, as white or pink spots appearing within a dark-colored mucosal background.

Heilbrun first described cathartic colon in 1943. It is a historic term referring to anatomic alterations of the colon secondary to chronic stimulant laxative use, and has been recognized as an infrequent, although severe, complication of laxative abuse. The diagnosis is most often considered when features such as loss of haustral markings, benign-appearing strictures, colonic dilatation, and a gaping ileocecal valve are seen on barium enema. The colon may be transformed into an inert tube, incapable of conducting its normal peristalsis or to propel the fecal stream (without the aid of large doses of laxatives). The mucosa appears smooth, thinned, and atrophic. Small submucosal retention cysts and punctuate superficial ulcerations may also be seen. If only a portion of the large bowel is affected, there is a predilection for the ascending colon, whereas the rectum may only be minimally affected. In advanced cases, a dilated terminal ileum may sometimes be seen (46).

The pathophysiology of a cathartic colon is poorly understood. Animal studies have suggested that chronic stimulant laxative intake results in degeneration of the colonic myenteric (Meisner's and Auerbach's) plexus (47). Little is known about its natural history after cessation of laxatives, but it is felt that many patients do not recover normal colonic function. Although some have undergone colectomy for this condition, there are occasional reports indicating a partial or near-complete resolution of findings after laxative use is stopped (48).

Among the renal electrolyte disturbances associated with laxative abuse are metabolic alkalosis or occasional metabolic acidosis, hyponatremia, hypovolemia, hypokalemia, hyperreninemia, hyperaldosteronism, hyperuricemia, hypocalcemia, hypercalcemia (rarely), and hypomagnesemia (49). Laxative abuse is a possible cause of chronic interstitial nephritis and may also contribute to the pathogenesis of analgesic abuse nephropathy.

Because the laxative abuse syndrome may account for as much as 3.5% to 7% of cases of chronic diarrhea of unknown origin, this diagnosis should be excluded before embarking on costly and invasive investigations (50). This may be accomplished by establishing definitive proof of laxative abuse as well as excluding any organic diseases. Common causes of chronic diarrhea should be evaluated by a combination of stool and plasma analysis, gastrointestinal endoscopy, and appropriate radiological investigation. The most important factor in diagnosing laxative abuse is a high level of suspicion on the part of the clinician.

Unfortunately, the majority of clinical and laboratory features of laxative abuse syndrome are nonspecific. Testing of stool and urine in a patient with suspected laxative abuse syndrome are perhaps the most useful studies. Sufficient phenolphthalein, senna, and bisacodyl are absorbed from the gastrointestinal tract and excreted by the kidney to make evaluation of the urine worthwhile. If the initial results are negative, testing should be repeated because the abuse can be intermittent, the excretion of drug rapid, and sometimes the patient may switch laxatives. Determination of the stool osmolarity is helpful to identify osmotically active substances such as magnesium sulfate or phosphosoda (which increase osmolarity) or surreptitious addition of water by the patient (which decreases osmolarity). A search of the hospitalized patient's belongings may be necessary to discover covert laxative abuse, but if found still requires confirmation by laboratory analysis.

The treatment of laxative abuse is extremely difficult and often very frustrating for the physician. Ideally, a team approach should be utilized, involving psychiatric input and direct support from the patient's family members. Relapses are unfortunately common, and complications, although rare, may be fatal if not recognized.

REFERENCES

1. Spira IA, Rodrigues R, Wolff WI. Pseudo-obstruction of the colon. Am J Gastroenterol 1976; 65:397–408.
2. Ogilvie H. Large-intestine colic due to sympathetic deprivation: a new clinical syndrome. Dis Colon Rectum 1987; 30:984–987.
3. Dorudi S, Berry AR, Kettlewell MGW. Acute colonic pseudo-obstruction. Br J Surg 1992; 79:99–103.
4. Nanni G, Garbini A, Luchetti P, Nanni G, Ronconi P, Castagneto M. Ogilvie's syndrome (acute colonic pseudo-obstruction). Dis Colon Rectum 1982; 25:157–166.
5. Strodel WE, Nostrant TT, Eckhauser FE, Dent TL. Therapeutic and diagnostic colonoscopy in nonobstructive colonic dilatation. Ann Surg 1983; 197:416–421.
6. Martin FM, Robinson AM Jr., Thompson WR. Therapeutic colonoscopy in the treatment of colonic pseudo-obstruction. Am Surg 1988; 54:519–522.
7. Turégano-Fuentes F, Muñoz-Jiménez F, Del Valle-Hernández E, et al. Early resolution of Ogilvie's syndrome with intravenous neostigmine. Dis Colon Rectum 1997; 40:1353–1357.
8. Alwan MH, Van Rij AM. Acute colonic pseudo-obstruction. Aust N Z J Surg 1998; 68:129–132.
9. Sloyer AF, Panella VS, Demas BE, et al. Ogilvie's syndrome: successful management without colonoscopy. Dig Dis Sci 1988; 33:1391—1396.
10. Jetmore AB, Timmcke AE, Gathright JB Jr., Hicks TC, Ray JE, Baker JW. Ogilvie's syndrome: colonoscopic decompression and analysis of predisposing factors. Dis Colon Rectum 1992; 35:1135–1142.
11. Vanek VW, Al-Salti M. Acute pseudo-obstruction of the colon (Ogilvie's syndrome) an analysis of 400 cases. Dis Colon Rectum 1986; 29:203–210.
12. Tenofsky PL, Beamer RL, Smith RS. Ogilvie syndrome as a postoperative complication. Arch Surg 2000; 135:682–687.
13. Geller A, Peterson BT, Gostout CJ. Endoscopic decompression for acute colonic pseudo-obstruction. Gastointest Endosc 1996; 44:144–150.
14. Paran H, Silverberg D, Mayo A, Shwartz I, Neufeld D, Freund U. Treatment of acute colonic pseudo-obstruction with neostigmine. J Am Coll Surg 2000; 190:315–318.
15. Gosche JR, Sharpe JN, Larson GM. Colonic decompression for pseudo-obstruction of the colon. Am Surg 1989; 55:111–115.
16. Abeyta BJ, Albrecht RM, Schermer CR. Retrospective study of neostigmine for the treatment of acute colonic pseudo-obstruction. Am Surg 2001; 67:265–268.
17. De Giorgio R, Barbara G, Stanghellini V, et al. Review article: the pharmacological treatment of acute colonic pseudo-obstruction. Aliment Pharmacol Ther 2001; 15:1717–1727.
18. Stephenson BM, Morgan AR, Salaman JR, Wheeler MH. Ogilvie's syndrome: a new approach to an old problem. Dis Colon Rectum 1995; 38:424–427.
19. Wojtalik RS, Lindenauer SM, Kahn SS. Perforation of the colon associated with adynamic ileus. Am J Surg 1973; 125:601–606.
20. Boley SJ, Agrawal GP, Warren AR, et al. Pathophysiologic effects of bowel distention on intestinal blood flow. Am J Surg 1969; 117:228–234.
21. Fiorito JJ, Schoen RE, Brandt LJ. Pseudo-obstruction associated with colonic ischemia: successful management with colonoscopic decompression. Am J Gastroenterol 1991; 86:1472–1476.
22. Kozarek RA, Earnest DL, Silverstein ME, Smith RG. Air-pressure-induced colon injury during diagnostic colonoscopy. Gastroenterology 1980; 78:7–14.
23. Schermer CR, Hanosh JJ, Davis M, Pitcher DE. Ogilvie's syndrome in the surgical patient: a new therapeutic modality. J Gastrointest Surg 1999; 3:173–177.
24. Trevisani GT, Hyman NH, Church JM. Neostigmine: safe and effective treatment for acute colonic pseudo-obstruction. Dis Colon Rectum 2000; 43:599–603.
25. Johnson CD, Rice RP, Kelvin FM, Foster WL, Williford ME. The radiologic evaluation of gross cecal distention: emphasis on cecal ileus. AJR Am J Roentgenol 1985; 145:1211–1217.
26. Kukora JS, Dent TL. Colonoscopic decompression of massive nonobstructive cecal dilation. Arch Surg 1977; 112:512–517.
27. Macrae FA, Tan KG, Williams CB. Towards safer colonoscopy: a report on the complications of 5000 diagnostic or therapeutic colonoscopies. Gut 1983; 24:376–383.
28. Pham TN, Cosman BC, Chu P, Savides TJ. Radiographic changes after colonoscopic decompression for acute pseudo-obstruction. Dis Colon Rectum 1999; 42:1586–1591.
29. Stephenson KR, Rodriguez-Bigas MA. Decompression of the large intestine in Ogilvie's syndrome by a colonoscopically placed long intestinal tube. Surg Endosc 1994; 8:116–117.
30. Catchpole BN. Ileus: use of sympathetic blocking agents in its treatment. Surgery 1969; 66:811–820.
31. Neely J, Catchpole B. Ileus: the restoration of alimentary-tract motility by pharmacological means. Br J Surg 1971; 58:21–28.

32. Hutchinson R, Griffiths C. Aute colonic pseudo-obstruction: a pharmacological approach. Ann R Coll Surg Engl 1992; 74:364–367.

33. Stephenson BM, Morgan AR, Drake N, Salaman JR, Wheeler MH. Parasympathomimetic decompression of acute colonic pseudo-obstruction. Lancet 1993; 342:1181–1182.

34. Ponec RJ, Saunders MD, Kimmey MB. Neostigmine infusion: new standard of care for acute colonic pseudo-obstruction? Am J Gastroenterol 2000; 95:304–305.

35. Duh QY, Way LW. Diagnostic laparoscopy and laparoscopic cecostomy for colonic pseudo-obstruction. Dis Colon Rectum 1993; 36:65–70.

36. Crass JR, Simmons RL, Frick MP, Maile CW. Percutaneous decompression of the colon using CT guidance in Ogilvie syndrome. AJR Am J Roentgenol 1985; 144:475–476.

37. Binder HJ. Use of laxatives in clinical medicine. Pharmacology 1988; 36(suppl 1):226–229.

38. Xing JH, Soffer EE. Adverse effects of laxatives. Dis Colon Rectum 2001; 34(suppl 8):1201–1208.

39. Ghadially FN, Walley VM. Melanosis of the gastrointestinal tract. Histopathology 1994; 25:197–207.

40. Byers RJ, Marsh P, Parkinson D, Haboubi NY. Melanosis coli is associated with an increase in colonic epithelial apoptosis and not with laxative use. Histopathology 1997; 30:160–164.

41. Lestina LS. An unusual case of melanosis coli. Gastrointest Endosc 2001; 54:119–121.

42. Lee FD. Importance of apoptosis in the histopathology of drug related lesions in the large intestine. J Clin Pathol 1993; 46:118–122.

43. Balazs M. Melanosis coli: ultrastructural study of 45 patients. Dis Colon Rectum 1986; 29:839–844.

44. Koskela E, Kulju T, Collan Y. Prevalence distribution and histologic features in 200 consecutive autopsies at Kuopio University Central Hospital. Dis Colon Rectum 1989; 32:235–239.

45. Nusko G, Schneider B, Ernst H, et al. Melanosis Coli – a harmless pigmentation or a precancerous condition? Z Gastroenterol 1997; 35:313–318.

46. Joo JS, Ehrenpreis ED, Gonzalez L, et al. Alterations in colonic anatomy induced by chronic stimulant laxatives. J Clin Gastroenterol 1998; 26(suppl 4):283–286.

47. Muller-Lissner S. What has happened to cathartic colon? Gut 1996; 39:486–488.

48. Urso FP, Urso MJ, Lee CH. The cathartic colon: pathological findings and radiological/pathological correlation. Radiology 1975; 116:557–559.

49. Baker EH, Sandle GI. Complications of laxative abuse. Annu Rev Med 1996; 47:127–134.

50. Campbell WL. Cathartic colon. Reversibility of roentgen changes. Dis Colon Rectum 1983; 26: 445–448.

22 | Volvulus

Johann Pfeifer
Department of General Surgery, University Clinic Medical School Graz, Graz, Austria

Heinz Hammer
Department of Gastroenterology, University Clinic Medical School Graz, Graz, Austria

DEFINITION

Volvulus refers to a torsion or twist of an organ on a pedicle. In the gastrointestinal tract, it can involve the stomach, spleen, gallbladder, small bowel, or large bowel (1), but it is by far most likely to occur in the colon. Clinically, there are differences in presentation and treatment depending on grade of obstruction (partial, complete) and the segment involved. Furthermore, colonic volvulus can be classified as common (sigmoid, cecum) or uncommon (splenic flexure, transverse colon). Sigmoid volvulus is most common and accounts for more than 75% of all cases reported (2).

HISTORICAL BACKGROUND

Volvulus of the colon was recognized in antiquity. The Ebers Papyrus from the period of the 17th Egyptian dynasty (1650–1552 B.C.) describes the development of sigmoid volvulus. According to Ballantyne's translation, the ancient Egyptians realized that if a volvulus did not reduce spontaneously, the sigmoid colon would "rot" (3). Hippocrates suggested insufflation of air per anum or the insertion of 10-digit-long suppositories to relieve obstruction. During the period of the Roman Empire, Aulus Cornelius Celsus (25 B.C.–A.D. 50) wrote an eight-volume medical compendium, "De Medicine," in which he classified diseases according to whether they were best treated by diet, medication, or surgery. He stated that the treatment regimen for volvulus (ileus) includes nothing by mouth, bloodletting, clysters, massage of the abdomen, application of hot plasters, hot oil baths, and hot oil enemas. Treatments proposed by Hippocrates and Celsus were used until the 19th century, when in 1883, Atherton reported the first operative detorsion for sigmoid volvulus (3). Since then, several surgical treatment forms have been developed including resection, shortening of the mesentery, mesosigmoidoplasty, and colopexy. From the beginning of the 20th century until 1947, surgery became the dominant treatment form. After Bruusgard published lower mortality rates with conservative treatments, there was a return to a more conservative approach (4). Currently, conservative and surgical treatment modalities both have their place in the treatment of volvulus.

CLASSIFICATION

Volvulus can involve the cecum, the transverse colon, the splenic flexure, and the sigmoid colon. Rarely, a compound volvulus of small and large bowel (ileosigmoid knot) has been reported. Ballantyne reported the various frequencies as follows: sigmoid colon 60.9%, cecum 34.5%, transverse colon 3.6%, and splenic flexure 1% (5).

EPIDEMIOLOGY

The incidence of colonic volvulus differs greatly in different parts of the world. In Western Europe and United States, the incidence is about 5% or less of intestinal obstructions (1,6), compared with the Middle East and Africa, where up to 75% of all intestinal obstructions have been reported to be caused by volvulus (Table 1).

True incidence rates were calculated in a population-based study in 1980 in Olmsted County, Minnesota, for the preceding 20 years with an average of 3/100,000 inhabitants/year.

Table 1 Incidence of Volvulus of Large Bowel Obstruction in Different Parts of the World

Continent	Country	Author	Year	Incidence (%)
North America	United States	Ballantyne (3)	1990	1–7
South America	Peru	Asbun et al. (8)	1992	79
Europe	United Kingdom	McConkey (9)	2002	3,5[a]
	Switzerland	Maurer et al. (10)	1998	13
Africa	South Africa	Mokoena and Madiba (11)	1995	8
	Guinea	Bagarani et al. (12)	1993	8
	Nigeria	Adensunkanmi and Agbakwuru (13)	1996	25.4
Asia	Turkey (West)	Fuzun et al. (14)	1991	12.7
	Turkey (East)	Gurleyik et al. (7)	2002	80.2
	Iran	Saidi (15)	1969	42
	India	de U (16)	2002	44.97

[a]Mortality rate for patients with decompression and observation alone.

Interestingly, there is a significant difference in the incidence in patients under 60 years (1/100,000 inhabitants/year), and for patients over 60 years (14/100,000 inhabitants/year). The patient's average age is about 60 to 65 years, whereby 80% are older than 50, and 45% are older than 70 years (5). There are conflicting results on the distribution by sex.

While no sex differences are noted in some American and Western European series, most series from the Middle East, South America, and Africa report a male preponderance of 70% to 90% (2,7,12,15). A significant number of psychiatric patients in Western Europe and United States are at risk of a volvulus (1–3). Blacks are more often affected than Caucasians (2,3). In the United States, the incidence of sigmoid volvulus is slightly higher than cecal volvulus, with a ratio of 60% to 40% (5). Splenic and transverse colon volvulus are responsible for less than 5% of all cases. In general, children are very rarely affected by colonic volvulus (17).

SIGMOID VOLVULUS
Etiology

The exact etiology of sigmoid volvulus is obscure, but several predisposing factors have been identified in recent decades. Two essential anatomical preconditions must be present: (i) a long, mobile sigmoid colon with a long, free mesosigmoid, and (ii) a close proximity of the limbs of the colon at a "fixed point" around which the colon can twist. It is thought that due to increased sigmoid load and gas distension, a high-fiber diet predisposes to colon prolongation and subsequent twisting on its mesentery. A similar mechanism is hypothesized in patients suffering from neuropsychiatric disorders, Parkinson's disease, stroke, and long-standing constipation leading to changes in bowel motility and chronic sigmoid overload with feces, followed by colon elongation and relative narrowing of the distance between the "fixed points." However, many other etiologies have also been reported as contributing to sigmoid volvulus formation; these include Chagas' disease (18), Hirschsprung's disease (17,19), megacolon (20), diabetes (21), adhesions (22), lead poisoning (23), pregnancy (24), vitamin B deficiency (23), ischemic colitis (25), peptic ulcer (2), tuberculosis (2), cardiovascular disease (26), sprue (27), hypokalemia (28), and excessive use of enemas (29).

Pathogenesis

The sigmoid colon may twist clockwise or counterclockwise, but the latter direction is more common; the mesocolon is twisted around its axis by varying degrees of rotation. To produce symptoms of obstruction, the volvulus must be rotated by more than 180°. Groth demonstrated that the twisting of the sigmoid on the mesentery is accompanied by an axial torsion on the bowel wall, which is twice as great as the torsion of the mesentery (30). This is because the sigmoid colon is fixed to the posterior peritoneal wall. Thus, an axial torsion of the bowel wall of 360° produces a 180° volvulus. Typically, sigmoid volvulus is a closed-loop colonic obstruction. In the early stages of obstruction, gas and fluid can enter the loop from the proximal colon and occasionally, due to trapped gas and air, diarrheal stools can occur. As the loop distends, the proximal influx also becomes obstructed. With simple obstruction, the bowel wall generally remains viable for a few days. This is because the sigmoid colon itself can tolerate more intraluminal pressures than other segments of the colon before a vascular compromise occurs. When the intraluminal pressure exceeds capillary pressure, occlusion of the veins comes first, followed by mesocolic thrombosis, which in turn is followed by arterial thrombosis leading to infarction. Necrosis begins usually at the point of twisting, and may advance to total bowel loop gangrene. Another more rapid and clinically more urgent event can occur due to twisting and compression of the mesenteric vessels. Ischemia, necrosis, and rapid distension of the bowel lumen occur much more rapidly under these circumstances.

Clinical Presentation

Sigmoid volvulus can be presented clinically in three different ways: as the more common subacute and the uncommon acute volvulus as well as the rare compound volvulus. The common subacute type occurs frequently in adult males, whose typical first symptom is difficulty in passing flatus. Distension of the abdomen and the tympanitic (drum-like) percussive note may increase. Interestingly, the abdomen is often not very tender and painful, and the patient's main problem may be dyspnea due to elevation of the diaphragm. Sometimes a gas-distended loop can be felt on the left side up to the costal margin. Vomiting is unusual, except perhaps once at the start of the attack. The patient's general condition is usually good, unless he presents late and in severe shock. The patient may mention previous mild attacks, during which twisting and subsequent release of the colon caused pain and constipation followed by diarrhea with passage of copious flatus. Surgery often reveals a thick-walled colon on the left side.

The uncommon acute volvulus seems more frequent in the Western world where a high-fiber diet is more uncommon. Typically, onset is rapid with colicky pain. Severe pain, tenderness, and vomiting are frequent, progressing to early peritonitis. The abdomen is not excessively distended, and colon loops can seldom be palpated. At the onset, the patient may have the urge to defecate and may pass a small amount of stool, sometimes mixed with blood. The chance of gangrene, peritonitis, and shock within 24 hours is about 50% (31). Upon operation, the wall of the colon is usually found to be thin and ischemia followed by gangrene is frequent. Some patients may fall between these two extremes. It should be noted that even after the subacute form which may last several days, gangrene and peritonitis can occur.

The third form is the rare compound small and large bowel ileus or ileosigmoid knot. The patient may present with mixed symptoms, either with constipation and vomiting or with an acute abdomen and shock. Surgery reveals a small bowel segment twisted around the base of the sigmoid loop, often requiring sigmoid and small bowel resection.

Diagnosis

In most cases, a preliminary clinical diagnosis is confirmed with a plain abdominal X-ray. The distended sigmoid loop is usually ahaustral and predominant in the abdomen, and has an inverted U-shape. A Gastrografin enema may help to differentiate among pseudo-obstruction, tumor obstruction, and volvulus. The "bird's beak" deformity of the contrast column is a typical feature at the site of the torsion, representing twisting of the bowel wall (2,3). Another typical radiological feature is the "coffee bean" sign (Fig. 1). When volvulus is suspected, endoscopy is generally indicated, both for diagnostic and therapeutic purposes; a rigid sigmoidoscope is often used. Typically, the rectum is normal and the mucosa forms spiral folds at the rectosigmoid junction. If the sigmoid mucosa is not ischemic, the mucosa will appear endoscopically normal.

Treatment
Rationale of Definitive Treatment
The treatment of sigmoid volvulus has changed in recent years from an immediate surgical correction with a high-mortality rate to a more conservative approach with immediate decompression of the volvulus followed by elective surgery. Historically, emergency sigmoid resections carried a mortality rate of more than 50% (2,3), which explains the rapid adoption of the conservative approach published by Bruusgard in 1947. He suggested a sigmoidoscopic deflation of the volvulus followed by stenting of the colon with a rectal tube. The procedure

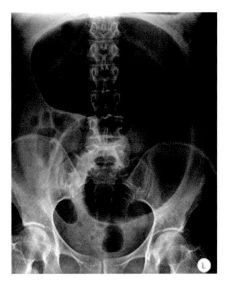

Figure 1 The coffee-bean sign on a plain abdominal X-ray in a patient with sigmoid volvulus.

was performed on 136 patients with a 90% success rate (123 patients). Four patients died, giving a mortality rate of 2.9% (4). In subsequent decades, several larger series showed similarly low mortality and a high success rate (Table 2). As technology advanced, colonoscopic rather than sigmoidoscopic decompression came to be used. The advantage is that the flexible colonoscope can be passed gently through the site of twisting and further on into the proximal colon. Thereafter, it is easier to suction liquid feces out of the proximal bowel and insert longer decompression tubes to diminish recurrence (Fig. 2). With the rigid sigmoidoscope, decompression is successful in 59%, compared with 90% with the flexible colonoscope in cases of nonstrangulated sigmoid volvulus (3). In spite of the good results with acute volvulus, the problem of recurrence remained. Bruusgard reported 31 recurrences in 91 patients, i.e., a recurrence rate of 34% (4). Further studies confirmed this observation, with recurrence rates up to 90% (Table 3). There was an obvious need for definitive treatment after successful conservative decompression and resuscitation of the patient, and elective surgery was proposed. The timing of elective surgery is, however, still a matter of discussion. Bak and Boley suggested elective surgery during the same hospital stay. They cited mortality rates of 6% compared to 30% for recurrent episodes (35). Shepherd reported 74 elective resections performed five to eight days after conservative treatment with a mortality rate of 2.8% (33). Arnold and Nance challenged this performance with a 15% mortality rate after the first volvulus episode, and 9% after recurrent episodes. Furthermore, the latter reported a poorer outcome of surgery in patients over 70 years of age, and suggested deferral of the operation in patients over 70 years of age (26). In clinical practice, the first presentation of volvulus to the physician

Table 2 Sigmoid Volvulus—Success and Mortality Rates for Conservative Treatment Endoscopic Decompression

Author	Year	N	N of decompression	Success rate (%)	Mortality rate (%)
Bruusgard (4)	1947	136	123	90	2.9
Drapanas and Stewart (32)	1961	98	82	84	1.2
Shepherd (33)	1968	89	78	88	3.4
Arnold and Nance (26)	1973	114	87	77	—
Arigbabu et al. (34)	1985	92	92	90.2	—
Bak and Boley (35)	1986	51	43	91	15.1
Friedman et al. (36)	1989	58	31	81	7,4[a]
Chung et al. (37)	1999	35	29	91	0[b]
Dulger et al. (38)	2000	61	24	100	7,6[b]
Grossmann et al. (39)	2000	228	189	81	16[a]
Renzulli et al. (40)	2002	20	19	58	0[b]

[a]Mortality rate for patients with decompression and observation alone.
[b]Mortality rate after decompression plus elective surgery.

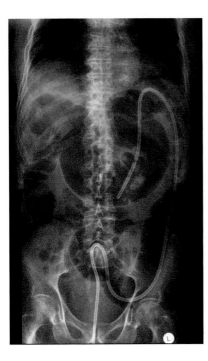

Figure 2 Decompression tube in place after acute attack of a sigmoid volvulus.

may not be the first episode of volvulus to the patient as some 50% of all patients report prior self-resolving episodes of presumptive volvulus (2,3,33,39,42). This may be important considering that subsequent volvulus episodes may have a lower mortality than the first episode.

Conservative Treatment

Initial management depends whether the surgeon believes that the bowel is viable or nonviable. The goals of treatment in a nonstrangulated viable bowel are primarily de-torsion, decompression, and prevention of recurrence. This means that proctosigmoidoscopy is indicated as an initial treatment. This can be done with a rigid, or ideally, flexible sigmoidoscope, often followed by a flexible tube left in place for about 48 hours. The patient is placed in the left lateral position and the rigid endoscope is inserted into the rectum. Frequent air insufflation is necessary to maintain a good view of the apex and to expand the rectal ampulla to prevent inadvertent perforation. Sometimes reduction of the volvulus can be achieved with air pressure alone. Spiraling mucosal folds are visible at the apex of the volvulus. While the endoscope is held there, a well-lubricated rectal tube is inserted via the endoscope over the apex of the volvulus. If this is not possible, a tube with a larger diameter should be used. Sometimes it is also helpful to change the patient's position, for example, the knee–elbow position. It is of utmost importance to avoid blind or forceful insertion. If the volvulus can be reduced, there is a sudden noisy discharge of gas and stool, and care must be taken to avoid the explosive

Table 3 Sigmoid Volvulus—Recurrence Rates for Endoscopic Decompression

Author	Year	*N*	Recurrence (n)	Recurrence (%)
Bruusgard (4)	1947	91	31	34
Drapanas and Stewart (32)	1961	40	24	60
Hines et al. (41)	1967	31	28	90
Shepherd (33)	1968	225	87	39
Arnold and Nance (26)	1973	55	30	55
Bak and Boley (35)	1986	33	23	70
Friedman et al. (36)	1989	7	3	43
Chung et al. (37)	1999	14	12	85.7
Grossmann et al. (39)	2000	44	10	23

evacuation. Flexible colonoscopic decompression has the advantage that a larger area of mucosa can be assessed for viability, but care must be taken to avoid perforation of the distended and edematous bowel segment. If a strangulated bowel is suspected, or if there is bloody discharge or necrotic bowel mucosa, emergency explorative laparotomy is indicated.

Surgical Treatment
Resection

Apart from failed endoscopic or radiologic decompression, indications for urgent surgical intervention are signs and symptoms suggesting intestinal ischemia, perforation, or peritonitis. The actual treatment depends on whether the colon is gangrenous or not. The frequency of gangrene in Western countries is about 10%, but it reaches 25% in underdeveloped countries (2,3,29,33). A gangrenous colon demands immediate excision (2,3,42). In these cases, untwisting is not wise as it can result in septic shock. The surgical possibilities are (i) resection and end colostomy plus mucus fistula, or (ii) resection, colostomy, and rectal stump closure (Hartmann's procedure). In these severely ill and often acidotic patients, an anastomosis is not advisable due to the high risk of anastomotic dehiscence. This is supported by Taha and Suleman, who in 46 patients reported a mortality rate of 60% for primary anastomosis for gangrenous bowel (43). Bagarani et al. reported similar results with a 50% morbidity and 33% mortality rate in patients with gangrenous bowel and primary anastomosis, whereas there was a zero percent mortality in patients with viable bowel and primary anastomosis. For the eight patients who underwent Hartmann's procedure, morbidity and mortality rates were 13% and 9%, respectively (12). In summary, mortality rates after resection of gangrenous bowel are eight times higher than emergency resection of viable bowel (Table 4). It is speculated that the gangrene itself is more likely to be responsible for the high-mortality rate than the surgical procedure chosen. If the bowel is viable, primary resection and anastomosis in an unprepped bowel is controversial. The trauma surgery literature, as well as other clinical studies, have shown that primary anastomosis, sometimes with the help of on-table lavage, can be done with low morbidity and mortality rates (46,47). Sule et al. reported on 27 patients with sigmoid volvulus who underwent emergency resection with a primary anastomosis, after an on-table wash out. There was no anastomotic leakage and no mortality (47). Generally, there is a trend toward primary anastomosis in left-sided bowel obstruction (42,45–47).

The surgeon's main goal should be to perform an elective procedure, with lower morbidity and mortality rates rather than an emergency operation, if possible (Table 5). The traditional elective procedure for decompressed sigmoid volvulus is sigmoid resection. However, subtotal or total colectomy is advised for patients with sigmoid volvulus and megacolon because only patients with additional megacolon who had undergone sigmoid resection tended to have recurrences (37). Laparoscopic colon resection is very attractive in volvulus patients, but due to distension, the laparoscopic technique may not be helpful in the acute situation. After decompression, laparoscopic surgery seems advantageous. While the published experience is limited, no complications have been reported (Table 6).

Table 4 Sigmoid Volvulus—Mortality Rates After Emergency Resection With/Without Gangrene

Author	Year	Viable bowel		Gangrenous bowel	
		N	Mortality (%)	*N*	Mortality (%)
Drapanas and Stewart (32)	1961	18	17	5	60
Shepherd (33)	1969	389	8	36	47
Arnold and Nance (26)	1973	85	23.5	14	57
Schagen van Leeuen (29)	1985	116	1.7	22	18
Bak and Boley (35)	1986	18	5,6[a]	11	36
Peoples et al. (44)	1990	50	0	4	75
Bagarani et al. (12)	1993	17	5.8	14	21.4
Grossmann et al. (39)	2000	20	24[b]	59	24[b]
Kuzu et al. (45)	2002	88	5.7	18	11.1
Renzulli et al. (40)	2002	9	0	?	12[c]

[a]Including some recurrent cases.
[b]Overall mortality rate for all emergency operations (viable plus gangrenous bowel).
[c]Overall mortality rate for emergency operations.

Table 5 Mortality Rates for Sigmoid Volvulus—Emergency Versus Elective Resection

Author	Year	Emergency operation		Elective operation	
		N	Mortality (%)	N	Mortality (%)
Arnold and Nance (26)	1973	25	44	74	15
Ballantyne (1)	1982	195	37	129	8.5
Schagen van Leeuen (29)	1985	22	18	116	0
Bak and Boley (35)	1986	14	36	18	5.6
Pahlman et al. (48)	1989	47	15	13	0
Bagarani et al. (12)	1993	14	21	17	5.8
Mokoena and Madiba (11)	1995	27	30	55	3.6
Grossmann et al. (39)	2000	79	24	99	6
Kuzu et al. (45)	2002	106	6.6	–	–

Nonresectional Procedures

A large variety of nonresection options for nonstrangulated bowel have been described. The most important procedure used to be operative detorsion of the volvulus and sigmoidopexy without resection to minimize morbidity and mortality. However, during reexploration after volvulus recurrence, unsuccessful fixation was often noticed. With recurrence rates of more than 40%, this method is now considered obsolete (2,3,33). Mesosigmoidoplasty is another method, whereby one leaf of the mesosigmoid is incised longitudinally and sutured transversely. It is a simple operation with low morbidity and mortality rates. The largest series, published by Subrahmanyam including 126 patients, reported a recurrence rate of 1.6% and 0% mortality with a documented mean follow-up of 8.2 years (54). There are, however, no other larger series on mesosigmoidoplasty. Furthermore, this operation can be difficult when the mesosigmoid is thickened and edematous. In 1991, Salim reported a new technique involving percutaneous decompression of the sigmoid volvulus followed by sigmoidoscopic decompression, which was successful in 27 of 38 patients, with a success rate of 71% (55). Due to the potential risk of peritoneal contamination and infection, we do not recommend this approach. Another therapeutic option in patients unfit for surgery, which was suggested recently, is endoscopic decompression followed by percutaneous endoscopic sigmoidopexy with T-fasteners (56). These authors feel that the long-term success is unlikely with this method, as even with surgery it is often difficult to fix the elongated bowel. Longer follow-up is needed to judge the efficacy of this approach in patients who might benefit from it.

CECAL VOLVULUS
Etiology

Cecal volvulus is responsible for about 1% of all intestinal obstructions or 10% to 40% of all cases of colonic volvulus. It occurs less commonly than sigmoid volvulus. The average cecal volvulus sufferer is much younger (30–60 years) than the typical sigmoid volvulus patient. Most studies report a predominance of female patients. The anatomic prerequisite is a congenital mobile cecum resulting from a lack of fixation of the mesentery of the right colon to the posterior parietal peritoneum of the right gutter. This anomaly was observed in a cadaver study in as many as 22% of the normal population (57).

Pathogenesis

Clinically, two different forms of cecal volvulus can be observed. An axial ileocolic volvulus accounts for about 90%; in 10% a so-called cecal bascule is seen (58). The first kind is in general

Table 6 Sigmoid Volvulus—Laparoscopic Sigmoid Resection

Author	Year	N	Complications (%)
Sundin et al. (49)	1992	1	0
Pruett (50)	1993	1	0
Mariette et al. (51)	1996	2	0
Chung et al. (52)	1997	5	0
Chung (53)	1997	4	0

a volvulus in clockwise or anticlockwise direction including rotation of the distal ileum. Other associated factors mentioned in the literature are adhesions from previous surgery (58,59), congenital bands (60), nonrotation of the midgut (61), torsion around a vitelline duct remnant (62), high-fiber diet (60), increased peristalsis from diarrhea or cathartics (63), and overeating (64). Displacement of the cecum out of the pelvis due to pelvic tumor (65) and pregnancy are other reported causes (66). Interestingly, in as many as one-third to one-half of the patients, a concomitant distal bowel obstruction can be seen (2). The second form is the cecal bascule. This involves folding of the ascending colon so that the cecum moves anteriorly and superiorly causing obstruction through a transverse fold. This form involves no axial twisting of the mesentery, and therefore strangulation and gangrene are rare.

Clinical Presentation

Three different clinical presentations of cecal volvulus are described in the literature: an acute fulminating type, an acute obstructing form, and an intermittent or recurrent form. The acute fulminating type is characterized by the clinical picture of the acute abdomen. Severe pain is typical for a vascular obstruction due to twisting of the mesentery.

The acute obstructed form is due to the fact that cecal volvulus often involves rotation of the ileum, and signs of distal small bowel obstruction are therefore present. Severe, intermittent colicky pain begins in the right abdomen. Pain eventually becomes continuous, vomiting may occur, and passage of gas and feces per anum decreases. Abdominal distension is variable.

The last form, which is intermittent or recurrent, can present uncharacteristically. There are either mild attacks of cramping or severe colicky pain lasting for only short periods. In such cases, identifying the correct diagnosis can be challenging.

Diagnosis

On a plain X-ray, cecal volvulus typically shows a single fluid level in the dilated cecum, which may be seen anywhere in the abdomen, depending on its position, site, and degree of twisting. Often, it is in the left-upper quadrant. Additional distended small bowel loops are frequently seen, along with a relative lack of gas in the large bowel. On Gastrografin enema, only 50% show a coffee-bean sign (cecal volvulus) or a teardrop (cecal bascule) (67). The whirl sign is usually present on the computed tomography scan (68). With radiological methods, a preoperative diagnosis is possible in 90% of cases (58,69). Diagnostic colonoscopy reveals a cul-de-sac at the hepatic flexure in cases of volvulus, and an obstructing fold in cecal bascule (3). Due to the hazard of iatrogenic perforation, the role of colonoscopy in cecal volvulus is somewhat debatable (3,5,58,70,71).

Treatment

Unlike sigmoid volvulus, conservative treatment of cecal volvulus with colonoscopy is often unsuccessful. This is mainly due to the longer distance from the anus to the site of the twist. Although successful decompression has been reported (71,72), it has not become popular due to the high-failure rate and the risk of perforation (5,59,70). Percutaneous deflation of the cecum was described by Patel et al. in 1987 (73). A simple intravenous cannula was inserted in the distended bowel. The cecum was deflated, and then the needle removed after a few minutes. Although successful, due to the risk of leakage, this procedure may be useful only as an alternative in patients at prohibitive surgical risk.

At laparotomy, the first step is evaluation of the bowel's viability. If the bowel is gangrenous, immediate resection with a right hemicolectomy is mandatory. Detorsion in nonviable bowel should be avoided as irreversible septic shock has been described (74,75). Most authors prefer a primary anastomosis, although ileostomy and mucus fistula remains an option (2,58).

When the bowel is viable, several options are available: nonresectional procedures such as detorsion and cecopexy or cecostomy, or resection of the mobile, distorted segment. The advantage of resection is that it prevents recurrence. The rationale for cecopexy is to anchor the mobile cecum and ascending colon to the parietal peritoneum, thus decreasing recurrences. The method of cecopexy varies from creating a peritoneal flap (76) to simple plication (77). The latter has also been done laparoscopically (78). Nonetheless, recurrences for cecopexy average 16% (range 0–40%) (5,48,70,79,80), and mortality rates are as high as 18% (48). Cecostomy was often done in the past. The advantage was that on one hand, the bowel was fixed by a tube to the anterior abdominal wall, and that on the other hand, a continuous decompression

Table 7 Cecal Volvulus—Mortality Rates After Emergency Resection With/Without Gangrene

Author	Year	N	Overall mortality	Viable bowel		Gangrenous bowel	
				N	Mortality (%)	N	Mortality (%)
Ballantyne et al. (5)	1985	39	17	24	12	15	33
Anderson and Welch (82)	1986	33	32	14	21	19	37
Pahlman et al. (48)	1989	17	24	14	4	3	60
Hiltunen et al. (80)	1992	11	9	2	0	9	9
Gupta and Gupta (70)	1993	11	18	2	0	9	17
Isbister (83)	1996	5	0	NS	NS	NS	NS
Remes-Troche et al. (84)	1997	7	21[a]	3	NS	4	NS
Grossmann et al. (85)	1999	55	18[b], 31[c]	NS	NS	NS	NS
Tuech et al. (86)	1996	22	9	10	0	12	17
Tuech et al. (87)	2002	45	6.6	22	4.5	23	8.7

Note: NS, not stated.
[a]Overall mortality including 25 cases of sigmoid volvulus and 1 case of transverse colon volvulus.
[b]For colectomy and primary anastomosis.
[c]For colectomy and stoma (Hartmann's procedure).

could be achieved. The main problem was leaking around the cecostomy tube, leading to life-threatening complications such as gangrene, cecal necrosis, intraperitoneal leakage, and fistula. Furthermore, it should not be done through a perforation due to the associated high morbidity and mortality (58,81). Only seven patients are reported to have undergone combined cecopexy and cecostomy, without mortality or recurrences. Nonetheless, this combined procedure cannot be recommended due to the small number of patients so treated (81). More recent literature demonstrates that mortality rates for nonresectional and resectional procedures are much better than in the previous decades (Table 7). This may be due at least in part to better diagnostic and therapeutic tools, especially in anesthesia and intensive care.

TRANSVERSE VOLVULUS
Etiology

Approximately 4% of all volvulus cases involve the transverse colon. Patients are often younger and female. Normally, a firm and far distant fixation of the hepatic and the splenic flexure as well as a short mesocolon transversum prevent the transverse colon from twisting.

Pathogenesis

Congenital abnormalities predisposing to twisting include a freely movable right colon, long mesocolon, close proximity of fixation or the Chilaiditi syndrome (hepatodiaphragmatic interposition of the colon) (88). Physiologic factors include constipation from various causes such as high-fiber diet (89), megacolon from Hirschsprung's disease (90), and scleroderma (91). Often distal colonic obstruction due to adhesions, strictures, neoplasm, or sigmoid volvulus elongates and expands the transverse colon and can lead to volvulus formation (2,89). Many patients have undergone previous upper abdominal surgery that has disrupted normal bowel fixation (2).

Clinical Presentation

Similar to sigmoid and cecal volvulus, an acute fulminant type with sudden, severe pain, little distension, and rapid development of shock must be distinguished from a subacute type with cramping, vomiting, distension, and gradual deterioration.

Diagnosis

Diagnosis is suspected based on clinical impression and confirmed by plain abdominal X-rays. A middle colonic obstruction, particularly distension of the proximal large bowel and two air-fluid levels representing proximal and distal transverse limbs are seen (67,92). However, this diagnosis is often only made during laparotomy (2).

Treatment

In a viable bowel endoscopic decompression and detorsion have been reported (93). However, recurrence rates of up to 75% mandate a subsequent definitive procedure (5,40,89,92,94). Nonresectional procedures include various forms of colopexy including suturing of the transverse mesocolon to the mesocolon of the ascending and descending colon (94).

In patients with good clinical condition or with a gangrenous bowel, resection (usually extended right hemicolectomy or partial left colectomy) is advised (95,96). Another option is creation of a colostomy and mucus fistula. The reported high-mortality rate of 33% reflects late diagnosis of volvulus (67).

SPLENIC FLEXURE VOLVULUS
Etiology and Pathogenesis

Splenic flexure volvulus is a rare entity and less than 30 cases have been reported in the literature. Female-to-male ratio is 2:1, and the average age is 50 years (2,3). A mobile splenic flexure, either due to congenital anomaly or postsurgical alterations, predisposes to volvulus. Constipation and psychiatric conditions may also contribute to this condition.

Clinical Presentation and Diagnosis

Similar to transverse volvulus, the clinical picture of colon obstruction is the leading symptom. Diagnosis is made clinically in conjunction with the X-ray findings; again, the correct diagnosis is often only made at laparotomy (97).

Treatment

Due to the technical problems of refixation of the left colonic flexure, resection is recommended (97–100).

REFERENCES

1. Ballantyne GH. Review of sigmoid volvulus: clinical patterns and pathogenesis. Dis Colon Rectum 1982; 25:823–830.
2. Bubrick MP. Volvulus of the colon. In: Gordon PH, Nivatvongs S, eds. Principles and Practice of Surgery for the Colon, Rectum, and Anus. St. Louis, Missouri: Quality Medical Publishing Inc, 1992:799–816.
3. Ballantyne GH. Volvulus of the colon. In: Fazio VW, ed. Current Therapy in Colon and Rectal Surgery. Philadelphia: BC Decker, 1990:254–265.
4. Bruusgard C. Volvulus of the sigmoid colon and its treatment. Surgery 1947; 22:466–478.
5. Ballantyne GH, Brandner MD, Beart RW Jr., Ilstrup DM. Volvulus of the colon. Incidence and mortality. Ann Surg 1985; 202:83–92.
6. Jones-Ian T, Fazio VS. Colonic volvulus, etiology and management. Dig Dis 1989; 7:203–209.
7. Gurleyik G, Kotan C, Dulundu E, Ozturk E, Sonmerz R, Saglam A. Clinical differences between surgically treated patients with large bowel obstruction in the cities of Van and Istanbul. Ulus Travma Derg 2002; 8:38–42.
8. Asbun HJ, Castellanos H, Balderrama B, et al. Sigmoid volvulus in the high altitude of the Andes: review of 230 cases. Dis Colon Rectum 1992; 35:350–353.
9. McConkey SJ. Case series of acute abdominal surgery in rural Sierra Leone. World J Surg 2002; 26:509–513.
10. Maurer CA, Renzulli P, Naef M, et al. Surgical therapy of ileus of the large intestine. Zentralbl Chir 1998; 123:1346–1354.
11. Mokoena TR, Madiba TE. Sigmoid volvulus among Africans in Durban. Trop Geogr Med 1995; 47:216–217.
12. Bagarani M, Conde AS, Longo R, Italiano A, Terenzi A, Venuto G. Sigmoid volvulus in West Africa: a prospective study on surgical treatments. Dis Colon Rectum 1993; 36:186–190.
13. Adensunkanmi AR, Agbakwuru EA. Changing pattern of acute intestinal obstruction in a tropical African population. East Afr Med J 1996; 73:727–731.
14. Fuzun M, Kaymak E, Harmancioglu O, Astarcioglu K. Principal causes of mechanical bowel obstruction in surgically treated adults in western Turkey. Br J Surg 1991; 78:202–203.
15. Saidi F. The high incidence of intestinal volvulus in Iran. Gut 1969; 10:838–841.
16. de U. Sigmoid volvulus in rural Bengal. Trop Doct 2002; 32:80–82.

17. Chirdan LB, Ameh EA. Sigmoid volvulus and ileosigmoid knotting in children. Pediatr Surg Int 2001; 17:636–637.
18. Habr-Gama A, Haddad J, Simonsen O, et al. Volvulus of the sigmoid colon in Brazil: report of 230 cases. Dis Colon Rectum 1976; 19:314–320.
19. Shepherd JJ. The epidemiology and clinical presentation of sigmoid volvulus. Br J Surg 1969; 56: 353–359.
20. Pfeifer J, Agachan F, Wexner SD. Surgery for constipation. Dis Colon Rectum 1996; 39:444–460.
21. Berenyl MR, Schwartz GS. Megasigmoid syndrome in diabetes and neurologic disease: review of 13 cases. Am J Gastroenterol 1967; 47:310–320.
22. String ST, DeCosse JJ. Sigmoid volvulus: an examination of the mortality. Am J Surg 1971; 121: 293–297.
23. Berger KE, Lundberg EZ. Intestinal volvulus precipitated by lead poisoning. JAMA 1951; 147: 13–16.
24. Stone K. Acute abdominal emergencies associated with pregnancy. Clin Obstet Gynecol 2002; 45: 553–561.
25. Meyers MS, Ghahremani GG, Govone AF. Ischemic colitis associated with sigmoid volvulus: new observations. Am J Radiol 1977; 128:591–595.
26. Arnold GJ, Nance FC. Volvulus of the sigmoid colon. Ann Surg 1973; 177:527–531.
27. Glazer IM, Aldersberg D. Volvulus of the colon: a complication of sprue. Gastroenterology 1953; 24:159–172.
28. Forward AD. Hypokalemia associated with sigmoid volvulus. Surg Gynecol Obstet 1966; 123:35–42.
29. Schagen van Leeuwen JH. Sigmoid volvulus in a West African population. Dis Colon Rectum 1985; 28:712–716.
30. Groth KE. The axial torsion of the colon through so-called physiologic volvulus. Acta Radiol 1934; 15:153–168.
31. Hinshaw DB, Carter R. Surgical management of acute volvulus of the sigmoid colon. A study of 55 cases. Ann Surg 1957; 146:52–60.
32. Drapanas T, Stewart JD. Acute sigmoid volvulus: concepts in surgical treatment. Am J Surg 1961; 101:70–77.
33. Shepherd JJ. Treatment of volvulus of sigmoid colon. A review of 425 cases. Br Med J 1968; 1:280–283.
34. Arigbabu AO, Badejo OA, Akinola DO. Colonoscopy in the emergency treatment of colonic volvulus in Nigeria. Dis Colon Rectum 1985; 28:795–798.
35. Bak MP, Boley SJ. Sigmoid volvulus in elderly patients. Am J Surg 1986; 151:71–75.
36. Friedman JD, Odland MD, Bubrick MP. Experience with colonic volvulus. Dis Colon Rectum 1989; 32:409–416.
37. Chung YF, Eu KW, Nyam DC, Leong AF, Ho YH, Seow-Choen F. Minimizing recurrence after sigmoid volvulus. Br J Surg 1999; 86:231–233.
38. Dulger M, Canturk NZ, Utkan NZ, Gonullu NN. Management of sigmoid colon volvulus. Hepato-gastroenterology 2000; 47:1280–1283.
39. Grossmann EM, Longo WE, Stratton MD, Virgo KS, Johnson FE. Sigmoid volvulus in Department of Veterans Affairs Medical Centers. Dis Colon Rectum 2000; 43:414–418.
40. Renzulli P, Maurer CA, Netzer P, Buchler MW. Preoperative colonoscopic derotation is beneficial in acute colonic volvulus. Dig Surg 2002; 19:223–229.
41. Hines JR, Geurkink RE, Bass RT. Recurrence and mortality rates in sigmoid volvulus. Surg Gynecol Obstet 1967; 124:567–570.
42. Madiba TE, Thomson SR. The management of sigmoid volvulus. J R Coll Surg Edinb 2000; 45:74–80.
43. Taha SE, Suleman SI. Volvulus of the sigmoid colon in Gezira. Br J Surg 1980; 67:433–435.
44. Peoples JB, McCafferty JC, Scher KS. Operative therapy for sigmoid volvulus. Identification of risk factors affecting outcome. Dis Colon rectum 1990; 33:643–646.
45. Kuzu MA, Aslar AK, Soran A, Polat A, Topcu Ö, Hengirmen S. Emergent resection for acute sigmoid volvulus: results of 106 consecutive cases. Dis Colon Rectum 2002; 45:1085–1090.
46. Naaeder SB, Archampong EQ. One-stage resection of acute sigmoid volvulus. Br J Surg 1995; 82: 1635–1536.
47. Sule AZ, Iya D, Obekpa PO, Ogbonna B, Momoh JT, Ugwu BT. One-stage procedure in the management of acute sigmoid volvulus. J R Coll Surg Edin 1999; 44:164–166.
48. Pahlman L, Enblad P, Rudberg C, Krog M. Volvulus of the colon: a review of 93 cases and current aspects of treatment. Acta Chir Scand 1989; 155:53–56.
49. Sundin JA, Wasson D, McMillen MM, Ballantyne GH. Laparoscopic-assisted sigmoid colectomy for sigmoid volvulus. Surg Laparosc Endosc 1992; 2:353–358.
50. Pruett B. Laparoscopic colectomy for sigmoid volvulus. J Miss State Med Assoc 1993; 34:73–75.
51. Mariette D, Sbai-Idrissi S, Bobocescu E, Vons C, Franco D, Smadja C. Laparoscopic colectomy: technique and results. J Chir (Paris) 1996; 133:3–5.
52. Chung CC, Kwok SP, Leung KL, Kwong KH, Lau WY, Li AK. Laparoscopy-assisted sigmoid colectomy for volvulus. Surg Laparosc Endosc 1997; 7:423–425.
53. Chung RS. Colectomy for sigmoid volvulus. Dis Colon rectum 1997; 40:363–365.
54. Subrahmanyam M. Mesosigmoidoplasty as a definitive operation for sigmoid volvulus. Br J Surg 1992; 79:683–684.

55. Salim AS. Management of acute volvulus of the sigmoid colon: a new approach by percutaneous deflation and colopexy. World J Surg 1991; 15:68–73.

56. Pinedo G, Kirberg A. Percutaneous endoscopic sigmoidopexy in sigmoid volvulus with T-fasteners. Dis Colon Rectum 2001; 44:1867–1870.

57. Donhauser JL, Atwell S. Volvulus of the cecum. Arch Surg 1949; 58:129–148.

58. Madiba TE, Thomson SR. The management of cecal volvulus. Dis Colon Rectum 2002; 45:264–267.

59. Burke JB, Ballantyne GH. Cecal volvulus: low mortality at a city hospital. Dis Colon Rectum 1984; 27:737–740.

60. Wolfer JA, Beaton LE, Anson BJ. Volvulus of the cecum: anatomic factors in its etiology. Report of a case. Surg Gynecol Obstet 1942; 74:882–894.

61. Berger RB, Hillemeier AC, Stahl RS, Markowitz RI. Volvulus of the ascending colon: an unusual complication of non-rotation of the midgut. Pediatr Radiol 1982; 12:298–300.

62. Bedard CK, Ramirez A, Holsinger D. Ascending colon volvulus due to a vitelline duct remnant in an elderly patient. Am J Gastroenterol 1979; 71:617–620.

63. Grover NK, Gulati SM, Tagore NK, Taneja OP. Volvulus of the cecum and ascending colon. Am J Surg 1973; 125:672–675.

64. Rehbar A, Easley GW, Mendoza CB Jr. Volvulus of the cecum. Am Surg 1973; 39:325–330.

65. Natarajan A, D'Souza RE, Lahoti NG. A rare case of dual obstruction of the colon. Trop Gastro-enterol 2001; 22:215–216.

66. Sorg J, Whitaker WG Jr., Richmond L. Volvulus of the right colon in the postpartum and postoper-ative period. JMA Ga 1977; 66:519–523.

67. Kerry RL, Lee F, Ransom HK. Roentgenologic examination in the diagnosis and treatment of colonic volvulus. AJR 1971; 113:343–348.

68. Frank AJ, Goffner LB, Fruauff AA, Losada RA. Cecal volvulus: the CT whirl sign. Abdom Imaging 1993; 18:288–289.

69. Anderson JR, Mills JO. Caecal volvulus: a frequently missed diagnosis. Clin Radiol 1984; 35:65–69.

70. Gupta S, Gupta SK. Acute caecal volvulus: report of 22 cases and review of the literature. Ital J Gastroenterol 1993; 25:380–384.

71. Orchard JL, Mehta R, Khan AH. The use of colonoscopy in the treatment of colonic volvulus. Am J Gastroenterol 1984; 79:864–867.

72. Anderson MJ Sr., Okike N, Spencer PJ. The colonoscope in cecal volvulus: report of three cases. Dis Colon Rectum 1978; 21:71–74.

73. Patel D, Ansari E, Berman MD. Percutaneous decompression of cecal volvulus. Am J Radiol 1987; 148:747–748.

74. Gordon R, Watson K. Ileosigmoid knot. J R Coll Surg Edinb 1984; 29:100–102.

75. Shepherd JJ. Ninety two cases of ileosigmoid knotting in Uganda. Br J Surg 1967; 54:561–566.

76. Smith WR, Goodwin JH. Cecal volvulus. Am J Surg 1973; 126:215–222.

77. Howard RS. Caecal volvulus. Arch Surg 1980; 115:274–277.

78. Shoop SA, Sackier JM. Laparoscopic cecopexy for cecal volvulus. Case report and review of the literature. Surg Endosc 1993; 7:450–454.

79. Todd GH, Forde KA. Volvulus of the caecum. Choice of operation. Am J Surg 1979; 138:632–634.

80. Hiltunen K, Syrjaö H, Matikainen M. Colonic volvulus. Diagnosis and results of treatment in 82 patients. Eur J Surg 1992; 158:607–611.

81. Rabinovici R, Simansky DA, Kaplan O, Mavor E, Manny J. Cecal volvulus. Dis Colon Rectum 1990; 33:765–769.

82. Anderson JR, Welch GH. Acute volvulus of the right colon. An analysis of 69 patients. World J Surg 1986; 10:336–342.

83. Isbister WH. Large bowel volvulus. Int I Colorectal Dis 1996; 11:96–98.

84. Remes-Troche JM, Perez-Martinez C, Rembis V, Arch Ferrer J, Ayala Gonzales M, Takahashi T. Surgical treatment of colonic volvulus. 10-year experience at the Instituo Nacional de la Nutricion Salvador Zubiran. Rev Gastroenterol Mex 1997; 62:276–280.

85. Grossmann EM, Johnson FE, Enger KT, Leake BA, Virgo KS, Longo WE. Cecal volvulus: outcome of management by celiotomy. Tech Coloproctol 1999; 3:139–143.

86. Tuech JJ, Becouarn G, Cattan F, Arnaud JP. Volvulus of the right colon. Plea for right hemicolectomy. Apropos of a series of 23 cases. J Chir (Paris) 1996; 133:267–269.

87. Tuech JJ, Pessaux P, Regenet N, Derouet N, Bergamaschi R, Arnaud JP. Results of resection for volvulus of the right colon. Tech Coloproctol 2002; 6:97–99.

88. Orangio GR, Fazio VW, Winkelman Em, McGonagle BA. The Chiliaditi syndrome and associated volvulus of the transverse colon: an indication for surgical therapy. Dis Colon Rectum 1986; 29:653–656.

89. Eisenstat TE, Raneri AJ, Mason GR. Volvulus of the transverse colon. Am J Surg 1977; 134:396–399.

90. Martin JD Jr., Ward CS. Megacolon associated with volvulus of the transverse colon. Am J Surg 1944; 64:412–416.

91. Budd DC, Nirdlinger EL, Sturtz DL, Fouty WJ Jr. Transverse colon volvulus associated with scleroderma. Am J Surg 1977; 133:370–372.

92. Newton NA, Reines HD. Transverse colon volvulus: case reports and review. Am J Roentgenol 1977; 128:69–72.

93. Joergensen K, Kronborg O. The colonoscope in volvulus of the transverse colon. Dis Colon Rectum 1980; 23:357–358.

94. Mortensen NJM, Hoffmann G. Volvulus of the transverse colon. Postgrad Med J 1979; 55:54–57.

95. Gumbs MA, Kashan F, Shumofsky E, Yerubandi SR. Volvulus of the transverse colon. Reports of cases and review of the literature. Dis Colon Rectum 1983; 26:825–828.

96. Asabe K, Ushijima H, Bepu R, Shirakusa T. A case of transverse colon volvulus in a child and a review of the literature in Japan. J Pediatr Surg 2002; 37:1626–1628.

97. Welch GH, Anderson JR. Volvulus of the splenic flexure of the colon. Dis Colon Rectum 1985; 28: 592–593.

98. Hajivassiliou CA, Farrow G, Harvey J. Splenic flexure volvulus presenting as proximal small intestinal obstruction. Aus N Z J Surg 1999; 69:318–319.

99. Mahajan R, Seth S, Braithwaite PA. Volvulus of the splenic flexure of colon: a case report and review. Int J Colorectal Dis 2000; 15:182–184.

100. Echenique Elizondo M, Amondarain Arratibel JA. Colonic volvulus. Rev Esp Enferm Dig 2002; 94:201–210.

23 | Adenoma/Adenocarcinoma (Excluding Adenomatous Polyposis)

David Weinberg
Gastroenterology Section, Divisions of Medical and Population Sciences, Fox Chase Cancer Center, Philadelphia, Pennsylvania, U.S.A.

Nancy Lewis and Elin Sigurdson
Division of Medical Sciences, Fox Chase Cancer Center, Philadelphia, Pennsylvania, U.S.A.

Michael Meyers
Department of Surgery, University of North Carolina, Chapel Hill, North Carolina, U.S.A.

INTRODUCTION

Colorectal cancer (CRC) is the third most commonly diagnosed cancer in the United States for both men and women. Only lung cancer exceeds it as a cause of cancer-related mortality (1). Through the identification and removal of adenomatous colorectal polyps, opportunities exist not just for early detection, but also for disease prevention. The adenoma–carcinoma sequence remains a paradigm of stepwise human carcinogenesis. The molecular and genetic alterations that characterize this progression, its time course, and phenotypic correlates are increasingly understood. Most CRCs develop in previously benign adenomas. Interruption of this sequence, through screening and mechanical intervention (polypectomy) reduces subsequent CRC incidence (2,3). It is hoped that chemoprevention for persons at average (4,5) and higher risk (6) will also prove beneficial. Unfortunately, neither screening nor chemoprevention is at present widely utilized in the general population (7).

Overall CRC incidence rates have modestly declined in the past 25 years, although this change is not equally shared by all segments of the population (Table 1) (8). Surgery remains the mainstay of curative therapy, although significant therapeutic advances for persons with locoregional or metastatic disease have been made in the last decade. The present chapter addresses the epidemiology of colon adenomas and cancer, current recommendations for screening persons at average risk for disease, and medical and surgical therapies for patients with CRC. While briefly mentioned, the molecular biology of CRC is more fully discussed in the chapter on polyposis syndromes and hereditary colon cancer, as are screening and treatment recommendations for persons at substantially elevated risk to develop CRC.

EPIDEMIOLOGY
General Trends

The epidemiology of colon adenomas and CRC is very similar. Unless stated otherwise, they will be considered together. The prevalence of colonic neoplasia varies widely around the world (9). In general, incidence rates are highest in developed countries. Such patterns are maintained even when age-related incidence is standardized, suggesting that environmental variations, particularly diet, underlie these patterns.

Age, Gender, and Ethnicity

Sporadic CRC is an age-related process. The prevalence of both colonic adenomas and CRC increases with age for both men and women. The development of adenomatous polyps generally precedes that of cancer by five to ten years (10); all ethnic groups in the United States are

Table 1 Age-Adjusted Colorectal Cancer Incidence and Mortality Rates 1992–1999[a]

	Incidence		Mortality	
Race/ethnicity[b]	Rate/100,000	Estimated annual percent change (%)	Rate/100,000	Estimated annual percent change (%)
All	54.3	−0.6	22.3	−1.7[c]
White (non-Hispanic)	55.2	−0.6	22.0	−1.8[c]
White (Hispanic)	37.5	−0.4	13.7	−0.7[c]
Black	61.9	−0.5	29.1	−0.5[c]
Asian/Pacific Islander	47.9	−0.2	13.7	−2.3[c]
American Indian/Alaska Native	35.2	1.7	12.8	2.8
Hispanic	35.7	−0.4	13.2	−0.7[c]

[a]Incidence and mortality trends are based on published surveillance, epidemiology, and end results (SEER) data (8).
[b]Race/ethnicity definitions based on National Institutes of Health (NIH) defined criteria.
[c]Trend is significantly different from zero ($p < 0.05$).

affected by CRC. Overall incidence and mortality rates for CRC have declined modestly since 1985, although this benefit has been less pronounced for African-Americans in the United States than for other race or ethnic groups (Table 1) (8). Declines in overall mortality may be due to greater population screening and improved diagnostic tools as well as treatment advances, particularly adjuvant chemotherapy (8,11).

Subsite Location

Within the colon itself, there appears to have been a "shift to the right" over time in terms of segmental location of neoplasia (12). The basis for this shift is unknown, but may reflect variable disease susceptibility of the left (descending, rectosigmoid) versus right colon. Interestingly, women appear more prone than men to right-sided cancers (13).

Physical Activity and Obesity

Substantial observational data suggest that regular physical activity may reduce CRC risk (14). In most studies, CRC risk decreased in a graded fashion relative to qualitative assessment of increasing exercise. Those individuals engaged in moderate or heavy activity had less than half the risk of those people who did not exercise. The mechanism for the apparent protective effect of physical activity is not known. Body mass has also been linked to CRC risk (15); as with physical activity, there is a direct relationship between progressive obesity and cancer risk (16). Because of the potential link between exercise and body mass, presumably these findings reflect similar root causes that require further exploration, because additional studies have linked total energy intake, glycemic load, and other related factors to CRC risk (17,18).

SPECIFIC ENVIRONMENTAL ASSOCIATIONS
Diet

The broadest support for the important role of diet in CRC comes from multiple observational studies demonstrating altered CRC risk profiles with migration or dietary change (9,19).

Fat

In general, diets high in fat are thought to increase cancer risk. Although the specific mechanisms relating dietary fat to CRC are unknown, multiple hypotheses have been advanced, linking cholesterol or bile acid and their metabolites with colon carcinogenesis (20). Additional theories regarding prostaglandin synthesis or the incorporation of fatty acids into cell membranes have been posited (21). Clinical studies of dietary fat alone reveal only a modest increase in CRC risk. After controlling for total energy intake (see section "Physical Activity and Obesity" above), women in the highest quintile of animal fat intake had a relative risk approximately twice that of women in the lowest quintile (22). Fat derived predominantly from red meat, rather than other animal sources increased risk slightly more. However, recent studies employing cohort or case–control designs have not identified a similar relationship (23,24).

From the perspective of cancer control, interventional studies aimed at reducing CRC via low fat diets have demonstrated no benefit (25). Further complicating the issue, specific types of dietary fat may prove beneficial. Marine fish oils are rich in unsaturated fatty acids, particularly n-3 and ω-3. The incidence of CRC is lower in areas where fish consumption is high (9). Animal studies of fish oils supplements demonstrate a reduction in crypt proliferative indices and beneficial effects on arachidonic acid concentration, both of which theoretically could reduce CRC risk (26).

Fiber

The majority of published studies support the contention that high fiber intake reduces CRC risk. A meta-analysis demonstrated a 47% risk reduction for persons consuming the greatest amounts of fiber relative to those subjects consuming the least (23). Mechanistically, fiber increases stool bulk and reduces bowel transit time, both of which result in reduced contact time between the bowel wall and potential intraluminal carcinogens. However, a high fiber diet emphasizing fruits and vegetables is also generally one rich in nonfiber nutrients. Differentiating which constituents are beneficial is difficult.

While primary prevention trials are encouraging, fiber supplementation to prevent adenoma recurrence has shown little benefit (25,27). At present, it remains an open question whether diets historically rich in fiber can minimize initial polyp (and by extension CRC) development. Initiation of high fiber diets later in life after the development of polyps, at least at present, seems less valuable.

Fruits and Vegetables

As suggested above, fruits and vegetables may contain high amounts of fiber and other protective nutrients. Which of the many constituents of these foods is active is unclear. At the most general level, diets rich in vegetables reduce CRC more than diets emphasizing fruit (28). Risk reductions of up to 40% have been described in observational studies for persons with the highest vegetable intake compared to the lowest intake (29). However, despite this information, data from controlled trials is lacking.

OTHER RISK FACTORS

Several diseases are associated with excess CRC risk; the most common of which is inflammatory bowel disease, where CRC risk parallels the extent and duration of colonic involvement (30). Endometrial or ovarian cancer predisposes women to colon cancer risk two to three times more than similarly aged women, but only if these gynecological cancers developed before age 50 to 60 (31). Previous breast cancer appears to confer little or no increased risk (32). Unlike other major cancers, there are little data regarding the role of occupational or toxic environmental exposure in the development of CRC (33). There are multiple small studies that attempt to link CRC with various infections and prescription medications. Unfortunately, effect sizes are small and the results inconsistent.

PATHOGENESIS OF COLONIC NEOPLASIA

Transformation of normal colonic mucosa to cancer occurs through several unique pathways with a similar end point. It is currently accepted that, in most cases, there is a stepwise progression from normal colonocyte to adenoma to carcinoma accompanied by progressively greater genetic alteration (34). This well-established paradigm applies to sporadic CRC as well as to hereditary syndromes such as familial adenomatous polyposis (FAP) (35,36). The contribution of various mechanisms—loss or mutation of chromosomal material, infidelity of DNA replication, and a growing awareness of the impact of epigenetic factors such as aberrant methylation—continue to be described (35,37).

Adenomatous polyposis coli (APC) gene mutations generally initiate the neoplastic process and allow adenoma formation (38–40). While a rough order of mutations is often observed, their aggregate presence, rather than the order of acquisition may play a greater role (Fig. 1).

Although a stepwise genetic pathway can be applied to the majority of sporadic colon cancers, evidence to support alternative pathways has also been described (3,41). Other proposed mechanisms include de novo carcinomas and lesions arising via the so-called serrated pathway

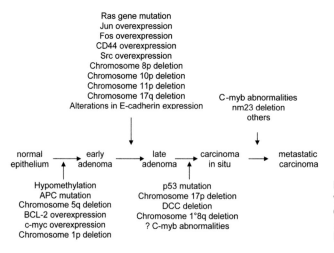
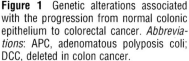

Figure 1 Genetic alterations associated with the progression from normal colonic epithelium to colorectal cancer. *Abbreviations*: APC, adenomatous polyposis coli; DCC, deleted in colon cancer.

(34). De novo carcinoma has been associated with the dome epithelium that overlies mucosa-associated lymph tissue in both experimental models and human subjects (42,43).

Malignant transformation does not necessarily appear associated only with adenomatous polyp formation. Serrated polyps include hyperplastic and mixed polyps and serrated adenomas (44). Recent evidence suggests that these polyps have a variety of genetic alterations that have previously been associated with adenomatous polyps and cancers including K-*ras* mutations, microsatellite instability (particularly microsatellite instability (MSI) MSI-high lesions), and loss of heterozygosity (45,46). Additional evidence for this alternate pathway is suggested by the findings of absent MSI-H expression in adenomatous polyps, the high degree of MSI-H expression in hyperplastic polyps, and the absence of classic genetic alterations associated with CRC (*APC, ras*, etc.) in MSI-H cancers (47,48).

Several other factors have been implicated in the development of colon cancer. A number of proangiogenic regulators have been associated with both transformation to cancer and development of metastasis. Among these agents are several small molecule growth factors, including basic fibroblast growth factor (bFGF), platelet-derived growth factor (PDGF), and vascular endothelial growth factor (VEGF) (49). VEGF remains the best characterized. It has been implicated in the progression of adenoma to carcinoma, but appears particularly important in metastasis, having been expressed in higher levels in tumors associated with metastatic disease than those without (50,51).

Cyclooxygenase (COX), in particular COX-2, has also been implicated in colon cancer development. COX-2 is detectable in 80% to 90% of colorectal adenocarcinomas, and expression is increased in colorectal adenomas when compared to normal mucosa (52,53). COX-2 expression has also correlated with invasiveness of CRC cell lines in vitro (54). This enzyme is of particular interest as a target for therapeutic intervention as well as chemoprevention.

Abnormalities in multiple genetic pathways can lead to CRC. The very brief discussion above highlights the heterogeneity of the transformation of normal mucosa to a malignant one. Interested readers should refer to the chapter on hereditary colon cancer and polyposis syndromes for a more complete review of the biology of colorectal neoplasia.

SCREENING FOR COLORECTAL NEOPLASIA

CRC screening reduces cancer-related incidence and mortality (2,55). Multiple authorities now recommend CRC screening as basic, preventive health care for persons 50 years and older at average risk (56,57). Average risk is assumed for any person free of signs or symptoms suggestive of CRC, without a personal or family history of the disease and without any concomitant diseases that might increase risk (Table 2).

The aim of screening is to sort asymptomatic persons into high-risk versus low-risk categories. It is important to emphasize the silent nature of most colon polyps and early colon cancers. Patients with CRC who develop anemia, abdominal pain, change in bowel habits, weight loss, or visible blood in stools are more likely to have an advanced neoplasm (21). Once

Table 2 Factors that Increase or Decrease Risk for Colorectal Cancer

Increased risk	Reduced risk
Age	Long-term use of aspirin or other nonsteroidal
Personal history of colorectal adenomas or cancer	anti-inflammatory drugs
Family history of colorectal adenomas or cancer	Long-term use of folic acid and calcium (?) supplements
Ulcerative colitis or Crohn's disease with substantial colonic	Hormone replacement therapy
involvement	Regular exercise
Prior endometrial or ovarian cancer	

signs or symptoms have arisen, "screening" for colon cancer is no longer appropriate. Specific complaints warrant expedient evaluation, optimally as thorough endoscopic assessment.

Multiple methods for screening have been advocated, including fecal occult blood testing (FOBT), flexible sigmoidoscopy (FS), barium enema (BE), and colonoscopy (Table 3) (57). Specific details of each are described below. FOBT is the most rigorously studied of the group, and the only modality with direct evidence from controlled, prospective trials that document clinical effectiveness (55). Because colonoscopy combines diagnostic accuracy with therapeutic capability, it is the present screening gold standard. However it is the most expensive option and the one with the greatest potential for complication. For persons at average risk, the "best test" is uncertain. Lacking compelling data, at present, it seems most appropriate for healthcare providers to concentrate on increasing screening by their patients through periodic use of any of the recommended techniques (58). All have been demonstrated as cost-effective (59). The availability of a number of acceptable options should be promoted as a positive aspect of CRC screening, not an excuse for the lack of performance.

Despite increased public awareness of CRC and greater willingness by insurers to cover screening costs, CRC screening rates remain low. Recent surveys suggest that less than 40% of the eligible population has ever completed a fecal occult blood test or FS, two screening mainstays (60). Less than 10% of the average risk populations have completed both of these tests within the recommended screening intervals. Participation in CRC screening lags behind screening for other malignancies such as breast and cervical cancer (7).

Specific CRC Screening Methods
Fecal Occult Blood Testing
FOBT is the most commonly used screening technique. It is simple to employ, inexpensive, and noninvasive. The best studied of several FOBT methods is the guaiac impregnated slide test. The pseudoperoxidase activity of hemoglobin is the basis for a true-positive result. It is important to emphasize that FOBT is a method to test the stool for blood, not for cancer. Hence, there are many causes of both false-positive and false-negative tests (Table 4).

Table 3 Representative Colorectal Cancer Screening Recommendations for Persons 50 Years and Older at Average Risk

Test	American Cancer Society	American College of Gastroenterology	U.S. Preventive Services Task Force
FOBT	Annually + flexible sigmoidoscopy every 5 yr	Annually + flexible sigmoidoscopy every 5 yr	Annually
Sigmoidoscopy	Every 5 yr	Every 5 yr	"Fair" evidence supporting use, but frequency not specified
FOBT + sigmoidoscopy	Annual FOBT + flexible sigmoidoscopy every 5 yr	Annual FOBT + flexible sigmoidoscopy every 5 yr	No clear evidence that combination is better than either test alone
Barium enema	Every 5 yr	Every 5–10 yr	No evidence of mortality reduction
Colonoscopy	Every 10 yr	Every 10 yr	Only indirect evidence of mortality reduction

Abbreviation: FOBT, fecal occult blood testing.

Table 4   Common Causes of False-Positive and False-Negative Fecal Occult Blood Testing

False positive	False negative
Non-neoplastic causes of gastrointestinal bleeding	Intermittent blood loss from neoplasia
Oral or nasal bleeding	Incorrect sampling or development
Exogenous peroxidase activity (red meat, some uncooked fruits, or vegetables)	Prolonged slide storage
	Vitamin C consumption
Medications [anticoagulants, nonsteroidal anti-inflammatory drugs (?)]	

False-positive tests result most often from non-neoplastic sources of gastrointestinal (GI) bleeding. Intermittently bleeding or nonbleeding polyps or cancers are the most frequent reason for falsely negative tests. Bleeding from the GI tract must generally be 5-fold to 10-fold greater than normal physiologic blood loss for a positive test (61). Thus, many patients with CRC will have a false-negative FOBT (62). While it is recommended that patients be counseled to alter their diet and to limit their intake of various medications, particularly nonsteroidal anti-inflammatory drugs (NSAIDs) for several days prior to FOBT use, there is little evidence these maneuvers are clinically meaningful (63,64).

Of greater practical concern is the frequent lack of follow-up of positive FOBT results. Only 50% of persons with a positive test performed for screening undergo a complete radiographic or endoscopic evaluation of their colon (65). A recent study documented that FOBT(+) patients were nearly fourfold more likely to have CRC or a worrisome adenomatous polyp than FOBT(−) patients (30.5% vs. 8.8%), strongly supporting complete colonic evaluation for any FOBT(+) patient (66).

Test Characteristics of FOBT

Although of primary importance for population-based screening, the sensitivity of FOBT testing in the asymptomatic population is not clear. Estimates have been derived largely from studies of symptomatic persons with known polyps or colon cancer. These estimates range from 10% to 39% for polyps and 50% to 92% for malignancy. The specificity of FOBT in this setting is greater than 95% (56).

The more clinically relevant positive predictive value (PPV) of FOBT is better described (Table 5). PPV reflects the likelihood that a person with a positive test has the target disease (adenomatous polyp or CRC). The PPV for any test depends in part on the prevalence of the disease (colonic neoplasia) in the screened population. The PPV of FOBT in population-based screening has been 2.5% to 50% for carcinomas and 16% to 40% for adenomas (56). This low PPV is virtually inevitable in the general population because most people do not have CRC.

Because of the limitations of FOBT testing, efforts have been made to develop other methods of detecting blood in stool, including tests based on the porphyrin-like moiety of hemoglobin (HemoQuant) as well as a human hemoglobin assay. While they may ultimately prove more useful than standard FOBT, they have not yet been the subjects of large-scale clinical testing (9).

FOBT Trials in Average Risk Persons

Several large prospective studies of FOBT have been completed (67–69). They document a reduction in CRC mortality of 15% to 33% depending on whether FOBT was performed

Table 5   Selected Results from Controlled Fecal Occult Blood Testing Screening Trials

Site	FOBT (+) rate (%)	PPV (%)	Dukes A or B colorectal cancer at diagnosis (%)	
			Screened	Unscreened
Sweden	1.9	22	65	33
United States	2.4	31	78	35
Denmark	1.0	58	81	55
England	2.1	53	90	40

Abbreviations: PPV, positive predictive value; FOBT, fecal occult blood testing.
Source: From Ref. 56.

annually or every other year. More recently, continued follow-up of the Minnesota cohort also demonstrated that regular use of FOBT led to a reduction in CRC incidence (2).

Periodic FOBT use is likely to reduce CRC incidence and mortality for two reasons. First, it allows the detection of adenomas prior to malignant transformation. Many polyps, particularly those lesions greater than 1 cm in diameter, bleed sufficiently for detection (70). The second reason is earlier cancer detection—people with regular exposure to FOBT tend to have earlier stage lesions than those persons whose cancers are detected because of symptom development. All major studies reveal that at least 70% of cancers in the "screened" group are confined to the bowel wall at diagnosis, compared to about 33% of persons presenting with symptoms. As CRC survival closely parallels cancer stage at diagnosis, these findings are not surprising.

In summary, FOBT is a potentially beneficial, but underutilized method of CRC screening. A recent meta-analysis demonstrates that the overall mortality reduction with FOBT use is 16% (71). The analysis further suggested that with optimal use of FOBT, a 23% reduction in mortality is possible. Such reductions would only be seen with wider use of screening and appropriate follow-up of positive examinations.

Flexible Sigmoidoscopy

Unlike FOBT, FS offers the opportunity to visualize the lower-third of the colon and to biopsy or remove polyps when found. Current average risk-screening guidelines recommend sigmoidoscopy every three to five years beginning at the age of 50, alone or with annual FOBT (57).

Many patients view sigmoidoscopy as embarrassing and physically uncomfortable. Physician reluctance stems from several issues: The continued absence of any prospective data suggesting that sigmoidoscopy reduces colon cancer morbidity or mortality and concerns about patient acceptability and lack of adequate reimbursement (72). As a result, only 15% to 30% of eligible persons undergo such testing (60).

Screening sigmoidoscopy theoretically offers substantial benefits; however its effectiveness has not been documented in randomized clinical trials. Sigmoidoscopy allows the detection and removal of adenomas prior to malignant transformation. In addition, it may offer a method of CRC risk stratification, if sigmoidoscopic results offer reliable predictive information about the likelihood of polyps or cancers in the nonvisualized colon. Such knowledge could modify the intensity of immediate follow-up (i.e., colonoscopy) and subsequent screening (73,74). As discussed below, the significance of distal polyps found on sigmoidoscopy remains uncertain (73–75).

Understanding the average distribution of polyps throughout the colon is essential to the evaluation of sigmoidoscopy as a screening tool. However, this information is generally lacking, because studies in asymptomatic, randomly selected individuals are limited. In the few studies of colonoscopy in healthy populations older than 50 years, nearly 25% of all persons had adenomas, with the majority (greater than 70%) distal to the transverse colon (76). Other studies suggest that approximately 40% of the adult population will develop an adenoma at some point, whereas only 5% to 6% of individuals develop colon cancer; therefore few adenomas progress to carcinoma (77).

Hyperplastic (nonadenomatous) polyps are frequent findings in the distal colon. While there may be occasional exceptions (78), the great majority of hyperplastic polyps pose no significant risk to progress to colon cancer, nor do they serve as "sentinel" lesions for more dangerous proximal adenomas. Sigmoidoscopy has a sensitivity and specificity for distal colonic polyps of both 95% or greater. However, sigmoidoscopy produces frequent false-positive results if one considers the detection of polyps with no or little malignant potential as test failures. As noted above, most polyps detected on routine examination will not progress to clinically significant neoplasia over time. At endoscopy, however, it is currently impossible to differentiate the fate of individual polyps. Because standard practice is to remove all polyps at the time of detection, it would be unethical to leave polyps in place for observation in some individuals. However, when the cost of sigmoidoscopy-based screening programs are calculated, consideration should be given to the number and cost of follow-up colonoscopies in persons very unlikely ever to develop significant colonic pathology (11,72). Ongoing studies of sigmoidoscopy in the United States and the United Kingdom may shed information in this regard (79).

To date, there have been no prospective, randomized trials evaluating the possible benefits of sigmoidoscopy. However, two well-done case-control studies provide good evidence that sigmoidoscopy is an effective screening technique (80,81). Selby retrospectively studied CRC-related mortality for patients whose cancers arose within 20 cm of the anus. Compared to controls, significantly fewer cases had undergone rigid sigmoidoscopy within the previous 10 years. Exposure to sigmoidoscopy was associated with a 70% reduction in cancer mortality resulting from tumors within reach of the endoscope. Sigmoidoscopy yielded no mortality benefit for patients with tumors beyond the reach of the endoscope, arguing against significant biases between cases and controls. A similar, but smaller study, reported an 80% reduction in CRC mortality for those individuals who had a sigmoidoscopy compared with those persons not examined (81).

If the benefit of FS screening were limited only to that gathered through the performance of a single endoscopy, detection of colonic polyps and cancers would still be greatly improved relative to no screening or to FOBT alone. By definition, sigmoidoscopy will miss proximal colonic lesions. Because most positive sigmoidoscopic examinations are followed by the evaluation of the remaining colon, prevention of colon cancer as a result of sigmoidoscopy would exceed the 50% predicted based on the percentage of potential cancers accessible to the flexible endoscope. However what characteristics of the distal polyp are sufficient to constitute a "positive" sigmoidoscopy and prompt a full colonic evaluation remain unclear. If any adenoma is an acceptable indication, then about 70% of important neoplastic lesions (cancers and advanced adenomas, i.e., adenomas greater than 1 cm or those with villous histology or dysplasia) will be detected using a sigmoidoscopy-based screening mechanism. However, it has been estimated that about 25% of persons with a normal sigmoidoscopy will harbor significant proximal adenomas (73–75).

Stratification of risk based upon "distal" colonic findings could be an important method to increase the utility of sigmoidoscopy if distal results could reliably predict the presence or absence of important proximal lesions. In existing studies, the presence of multiple distal adenomas, any distal adenoma with a villous component, or one with dysplasia were each important predictors of proximal disease (82). Other variables include age greater than 65 years, male gender, more than one adenoma, and a family history of CRCs were also predictors (74). Future, prospective studies are required, however, to determine the utility of these types of clinical variables.

Barium Enema

Methodologically rigorous studies of the role of BE in CRC screening are limited. Single-contrast BE is an inadequate method to detect polyps in most cases. Double-contrast (air and barium) techniques improve the ability of BE to detect colonic neoplasia. Early studies suggested that the accuracy of double-contrast BE in screening for polyps and cancers greater than 1 cm was greater than 90% (11). Proponents of radiographic screening argue that the great majority of cancers originate in these larger polyps; therefore barium-based studies are a useful method to identify patients most in need of colonoscopy and polypectomy. However, more recent direct comparisons of BE and colonoscopy suggest that the former identifies only 50% of polyps 1 cm or more in size seen on colonoscopy (83).

BE remains an alternative for average risk screening, although in the United States, interest is clearly shifting to colonoscopy as a method to visualize the entire large bowel, despite its greater expense and potential for complication.

Colonoscopy

Increasingly, colonoscopy is advocated as the optimal mode of CRC screening, combining diagnostic and therapeutic capability into one examination. While clearly and irrefutably increasing the detection of colonic neoplasia, wide adoption would entail substantially higher cost and risk compared with FOBT or sigmoidoscopy. The risk of significant complication from colonoscopy is estimated at <1/1500 procedures, while the charge per procedure is generally $1000 or greater (84–86). By comparison, sigmoidoscopy charges are approximately $150, with a significant complication rate of 1/2000 procedures.

While it is a reasonable supposition, there are no data from randomized clinical trials demonstrating the superiority of colonoscopy to other screening techniques, nor is there any information directly indicating that a program of periodic colonoscopy results in a reduction in CRC incidence or mortality for persons at average risk. The National Polyp Study compared the cancer risk for persons with known adenomas whose polyps were removed, to those in whom polyps were left in place (3). Colonoscopy-based primary prevention trials would be very expensive and time consuming, although efforts to arrange such trials are underway (11).

Two studies recently published provide some valuable information comparing colonoscopy with FS (73–75). Overall, approximately 40% of patients had an adenoma, and 10% of all persons undergoing average risk screening colonoscopy harbored either a cancer or an advanced adenoma (definition above) at the time of their colonoscopy. In these studies, any findings distal to the splenic flexure were taken as a proxy for those that hypothetically would be identified by sigmoidoscopy. Clearly this represented a best-case scenario, not likely achieved in standard clinical practice. Under these conditions, one-third of cancers and 40% of advanced neoplasia would have been missed by sigmoidoscopy.

A substantial advantage of colonoscopy compared to FOBT or FS is the interval between examinations. The high prevalence and slow growth rate of colonic polyps have prompted suggestions of screening strategies using a single colonoscopy at the age of 55 to 60. Cancer incidence rates increase markedly from approximately 50/100,000 to 244/100,000 at age 65 and 415/100,000 by age 75 (8). A negative examination at age 60 would not only screen for neoplasia, but may also contribute important prognostic information regarding a given individual's propensity for colonic neoplasia. Given the natural history of polyps, presumably 7 to 10 years could elapse between normal examinations for most persons at average risk.

Others have argued that if the cost of colonoscopy were decreased, it would be more cost-effective than any other screening procedure because of better colon visualization, the opportunity for concurrent polypectomy, and the savings from colon cancer averted by early removal of polyps. However, endoscopic availability may limit the feasibility of widespread screening with colonoscopy. Colonoscopy is more difficult to learn and to perform than FS. Although nonphysician providers have been recruited to perform sigmoidoscopy (87), it is unlikely that they could easily be trained to perform colonoscopy and polypectomy. Who would perform all these procedures, and at what interval, would need to be determined.

Cost-Effectiveness of CRC Screening

It is unlikely there will ever be a clinical trial directly comparing the various modes of CRC screening for clinical or cost-effectiveness. In lieu of such trials, researchers have constructed several computer models (86,88). The most obvious drawback of modeling is the possibility for error in the various assumptions about the natural history of colon polyps or cancer, the screening tests themselves, or compliance with testing. Allowing for these potential shortcomings, available models reach several conclusions. First, population-based CRC screening would be expensive. The screening of 60 million average-risk Americans older than 50 with FOBT/FS could cost in excess of three billion dollars annually; this does not include the cost of follow-up colonoscopies. Despite this impressive figure, CRC screening by any standard technique is cost-effective. All screening modalities would cost less than $25,000 per year of life saved. This figure compares favorably to the cost-effectiveness of other widely practiced cancer-screening strategies such as mammography.

It is valuable to recognize that the annual direct costs of colon cancer care were recently estimated to be over five billion dollars (89). Any calculation of the overall financial burden posed by CRC needs to consider associated costs ranging from screening through therapy. While each screening modality is essentially equally cost-effective, the basis for cost savings varies with each modality (90). FOBT is the single least expensive test. It prevents the fewest cancers and therefore has the greatest associated treatment costs. Conversely, colonoscopy on the other extreme is the most expensive screening test, but also prevents the greatest number of cancers. Ultimately, decisions about cost-effectiveness are societal ones. At present, most screening programs emphasize the immediate costs of testing, neglecting to consider longer-term concerns.

Novel Forms of CRC Screening
Virtual Colonoscopy

Rapidly evolving computer hardware and software permit computed tomographic colonography (CTC) and magnetic resonance colonography (MRC) imaging. Growing facility with image interpretation has yielded several intriguing early reports regarding the detection of colonic masses (91–93). Public interest in virtual colonoscopy is substantial, although at present, patients are still required to undergo a laxative-based bowel preparation. False-positive and false-negative rates, especially for smaller lesions, remain too high for broad-based screening. Because these techniques cannot offer therapeutic capacity, virtual colonoscopy may find its place as part of a two-step screening where patients with positive studies proceed to conventional colonoscopy (10). The cost-effectiveness of such an approach requires careful scrutiny before broad adoption. These imaging techniques are also discussed in more detail in the chapter on radiology of the colon.

Fecal DNA screening

The inherent appeal of noninvasive testing has driven studies of other methods to analyze stool samples, beyond the nonspecific finding of occult blood. More precise stool-based testing would represent an advance that may attract broader population-based screening participation. Early studies assessing at the detection of altered DNA in stool are promising as are studies of other markers (94–96). As with virtual colonoscopy, stool-based molecular testing may be too expensive for broad adoption under current conditions.

CRC Risk Assessment

Age, personal, or family history of colorectal neoplasia, and the presence of selected other diseases are the main features affecting risk stratification for CRC (Table 2). At present, risk assessment employs epidemiological associations to identify individual risk. Recent advances have yielded promising genetic testing for persons at higher risk, for example, in FAP. Similar progress, albeit slower, may soon allow for improved, individualized risk assessment for persons at average risk. Early examples include assays for loss of imprinting (97) or the I1307K mutation seen predominantly in Ashkenazi Jews (98).

Until more individualized risk assessment tools become available, application of standard risk criteria suggest that 5% to 10% of the population is at high risk, 15% to 20% at moderate risk, and 70% to 80% at average risk.

High Risk

Family history is the key factor for CRC risk assessment. Approximately 5% of persons with CRC suffer from FAP or hereditary nonpolyposis colon cancer (HNPCC). Early development of CRC in 80% (HNPCC) to 100% (FAP) of affected persons characterizes these autosomal dominant diseases (77). Other characteristics typical of FAP are the presence of hundreds to thousands of colonic polyps as well as a propensity for polyp formation elsewhere in the GI tract. HNPCC or Lynch syndrome is notable for proximal CRCs, fewer polyps, and strong association with extracolonic malignancy. Screening for persons known or suspected to have these syndromes is different than for persons of average risk. Early, periodic endoscopic evaluation is the standard of care for these persons. Referral to centers that are equipped to provide molecular diagnostics and genetic counseling should be considered for all patients with these diseases. As noted, the hereditary colon cancer chapter provides an expanded discussion of this topic.

Moderate Risk

Far more common are patients with a less extensive family history of colon cancer, for instance, a single first-degree relative. "Familial" colon cancer represents about 25% of new colon cancer cases. Individual risk rises stepwise with increasing numbers of affected relatives. In general, a single first-degree relative with CRC increases personal risk by approximately two to three times relative to the general population (99). Associated risk is greatest when the affected relative is less than 50 years of age at diagnosis (100).

It is also important to note that the first-degree relatives of persons with adenomatous polyps exhibit approximately the same degree of cancer risk as the first-degree relatives of persons with CRC (101). However, studies describing this association were more likely to include persons with large or symptomatic polyps. Extrapolating these data to the more common scenario of risk assessment for a patient with a first-degree relative with small polyps is difficult.

Until studies that stratify risk by polyp size (or other factors) are available, it is reasonable to consider polyps in relatives greater than 1 cm to confer a risk similar to CRC.

Persons with a prior history of colonic adenomas intuitively are at elevated risk to develop more adenomas in the future. Exact figures are lacking, but most studies suggest up to a 50% recurrence rate within 15 years (102). These subsequent polyps tend to be smaller and less histologically advanced than the index polyps. In the National Polyp study, adenomas with worrisome histological features (advanced size, villous component, dysplasia, etc.) were seen in approximately 3% of colonoscopies performed three years after the initial study, although it was impossible to determine if these were lesions missed on the prior exam or were de novo adenomas (3).

A prior history of CRC also clearly influences the likelihood of developing a second CRC over time. Metachronous CRC has been described in up to 4.7% of patients (9). The utility of postoperative surveillance is described elsewhere in this chapter.

Finally, as noted above, several common diseases are associated with excess CRC risk. These include inflammatory bowel disease, particularly persons with longstanding pancolitis (30). Early-onset (before the age of 60) endometrial or ovarian cancer increases risk two to three times (31). Finally, there are less compelling data suggesting that a host of conditions such as cholecystectomy, pernicious anemia, type 2 diabetes, and immunosuppression following organ transplantation may all modestly increase CRC risk (33). Table 6 summarizes screening recommendations for these higher-risk populations.

CHEMOPREVENTION

Numerous compounds have been suggested as potential chemopreventive agents for CRC. Cancer chemoprevention relies on the use of agents to prevent, inhibit, or reverse carcinogenesis (103). These agents can be used to intervene at any point in the process of carcinogenesis ranging from before the development of any abnormality until the development of invasive disease.

Table 6 Screening and Surveillance Recommendations for Persons at Moderate and Greater Risk for Colorectal Cancer but Without Prior History Consistent with Hereditary Nonpolyposis Colon Cancer or Familial Adenomanous Polyposis

Personal history	Initial screening	Subsequent screening or surveillance
Adenomatous polyps		
Exam reveals adenoma with any of the following: ≥1 cm, high grade dysplasia, villous component, number greater than 3	Colonoscopy at time of polyp identification	Repeat colonoscopy within 3 yr. If normal, repeat in 3 yr. If normal again, revert to average screening recommendations
Exam reveals <3 adenomas, all <1 cm, all with tubular histology	Colonoscopy at time of polyp identification	Repeat colonoscopy within 5 yr. If normal, revert to average screening recommendations
More than 10 adenomas	Colonoscopy at time of polyp identification	Repeat colonoscopy within 1 yr. Consider genetic testing if clinically appropriate
CRC resected for cure	Preoperative or perioperative clearing colonoscopy	Repeat colonoscopy within 1 yr. If negative, repeat in 3 yr
Family history		
Adenomatous polyps or CRC in first degree relative: prior to age 60 *or* in 2 first-degree relatives of any age	Colonoscopy at 40 or 10 yr earlier than youngest affected relative	Repeat colonoscopy within 5 yr
Other risk factors		
Personal history of inflammatory bowel disease	8 yr after diagnosis (UC or CD) if pancolitis; 15 yr if left-sided colitis only	Repeat colonoscopy every 1–2 yr
Ovarian or endometrial cancer prior to age 60	Colonoscopy within 1 yr of diagnosis	Repeat colonoscopy every 5 yr

Abbreviations: CRC, colorectal cancer; UC, ulcerative colitis; CD, Crohn's disease.
Source: From Refs. 11, 228.

Calcium

The majority of human studies suggest that regular calcium supplementation reduces adenoma formation and recurrence, although variation in duration of use and dose of calcium supplements confounds the overall picture (104). Calcium's benefit is thought to result from reduced colonic epithelial proliferation, perhaps by binding to fatty and bile acids in the fecal stream, thereby reducing toxic exposure to the colonic epithelium (105). A Women's Health Initiative study is randomizing women to receive calcium and Vitamin D or placebo. Results from this study may yield valuable information with respect to this issue.

Antioxidant Vitamins (A, C, E, and Selenium)

Large numbers of studies have addressed the relationship between various vitamins with anti-oxidant potential and CRC (106). It is hypothesized that antioxidants reduce carcinogenesis through neutralization of toxic free radicals. Early enthusiasm about beta carotene (a vitamin A precursor) and the retinoids (vitamin A) have been dampened by the lack of substantial benefit in more recent investigation (107). Unfortunately, adequately powered studies have also demonstrated little benefit from α-tocopherol (vitamin E) (108). While larger studies are ongoing, there appears at present to be little reason to promote these agents for colon cancer prevention (109).

Folate

Folate is central to methyl group metabolism. It is crucial for DNA methylation while also influencing the availability of nucleotides for DNA replication and repair. Adequate intracellular levels of folate are required for DNA synthesis and the production of S-adenosylmethionine, the universal methyl donor important in DNA (and RNA) methylation (110).

Epidemiological studies have linked inadequate folate stores with many human cancers, including CRC (111–113). The strongest data come from the Nurses' Health Study, where more than 88,000 women were followed prospectively for over 15 years. Women in the highest quartile of folate use had a relative risk of 0.69 (95% CI 0.52–0.91) of CRC compared to those in the lowest quartile. Those women who regularly used multivitamin supplements (containing >100 μg of folate) for more than 15 years and did not consume excess alcohol had the greatest decrease of all, with a relative risk of 0.21 for proximal colon cancer and 0.37 for distal malignancy (5).

Nonsteroidal Anti-inflammatory Drugs

The observation that sulindac caused the partial regression of existing polyps in patients with FAP (6) has spurred on extensive investigation of this class of drugs as potential chemopreventive agents in CRC (114). Animal studies and observational epidemiological reports strongly support the protective effect of NSAIDs.

These agents have a myriad of effects including slowing of the cell cycle, stimulation of apoptosis, an antiangiogenic effect, and overall reduction of cellular proliferation (115). Antineoplastic effects operate, at least in great part, via inhibition of COX, an enzyme that facilitates the conversion of arachidonic acids into a variety of bioactive substances (prostaglandins, prostacyclins, and thromboxanes) that can promote carcinogenesis. Two isoforms of COX, COX-1 and COX-2, have been described. COX-1 is constitutively expressed by all cells, and plays an important regulatory role in a number of cellular functions. It is also thought that the clinically undesirable side effects of NSAIDs on platelets, kidneys, and the GI tract result from COX-1 inhibition. In contrast, COX-2 production is induced by a number of cellular growth factors and cytokines associated with neoplasia, inflammation, and other stimuli. Expression of COX-2 is increased in up to 90% of CRCs and more than 50% of colonic adenomas (116).

Multiple observational studies have documented a reduction in CRC for long-term, regular users of aspirin. Risk reduction appears to be as great as 50% (117,118). It is important to note that large trials usually do not demonstrate any substantial benefit until aspirin was regularly consumed for 10 years (117). Because of the apparently long time-frame required to demonstrate benefit in terms of cancer prevention (similar effects are seen with other potential chemopreventive agents such as folate), many studies have employed intermediate markers such as adenoma formation or regression of existing adenomas to document the benefit of

NSAID-based chemoprevention. Both sulindac and more recently, a COX-2 specific inhibitor, celecoxib, have been shown to reduce the number and size of adenomas in randomized trials of FAP patients (6,119). There appears to be less efficacy when NSAIDs were used as a primary preventive technique (120). While the molecular basis for FAP likely shares many characteristics with sporadic adenomas (and cancer), comparable data does not exist for sporadic polyps or cancer. Trials are ongoing to demonstrate the effectiveness of NSAIDs in this setting.

Hormone Replacement Therapy

Numerous observational and case–control studies have documented the protective effect of hormone replacement therapy (HRT) against CRC in women. Meta-analyses of these studies suggest a 20% risk reduction for CRC, particularly for long-term and current users of HRT (121). The basis for this protection is speculative and typically hinges on the role of bile salt pool alteration, although more recent evidence suggests that estrogen can reduce the age-related methylation-based silencing of estrogen receptor expression and it may also limit IGF-1 expression (122,123). Any of these mechanisms theoretically could inhibit carcinogenesis.

Recently, results from the prospective Women's Health Initiative trial reported a 40% reduction in CRC risk for HRT users versus nonusers (124). However, this trial also documented unwanted side effects including an increased risk of breast cancer and no apparent cardioprotective effect from HRT. At present, recommendations about HRT for chemoprevention are unclear, as there are many potential issues to consider.

CLINICAL PRESENTATION AND DIAGNOSIS

The progression from adenoma to carcinoma is generally slow. It is currently thought that 5 to 10 years are typically required for a small adenoma to progress to cancer. While this large window facilitates screening, it tends to limit the acute onset of dramatic or characteristic signs or symptoms. In asymptomatic adults of age 50 and older, up to 40% may develop colonic neoplasia at some point. About 3% to 8% will have advanced lesions (adenomas >1 cm or cancer) (75,125,126). The nonspecific symptoms or signs that lead most often to diagnostic evaluation include intermittent lower GI bleeding or occult fecal blood, change in bowel habits, and abdominal pain (126). These findings tend to be more prominent in those with lesions larger than 1 cm, but even these are usually clinically silent (75).

Manifestations of colonic blood loss range from acute hemorrhage to asymptomatic anemia. Abrupt discharge of large volumes of blood per rectum suggests alternative diagnoses. Hematochezia is more common with left-sided lesions while detection of occult blood loss more often characterizes more proximal lesions. Gradual blood loss is often missed by fecal occult blood tests, but may come to light when anemia (and often iron deficiency) is revealed through standard blood tests. If symptomatic, this microcytic anemia may be accompanied by weakness, dizziness, generalized malaise, or exacerbation of underlying conditions such as ischemic heart disease.

As colon cancers grow, change in bowel habits or crampy abdominal pain may occur as the bowel lumen becomes compromised. This is particularly true for lesions in the left colon where the lumen is of smaller caliber. Colon cancer remains a common cause of bowel obstruction despite increased diligence to screening and early detection. Uncommonly, tumors may progress and present with perforation. This can occur at the site of tumor as a result of tumor penetration though the bowel wall or at a proximal site (most commonly the cecum) secondary to distal obstruction. Both findings are negative prognostic indicators.

Locally advanced tumors may present with other findings less commonly seen, particularly symptoms suggesting invasion of nearby organs or other soft-tissue structures. Symptoms of a colovesical or colovaginal fistula, for example, pneumaturia or fecaluria, may be presenting complaints and are indicative of significant local progression, as is hydronephrosis. Some patients may also present with weight loss and nutritional compromise. Most commonly seen with advanced disease, the latter is likely multifactorial and not simply associated with decreased nutritional intake.

Physical examination is of modest benefit in the diagnosis of colorectal neoplasms. However, a complete examination, including digital rectal examination, is important. Stool should be tested for the presence of occult blood.

ADENOMATOUS POLYPS: THE ROLE OF SIZE AND HISTOLOGY

Colorectal polyps can be divided into those with ultimate malignant potential and those without. Most polyps with malignant potential are adenomatous and can be further subdivided to include tubular, tubulovillous, and villous adenomas.

Adenomatous Polyps

The cancer risk of adenomatous polyps is associated with two factors: the size of the lesion and the degree of villous features histologically. The majority of colorectal adenomas are small, with roughly 95% less than 2 cm in greatest diameter. However, there is a correlation between the degree of villous component and polyp size at diagnosis. Only 4% to 14% of tubular adenomas, but 30% to 60% of tubulovillous and villous adenomas, exceed 2 cm in one series (37,127).

Adenomas smaller than 5 mm confer almost no risk of harboring cancer, while increasing size and villous component have positive linear relationships with invasive capacity. Polyps greater than 2 cm appear to have the greatest risk with more than 6% of tubular adenomas, 11% of tubulovillous adenomas, and 17% of villous adenomas associated with invasive cancer in one series (127). Muto et al. found an even stronger correlation between size and invasive cancer, with 35% of tubular, 46% of tubulovillous, and 53% of villous adenomas greater than 2 cm associated with cancer (37).

Tubular Adenomas

Tubular adenomas are more frequently pedunculated lesions. They represent the majority of adenomatous polyps, accounting for nearly two-thirds of lesions identified (125,127). The majority of tubular adenomas are small, with recent reports suggesting that most are less than 1 cm at detection (75,127). Histologically, these lesions have a predominantly tubular configuration with glands embedded in the lamina propria and infolding of tubules. While the percentage of specific tubular versus villous elements required to define adenoma type is subject to individual definition, it is generally accepted that tubular adenomas must contain greater than 75% tubular features to meet criteria (127). Early lesions generally show minimal atypia, but tubular adenomas can display a wide range of dysplasia. Larger lesions, in particular, can have mild-to-severe dysplasia or harbor invasive carcinoma.

Tubulovillous Adenomas

Tubulovillous adenomas are characterized by a combination of both tubular and villous elements. One definition suggests that a polyp should contain at least 25% of both tubular and villous features to meet criteria (127). However, in practice definitions may be less precise. These lesions occur less frequently than tubular adenomas but harbor malignancy more commonly, with a risk, i.e., 1.5 to 2 times greater than that of tubular adenomas depending on size (127).

Villous Adenomas

Villous adenomas are the least common type of adenomatous polyp, comprising only 5% to 10% of all adenomas. They are more often sessile than other polyps and commonly appear multilobulated and friable with a "cauliflower-like" appearance. Histologically, epithelial fronds that may be single or branched are characteristic. While variable, a lesion with greater than 75% villous morphology meets most definitions for villous adenoma (127). Relative to other adenomatous polyps, villous lesions have the most pronounced association with carcinoma. Importantly, sampling error with endoscopic biopsy may occur, particularly, with larger lesions, and all villous adenomas should be removed completely because of the high rate of associated cancer.

CRC STAGING

A number of staging systems have been described for CRC. From the original description by Dukes more than 70 years ago, staging has evolved in an effort to best reflect prognosis. Ongoing questions about the clinical utility of micrometastatic disease as well as reliable

Table 7 TNM Staging Definitions

TX	Primary tumor cannot be assessed
T0	No evidence of primary tumor
Tis	Carcinoma in situ: intraepithelial or invasion of lamina propria
T1	Tumor invades submucosa
T2	Tumor invades muscularis propria
T3	Tumor invades through the muscularis propria into the subserosa, or into nonperitonealized pericolic or perirectal tissues
T4	Tumor directly invades other organs or structures, and/or perforates visceral peritoneum
Regional lymph nodes (N)	
NX	Regional lymph nodes cannot be assessed
N0	No regional lymph node metastasis
N1	Metastasis in 1 to 3 regional lymph nodes
N2	Metastasis in 4 or more regional lymph nodes
Distant metastasis (M)	
MX	Distant metastasis cannot be assessed
M0	No distant metastasis
M1	Distant metastasis

Stage grouping			
Stage	T	N	M
0	Tis	N0	M0
I	T1	N0	M0
	T2	N0	M0
IIA	T3	N0	M0
IIB	T4	N0	M0
IIIA	T1–T2	N1	M0
IIIB	T3–T4	N1	M0
IIIC	Any T	N2	M0
IV	Any T	Any N	M1

Source: From Ref. 229.

methods to detect it continue to place a high premium on accurate histological staging. In most cases, staging determines not only prognosis, but also therapy.

The combined American Joint Committee on Cancer and International Union Against Cancer system for staging is currently the most widely used. It provides more detail than previous staging systems while adding greater precision in the identification of prognostic groups (128). This system takes into account the primary tumor (T), lymph-node status (N), and the presence of distant metastasis (M) in classifying the extent of disease (Table 7). The tumor node metastasis (TNM) system applies to both clinical and pathologic staging, but the majority of lesions are staged after pathologic review. Five-year survival rates (without treatment) range from 85% to 90% for stage I to less than 5% for stage IV disease. Preoperative staging should consist of routine laboratory studies, including liver function tests and a carcinoembryonic antigen (CEA) level. A preoperative computed tomography (CT) scan should be considered if one is willing to attend to liver metastases surgically at the time of primary colon resection or if liver function tests are abnormal. Positron-emission tomography scan is gaining favor in the staging of CRC, but as yet should be reserved for the evaluation of metastatic disease and not for primary staging.

SURGICAL MANAGEMENT OF COLON CANCER
Principles of Management

The surgical resection of a primary colon cancer entails removal of the tumor with adequate margins and removal of the draining lymph nodes. In most cases, bowel continuity is restored at the time of resection. The lymphatic drainage of the colon has been studied and provides

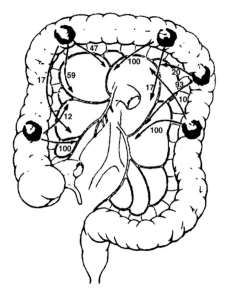

Figure 2 The arterial blood supply of the colon.

the rationale for the appropriate resection for colon cancer depending on the site (Fig. 2) (129). The extent of resection is determined by the need to achieve a 5-cm margin of resection around the tumor, and the viability of the colon after ligation of blood vessels during the lymphadenectomy.

Surgical technique significantly affects cancer outcome. Evidence-based recommendations for various aspects of CRC surgical therapies were published in 2001 following a National Cancer Institute conference (130). More recent efficacy data suggest that the number of lymph nodes resected and analyzed correlates strongly with overall and disease-free survival (DFS) (131). Analysis of more than 3400 colon cancer patients treated in an intergroup adjuvant chemotherapy study demonstrated that after controlling for the number of nodes involved with cancer, survival rose as the number of recovered nodes increased. Even with no nodal metastases, overall survival (OS) improved as more nodes were recovered. When more than 40 lymph nodes were examined, as opposed to less than 10, there was a 23% improvement in five-year survival.

Detection and Diagnosis

Colonoscopy has become the standard for identifying the primary cancer and identifying and removing synchronous polyps or cancers. Additional diagnostic procedures include digital rectal examination (in the case of rectal cancers), sigmoidoscopy, and BE. If a full colonoscopy is not technically possible, the nonvisualized colon may be examined with an air-contrast BE. When preoperative visualization is not possible, colonoscopy should be performed after recovery from the primary resection. An alternative method for the evaluation of the proximal colon in these cases is intraoperative colonoscopy—a very important component of laparoscopic colectomy. In the future, virtual colonography may supplant BE or traditional colonoscopy in some of these circumstances.

Preoperative Evaluation

In preparing for a laparotomy, the patient should undergo a complete history and physical examination, blood tests (including complete blood count, liver and renal function assessment, coagulation profile, and CEA), and a chest X ray. Tumor markers are used to preoperatively follow patients and should be measured before the operation. About 44% of patients with normal CEAs preoperatively will still have a rise in CEA with a recurrence (132).

Preparing a patient for laparotomy includes evaluating the patient's cardiopulmonary reserve (to optimize the risk factors associated with the operation), mechanical bowel preparation, prophylactic antibiotics, and thromboembolic prophylaxis. In the absence of the need for emergent surgery, maximizing the patient's cardiac and pulmonary status is worthwhile.

A mechanical bowel preparation purges the colon in order to diminish the incidence of wound and intra-abdominal infectious complications. A number of formulations are available, which may be administered to the patient at home. Polyethylene glycol solutions or phospho-soda preparations are safe and effective, and can be managed by most as outpatients. Sodium phosphate is the preferred and superior method (133,134). Oral tablet preparations are available and appear to be equally effective. If a patient is partially obstructed, an in-patient preparation with enemas and mild oral cathartics may be preferred. Several recent prospective randomized trials and meta-analyses have challenged the need for mechanical bowel preparation (135,136). Despite the high scientific level of evidence of these studies, preoperative mechanical bowel preparation remains the standard of care.

Mechanical bowel preparations began in the era before broad-spectrum intravenous antibiotics were available. Several institutions have studied the need for a mechanical bowel preparation. These studies, while small, do not demonstrate an increased risk of infection when the mechanical preparation is omitted, but broad-spectrum intravenous antibiotics were given (137,138). Nonetheless, a survey of the American Society of Colon and Rectal Surgeons shows that most surgeons continue to employ a mechanical preparation with an intravenous antibiotic coverage, and some still use oral antibiotics (139).

Prophylactic intravenous antibiotics reduce the wound infection rate in patients undergoing elective colon resection from about 30% to 15% (140). The intravenous antibiotic must be delivered before the incision is made to be effective. Historically, oral antibiotics were given with the mechanical bowel preparation, and decreased the wound infection rate. With modern systemic antibiotics, the contribution of oral antibiotics is uncertain, and their use is diminishing.

Venous thrombosis and pulmonary emboli remain a problem. Patients with malignancies and those undergoing pelvic operations are felt to be at increased risk. Intermittent pneumatic compression devices are now widely used, and have been shown to decrease the incidence of thromboembolic complications. Subcutaneous heparin appears to decrease further the risk, although this has not been demonstrated specifically in colon cancer patients. It may increase the risk of hemorrhagic complications slightly. More recently, low-molecular-weight heparin preparations such as enoxaparin (Lovenox®) have been used, but they have not proven any more efficacious than heparin (141). Studies using low-molecular-weight dextran have not shown a significant benefit over subcutaneous heparin (142).

The use of perioperative blood transfusions in patients with CRC is controversial. There is evidence that suggests the immunosuppressive effect of blood products may have an effect on tumor recurrence and survival (143,144). This remains controversial and other authors have not seen a similar effect (145). It is possible that any effect on survival and tumor recurrence may be related to other unevaluated tumor variables or underlying illness as opposed to perioperative immunosuppression.

Preoperative and Intraoperative Staging Techniques

Considerable debate surrounds the need for extensive preoperative staging. There are few situations in which the primary tumor should not be resected; so many surgeons do not advocate preoperative staging scans. However, if the surgeon is prepared to address liver metastases during the operation to resect the primary tumor, it is important to perform cross-sectional liver imaging preoperatively, regardless of whether there are any abnormalities in liver function tests.

Intraoperative staging includes the complete assessment of the peritoneal cavity for tumor implants, assessment of adherence of the primary tumor to adjacent organs, and examination of the liver. Bimanual palpation of the liver is not adequate to accomplish this latter task. Intraoperative ultrasound can identify small metastases within the liver and, while not the standard of care, is becoming more widely used because of the increase in sensitivity over other imaging modalities (146).

SURGICAL RESECTION
Surgical Management of Polyps

The great majority of colorectal polyps can be completely removed endoscopically. However, because of size, position, or concern about bowel wall invasion, some polyps may require surgical excision.

All polyps containing invasive cancer should be completely excised with an adequate margin. The size of the margin has been the subject of debate; however, size greater than 2 mm appears sufficient (147). If an adequate margin cannot be achieved endoscopically, a segmental colectomy should be performed.

While determining the completeness of endoscopic polypectomy is relatively straight forward, it is more difficult to identify those patients who require further treatment due to risk of lymph-node metastasis. Haggitt has described a morphologic staging system based on the depth of penetration by invasive cancer in the polyp (148). This system correlates depth of invasion with lymph-node involvement and outcome. Five levels of invasion have been defined (Fig. 3): level 0, carcinoma in situ or intramucosal carcinoma (not invasive); level 1: invasion into the head of the polyp; level 2, invasion into the neck of the polyp; level 3, invasion into the stalk; level 4, invasion into the submucosa of the bowel wall below the stalk of the polyp, but above the muscularis propria. In this system, all sessile polyps with invasive cancer are defined as having level 4 invasion.

Based on this staging system, several series have defined the appropriate management of patients with polyps-harboring cancer. Lesions of Haggitt level 1 to 3 have a very small risk of lymph-node metastasis (<1%) and can be safely treated by complete endoscopic excision (148–150). Level 4 lesions have a significant risk of lymph-node metastasis, ranging from 15% to 25% (148,149). These lesions require surgical resection with appropriate margins. One potential flaw in this system is that all sessile polyps are categorized as level 4 and require a colectomy. Presumably, all sessile polyps do not pose the same risk of lymph-node metasta- sis. Many can be resected safely by endoscopic means, which, in some patients, may represent the best treatment alternative.

A separate system for staging of sessile polyps has been proposed (151). This system emphasizes the depth of submucosal invasion by the sessile polyp. Polyps are divided into three categories: Sm1, invasion into the upper-third of the submucosa; Sm2, invasion into the middle-third of the submucosa; and Sm3, invasion into the lower-third of the submucosa. Several series have suggested that sessile polyps with Sm1 and Sm2 invasion have little risk of lymph-node metastasis and require no further treatment which resected with an adequate margin and in the absence of other poor prognostic features (152–154). Sm3 lesions have a greater propensity for lymph-node metastasis and require an oncologic resection (152–154). While this system is not widely used, it may provide a means of better determining those patients with sessile polyps, who require further therapy.

Other prognostic factors that influence the management of malignant polyps include the presence of lymphatic or vascular invasion within the cancer and poor histologic grade. Vascular invasion has been associated with increased rates of lymph-node metastasis in polyps-harboring invasive cancer independent of the level of invasion (147,153,155,156). Patients with lymphovascular invasion require definitive surgical treatment regardless of

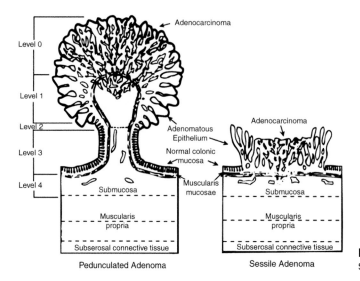

Figure 3 Proposed polyp staging system.

the depth of invasion. Similarly, poorly differentiated cancers, while accounting for only a small portion of malignant polyps, have been associated in some reports with an increased incidence of lymph-node metastasis (147,153,155–157). Most surgeons would favor definite resection for any patient with a poorly differentiated cancer arising in a polyp.

In the absence of additional information, majority opinion would favor the following indications for oncologic surgical resection of malignant polyps: margin <2 mm, Haggitt level 4 invasion for pedunculated polyps, deep submucosal invasion for sessile polyps, poorly differentiated cancers regardless of depth of invasion, and lymphovascular invasion regardless of depth of invasion.

Localized Colon Cancer
Asymptomatic Primary Tumor

The goal of surgical resection of the primary tumor whether adenomatous or cancerous is complete removal of the primary tumor, removal of the lymphatic drainage bed, and en bloc removal of adherent structures (Fig. 4). Tumors located in the retroperitoneal portion of the colon (the right colon, hepatic flexure, splenic flexure, and descending colon) are at risk for local recurrence in the retroperitoneum, and wide soft-tissue margins are necessary to decrease this risk. With the intraperitoneal colon, local recurrence is increased with inadequate

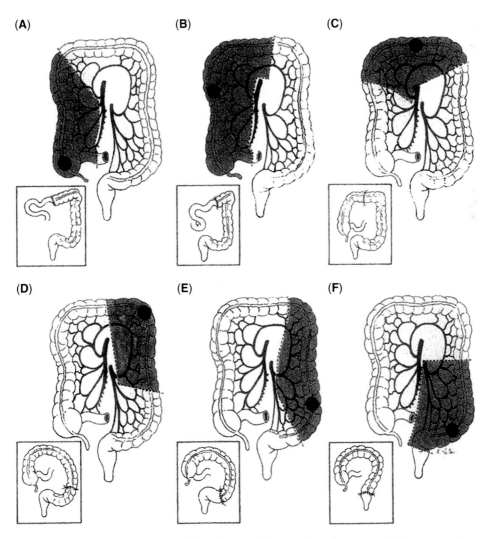

Figure 4 The extent of resection for (**A**) cecal cancer, (**B**) ascending colon cancer, (**C**) transverse colon cancer, (**D**) splenic flexure cancer, (**E**) descending colon cancer, and (**F**) sigmoid colon cancer.

margins proximally and distally. Removal of at least 5 cm of bowel proximal and distal to the tumor is recommended. The extent of resection is often larger than 5 cm and is dictated by the lymphatic drainage of the bowel. The arterial blood supply of the right colon is from the ileocolic, right colic, and right branch of the middle colic artery from the superior mesenteric artery (Fig. 5). The blood supply of the left colon is from the left colic and sigmoid vessels. The marginal artery from the left colic artery supplies the splenic flexure and transverse colon. The lymphatic drainage follows the vascular supply of the colon. Tumors spread through the epicolic, paracolic, intermediate, and principal nodes. The removal of these nodes, with the concomitant ligation of vessels, defines the extent of colon resection to encompass the tumor and lymphatic drainage bed. Tumors arising between major vascular pedicles (such as those in the hepatic flexure) generally require a more extensive resection, in order to encompass both drainage areas.

For tumors of the splenic flexure, many authors advocate ligation of the inferior mesenteric artery (IMA) at its origin at the aorta. In a randomized trial, this maneuver had no significant effect on long-term survival (158). Retrospective studies suggest an improved survival with high ligation of the IMA (compared to taking sigmoid vessels and sparing the left colic artery), but it is difficult to separate the impact of the surgeon himself and improved pathologic staging (with an increased number of nodes examined), from the benefit of the improved node dissection on outcome (159,160).

In the absence of obstruction, patients need not generally fear a colostomy. The surgeon has the choice of end-to-end, end-to-side, and side-to-side anastomosis, any of which can be either hand sewn or stapled. There is no evidence to indicate that any one technique is superior, provided care is taken to assure that the anastomosis is performed without tension, and with good blood supply (161). The most common causes for an anastomotic leak are poor blood supply or tension on the anastomosis. A surgeon should be prepared to employ all techniques of anastomoses, and should select the appropriate operation that will minimize risks for anastomotic leak in a given situation.

Sentinel Node Evaluation

The role of sentinel node biopsy in colon resection is being studied in many centers (162). In most cases, it does not change the operation performed. In a small number of cases, it appears to be helpful in identifying aberrant drainage of the colon. However, it is likely to improve staging of the cancer (as it has done in both breast cancer and melanoma). The use of Lymphazurin injection to the circumference of the colon at the site of the tumor is common. Some authors have described the combination of Lymphazurin and fluorescein, with the use of a Woods' lamp to identify the sentinel nodes. The first nodes to appear are marked by the

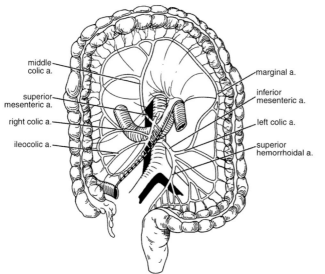

Figure 5 Arterial supply of the colon.

surgeon for the pathologist. Reports indicate increased detection of micrometastases (163). The impact of micrometastases on survival is unknown, as is the role of selecting patients for adjuvant therapy based on micrometastatic disease (164).

Involvement of Adjacent Organs

Direct involvement of colon cancer with small bowel, bladder, uterus, fallopian tubes and ovaries, kidney, stomach, duodenum, pancreas, gallbladder, and spleen has been described (165). Such local involvement occurs in less than 15% of colon cancer cases. More than half of the adjacent organ involvement is malignant (166). While not always predicted preoperatively, a CT scan often helps the surgeon and the patient prepare for a more extensive operation. Hematuria should alert the clinician to possible involvement of the kidneys or bladder. Abnormal vaginal bleeding should be assessed preoperatively, especially if the patient has a bulky cecal or sigmoid cancer. Unexplained weight loss is a potential indication of involvement of the stomach or duodenum or the presence of a malignant fistula to the small bowel.

If a tumor adheres to an adjacent organ, the organ must be removed en bloc with the primary tumor. It is impossible to determine at the time of operation whether the organ is attached by inflammatory or by malignant adhesions. The surgeon should assume that the adhesions are malignant and perform the appropriate cancer operation (167). Failure to do so is a common cause of locoregional recurrence (168).

Adjacent organ involvement does not significantly decrease survival if the appropriate operation is performed. Such primary tumors are not incurable and indeed are often node negative, with a high expectation of survival.

Multiple Primary Tumors

Complete preoperative assessment of the colon is preferable as up to 5% of patients have a second primary cancer, and over 25% will have additional polyps (169). As noted above, preoperative colonoscopy should be performed to identify, and, if possible, remove other neoplastic lesions. Benign polyps that cannot be removed endoscopically should be removed by colotomy and polypectomy during the operation. If a second cancer is found in the same region as the first, a hemicolectomy can be performed to encompass the tumors and both drainage areas. If the sites are further apart, two partial colectomies or a subtotal colectomy can be performed.

Special attention should be addressed to younger patients with two cancers, a cancer with synchronous polyps, patients with a strong family history of colon cancer, or those with known hereditary colon cancer syndromes.

Obstructing Colon Cancer

The overall outcome of patients with obstructing tumors is worse than that of nonobstructing colon cancers (170). Patients who present to the emergency room with a large-bowel obstruction are at heightened risk for surgical complications including infection, need for a temporary colostomy, and perioperative mortality. Because of the inability mechanically to prepare and to clean the colon, there is an increased bacterial load in an obstructed bowel, and a decreased time to prepare the patient for surgery.

Obstructing right colon cancer can often be managed without a colostomy. The bowel can be cleansed with enemas, and a primary anastomosis performed if the small bowel is viable and the patient stable. Historically, obstructing left colon cancer was managed with a transverse loop colostomy to allow the patient to be stabilized and prepared for surgery. The left colon cancer was resected in a second stage and, after several weeks of healing, the colostomy would be closed in a third stage. This approach has been supplanted by a two-stage operation for stable patients. The first operation removes the left colon cancer and an end colostomy with mucous fistula or Hartmann pouch created. A second operation is performed several weeks later (when the patient was stable), and the bowel had been mechanically cleansed. The colostomy is then closed and bowel continuity restored. Compared to a three-stage procedure, this paradigm has a lower morbidity and mortality.

Today, additional options include the following: (i) a subtotal colectomy with an ileorectal anastomosis, (ii) removing the entire obstructed, contaminated colon, (iii) a hemicolectomy with on-table lavage to clean the colon prior to anastomosis, and (iv) preoperative endoscopic stent placement with subsequent bowel prep and resection. These procedures should be reserved for patients who are healthy, stable, and without evidence of perforation. If the surgeon has any concerns that an anastomosis might leak (due to poor nutrition, peritonitis, immunosuppression or hemodynamic instability), a colostomy should be performed. For gravely ill patients, a transverse loop colostomy remains an appropriate option for a patient without evidence of a perforation.

Perforated Colon Cancer

Two types of colon perforation can occur in association with colon cancer. Both are life-threatening emergencies. The most common is perforation of the colon cancer itself with fecal peritonitis. The second is a cecal perforation from an obstructing distal colon cancer. After resuscitating the patient and treating with broad-spectrum antibiotics, an emergency operation is undertaken. Perforation of the primary tumor is treated with colon resection and an end colostomy or ileostomy. The distal end of the colon is brought to the skin as a mucous fistula or oversewn and left in the pelvis (a Hartmann procedure).

In contrast, if an obstructing colon cancer presents with fecal peritonitis from a proximal perforation, then a subtotal colectomy, with ileostomy and a Hartmann procedure can be performed if the patient is stable. If the patient is gravely ill, a limited resection of the perforated colon (usually the cecum) with ileostomy and mucous fistula can be performed to save the patient's life. The cancer is resected when the patient has recovered and can tolerate a more extensive operation.

Laparoscopic Colon Resection

For more than a decade, surgeons have studied the role of laparoscopy in the conduct of a colectomy. During this time, the instrumentation has improved considerably, making operations easier and safer to perform. Initial enthusiasm was dampened by reports of port-site implants, and one series suggested an alarmingly high rate of port-site recurrence (171). There were strong concerns that an inadequate cancer operation might result. It now seems that port-site implants can be prevented with appropriate care, and the rate of such metastasis in recent series is acceptably low, comparable to the wound recurrence rate in open colectomy (172).

Two randomized phase III studies have now been reported, which compare laparoscopic-assisted colectomy (LAC) with open colectomy (OC) for colon cancer (173,174). The first reported study from Barcelona randomized 219 patients to LAC or OC (173). Eleven percent of patients in the LAC arm were converted to OC. Duration of the operation was considerably higher in the LAC group, but complications were significantly higher in the OC group (including an 18% wound infection rate and a 2% evisceration rate). Duration of hospital stay was 5.2 days in the LAC group compared to 7.9 days in the OC group. OS was not significantly different between the two groups, but cancer-related survival was higher in the LAC group, predominantly in stage III disease. Sites of recurrence were statistically similar, although there were twice as many locoregional relapses in the OC group. Survival advantage accrued to Stage III patients is predominantly due to the very poor prognosis of OC stage III patients compared to historical controls.

The largest phase III randomized study by the Clinical Outcomes of Surgical Therapy Study Group randomized 872 patients to LAC or OC (174). This study included detailed quality of life (QOL) outcomes as well as cancer-specific outcomes. The rates of recurrent cancer were similar after LAC and OC, suggesting that laparoscopic approach was not inferior to open surgery for colon cancer. Only minimal short-term QOL benefits, however, accrued to patients with LAC compared to OC, although conversion to OC was 21% in the LAC group, which may mask the benefit of LAC.

Prospective studies have compared the length of colon and mesentery removed, the proximal and distal margins achieved, and number of lymph nodes retrieved in open and LAC. They appear to be similar (175–177). A large randomized phase III study in the United States and several in Europe are examining the OS, the cancer-specific survival, and the local recurrence rate of laparoscopic-assisted colectomies in comparison to conventional colectomies. The one study that has been reported does not show a difference in cancer-specific outcomes (173). Interestingly, it is not clear that time in the hospital or time to return to normal activity differs between these two groups.

As with all new techniques, there is a learning curve. In most studies, the average time to complete a laparoscopic colectomy decreased from four hours to two and a half hours with experience. Most surgeons will require between 20 and 100 cases to achieve technical proficiency.

Potential contraindications to laparoscopic colectomy include major cardiopulmonary disease, coagulopathy, portal hypertension, severe obesity, and pregnancy. Operations in patients who have undergone extensive abdominal surgery in the past or who have significant adhesions are more difficult. Patients with large tumors or adjacent organ involvement should have an open colectomy. Tumors of the transverse colon (where both flexures must be mobilized and the omentum removed) can be laparoscopically difficult to address.

Intraoperatively, identifying a very small tumor can be difficult, due to the inability to palpate the colon. A preoperative BE or intraoperative colonoscopy can assist in determining the appropriate segment of colon to be removed. Nonetheless, it is plausible that the wrong segment of colon would be removed on the basis of erroneous colonoscopy reports of the tumor location. Preoperative endoscopic tattooing of the lesion is very helpful in preventing problems such as this, and intraoperative examination of the specimen is also mandatory to definitively identify the lesion. For all these reasons, the appropriate role of laparoscopic resections in the management of patients with colon cancer remains controversial, and is discussed in further detail in the chapter on laparoscopy of the colon.

In conclusion, laparoscopic colectomy is often an ideal option for patients with colonic adenoma particularly in the right or sigmoid colon. The laparoscopic approach for malignancy, when employed by well-trained surgeons and applied in appropriately selected patients, offers equivalent or even potentially superior outcomes. Regardless of which approach is selected, an identical cancer operation should be performed by laparoscopic, laparoscopic-assisted, or laparotomy techniques in both adenomatous and carcinomas.

Surgical Management of Stage IV Disease

Even in patients with metastatic colon cancer, a formal hemicolectomy to remove the primary tumor and its lymphatic drainage should be performed in most cases. Historically, the median survival of patients with unresectable metastases is 7 to 12 months with 5-fluorouracil (5-FU)-based chemotherapy (177,178). In patients with resectable liver metastases, median survival ranges from 30 to 40 months, and five-year survival is 27% to 37% (179–181). Survival has increased with the availability of newer agents such as CPT-11 and oxaliplatin (182,183).

These intervals are thus sufficient for patients to develop complications from primary tumor progression. The exception to this rule is the patient with an asymptomatic primary tumor and malignant ascites. Such patients almost never develop obstructive symptoms before they succumb to their disease.

There is growing evidence that resection of selected hepatic and pulmonary metastases can prolong life in some settings. There is wide agreement that extrahepatic disease is a contraindication to resection of hepatic metastases. In the absence of such clinical circumstances, the prognostic factors that predict survival after resection of hepatic metastasis are controversial. Frequently cited considerations include number and size of metastases, extent of liver involvement, presence of bilobar metastatic disease, if the primary cancer was node-positive, and the ability to obtain clean surgical margins at the time of hepatic resection (184,185).

Less is known about the utility of resection of isolated lung metastasis (186,187). Small series suggest some survival benefit. As perhaps expected, this benefit seemed concentrated most in those patients with few, small metastases.

CHEMOTHERAPY FOR CRC
Adjuvant Therapy for Locoregional Colon Cancer

Detection of early-stage CRC frequently results in cure with surgery alone. The five-year survival rate for surgically resected, node-negative colon cancer invading the mucosa or submucosa only exceeds 90%. When the tumor invades the muscularis propria or penetrates the wall, but does not involve the regional lymph nodes, the five-year survival falls to 80% and 70%, respectively. Unfortunately, most patients with newly diagnosed CRC have either locally advanced or metastatic disease at presentation. The five-year OS of patients who present with colonic obstruction, bowel perforation, or lymph-node involvement falls dramatically to 50% or less (188). Further, many patients with resectable disease at presentation are not cured with surgery alone, ultimately suffering tumor recurrence due to undetected micrometastases. Such disease might be eradicated with the use of adjuvant therapy, with ample evidence demonstrating a reduction in local and/or distant recurrence in patients treated with chemotherapy in this setting.

Although newer agents have recently been approved for the treatment of metastatic CRC, 5-FU remains the backbone of therapy. 5-FU exerts its effect through several mechanisms. Primarily, 5-FU impairs DNA synthesis by inhibiting thymidylate synthase, but it is also directly incorporated into RNA and DNA (Fig. 6). 5-FU has a half-life of less than 15 minutes and is rapidly degraded by endogenous dihydropyrimidine dehydrogenase. 5-FU is commonly administered with leucovorin (folinic acid). The latter exercises its modulating effect by binding to thymidylate synthase and potentiating the inhibition of this enzyme by fluorodeoxyuridine monophosphate.

Several trials have established adjuvant therapy with 5-FU and leucovorin (LV) as the standard of care in patients with node-positive (stage III) colon carcinoma (189,190). In metastatic colon cancer, the addition of leucovorin as a biochemical modulator greatly improved response rates compared with 5-FU alone (177); hence this combination was further evaluated in the adjuvant setting. The North Central Cancer Treatment Group (NCCTG) (191) and the IMPACT groups (190) compared 5-FU/LV versus surgery alone. Each study showed a benefit to adjuvant chemotherapy. The National Surgical Adjuvant Breast and Bowel Project (NSABP) conducted a follow-up study CO-3 (192) comparing 5-FU/LV to 5-FU, vincristine, and methyl-CCNU. Again, a survival benefit was noted for patients in the 5-FU/LV arm. Taken together, over 4000 patients have participated in randomized trials comparing adjuvant therapy to surgery alone, with a relative mortality reduction of 22% to 33%.

Several studies have been completed demonstrating the benefits of leucovorin, levamisole, or both in combination with 5-FU. A four-arm study compared 5-FU/levamisole to 5-FU/levamisole/leucovorin for 6 or 12 months (193). This study showed that six months of 5-FU/levamisole was inferior to the other arms. The intergroup study INT-0089 (194) compared one year of 5-FU/levamisole with six months of 5-FU/LV (Mayo regimen) versus 5-FU/LV weekly (Roswell Park regimen) to six months of 5-FU/LV/levamisole. There were no significant differences between the arms, with a five-year DFS of 56% to 60% and OS of 63% to 67%. This established 5-FU/LV for six months to be equivalent to 5-FU/levamisole for one year. The NSABP CO-4 (195) also compared 5-FU/levamisole with 5-FU/LV and the three-drug combination. The conclusions drawn from this study were that 5-FU/LV for six months was at least as effective, if not better than 5-FU/levamisole for 12 months, with a five year DFS of 65 and 60%, respectively. The addition of levamisole to 5-FU/LV did not provide additional benefit.

More recently, the X-ACT trial compared capecitabine, an oral analogue of 5-FU, to bolus 5-FU/LV in patients with stage III colon cancer. Capecitabine is initially metabolized in the liver to 5′-deoxy-5-fluorocytidine, and then converted in peripheral tissues to

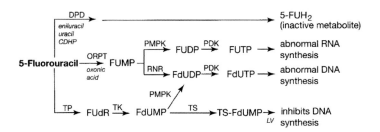

Figure 6 5-Fluorouracil metabolism. *Abbreviations*: TS, thymidylate synthase; DPD, dihydropyrimidine dehydrogenase; TP, thymidine phosphorylase; TK, thymidine kinase; PMPK, pyrimidine monophosphate kinase; OPRT, orotate phophoribosyltransferase; RNR, ribonucleotide reductase; PDK, pyrimidine diphosphate kinase.

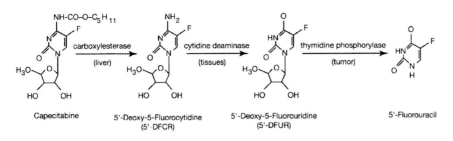

Figure 7 Metabolism of capecitabine.

5'-deoxy-5-fluorouridine. The final conversion to active 5-FU involves thymidine phosphoryl-ase, an enzyme found in higher concentrations in tumor tissue than in surrounding normal tissue (Fig. 7). Capecitabine resulted in a superior relapse-free survival at three years (65.5% vs. 61.9%) and a trend toward improved three-year OS (81.3% vs. 77.6 %) when compared to 5-FU/LV administered intravenously. As a result, capecitabine is a reasonable alternative in the adjuvant setting (196).

Studies combining 5-FU with newer agents such as oxaliplatin are ongoing. The MOSAIC trial is the first randomized trial to show benefit of a triple-drug therapy in the adjuvant setting. Over 220 patients with stage II and stage III colon cancer were randomized to receive infusional 5-FU/LV with or without oxaliplatin. There was an improvement in three-year DFS and OS in the oxaliplatin-containing arm (197).

Adjuvant therapy for stage III colon cancer is considered standard today. The most com-monly used intravenous 5-FU adjuvant regimens are the Mayo Clinic and the Roswell Park regimens, with oral capecitabine, a reasonable alternative (Table 8). Additional data with newer agents is maturing.

Adjuvant therapy for stage II colon cancer remains controversial. While there is no clear biological reason not to expect a treatment benefit, patients with stage II disease have a smaller number of cancer-related events. As such, the number of patients needed to detect a treatment benefit is much larger than studies enrolling patients with node-positive disease. While many of the trials discussed above included patients with stage II colon cancer, these trials were not individually powered to detect a survival difference for the node-negative group. A pooled analysis of four adjuvant trials noted an overall mortality reduction of 30% in stage II compared with 18% in stage III patients (198). In contrast, a second pooled analysis of 1016 stage II patients with T3 to T4, NO, MO disease entered into five randomized clinical trials failed to show any significant benefit to treatment with 5-FU/LV compared with observation alone (199).

At present, the utility of adjuvant therapy for patients with stage II colon cancer remains somewhat unclear. Because the OS for certain subsets of patients (i.e., those with obstruction or perforation or those with molecular genetic factors, which portend a poorer prognosis) is equivalent to that of node-positive patients, many oncologists recommend 5-FU based adju-vant therapy to this group of higher risk patients routinely.

Adjuvant Therapy for Locoregional Rectal Cancer

Stage for stage, the mortality rate for rectal cancer is slightly higher than colon cancer. Because of the increased risk of local recurrence, perhaps due to more limited surgical resection mar-gins, adjuvant treatment is typically prescribed. The intent of adjuvant treatment for rectal cancer, usually the combination of radiation and chemotherapies, is to minimize the risk of local

Table 8 Adjuvant Chemotherapeutic Regimens for Colon Cancer

Mayo Clinic regimen	5-FU 425 mg/m² IV bolus following LV 20 mg/m² IV bolus daily × 5 days Repeat for 6 cycles at 28–35 day intervals
Roswell Park regimen	LV 500 mg/m² IV over 2 hr weekly for 6 wks 5-FU 500 mg/m² IVP one hour into leucovorin infusion Repeat 4 cycles at 8-wk intervals

as well as distant recurrence. This is an extremely important issue given the morbidity associated with pelvic recurrence. About 76% of patients with fatal rectal cancer die with local failure.

Role of Radiotherapy in Local Rectal Cancer

The utility of radiotherapy either prior to or after surgical resection in rectal cancer is well described. In order to decrease exposure of the small bowel, paired lateral fields are combined with a posteroanterior field. Additional maneuvers include the displacement of the small bowel with the insertion of surgical mesh at the time of surgical resection. Typically, a total of 4500 cGy in 180 cGy daily fractions is delivered over a five-week period. The targeted area encompasses the whole pelvis including the tumor bed and nodal groups with a boost of 540 cGy to 900 cGy in 180 cGy fractions to a smaller pelvic field without small bowel.

While adjuvant radiation therapy decreases the rate of local recurrence, most studies have failed to show that alone it provides any OS benefit. These findings have prompted exploration of combined chemotherapy and radiation. The Gastrointestinal Tumor Study Group conducted a small four-arm trial randomizing 200 patients to undergo surgery alone versus surgery followed by radiotherapy, 5-FU/methyl-CCNU, or combined chemotherapy and radiation (200,201). DFS improved with combined-modality therapy compared to surgery alone (67% vs. 45%). By comparison, the chemotherapy arm showed an improvement in OS (202). The NCCTG compared adjuvant radiation to combined modality therapy where 5-FU/methyl CCNU were administered during and after radiation. Chemoradiation decreased local recurrence by 46%, distant failure by 73%, and improved OS by 29% (203). xS did not improve with the addition of radiation, radiotherapy did improve local control (204).

Finally, INT-0114 randomized 1696 patients with stage II or III surgically resected rectal cancer patients to one of four arms: bolus 5-FU alone, with LV, with levamisole, or both. Chemotherapy was administered before and after radiation. All four arms had similar five-year DFS and OS rates (62–68% and 78–80%, respectively). No beneficial effects were noted with the addition of levamisole to systemic therapy or with the addition of LV during radiation (205). Combined-modality therapy with 5-FU has become an accepted standard for both stage II and stage III rectal cancer.

Adjuvant vs. Neoadjuvant Therapy for Local Rectal Cancer

It is unknown whether neoadjuvant (preoperative) or adjuvant (postoperative) therapy yields the greatest benefit. There are theoretical advantages to both. Preoperatively, the radiated area is smaller and does not require coverage of the perineum, thereby decreasing radiation toxicity to the small bowel. Without disturbing the blood supply, increased delivery of chemotherapy to the tumor bed and increased oxygen tension within the tumor may occur. There is less risk of dissemination of viable tumor cells during surgery, and the use of neoadjuvant treatment may result in more frequent sphincter-sparing procedures.

In contrast, the benefits to postoperative adjuvant therapy include a more accurate surgical and pathologic staging. Omental slings and tissue expanders placed intraoperatively can decrease the risk of radiation toxicity to the small bowel, and clips placed during surgery can help accurately identify clinical target volumes.

A phase III randomized trial (NSABP-R03) comparing preoperative to postoperative chemotherapy with radiation closed in 1999 due to poor accrual. The DFS at one year was 83% in the preop arm compared to 78% in the postop arm ($p = 0.29$) (206). More recent randomized trial data suggests that preoperative or postoperative adjuvant combined-modality therapy results in similar five-year DFS, OS, and distant recurrence rates. However, there were fewer pelvic recurrences, fewer anastomotic stenoses, and a greater ability to perform sphincter-sparing surgery in the patients treated preoperatively (207).

Given the currently available data, combined-modality treatment with 5-FU and radiation therapy either preoperatively or postoperatively, in conjunction with four cycles of systemic 5-FU/LV, is considered standard treatment for stage II and stage III rectal cancer.

The Future

Oral fluoropyrimidines and newer agents such as irinotecan and oxaliplatin may play an important role in the future management of resectable CRC. Several ongoing cooperative group studies may soon provide relevant data. Neoadjuvant therapy has the added benefit of "downstaging" the tumor and therefore potentially increasing the opportunity of resection for cure and possibly also of anastomosis. It has become favored over postoperative adjuvant therapy by many surgeons for these reasons.

Chemotherapeutic Options for Metastatic Colorectal Cancer

Until recently, 5-FU in combination with modulating agents such as leucovorin was the mainstay of chemotherapy for metastatic CRC. There are now several newer chemotherapeutic agents that are frequently used, either alone or in combination including capecitabine, irinotecan, and oxaliplatin. Furthermore, new monoclonal antibodies targeting the VEGF and the epidermal growth factor receptor (EGFR) have been Food and Drug Administration (FDA) approved for use in the metastatic setting. Some of the combination regimens discussed below are listed in Table 9.

Irinotecan (Camptosar, Pharmacia Corporation) is a prodrug of SN-38 that exerts its antitumor activity by inhibiting topoisomerase I, an enzyme required for unwinding of double-stranded DNA during replication (Fig. 8). In several phase II trials, the response rate of single agent irinotecan in previously untreated patients with CRC ranges from 19% to 32% (208–210). As a second-line agent in patients who were 5-FU refractory, irintoecan improved OS when compared to best supportive care (211,212).

Given irinotecan's single-agent activity, investigators at Memorial Sloan Kettering developed a weekly regimen, combining it with 5-FU and leucovorin (IFL). Two randomized studies compared IFL to 5-FU/LV. The first compared IFL to 5-FU/LV to single-agent irinotecan. The triple-drug combination demonstrated a superior response rate and OS (183). Similarly, European investigators demonstrated better response rate and OS rates with combination therapy, leading to a new standard of care for first-line treatment of metastatic CRC (213).

Table 9 Chemotherapeutic Regimens for Metastatic Colorectal Cancer

Capecitabine	1250 mg/m^2 b.i.d. po × 14 d q 3 wks
IFL	Irinotecan 125 mg/m^2 IV over 90 min
	LV 20 mg/m^2 IV bolus
	5-FU 500 mg/m^2 IV bolus
	Repeat weekly × q 6 wks
OR	Irinotecan 80 mg/m^2 IV over 90 min
	LV 500 mg/m^2 IV over 2 hrs
	5-FU 2300 mg/m^2 continuous infusion (CIV) over 24 hrs
	Repeat weekly × 6 q 7 wks
OR	Irinotecan 180 mg/m^2 IV over 90 min d1
	LV 200 mg/m^2 IV over 2 hrs, d1, d2
	5-FU 400 mg/m^2 IV bolus d1, d2, followed by
	5-FU 600 mg/m^2 CIV over 22 hrs, d1, d2
	Repeat every 2 wks
LV5FU2	LV 200 mg/m^2 over 2 hrs
	5-FU 400 mg/m^2 bolus
	5-FU 600 mg/m^2 CIV over 22 hrs, d1, d2
	Repeat every 2 wks
FOLFOX4	Oxaliplatin 85 mg/m^2 over 2 hrs d1
	LV 200 mg/m^2 over 2 hrs
	5-FU 400 mg/m^2 bolus
	5-FU 600 mg/m^2 CIV over 22 hrs, d1, d2
	Repeat every 2 wks
FOLFOX6	Oxaliplatin 100 mg/m^2 over 2 hrs
	L-isomer of folinic acid 200 mg/m^2 IV over 2 hrs
	5-FU 2.4–3 g/m^2 CIV over 46 hrs
	Repeat every 2 wks
FOLFIRI	Irinotecan 180 mg/m^2 IV over 90 min
	L-isomer of folinic acid 200 mg/m^2 IV over 2 hrs
	5-FU 2.4–3 g/m^2 CIV over 46 hrs
	Repeat every 2 wks

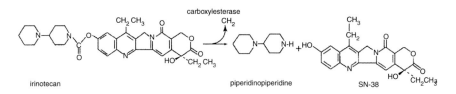

Figure 8 Metabolism of irinotecan.

One of the newer FDA-approved agents for CRC is oxaliplatin (Eloxatin, Sanofi-Synthelabo). Oxaliplatin, a platinum compound with a diaminocyclohexane (DACH)-carrier ligand, has a different spectrum of activity and toxicity profile than other platinum compounds such as cisplatin and carboplatin. The DACH-platinum adducts formed by oxaliplatin are bulkier, more effective inhibitors of DNA synthesis than similar agents. These adducts also inhibit the binding of DNA repair enzymes. Common oxaliplatin-related toxicities include a cold-induced dysesthesia, frequently presenting as a sensation of laryngospasm, a cumulative dose-related peripheral neuropathy and neutropenia. The renal and auditory toxicities frequently seen with cisplatin and carboplatin are rarely encountered.

As a single agent, oxaliplatin has a response rate of 12% to 27% in previously untreated patients with CRC and a response rate of 7.8% to 10.3% in patients who have failed prior therapies. Preclinical evidence suggests a synergistic effect when oxaliplatin is combined with 5-FU. Response rates for this combination range from 17.5% to 22.8 % when used as second-line therapy (214–217).

Two multicenter randomized phase III trials comparing oxaliplatin/5-FU/LV to 5-FU/LV as first-line therapy have been conducted (216,217). Giachetti et al. randomized 200 patients to receive a five-day course of 5-FU/LV with or without oxaliplatin on the first day of each course, which was repeated every three weeks (217). In a larger study, deGramont et al. randomized 420 patients to receive LV5-FU2 with or without oxaliplatin on day 1 (216). In both studies, the response rate and progression-free survival was significantly better in the oxaliplatin-containing arm, with response rates of 50.7% to 53% compared to 16% to 22.3%. OS, however, was not significantly different.

The final results of the Intergroup N9741 study have been published. This trial initially had a six-arm design, but the original control arm of bolus 5-FU/LV was dropped when the superiority of the IFL regimen became apparent. The bolus 5-FU/LV/oxaliplatin and the bolus 5-FU/LV/irinotecan arms were also dropped due to excessive toxicity. The remaining three arms included IFL, oxaliplatin plus infusional 5-FU/LV (FOLFOX4), and irinotecan plus oxaliplatin (IROX). The FOLFOX4 arm showed an improved response rate (45% vs. 31%), an improvement in time to progression (TTP) (8.7 months vs. 6.9 months), an improvement in median survival (19.5 months vs. 15 months) and one year survival (71% vs. 58%) when compared to the newest standard therapy with IFL (184,218).

It is important to note that this trial was conducted in the United States at a time when oxaliplatin was not yet available off-study. As a result, 52% of patients who progressed on the FOLFOX arm went on to receive irinotecan, whereas only 17% of those patients who progressed on the IFL arm received oxaliplatin as second-line therapy, making interpretation of the survival data difficult.

The optimal regimen or the best sequence to administer these agents remained undetermined. A subsequent study by Tournig et al. randomized patients to receive 5-FU, LV, irinotecan (FOLFIRI), or FOLFOX6 initially, and upon progression, cross to the other arm. The primary end point was overall time to progression after second-line treatment. The initial response rate of both sequences was similar (54–56%), with a median OS of 20.6 to 21.5 months (219,220).

Clearly oxaliplatin is an active agent against CRC, and these studies have led to the FDA approval of this drug in August 2002. Multiple trials of combination regimens in metastatic CRC are ongoing and include oxaliplatin plus irinotecan, capecitabine plus oxaliplatin (CAPOX) and capecitabine plus irinotecan (CAPIRI). Early results of several phase II studies of CAPOX and CAPIRI have been reported. Response rates range from 38% to 55%, making these regimens attractive combinations for phase III study (221–223).

Targeted Therapies for CRC

Expanding knowledge of cancer molecular biology has led to new classes of antitumor agents. Identification of novel tumor-specific targets has the potential to guide the development of agents that are more selective, tolerable, and effective.

Vascular Endothelial Growth Factor

VEGF is the predominant angiogenic factor in human CRC. VEGF expression levels correlate with advanced metastatic disease and a poor prognosis in earlier stages (224–226). A recombinant humanized monoclonal antibody against VEGF (rhuMab VEGF; bevacizumab, Avastin[TM] Genentech) has been developed. This antibody competitively inhibits the binding of VEGF to its endothelial cell receptors and limits tumor-associated angiogenesis in animal models (227,228). In humans, bevacizumab doses up to 10 mg/kg administered intravenously every 14 days were well tolerated and demonstrated antitumor activity in phase II studies (229). The most serious toxicity of this agent is arterial and venous thrombosis.

The results of a randomized phase II study evaluating two different doses of bevacizumab with 5-FU/LV was recently reported (230). One hundred and four previously untreated patients with metastatic CRC were randomized to one of three arms: weekly 5-FU/LV alone, weekly 5-FU/LV with bevacizumab 5 mg/kg every two weeks, or weekly 5-FU/LV with bevacizumab 10 mg/kg every two weeks. Higher response rates were seen in the bevacizumab arms (17%, 40%, and 24%, respectively). Longer-median TTP and OS were noted as well.

A phase III trial comparing IFL versus IFL/bevacizumab versus 5-FU/LV/ bevacizumab has been completed. The addition of bevacizumab to IFL improved RR (44.8% vs 34.8%), median survival (20.3 months vs. 15.6 months), leading to its recent FDA approval (231). The Eastern Cooperative Oncology group conducted a phase III study in patients who progressed on 5-FU and irinotecan, randomizing patients to receive 5-FU/LV/Oxaliplatin/bevacizumab or bevacizumab alone. This trial has completed accrual, and results are eagerly awaited.

Epidermal Growth Factor Receptor

One example relevant to the development and progression of many solid tumors, including CRC, is overexpression of protein kinases, such as the EGFR. Approximately 80% of colorectal tumors overexpress this receptor. Ligand binding results in EGFR dimerization, which activates intrinsic protein tyrosine kinase autophosphorylation. This in turn, initiates a series of signals to the nucleus stimulating DNA synthesis and cell division. In addition, receptor ligands including epidermal growth factor (EGF) and transforming growth factor alpha (TGF-α) have been shown to induce production of VEGF, which, in turn, stimulates angiogenesis. Neutralizing antibodies against EGFR can block EGF and TGF-α binding and down-regulate VEGF production.

In addition to decreased angiogenesis, other cellular results include inhibition of cell-cycle progression and increased apoptosis. Clinically, overexpression of the EGFR is associated with poor prognosis and an increased resistance to chemotherapy and radiotherapy. There are now three monoclonal antibodies targeting the EGFR in clinical trials: Cetuximab, ABX-EGF, and EMD 72000. Cetuximab (IMC-C225; Erbitux[TM]), a chimerized murine antibody, has activity against CRC as a single agent (231–233) and in combination with chemotherapy (234–236). Although relatively well tolerated, toxicities include an acneiform rash. In a single-agent trial, patients with metastatic disease, who failed prior therapy with irinotecan, there was a 10.5% response rate with 36.8% of patients having prolonged stable disease (232). In another phase II trial of 121 patients with irinotecan-refractory disease, there was a 22.5% response rate in patients who received irinotecan in combination with C225 (235). Interestingly, there was a correlation between the grade of skin rash and tumor inhibition, and median duration of survival. Phase I and II trials evaluating two humanized monoclonal antibody EGFR antagonists, ABX-EGF and EMD 72000, are also underway.

In summary, there is strong preclinical rationale and positive clinical trials to support the idea that these new targeted therapies represent the dawn of a new era in cancer treatment. Over the past decade we have gone from having only one active agent for the treatment of CRC to an additional five new agents. This has resulted in nearly doubling the median OS of patients with metastatic CRC and will hopefully translate into improved cure rates for those with resectable disease.

POSTOPERATIVE SURVEILLANCE FOR CRC

The goal of postoperative surveillance is to detect disease recurrence at the earliest time, to maximize the possibility that intervention will be clinically beneficial (237,238). Up to 39% of patients with recurrent disease could experience an increase in OS if surgical intervention could be applied at an appropriately early stage (182,238).

All strategies for postoperative surveillance stress regular follow-up employing clinical, radiological, endoscopic, and laboratory data to facilitate earlier detection of recurrent disease (238–240). Prompt identification of tumor recurrence is important for several reasons. First, metastatic cancer cells appear to be more sensitive to chemotherapeutic agents after resection. Also, initiating treatment at an early stage permits eradication of tumor prior to the development of chemotherapy-resistant clones. In addition, assuming that recurrence is initially localized, early detection and treatment may prevent dissemination. Furthermore, micrometastatic tumors are particularly well suited as targets for chemotherapy (241).

The reduction in mortality in CRC patients undergoing intensive postoperative surveillance highlights the importance of early detection of disease recurrence (242,243).

Limitations in Current Postoperative Surveillance Programs

Current surveillance protocols have not been uniformly successful in improving the OS of patients with recurrent CRC (237,239,244). Components of a postoperative surveillance program (CEA and other laboratory tests, colonoscopy, CT scans, and chest X-ray) together or separately are insensitive for detecting most early recurrences (238,239). The first major hurdle to overcome is the absence of a sensitive, responsive marker for early, potentially treatable, recurrent disease.

CEA for Postoperative Surveillance

Although all follow-up programs emphasize the need for multiple modalities, one consistent element of post-operative surveillance is serial measurement of serum CEA. Most reports suggest that periodic measurements postoperatively can detect recurrent disease at a surgically treatable stage (237,238,245,246).

Increasing CEA levels are associated with an increased risk for disease recurrence, tumor progression, tumor burden, and mortality (236,237). However, the sensitivity and specificity of CEA to detect recurrent CRC early remain limited because (i) CEA is produced by <80% of colorectal tumors, (ii) it is generated by other tumors and some normal extraintestinal tissues, and (iii) conditions other than CRC can cause elevated serum CEA levels (237,247). Overall, the sensitivity and specificity of this test for recurrence are 36% to 75% and 62% to 99%, respectively (245,248). Although the test detects tumor recurrence in the liver, it is less sensitive in detecting local, regional, or pulmonary metastases (237,245). Unfortunately, in most cases, CEA fails to detect recurrent disease at a point where cure can be improved (248,249).

At present, there is little data to support aggressive surveillance programs. Despite a lack of effective therapies in the face of recurrence, the concept of early detection is attractive. Identification of a sensitive and specific postoperative surveillance test(s) will be of value, particularly as therapeutic options evolve.

REFERENCES

1. American Cancer Society. Cancer Facts Figures 2002.
2. Mandel JS, Church TR, Bond JH, et al. The effect of fecal occult-blood screening on the incidence of colorectal cancer. N Engl J Med 2000; 343(22):1603–1607.
3. Winawer SJ, Zauber AG, Ho MN, et al. Prevention of colorectal cancer by colonoscopic polypectomy. The National Polyp Study Workgroup. N Engl J Med 1993; 329(27):1977–1981.
4. Thun MJ. Aspirin, NSAIDs, and digestive tract cancers. Cancer Metastasis Rev 1994; 13(3–4): 269–277.
5. Giovannucci E, Stampfer MJ, Colditz GA, et al. Multivitamin use, folate, and colon cancer in women in the Nurses' Health Study. Ann Intern Med 1998; 129(7):517–524.
6. Steinbach G, Lynch PM, Phillips RK, et al. The effect of celecoxib, a cyclooxygenase-2 inhibitor, in familial adenomatous polyposis. N Engl J Med 2000; 342(26):1946–1952.

7. Shapiro JA, Seeff LC, Nadel MR. Colorectal cancer-screening tests and associated health behaviors. Am J Prev Med 2001; 21(2):132–137.

8. Ries L, Eisner M, Kosary C, et al. eds. SEER Cancer Statistics Review, 1973–1999. Bethesda: National Cancer Institute, 2002.

9. Bresalier R. Malignant neoplasms of the large intestine. In: Sleisenger M, ed. Gastrointestinal and Liver Disease. 7th ed. Philadelphia: Saunders, 2002.

10. Winawer SJ. A quarter century of colorectal cancer screening: progress and prospects. J Clin Oncol 2001; 19(suppl 18):6S–12S.

11. Levin B. Colorectal cancer: screening and surveillance. In: Tepper J ed. Gastrointestinal Oncology. Philadelphia: Lipincott, 2002.

12. Bufil J. Evidence for distinct genetic categories based on proximal or distal location. Ann Intern Med 1990; 113:779.

13. Devesa SS, Chow WH. Variation in colorectal cancer incidence in the United States by subsite of origin. Cancer 1993; 71(12):3819–3826.

14. Colditz GA, Cannuscio CC, Frazier AL. Physical activity and reduced risk of colon cancer: implications for prevention. Cancer Causes Control 1997; 8(4):649–667.

15. Murphy TK, Calle EE, Rodriguez C, Kahn HS, Thun MJ. Body mass index and colon cancer mortality in a large prospective study. Am J Epidemiol 2000; 152(9):847–854.

16. Calle E, Rodriguez C, Walker Thurmond K, Thun M. Overweight, obesity, and mortality from cancer in a prospectively studied cohort of U.S. adults. N Engl J Med 2003; 348:1625–1638.

17. Franceschi S, Dal Maso L, Augustin L, et al. Dietary glycemic load and colorectal cancer risk. Ann Oncol 2001; 12(2):173–178.

18. Giacosa A, Franceschi S, La Vecchia C, Favero A, Andreatta R. Energy intake, overweight, physical exercise and colorectal cancer risk. Eur J Cancer Prev 1999; 8(suppl 1):S53–S60.

19. Willett W. The search for the causes of breast and colon cancer. Nature 1989; 338(6214):389–394.

20. Giovannucci E, Goldin B. The role of fat, fatty acids, and total energy intake in the etiology of human colon cancer. Am J Clin Nutr 1997; 66(suppl 6):1564S–1571S.

21. Boland C. Malignant tumors of the colon. In: Powell D, ed. Textbook of Gastroenterology. 3rd ed. Philadelphia: Lipincott, 1999.

22. Willett WC, Stampfer MJ, Colditz GA, Rosner BA, Speizer FE. Relation of meat, fat, and fiber intake to the risk of colon cancer in a prospective study among women. N Engl J Med 1990; 323(24):1664–1672.

23. Howe GR, Aronson KJ, Benito E, et al. The relationship between dietary fat intake and risk of colorectal cancer: evidence from the combined analysis of 13 case-control studies. Cancer Causes Control 1997; 8(2):215–228.

24. Gaard M, Tretli S, Loken EB. Dietary factors and risk of colon cancer: a prospective study of 50,535 young Norwegian men and women. Eur J Cancer Prev 1996; 5(6):445–454.

25. Schatzkin A, Lanza E, Corle D, et al. Lack of effect of a low-fat, high-fiber diet on the recurrence of colorectal adenomas. Polyp Prevention Trial Study Group. N Engl J Med 2000; 342(16):1149–1155.

26. Anti M, Marra G, Armelao F, et al. Effect of omega-3 fatty acids on rectal mucosal cell proliferation in subjects at risk for colon cancer. Gastroenterology 1992; 103(3):883–891.

27. Alberts DS, Martinez ME, Roe DJ, et al. Lack of effect of a high-fiber cereal supplement on the recurrence of colorectal adenomas. Phoenix Colon Cancer Prevention Physicians' Network. N Engl J Med 2000; 342(16):1156–1162.

28. Potter JD. Colorectal cancer: molecules and populations. J Natl Cancer Inst 1999; 91(11):916–932.

29. Sellers TA, Bazyk AE, Bostick RM, et al. Diet and risk of colon cancer in a large prospective study of older women: an analysis stratified on family history (Iowa, United States). Cancer Causes Control 1998; 9(4):357–367.

30. Bernstein CN, Blanchard JF, Kliewer E, Wajda A. Cancer risk in patients with inflammatory bowel disease: a population-based study. Cancer 2001; 91(4):854–862.

31. Weinberg DS, Newschaffer CJ, Topham A. Risk for colorectal cancer after gynecologic cancer. Ann Intern Med 1999; 131(3):189–193.

32. Newschaffer CJ, Topham A, Herzberg T, Weiner S, Weinberg DS. Risk of colorectal cancer after breast cancer. Lancet 2001; 357(9259):837–840.

33. Ahlquist D, Pasha T. Clinical aspects of sporadic colorectal cancer. In: Rustgi A, ed. Gastrointestinal Cancers. Philadelphia: Saunders, 2003.

34. Jass JR. Pathogenesis of colorectal cancer. Surg Clin North Am 2002; 82(5):891–904.

35. Vogelstein B, Fearon ER, Hamilton SR, et al. Genetic alterations during colorectal-tumor development. N Engl J Med 1988; 319(9):525–532.

36. Kinzler KW, Vogelstein B. Lessons from hereditary colorectal cancer. Cell 1996; 87(2):159–170.

37. Muto T, Bussey HJ, Morson BC. The evolution of cancer of the colon and rectum. Cancer 1975; 36(6):2251–2270.

38. Kinzler KW, Nilbert MC, Su LK, et al. Identification of FAP locus genes from chromosome 5q21. Science 1991; 253(5020):661–665.

39. Nishisho I, Nakamura Y, Miyoshi Y, et al. Mutations of chromosome 5q21 genes in FAP and colorectal cancer patients. Science 1991; 253(5020):665–669.

40. Groden J, Thliveris A, Samowitz W, et al. Identification and characterization of the familial adenomatous polyposis coli gene. Cell 1991; 66(3):589–600.

41. Citarda F, Tomaselli G, Capocaccia R, Barcherini S, Crespi M. Efficacy in standard clinical practice of colonoscopic polypectomy in reducing colorectal cancer incidence. Gut 2001; 48(6):812–815.

42. Jass JR, Constable L, Sutherland R, et al. Adenocarcinoma of colon differentiating as dome epithelium of gut-associated lymphoid tissue. Histopathology 2000; 36(2):116–120.

43. Shimoda T, Ikegami M, Fujisaki J, Matsui T, Aizawa S, Ishikawa E. Early colorectal carcinoma with special reference to its development de novo. Cancer 1989; 64(5):1138–1146.

44. Jass JR. Serrated adenoma and colorectal cancer. J Pathol 1999; 187(5):499–502.

45. Jass JR. Towards a molecular classification of colorectal cancer. Int J Colorectal Dis 1999; 14(4–5): 194–200.

46. Rashid A, Houlihan PS, Booker S, Petersen GM, Giardiello FM, Hamilton SR. Phenotypic and molecular characteristics of hyperplastic polyposis. Gastroenterology 2000; 119(2):323–332.

47. Jass JR, Iino H, Ruszkiewicz A, et al. Neoplastic progression occurs through mutator pathways in hyperplastic polyposis of the colorectum. Gut 2000; 47(1):43–49.

48. Loukola A, Salovaara R, Kristo P, et al. Microsatellite instability in adenomas as a marker for hereditary nonpolyposis colorectal cancer. Am J Pathol 1999; 155(6):1849–1853.

49. Neufeld G, Kessler O, Vadasz Z, Gluzman-Poltorak Z. The contribution of proangiogenic factors to the progression of malignant disease: role of vascular endothelial growth factor and its receptors. Surg Oncol Clin N Am 2001; 10(2):339–356.

50. Takahashi Y, Tucker SL, Kitadai Y, et al. Vessel counts and expression of vascular endothelial growth factor as prognostic factors in node-negative colon cancer. Arch Surg 1997; 132(5):541–546.

51. Takahashi Y, Kitadai Y, Bucana CD, Cleary KR, Ellis LM. Expression of vascular endothelial growth factor and its receptor, KDR, correlates with vascularity, metastasis, and proliferation of human colon cancer. Cancer Res 1995; 55(18):3964–3968.

52. Hasegawa K, Ichikawa W, Fujita T, et al. Expression of cyclooxygenase-2 (COX-2) mRNA in human colorectal adenomas. Eur J Cancer 2001; 37(12):1469–1474.

53. Williams CS, Smalley W, DuBois RN. Aspirin use and potential mechanisms for colorectal cancer prevention. J Clin Invest 1997; 100(6):1325–1329.

54. Tsujii M, Kawano S, DuBois RN. Cyclooxygenase-2 expression in human colon cancer cells increases metastatic potential. Proc Natl Acad Sci USA 1997; 94(7):3336–3340.

55. USPSTF. Screening for colorectal cancer: recommendation and rationale. Ann Intern Med 2002; 137(2):129–131.

56. Winawer SJ, Fletcher RH, Miller L, et al. Colorectal cancer screening: clinical guidelines and rationale. Gastroenterology 1997; 112(2):594–642.

57. Smith RA, Cokkinides V, von Eschenbach AC, et al. American Cancer Society guidelines for the early detection of cancer. CA Cancer J Clin 2002; 52(1):8–22.

58. Ransohoff DF, Sandler RS. Clinical practice. Screening for colorectal cancer. N Engl J Med 2002; 346(1):40–44.

59. Pignone M, Saha S, Hoerger T, Mandelblatt J. Cost-effectiveness analyses of colorectal cancer screening: a systematic review for the U.S. Preventive Services Task Force. Ann Intern Med 2002; 137(2):96–104.

60. Nadel MR, Blackman DK, Shapiro JA, Seeff LC. Are people being screened for colorectal cancer as recommended? Results from the National Health Interview Survey. Prev Med 2002; 35(3):199–206.

61. Macrae FA, St John DJ. Relationship between patterns of bleeding and Hemoccult sensitivity in patients with colorectal cancers or adenomas. Gastroenterology 1982; 82(5 Pt 1):891–898.

62. Wexner SD, Brabbee GW, Wichem WA Jr. Sensitivity of hemoccult testing in patients with colorectal carcinoma. Dis Colon Rectum 1984; 27(12):775–776.

63. Pye G, Ballantyne KC, Armitage NC, Hardcastle JD. Influence of non-steroidal anti-inflammatory drugs on the outcome of faecal occult blood tests in screening for colorectal cancer. Br Med J (Clin Res Ed) 1987; 294(6586):1510–1511.

64. Thomas WM, Pye G, Hardcastle JD, Chamberlain J, Charnley RM. Role of dietary restriction in Haemoccult screening for colorectal cancer. Br J Surg 1989; 76(9):976–978.

65. Lurie JD, Welch HG. Diagnostic testing following fecal occult blood screening in the elderly. J Natl Cancer Inst 1999; 91(19):1641–1646.

66. Lieberman DA, Weiss DG. One-time screening for colorectal cancer with combined fecal occult-blood testing and examination of the distal colon. N Engl J Med 2001; 345(8):555–560.

67. Mandel JS, Bond JH, Church TR, et al. Reducing mortality from colorectal cancer by screening for fecal occult blood. Minnesota Colon Cancer Control Study. N Engl J Med 1993; 328(19):1365–1371.

68. Kronborg O, Fenger C, Olsen J, Jorgensen OD, Sondergaard O. Randomised study of screening for colorectal cancer with faecal-occult-blood test. Lancet 1996; 348(9040):1467–1471.

69. Hardcastle JD, Chamberlain JO, Robinson MH, et al. Randomised controlled trial of faecal-occult-blood screening for colorectal cancer. Lancet 1996; 348(9040):1472–1477.

70. Young GP, St John DJ, Winawer SJ, Rozen P. Choice of fecal occult blood tests for colorectal cancer screening: recommendations based on performance characteristics in population studies: a WHO (World Health Organization) and OMED (World Organization for Digestive Endoscopy) report. Am J Gastroenterol 2002; 97(10):2499–2507.

71. Towler B, Irwig L, Glasziou P. Screening for colorectal cancer using the fecal occult blood test, Hemoccult. Cochrane Library. Update Software, 2000 ed. Oxford; 2000.

72. Lewis JD, Asch DA. Barriers to office-based screening sigmoidoscopy: does reimbursement cover costs? Ann Intern Med 1999; 130(6):525–530.

73. Imperiale TF, Wagner DR, Lin CY, Larkin GN, Rogge JD, Ransohoff DF. Risk of advanced proximal neoplasms in asymptomatic adults according to the distal colorectal findings. N Engl J Med 2000; 343(3):169–174.

74. Levin TR, Palitz A, Grossman S, et al. Predicting advanced proximal colonic neoplasia with screening sigmoidoscopy. JAMA 1999; 281(17):1611–1617.

75. Lieberman DA, Weiss DG, Bond JH, Ahnen DJ, Garewal H, Chejfec G. Use of colonoscopy to screen asymptomatic adults for colorectal cancer. Veterans Affairs Cooperative Study Group 380. N Engl J Med 2000; 343(3):162–168.

76. Johnson DA, Gurney MS, Volpe RJ, et al. A prospective study of the prevalence of colonic neoplasms in asymptomatic patients with an age-related risk. Am J Gastroenterol 1990; 85(8):969–974.

77. Itzkowitz S. Colonic polyps and polyposis syndromes. In: Sleisenger M, ed. Gastrointestinal and Liver Disease. Philadelphia: Saunders, 2002.

78. Hamilton SR. Origin of colorectal cancers in hyperplastic polyps and serrated adenomas: another truism bites the dust. J Natl Cancer Inst 2001; 93(17):1282–1283.

79. UK Flexible Sigmoidoscopy Screening Trial Investigators. Single flexible sigmoidoscopy screening to prevent colorectal cancer: baseline findings of a UK multicentre randomised trial. Lancet 2002; 359(9314):1291–1300.

80. Selby JV, Friedman GD, Quesenberry CP Jr., Weiss NS. A case-control study of screening sigmoidoscopy and mortality from colorectal cancer. N Engl J Med 1992; 326(10):653–657.

81. Newcomb PA, Norfleet RG, Storer BE, Surawicz TS, Marcus PM. Screening sigmoidoscopy and colorectal cancer mortality. J Natl Cancer Inst 1992; 84(20):1572–1575.

82. Atkin WS, Morson BC, Cuzick J. Long-term risk of colorectal cancer after excision of rectosigmoid adenomas. N Engl J Med 1992; 326(10):658–662.

83. Winawer SJ, Stewart ET, Zauber AG, et al. A comparison of colonoscopy and double-contrast barium enema for surveillance after polypectomy. National Polyp Study Work Group. N Engl J Med 2000; 342(24):1766–1772.

84. Sonnenberg A, Delco F, Inadomi JM. Cost-effectiveness of colonoscopy in screening for colorectal cancer. Ann Intern Med 2000; 133(8):573–584.

85. Wexner SD, Garbus JE, Singh JJ. SAGES Colonoscopy Study Outcomes Group. A prospective analysis of 13,580 colonoscopies. Reevaluation of credentialing guidelines. Surg Endosc 2001; 15(3): 251–261.

86. Wexner SD, Forde KA, Sellers G, et al. How well can surgeons perform colonoscopy? Surg Endosc 1998; 12(12):1410–1414.

87. Shapero TF, Alexander PE, Hoover J, Burgis E, Schabas R. Colorectal cancer screening: video-reviewed flexible sigmoidoscopy by nurse endoscopists—a Canadian community-based perspective. Can J Gastroenterol 2001; 15(7):441–445.

88. Vijan S, Hwang EW, Hofer TP, Hayward RA. Which colon cancer screening test? A comparison of costs, effectiveness, and compliance. Am J Med 2001; 111(8):593–601; Group L. Gastrointestinal Cancers. American Gastroenterological Association, 2001.

89. Group L. (American Gastroenterological Association). Gastrointestinal Cancers, 2001.

90. Wagner J, Tunis S, Brown M, Ching A, Almeida R. Cost effectiveness of colorectal cancer screening in average risk adults. In: Levin B, ed. Prevention and Early Detection of Colorectal Cancer. Philadelphia: Saunders, 1996.

91. Rex DK, Vining D, Kopecky KK. An initial experience with screening for colon polyps using spiral CT with and without CT colography (virtual colonoscopy). Gastrointest Endosc 1999; 50(3):309–313.

92. Luboldt W, Bauerfeind P, Wildermuth S, Marincek B, Fried M, Debatin JF. Colonic masses: detection with MR colonography. Radiology 2000; 216(2):383–388.

93. Pickhardt PJ, Choi JR, Hwang I, et al. Computed tomographic virtual colonoscopy to screen for colorectal neoplasia in asymptomatic adults. N Engl J Med 2003; 349(23):2191–2200.

94. Traverso G, Shuber A, Olsson L, et al. Detection of proximal colorectal cancers through analysis of faecal DNA. Lancet 2002; 359(9304):403–404.

95. Jen J, Johnson C, Levin B. Molecular approaches for colorectal cancer screening. Eur J Gastroenterol Hepatol 1998; 10(3):213–217.

96. Ahlquist DA, Skoletsky JE, Boynton KA, et al. Colorectal cancer screening by detection of altered human DNA in stool: feasibility of a multitarget assay panel. Gastroenterology 2000; 119(5):1219–1227.

97. Cui H, Cruz-Correa M, Giardiello FM, et al. Loss of IGF2 imprinting: a potential marker of colorectal cancer risk. Science 2003; 299(5613):1753–1755.

98. Laken SJ, Petersen GM, Gruber SB, et al. Familial colorectal cancer in Ashkenazim due to a hypermutable tract in APC. Nat Genet 1997; 17(1):79–83.

99. Fuchs CS, Giovannucci EL, Colditz GA, Hunter DJ, Speizer FE, Willett WC. A prospective study of family history and the risk of colorectal cancer. N Engl J Med 1994; 331(25):1669–1674.

100. St John DJ, McDermott FT, Hopper JL, Debney EA, Johnson WR, Hughes ES. Cancer risk in relatives of patients with common colorectal cancer. Ann Intern Med 1993; 118(10):785–790.

101. Winawer SJ, Zauber AG, Gerdes H, et al. Risk of colorectal cancer in the families of patients with adenomatous polyps. National Polyp Study Workgroup. N Engl J Med 1996; 334(2):82–87.

102. Neugut AI, Jacobson JS, Ahsan H, et al. Incidence and recurrence rates of colorectal adenomas: a prospective study. Gastroenterology 1995; 108(2):402–408.

103. Kelloff GJ, Crowell JA, Steele VE, et al. Progress in cancer chemoprevention. Ann N Y Acad Sci 1999; 889:1–13.

104. Hyman J, Baron JA, Dain BJ, et al. Dietary and supplemental calcium and the recurrence of colorectal adenomas. Cancer Epidemiol Biomarkers Prev 1998; 7(4):291–295.

105. Martinez ME, Willett WC. Calcium, vitamin D, and colorectal cancer: a review of the epidemiologic evidence. Cancer Epidemiol Biomarkers Prev 1998; 7(2):163–168.

106. Patterson RE, White E, Kristal AR, Neuhouser ML, Potter JD. Vitamin supplements and cancer risk: the epidemiologic evidence. Cancer Causes Control 1997; 8(5):786–802.

107. Albanes D, Malila N, Taylor PR, et al. Effects of supplemental alpha-tocopherol and beta-carotene on colorectal cancer: results from a controlled trial (Finland). Cancer Causes Control 2000; 11(3): 197–205.

108. Malila N, Virtamo J, Virtanen M, Albanes D, Tangrea JA, Huttunen JK. The effect of alpha-tocopherol and beta-carotene supplementation on colorectal adenomas in middle-aged male smokers. Cancer Epidemiol Biomarkers Prev 1999; 8(6):489–493.

109. Hercberg S, Preziosi P, Galan P, et al. "The SU.VI.MAX Study": a primary prevention trial using nutritional doses of antioxidant vitamins and minerals in cardiovascular diseases and cancers. Supplementation on VItamines et Mineraux AntioXydants. Food Chem Toxicol 1999; 37(9–10):925–930.

110. Ryan BM, Weir DG. Relevance of folate metabolism in the pathogenesis of colorectal cancer. J Lab Clin Med 2001; 138(3):164–176.

111. Kim YI. Folate and cancer prevention: a new medical application of folate beyond hyperhomocysteinemia and neural tube defects. Nutr Rev 1999; 57(10):314–321.

112. Giovannucci E, Stampfer MJ, Colditz GA, et al. Folate, methionine, and alcohol intake and risk of colorectal adenoma. J Natl Cancer Inst 1993; 85(11):875–884.

113. Giovannucci E, Rimm EB, Ascherio A, Stampfer MJ, Colditz GA, Willett WC. Alcohol, low-methionine—low-folate diets, and risk of colon cancer in men. J Natl Cancer Inst 1995; 87(4):265–273.

114. Torrance CJ, Jackson PE, Montgomery E, et al. Combinatorial chemoprevention of intestinal neoplasia. Nat Med 2000; 6(9):1024–1028.

115. Williams CS, Mann M, DuBois RN. The role of cyclooxygenases in inflammation, cancer, and development. Oncogene 1999; 18(55):7908–7916.

116. Eberhart CE, Coffey RJ, Radhika A, Giardiello FM, Ferrenbach S, DuBois RN. Up-regulation of cyclooxygenase 2 gene expression in human colorectal adenomas and adenocarcinomas. Gastroenterology 1994; 107(4):1183–1188.

117. Giovannucci E, Rimm EB, Stampfer MJ, Colditz GA, Ascherio A, Willett WC. Aspirin use and the risk for colorectal cancer and adenoma in male health professionals. Ann Intern Med 1994; 121(4):241–246.

118. Thun MJ, Namboodiri MM, Calle EE, Flanders WD, Heath CW Jr. Aspirin use and risk of fatal cancer. Cancer Res 1993; 53(6):1322–1327.

119. Giardiello FM, Hamilton SR, Krush AJ, et al. Treatment of colonic and rectal adenomas with sulindac in familial adenomatous polyposis. N Engl J Med 1993; 328(18):1313–1316.

120. Giardiello FM, Yang VW, Hylind LM, et al. Primary chemoprevention of familial adenomatous polyposis with sulindac. N Engl J Med 2002; 346(14):1054–1059.

121. Nelson HD, Humphrey LL, Nygren P, Teutsch SM, Allan JD. Postmenopausal hormone replacement therapy: scientific review. JAMA 2002; 288(7):872–881.

122. Nanda K, Bastian LA, Hasselblad V, Simel DL. Hormone replacement therapy and the risk of colorectal cancer: a meta-analysis. Obstet Gynecol 1999; 93(5 Pt 2):880–888.

123. Newcomb PA, Taylor JO, Trentham-Dietz A. Interactions of familial and hormonal risk factors for large bowel cancer in women. Int J Epidemiol 1999; 28(4):603–608.

124. Rossouw JE, Anderson GL, Prentice RL, et al. Risks and benefits of estrogen plus progestin in healthy postmenopausal women: principal results from the Women's Health Initiative randomized controlled trial. JAMA 2002; 288(3):321–333.

125. Imperiale TF, Wagner DR, Lin CY, Larkin GN, Rogge JD, Ransohoff DF. Results of screening colonoscopy among persons 40 to 49 years of age. N Engl J Med 2002; 346(23):1781–1785.

126. Rex DK. Colonoscopy: a review of its yield for cancers and adenomas by indication. Am J Gastroenterol 1995; 90(3):353–365.

127. Shinya H, Wolff WI. Morphology, anatomic distribution and cancer potential of colonic polyps. Ann Surg 1979; 190(6):679–683.

128. Greene FL, Page DL, Fleming ID, et al. AJCC Cancer Staging Manual. 6th ed. New York: Springer-Verlag, 2002.

129. Hertzer F, Slanetz C. Patterns and significance of lymphatic spread from cancer of the colon and rectum. In: Ballon S, ed. Lymphatic System Metastasis. Boston, MA: GK Hall, 1980:283.

130. Nelson H, Petrelli N, Carlin A, et al. Guidelines 2000 for colon and rectal cancer surgery. J Natl Cancer Inst 2001; 93(8):583–596.

131. LeVoyer T, Sigurdson E, Hanlon A. Colon cancer survival is associated with increasing number of lymph nodes analyzed. A secondary survey of INT-0089. J Clin Onc 2003; In press.

132. Zeng Z, Cohen AM, Urmacher C. Usefulness of carcinoembryonic antigen monitoring despite normal preoperative values in node-positive colon cancer patients. Dis Colon Rectum 1993; 36(11):1063–1068.

133. Cohen SM, Wexner SD, Binderow SR, et al. Prospective, randomized, endoscopic-blinded trial comparing precolonoscopy bowel cleansing methods. Dis Colon Rectum 1994; 37(7):689–696.

134. Oliveira L, Wexner SD, Daniel N, et al. Mechanical bowel preparation for elective colorectal surgery. A prospective, randomized, surgeon-blinded trial comparing sodium phosphate and polyethylene glycol-based oral lavage solutions. Dis Colon Rectum 1997; 40(5):585–591.

135. Makhija R. Meta-analysis of randomized clinical trials of colorectal surgery with or without mechanical bowel preparation (Br J Surg 2004; 91:1125–1130). Br J Surg 2004; 91(11):1528.

136. Slim K, Vicaut E, Panis Y, Chipponi J. Meta-analysis of randomized clinical trials of colorectal surgery with or without mechanical bowel preparation. Br J Surg 2004; 91(9):1125–1130.

137. Zmora O, Mahajna A, Bar-Zakai B, et al. Colon and rectal surgery without mechanical bowel preparation: a randomized prospective trial. Ann Surg 2003; 237(3):363–367.

138. Miettinen RP, Laitinen ST, Makela JT, Paakkonen ME. Bowel preparation with oral polyethylene glycol electrolyte solution vs. no preparation in elective open colorectal surgery: prospective, randomized study. Dis Colon Rectum 2000; 43(5):669–675; discussion 675–677.

139. Zmora O, Wexner SD, Hajjar L, et al. Trends in preparation for colorectal surgery: survey of the members of the American Society of Colon and Rectal Surgeons. Am Surg 2003; 69(2):150–154.

140. Schoetz DJ Jr., Roberts PL, Murray JJ, Coller JA, Veidenheimer MC. Addition of parenteral cefoxitin to regimen of oral antibiotics for elective colorectal operations. A randomized prospective study. Ann Surg 1990; 212(2):209–212.

141. Anonymous. Efficacy and safety of enoxaparin versus unfractionated heparin for prevention of deep vein thrombosis in elective cancer surgery: a double-blind randomized multicentre trial with venographic assessment. ENOXACAN Study Group. Br J Surg; 84:1099–1103.

142. McLeod RS, Geerts WH, Sniderman KW, et al. Subcutaneous heparin versus low-molecular-weight heparin as thromboprophylaxis in patients undergoing colorectal surgery: results of the canadian colorectal DVT prophylaxis trial: a randomized, double-blind trial. Ann Surg 2001; 233(3):438–444.

143. Amato AC, Pescatori M. Effect of perioperative blood transfusions on recurrence of colorectal cancer: meta-analysis stratified on risk factors. Dis Colon Rectum 1998; 41(5):570–585.

144. Burrows L, Tartter P. Effect of blood transfusions on colonic malignancy recurrent rate. Lancet 1982; 2(8299):662.

145. Donohue JH, Williams S, Cha S, et al. Perioperative blood transfusions do not affect disease recurrence of patients undergoing curative resection of colorectal carcinoma: a Mayo/North Central Cancer Treatment Group study. J Clin Oncol 1995; 13(7):1671–1678.

146. Cervone A, Sardi A, Conaway GL. Intraoperative ultrasound (IOUS) is essential in the management of metastatic colorectal liver lesions. Am Surg 2000; 66(7):611–615.

147. Cooper HS, Deppisch LM, Gourley WK, et al. Endoscopically removed malignant colorectal polyps: clinicopathologic correlations. Gastroenterology 1995; 108(6):1657–1665.

148. Haggitt RC, Glotzbach RE, Soffer EE, Wruble LD. Prognostic factors in colorectal carcinomas arising in adenomas: implications for lesions removed by endoscopic polypectomy. Gastroenterology 1985; 89(2):328–336.

149. Nivatvongs S, Rojanasakul A, Reiman HM, et al. The risk of lymph node metastasis in colorectal polyps with invasive adenocarcinoma. Dis Colon Rectum 1991; 34(4):323–328.

150. Kyzer S, Begin LR, Gordon PH, Mitmaker B. The care of patients with colorectal polyps that contain invasive adenocarcinoma. Endoscopic polypectomy or colectomy? Cancer 1992; 70(8):2044–2050.

151. Nivatvongs S. Surgical management of early colorectal cancer. World J Surg 2000; 24(9):1052–1055.

152. Tanaka S, Haruma K, Teixeira CR, et al. Endoscopic treatment of submucosal invasive colorectal carcinoma with special reference to risk factors for lymph node metastasis. J Gastroenterol 1995; 30(6):710–717.

153. Nascimbeni R, Burgart LJ, Nivatvongs S, Larson DR. Risk of lymph node metastasis in T1 carcinoma of the colon and rectum. Dis Colon Rectum 2002; 45(2):200–206.

154. Kikuchi R, Takano M, Takagi K, et al. Management of early invasive colorectal cancer. Risk of recurrence and clinical guidelines. Dis Colon Rectum 1995; 38(12):1286–1295.

155. Brodsky JT, Richard GK, Cohen AM, Minsky BD. Variables correlated with the risk of lymph node metastasis in early rectal cancer. Cancer 1992; 69(2):322–326.

156. Blumberg D, Paty PB, Picon AI, et al. Stage I rectal cancer: identification of high-risk patients. J Am Coll Surg 1998; 186(5):574–579; discussion 579–580.

157. Coverlizza S, Risio M, Ferrari A, Fenoglio-Preiser CM, Rossini FP. Colorectal adenomas containing invasive carcinoma. Pathologic assessment of lymph node metastatic potential. Cancer 1989; 64(9): 1937–1947.

158. Rouffet F, Hay JM, Vacher B, et al. Curative resection for left colonic carcinoma: hemicolectomy versus segmental colectomy. A prospective, controlled, multicenter trial. French Association for Surgical Research. Dis Colon Rectum 1994; 37(7):651–659.

159. Slanetz CA Jr., Grimson R. Effect of high and intermediate ligation on survival and recurrence rates following curative resection of colorectal cancer. Dis Colon Rectum 1997; 40(10):1205–1218; discussion 1218–1219.

160. Grinnell R. Results of ligation of inferior mesenteric artery at the aorta in resections of carcinoma of the descending and sigmoid colon and rectum. Surg Gynecol Obstet 1965; 120:1031–1036.

161. Docherty JG, McGregor JR, Akyol AM, Murray GD, Galloway DJ. Comparison of manually constructed and stapled anastomoses in colorectal surgery. West of Scotland and Highland Anastomosis Study Group. Ann Surg 1995; 221(2):176–184.

162. Wood TF, Saha S, Morton DL, et al. Validation of lymphatic mapping in colorectal cancer: in vivo, ex vivo, and laparoscopic techniques. Ann Surg Oncol 2001; 8(2):150–157.

163. Saha S, Wiese D, Badin J, et al. Technical details of sentinel lymph node mapping in colorectal cancer and its impact on staging. Ann Surg Oncol 2000; 7(2):120–124.

164. Bilchik AJ, Nora D, Tollenaar RA, et al. Ultrastaging of early colon cancer using lymphatic mapping and molecular analysis. Eur J Cancer 2002; 38(7):977–985.

165. Kelley WE Jr., Brown PW, Lawrence W Jr., Terz JJ. Penetrating, obstructing, and perforating carcinomas of the colon and rectum. Arch Surg 1981; 116(4):381–384.

166. Gall FP, Tonak J, Altendorf A. Multivisceral resections in colorectal cancer. Dis Colon Rectum 1987; 30(5):337–341.

167. Davies GC, Ellis H. Radical surgery in locally advanced cancer of the large bowel. Clin Oncol 1975; 1(1):21–26.

168. Hunter JA, Ryan JA Jr., Schultz P. En bloc resection of colon cancer adherent to other organs. Am J Surg 1987; 154(1):67–71.

169. Arenas RB, Fichera A, Mhoon D, Michelassi F. Incidence and therapeutic implications of synchronous colonic pathology in colorectal adenocarcinoma. Surgery 1997; 122(4):706–709; discussion 709–710.

170. Carraro PG, Segala M, Cesana BM, Tiberio G. Obstructing colonic cancer: failure and survival patterns over a ten-year follow-up after one-stage curative surgery. Dis Colon Rectum 2001; 44(2): 243–250.

171. Berends FJ, Kazemier G, Bonjer HJ, Lange JF. Subcutaneous metastases after laparoscopic colectomy. Lancet 1994; 344(8914):58.

172. Reilly WT, Nelson H, Schroeder G, Wieand HS, Bolton J, O'Connell MJ. Wound recurrence following conventional treatment of colorectal cancer. A rare but perhaps underestimated problem. Dis Colon Rectum 1996; 39(2):200–207.

173. Lacy AM, Garcia-Valdecasas JC, Delgado S, et al. Laparoscopy-assisted colectomy versus open colectomy for treatment of non-metastatic colon cancer: a randomised trial. Lancet 2002; 359(9325): 2224–2229.

174. Weeks JC, Nelson H, Gelbert S, et al. Short-term quality of life outcomes following laparascopic-assisted colectomy vs. open colectomy for colon cancer JAMA 2002; 287:321–328; The Clinical Outcomes of Surgical Therapy Study Group. A comparison of laparoscopically assisted and open colectomy for colon cancer. N Engl J Med 2004; 350(20):2050–2059.

175. Leung KL, Yiu RY, Lai PB, Lee JF, Thung KH, Lau WY. Laparoscopic-assisted resection of colorectal carcinoma: five-year audit. Dis Colon Rectum 1999; 42(3):327–332; discussion 332–333.

176. Poulin EC, Mamazza J, Schlachta CM, Gregoire R, Roy N. Laparoscopic resection does not adversely affect early survival curves in patients undergoing surgery for colorectal adenocarcinoma. Ann Surg 1999; 229(4):487–492.

177. Poon MA, O'Connell MJ, Moertel CG, et al. Biochemical modulation of fluorouracil: evidence of significant improvement of survival and quality of life in patients with advanced colorectal carcinoma. J Clin Oncol 1989; 7(10):1407–1418.

178. Buroker TR, O'Connell MJ, Wieand HS, et al. Randomized comparison of two schedules of fluorouracil and leucovorin in the treatment of advanced colorectal cancer. J Clin Oncol 1994; 12(1): 14–20.

179. Fong Y, Fortner J, Sun RL, Brennan MF, Blumgart LH. Clinical score for predicting recurrence after hepatic resection for metastatic colorectal cancer: analysis of 1001 consecutive cases. Ann Surg 1999; 230(3):309–318; discussion 318–321.

180. Jamison RL, Donohue JH, Nagorney DM, Rosen CB, Harmsen WS, Ilstrup DM. Hepatic resection for metastatic colorectal cancer results in cure for some patients. Arch Surg 1997; 132(5):505–510; discussion 511.

181. Scheele J, Stang R, Altendorf-Hofmann A, Paul M. Resection of colorectal liver metastases. World J Surg 1995; 19(1):59–71.

182. Goldberg RM, Sargent DJ, Morton RF, et al. A randomized controlled trial of fluorouracil plus leucovorin, irinotecan, and oxaliplatin combinations in patients with previously untreated metastatic colorectal cancer. J Clin Oncol 2004; 22(1):23–30.

183. Saltz LB, Cox JV, Blanke C, et al. Irinotecan plus fluorouracil and leucovorin for metastatic colorectal cancer. Irinotecan Study Group. N Engl J Med 2000; 343(13):905–914.

184. Fong Y, Fortner J, Sun R, Brennan M, Blumgart L. Clinical score for predicting recurrence after hepatic resection for metastatic colorectal cancer: analysis of 1001 consecutive cases. Ann Surg 1999; 230(3):309–318.

185. Ambiru S, Miyazaki M, Isono T, et al. Hepatic resection for colorectal metastases: analysis of prognostic factors. Dis Colon Rectum 1999; 42(5):632–639.

186. Goya T, Miyazawa N, Kondo H, Tsuchiya R, Naruke T, Suemasu K. Surgical resection of pulmonary metastases from colorectal cancer. 10-year follow-up. Cancer 1989; 64(7):1418–1421.

187. Yano T, Hara N, Ichinose Y, Yokoyama H, Miura T, Ohta M. Results of pulmonary resection of metastatic colorectal cancer and its application. J Thorac Cardiovasc Surg 1993; 106(5):875–879.

188. Gunderson LL, Sargent DJ, Tepper JE, et al. Impact of T and N stage and treatment on survival and relapse in adjuvant rectal cancer: a pooled analysis. J Clin Oncol 2004; 22(10):1785–1796.

189. Efficacy of adjuvant fluorouracil and folinic acid in colon cancer. International Multicentre Pooled Analysis of Colon Cancer Trials (IMPACT) investigators. Lancet 1995; 345(8955):939–944.

190. Francini G, Petrioli R, Lorenzini L, et al. Folinic acid and 5-fluorouracil as adjuvant chemotherapy in colon cancer. Gastroenterology 1994; 106(4):899–906.

191. O'Connell MJ, Mailliard JA, Kahn MJ, et al. Controlled trial of fluorouracil and low-dose leucovorin given for 6 months as postoperative adjuvant therapy for colon cancer. J Clin Oncol 1997; 15(1):246–250.

192. Wolmark N, Rockette H, Fisher B, et al. The benefit of leucovorin-modulated fluorouracil as postoperative adjuvant therapy for primary colon cancer: results from National Surgical Adjuvant Breast and Bowel Project protocol C-03. J Clin Oncol 1993; 11(10):1879–1887.

193. O'Connell MJ, Laurie JA, Kahn M, et al. Prospectively randomized trial of postoperative adjuvant chemotherapy in patients with high-risk colon cancer. J Clin Oncol 1998; 16(1):295–300.

194. de Gramont A, Figer A, Seymour M, et al. A randomized trial of leucovorin (LV) and 5-fluorouracil (5FU) with or without oxaliplatin in advanced colorectal cancer (CRC). Proc Am Soc Clin Oncol 1998; 17:257a.

195. Wolmark N, Rockette H, Mamounas E, et al. Clinical trial to assess the relative efficacy of fluorouracil and leucovorin, fluorouracil and levamisole, and fluorouracil, leucovorin, and levamisole in patients with Dukes' B and C carcinoma of the colon: results from National Surgical Adjuvant Breast and Bowel Project C-04. J Clin Oncol 1999; 17(11):3553–3559.

196. Cassidy J. Capecitabine (X) vs bolus 5-FU/leucovorin (LV) as adjuvant therapy for colon cancer (the X-ACT) study): efficacy results of a phase III trial [abstr 3509]. Proc Am Soc Clin Oncol 2004; 23.

197. Andre T, Boni C, Mounedji-Boudiaf L, et al. Oxaliplatin, fluorouracil, and leucovorin as adjuvant treatment for colon cancer. N Engl J Med 2004; 350(23):2343–2351.

198. Mamounas E, Wieand S, Wolmark N, et al. Comparative efficacy of adjuvant chemotherapy in patients with Dukes' B versus Dukes' C colon cancer: results from four National Surgical Adjuvant Breast and Bowel Project adjuvant studies (C-01, C-02, C-03, and C-04). J Clin Oncol 1999; 17(5):1349–1355.

199. Efficacy of adjuvant fluorouracil and folinic acid in B2 colon cancer. International Multicentre Pooled Analysis of B2 Colon Cancer Trials (IMPACT B2) Investigators. J Clin Oncol 1999; 17(5):1356–1363.

200. Prolongation of the disease-free interval in surgically treated rectal carcinoma. Gastrointestinal Tumor Study Group. N Engl J Med 1985; 312(23):1465–1472.

201. Douglass HO Jr., Moertel CG, Mayer RJ, et al. Survival after postoperative combination treatment of rectal cancer. N Engl J Med 1986; 315(20):1294–1295.

202. Fisher B, Wolmark N, Rockette H, et al. Postoperative adjuvant chemotherapy or radiation therapy for rectal cancer: results from NSABP protocol R-01. J Natl Cancer Inst 1988; 80(1):21–29.

203. Krook JE, Moertel CG, Gunderson LL, et al. Effective surgical adjuvant therapy for high-risk rectal carcinoma. N Engl J Med 1991; 324(11):709–715.

204. Wolmark N, Wieand HS, Hyams DM, et al. Randomized trial of postoperative adjuvant chemotherapy with or without radiotherapy for carcinoma of the rectum: National Surgical Adjuvant Breast and Bowel Project Protocol R-02. J Natl Cancer Inst 2000; 92(5):388–396.

205. Tepper JE, O'Connell M, Niedzwiecki D, et al. Adjuvant therapy in rectal cancer: analysis of stage, sex, and local control–final report of intergroup 0114. J Clin Oncol 2002; 20(7):1744–1750.

206. Roh MS, Petrelli NJ, Wieand S, et al. Phase III randomized trial of preoperative versus postoperative multimodality therapy in patients with carcinoma of the rectum. Proc Am Soc Clin Oncol 2001; 20:123a.

207. Sauer R. Adjuvant versus neoadjuvant combined modality treatment for locally advanced rectal cancer: first results of the German rectal cancer study (CAO/ARO/AIO–94). Int J Radiat Oncol Biol Phys 2003; 57(suppl 2):S124–S125.

208. Conti JA, Kemeny NE, Saltz LB, et al. Irinotecan is an active agent in untreated patients with metastatic colorectal cancer. J Clin Oncol 1996; 14(3):709–715.

209. Pitot HC, Wender DB, O'Connell MJ, et al. Phase II trial of irinotecan in patients with metastatic colorectal carcinoma. J Clin Oncol 1997; 15(8):2910–2919.

210. Rougier P, Bugat R, Douillard JY, et al. Phase II study of irinotecan in the treatment of advanced colorectal cancer in chemotherapy-naive patients and patients pretreated with fluorouracil-based chemotherapy. J Clin Oncol 1997; 15(1):251–260.

211. Cunningham D, Pyrhonen S, James RD, et al. Randomised trial of irinotecan plus supportive care versus supportive care alone after fluorouracil failure for patients with metastatic colorectal cancer. Lancet 1998; 352(9138):1413–1418.

212. Rougier P, Van Cutsem E, Bajetta E, et al. Randomised trial of irinotecan versus fluorouracil by continuous infusion after fluorouracil failure in patients with metastatic colorectal cancer. Lancet 1998; 352(9138):1407–1412.

213. Douillard JY, Cunningham D, Roth AD, et al. Irinotecan combined with fluorouracil compared with fluorouracil alone as first-line treatment for metastatic colorectal cancer: a multicentre randomised trial. Lancet 2000; 355(9209):1041–1047.

214. Machover D, Diaz-Rubio E, de Gramont A, et al. Two consecutive phase II studies of oxaliplatin (L-OHP) for treatment of patients with advanced colorectal carcinoma who were resistant to previous treatment with fluoropyrimidines. Ann Oncol 1996; 7(1):95–98.

215. Becouarn Y, Ychou M, Ducreux M, et al. Phase II trial of oxaliplatin as first-line chemotherapy in metastatic colorectal cancer patients. Digestive Group of French Federation of Cancer Centers. J Clin Oncol 1998; 16(8):2739–2744.

216. de Gramont A, Figer A, Seymour M, et al. Leucovorin and fluorouracil with or without oxaliplatin as first-line treatment in advanced colorectal cancer. J Clin Oncol 2000; 18(16):2938–2947.

217. Giacchetti S, Perpoint B, Zidani R, et al. Phase III multicenter randomized trial of oxaliplatin added to chronomodulated fluorouracil-leucovorin as first-line treatment of metastatic colorectal cancer. J Clin Oncol 2000; 18(1):136–147.

218. Goldberg RM, Morton RF, Sargent DJ, et al. N9741: oxaliplatin (oxal) or CPT–11 + 5–fluorouracil (5FU)/leucovorin (LV) or oxal + CPT–11 in advanced colorectal cancer (CRC). Initial toxicity and response data from a GI intergroup study. Proc Am Soc Clin Oncol 2002; 21:128a.

219. Tournigand C, Andre T, Achille E, et al. FOLFIRI followed by FOLFOX6 or the reverse sequence in advanced colorectal cancer: a randomized GERCOR study. J Clin Oncol 2004; 22(2):229–237.

220. Tournigand C, Louvet C, Quinaux E, et al. FOLFIRI followed by FOLFOX versus FOLFOX followed by FOLFIRI in metastatic colorectal cancer (MCRC): final results of a phase III study. Proc Am Soc Clin Oncol 2001; 20:124a.

221. Borner MM, Dietrich D, Stupp R, et al. Phase II study of capecitabine and oxaliplatin in first- and second-line treatment of advanced or metastatic colorectal cancer. J Clin Oncol 2002; 20(7):1759–1766.

222. Shields AF, Zalupski MM, Marshall JL, Meropol NJ. A phase II trial of oxaliplatin and capecitabine in patients with advanced colorectal cancer. Proc Am Soc Clin Oncol 2002; 21:143a.

223. Scheithauer W, Kornek GV, Raderer M, et al. Intermittent weekly high-dose capecitabine in combination with oxaliplatin: a phase I/II study in first-line treatment of patients with advanced colorectal cancer. Ann Oncol 2002; 13(10):1583–1589.

224. Brown LF, Berse B, Jackman RW, et al. Expression of vascular permeability factor (vascular endothelial growth factor) and its receptors in adenocarcinomas of the gastrointestinal tract. Cancer Res 1993; 53(19):4727–4735.

225. Cascinu S, Staccioli MP, Gasparini G, et al. Expression of vascular endothelial growth factor can predict event-free survival in stage II colon cancer. Clin Cancer Res 2000; 6(7):2803–2807.

226. Kumar H, Heer K, Lee PW, et al. Preoperative serum vascular endothelial growth factor can predict stage in colorectal cancer. Clin Cancer Res 1998; 4(5):1279–1285.

227. Kim KJ, Li B, Houck K, Winer J, Ferrara N. The vascular endothelial growth factor proteins: identification of biologically relevant regions by neutralizing monoclonal antibodies. Growth Factors 1992; 7(1):53–64.

228. Kim KJ, Li B, Winer J, et al. Inhibition of vascular endothelial growth factor-induced angiogenesis suppresses tumour growth in vivo. Nature 1993; 362(6423):841–844.

229. Sledge G, Miller K, Novotny WF, Gaudreault J, Ash M, Colbleigh M. A phase II trial of single-agent rhuMAb VEGF (recombinant humanized monoclonal antibody to vascular endothelial cell growth factor) in patients with relapsed metastatic breast cancer. Proc Am Soc Clin Oncol 2000; 19:3a.

230. Kabbinavar F, Hurwitz HI, Fehrenbacher L, et al. Phase II, randomized trial comparing bevacizumab plus fluorouracil (FU)/leucovorin (LV) with FU/LV alone in patients with metastatic colorectal cancer. J Clin Oncol 2003; 21(1):60–65.

231. Hurwitz H, Fehrenbacher L, Novotny W, et al. Bevacizumab plus irinotecan, fluorouracil, and leucovorin for metastatic colorectal cancer. N Engl J Med 2004; 350(23):2335–2342.

232. Saltz LB, Meropol NJ, Loehrer PJ, Waksal H, Needle MN, Mayer RJ. Single agent IMC-C225 (Erbitux) has activity in CPT-11-refractory colorectal cancer (CRC) that expresses the epidermal growth factor receptor (EGFR). Proc Am Soc Clin Oncol. 2002; 21:127a.

233. Saltz LB, Meropol NJ, Loehrer PJ Sr., Needle MN, Kopit J, Mayer RJ. Phase II trial of cetuximab in patients with refractory colorectal cancer that expresses the epidermal growth factor receptor. J Clin Oncol 2004; 22(7):1201–1208.

234. Cunningham D, Humblet Y, Siena S, et al. Cetuximab monotherapy and cetuximab plus irinotecan in irinotecan-refractory metastatic colorectal cancer. N Engl J Med 2004; 351(4):337–345.

235. Saltz LB, Rubin M, Hochster H. Cetuximab (IMC-C225) plus irinotecan (CPT-11) is active in CPT-11 refractory colorectal cancer (CRC) that expresses epidermal growth factor receptor (EGFR). Proc Am Soc Clin Oncol 2001; 20(3a).

236. Rosenberg AH, Loehrer PJ, Needle MN, et al. Erbitux (IMC-C225) plus weekly irinotecan (CPT-11), fluorouracil (5FU) and leucovorin (LV) in colorectal cancer (CRC) that expresses the epidermal growth factor receptor (EGFr). Proc Am Soc Clin Oncol 2002; 21:135a.

237. Berman JM, Cheung RJ, Weinberg DS. Surveillance after colorectal cancer resection. Lancet 2000; 355(9201):395–399.

238. Renehan AG, Egger M, Saunders MP, O'Dwyer ST. Impact on survival of intensive follow up after curative resection for colorectal cancer: systematic review and meta-analysis of randomised trials. BMJ 2002; 324(7341):813.

239. Bruinvels DJ, Stiggelbout AM, Kievit J, van Houwelingen HC, Habbema JD, van de Velde CJ. Follow-up of patients with colorectal cancer. A meta-analysis. Ann Surg 1994; 219(2):174–182.

240. Virgo KS, Vernava AM, Longo WE, McKirgan LW, Johnson FE. Cost of patient follow-up after potentially curative colorectal cancer treatment. JAMA 1995; 273(23):1837–1841.

241. Pantel K, Cote RJ, Fodstad O. Detection and clinical importance of micrometastatic disease. J Natl Cancer Inst 1999; 91(13):1113–1124.

242. Kjeldsen BJ, Kronborg O, Fenger C, Jorgensen OD. A prospective randomized study of follow-up after radical surgery for colorectal cancer. Br J Surg 1997; 84(5):666–669.

243. Ohlsson B, Breland U, Ekberg H, Graffner H, Tranberg KG. Follow-up after curative surgery for colorectal carcinoma. Randomized comparison with no follow-up. Dis Colon Rectum 1995; 38(6): 619–626.

244. Green RJ, Metlay JP, Propert K, et al. Surveillance for second primary colorectal cancer after adjuvant chemotherapy: an analysis of Intergroup 0089. Ann Intern Med 2002; 136(4):261–269.

245. Northover J. Carcinoembryonic antigen and recurrent colorectal cancer. Gut 1986; 27(2):117–122.

246. Martin EW Jr., Minton JP, Carey LC. CEA-directed second-look surgery in the asymptomatic patient after primary resection of colorectal carcinoma. Ann Surg 1985; 202(3):310–317.

247. Schoemaker D, Black R, Giles L, Toouli J. Yearly colonoscopy, liver CT, and chest radiography do not influence 5-year survival of colorectal cancer patients. Gastroenterology 1998; 114(1):7–14.

248. Sugarbaker PH, Gianola FJ, Dwyer A, Neuman NR. A simplified plan for follow-up of patients with colon and rectal cancer supported by prospective studies of laboratory and radiologic test results. Surgery 1987; 102(1):79–87.

249. Moertel CG, Fleming TR, Macdonald JS, Haller DG, Laurie JA, Tangen C. An evaluation of the carcinoembryonic antigen (CEA) test for monitoring patients with resected colon cancer. JAMA 1993; 270(8):943–947.

24 | Other Benign and Malignant Colonic Tumors

David E. Milkes and Roy M. Soetikno
Department of Veterans Affairs, Palo Alto Health Care System, Stanford University School of Medicine, Stanford, California, U.S.A.

LIPOMA
Epidemiology

Lipomas are the most common, benign, nonepithelial tumors found in the colon. Although the most frequent site of gastrointestinal (GI) lipomas is the colon, the reported rates of colonic lipomas in autopsy and surgical series are low, ranging from 0.035% to 4% (1–4). There have been no malignant changes ever reported; therefore, colonic lipomas are considered to have no malignant potential (5–7). Of note, liposarcomas have been reported only in the small bowel (8–10).

The etiology of colonic lipomas is unknown. Lipomas have been associated with two rare syndromes, familial multiple lipomatosis and Weber-Christian disease (5,11,12). Although most series have reported an increased frequency of lipomas in the right colon as compared to the left, some older series may have included lipomatosis of the ileocecal valve as lipomas rather than true lipomas (5). Multiple lipomas may present in 10% to 24% of the cases (5,13–16). Most series also report that lipomas are 1.5 to 2 times more common in women than men (15–18). Colonic lipomas have been found in patients from the age of 10 months to 87 years with the mean age being 65 years (13,17,18). Lipomas can be very large: the largest reported colonic lipoma measured 16 cm (19).

Presentation

In general, colonic lipomas are asymptomatic and found incidentally (5). The size of the lesion appears to correlate with symptoms: lipomas larger than 2 cm are likely to produce symptoms (1,13,20), and 75% of lipomas larger than 4 cm produce symptoms (12,20). When signs and symptoms are present, they are usually vague and nonspecific. The most common symptoms are abdominal pain, GI bleeding, and change in bowel habits (17). Pain may be secondary to intermittent intussusceptions from prolapse of the mass or obstruction (21). Other symptoms and signs include weight loss, anemia, or palpable mass (caused by impacted stool proximal to the lipomas, intussusceptions, or the lipoma itself) (7,16,17,22). Rare presentations include massive GI bleeding, bowel perforation, extrusion through the anus, and self-amputation with recovery of the lipoma after spontaneous passage out of the rectum (22–26).

Diagnosis
Radiology

Characteristic findings on barium enema are of a smooth, ovoid, well-demarcated lesion (27). Lipomas may appear radiolucent due to the radiolucency of fat (7,28). Water enemas have been described as being useful in demonstrating this radiolucent characteristic by accentuating the difference in density between the fatty mass and surrounding tissue (29). The "squeeze" sign in which the shape of the mass on barium enema changes with external compression or peristalsis, is considered by some to be pathognomonic of lipomas (30). In atypical cases, the findings on barium may appear as an apple-core lesion, thereby mimicking malignant lesions (28,31).

Large colonic lipomas can be well demonstrated by computed tomography (CT) because of their characteristic fatty densitometric values (27,32,33). Magnetic resonance imaging (MRI) has also been shown to be useful in demonstrating large lipomas, chiefly on T1-weighted and fat-suppressing images (27). Radiographic images, however, may be misleading. A colonic lipoma at the leading edge of an intussusception may appear as soft tissue density on CT

(A)   (B)

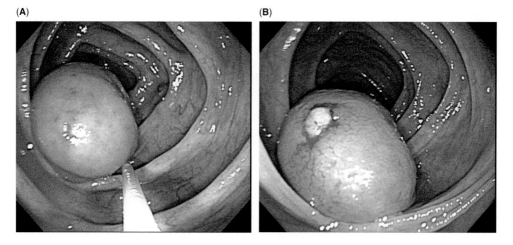

Figure 1 (*See color insert*) (**A**) Large submucosal lesion of the colon. (**B**) The naked fat sign. Diagnosis of lipoma is conclusive when fat extrudes from the biopsy-on-biopsy site of a submucosal colonic lesion.

rather than as a fat density due to infarction, edema, and fibrosis of the lipoma (34). Such findings have been attributed to adenocarcinoma, lymphoma, or metastatic tumors (34).

Endoscopy

The typical endoscopic appearance of a subepithelial lipoma is a smooth, yellowish hemispherical sessile polyp, although lipomas may also be pedunculated (35,36). The top of the polyp may appear reddish with a gradual change to yellow at the base, or there may be a speckling of red dots on the yellow surface (20,37). Probing a lipoma with a closed biopsy forceps demonstrates a soft, pliable lesion that is easily indented. Upon withdrawal of the forceps, the indented area quickly springs back to resume its original shape, much like a foam pillow. Therefore, the terms "pillow" or "cushion" signs have been widely used (20,26,36,38). In addition, the overlying mucosa can be grasped and pulled away from the submucosa to produce a tent-like appearance, the so-called "tenting sign" (20,36,38). Biopsy of the overlying mucosa only shows normal colonic mucosa and does not yield a histologic diagnosis of lipoma. But, repeated biopsy at the same site on the lesion can allow the underlying fat to protrude out, the so-called "naked fat sign," which is considered to be pathognomonic of a lipoma (Fig. 1) (36,37). Endoscopic ultrasonography (EUS) and chromoendoscopy have been utilized to assist in the assessment of lipomas (38). EUS findings typically demonstrate a hyperechoic lesion originating in the third or submucosal layer of the colonic wall, and as expected, chromoendoscopic findings typically demonstrate normal mucosal pit patterns (39).

The diagnosis of lipomas, however, can sometimes be challenging. In particular, lipomas that are ulcerated, necrotic, or firm may mimic malignant polyps (1,31); others may be mistaken for adenomatous polyps (13,36,40). The ileocecal valve can appear to have a soft, diffuse swelling referred to as a "fatty valve" (20). However, a "fatty" ileocecal valve does not necessarily represent a lipoma. Distinguishing a lipoma at the ileocecal valve from lipomatosis, a submucosal infiltration of adipose tissue without a distinct capsule, can be difficult (8,14).

Pathology

The typical histology of lipomas reveals a mass of mature adipose tissue surrounded by a fibrous capsule (8,16). Varying numbers of fibrous septa may penetrate the mass of adipose tissue (16). Within the colonic wall, 90% of lipomas are submucosal, 10% are subserosal, and very rare cases originate in the muscularis propria layer (1,41,42).

Necrosis, cystic degeneration, ulceration, and calcification are features that can be found on the pathologic specimen (12,22,25). Pseudomalignant features including nuclear atypia and atypical mitoses have been described in ulcerated lipomas, but these changes have been attributed to reactive changes of inflammation (8). True malignant degeneration to liposarcoma has not been reported in colon lipomas (7,8). Rare mixed lesions such as an adenolipoma with both adenomatous and lipomatous features, as well as a lipoma with overlying hyperplastic mucosa have been described (43,44).

Analysis of pathology specimens of resected lipomas has demonstrated that some pedunculated lipomas do not have a true stalk, but rather have a pseudopedicle: invaginated bowel wall with the serosa pulled inside to form the core of the stalk (20). It has been hypothesized that pseudopedicles are formed by repeated peristalsis activity with progressive extrusion of the submucosal mass into the bowel lumen (21,36). The resulting pseudopedicle is covered with normal overlying mucosa but has muscularis propria and serosa internally.

Management

Because colonic lipomas are benign lesions and largely asymptomatic, resection is indicated if clinical complications are present or the diagnosis of lipoma cannot be made with reasonable certainty such that a histologic diagnosis is necessary to rule out a potentially malignant lesion (6,20,36,45,46). In particular, small asymptomatic lipomas measuring less than 2 cm are unlikely to require treatment (6,36) because their growth rate is likely slow, and the risks of complications such as obstruction and bleeding are believed to be low (47,48).

The first endoscopic removal of a colonic lipoma was reported in 1973, and subsequently, numerous reports of the successful endoscopic removal of colonic lipomas have been reported (47,49–51). While pedunculated lipomas as large as 6×11 cm in size have been safely removed during endoscopy (52), endoscopic resection of lipomas may carry significant risk (6,36). In fact, the reported rate of perforation during snare polypectomy of lipomas is as high as 43% (36).

Large pedunculated lipomas may have "stalks" that are actually pseudopedicles. These "stalks" present a great danger for polypectomy because they consist of invaginated serosa (20). Reportedly, colonoscopic resection of colonic lipomas larger than 2.5 cm is associated with an increased risk of perforation (36). Piecemeal snare cautery resection of lipomas, which may improve the safety of polypectomy of large lesions, is not advocated because fatty tissue conducts electricity poorly, and snare entrapment therefore becomes a potential risk (6,40). Thus, proposed criteria for endoscopic resection in one study have included a pedunculated or sessile lesion with a base below 2 cm—determined to be mobile upon probing with a closed biopsy forceps (46). Immobile lesions were interpreted as involving deeper layers, such as the muscularis propria, whereby resection could increase the risk of perforation (46). The use of preoperative EUS to assess for pseudopedicles and depth of involvement has been proposed to improve the safety of endoscopic resection (40,46).

Lipomas that cannot be removed safely at endoscopy (and require removal for symptoms or complications) should be surgically resected. Surgery is also indicated when colonic lipomas present with acute intussusception or bowel obstruction (6,12). Although the endoscopic correction of an intussusception with subsequent endoscopic polypectomy of a large lipoma of the colon has been reported as feasible, surgery is still considered the primary modality for treating intussusception and bowel obstruction (44). The surgical options to resect lipomas include hemicolectomy, segmental resection, colotomy with enucleation, and local excision (1,17,20). Although laparoscopic colotomy has been reported (53), laparoscopic segmental resection is the preferred treatment. The technique is identical to the technique used for sequential resection of endoscopically irretrievable polyps or carcinomas. Successful laparoscopic colotomy and excision has been reported (54). Lipomas located at the subserosal surface may be removed with simple excision of the tumor without opening the bowel lumen (16). In addition, laparoscopic-guided colonoscopic snare incision may be possible.

Outcome

Clinical outcomes from lipomas are excellent. The majority is asymptomatic and found incidentally. The less common lipomas with associated morbidity, such as obstruction, pain, or bleeding may be readily treated with proper resection of the lesion. Once removed, colonic lipomas typically do not recur (47). Reports of mortality from colonic lipomas are lacking even in the rare dramatic cases with intussusception, obstruction, massive bleeding, or perforation (22).

Table 1 Dawson's Criteria for the Diagnosis of Primary Gastrointestinal Lymphoma

No palpable superficial lymphadenopathy
No obvious mediastinal lymph node enlargement on radiographic imaging
No abnormalities of the total white blood cell count or differential
At laparotomy, the bowel lesion predominates, and only regional draining lymph nodes are
   affected by disease
No involvement of the liver or spleen

COLORECTAL LYMPHOMA
Introduction

Summarizing the literature regarding colorectal lymphoma based on data from institutional case series and case reports is challenging. The difficulty can be appreciated by highlighting the following factors: primary and secondary colorectal lymphomas are not always distinguished; different nomenclatures and staging criteria are frequently used; pediatric and adult cases are combined; and practically all series are retrospective (53). Despite these difficulties, important information regarding colorectal lymphoma has been obtained.

An important initial distinction is to differentiate between primary and secondary colorectal lymphoma, because prognosis and treatment options differ (53). Primary lymphoma originates in the colon or rectum, whereas secondary lymphoma represents metastasis to the GI tract. Primary lymphoma, if detected early enough, is potentially curable, whereas secondary lymphoma is, by definition, a later stage occurrence and, typically, has a poor prognosis.

Dawson's criteria are widely used to define primary colorectal lymphoma (Table 1) (55). Furthermore, presenting symptoms should be attributable to colonic involvement, supporting that the colon and/or rectum is the primary organ affected (56). Additional criteria for primary colorectal lymphoma that have been proposed include a normal bone marrow biopsy and absence of lymphadenopathy on CT scan (53,57).

This section will focus mainly on primary colorectal lymphoma. Information regarding secondary colorectal lymphoma is summarized at the end of this section.

Epidemiology of Primary Colorectal Lymphoma

The GI tract is the most common site of extranodal lymphoma, representing about 50% of extranodal lymphoma cases (58–62). The majority of cases occur in the stomach and small bowel; the colon is the least commonly affected intestinal organ (3,62,63). Primary lymphoma originating in the colorectal segment is rare, representing only 0.16% to 2% of all malignancies in the colorectum (53,56,64,65).

The majority of studies have shown an increased incidence in males compared to females with a ratio of about 2:1 (53,64,66). Some studies suggest that the incidence of GI lymphoma is increasing, but this hypothesis is controversial (57,59). An increasing number of cases has been noted in patients with acquired immune deficiency syndrome (67,68). The age-range of affected patients is between 3 and 89 years, with the most commonly affected age group being 50 to 70 years (53,56,64,66). Ninety percent of the cases present with discrete lesions, whereas multiple or diffuse lesions may be found in up to 10% of the cases (53,66). Synchronous and metachronous colonic adenocarcinoma has been reported (53,62). Within the colon, the cecum is the usual site of involvement (60%), and then the rectum (20%) followed in decreasing order by the ascending, descending, sigmoid, and transverse colon (53,66). The abundant lymphoid tissue in the ileocecal region has been hypothesized to explain the greater frequency of occurrence there (56,64,66).

Studies from both Asia and India have reported a younger mean age of onset (69,70) and a higher proportion of T-cell lymphomas compared to Western populations (67,70,71). These observations suggest that environmental and/or ethnic differences may play a role (67).

Presentation

Vague symptoms may contribute to a delayed diagnosis of up to a year because both patient and physician may ignore nonspecific symptoms (57). Abdominal pain and weight loss are the most common presenting symptoms, followed by GI bleeding, and change in bowel habits

(53,56,62,64,66). Less common symptoms include indigestion, fever, abdominal fullness, vomiting, anorexia, and weakness (62,66,67,72). Rare presentations include appendicitis, acute bowel obstruction, intussusception, toxic megacolon, and bowel perforation (62,66,73,74). A palpable mass is the most common physical finding (56). Lymphoma is the second most common cause of acute lower GI tract bleeding in patients infected with HIV (75).

Presenting symptoms, such as bloody diarrhea, fever, and abdominal pain can be mistaken for either ulcerative colitis or Crohn's disease (76,77). Colonoscopy findings may be consistent with inflammatory bowel disease (IBD) contributing to a delay in diagnosis of up to eight years (78,79). Often, it is not until the development of peripheral lymphadenopathy that the diagnosis of colonic lymphoma is made (76).

Diagnosis

In majority of the cases, the diagnosis of colorectal lymphoma is made at laparotomy (53,56,66,80). However, radiographic findings may be suggestive of malignancy, and colonoscopy with biopsy is the most frequent modality used to make a preoperative diagnosis (57).

Radiology

Findings on barium enema in patients with colorectal lymphoma include intraluminal mass, mucosal nodularity, and annular stricture (53,56,81). In rare cases, barium enema may demonstrate numerous aphthous ulcers mimicking IBD or infectious colitis (71,81,82). CT scan imaging may show nonspecific colonic wall thickening (66). Abnormal radiographic findings usually prompt further investigation with colonoscopy.

Endoscopy

On colonoscopy, colorectal lymphomas exhibit a wide variation in gross morphological forms ranging from small superficial erosions to large masses (Fig. 2) (67,72,83). Colonoscopy with biopsy may be diagnostic in up to 83% of the cases (56,66). Failed diagnoses may occur because the biopsy is too superficial (66).

There is no known association between the endoscopic morphologic findings and the histopathology of the lymphoma (72). Even cases presenting with numerous polypoid lesions consistent with malignant lymphomatous polyposis may ultimately be diagnosed as mucosa-associated lymphoid tissue (MALT) lymphoma (84–88). The endoscopic findings of colorectal lymphomas may appear similar to those of IBD (76,78,79,82,89). Skip lesions, scattered superficial ulcers, or cobblestoning may be misinterpreted as Crohn's disease (78,79,82). In addition, lymphoma may be seen coexistent with Crohn's disease.

Although no universally accepted endoscopic classification of colorectal lymphoma is available, a recent classification scheme was proposed to facilitate communication among endoscopists (72). Accordingly, colorectal lymphomas are classified into five distinct morphologies: fungating, ulcerative, infiltrative, ulcerofungating, and ulceroinfiltrative (72).

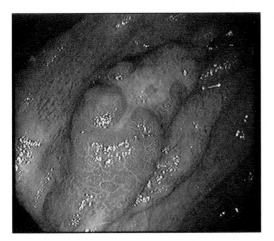

Figure 2 (*See color insert*) An example of primary colorectal lymphoma that presented as an ulcerated submucosal lesion.

In addition, multiple lymphomatous polyposes are reported as a polyposis type (72). EUS has been used in cases of colorectal lymphoma, but its role has not been clearly defined (90).

Pathology

Primary GI lymphoma is almost always non-Hodgkin's lymphoma. Hodgkin's lymphoma represents less than 4% of the cases of primary colorectal lymphoma (63,64). In fact, applying the strictest criteria for diagnosis of primary Hodgkin's lymphoma of the colon, its occurrence may be limited to five case reports (73,79). Overall, B-cell lymphomas are found more commonly than T-cell lymphomas (66). In several series, the most frequent type of colorectal lymphoma is diffuse large B-cell lymphoma (53,56,70).

Histologic Classifications

The nomenclature and terminology of colorectal lymphoma is confusing because a variety of different classifications have been used. Historically, classifications were based primarily on microscopic findings, whereas current classifications incorporate immunohistochemistry, flow cytometry, and cytogenetics. Early classifications include those developed by Rappaport, Kiel, and Lukes-Collins (91,92).

In 1982, the National Cancer Institute sponsored a meeting to unify the existing classification schemes into a single scheme. The resulting International Working Formulation allowed all the previous histologic terms to be compared using a single formulation. As immunohistologic staining became more advanced, the ability to identify and differentiate lymphocyte cell types improved and new guidelines were needed.

In 1994, the International Lymphoma Study Group established the Revised European-American Lymphoma (REAL) classification of lymphoid neoplasms (93,94). The REAL classification is the first to identify MALT lymphoma and peripheral T-cell lymphoma as separate clinicopathological entities (71). The REAL classification recognizes over 25 distinct types of non-Hodgkin's lymphoma based upon microscopic morphology, immunophenotype, genetic features, and clinical features (93). With the exception of primary cutaneous T-cell lymphoma, any one of the lymphomas described in the REAL classification may theoretically occur in the GI tract (95). The REAL classification also provides the synonymous terms for each type of lymphoma defined in previous classification schemes (93). Even more recently, a World Health Organization (WHO) classification of lymphomas has been developed (93). A basic histologic categorization of primary non-Hodgkin's lymphoma involving the colorectal region is shown in Table 2 (58).

Staging

Various staging systems have been used for primary colorectal lymphoma. The original system was the Ann Arbor staging classification; however this system did not differentiate locally draining intra-abdominal lymph nodes from distant, noncontiguous intra-abdominal lymph nodes. The Ann Arbor classification as modified by Musshoff and Schmidt-Vollmer allows for more accurate staging by differentiating intra-abdominal lymph nodes into three categories: regional, noncontiguous regional, and distant (Table 3) (57,96). The modified Ann Arbor classification also correlates better with prognosis (57). At presentation, 66% of the patients have an advanced stage of disease with regional spread (56,62).

Pathogenesis and Risk Factors

Conditions that result in chronic antigenic stimulation may predispose to the development of colorectal lymphoma. The basic pathogenesis model is that an antigenic stimulus causes

Table 2 Primary Colorectal Non-Hodgkin's Lymphoma

B-cell
Low or high grade lymphoma corresponding to lymph node equivalents
Mucosa-associated lymphoid tissue type
Low grade
High grade with or without low grade component
Mantle cell (malignant lymphomatous polyposis)
Burkitt's and Burkitt-like
T-cell

Source: Adapted from Ref. 58.

Table 3 Staging System for Primary Colorectal Lymphoma

Stage	Extranodal pattern
EI	Localized involvement of one or more colorectal sites without lymph node involvement, confined to the mucosa and submucosa (EI_1), or beyond the submucosa (EI_2)
EII	Localized involvement of one or more colorectal sites with lymph node infiltration and any depth of lymphoma infiltration into the gut wall, with regional lymph node (EII_1) or second contiguous extra lymphatic site (EII_{1E})
EII_2	Localized involvement of one or more colorectal sites with lymph node infiltration and any depth of lymphoma infiltration into the gut wall, extending beyond regional lymph nodes on the same side of the diaphragm (EII_2), including a second localized extra lymphatic site (EII_{2E})
EIII	Localized colorectal involvement and lymph node regions on both sides of the diaphragm, which may also be accompanied by a second localized involvement of an extra lymphatic site ($EIII_E$) or by involvement of the spleen (III_S), or both (III_{SE})
EIV	Localized colorectal bulk of lymphoma with or without infiltration of associated lymph nodes and diffuse or disseminated involvement of one or more non-GI tract organs or tissues
Modifiers	
A	Without general symptoms
B	With general symptoms according to the Ann Arbor definition
E	Extraintestinal involvement

Source: Adapted from Refs. 56, 60, 96.

proliferation of lymphocytes, eventually leading to a malignant transformation with clonal expansion (87,97). This hypothesis is analogous to that proposed for the development of T-cell lymphoma in celiac sprue and gastric MALT lymphoma associated with *Helicobacter pylori* infection (73,87). The antigenic stimuli involved in the development of colorectal lymphoma may be from an autoimmune disease, chronic infection, or chronic inflammation (73,98).

A different model hypothesizes that in an immunocompromised state, malignant transformation of lymphocytes results from viruses such as the Epstein-Barr virus (56,73). The commonly cited inflammatory and immunocompromised conditions associated with colorectal lymphoma include IBD, organ transplantation, HIV, and immunosuppressant drugs such as 6-mercaptopurine and azathioprine (57,73,99). Rarely cited associated conditions include celiac disease, *H. pylori*, chronic diverticulitis, and alpha-chain disease (73,97,98,100). Numerous reports of patients with either ulcerative colitis or Crohn's disease developing lymphoma in diseased segments of bowel initially suggested that IBD might be a risk factor for lymphoma (64,74,101–105). However, the association between IBD and lymphoma is controversial (106–110). Several studies from tertiary medical centers have reported an increased risk of lymphoma in patients with IBD, but large population-based studies have shown no associated risk (106,107,111). Other studies have concluded that it is the use of 6-mercaptopurine or azathioprine rather than IBD itself that increases the risk of lymphoma (106–108). However, cases of lymphoma associated with ulcerative colitis have also developed in the absence of immunomodulator therapy (101). Other factors in IBD patients that may predispose them to colorectal lymphoma include altered lymphoid populations and chronic inflammation (73,109,110). The average duration of colitis prior to the detection of lymphoma is 12 years (53,104). When lymphoma is found in a colitic colon, it may be rather large. The reason for the advanced stage may be that vague symptoms from the lymphoma were erroneously attributed to the IBD. The diagnosis is made only at the time of surgery or subsequently by the pathologist.

Organ transplantation, particularly renal and cardiac transplantation, has been associated with increased risk for colorectal lymphoma perhaps due to immunosuppression with cyclosporin (112–114). The dose, duration, and number of immunosuppressant drugs appear to be important factors in the development of lymphoma in transplant patients (115).

Management

Prospective, randomized trials to guide therapy of colorectal lymphomas are lacking. Most studies on treatment have combined patients with any type of primary GI lymphoma with various stages and types of lymphoma, and employing nonuniform surgical approaches (80).

Treatment options include surgery, chemotherapy, radiation therapy, various combinations of the above three, as well as conservative management with no specific therapy (72). The value of single or combined therapy is difficult, if not impossible, to be systematically assessed (53,80). Therefore, a multidisciplinary approach involving surgeons, gastroenterologists, and oncologists is typically warranted in the management of colorectal lymphoma.

Traditionally, surgical excision, when technically feasible, has been the mainstay of treatment (53). Some have suggested that surgery should be the primary treatment modality for colorectal lymphoma (62,66,109). The purported advantages of surgery are that it provides adequate tissue for accurate histopathologic analysis, staging, and prognosis (56,66,74). Surgery has been argued to offer a chance of cure and increased survival for early disease (56,66,74,80). Earlier reports suggested that surgical resection prevents complications such as perforation that may occur spontaneously or with chemotherapy (56,66,74). But with modern treatments, the incidence of perforation with chemotherapy appears rare (63,74,80). Surgery is usually warranted in patients with obstruction or intussusception (72). Obstructed patients with distal colonic lymphomas who are judged to be poor surgical candidates have been successfully palliated with colonic stenting (116). Right hemicolectomy is the most commonly performed surgery because the majority of colorectal lymphomas occur in the cecum (56,57). Resection usually includes regional lymph node dissection and can be achieved with primary anastomosis (57,62).

The current preferred for a right hemicolectomy for lymphoma would undoubtedly be a laparoscopic-assisted resection. The only reason not to perform a laparoscopic-assisted resection might be due to local tumor invasion into adjacent structures or to a very large tumor mass, necessitating a large incision for specimen extraction. In the absence of these few isolated circumstances, a three-or-four-port laparoscopic-assisted resection with either intracorporeal or extracorporeal vascular ligation, either intracorporeal or extracorporeal bowel division, and extracorporeal anastomosis is preferred. The technique is identical to that undertaken for other neoplasms of the right colon. Laparoscopic resection of rectal lymphoma might be technically challenging due to the large and often locally aggressive nature of the lesion, preventing optimal visualization during pelvic dissection. However, even in this instance, laparoscopic mobilization of the splenic flexure within intracorporeal vascular ligation might permit the abdominoperineal resection to be performed through a Pfannenstiel or small lower midline incision, rather than a standard midline incision.

Institutional experiences have led to recommendations for adjuvant chemotherapy to prevent disease relapse and improve survival (56,79,80,117). The most frequently used chemotherapy regiments are CHOP (cyclophosphamide, vincristine, doxorubicin, prednisone), MOPP (mechlorethamine, vincristine, procarbazine, and prednisone) and ABVD (doxorubicin, bleomycin, vinblastine, dacarbazine) (62,66,73). Trials of neoadjuvant chemotherapy are lacking (57). Adjuvant radiation therapy has been used for residual tumor after incomplete resection and in cases of advanced disease and high-grade lymphomas (56,57,61,62). Radiation therapy has been strongly advocated by some based on their institutional experience (62).

Treatment options for a few clinical settings of colorectal lymphoma deserve mention. The approach to organ transplant recipients with colorectal lymphoma includes stopping or reducing immunosuppression therapy, followed by surgical resection, and adjuvant chemotherapy (59,115). In some cases, a conservative approach with withdrawal of immunosuppression therapy may suffice (73). Several observations of colorectal MALT lymphoma regression after administration of antibiotic regiments used to eradicate *H. pylori* are provocative (88,98,118,119). Regression of colorectal MALT lymphoma with antibiotic therapy has also been reported in *H. pylori*–negative patients, suggesting that other causative organisms may play a role in colorectal MALT lymphomas (98,118,120). The finding of colorectal MALT should prompt screening for involvement of other GI sites with endoscopy and radiographic imaging because synchronous upper GI tract lesions have been reported (60,121). HIV testing of patients with primary colorectal lymphoma has been suggested, because there are several cases of patients in whom their diagnosis of colorectal lymphoma prompted determination of a positive HIV status (57).

Local relapse may occur as long as eight years after surgical resection, but generally occurs within two years (56,57,66). Recurrent disease may develop in the abdominal cavity or in extra-abdominal organs (57,66). Empiric long-term follow-up strategies have included annual colonoscopy and abdominal CT (56,66).

Outcome

Specific adverse prognostic factors cited in the literature include advanced age, inoperable tumor, tumor size above 5 cm, transmural invasion, regional lymph node involvement, advanced staging, high-grade histology, and the presence of B-symptoms (53,56,64,66,70).

Histologic type has been reported to affect survival (62). For example, malignant lymphomatous polyposis has a poor mean survival of three years whereas patients with low-grade colorectal MALT lymphoma have survived more than six years without surgery or chemotherapy (67,85).

Differences in treatment have been observed to affect outcomes. The 10-year survival rate of those receiving curative resection has been reported as high as 50%, and curative resection has been associated with better five-year survival compared to palliative resection (53,62). Trends toward improved median survival have been reported in patients treated with surgery and adjuvant chemotherapy when compared to surgery alone (56,70,80,117).

For patients treated with both surgery and adjuvant therapy, overall five-year survival is 20% to 55% (56,57,64,66,67,70). Five-year survival rates are lower for primary colorectal lymphoma compared to gastric lymphoma, small bowel lymphoma, and colorectal adenocarcinoma (53,61,66). There are reports of 27% five-year survival for locally advanced disease compared to 5% to 15% five-year survival for disseminated disease (66).

Secondary Lymphoma

Scant information is available regarding secondary colorectal lymphoma, although this entity is more common than primary colorectal lymphoma (53,56,122). The distribution is different from primary colorectal lymphoma in that secondary involvement more commonly affects the rectum and left colon (53). Autopsy series have shown an incidence of metastatic lymphoma involving the colon and rectum between 7% and 24.5% (123–125). More cases are identified at autopsy than are identified clinically, suggesting that the majority of cases of secondary colorectal lymphoma are asymptomatic or that colonic diagnostic workups are not pursued (53,125).

Secondary colorectal lymphomas are, by definition, advanced stage lymphomas, and have a poorer prognosis compared to primary colorectal lymphomas (53,56). Patients with secondary GI lymphoma who develop GI bleeding, obstruction, or perforation usually survive less than three months (53).

LEIOMYOMAS
Introduction

Leiomyomas and leiomyosarcomas are tumors thought to be of smooth muscle origin. The term GI stromal tumor has been suggested as the preferred terminology (126,127). As will be discussed later in this section, recent immunohistochemical advances and molecular genetic discoveries suggest that true smooth muscle tumors (leiomyomas and leiomyosarcomas) may be differentiated from GI stromal tumors. Past studies could not make such a distinction, and therefore, information from prior studies likely reflects smooth muscle tumors and GI stomal tumors having been considered as a single lesion.

Epidemiology

Leiomyomas are rare colonic lesions. Only 3% of all digestive tract leiomyomas are found in the colon (128,129). Within the colon, most are found within the transverse, descending, and sigmoid portions (127,128). More leiomyomas are found in the colon than the rectum (130). In only 1% of the cases are multiple colonic sites involved (127). In extremely rare cases, diffuse lesions may affect the colon, a condition referred to as leiomyomatosis (131,132).

Peak age of incidence from one study was between 30 and 39 years (127), although another study found the median age to be 65 years (130). The youngest reported patient with leiomyoma of the colon was 21 months, and the oldest, 79 years (127). Data on whether a higher incidence is found in males or females is inconclusive (127,130). Colonic leiomyomas have been associated with tuberous sclerosis (133,134).

Leiomyomas may exhibit a variety of growth patterns. Endocolic tumors are attached to the bowel wall and completely confined to the bowel lumen, whereas exocolic tumors are confined to the extraluminal space without bulging into the bowel lumen (135). A combined type has been described with growth into both the bowel lumen and the extraluminal space, a so-called dumbbell lesion (135). Finally, concentric lesions can results from circumferential intramuscular involvement (135). Exocolic and endocolic growth patterns are the most common, occurring at rates of 47% and 32%, respectively (127). The less common intramural and dumbbell tumors occur at rates of 15% and 6%, respectively.

Presentation

Leiomyomas are usually asymptomatic and discovered incidentally (128). Common presentations include pain, a palpable mass, and GI hemorrhage (127). Less common symptoms at presentation may include nausea and vomiting, weight loss, constipation, fever, diarrhea, iron deficiency anemia, and altered bowel habits (127). Rarely, bowel obstruction, intussusception, or perforation may occur (128,129,135). Most cases of colonic leiomyomas present with symptom duration of less than one year, but cases with symptoms for greater than 10 years have been reported (127). Patients preoperatively diagnosed with appendicitis have subsequently been diagnosed with leiomyoma of the appendix (127).

Diagnosis
Radiology

Barium enema findings reflect the type of tumor growth pattern. Endocolic lesions show a well-defined mass that does not interrupt haustral pattern or mucosal markings, although ulceration or perforation of the mucosa may be present (127,135). Exocolic lesions are difficult to differentiate from extrinsic compression or normal indentation (135,136). Concentric, intramuscular lesions can appear as apple-core lesions, especially if there is irregularity of the overlying mucosa (135).

On CT scan, colonic leiomyomas can be mistaken for prostatic, gynecological, or other colorectal tumors (135). Typical CT scan imaging demonstrates well-marginated lesions with homogenous enhancement after contrast injection (135,136). Leiomyomas may appear more heterogenous in cases of associated necrosis (127,136). Leiomyomas with calcifications have been reported (135).

Radiologic criteria to differentiate benign leiomyomas from malignant leiomyosarcomas are limited. Findings that favor leiomyosarcoma include lymphadenopathy, metastatic lesions, degenerative changes, and tumor size greater than 5 cm (135,137,138). Growth pattern is not useful in distinguishing tumor type. Some studies have associated exocolic lesions with leiomyosarcoma, whereas other studies have associated endocolic lesions with leiomyosarcoma (135,127,137,138).

Endoscopy

Colonoscopy is an increasingly important tool to diagnose colonic smooth muscle tumors (127,128). Most colonic leiomyomas appear as solitary lesions (128). They are smooth, reddish lesions with normal overlying mucosa (128). Their endoscopic appearance may also be a pedunculated intraluminal polyp mimicking an adenomatous polyp (129,139). The lesions are firm when probed with a biopsy forceps (128). Superficial biopsies are rarely diagnostic because only normal overlying mucosa is sampled (128). In rare cases, a diagnosis of leiomyoma may be accomplished with deep endoscopic biopsy, but determining the malignant potential of the lesion from the biopsy specimen may not be possible (139).

It is important to distinguish benign leiomyomas from malignant leiomyosarcomas as prognosis and treatment differ. EUS can be useful in assessing leiomyoma tumor size, location within the bowel wall, and extent of the disease (140). Benign leiomyomas typically appear as homogenous, hypoechoic masses within the fourth layer of the bowel wall (141). Using EUS to make a distinction between benign and malignant stromal tumors remains difficult because experience and interobserver variability are the factors (126,129,139). Findings on EUS of tumor invasion through the bowel wall or evidence of lymph node involvement are suggestive of leiomyosarcoma (140). Other EUS findings associated with malignant stromal tumors are tumor size greater than 4 cm, irregular borders, echogenic foci, and anechoic cystic spaces (126,141,142).

Pathology

Characterization of smooth muscle tumors and stromal tumors is advancing. Earlier literature did not differentiate GI stromal tumors from smooth muscle tumors such as leiomyomas, leiomyosarcomas, and leiomyoblastomas (130). But current evidence suggests that GI stromal tumors are mesenchymal tumors and not true smooth muscle tumors (130).

As true smooth muscle tumors, leiomyomas stain positive for smooth muscle actin, desmin, or both (143), and are negative for CD117 or KIT protein (130). Leiomyomas can be distinguished from GI stromal tumors by low cellularity, eosinophilic cytoplasm, consistently positive for smooth muscle actin and desmin, and negative for CD34 and CD117 (130). The expression of CD117 is the most specific marker of GI stromal tumors to separate them from true smooth muscle tumors (130).

The usual histologic appearance of leiomyomas is a well-circumscribed, whorled bundle of smooth muscle cells arising from the muscularis that is sparsely cellular and without mitotic figures (128). Leiomyomas may arise from muscularis propria, muscularis mucosa, or vessel-related smooth muscle (139). The majority of colonic leiomyomas originate in the muscularis mucosa (130). True intramural colonic leiomyomas from the muscularis propria are considered rare (130). Leiomyomas are usually below 5 cm, but lesions above 29 cm have been reported (127,144).

Few reliable histologic criteria are available to determine malignancy, although a number of mitotic figures and nuclear abnormalities have been proposed to distinguish benign leiomyomas from malignant leiomyosarcomas (128). The presence of mitoses is the hallmark of malignancy such that tumors with five or more mitoses per 50 high power fields are generally considered malignant (127,135,140,145–147). Other microscopic criteria suggestive of malignancy include increased cell size, increased irregularity of cell size and shape, diminished and disorganized bundles of myofilament, reduction of collagen stroma, presence of short, plump cells with oval nuclei, and nuclear pleomorphism (71,127,148). Electron microscopy can be helpful in making a distinction between benign and malignant lesions (135). This is rapidly becoming better understood in the proximal GI tract, and the authors suspect they can generalize at least some of that terminology/classification.

Treatment

The natural history of leiomyomas in the colon and rectum is unknown due to the rarity of the lesion (128). Some authorities have argued that leiomyomas may be precursor lesions of malignant leiomyosarcomas, and therefore, they recommend approaching leiomyomas as potentially malignant lesions (128). In support of this argument are case reports of patients who initially present with benign leiomyomas but present later with metastatic disease (147). Surgery is the treatment of choice for most leiomyomas (139).

The endoscopic removal of leiomyomas is controversial and large submucosal lesions suspected of being leiomyomas are best removed surgically to ensure adequate excision and complete tissue diagnosis (129). Safe colonoscopic removal of pedunculated and sessile leiomyomas up to 1.5 cm has been reported (77,128,129). Endoscopic removal of large leiomyomas measuring 4 cm has resulted in colonic perforation (149). Small, benign-appearing tumors may be removed by excisional biopsy or partial resection of the colon. As for all colorectal neoplasia, enucleation is not advised. For pedunculated polyps removed by division of the stalk, it is important to make sure that surgical margins are clear of tumor (127). Although colotomy and polypectomy have been described, the preferred surgical option is a standard resection. If an anatomic segmental colectomy or anterior resection or abdominoperineal resection are performed, then lack of involvement of the proximal and distal surgical margins should be virtually assured. Contingent upon the degree of invasion of the local lesion, the radial margins could potentially be involved, especially in rectal lesions. Standard laparoscopic-assisted surgical approaches are generally acceptable.

In the case of leiomyosarcoma, treatment involves surgical resection and an assessment for peritoneal and visceral metastases (150). Leiomyosarcomas typically metastasize to the liver, lung, and peritoneum, suggesting that spread is typically hematogenous and not via the lymphatics (140,150). The liver is the most common site of metastasis, followed by lungs, peritoneum, and other parts of the GI tract, then the mesenteric lymph nodes (127). If a primary lesion is symptomatic and distant metastasis are noted, surgical resection of the primary lesion can still result in long-term survival because some leiomyosarcomas are slow growing (127). Reporting on their experience from 22 cases, Randleman et al. suggested adjusting surgical treatment of leiomyosarcomas to the size of the tumor (151). Accordingly, tumors below 2.5 cm and confined to the bowel wall are treated by wide local excision, whereas tumors above 2.5 cm are treated with more radical surgery such as abdominoperineal excision (151). Because leiomyosarcomas can recur at the surgical anastomosis, periodic surveillance colonoscopy and CT scanning have been recommended (127,152–154).

Besides surgical resection, other modalities have been used to treat leiomyosarcomas. Mixed results have been reported with radiation therapy (154,155). There is limited success with chemotherapy for metastatic leiomyosarcoma. Doxorubicin, dacarbazine, and ifosfamide have been used alone or in combination with response rates reported between 15% and 48% (127). The same results should be anticipated whether the resection is done by laparotomy, laparoscopy, or a laparoscopic-assisted approach.

Outcomes

Prognosis of leiomyomas of the colon is good. There are no reported cases of recurrence after surgical resection (127). The overall five-year survival rate for colorectal leiomyosarcoma is 20% to 50% (71,135,156,157).

CARCINOIDS

As clinical and basic science has evolved, carcinoid tumors have become better understood. The term "karzinoid," meaning "carcinoma-like," originated in 1907 and was intended to emphasize the benign nature of the lesion (158). Subsequently, the malignant potential of carcinoid tumors has been well recognized, and now carcinoids are considered malignant neoplasms (159). As with other tumors with the ability for *a*mine *p*recursor *u*ptake and *d*ecarboxylation, carcinoids are sometimes referred to as APUDomas (160,161). Advances in cell biology and cytochemistry have cast doubt on the original concept of APUDomas, and the term is currently considered inadequate (160). The favored terminology groups carcinoids with neuroendocrine tumors, with the ability to synthesize and secrete neuroamines and neuropeptides (160,162).

When considering carcinoids of the colorectal segment, there are obvious differences between rectal and colonic carcinoids in epidemiology, clinical presentation, biology, treatment, and prognosis (Table 4). These differences may relate in part to the embryological development of the gut. In 1963, a classification of carcinoid tumors based, in part, on embryological development, divided tumors into foregut, midgut, and hindgut (159). Accordingly, carcinoids in the jejunum, ileum, appendix, cecum, ascending, and transverse colon are midgut tumors, whereas carcinoids in the descending, sigmoid, and rectum are hindgut

Table 4 Differences Between Rectal Carcinoids and Colonic Carcinoids

	Rectal	**Colonic**
Mean age at diagnosis (years)	Younger	Older
Ratio M:F	M > F	M < F
% of GI carcinoids	13–30%	0.6–7%
Stage at presentation	Early	Late
Incidence of metastases	Low	High
Presentation	Usually asymptomatic	Usually symptomatic
Common treatment	Endoscopic resection	Surgical resection
5-year survival	Fair to good	Poor to fair
Factors secreted	Somatostatin, peptide YY, glicentin, neurotensin, 5-hydroxytryptophan	5-hydroxytryptamine, tachykinins, bradykinin, prostaglandins

Abbreviation: GI, gastrointerstinal.

tumors (159). Simply comparing midgut and hindgut carcinoids does not enable an informative distinction between colonic and rectal carcinoids, because colonic carcinoids are divided between midgut and hindgut lesions. Therefore, to enable a comparison, colonic carcinoids are defined as those arising in the colon, excluding the appendix and the rectum (158,159,163,164).

Epidemiology
Rectal Carcinoids
Rectal carcinoids are rare and comprise 0.7% to 1.3% of all rectal tumors (161,165). However, the rectum is the third most common location of carcinoid tumors (161). Data from over 8000 cases of carcinoid tumors compiled from the National Cancer Institute databases reveal that 74% of carcinoids occur in the GI tract with the highest incidence found in the small bowel (28.7%), appendix (19%), and rectum (13%) (159). Only one study, an institutional case series, has suggested that the rectum is the most common location of carcinoids (166). Excluding non-GI tract tumors, rectal carcinoids represent 20% to 30% of all GI carcinoids (165,167).

Slightly more men than women are affected, with the mean age at diagnosis between 48 and 59 years (159,161,166–169). Rectal carcinoids have been found in patients with a wide age-range from 20 to 85 years (161,169). Racial differences are difficult to assess, but the collective literature supports a relatively high incidence of rectal carcinoids in Japanese, South Asian, and non-Caucasian groups (165), and a three- to fourfold higher age-adjusted incidence in African-Americans (159). The incidence of rectal carcinoids in patients undergoing screening sigmoidoscopy examinations varies between 0.014% and 0.04% (164). The rate of detection of rectal carcinoids is about 1 per 1400 proctosigmoidoscopies, so physicians performing screening are likely to see a few cases in their career (159,168). Autopsy series have reported higher incidence of carcinoids compared to population-based series, suggesting that a significant number of carcinoids remain asymptomatic and undetected during life (159). The numbers of reported rectal carcinoids is increasing, probably due to the increased number of screening endoscopic examinations being performed (159,166).

The most well-described association of rectal carcinoids occurring in 4% to 32% cases, are synchronous and metachronous neoplasms (159,161,169,170). Colorectal adenocarcinomas in particular, as well as malignancies of the breast, lung, and female genitourinary tract, have been associated with rectal carcinoids (159,161,170). An association of rectal carcinoids and ulcerative colitis has been uncommonly appreciated, and no proposed pathogenic mechanism exists (165,167). Rare cases arising in rectal duplication cysts or postcolectomy rectal stumps have been described (167,169).

Colonic Carcinoids
Colonic carcinoids, excluding those arising in the appendix and rectum, are extremely rare (158). Carcinoids represent 0.3% of all cancers found in the colon (159). Colonic carcinoids comprise 0.6% to 7% of all GI carcinoids (158,159,162,170,171). The mean age at diagnosis is 64 to 68 years with a wide age range of 12 to 89 years (125,158,164). Colonic carcinoids predominate in females with the female:male ratio as high as 2:1 (158,159,163,164). The age-adjusted incidence of colonic carcinoids is up to 0.31 cases per 100,000 population per year (164). Age-adjusted incidence rates are similar in Whites and African-Americans (159). Up to 19% of colonic carcinoids are associated with another malignancy (159).

Within the colon, most carcinoids are found in the cecum (39–50%) (158,163,164). The incidence at other sites is ascending by 13% to 16%: transverse, 10% to 17%; descending, 13%; and sigmoid, 15% to 17% (125,158,164). Simultaneous adenocarcinomas of the GI tract are found in 7% to 9% of rectal carcinoids, and 3% to 10% of colonic carcinoids (166,170,172).

Presentation
Rectal Carcinoids
The majority of rectal carcinoids are asymptomatic and discovered incidentally (161,162,166,169). Larger tumor size and metastases are associated with symptomatic rectal carcinoids (166,167). The most common symptoms attributable to rectal carcinoids are rectal bleeding, constipation, change in bowel habits, and rectal pain (161,166,167). Other less common symptoms include tenesmus, pain with defecation, pruritus ani, and weight loss (161,166,167). In very rare instances, rectal carcinoids may present with perforation (161). The median duration of

symptoms is three months (167). When metastasis occurs, it is usually to the liver (167). Rectal carcinoids cause carcinoid syndrome in only extremely rare cases (173).

Colonic Carcinoids

More that 90% of patients with colonic carcinoids are symptomatic at the time of initial presentation (158,163). Symptom duration is usually less than three months (158). The most common presenting symptoms are abdominal pain, weakness/malaise, anorexia, and weight loss (125,158). Less common symptoms include diarrhea, GI bleeding, and nausea/vomiting (158,163). Rare cases may present with bowel obstruction (163). In approximately 40% of the cases, a palpable abdominal mass is noted on physical examination (163). Up to 86% of colonic carcinoids present at a late stage with either local or distant metastases (158,163,164).

A few patients with colonic carcinoids have symptoms secondary to carcinoid syndrome. Carcinoid syndrome complicates up to 10% of midgut cases and is associated with 3% of colonic carcinoids (158,162,173). Patients with carcinoid syndrome most commonly have flushing and diarrhea (160,162). Dyspnea and abdominal pain are less common symptoms (160,162). Rare manifestations of carcinoid syndrome include wheezing, proximal myopathy, dermatosis, right-sided heart lesions, and arthropathy (160,162). Carcinoid syndrome only complicates cases with liver metastases or extensive nodal metastases without liver involvement (165).

Diagnosis
Rectal Carcinoids

Most rectal carcinoids are diagnosed during screening proctosigmoidoscopy and colonoscopy. Proper recognition by physical examination characteristics and endoscopic appearance can lead to a high preoperative diagnosis in up to 73% of the cases (166). Many rectal carcinoids can be detected on digital rectal examination because the majority is found between 5 and 10 cm of the anal verge (166). They feel firm, nodular, smooth, and rubbery on digital rectal examination. During endoscopy, they typically appear yellow, submucosal, firm, and sessile. Less commonly, rectal carcinoids may appear whitish, reddish, semipedunculated, pedunculated, or depressed (166,174). Preoperative endoscopic biopsy is diagnostic in 50% to 88% of the cases (174,175). On EUS, rectal carcinoids appear as hypoechoic, homogenous, smooth-contoured lesions, sometimes with a hyperechoic central area (176). Routine testing of urine 5-hydroxyindolacetic acid (5-HIAA) is not useful in rectal carcinoids (166,177).

Colonic Carcinoids

A variety of modalities are usually used to diagnose colonic carcinoids including barium enema, CT scan, colonoscopy, laparoscopy, and even liver biopsy (158). Urinary 5-HIAA levels are elevated in a minority of the patients (163). Barium enema findings of colonic carcinoids usually show annular lesions, large ulcerating lesions, or obstruction (163).

Metastases may be detected by CT, MRI, or nuclear scintigraphy (162). On CT scan, liver metastases from carcinoids are hypervascular and best depicted on the arterial phase (178). The preferred radiopharmaceutical to identify carcinoids is Indium-labeled (111) octreotide (162). Octreotide scintigraphy has a sensitivity of 86% and specificity of 100% (162). Octreotide scintigraphy can be used to identify unsuspected metastatic lesions (162).

Overproduction of serotonin has been implicated in the pathogenesis of carcinoid syndrome (160). Serotonin is metabolized in the liver to 5-HIAA and excreted in the urine (160). Therefore, carcinoids that drain into the portal circulation can secrete large amounts of serotonin without causing the carcinoid syndrome. Carcinoid syndrome results from tumor secretion into the systemic circulation that bypasses hepatic degradation. This occurs with hepatic metastases or occasionally peritoneal or retroperitoneal metastases.

In the rare patients who present with flushing or diarrhea, measurement of 24-hour urinary 5-HIAA is the typical screening test for carcinoid syndrome with a sensitivity of 75% and specificity of over 90% (162). In cases with a high clinical suspicion and borderline urinary 5-HIAA results, pentagastrin provocation testing may be used cautiously with an awareness that hazardous flushing may be provoked (160,162). False-negative urinary 5-HIAA results may occur in patients on L-dopa or salicylates (162).

Table 5 T-Staging of Carcinoid Tumors

T1	Tumor within mucosa and submucosa
T2	Tumor invasion to the muscularis propria
T3	Tumor penetrating the full rectal wall to the subserosa
T4	Tumor spreading to perirectal tissue beyond the subserosa
N0	No lymph node involvement
N1	Lymph node involvement
M0	No distant metastases
M1	Distant metastases

Source: From Refs. 167, 173.

Staging
Rectal Carcinoids

Some studies have used a tumor/node/metastasis (TNM) system for staging rectal carcinoids (Table 5) (167). EUS has been shown to be helpful in assessing the depth of invasion of rectal carcinoids prior to resection (176). In a small case series, high-frequency ultrasound probes had a 100% accuracy at staging rectal carcinoids confined to the submucosa when compared with resected tissue specimens (176). Tumor size is correlated with depth of invasion of the bowel wall (167). In general, tumors less than 2 cm are not associated with lymph node metastasis (167).

Colonic Carcinoids

The Dukes' classification as modified by Turnbull has been used for staging colonic carcinoids (158,163,179) (Table 6). Colonic carcinoids vary from 2 to 10 cm, with an average of 5.8 cm (158). There is a poor correlation between size and depth of invasion (158). Involvement of the pericolic fat is noted in over 85% colonic carcinoids (158). Metastatic disease presents in 64% of colonic carcinoids, compared to only 3% to 5% of appendix, and 14% to 34% of rectum (158). Neuron-specific enolase and serotonin are the most common positive stains in colonic carcinoids (158).

Pathology

The typical histologic appearance of carcinoids is uniformly arranged ovoid cells with a round, moderately hyperchromatic nucleus, rare mitotic activity, and a granular cytoplasm (161,165,173). Different patterns of cell arrangements have been described such as insular (nests), trabecular (ribbon-like), glandular (rosette-like), and uniform sheets (158,161). Rare cases of composite adenocarcinomas and carcinoids, so-called adenocarcinoid tumors, have been reported in the colon and rectum and should be distinguished from carcinoids (165,180).

Carcinoid tumors have an affinity for silver salts and two silver staining reactions are available for cases with ambiguous histology (160,165). The argentaffin reaction relies on exposing cells to silver salts with the endogenous reduction of silver salts to metallic silver (160,165). The argyrophil reaction relies on the addition of a reducing agent followed by exposure to silver salts (160,165). As a general rule, midgut carcinoids exhibit both argentaffin and argyrophil reactions, but hindgut carcinoids primarily exhibit the argyrophil reaction (160,162). Seventy percent of rectal carcinoids are argyrophil reactive, but only 8% to 16% are argentaffin positive (165).

Staining for hormones as well as endocrine markers may be helpful. Stains with positive rates of at least 70% to 80% include chromogranin, neuron-specific enolase, and prostate-specific

Table 6 Modified Dukes' Staging of Turnbull

Stage A	Tumor confined to the colon and bowel wall
Stage B	Tumor extension into pericolic fat
Stage C	Tumor metastasis to regional mesenteric lymph nodes, but no evidence of distant spread
Stage D	Parietal invasion, adjacent organ invasion, or tumor metastasis to distant organs

acid phosphatase (165,169,173). Stains less likely to be positive include S-100 protein, leu 7, human islet cell antibody, serotonin, human pancreatic polypeptide, and glucagon (165,169,173).

In difficult cases, when histology and staining results are still questionable, findings on electron microscopy can aid in diagnosis (165). Electron microscopy can reveal large, uniform neurosecretory granules in the cytoplasm (161,163,165).

Determining the malignant potential of carcinoid lesions is controversial. Past studies have emphasized that certain criteria are useful in differentiating benign from malignant carcinoids, but more recent studies have concluded that all carcinoids should be considered potentially malignant lesions (159–161,166). No single criterion, other than the documented spread of tumor, can predict the behavior of carcinoids (162,166). In particular, histologic criteria, including tumor size, fail to precisely distinguish the malignant potential of carcinoids (159,162,165).

Tumor size and depth of invasion do correlate with the incidence of metastatic disease (161,165–167). For rectal carcinoids below 1 cm, the risk of metastasis is below 3%; for lesions 1 to 1.9 cm, the risk is 7% to 15%, and those above 2 cm nearly always metastasize at above 80% (161,162,165–167). Controlling for tumor size, depth of invasion also correlates strongly with metastases. For rectal tumors above 2 cm, those confined to submucosa have a 12% chance of metastasis compared to 88% chance for those invading the muscularis propria (161,165). A similar difference is found for rectal lesions below 2 cm compared by depth of invasion (161,165). There is a relationship between tumor size and the probability of metastatic disease: 1 cm or less, 3%; 1.1 cm to 1.9 cm, 11% to 25%; 2 cm or greater, 74% (161,173). Invasion through the muscularis propria is associated with metastatic disease (161). Also for colonic carcinoids, the presence of metastatic disease is correlated with size of tumor (164).

Other factors shown to be associated with an increased risk for metastases are DNA aneuploidy, above two mitoses in 10 high-powered fields, and atypical features on histology (169,177,181).

Treatment
Rectal Carcinoids
Traditionally, a therapeutic approach to rectal carcinoids based on tumor size alone was followed because mainly lesions larger than 2 cm were believed to have a high risk for malignant behavior (161), and in most cases, treatment decisions can still be based on tumor size (172). In general, rectal carcinoids below 1 cm may be removed by local resection, those between 1 and 2 cm, with transmural resection, and those above 2 cm, with extended surgical resection (172). Because the pathologist may have difficulty determining whether or not the margin is free from carcinoid, an effort should be made during endoscopic biopsy to ink-mark the area surrounding any carcinoid lesion. Because these lesions are often small and, in fact, removal is usually surmised, surgical resection is certainly facilitated by endoscopic ink-marking. However, a small portion of lesions measuring less than 2 cm exhibit malignant behavior and, therefore, additional factors should be included in making treatment decisions (161). Tumor size, depth of invasion, lymph node involvement, and distant metastatic disease will influence treatment decisions.

Determination of pretreatment serum levels of serotonin and gastrin, as well as 24-hour 5-HIAA, and following these levels posttreatment has no proven utility (173).

Size up to 1 cm
Small lesions up to 1 cm without lymph node involvement or distant metastases should be treated by complete local excision (162,167,173,174,182,183). Curative local resection may be achieved either surgically or endoscopically. Patients should be informed that even small carcinoids carry a 1% to 3% risk of malignant disease (166). Successful surgical approaches include local biopsy forceps excision with fulguration or local transanal excision (166). Transanal excision has the advantage of a complete pathology specimen for accurate assessment of muscularis propria involvement (166). Transanal excision is certainly facilitated if during endoscopic biopsy or endoscopic removal, the area was ink marked.

Various endoscopic mucosal resection (EMR) techniques have been effective for rectal carcinoids including strip biopsy, aspiration resection, band-snare resection, and endosonography probe-guided band ligation (174). Standard polypectomy and standard EMR are associated with high rates of positive margins, 56% and 20%, respectively. Therefore,

(A)   **(B)**   **(C)**

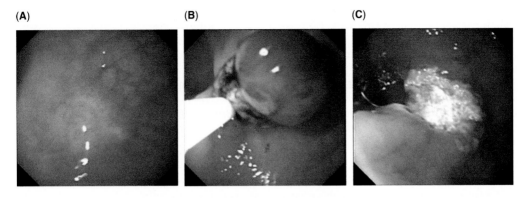

Figure 3 (*See color insert*) An example of a rectal carcinoid lesion. (**A**) The lesion was submucosal; previous biopsy of the site showed carcinoid. (**B**) Rubber band placement at the lesion base to protrude the submucosa. A snare loop has been positioned below the rubber band. (**C**) Lesion following complete resection.

specialized EMR techniques are favored. Aspiration techniques, such as EMR with a ligation device, can achieve wider and deeper resection margins, with an associated rate of negative margins of 100% for rectal carcinoids (Fig. 3) (183).

Prior to local excision, a colonoscopy is warranted to exclude synchronous lesions (162,166,174). Some investigators advocate a preoperative assessment with some combination of EUS, abdominal ultrasound, abdominal CT, and octreotide scintigraphy to confirm that lesions are confined to the submucosal without local or distant metastases (173,174). Other investigators proceed directly to endoscopic resection in suspected cases with lesions measuring up to 1 cm (182). Perforation and bleeding rates are less than 1% after either EMR or local surgical excision (107,166,174,182). As most rectal carcinoids treated by EMR are in the extra-peritoneal segment, the risk of perforation is considerably low (174,182,183). Follow-up with annual colonoscopy, EUS, chest X ray, and abdominal CT has been advocated (166).

Size Between 1 and 2 cm
In the absence of loco-regional spread or distant metastases, intermediate-size rectal carcinoids should be resected with transanal excision (161,166,172,173). Such a surgical approach provides an adequate pathologic specimen to assess depth of invasion. Long-term survival after resection of intermediate-sized tumors confined to the submucosa is excellent (161,166). However, up to 47% of intermediate-sized rectal carcinoid with atypical histology or invasion of the muscularis propria are associated with metastases at presentation or develop metastatic disease after resection (161,177). Therefore, further extensive resection may be warranted if such findings are demonstrated after transanal excision (161,172,177). But as is discussed below, further extensive surgical resection in this setting is controversial (177).

Size Greater than 2 cm or Presence of Locoregional Spread
Treatment recommendations for rectal carcinoids that involve the muscularis propria, have spread to local lymph nodes, or measure more than 2 cm are difficult to make, as the data are inconclusive. Due to conflicting results in these cases, extensive surgery with either abdominal perineal resection or low anterior resection is controversial.

Some studies have noted that no patients with T3 or T4 lesions, or positive lymph nodes, or tumor size greater than 2 cm were cured by radical surgery (167,177). The authors concluded that there is no apparent role for radical surgery if the entire tumor can be removed by local excision because more extensive surgery does not result in cure or a survival benefit (167,177). Because these studies have included only small numbers of patients, there are insufficient data to conclude that radical surgery is indicated in such settings (166). The majority of reports recommend radical surgery for tumors greater than 2 cm or those with locoregional spread in the absence of distant metastases (161,166,172,173). These reports acknowledge that although the risk of tumor recurrence or future development of metastatic disease may approach 100%, surgery still remains the only potential curative option for these patients (166). Furthermore, several cases of patients with advanced lesions, without distant metastases being cured with radical surgery, have been documented (173). Laparoscopic approaches should be perfectly acceptable in most cases. Both laparoscopic anterior resection and laparoscopic abdominoperineal resection are feasible. If a laparoscopic anterior resection is performed, it may be preferable to perform a coloanal anastomosis with a colonic J pouch than a straight low anterior anastomosis.

A reasonable approach for these tumors is to attempt sphincter-sparing low anterior resection with an understanding that the risk of recurrent disease is still high (173,177). Otherwise, if abdominal perineal resection is required, quality of life issues should be addressed with patients prior to permanent colostomy with a high risk of recurrent disease (177).

Distant Metastases

For rectal carcinoids with distant metastases, surgery should only be performed with palliative intent to control local complications such as obstruction or bleeding (172,173). Aggressive surgery in this setting does not alter the natural history of the disease or the life expectancy of the patient (172). Adjuvant chemotherapy and radiation therapy have been used, but data on significant benefit from this approach are lacking (166).

Colonic Carcinoids

Colonic carcinoids are generally treated surgically. The type of operation depends on the location of the tumor. Surgical approaches include right hemicolectomy, left hemicolectomy, and segmental resection (158). Right hemicolectomy is the most commonly performed surgery because most colonic carcinoids present in the right colon (163). Because the risk of lymph node involvement is low for lesions less than 2 cm in size, some have suggested that local resection is adequate (164). Others note that because 20% of colonic carcinoids below 2 cm have lymph node involvement, a standard resection can be performed either by laparotomy or by laparoscopy (172). Whether the resection is performed by laparoscopy, laparoscopic–assisted, or by laparotomy techniques, a "cancer type" resection should be undertaken with complete lymph node harvest. After surgical resection, vigorous surveillance for metastatic disease is recommended (164).

Radiation therapy has been used in patients with stage D colonic carcinoid (164). Chemotherapies used are usually a combination of 5-fluorouracil and streptozotocin (158), although 5-fluorouracil alone has been used (125).

Carcinoid Syndrome and Metastatic Disease

A variety of palliative medical and surgical therapies are available for patients with carcinoid syndrome and metastatic disease. Partial liver resection to remove metastatic disease may alleviate symptoms of carcinoid syndrome (160). If liver resection is not possible, hepatic artery embolization or ligation may result in long-term remission and symptom relief (160,162,184). In rare instances, liver transplantation has been used to treat metastatic carcinoid to the liver with posttransplant survival of 13 months (185).

Right heart failure, mainly related to tricuspid valve regurgitation, is the cause of death in up to one-third of the patients with carcinoid syndrome (162). Reconstructive valvular surgery has been employed to achieve long-lasting symptomatic relief (186). Tricuspid valve replacement may be appropriate in carefully selected patients with carcinoid syndrome (162).

Medical treatments for carcinoid syndrome include octreotide, interferon, and chemotherapy (162). External bean radiation therapy is reserved for cord compression and painful bone metastases (162). A positive octreotide scintigraphy study correlates with the presence of tumor cell somatostatin receptors, and is therefore, predictive of a clinical response to prolonged octreotide administration (162).

Octreotide is effective for relieving diarrhea and flushing. Over two-thirds of the patients treated with octreotide have symptom-improvement for a median duration of 12 months (187). The initial loss of therapeutic response is due to tumor cell down-regulation of somatostatin receptors, which can be restored by a drug-free period (162). But eventually, receptor-negative cells arise such that further administration of octreotide is not helpful (162). Another consequence of prolonged octreotide administration is gallstone formation, which occurs in about 20% of the patients (188).

Octreotide has a limited antiproliferative effect that causes the primary and metastatic carcinoid lesions to temporarily diminish in size (162). This antiproliferative effect may account for the improved survival in patients receiving octreotide compared to chemotherapy (162,187).

An initial dose of 100 µg of subcutaneous octreotide given three times per day may be used, but most patients eventually require escalating doses up to a maximum daily dose of 1500 µg (162). Long-acting octreotide analogues offer more convenient dosing schedules. Lanreotide 20 mg intramuscularly every 10 days affords equivalent control of carcinoid syndrome symptoms compared to standard daily octreotide (189). And intramuscular octreotide LAR 20 mg once per month is another equally effective alternative (190).

Interferon can improve diarrhea and flushing in 66% of the patients, but has more side effects than octreotide (162). Interferon may diminish the tumor-size and retard tumor growth better than octreotide (162). The median duration of response to interferon is 34 months (191).

Other medications have limited benefit to treat carcinoid syndrome. Serotonin antagonists such as methysergide, cyproheptadine, ondansetron, and ketanserine may be used to treat diarrhea and flushing (160,162). Codeine and loperamide have been used to control diarrhea (162). Agents to control flushing include histamine receptor antagonists, kallikrein inhibitors, alpha-adrenergic blockers, beta-adrenergic blocking agents, and phenothiazine derivatives (160,162).

Chemotherapy results for treating metastatic carcinoid tumors are disappointing with median survival times less than those achieved with octreotide or interferon (192). The best response rates, between 22% and 33%, were achieved with streptozotocin-containing combinations (193). Chemotherapy alone does not improve survival and should be reserved for those cases in which other measures to control symptoms have failed (162).

Carcinoid Crisis

Carcinoid crisis is a life-threatening condition that may occur after induction of anesthesia or with tumor manipulation (162). Massive amounts of secreted hormones may produce severe hypotension, bronchospasm, and metabolic instability (162,172). Successful preoperative prophylaxis against carcinoid crisis can be achieved with 100 to 400 µg of subcutaneous octreotide (162,172).

Outcomes

For both colonic and rectal carcinoids, the stage of disease correlates with survival, such that more advanced stages have worse prognoses (159). The classification of carcinoids into foregut, midgut, and hindgut is not useful in determining prognosis because five-year survival rates do not significantly differ between these groups (159). The overall five-year survival is worse for colonic carcinoids compared to rectal carcinoids, 42% and 72%, respectively (159).

Rectal Carcinoids

For rectal carcinoids, both tumor size and stage of disease correlate with survival. Long-term survival after resection of small lesions up to 1 cm in size approaches 100% (161). The mortality rate of tumors between 1 and 2 cm is 13%, compared with nearly 100% mortality for tumors greater than 2 cm (167).

T1 lesions up to 1 cm have excellent long-term survival of about 100% (161,167,169,173). Even larger T1 lesions up to 1.9 cm have excellent disease-free survival between 10 and 27 years after resection (161). Long-term survival of T2 rectal carcinoids decreases to 75% (167). T3 and T4 lesions in some studies are universally fatal, with median survival of only seven months (167). The five-year survival rate of patients with positive lymph nodes is 44%, and those with distant metastases is only 7% (161,170).

The presence of symptoms attributable to the rectal carcinoid is associated with worse outcome (167). Median survival of patients with symptoms is only 19 months compared to 38 months for asymptomatic patients (167). The presence of tumor ulceration or umbilication is also an ominous finding regardless of tumor size (166).

Colonic Carcinoids

Colonic carcinoids have the worst five-year survival amongst all the GI carcinoids (159). The five-year survival of colonic carcinoids ranges from 20% to 37%, which is lower than the five-year survival rate of colonic adenocarcinoma at 58% (158,159,163,164). The median survival after diagnosis is 4.5 months. The 10-year survival is 10%, although survival up to 28 years has been reported (163).

Survival is directly correlated with stage of disease such that patients with distant metastases have the lowest survival (158). The five-year survival rate for stage A colonic carcinoids is statistically significant compared to stage D, 83% and 21%, respectively (164). Smaller tumor size and a left-sided colon location show a trend toward improved survival (164). The improved survival for left-sided lesions is likely due to earlier detection and, therefore, earlier stage of disease.

Unfavorable prognostic indicators for colonic carcinoids associated with worse outcomes include poor differentiation, a high nuclear grade, or a tumor mitotic rate of greater than 20 mitoses per 10 high-power fields (158). Malnutrition and widespread metastatic disease contribute to 22% operative mortality and 20% mortality during initial hospitalizations (125,158).

Carcinoid Syndrome

The development of carcinoid syndrome carries a poor prognosis (162). Mean survival after the first flushing episode is 36 months, and six-year survival is 25% (162,170). Octreotide and interferon may improve survival (162,187,192). Survival times reported for carcinoid syndrome are generally from studies that predate the use of octreotide (162).

REFERENCES

1. Ryan J, Martin JE, Pollock DJ. Fatty tumours of the large intestine: a clinicopathological review of 13 cases. Br J Surg 1989; 76(8):793–796.
2. Haller JD, Roberts TW. Lipomas of the colon: a clinicopathologic study of 20 cases. Surgery 1964; 55:773–781.
3. Weinberg T, Feldman M. Lipomas of the gastrointestinal tract. Am J Clin Pathol 1955; 25:272–281.
4. Mayo CW, Pagtalunan RJ, Brown DJ. Lipoma of the alimentary tract. Surgery 1963; 53:598.
5. Taylor BA, Wolff BG. Colonic lipomas. Report of two unusual cases and review of the Mayo Clinic experience 1976–1985. Dis Colon Rectum 1987; 30(11):888–893.
6. Christie JP. The removal of lipomas. Gastrointest Endosc 1990; 36(5):532–533.
7. Siegal A, Witz M. Gastrointestinal lipoma and malignancies. J Surg Oncol 1991; 47(3):170–174.
8. Snover DC. Atypical lipomas of the colon. Report of two cases with pseudomalignant features. Dis Colon Rectum 1984; 27(7):485–488.
9. Mohandas D, Chandra RS, Srinivasan V, Bhaskar AG. Liposarcoma of the ileum with secondaries in the liver. Am J Gastroenterol 1972; 58(2):172–176.
10. Atik M, Whittlesey RH. Liposarcoma of jejunum. Ann Surg 1957; 146:837–842.
11. McGrew W, Dunn GD. Colonic lipomas: clinical significance and management. South Med J 1985; 78(7):877–879.
12. Gordon RT, Beal JM. Lipoma of the colon. Arch Surg 1978; 113(7):897–899.
13. Rogy MA, Mirza D, Berlakovich G, Winkelbauer F, Rauhs R. Submucous large-bowel lipomas—presentation and management. An 18-year study. Eur J Surg 1991; 157(1):51–55.
14. Ackerman NB, Chughtai SQ. Symptomatic lipomas of the gastrointestinal tract. Surg Gynecol Obstet 1975; 141(4):565–568.
15. Castro EB, Stearns MW. Lipoma of the large intestine: a review of 45 cases. Dis Colon Rectum 1972; 14:441–444.
16. Michowitz M, Lazebnik N, Noy S, Lazebnik R. Lipoma of the colon: a report of 22 cases. Am Surg 1985; 51(8):449–454.
17. Hancock BJ, Vajcner A. Lipomas of the colon: a clinicopathologic review. Can J Surg 1988; 31(3): 178–181.
18. D'Javid IF. Lipomas of the large intestines: review of the literature and report of a case. J Int Coll Surg 1960; 33:639–668.
19. Alponat A, Kok KY, Goh PM, Ngoi SS. Intermittent subacute intestinal obstruction due to a giant lipoma of the colon: a case report. Am Surg 1996; 62(11):918–921.
20. Khawaja FI. Pedunculated lipoma of the colon: risks of endoscopic removal. South Med J 1987; 80(9):1176–1179.
21. Fernandez MJ, Davis RP, Nora PF. Gastrointestinal lipomas. Arch Surg 1983; 118(9):1081–1083.
22. Franc-Law JM, Begin LR, Vasilevsky CA, Gordon PH. The dramatic presentation of colonic lipomata: report of two cases and review of the literature. Am Surg 2001; 67(5):491–494.
23. Key JC, Roberts JW. Massive bleeding from colonic lipomas. Arch Surg 1980; 115:889–890.
24. Kabaalioglu A, Gelen T, Aktan S, Kesici A, Bircan O, Luleci E. Acute colonic obstruction caused by intussusception and extrusion of a sigmoid lipoma through the anus after barium enema. Abdom Imaging 1997; 22(suppl 4):389–391.

25. Radhi JM, Haig TH. Lipoma of the colon with overlying hyperplastic epithelium. Can J Gastroenterol 1997; 11(8):694–695.
26. Zamboni WA, Fleisher H, Zander JD, Folse JR. Spontaneous expulsion of lipoma per rectum occurring with colonic intussusception. Surgery 1987; 101(1):104–107.
27. Liessi G, Pavanello M, Cesari S, Dell'Antonio C, Avventi P. Large lipomas of the colon: CT and MR findings in three symptomatic cases. Abdom Imaging 1996; 21(2):150–152.
28. Notaro JR, Masser PA. Annular colon lipoma: a case report and review of the literature. Surgery 1991; 110(3):570–572.
29. Margulis AR, Jovanovich A. Roentgen diagnosis of submucous lipoma of the colon. Am J Roentgen 1960; 84:1114–1119.
30. Hurwitz MM, Redleaf PD, Williams HJ, Edwards JE. Lipomas of the gastrointestinal tract. An analysis of seventy-two tumors. Am J Roentgenol Radium Ther Nucl Med 1967; 99(1):84–89.
31. LoIudice TA, Lang JA. Submucous lipoma simulating carcinoma of the colon. South Med J 1980; 73(4):521–523.
32. Heiken JP, Forde KA, Gold RP. Computerized tomography as a definite method for diagnosing gastrointestinal lipomas. Radiology 1982; 142:409–414.
33. Ho KJ, Shin MS, Tishler JM. Computed tomographic distinction of submucosal lipoma and adenomatous polyp of the colon. Gastrointest Radiol 1984; 9(1):77–80.
34. Buetow PC, Buck JL, Carr NJ, et al. Intussuscepted colonic lipomas: loss of fat attenuation on CT with pathologic correlation in 10 cases. Abdom Imaging 1996; 21(2):153–156.
35. Hall PA, Murfitt J, Pollock DJ. Caecal lipomas mimicking colonic angiodysplasia. Br J Radiol 1985; 58(696):1213–1214.
36. Pfeil SA, Weaver MG, Abdul-Karim FW, Yang P. Colonic lipomas: outcome of endoscopic removal. Gastrointest Endosc 1990; 36(5):435–438.
37. Messer J, Waye JD. The diagnosis of colonic lipomas— the naked fat sign. Gastrointest Endosc 1982; 28:186–188.
38. DeBeer RA, Shinya H. Colonic lipomas. An endoscopic analysis. Gastrointest Endosc 1975; 22:90–91.
39. Tamura S, Yokoyama Y, Morita T, Tadokoro T, Higashidani Y, Onishi S. "Giant" colon lipoma: what kind of findings are necessary for the indication of endoscopic resection? Am J Gastroenterol 2001; 96(6):1944–1946.
40. Chase MP, Yarze JC. "Giant" colon lipoma—to attempt endoscopic resection or not? Am J Gastroenterol 2000; 95(8):2143–2144.
41. Alkim C, Sasmaz N, Alkim H, Caglikulekci M, Turhan N. Sonographic findings in intussusception caused by a lipoma in the muscular layer of the colon. J Clin Ultrasound 2001; 29(5):298–301.
42. Zeebregts CJ, Geraedts AA, Blaauwgeers JL, Hoitsma HF. Intussusception of the sigmoid colon because of an intramuscular lipoma. Report of a case. Dis Colon Rectum 1995; 38(8):891–892.
43. Radhi JM. Lipoma of the colon: self-amputation. Am J Gastroenterol 1993; 88(11):1981–1982.
44. Kunimura T, Ooike N, Sasajima Y, Inagaki T, Morohoshi T. A resected case of adenolipoma of the colon: is it a new entity of the colonic tumor? Am J Gastroenterol 2001; 96(2):611–612.
45. Marin GA, Villa GL. Colonic lipomas. Endoscopic and radiologic characteristics. N J Med 1990; 87(4):301–303.
46. Yu JP, Luo HS, Wang XZ. Endoscopic treatment of submucosal lesions of the gastrointestinal tract. Endoscopy 1992; 24(3):190–193.
47. Papp JP, Haubrich WS. Endoscopic removal of colon lipomas. Gastrointest Endosc 1973; 20(2):66–67.
48. Welen S, Youher J, Spratt JS. The rates and patterns of growth of 375 tumours of the large intestines and rectum observed serially by double contrast enema study (Malmo technique). Am J Roentgend 1963; 90:673.
49. Waye JD, Frankel A. Removal of pedunculated lipoma by colonoscopy. Am J Gastroenterol 1974; 61:221–222.
50. Shapiro PD, Michas CA. Endoscopic removal of submucosal colonic lipomas. Arch Surg 1976; 111(1):89.
51. Bar-Meir S, Halla A, Baratz M. Endoscopic removal of colonic lipomas. Endoscopy 1981; 13:135–136.
52. Kitamura K, Kitagawa S, Mori M, Haraguchi Y. Endoscopic correction of intussusception and removal of a colonic lipoma. Gastrointest Endosc 1990; 36(5):509–511.
53. Richards MA. Lymphoma of the colon and rectum. Postgrad Med J 1986; 62(729):615–620.
54. Scoggin SS, Frazee RC. Laparoscopically assisted resection of a colonic lipoma. J Laparoendosc Surg 1992; 2:185–189.
55. Dawson IMP, Cornes JS, Morson BC. Primary malignant lymphoid tumors of the intestinal tract. Report of 37 cases with a study of the factors influencing prognosis. Br J Surg 1961; 40:80–89.
56. Zighelboim J, Larson MV. Primary colonic lymphoma. Clinical presentation, histopathologic features, and outcome with combination chemotherapy. J Clin Gastroenterol 1994; 18(4):291–297.
57. Doolabh N, Anthony T, Simmang C, et al. Primary colonic lymphoma. J Surg Oncol 2000; 74(4): 257–262.
58. Isaacson P. Gastrointestinal lymphoma. Hum Path 1994; 25:1020–1029.
59. Crump M, Gospodarowicz M, Shepherd FA. Lymphoma of the gastrointestinal tract. Semin Oncol 1999; 26(3):324–337.

60. Radaszkiewicz T, Dragosics B, Bauer P. Gastrointestinal malignant lymphomas of the mucosa-associated lymphoid tissue: factors relevant to prognosis. Gastro 1992; 102:1628–1638.

61. Rao AR, Kagan AR, Potyk D, et al. Management of gastrointestinal lymphoma. Am J Clin Oncol 1984; 7:213–219.

62. Contreary K, Nance FC, Becker WF. Primary lymphoma of the gastrointestinal tract. Ann Surg 1980; 191:593–598.

63. Lewin KJ, Ranchod M, Dorfman RF. Lymphomas of the gastrointestinal tract: a study of 117 cases presenting with gastrointestinal disease. Cancer 1978; 42:693–707.

64. Henry CA, Berry RE. Primary lymphoma of the large intestine. Am Surg 1988; 54(5):262–266.

65. Dragosics B, Bauer P, Radaszkiewicz T. Primary gastrointestinal non-Hodgkin's lymphomas: a retrospective clinicopathologic study of 150 cases. Cancer 1985; 55:1060–1073.

66. Waisberg J, Bromberg SH, Franco MI, et al. Primary non-Hodgkin lymphoma of the right colon: a retrospective clinical-pathological study. Int Surg 2001; 86(1):20–25.

67. Wang MH, Wong JM, Lien HC, Lin CW, Wang CY. Colonoscopic manifestations of primary colorectal lymphoma. Endoscopy 2001; 33:605–609.

68. Ziegler H, Beckstead JA, Volberding PA. Non-Hodgkin's lymphoma in homosexual men. N Engl J Med 1984; 311:565–570.

69. Nirmala V, Thomas JA, Anthony AJ. Primary malignant lymphoma of colon. Indian J Cancer 1981; 18(1):47–50.

70. Hwang WS, Yao JC, Cheng SS, Tseng HH. Primary colorectal lymphoma in Taiwan. Cancer 1992; 70(3):575–580.

71. Lee HJ, Han JK, Kim TK, Kim YH, Kim KW, Choi BI. Peripheral T-cell lymphoma of the colon: double-contrast barium enema examination findings in six patients. Radiology 2001; 218(3): 751–756.

72. Myung SJ, Joo KR, Yang SK, et al. Clinicopathologic features of ileocolonic malignant lymphoma: analysis according to colonoscopic classification. Gastrointest Endosc 2003; 57(3):343–347.

73. Kumar S, Fend F, Quintanilla-Martinez L, et al. Epstein-Barr virus-positive gastrointestinal Hodgkin's disease: association with inflammatory bowel disease and immunosuppression. Am J Surg Path 2000; 24:66–73.

74. Sanz AM, Codine JG, MP R, et al. Toxic megacolon: a rare presentation of primary lymphoma of the colon. Eur J Gastroenterol Hepatol 2000; 12:583–586.

75. Bini EJ, Weinshel EH, Falkenstein DB. Risk factors for recurrent bleeding and mortality in human immunodeficiency virus-infected patients with acute lower GI hemorrhage. Gastroinest Endosc 1999; 49:748–753.

76. McCullough JE, Kim CH, Banks PM. Mantle zone lymphoma of the colon simulating diffuse inflammatory bowel disease. Role of immunohistochemistry in establishing the diagnosis. Dig Dis Sci 1992; 37(6):934–938.

77. Friedman CJ, Cunningham WM, Sperling MH. Colonoscopic removal of a colonic leiomyoma. Gastrointest Endosc 1979; 25:107–108.

78. Weir AB, Poon MC, Groarke JF, Wilkerson JA. Lymphoma simulating Crohn's colitis. Dig Dis Sci 1980; 25(1):69–72.

79. Vadmal MS, LaValle GP, DeYoung BR, Frankel WL, Marsh WL. Primary localized extranodal Hodgkin disease of the transverse colon. Arch Pathol Lab Med 2000; 124:1824–1827.

80. Aviles A, Neri N, Huerta-Guzman J. Large bowel lymphoma: an analysis of prognostic factors and therapy in 53 patients. J Surgic Oncol 2002; 80:111–115.

81. O'Connell DJ, Thompson AJ. Lymphoma of the colon: the spectrum of radiologic changes. Gastrointest Radiol 1978; 2(4):377–385.

82. Gedgaudas-McClees RK, Maglinte DD. Aphthous lesions in nodular lymphoma of the colon. South Med J 1986; 79(7):907–908.

83. Chiu KW, Changchien CS, Chuah SK, Chen CL. Endoscopic and image features in primary gastrointestinal lymphoma: a 7-year experience. Hepatogastroenterology 1995; 42(4):367–370.

84. Gloeckner K, Leithaeuser F, Lang W, Merz H, Feller AC. Colonic primary large cell lymphoma with marginal zone growth pattern presenting as multiple polyps. Am J Surg Path 1999; 23: 1149–1153.

85. Telford JJ, Ruymann FW. Image of the month: malignant lymphomatous polyposis. Gastroenterology 2001; 121:1274.

86. Yatabe Y, Nakamura S, Nakamura T, et al. Multiple polypoid lesions of primary mucosa-associated lymphoid-tissue lymphoma of colon. Histopathology 1998; 32(2):116–125.

87. Breslin NP, Urbanski SJ, Shaffer EA. Mucosa-associated lymphoid tissue (MALT) lymphoma manifesting as multiple lymphomatosis polyposis of the gastrointestinal tract. Am J Gastroenterol 1999; 94(9):2540–2545.

88. Auner HW, Beham-Schmid C, Linder G, Fickert P, Linkesch W, Sill H. Successful nonsurgical treatment of primary mucosa-associated lymphoid tissue lymphoma of colon presenting with multiple polypoid lesions. Am J Gastroenterol 2000; 2000:2387–2388.

89. Friedman HB, Silver GM, Brown CH. Lymphoma of the colon simulating ulcerative colitis. Report of four cases. Am J Dig Dis 1968; 13(10):910–917.

90. Yoshimura D, Maruoka A, Maekawa S, Yao T, Harada N, Nawata H. Transverse colon malt lymphoma with nodal metastasis. Gastrointest Endosc 2002; 55(2):238–239.
91. Group ILS. A clinical evaluation of the international lymphoma study group classification of non-Hodgkin's lymphoma. The non-Hodgkin's lymphoma classification project. Blood 1997; 89: 3909–3918.
92. Lukes R, Collins R. Immunologic characterization of human malignant lymphomas. Cancer 1974; 34:1488.
93. Harris NL, Jaffe ES, Stein P, et al. A revised European-American classification of lymphoid neoplasms: a proposal from the international lymphoma study group. Blood 1994; 84:1361–1392.
94. Herrington LJ. Epidemiology of the revised European-American lymphoma classification subtypes. Epidemiol Rev 1998; 20:187–203.
95. Sallach S, Schmidt T, Pehl C, et al. Primary low-grade B cell non-Hodgkin's lymphoma of MALT type simultaneously arising in the colon and in the lung: report of a case. Dis Colon Rectum 2001; 44(3):448–452.
96. Musshoff K, Schmidt-Vollmer H. Prognosis of non-Hodgkin's lymphomas with special emphasis on the staging classification. Z Krebsforsch Klin Onkol Cancer Res Clin Oncol 1975; 83:323–341.
97. Pulte D, Murray J. Celiac disease and diffuse T-cell lymphoma of the colon. Gastrointest Endosc 2001; 53(3):379–381.
98. Raderer M, Pfeffel F, Pohl G, Mannhalter C, Valencak J, Chott A. Regression of colonic low grade B cell lymphoma of the mucosa associated lymphoid tissue type after eradication of *Helicobacter pylori*. Gut 2000; 46(1):133–135.
99. Parente F, Rizzardini G, Cernuschi M, Antinori S, Fasan M, Bianchi-Porro G. Non-Hodgkin's lymphoma and AIDS: frequency of gastrointestinal involvement in a large Italian series. Scand J Gastroenterol 1993; 28:315–318.
100. Cho C, Linscheer WG, Bell R, Smith R. Colonic lymphoma producing alpha-chain disease protein. Gastroenterology 1982; 83(1 Pt 1):121–126.
101. Khan S, Anderson GK, Eppstein AC, Eggenberger JC, Margolin DA. Ulcerative colitis and colonic lymphoma: a theoretical link. Am Surg 2001; 67(7):654–656.
102. Hope-Ross M, Magee DJ, O'Donoghue, Murphy JJ. Ulcerative colitis complicated by lymphoma and adenocarcinoma. Br J Surg 1985; 72:22.
103. Glick SN, Roth T, Teplick SK. Development of non-Hodgkin's lymphoma of the colon after radiation therapy for Hodgkin's disease. Dig Dis Sci 1991; 36(10):1491–1494.
104. Renton P, Blackshaw AJ. Colonic lymphoma complicating ulcerative colitis. Br J Surg 1976; 63: 542–545.
105. Wagonfeld JB, Platz CE, Fishman FL, Sibley RK, Kirsner JB. Multicentric colonic lymphoma complicating ulcerative colitis. Am J Dig Dis 1977; 22(6):502–508.
106. Loftus EV, Tremaine WJ, Habermann TM, Harmsen WS, Zinmeister AR, Sandborn WJ. Risk of lymphoma in inflammatory bowel disease. Am J Gastroenterol 2000; 95:2308–2312.
107. Lewis JD, Bilker WB, Brensinger C, Deren JJ, Vaughn DJ, Strom BL. Inflammatory bowel disease is not associated with an increased risk of lymphoma. Gastroenterology 2001; 121:1080–1087.
108. Dayharsh GA, Loftus EV, Sanborn WJ, et al. Epstein-Barr virus-positive lymphoma in patients with inflammatory bowel disease treated with azathioprine or 6-mercaptopurine. Gastroenterology 2002; 122:72–77.
109. Shepherd NA, Hall PA, Williams GT, et al. Primary malignant lymphoma of the large intestine complicating chronic inflammatory bowel disease. Histopathology 1989; 15(4):325–337.
110. Grenstein AJ, Mullin GE, Strauhen JA, et al. Lymphoma in inflammatory bowel disease. Cancer 1992; 69:1119–1123.
111. Farrell RJ, Ang Y, Kileen P, et al. Increased incidence of non-Hodgkin's lymphoma in inflammatory bowel disease patients on immunosuppressive therapy but overall risk is low. Gut 2000; 47:514–519.
112. Phillips DL, Keeffe EB, Benner KG, Braziel RM. Colonic lymphoma in the transplant patient. Dig Dis Sci 1989; 34(1):150–154.
113. Coggon DN, Rose DH, Ansell ID. A large bowel lymphoma complicating renal transplantation. Br J Radiol 1981; 54:418–420.
114. Stylianos S, Chen MH, Treat MR, LoGerfo P, Rose EA. Colonic lymphoma as a cause of massive rectal bleeding in a cardiac transplant recipient. J Cardiovasc Surg (Torino) 1990; 31(3):315–317.
115. Roca-Tey R, Borrellas X, Cantarell C, Capdevila L, Piera L. Immunoblastic lymphoma of the colon in a renal transplant patient presenting with autoimmune haemolytic anaemia of the cold antibody type. Nephrol Dial Transplant 1997; 12(9):2000–2001.
116. Arnell T, Stamos MJ, Takahashi P, Ojha S, Sze G, Eysselein V. Colonic stents in colorectal obstruction. Am Surg 1998; 64:986–988.
117. Auger MJ, Allan NC. Primary ileocecal lymphoma: a study of 22 patients. Cancer 1990; 65:358–361.
118. Inoue F, Chiba T. Regression of MALT lymphoma of the rectum after anti-*H. pylori* therapy in a patient negative of H. pylori. Gastroenterology 1999; 117:514–515.
119. Matsumoto T, Iida M, Shimizu M. Regression of mucosa-associated lymphoid-tissue lymphoma of rectum after eradication of *Helicobacter pylori*. Lancet 1997; 350:115–116.

120. Hoption Cann SA, Van Netten JP, Van Netten C. Malt lymphomas and *Helicobacter pylori*? Gut 2001; 48:283.

121. Nakagawara M, Kajimura M, Hanai H, Simizu S, Kobayashi H, Kaneko E. Simultaneous mucosa-associated lymphoid tissue lymphoma of the stomach and colon. Gastrointest Endosc 1999; 50:414–415.

122. Jones SE, Fuks Z, Bull M, et al. Non-Hodgkin's lymphomas IV. Clinicopathological correlation in 405 cases. Cancer 1973; 31:806–823.

123. Peters MV, Hasselback R, Brown TC. The natural history of the lymphomas related to the clinical classification. Proceedings of the International Conference on Leukaemia-Lymphoma 1968; 357.

124. Ehrlich AN, Stalder G, Geller W, Sherlock P. Gastrointestinal manifestations of malignant lymphoma. Gastroenterology 1968; 54:1115–1121.

125. Rosenberg SA, Diamond HD, Jaslowitz B, Craver LF. Lymphosarcoma: a review of 1269 cases. Medicine 1961; 40:31.

126. Chak A. EUS in submucosal tumors. Gastrointest Endosc 2002; 56:S43–S48.

127. Hatch KF, Blanchard DK, Hatch GF, et al. Tumors of the appendix and colon. World J Surg 2000; 24:430–436.

128. Bjorsdottir H, Bjornsson J, Gudjonsson H. Leiomyomatous colonic polyp. Dig Dis Sci 1993; 38: 1945–1947.

129. Kadakia SC, Kadakia AS, Seargent K. Endoscopic removal of colonic leiomyoma. J Clin Gastroenterol 1992; 15:59–62.

130. Miettinen M, Sarlomo-Rikala M, Sobin LH. Mesenchymal tumors of masacularis mucosae of colon and rectum are benign leiomyomas that should be separated from gastrointestinal anomal tumors-a clinicopathologic and immunohistochemical study of eighty-eight cases. Mod Path 2001; 14:950–956.

131. Spaun E, Nielsen L. Leiomyomatosis of the colon and mesentery: report of a case. Am J Gastroenterol 1986; 81:385–388.

132. Freni SC, Keeman JN. Leiomyomatosis of the colon. Cancer 1977; 39:263–266.

133. Hizawa K, Iida M, Matsumoto T, et al. Gastrointestinal involvement in tuberous sclerosis: two case reports. J Clin Gastroenterol 1994; 19:46–49.

134. Byard RW, Phillips GE, Dardick I, Robertson E, Carter RF, Bourne AJ. Two unusual tumours of the gastrointestinal tract in a patient with tuberous sclerosis. J Paediatr Child Health 1991; 27:116–119.

135. Lee SH, Ha HK, Byun JY, et al. Radiological features of leiomyomatous tumours of the colon and rectum. J Comput Assist Tomagr 2000; 24:407–412.

136. Goodman P, Raval B, Bonnati C, Schmidt WA. Leiomyoma involving the gastrocolic ligament: CT demonstration. Comput Med Imaging Graph 1990; 14:431.

137. Megibow AJ, Balthazar EJ, Hulnick DH, Naidich DP, Bosniak MA. CT evaluation of gastrointestinal leiomyoma and leiomyosarcomas. AJR 1985; 144:727–731.

138. Chun HJ, Byun JY, Chun KA, et al. Gastrointestinal leiomyoma and leiomyosarcoma: CT differentiation. J Comput Assist Tomagr 1998; 22:69–74.

139. Chow WH, Kwan WK, Ng WF. Endoscopic removal of leiomyoma of the colon. HKMJ 1997; 3:325–327.

140. Wolf O, Glaser F, Kuntz C, Lehnert T. Endorectal ultrasound and leiomyosarcoma of the section. Clin Investig 1994; 72:381–384.

141. Chak A, Canto MI, Rosch T, et al. Endosonographic differentiation of benign and malignant stromal tumors. Gastrointest Endosc 1997; 45:468–473.

142. Palazzo L, Landi B, Cellier C, Cuillerier E, Roseau G, Barbier JP. Endosonographic features predictive of benign and malignant gastrointestinal stromal cell tumors - definition, clinical, biological, immunohistochemical, and molecular genetic features and differential diagnosis. Virchows Arch 2000; 438:1–12.

143. Miettinen M, Sarlomo-Rikala M, Sobin LH, Lasota J. Gastrointestinal stromal tumors and leiomyosarcomas in the colon: a clinicopathologic immunohistochemical and molecular genetic study of 44 cases. Am J Surg Path 2000; 24:1339–1352.

144. Weston PM, Travis R, Thompson HH. Giant cystic leiomyoma of the sigmoid colon. Compt Med Imaging Graph 1991; 15:41.

145. Nemer FD, Soeckinger JM, Evans OT. Smooth-muscle rectal tumors: a therapeutic dilemma. Dis Colon Rectum 1977; 20:405–413.

146. Ranchod M, Kempson RL. Smooth-muscle tumors of the gastrointestinal tract and retroperitoneum. Cancer 1977; 39:255–262.

147. Plukker JT, Blomjous EM, Wagstaff J, Meijer S. Primary leiomyosarcoma of the rectum: report of two cases and review of the literature. Neth J Surg 1989; 41:88–91.

148. Evans RW. Histological appearance of tumors with a consideration of their histogenesis and certain aspects of their clinical features and behavior. Edinburgh, UK: Livingstone, 1956:773.

149. Cummings SP, Lally KP, Pineoro-Carrero V, Beck DE. Colonic leiomyoma—an unusual cause of gastrointestinal hemorrhage in childhood. Dis Colon Rectum 1990; 33:511–514.

150. Stavorovsky M, Jaffa AJ, Papo J, Baratz M. Leiomyosarcoma of the colon and rectum. Dis Colon Rectum 1980; 23:249–254.

151. Randleman CD, Wolff BG, Dozois RR, Spencer RJ, Weiland LH, Ilstrup DM. Leiomyosarcoma of the rectum and the anus: a series of 22 cases. Int J Colorectal Dis 1989; 4:91–96.

152. Scott CR. Myoma malignum particularly other than uterine. Northwest Med 1923; 22:436.
153. Stair JM, Stevenson DR, Scheafer RF, Lang NP. Leiomyosarcoma of the rectum: report of three cases. J Surg Oncol 1983; 24:180–183.
154. Minsky BD, Cohen AM, Hajdu SI. Conservative management of anal leiomyosarcoma. Cancer 1990; 33:319.
155. Consentino B, Arnaud A, Sarles JC. Leiomyosarcoma of the anal canal. J Chir 1988; 125:245.
156. Anderson PA, Dokerty MB, Luie LA. Myomatous tumors of the rectum (leiomyosarcoma and leiomyoma). Surgery 1950; 28:642–650.
157. Friesen R, Mooyana MB, Murray RB, Murphy F, Inglis FG. Colorectal leiomyosarcomas: a pathologic study with long-term follow-up. Can J Surg 1992; 35:505.
158. Spread C, Berkel H, Jewell L, Jenkins H, Yakimets W. Colon carcinoid tumors: a population-based study. Dis Colon Rectum 1994; 482–491.
159. Modlin IM, Sandor A. An analysis of 8305 cases of carnoid tumors. Cancer 1997; 79:813–829.
160. Delcore R, Friesen SR. Gastrointestinal neuroendocrine tumors. J Am Coll Surg 1994; 178: 187–211.
161. Naunheim KS, Zeitels J, Kaplan EL, et al. Rectal carcinoid tumors: treatment and prognosis. Surgery 1983; 94:670–676.
162. Janmohamed S, Bloom SR. Carcinoid tumors. Postgrad Med J 1997; 73:207–214.
163. Rosenberg JM, Welch JP. Carcinoid tumors of the colon: a study of 72 patients. Am J Surg 1985; 149:775–779.
164. Ballantyne GH, Savoca PE, Flannery JT, Ahlman MH, Modlin IM. Incidence and mortality of carcinoids of the colon. Cancer 1992; 69:2400–2405.
165. Mani S, Modlin IM, Ballantyne GH, Ahlman H, West B. Carcinoids of the rectum. J Am Coll Surg 1994; 179:231–247.
166. Jetmore AB, Ray JE, Gartright JB, McMullen KM, Hicks TC, Timmcke AE. Rectal carcinoids: the most frequent carcinoid tumor. Dis Colon Rectum 1992; 35:717–725.
167. Sauven P, Ridge JA, Quan SH, Sigurdson ER. Anorectal carcinoid tumors: is aggressive surgery warranted? Ann Surg 1990; 211:67–71.
168. Matsui K, Jwase T, Kitagawa M. Small, polypoid-appearing carcinoid tumors of the rectum: clinico-pathologic study of 16 cases and effectiveness of endoscopic treatment. Am J Gastroenterol 1993; 88:1949–1953.
169. Federspiel BH, Burke AP, Sobin LH, Shekitka KM. Rectal and colonic carcinoids: a clinicopathologic study of 84 cases. Cancer 1990; 65:135–140.
170. Godwin JD. Carcinoid tumors: an analysis of 2,837 cases. Cancer 1975; 36:560–569.
171. Vinik AI, McLeod MK, Fig LM, Shapiro B, Llyod RV, Cho K. Clinical features, diagnosis and localization of carcinoid tumors and their management. Gastrointest Endocrinol 1989; 18:865.
172. Stinner B, Kisker O, Zielke A, Rothmund M. Surgical management for carcinoid tumors of small bowel, appendix, colon, and rectum. World J Surg 1996; 20:183–188.
173. Schindl M, Niederle B, Hafner M, et al. Stage-dependent therapy of rectal carcinoid tumors. World J Surg 1998; 22:628–634.
174. Imada-Shirakata Y, Sakai M, Kajiyama T, et al. Endoscopic resection of rectal carcinoid tumors using aspiration lumpectomy. Endoscopy 1996; 28:34–38.
175. Yamauchi H, Hirata A, Sasaki S, et al. Heal carcinoid tumor with a rose-shaped appearance by dye-spraying diagnosis at colonoscopy. Gastrointest Endosc 2001; 54:267–268.
176. Yoshida M, Tsukamoto Y, Niwa Y, et al. Endoscopic assessment of invasion of colorectal tumors with a new high-frequency ultrasound probe. Gastrointest Endosc 1995; 41:587–592.
177. Koura AN, Giacco GG, Curley SA, Skibber JM, Feig BW, Ellis LM. Carcinoid tumors of the rectum: effect of size, histopathology, and surgical treatment on metastasis free survival. Cancer 1997; 79:1294–1298.
178. Pelage JP, Soyer P, Bondiaf M, et al. Carcinoid tumors of the abdomen: CT features. Abdom Imaging 1999; 24:240–245.
179. Turnbull RB, Kyle K, Watson FR. Cancer of the colon: the influence of the no-touch isolation technique on survival rates. Ann Surg 1967; 166:420–427.
180. Bates HRJ, Belter LF. Composite carcinoid tumor (argentaffinoma-adenocarcinoma) of the colon: report of two cases. Dis Col Rectum 1967; 10:467–470.
181. Tsioulias G, Muto T, Kubota Y, et al. DNA ploidy pattern in rectal carcinoid tumors. Dis Colon Rectum 1991; 34:31–36.
182. Berkelhammer C, Jasper I, Kirvaitis E, Schreiner S, Hamilton J, Walloch J. "Band-snare" resection of small rectal carcinoid tumors. Gastrointest Endosc 1999; 50(4):582–585.
183. Ono A, Fujii T, Saito Y, et al. Endoscopic submucosal resection of rectal carcinoid tumors with a ligation device. Gastrointest Endosc 2003; 57(4):583–587.
184. Mitty HA, Warner RRP, Newman LH, Trains JS, Parnes IH. Control of carcinoid syndrome with hepatic artery embolization. Radiology 1985; 155:623–626.
185. Frilling A, Rogiers X, Broelsch CE. Liver transplantation for metastatic carcinoid tumors. Digestion 1994; 55:104–106.
186. Connolly HM, Nishimura RA, Smith HC, Pellikka PA, Mullany CJ, Kvols LK. Outcome of cardiac surgery for carcinoid heart disease. J Am Coll Cardiol 1995; 25:410–416.

187. Kvols LK. Metastatic carcinoid tumours and the malignant carcinoid syndrome. Ann NY Acad Sci 1994; 733:464–470.
188. Lamberts SWJ, Van der Lely A, De Herder WW, Hofland LJ. Octreotide. N Eng J Med 1996; 334: 246–254.
189. O'Toole D, Ducreux M, Bommelaer G, Wemeau JL, Bouche O, Catus F, et al. Treatment of carcinoid syndrome: a prospective crossover evaluation of lanreotide versus octreotide in terms of efficacy patient acceptability and tolerance. Cancer 2000; 88:770–776.
190. Rubin J, Ajani J, Schirmer W, et al. Octreotide acetate long-acting formulation versus open-label subcutaneous octreotide acetate in malignant carcinoid syndrome. J Clin Oncol 1999; 17:600–606.
191. Oberg K, Eriksson B. The role of interferons in the management of carcinoid tumours. Br J Haematol 1991; 79(suppl 1):74–77.
192. Oberg K. The use of chemotherapy in the treatment of neuroendocrine tumors. Endocrinal Metab Clin North Am 1993; 22:941–952.
193. Oberg K. Medical treatment of neuroendocrine gut and pancreatic tumors. Acta Oncol 1989; 28: 425–431.

25 | Intestinal Polyposis Syndromes and Hereditary Colorectal Cancer

Jonathan P. Terdiman
Department of Medicine, University of California–San Francisco, San Francisco, California, U.S.A.

Madhulika G. Varma
Department of Surgery, University of California–San Francisco, San Francisco, California, U.S.A.

INTRODUCTION

Colorectal cancer (CRC) is the second leading cause of cancer death in the United States. Each year approximately 130,000 Americans are diagnosed with the disease and 50,000 will die of it (1). The cumulative lifetime risks of CRC and mortality from CRC are approximately 3% to 6% and 2%, respectively. The majority of CRCs occur in individuals over 60 years old, who have no previous personal or family history of the disease. Although the major risk factors for these sporadic cases are advancing age and environmental exposures, most importantly diet, approximately 20% to 25% of CRCs are in younger individuals or in those people with a personal or family history of cancer, suggesting a heritable susceptibility (2).

The genetic predisposition to CRC falls into two major groups, common familial CRC (15–20% of CRC) and hereditary CRC (5% of CRC)(Fig. 1) (3). In common familial CRC, first-degree relatives of persons with CRC or adenomatous polyps have an approximately twofold risk of developing CRC, and the risk increases with the number of relatives affected and the earlier the age of onset in the family (4). A family history of extracolonic cancers (e g , uterine), or the presence in individual family members of multiple colorectal or other cancers, also increases the risk. Increased risk for CRC in common familial CRC is conveyed by the inheritance of one or more, of likely many possible, low penetrance susceptibility alleles, most of which have yet to be identified (5). Carriage of these susceptibility alleles increases the risk of acquiring CRC, but by no means is the development of CRC certain. In fact, in the large majority of allele carriers, CRC does not occur. Common familial CRC will be discussed in greater detail in a subsequent part of this chapter.

Upwards of 5% of CRCs are hereditary in etiology, meaning that they are caused by carriage of a highly penetrant, dominantly inherited, susceptibility allele. Hereditary CRC is conventionally divided between the polyposis syndromes and hereditary nonpolyposis CRC (Table 1) (3). The polyposis syndromes are defined by the presence of multiple polyps in the gut lumen and have conventionally been categorized by polyp histology. The most common and important of the polyposis syndromes is familial adenomatous polyposis (FAP). FAP carries a lifetime risk of CRC, approaching 100% if the colon is not prophylatically removed (6). The other major categories of hereditary polyposes are the hamartomatous polyposis syndromes, most importantly Peutz–Jeghers syndrome (PJS), hereditary juvenile polyposis, and Cowden syndrome. There are a number of other very rare hereditary polyposis syndromes, as well as several nonhereditary polyposis syndromes, that may or may not confer an increased risk for CRC.

Much more common than any of the polyposis syndromes is hereditary nonpolyposis colorectal cancer (HNPCC). At least 2% to 3% of all CRC is secondary to HNPCC (7,8). In HNPCC, the lifetime risk of CRC approaches 70% to 80%, but not as a consequence of an increased number of colorectal adenomas (6).

The primary importance of familial and hereditary CRC is the increased risk of CRC, and often, other cancers, for individuals with these conditions. Failure to recognize common familial CRC, or more importantly, one of the hereditary syndromes, will lead to inadequate cancer screening and surveillance in individuals at risk, with subsequent premature loss of life. Recently, the elucidation of the genes responsible for many of these syndromes has revolutionized the care of at-risk individuals and families. Genetic testing has the potential

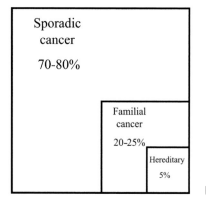

Figure 1 Frequency of sporadic, familial, and hereditary colorectal cancer.

to greatly improve the efficiency and reduce the costs and morbidity of cancer screening and surveillance. Genetic testing is now commercially available and is the standard of care for individuals and families with, or suspected of having, FAP or HNPCC (9,10). Genetic testing will ultimately make an impact on the management of individuals at risk for common familial CRC as well. However, genetic testing raises a number of vexing clinical, ethical, legal, and psychosocial questions.

This chapter will discuss the clinical features, genetics, and management of common familial and hereditary CRC, specifically the polyposis syndromes and HNPCC. Attention will be paid to the appropriate indications and methods for genetic testing in hereditary CRC.

POLYPOSIS SYNDROMES
Adenomatous Polyposis Syndromes
Familial Adenomatous Polyposis
Clinical Features: Intestinal
FAP is an autosomal dominant disorder that affects about 1 in 10,000 to 15,000 individuals and accounts for probably less than 0.1% of CRCs (11). In classic FAP, affected individuals develop hundreds to thousands of colonic adenomas by the mid to late teens, with over 95% of affected individuals demonstrating polyposis by age 35. CRC is inevitable in untreated patients, with the majority of cancers appearing by age 40 and over 90% by age 45 (12,13). Variants of FAP are now recognized in which polyps are greatly reduced in number, are predominantly or exclusively located in the right colon, and occur approximately a decade later than in classic FAP.

Table 1 Classification of Hereditary Colorectal Cancer Syndromes

Polyposis syndromes (< 1% of all colorectal cancers)
Adenomatous polyposis syndromes
Familial adenomatous polyposis
Gardner syndrome
Turcot syndrome
Attenuated adenomatous polyposis coli
Hamartomatous polyposis syndromes
Peutz–Jeghers syndrome
Juvenile polyposis
Hereditary mixed polyposis syndrome
Cowden syndrome
Bannayan–Riley–Ruvalcaba syndrome
Ruvulcaba–Myhre syndrome
Bannayan–Zonana syndrome
Soto syndrome
Lhermitte–Duclos disease
Gorlin syndrome
Hereditary nonpolyposis colorectal cancer (3–5% of all colorectal cancers)
Lynch syndrome
Muir–Torre syndrome
Turcot syndrome

This latter condition has been termed attenuated adenomatous polyposis coli (AAPC) or attenuated FAP (14,15).

In addition to colonic polyps, up to 90% of individuals with FAP will develop small bowel adenomas, most commonly at or near the ampulla of Vater (16–19). These lesions are usually multiple and sessile, often forming carpet-like lesions. Because the ampulla of Vater is almost invariably involved, to assess the full extent of duodenal polyposis, duodenoscopy, in addition to routine upper endoscopy, is required (20). The burden of duodenal polyposis can be rated by the Spigelman classification (21). The lifetime risk for small bowel carcinoma is approximately 5%, and duodenal cancer is the leading cause of cancer death in FAP patients that have undergone a colectomy (13,22–24). Individuals with stage III or IV polyposis as per the Spigelman classification, based on size and number of polyps and degree of dysplasia, are at greatest risk for periampullary/duodenal carcinoma (25).

Most FAP patients also will develop gastric polyposis. Gastric polyps are usually of the fundic-gland histological type, but adenomas rarely do occur (19). Gastric carcinoma risk is not much increased in Western families, but is reported to be increased three- to fourfold in Japanese and Korean families with FAP. Overall the lifetime risk of gastric cancer in individuals with FAP has been reported at 0.5% (19). The gastric adenoma is felt to be the precursor lesion for gastric cancer, as fundic-gland polyps are considered to have almost no malignant potential. There has, however, been a case reported of gastric cancer arising in an area of fundic-gland polyposis (26).

Clinical Features: Extra-Intestinal

Approximately two-thirds of FAP patients will have congenital hypertrophy of the retinal pigment epithelium (CHRPE), which are typically are flat, oval, and pigmented lesions and are best detected by opthalmoscopy after pupillary dilation. In FAP, the lesions are usually multiple ($\geq$4), bilateral, or large (27,28). Although CHRPE does not affect vision, or have any malignant potential, it is important as an early marker to identify susceptible individuals, as it can be detected at birth. In CHRPE-positive families, nearly all individuals with FAP in the family will have CHRPE. Thus, an examination of the fundus can identify susceptible family members at a young age (28).

Other benign extra-intestinal manifestations of FAP include dental abnormalities, osteomas, lipomas, epidermoid cysts, and desmoid tumors (12,17). Desmoids develop in about 9% to 17% of individuals with FAP, approximately half are intra-abdominal, involving the small bowel and its mesentery, and the rest occur in the abdominal wall or other extra-abdominal sites such as the neck, thigh, breast, axilla, or back. Surgical trauma is clearly implicated in the development of desmoid tumors, as about 70% to 80% occur in patients who have had prior abdominal surgery (17,29). Other factors that may predispose patients to develop desmoids are a family history of desmoids, female gender, and pregnancy or hormone use. The role of pregnancy remains unclear, however, as different studies have reported conflicting results; one study concluding that pregnancy ameliorates the course of desmoid tumors, whereas the other study reached the opposite conclusion finding an exacerbation of the growth of desmoids after pregnancy (30,31). Although desmoids are not malignant they may cause considerable morbidity and mortality by local invasion. Surgical treatment of intra-abdominal desmoids also results in a very high morbidity and mortality and is therefore reserved for those patients who have severe symptoms. Abdominal wall desmoids are more likely to be amenable to curative resection with less morbidity but unfortunately still have a high recurrence rate of up to 70% (29,32). FAP in conjunction with soft tissue tumors, osteomas, and dental abnormalities was once referred to as the Gardner syndrome.

Individuals with FAP are at increased risk for cancer at sites other than the colon and rectum and small bowel. Malignancies associated with FAP include hepatoblastoma in young children, medulloblastoma, papillary carcinoma of the thyroid, and pancreatic cancer (12,33,34). The association of FAP and central nervous systems tumors, primarily medulloblastoma, has been termed Turcot syndrome (35,36).

Genetics

The great majority of cases of FAP are caused by a germ-line mutation of the tumor supressor *APC* gene located on chromosome 5q21 (37–39). Normally each individual has two functional copies of *APC* in all cells. Loss of *APC* function in a colonic epithelial cell by mutation of one gene copy and loss of the other is an early and critical genetic step in the development of most sporadic colorectal neoplasms. Owing to a germline mutation of *APC*, which usually is inherited from a parent but can occur spontaneously in about one-third of cases, individuals with FAP only have one functional copy of the *APC* per cell, and initiation of colonic neoplasia is far more likely to occur, resulting in a dramatic increase in the number of colorectal adenomas and cancers. Data suggest that in some circumstances mutation of one gene copy alone may be enough to eliminate *APC* function in a cell because the mutant *APC* gene product can interfere with the function of the wild-type gene product (40,41).

APC is a large gene containing 15 exons and 2843 codons (40). The APC protein is involved in the control of cellular proliferation and apoptosis, as well as cellular adhesion. APC mutations are most commonly single base pair substitutions or short deletions or insertions that result in a truncated protein that loses all but one or two of seven β-catenin binding/degradation sites. Without this functional domain, APC cannot participate in the regulation of cytoplasmic β-catenin levels via APC-mediated degradation (in coordination with axin/conductin and glycogen synthase kinase 3β) (42–44). Degradation of β-catenin prevents its translocation into the nucleus where it binds one of the T-cell factors to initiate transcription of genes that promote cellular proliferation and prevent cell death such as *cyclin D* and *c-myc* (45,46).

The specific location of a germline mutation in *APC* may determine in part the disease phenotype (47). Mutations at either end of the gene (for example proximal to codon 158 or distal to codon 1900) are associated with an attenuated variant of the FAP characterized by sparse polyposis and a lack of desmoids, osteomas, or CHRPE (48), though phenotypic variation occurs in these families, with some family members still demonstrating a classic phenotype (49–53). Mutations between codons 1250 and 1330 are linked with profuse polyposis (54). CHRPE is present in patients in whom the mutation lies downstream to codon 463 but proximal to codon 1444 (55,56). Severe periampullary polyposis is associated with mutations downstream from codon 1051 (57), and desmoid tumors tend to occur with mutations between codons 1445 and 1578 (58,59). Such genotype–phenotype correlation will prove useful in increasing the accuracy and effectiveness of screening, surveillance, and treatment (60–62).

Genetic testing for FAP is commercially available and is the standard of care for families suspected of having the syndrome (see below) (9,10). Testing starts with a family member suspected of having FAP based on clinical presentation. If the disease-causing mutation can be identified, nonaffected family members can then be tested to determine if they too carry the mutation. Family members proven not to have inherited the respective mutation are spared screening and surveillance.

Recently, a small number of cases of FAP have been attributed to inherited defects of the base excision repair gene *MYH* (63,64). *MYH* is responsible for repair of G:C to T:A mutations that occur as a consequence of oxidative DNA damage (63). Germline *MYH* mutations must be biallelic to cause polyposis, so in this circumstance the adenomatous polyposis is the consequence of recessive rather than dominant inheritance as it is with germline *APC* mutations. Mutations in *MYH* may account for some of the cases of FAP that occur without a family history that had previously been felt to be secondary to spontaneous germline mutations of *APC*.

Surveillance and Treatment

Colonic and extracolonic screening and surveillance recommendations for FAP are summarized in Table 2 (3,65). Endoscopic surveillance will reduce rates of CRC and mortality in FAP patients (66). Individuals at risk for FAP should undergo annual flexible sigmoidoscopy beginning at age 10 to 12 years. Once adenomas have been identified, yearly colonoscopy is required. Colectomy should be undertaken once any of the polyps is ≥5 mm, or if any biopsies of any of the polyps demonstrate villous features or high-grade dysplasia. In families with suspected AAPC, surveillance should be undertaken with complete colonoscopy rather than sigmoidoscopy because of the proximal location of the polyps. Owing to the later onset of polyposis in these families, some experts recommend that surveillance can sometimes be safely deferred until approximately age 20. However, in the author's opinion, delaying the onset of surveillance in AAPC families can be problematic because of the phenotypic variability in such families.

Surveillance for upper tract adenomas is indicated in patients with FAP as well (20). Upper gastrointestinal (GI) endoscopy and duodenoscopy, with biopsy of the ampulla of

Table 2 Options for Cancer Prevention in FAP for Known or Suspected Gene Mutation Carriers

Primary recommendations
  Annual flexible sigmoidoscopy beginning by age 10–12 yr
  Annual colonoscopy, beginning by age 20 yr, when attenuated FAP suspected
  Prophylactic colectomy in teen years or when polyps detected at colonoscopy
  Endoscopic surveillance every 4–6 mo after ileorectal anastomosis and annually after ileoanal anastomosis
  Upper endoscopy, including duodenoscopy, every 6 mo to 3 yr starting by age 20–25 yr
Secondary recommendations
  Annual thyroid exam beginning by age 10–12 yr
  Annual palpation of liver during first decade of life (consider annual hepatic ultrasound and measure of alpha feto-protein)
  Consider serial MRI of brain in families with Turcot syndrome
  Consider serial MRCP or endoscopic ultrasound in families with multiple pancreatic cancers
  Consider use of sulindac or celecoxib chemoprevention in individuals with colorectal adenomas

Abbreviations: FAP, familial adenomatous polyposis; MRI, magnetic resonance imaging; MRCP, magnetic resonance cholangiopancreatography.

Vater, should be initiated once colonic adenomas have been identified, and no later than age 25 (65). Enteroscopy and/or enteroclysis also are advocated by some experts to exclude small bowel adenomas distal to the duodenum. However, significant lesions in the middle or distal small bowel are rare. The upper GI surveillance interval remains empirical, but generally screening should be undertaken every one to three years depending on the polyp burden encountered. Once detected, upper tract adenomas can be removed or ablated by a variety of methods, though there are no data to show that this regimen will improve long-term outcomes (67–69). If invasive cancer or high-risk adenomas are encountered (Spigelman stage IV) then operative resection is indicated. Unfortunately, surgical treatment of duodenal cancers still results in high mortality from metastatic disease (46%) and even those with severe adenomatosis are susceptible to death from metastatic disease (9%). Recurrence rates are also high unless pancreas-sparing duodenectomy is performed. It is therefore important to treat these lesions prior to the detection of invasive cancer and to follow carefully for recurrences (70).

All patients with FAP are destined to develop cancer of the colon or rectum. However, three crucial factors have led to a significant improvement in prognosis of these patients. They include the earlier identification of at-risk family members, endoscopic screening of colonic polyps in the premalignant stage, and definitive surgical treatment to eradicate the progression of colorectal polyposis to cancer. Although the use of chemoprevention has been shown to be beneficial in the reduction of the number and size of colorectal polyps (71,72), its use does not in any way replace surgery as definitive treatment.

Choice of Operation

Undoubtedly, the only way to completely eliminate the risk of cancer is to perform a total proctocolectomy with a permanent Brooke or Kock's ileostomy. These options were originally the only ones available to a patient population of young men and women, usually in their teens or twenties with normal preoperative bowel function. This limited choice resulted in some patients avoiding surgery because of fear of a lifelong stoma. Because of issues of self-image, sexuality, and quality of life, a total abdominal colectomy with an ileorectal anastomosis (IRA) became a more popular surgical alternative during the 1940s. The colon was removed, leaving only 15 cm of rectum for the anastomosis to the terminal ileum. The advantages of this procedure included the maintenance of intestinal continuity and avoided pelvic dissection, thus eliminating nerve damage affecting urinary and sexual function. The primary disadvantage, however, was the risk of developing severe polyposis or even cancer in the retained rectal stump. It was therefore only performed in patients who had rectal polyps that were amenable to endoscopic surveillance and removal. With the introduction of the total proctocolectomy with ileal pouch-anal anastomosis (IPAA) in 1979, patients had the option of eradicating almost all of the tissue at risk and still maintaining intestinal continuity. This operation involved removal of the entire abdominal colon and rectum with creation of a J, S, or W or lateral pouch from the terminal ileum. This ileal pouch was then anastomosed to the anal canal as a rectal reservoir. However, the disadvantages of this operation were the higher early and late complication rates associated with a procedure that was much more complex than the IRA. These young patients were subjected to the possibility of sexual dysfunction, pelvic sepsis, fecal incontinence, and a temporary or even a permanent ileostomy.

Recent studies evaluating the morbidity of IRA and IPAA show that they are comparable with overall complication rates for IRA ranging from 7% to 25% and those of IPAA from 24% to 60% (73–77). The most significant complications included anastomotic leak with associated pelvic abscess, wound infections, anastomotic strictures, and small bowel obstructions. Complications specific to IPAA included fistula formation, pouchitis and pouch failure, and urinary and sexual dysfunction. Complication rates have also been found to be worse in those patients converted from an IRA to IPAA as opposed to having an IPAA as their initial operation, 54% to 60% versus 34% to 40%, respectively (73,78).

The comparison of functional outcomes for these two operations is also an important consideration. The total number of stools per day (four to eight vs. three to five), the incidence of incontinence (2–25% vs. 0–15%), seepage (12–25% vs. 11%), urgency (21% vs. 8%), pad usage, and nighttime stools is higher in the IPAA patients (75,78–82). Yet the quality of life has frequently been reported as the same for both groups, indicating that patients are able to accept the slightly increased morbidity and poorer functional outcome of the IPAA in exchange for the diminished cancer risk.

The incidence of rectal cancer in the retained rectum also must be balanced with the morbidity of proctectomy. In patients who have had a total abdominal colectomy and IRA, the age-dependent risk of carcinoma in the retained rectal stump was originally reported to be between 10% and 18% up to the age of 50. It then rose sharply to 25% to 30% at age 60 (83,84). The cumulative incidence of rectal carcinoma in the retained rectal stump has also been shown to increase with time from the original operation as well as advancing age. In a large study of 659 patients from a Scandinavian registry, the cumulative incidence after an IRA was reported to be 4%, 12%, 17%, and 32% at 10, 20, 30, and 40 years after the operation, respectively (84). Interestingly, in a decision analysis using the same patients, the 10-year incidence was examined in those patients undergoing IRA both before and after 1980, the year the IPAA was introduced. The incidence of rectal cancer decreased from 5.1% to 2.1% in the patients who had IRA in the era of IPAA, indicating that patients were more appropriately selected for this surgical option (85). Other recent data have confirmed this significant decrease in the risk of carcinoma in the retained rectal stump. Other risk factors for rectal cancer after IRA include having greater than 20 polyps in the rectum, severe colonic polyposis at initial presentation, presence of CRC at time of IRA, and location of APC mutation between codons 1250 and 1464 (61,86–88). Surveillance of the residual rectum is also a factor that must be considered when choosing an operation. Two studies have demonstrated the difficulty in identifying patients who develop cancer in the setting of regular surveillance. As many as 75% of those diagnosed with rectal cancer have undergone endoscopy within the past 12 months (85,87). Therefore, this operation should only be performed if patients have less than 20 polyps in the rectum, no evidence of CRC, and most importantly, can be relied upon to comply with routine endoscopic surveillance of their rectum.

In consideration of the high risk of rectal cancer with IRA, a restorative proctocolectomy with IPAA has increasingly become the operation of choice for FAP. This operation theoretically removes almost all of the mucosa at risk and obviates the need for a possible proctectomy in the future. However, the incidence of cancer or adenomas after IPAA remains an important consideration and the role of mucosectomy to eliminate all residual rectal mucosa has been widely debated. When the procedure was first performed, all proctectomies involved transanal mucosectomy with a hand sewn anastomosis of the pouch to the anal canal. With the advent of the circular stapler, the double-stapled technique became widely popular because of the reduced incidence of operative and postoperative complications and the improved functional results. However, it was understood that to resect all of the rectum via the abdomen, a small amount of mucosa above the dentate line, known as the anal transition zone, would remain. This zone has been found to play a role in continence and the ability to discriminate gas and stool (89). It was also felt that the functional outcome was superior due to less manipulation of the anal canal during the operation (90). Comparison of the two techniques indicate that anastomotic stricture, sepsis, incontinence, daytime and nighttime seepage, pad usage, and need for an ileostomy are all higher in the mucosectomy group (91).

Yet the issue of residual mucosa that was at risk of developing cancer remained. Interestingly, the first case of cancer at the IPAA was reported in a patient 20 years after IPAA with mucosectomy (92). Since then a number of cases have been reported in patients who had mucosectomies (93), and a study done at the Mayo Clinic described residual rectal mucosa embedded within the rectal muscular cuff and the pouch in 4 of 26 pouches that were excised in patients who had mucosectomies performed, indicating that mucosectomy does not completely remove all the mucosa at risk. Additionally, reports of cancer arising in the anal transition zone and even the ileal pouch have now been described (94). Neoplastic polyps have also been noted in the pouch and anal canal and do not appear to be related to the degree of colonic polyposis or the presence of adenomas at the resection margins of the original surgery (95,96). Two studies comparing mucosectomy and hand sewn anastomosis with a double-stapled anastomosis found an increased incidence of adenomas at the anal transition zone in the latter group, with similar development of polyps within the pouch. The seven-year risk of anastomotic polyp development was 10% versus 31% for the two groups. None of these studies reported the presence of a cancer and so the actual risk of malignant transformation of pouch and anal canal polyps is unclear. Since the absolute risk estimate of developing polyps or cancer in the ileal pouch, ileoanal anastomosis, or anal transition zone is still not known, whether or not mucosectomy is performed, patients should undergo routine pouch and anal transition zone surveillance (91,97).

Other surgical controversies relating to IPAA include the role of laparoscopic surgery and the need for temporary diversion. As laparoscopic surgery of the colon is discussed in detail in another chapter it will not be included here. However, the use of a temporary diverting loop ileostomy to protect the IPAA and theoretically minimize the risk of pelvic sepsis and future pouch function is still ardently debated. Historically all patients undergoing IPAA had a temporary loop ileostomy created at the time of surgery. The pouch was then radiographically examined for leaks approximately six weeks after surgery and, if normal, the ileostomy was reversed. This method required a second surgery and hospitalization with their attended associated potential complications. When all pouches were hand sewn, this strategy seemed most sensible because the anastomosis was often technically difficult to perform with multiple suture lines creating ischemia and tension; anastomotic stenosis was expected. With the advent of circular staplers, the anastomosis became technically easier to perform and so avoidance of routine diversion was considered. Many studies have been done to compare the two techniques, and pelvic sepsis rates have ranged from 4% to 22% in the nondiverted population, which is comparable to the rate in patients who are diverted. However, all studies have concluded that patients must be carefully selected to achieve the best outcome (98,99). Advocates of nondiversion emphasize that patients undergoing restorative proctocolectomy for FAP, unlike patients with ulcerative colitis, are healthy, well nourished, with nondiseased colons and, not on steroids or immunosuppressive medications that would predispose them to anastomotic complications. However, the converse argument is that if postoperative sepsis results in pouch failure, the patient with mucosal ulcerative colitis (MUC) would more easily accept a permanent ileostomy than would the patient with FAP. Thus, the desire to avoid a second operation and three months of fecal diversion must be balanced against the potentially increased chance of inferior function and/or pouch excision due to postoperative pelvic sepsis. Only a thorough and well-detailed informed consent will allow selection of the appropriate choice in an individual patient. No study has compared diversion to nondiversion specifically in this population; however, one can extrapolate from the studies done in all patients with IPAA that FAP patients may be candidates for a one-stage operation.

Since the introduction of the ileal-pouch anal anastomosis in 1979, and continued selected use of IRA, ileostomies are infrequently used in FAP (100). End ileostomies are now reserved for those patients who have problems with fecal incontinence, who have advanced stage rectal cancers, who request this option, or in whom a restorative proctocolectomy was technically impossibly or failed.

After colectomy ongoing surveillance is required; if the rectum was retained, endoscopic examination should be performed approximately every 6 to 12 months to remove or ablate any adenomas found. The risk of rectal cancer in individuals with FAP with an IRA exceeds 10%, and upwards of 20% of patients who undergo a colectomy with IRA will ultimately require completion proctectomy (86). However, many of these patients can undergo conversion of an IRA to an IPAA. Nonetheless, even after IPAA, a substantial risk of the development of pouch adenomas exists, though the risk of developing invasive cancer appears to be low (95,97). Therefore, endoscopic examination of the ileal pouch is recommended every one to two years.

In addition to endoscopic screening, cancer prevention efforts in FAP may be augmented by chemoprevention with use of nonsteroidal anti-inflammatory drugs (NSAIDs) or cyclo-oxygenase 2 (COX-2)–selective inhibitors. Both the NSAID, sulindac, and the COX-2 inhibitor, celecoxib, have been demonstrated to reduce the size and number of adenomas in individuals with FAP (71,72). Unfortunately, in one study, the use of sulindac did not prevent the development of adenomas (101), but sulindac, celecoxib, and like drugs may slow polyp progression (102). They are unlikely to obviate the need for surgery in patients, as rectal cancer has been found to develop after the regression of polyps with continuous sulindac therapy (103) but may serve to delay the timing or prevent the need for a second operation in those with retained rectums. However, rectal carcinoma has been reported in a patient with IRA on local sulindac therapy (104). The exact role of these medications in the management of FAP remains to be elucidated.

Hereditary Hamartomatous Polyp Syndromes
Peutz–Jeghers Syndrome
Clinical Features

PJS is an autosomal dominantly inherited cancer predisposition syndrome characterized by the presence of numerous hamartomatous polyps in the GI tract and mucocutaneous pigmentation (105). This syndrome is rare, occurring in approximately 1 in 200,000 births (12). The classic mucocutaneous melanin pigment spots occur on the lips and buccal mucosa, but can also be found on other areas of the skin, such as the dorsal and volar aspects of the hands and feet (106). The spots are often most obvious among affected Caucasians with dark hair and skin tones, though PJS occurs among all races and skin types. Pigment spots can be identified in 95% of PJS patients, often from birth or early infancy. However, the spots can fade with age, and therefore the absence of typical pigmentation does not exclude the diagnosis. No malignant potential has been ascribed to the hyperpigmentation of PJS.

The predominant clinical feature of PJS is the presence of numerous GI harmartomatous polyps. The polyps have a distinctive histology with an arborizing pattern of smooth muscle in the lamina propria that distinguishes them from the hamartomas seen in juvenile polyposis or Cowden syndrome (107). The polyps can be pedunculated or sessile, and they range in size from several millimeters to giant polyps, 3–4 cm in size. The polyps occur throughout the GI tract, from esophagus to rectum. Polyps are seen in the stomach in approximately 40% of cases, in the small bowel in 80%, especially the jejunum, and in the colon and rectum in 40% (106,107). The polyps occur at a young age, and the typical age of diagnosis of PJS secondary to polyp complications is in the mid-20s. One-third of PJS patients will experience polyp-related symptoms by age 10, and 50% to 60% will have symptoms before the age 20 (108). The major complications related to PJS polyps are recurrent GI bleeding and obstruction, often secondary to intussusception. Upwards of 40% to 50% of PJS patients will require operation for polyp-related bowel obstruction at some point in time (106,109).

Although the typical PJS polyp is benign and without dysplasia, there is no doubt that PJS is associated with very high rates of intestinal and extra-intestinal cancer (110,111). The majority of PJS-related deaths after age 30 are secondary to malignancy, and the lifetime risk of cancer in PJS approaches 90% (111). Intestinal cancers may be secondary to the malignant degeneration of the hamartomatous polyps, and foci of dysplasia can sometimes be found in large PJS polyps (112). The majority of intestinal cancers are adenocarcinomas, though an increased risk for malignant GI stromal tumors, such as leiomyosarcoma, exists as well. Extra-intestinal cancers are also very common in PJS and, in fact, are more common than intestinal cancers. The most common extra-intestinal cancer is cancer of the pancreas. Increased risk for cancer of the breast, ovary, lung, cervix, uterus, and testes has been documented, as well as others (Table 3) (106,111). In addition to the more common intestinal and extra-intestinal cancers, PJS is associated with an increased frequency of unusual neoplastic and non-neoplastic tumors of the genital tract. Most of these lesions occur in women, and they are often small, bilateral, multifocal, and frequently benign. The lesions include ovarian sex cord tumors with annular tubules, mucinous neoplasms of the ovary, mucinous metaplasia of the fallopian tube, and extremely well-differentiated adenocarcinoma (adenoma malignum) of the cervix (12). Like women, men can also develop rare Sertoli cell or testicular tumors of the seminiferous tubules.

Table 3 Cancer Risk in Peutz–Jeghers Syndrome

Cancer site	Approximate lifetime risk (%)
All cancers	93
Gastrointestinal cancers	
Colorectal	39
Pancreas	36
Stomach	29
Small bowel	13
Esophagus	0.5
Nongastrointestinal cancers	
Breast	54
Ovary	21
Lung	15
Cervix	10
Uterus	9
Testes	9

Genetics

PJS is caused by a germ line mutation in the tumor-supressor *STK11* gene (also called *LKB1*) located on 19p. The *STK11* gene product is a serine-threonine kinase involved in the transduction of intracellular growth signals (113,114). Mutations in *STK11* can be documented in about one-half of PJS families. Some mutations may not be readily detectable by the methods generally employed, but it also is possible that some PJS families may be the consequence of germline mutations in other genes, possibly one or more of those in the *STK11* molecular pathway (115). As with FAP testing, if a pathogenic gene alteration can be detected in an affected family member, nonaffected family members can then be tested with essentially 100% accuracy.

Surveillance and Treatment

Although the lifetime risk of cancer in PJS is extremely high, the ability to reduce cancer incidence and cancer-related mortality in PJS patients through intensive surveillance remains unproved. Surveillance guidelines for PJS remain empirical and have not been formally adopted by any of the major professional organizations (Table 4) (65,106,116). However, most experts recommend surveillance and they further recommend that any intestinal polyps encountered, especially those greater than 1–1.5 cm in size be removed, even if that requires exploratory laparotomy and intraoperative endoscopy (117).

Juvenile Polyposis

Clinical Features

Juvenile polyps are common, occurring in about 2% of children. Typically, the polyps are few in number, with juvenile polyposis defined as the presence of 10 or more juvenile polyps. Approximately one-third of cases of juvenile polyposis have a hereditary etiology, whereas the remainder are sporadic. Hereditary juvenile polyposis is rare, occurring in roughly 1 in 100,000 individuals (116). Histologically juvenile polyps are hamartomas with a characteristic hyperplastic appearance of the surface epithelium, expansion of the lamina propria and frequent cyst formation with mucus engorgement. The characteristic cystically dilated glands have led these polyps also to be termed juvenile retention polyps (118). The polyps can range in size from several millimeters to

Table 4 Cancer Prevention Options in Peutz–Jeghers Syndrome

Upper endoscopy every 2 yr starting at age 10–15 yr
Enteroscopy/small bowel X-ray (small bowel follow through or enteroclysis) every 2 yr starting at age 10–15 yr
Colonoscopy every 3 yrs starting at age 15–20 yr
Removal of all polyps found > 1–1.5 cm (either by endoscopy methods or at laparotomy with intraoperative endoscopy)
Endoscopic ultrasound or MRCP every 1–2 yr starting at age 30 yr
Annual breast exam and mammography starting at age 25 yr
Annual pelvic exam, pap smear, transvaginal ultrasound, and CA-125 levels starting at age 20–25 yr
Annual testicular exam starting at age 10, with testicular ultrasound for onset of feminizing features

Abbreviation: MRCP, magnetic resonance cholangiopancreatography.

several centimeters, and they may be sessile or pedunculated, more often the latter. Juvenile polyps are most commonly found in the colon and rectum, but in hereditary juvenile polyposis, the polyps can be found throughout the GI tract, as well as in the colon and rectum (119). In contrast to individuals with sporadic juvenile polyps, those with hereditary juvenile polyposis will continue to form polyps throughout their lifetime.

The primary clinical manifestation of juvenile polyposis is colorectal bleeding. The blood loss may be occult, with subsequent development of iron deficiency anemia, or overt GI bleeding may occur (116). Bleeding from juvenile polyps is one of the leading causes of lower GI hemorrhage among children.

As with the other hereditary hamartomatous polyp syndromes, juvenile polyposis is associated with an increased risk for CRC (120,121). Increased cancer risk is not seen among individuals with sporadic juvenile polyps. The exact magnitude of the risk in hereditary juvenile polyposis remains uncertain, but may approach that seen in FAP. Cancer risk is certainly increased manyfold (122). CRC occurs in juvenile polyposis patients at a young age, often in the mid-30s (119,120). Cancer will arise from a juvenile polyp that has developed dysplastic/adenomatous features, and therefore, increased cancer risk can extend to other segments of the bowel involved with polyps. Individuals with many polyps with mixed histological features of juvenile polyps and adenomas are termed as having hereditary mixed polyposis syndrome. However, CRC can occur in individuals with no prior evidence of dysplastic polyps (116). It is not clear if there is an increased risk for extracolonic cancer in the absence of polyps in that segment of bowel, or if there is an increased risk of extra-intestinal cancer, such as pancreatic cancer.

Genetics

Hereditary juvenile polyposis is an autosomal dominant disorder, and disease-causing germline mutations can be found in about 50% of patients. The majority of mutations are found in *SMAD4*, located on 18q, and commercial genetic testing is available (119,123–125). *SMAD4* is a tumor suppressor gene of importance in the development of sporadic pancreatic and CRC, among others (126). *SMAD4* is a critical component of the growth inhibitory *TGFβ* signaling pathway (127). Some juvenile polyposis families are found to have disease-causing mutations in the *PTEN* gene (see below) (128) or in the bone morphogenetic protein receptor 1A (*BMPR1A*) gene (129). *BMPR1A* is a serine-threonine kinase type receptor belonging to the superfamily of *TGFβ* receptors involved in growth inhibitory signaling.

Surveillance and Treatment

There are no formal screening or surveillance recommendations for hereditary juvenile polyposis. In asymptomatic children from families with the syndrome, complete colonoscopy should commence in the early teen years and should be repeated every one to three years depending on the size and number of polyps found (65,116). Polyps found should be removed. In hereditary juvenile polyposis, as with all the hereditary polyposis syndromes, polyps will continue to recur throughout the patient's lifetime, and intensive surveillance should continue until age 70 (65). If the number of polyps is great, especially if polyps with dysplastic features are encountered, colectomy is indicated. At the time that colonic polyps are detected, upper endoscopy and small bowel contrast X rays should be performed to look for extracolonic polyps. If none are found, repeat upper GI screening exams may be performed approximately every one to three years (65,116).

Cowden Syndrome
Clinical Features

Cowden syndrome, also termed the gingival multiple hamartoma syndrome, is a rare syndrome (1 in 200,000 individuals) characterized by skin lesions, intestinal hamartomas, and an increased risk of cancer (12). The syndrome is hereditary with an autosomal dominant means of transmission. The syndrome is most widely recognized on the basis of characteristic mucocutaneous lesions that include facial trichilemmomas, acral keratoses, café au lait spots, and verrucous papules of the oral mucosa, gingiva, and tongue. Subcutaneous lipomas and fibromas are common, as are benign thyroid nodules, uterine leiomyomas, and fibrocystic disease of the breast. The characteristic cutaneous lesions are found in approximately 85% of Cowden syndrome patients. Sixty percent of Cowden patients develop hamartomatous polyps of the GI tract (116,130). The GI polyps most often resemble juvenile polyps, but other benign GI tract polyps can occur as well, including lipomas, ganglioneuromas, inflammatory polyps, and lymphoid hyperplasia (118). Juvenile-type polyps that contain some neural elements are particularly characteristic of the syndrome.

The syndrome is often associated with congenital abnormalities (50% of the time) that include craniomegaly and mental retardation. Families with macrocephaly, lipomas, and pigmentation of the glans penis belong to the Bannayan–Ruvalcaba–Riley syndrome (syndrome variations have been termed Soto syndrome, Ruvalcaba–Myhre syndrome, and Bannyan–Zonana syndrome), whereas those with glial mass in the cerebellum leading to altered gait and seizures belong to the subsyndrome called Lhermitte–Duclos disease (12).

Cowden syndrome is a cancer susceptibility syndrome, and cancer is the primary source of morbidity and mortality among affected individuals. The lifetime incidence of breast cancer among women with Cowden syndrome is 25% to 50%, and the cancer often is bilateral and with an early age of onset (median age 41 years) (12). Individuals with Cowden syndrome also have a lifetime risk of follicular carcinoma of the thyroid that approaches 10%. Though many affected individuals have GI tract hamartomas, an excess of GI cancer risk has not been clearly described (116,130). There is probably a modest increased risk for CRC among individuals with colorectal hamartomas. Increased risk for other cancers is also likely present, including skin, ovary, uterus, lung, and kidney.

Genetics
Cowden syndrome, and its associated subsyndromes, are caused by a germ-line mutation in the tumor supressor gene *PTEN* on 10q (131,132). *PTEN* is an intracellular tyrosine phosphatase that has been shown to be mutated in a significant percentage of sporadic tumors, including glioblastomas, prostate, thyroid, and kidney cancers. *PTEN* mutation testing is commercially available, and mutations can be detected in about 90% of affected individuals (12). The principles of clinical genetic testing would mirror those in FAP, PJS, and hereditary juvenile polyposis.

Screening, Surveillance, and Treatment
The major cancer morbidity from Cowden syndrome is secondary to breast cancer. Breast cancer surveillance should commence at age 20 (monthly self-exam and yearly physician exam and mammography) (12). Annual thyroid exams are recommended to start in the teens. No guidelines regarding GI screening or surveillance have been established (130). Upon diagnosis, it makes sense to perform upper and lower GI endoscopy to look for GI polyps. Among individuals with GI polyps, regular surveillance and polypectomy is likely wise. Those without polyps initially might undergo screening colonoscopy starting at age 40, with repeat exams every three to five years.

Gorlin Syndrome
Gorlin syndrome is a rare autosomal dominantly inherited condition (1 in 55,000 people) characterized by multiple basal cell nevi and carcinomas (12). The condition is also called the basal cell nevus syndrome and accounts for about 0.5% of persons with basal cell carcinoma. The carcinomas often first occur before 30 years of age, with 90% of affected individuals with cancer by age 40. Other features of the syndrome include odontogenic or polyostotic bone cysts, facial congenital defects including macrocephaly, cleft lip or palate, congenital skeletal abnormalities of the ribs and/or spine, ectopic calcification of the falx cerebri, cardiac, or ovarian fibromas, medulloblastoma, and characteristic pits of the skin of the palms and soles (three or more pits). Rarely, GI hamartomas occur (12,130). The syndrome is caused by a germline mutation in the *PTC* gene on 9q (12). Spontaneous germline mutations of PTC are the cause of Gorlin syndrome in greater than 50% of cases.

Hereditary Neural Polyposis Syndromes
Neurofibromatosis Type 1
Neurofibromatosis type 1 (NF1), also called von Recklinghsausen disease, is defined by the presence of café-au-lait spots (5 or >0.5 cm), multiple cutaneous or subcutaneous neurofibromas, multiple axillary or inguinal freckles, bilateral optic nerve gliomas, multiple hamartomas of the iris, and congenital abnormalities of the long bones (bowing or thinning of the cortex)

(12,130). Seizures are reported in 3% to 5% of affected individuals and learning disabilities in 25% to 40%. This condition is caused by the autosomal dominant inheritance of a mutated *NF1* gene located on 17q (12). *NF1* encodes a guanosine triphosphatase–activating protein. Approximately 25% of patients with *NF1* have intestinal polypoid neurofibromas or ganglioneuromas (130). The polyps are most commonly found in the small bowel, but can occur in the stomach and colon as well. In most cases, the polyps are clinically silent, but can rarely cause abdominal pain or hemorrhage.

Multiple Endocrine Neoplasia Type 2

Multiple endocrine neoplasia type 2 (MEN2) is characterized by the presence of medullary carcinoma of the thyroid, pheochromocytoma, parathyroid hyperplasia or adenomas, marfanoid habitus, and ganglioneuromas of the GI tract (12). The ganglioneuromas occur in nearly all patients with MEN2B, and they occur throughout the GI tract, but are most common in the colon and rectum (130). The polyps are often clinically silent. However, generalized dysmotility of the GI tract is often associated with the disease and may be in part secondary to the intestinal ganglioneurons. MEN2 is caused by a germline mutation in the *RET* proto-oncogene (12). The condition is transmitted in autosomal dominant fashion, though about 50% of cases are secondary to a spontaneous, new germline mutation.

Sporadic (Nonhereditary) Polyposis Syndromes
Hyperplastic Polyposis

Hyperplastic polyposis is defined as the presence of 10 or more typical colorectal hyperplastic polyps. Most cases of hyperplastic polyposis involve the occurrence of diminutive (one to several millimeters) polyps located in the rectum and left colon. This phenomenon likely is sporadic in etiology and not associated with an increased risk for CRC. Rarely patients may have tens to hundreds of diminutive hyperplastic polyps throughout the colon, simulating FAP (133,134). Whether or not cancer risk is increased in these patients is unclear. Very rarely, patients with hyperplastic polyposis have giant (up to 2–3 cm) polyps, often found in the proximal colon (133–135). In this circumstance an increased risk for CRC is likely (133,134,136), though the magnitude of the risk remains uncertain. Some experts recommend polypectomy for these large hyperplastic polyps and increased colonic surveillance in these patients (133). However, the risks and benefits of this approach are unknown and such recommendations remain controversial. If the hyperplastic polyps have a mixed hyperpastic/adenomatous histology, the polyps are properly classified as being serrated adenomas. When serrated polyposis is present, the increased risk for CRC is clear, and the polyps must be removed, if possible by endoscopy, or if necessary, by colectomy. The genetic basis of hyperplastic or serrated polyposis is uncertain, but likely involves a type of mutator pathway (134,137–140). The molecular pathway to the giant hyperplastic polyp and/or serrated adenoma may be the consequence of the CpG island methylator phenotype, with promoter methylation and inactivation of the hyperplastic polyposis 1 (*HPP1*) gene on 2q (139,141,142). Whether or not some cases of hyperplastic polyposis are hereditary is unclear. Most cases appear to be sporadic, however, the hyperplastic/serrated polyposis has been described in families, suggesting a hereditary component in a minority of cases (130,134).

Cronkhite-Canada Syndrome

Cronkhite-Canada syndrome is an acquired condition with an average age of onset during the sixth to seventh decade of life (133,143). No familial occurrences of Cronkhite-Canada syndrome have been reported. The syndrome is extremely rare, with a worldwide distribution, and has no known cause. Cronkhite-Canada is more common in men (60%) than women and is characterized by the onset of generalized GI polyposis, with esophageal sparing, in association with cutaneous hyperpigmentation, hair loss, nail atrophy, and hypogeusia (133). The polyps are sessile and innumerable, and range in size from several millimeters to several centimeters. On histological examination the polyps resemble juvenile polyps, though dysplastic changes do rarely occur (144).

Cronkhite-Canada syndrome has an acute onset and is progressive, though symptomatic remission does occur in a minority of cases (130,133,145). The primary clinical manifestations are that of progressive diarrhea, often with significant malabsorption and protein-losing enteropathy (133). Malnutrition is common, and the condition can be fatal. For those with a more protracted course of illness, the lifetime incidence of CRC exceeds 10% (146,147). The primary therapy is supportive care (130). Patients often require nutritional support and may require total parenteral nutrition to prevent severe dehydration and malnutrition (148). If a particular segment of the GI tract is heavily involved with polyps, then operative resection may be helpful (133). Other interventions that have been tried with uncertain efficacy include administration of corticosteroids and antibiotics (148).

Inflammatory Polyposis

Inflammatory polyps, often called pseudopolyps, can occur during the healing phase of any inflammatory injury to the GI tract. Inflammatory polyps are most commonly seen in individuals with ulcerative colitis or Crohn's disease affecting the colon (149). They can also occur during the healing phase of other colitides, such as ischemic colitis (133). The polyps have a characteristic filiform appearance and on histological examination represent tissues with inflammatory elements that persist during healing (150). Inflammatory polyps may be few in number, or they may be innumerable, and their size ranges from several millimeters to several centimeters (133). The polyps have no malignant potential themselves, though they are often associated with longstanding chronic colitis and its attendant risk of colitis-related dysplasia and cancer.

Inflammatory polyposis is an acquired condition. However, a case of familial inflammatory intestinal polyposis has been described and termed Devon polyposis (130).

Lipomatous Polyposis

Intestinal lipomas are benign tumors consisting of collections of adipose tissue in the submucosa. Solitary lipomas are common in the intestine, most often occurring in the vicinity or involving the ileocecal valve. Diffuse lipomatous polyposis is an extremely rare condition (133,151). The polyps may occur in the small bowel, large bowel, or both. There is an association of diffuse intestinal lipomatous polyposis and lipomatosis or hypertrophy of the appendices epiploicae of the colon (152). Diffuse lipomatous polyposis is usually asymptomatic, but patients may present with GI bleeding, diarrhea, intussusception, or obstruction (133,153).

Nodular Lymphoid Hyperplasia

Nodular lymphoid hyperplasia refers to a condition in which numerous lymphoid nodules are found in the small intestine, large intestine, or both (154). Histologically, the nodules are enlarged lymphoid clusters with germinal centers in the lamina propria or submucosa (154). Lymphoid hyperplasia occurs most frequently in individuals with immune deficiencies such as common variable immune deficiency (CVID) or the acquired immune deficiency syndrome (133,155). Nodular plymphoid hyperplasia can also occur in individuals without immune system dysfunction and may be identified at as many as 3% of autopsies (133). In most cases, nodular lymphoid hyperplasia is asymptomatic, but it can be associated with diarrhea and malabsorption. This is especially true among those individuals with CVID (133,156). CVID patients will often have Giardiasis that must be treated. The mucosal disease associated with CVID can respond to treatment with corticosteroids or immune modulators, such as azathioprine (133,156).

Lymphomatous Polyposis

Multiple lymphomatous polyposis (MLP) is a rare manifestation of intestinal lymphoma. MLP is a non-Hodgkin B-cell lymphoma that appears to be the GI counterpart of mantle cell lymphoma, and extra-intestinal lymphoma is often present (130,133). Multiple nodular/polypoid lesion of the GI tract also may be seen in Mediterranean-type lymphoma. Mediterranean-type lymphoma of the gut begins as an intense proliferation of plasma cells in the lamina propria, with eventual malignant transformation (130). This lymphoma is almost always associated with production of an abnormal IgA paraprotein (130).

Hereditary Nonpolyposis Colorectal Cancer

Clinical Features

HNPCC, like FAP, is an autosomal dominant disorder characterized by the occurrence of multiple CRCs in a family. HNPCC is also called the Lynch syndrome after Henry Lynch (157) a pioneer in the field of familial cancer, who has devoted much of his career to the description of the syndrome and the care of affected families. HNPCC accounts for approximately 1% to 5%

of all CRC cases (7,8,158–161). Hereditary nonpolyposis CRC is a misnomer because adenomatous polyps are the precursor of CRC in the syndrome. Unlike FAP, the number of polyps appears not much greater than in the general population, but the polyps are far more likely to be flat, to have villous features or high-grade dysplasia, and more importantly, to grow rapidly and progress to invasive cancer (162–167). Population-based data on HNPCC gene carriers are few, but individuals with HNPCC appear to have a lifetime risk of CRC of about 80% (168–171). The mean age of onset of CRC in HNPCC is approximately 45, but may appear in the teens (157,163). Furthermore, synchronous and metachronous CRC is far more common in HNPCC than in sporadic CRC. Synchronous cancers are present in 5% to 20% of patients and the rate of metachronous cancers approaches 1% to % per year, depending on the length of colon remaining after initial resection (172). This represents a manyfold increase in the rate of metachronous cancers compared with the sporadic CRC (173). Also, compared with sporadic CRC, HNPCC cancers are more commonly on the right side of the colon, more poorly differentiated, and have other unusual histological characteristics, most importantly, the presence of tumor infiltrating lymphocytes (174–176). Nonetheless, several studies have found that survival is better than in sporadic cancer when matched for stage (177–181).

The risk for other cancers in HNPCC is greatly increased. For example, endometrial cancer will occur in 20% to 60% of women with HNPCC, as compared with 3% in the general population (168). Individuals with HNPCC also are at an increased risk of gastric, ovarian, small bowel, transitional cell (renal pelvis and ureter), sebaceous, central nervous system, and possibly other cancers (Table 5) (168,169,171,182). When HNPCC was first described in the 1920s, gastric cancer was the primary malignancy. The decreasing frequency of gastric cancers and increasing frequency of CRCs in HNPCC kindred has mirrored this change in the general population in Western Europe and the United States (163,183). Gastric cancer is still an important part of HNPCC in regions in which that cancer is endemic, such as Korea (184,185). The occurrence of sebaceous adenomas, carcinomas, and keratoacanthomas in conjunction with HNPCC-related visceral malignancies define the Muir-Torre syndrome, a variant of HNPCC (186,187). Some cases of Turcot syndrome are also variants of HNPCC, with glioblastoma as the associated central nervous system cancer (35,36).

Diagnostic Criteria
Obtaining a personal and family cancer history from all patients is critical, and a high index of suspicion needs to be maintained if individuals with HNPCC are to be detected. Many diagnostic criteria have been proposed for HNPCC, the best known of which are the Amsterdam criteria (188). The criteria are (i) histologically verified CRC in three or more relatives, one of whom is a first-degree relative of the other two, having excluded FAP; (ii) CRC involving at least two generations; and (iii) one or more of the CRCs diagnosed before age 50. The criteria were designed specifically to facilitate research on HNPCC before the mutations responsible for the syndrome had been identified, but are felt to be overly restrictive and insensitive (189–192). In response to this problem, a number of other less stringent diagnostic criteria and guidelines for HNPCC have been promulgated, including the Amsterdam II criteria and the Bethesda guidelines (Table 6) (193,194). The Bethesda guidelines have been modified (10) and are currently in the process of being further modified. At the heart of all of these criteria are certain basic features that are typical of HNPCC: early age of onset of colorectal or endometrial cancer (<50 years of age), multiple family members with colorectal,

Table 5 Lifetime Risk for Cancer Among Hereditary Nonpolyposis Colorectal Cancer Gene Carriers

Cancer type	Lifetime risk (%)
Colorectal	70–80
Endometrial	20–60
Ovarian	10–12
Gastric	5–13
Renal pelvis/ureter/kidney	4–10
Biliary tract/gallbladder/pancreas	2–18
Small bowel	1–4
CNS (usually glioblastoma)	1–4

Abbreviation: CNS, central nervous system.

Table 6 Clinical Criteria for HNPCC

Name	Criteria
Amsterdam	There should be at least three relatives with CRC; all the following criteria should be present One should be the first-degree relative of the other two At least two successive generations should be affected At least one CRC should be diagnosed before age 50 Familial adenomatous polyposis should be excluded
Amsterdam II	There should be at least three relatives with an HNPCC-associated cancer (CRC, cancer of the endometrium, small bowel, ureter, or renal pelvis); all the following criteria should be present: One should be the first-degree relative of the other two At least two successive generations should be affected At least one CRC should be diagnosed before age 50 Familial adenomatous polyposis should be excluded
Bethesda (modified)	Individuals with cancer in families that fulfill the Amsterdam criteria Individuals with two HNPCC-related cancers, including synchronous or metachronous CRCs or associated extra-colonic cancers Individuals with CRC and a first-degree relative with CRC and/or HNPCC-related extracolonic cancer and/or colorectal adenoma; one of the cancers diagnosed at < 50 yr and the adenoma diagnosed at < 40 yr Individuals with CRC or endometrial cancer diagnosed at < 50 yr Individuals with right-sided CRC with an undifferentiated pattern (solid/cribriform) on histopathology diagnosed at < 50 yr Individuals with signet-ring-cell-type CRC diagnosed at < 50 yr Individuals with adenomas diagnosed at < 40 yr

Abbreviations: CRC, colorectal cancer; HNPCC, hereditary nonpolyposis colorectal cancer.

endometrial, or another HNPCC-related cancer, and multiple HNPCC-related cancers in the same individual. If one or more of these features is identified, the diagnosis of HNPCC should be considered. It should be pointed out, however, that the personal and family cancer history need not be very striking in cases of HNPCC detected in the general population, so vigilance is required.

Genetics

The genetic basis of HNPCC is a germline mutation in one of a set of genes responsible for DNA mismatch repair (MMR), and the syndrome might be best termed the hereditary deficient MMR syndrome (195). The growing number of MMR genes include *MSH2, MLH1, PMS1, PMS2, MSH3, MSH6,* and others (196–201). Over 90% of the identified mutations are in two genes, *MSH2* and *MLH1*, located on chromosome 2p and 3p, respectively (202). Upwards of 5% to 10% of HNPCC families, often with some atypical or attenuated features, will be accounted for by a germline mutation in *MSH6* (201,203–208). Persons with HNPCC have a nonfunctioning copy of the gene in the germ line, usually through an inherited, or occasionally spontaneous, germline mutation. When the remaining working copy of the gene is inactivated by mutation, loss, or other mechanisms, the cell loses the ability to repair the inevitable mismatches of DNA base pairs during DNA replication, as well as short insertion and deletion loops (209,210).

Particularly vulnerable to mutation during replication are DNA regions in which nucleotide bases are repeated several or many times. Such DNA-repeat sequences are distributed throughout the genome (most commonly A_n/T_n or CA_n/GT_n) and are called microsatellites. Greater than 90% of CRCs in HNPCC demonstrate multiple change-of-length mutations of these microsatellites, termed microsatellite instability (MSI) (211–213). MSI is classified as being absent, low, or high depending on the frequency of microsatellite mutation. The instability of HNPCC tumors is almost always high frequency (214,215). Microsatellites are found in the coding regions of genes involved in growth regulation such as the gene for the transforming growth factor β (TGF-β) receptor type II and *BAX* (216–220). Mutations of these genes are common in tumors with high-frequency MSI. The binding of TGFβ with its receptor is important in inhibition of cellular proliferation, and *BAX* is important in the induction of programmed cell death (apoptosis). A simple laboratory assay can detect the presence or absence and degree of MSI in tumor tissue using a standard set of microsatellite markers. The optimal choice of markers remains an area of investigation, and the National Cancer Institute recently convened a workshop to determine if the recommended marker set should be changed. In addition, tumors that have lost the function of one of the MMR genes show negative staining for the protein product of that gene by immunohistochemistry. Staining tumors for MSH2 or MLH1 also may aid in the diagnosis of HNPCC (221–224).

As with *APC*, the specific mutations in the MMR genes (genotype) correlates with the observed phenotype. For example, extracolonic tumors are more common with *MSH2* mutation than *MLH1* mutation. Families with an *MSH6* mutation tend to have a more attenuated phenotype (later age of onset and lower percentage of gene carriers developing cancer) and an abundance of endometrial cancers when compared with *MSH2* or *MLH1* gene-carrying families (171,225,226). As in FAP, a better understanding of genotype–phenotype correlation will lead to improved HNPCC screening, surveillance, and treatment.

Genetic testing for HNPCC, as well as tumor analysis for MSI and MMR protein immunostaining, is commercially available. Molecular diagnostics for HNPCC is now recommended (9) and, in the correct circumstances, can greatly facilitate the care of individuals and families suspected of having the syndrome (see below) (227).

Surveillance and Treatment

Recommendations for surveillance in individuals with known or suspected HNPCC are summarized in Table 7. Colonoscopy is recommended every one to three years starting at age 20, or at least 10 years before the earliest age of cancer in the family (228). Some experts have recommended more frequent surveillance (65,229), e.g., that the surveillance frequency be increased to yearly starting at age 40 (230). Complete colonoscopy is essential because of the preponderance of right-sided tumors in HNPCC. Colonoscopy needs to be repeated frequently because of accelerated rate at which adenomas transform into invasive cancer in HNPCC. Colonoscopic surveillance is of demonstrated efficacy in HNPCC. Individuals that undergo regular total colonic surveillance have a markedly lower incidence of CRC, CRC-related mortality, and all-cause mortality, than those not undergoing regular surveillance (231), and surveillance is cost effective (232,233).

In addition to CRC surveillance, endometrial cancer surveillance is recommended for individuals at risk for HNPCC (228). There is no consensus on the optimal method of surveillance, but choices include yearly endometrial biopsy or yearly transvaginal ultrasound, which also serves as a surveillance test for ovarian cancer, especially if coupled with regular (every 6–12 months) determination of CA-125 levels. Surveillance for other HNPCC-related cancers is not generally recommended. However, recommendations should be tailored to the tumors appearing in the family being treated. For example, genitourinary cancers may be screened by periodic urine cytology and gastric cancer by upper GI endoscopy. The need for and efficacy of surveillance for extracolonic cancer in HNPCC remains unproved (234,235).

With respect to treatment for colon cancers associated with HNPCC, many experts advocate total abdominal colectomy with IRA at the time of the initial cancer resection because of the high rate of metachronous tumors (65,236). However, what appears to be most important is adequate postoperative surveillance, rather than the extent of the initial resection (233). Unless patients are diagnosed with synchronous cancers, or they cannot be relied upon to follow up

Table 7 Options for Cancer Prevention in Hereditary Nonpolyposis Colorectal Cancer for Known or Suspected Gene Mutation Carriers

---

Primary recommendations

    Colonoscopy every 1–2 yr beginning at age 20–25 (or 10 yr before the earliest diagnosis of colorectal cancer in the family, whichever comes first) until age 40 and then annual colonoscopy

    Annual transvaginal ultrasound with color Doppler and/or endometrial aspirate beginning at age 25–35

Secondary recommendations

    Consider total abdominal colectomy with ileorectal anastomosis at diagnosis of colorectal cancer

    Consider prophylactic hysterectomy and oopherectomy in known gene carriers at time of colonic operation or after childbearing complete

    Consider annual measure of CA-125 level

    Consider serial upper endoscopy among families with gastric cancer

    Consider annual urine cytology among families with urinary tract cancers

---

for colonoscopic surveillance, a partial colectomy can be offered. As with FAP, the rate of rectal cancer in HNPCC can exceed 10% over an extended follow up period, so ongoing surveillance is essential, even if an IRA is performed (237). When adenomas are encountered during surveillance colonoscopy, they are removed endoscopically using standard techniques, and in general, colonoscopic surveillance is continued. However, HNPCC-related polyps are often sessile, so adequate endoscopic resection can be difficult to perform. If there is any doubt, one should proceed with operative resection. Because of the high risk of endometrial and ovarian cancer, some experts have advocated prophylactic hysterectomy and oophorectomy for women beyond childbearing age, especially if they are undergoing a colonic resection for CRC. A recent consensus, however, found insufficient evidence to recommend for or against prophylactic hysterectomy and oophorectomy (228).

Common Familial CRC

Clinical Features

The rare hereditary syndromes such as FAP and HNPCC, confer the highest risks of colon cancer; however, these entities account for no more than 5% of all CRCs. Nevertheless, familial history is an important risk factor in the development of CRC, suggesting a critical hereditary component in upwards of 25% of cases (3,238). The magnitude of the risk depends on the number of first-degree relatives affected and the age at diagnosis (Table 8) (4). In a recent meta-analysis, individuals with a single first-degree relative with CRC have a risk about 2.25 times that in the general population. Individuals with more than one first-degree relatives with CRC have a risk about 4.25 times that in the general population, and individuals with a relative diagnosed with CRC before the age of 45 have a risk about four times higher than the general population (4). Individuals with a first-degree relative with colorectal adenoma also have a risk of colon cancer about twice that in the general population (239). Colon cancer in a second- or third-degree relative increases colon cancer risk, but only about 50% above average risk (230). Importantly, individuals with a first-degree relative with a family history of colon cancer have a colon cancer risk at age 40, which is similar to the general population risk at age 50 (Fig. 2) (230,240). Though family history of CRC increases an individual's risk for the disease, especially at a younger age than seen in pure sporadic cancer, there is no convincing evidence yet that the clinical presentations of these common familial CRCs differ in important ways from sporadic CRC with respect to features such as tumor location or aggressiveness.

Genetics

The gene alterations responsible for common familial CRC are being discovered in increasingly greater numbers, though for the most part these cancer susceptibility alleles remain unknown (2,5). Kindred studies suggest that these genes are dominantly inherited, but unlike in true hereditary CRC, the altered genes that cause familial CRC are generally low penetrance (241). Thus, inheriting a disease susceptibility gene increases one's risk for CRC, but by no means guarantees that the disease will occur. Candidate susceptibility alleles are many and include minor mutations in the same genes that cause hereditary CRC. An example of this is the *I1307K* allele of *APC* found in Ashkenazi Jews (242). The protein product of the allele is full length and functional, but 30 times more likely to mutate than the wild-type allele, most commonly through an insertion that leads to APC protein truncation (243,244). Inheritance of this unstable *APC* allele increases the chance of developing CRC by approximately

Table 8 Risk for CRC Based on Family History

Family history	Lifetime risk for colorectal cancer
No family history	3–6%
One first-degree relative with CRC	2–3-fold increased risk
One first-degree relative with CRC < age 50	3–5-fold increased risk
Two first-degree relatives with CRC	3–5-fold increased risk
One second- or third-degree relative with CRC	1.5-fold increased risk
Two second- or third-degree relatives with CRC	2–3-fold increased risk
One first-degree relative with adenoma	1.5–2-fold increased risk

Abbreviation: CRC, colorectal cancer.

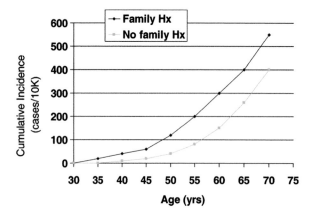

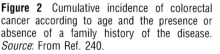

Figure 2 Cumulative incidence of colorectal cancer according to age and the presence or absence of a family history of the disease. *Source*: From Ref. 240.

one-and-a-half to twofold, rather than the near 100% risk of CRC that occurs in classic FAP (245). A recent large community-based study of Ashkenazi Jews was estimated that by age 70, 5.1% of allele carriers will develop CRC compared with 3.1% of noncarriers (245). It appears that the magnitude of increased risk conferred by carriage of *APC I1307K* is low to modest, and there is still little evidence that the adenomas or CRC in those with *I1307K* appears at an earlier age or differs presentation or prognosis from sporadic (246–252). Nevertheless, even a small increase in CRC risk conferred by a gene that is common in a particular population will have important implications for that population.

The *I1307K APC* allele is only one example of the minor CRC susceptibility genes that will be identified with increasing frequency in the future. Other CRC predisposition alleles likely include one of a number of variants of genes involved in carcinogen metabolism, or certain inherited alleles of many of the oncogenes and tumor suppressor genes involved in the molecular progression of sporadic CRC (2,5,253). CRC resistance genes will likely be described as well. The particular combination of minor susceptibility and resistance genes a person inherits will prove to be a major determinant of the differing risk of CRC between individuals.

Surveillance and Treatment

Several different screening recommendations for individuals with familial risk have been published. A recent task force, comprising several different professional organizations, recommended that CRC screening in individuals with a family history of CRC be the same as the screening recommended for the general public, but that this screening start at age 40 (230). Screening options for the general population include yearly fecal occult blood testing or flexible sigmoidoscopy every five years, or both, or air-contrast barium enema every 5 to 10 years, or colonoscopy every 10 years. The task force also recommends that special efforts be made to ensure compliance particularly for those in whom the relative had an adenomatous polyp before the age of 60 or colon cancer before the age of 55. In contrast, the American College of Gastroenterology recommends that individuals with a strong family history of colon cancer, e. g. , those with multiple first-degree relatives with CRC, or a single first-degree relative with cancer diagnosed age less than 60, should undergo screening colonoscopy starting at age 40, or 10 years younger than the age at diagnosis of the youngest affected relative. They then recommend that colonoscopy be repeated at three- to five-year intervals (254). The U.S. Preventive Services Task Force does not address familial risk outside of the hereditary syndromes (255). Treatment of colon and rectal cancer in this setting involves partial colectomy with close surveillance of the residual colon and rectum thereafter.

Genetic Testing for Hereditary CRC

Available Tests

Genetic tests are commercially available for FAP, HNPCC (*MSH2* and *MLH1*), and the *I1307K APC* allele. Testing for PJS, juvenile polyposis, and Cowden syndrome also is becoming available through commercial laboratories (256–258). Genetic testing for common familial CRC will certainly become common in the near future. The germline genetic tests typically are performed on DNA extracted from white blood cells obtained from a blood sample. The laboratories that provide these tests, the tests themselves, and their costs are constantly changing. An online reference for genetic testing laboratories and location of genetics professionals can be found (259).

Methods of Mutation Detection

Commercial laboratories employ various methods of mutation detection in FAP and HNPCC, which is made difficult because the genes are large and the known mutations are scattered throughout the genes. Further, many families harbor their own unique mutation. Unlike many other genetic disorders, a single or a few very common mutations cannot be easily and rapidly detected (2,6). Direct gene sequencing remains the most precise method for mutation detection, but is time consuming and expensive even with robotics (260). To circumvent searching for all mutations by sequencing, other techniques for screening mutations are employed, such as single-strand conformational polymorphism and denaturing gradient gel electrophoresis, or the in vitro synthesized protein assay, also called the protein truncation test. Even sequencing is not 100% sensitive, as it can miss certain mutations, such as large genomic deletions or rearrangements, and high specificity can be difficult to achieve because of the detection of numerous simple amino acid alterations (missense changes) that are often harmless polymorphisms but may be deleterious mutations. Because of insufficient data, these DNA alterations are often labeled variants of uncertain significance (2,6,260). Because the sensitivity of sequencing is less than 100% some laboratories also offer other techniques, such as haploconversion or Southern blot analysis, in an effort to detect mutations, such as gene promoter mutations or large deletions that would be missed by sequencing (261,262).

Once a particular mutation has been identified in a family, the search for that mutation in other family members can be accomplished rapidly, accurately, and inexpensively. The most commonly used technique relies on the detection of hybridization between the DNA to be tested and a DNA sequence that carries the known mutation. The *APC I1307K* allele also can be detected in this fashion.(2,260).

Microsatellite Instability Testing and Protein Immunohistochemistry in HNPCC

Since the large majority of HNPCC-related tumors (90–100%) demonstrate high-frequency instability (MSI-H), MSI testing of tumors is advocated as a way of screening for HNPCC (10,192,194). The MSI assay can be performed on tissues that have been formalin-fixed and embedded in paraffin. In unselected colorectal tumors the specificity of MSI-H for HNPCC is low because 10% to 15% of all CRCs will demonstrate MSI-H but only 10% to 15% of these are due to a germline HNPCC mutation (263). As the sensitivity of MSI-H in HNPCC-related tumors is not 100%, some investigators caution that germline HNPCC testing should not be abandoned if MSI-H is not found when the clinical history is compelling (190). Immunostaining for the MMR gene proteins in tumors has also been advocated as a method of screening for HNPCC prior to germline genetic testing (221,224). As with MSI testing, the absence of protein staining, especially *MLH1*, does not guarantee HNPCC. This is because the MMR gene proteins may be inactivated solely within the tumor (somatic inactivation) in a minority of sporadic cancers (264). Furthermore, as with MSI testing, the sensitivity of protein staining is not 100% because gene inactivation can occur, but protein staining may still be present in the tumor. In fact, protein immunostaining is less sensitive than MSI testing as a screening test for HNPCC (192). Both tumor MSI analysis and tumor *MSH2* and *MLH1* protein immunohistochemistry are commercially available.

Genetic Counseling and Informed Consent

Prior to genetic testing for hereditary CRC, genetic counseling and informed consent are essential (265). Genetic counseling for hereditary cancer is best performed by trained genetic counselors in conjunction with physicians who are experts on the disease, such as a gastroenterologist, oncologist, or surgeon (256). Genetic counselors are master's degree–level health care professionals with training in both the psychosocial and medical aspects of inherited disease, and now, with specific training in adult hereditary cancer syndromes. The role of the counselor can be filled by other trained professionals, such as nurses or physicians, with a special interest and expertise in hereditary cancer.

The genetic counseling process includes constructing and evaluating a pedigree; eliciting and evaluating personal and family medical history; and providing information about genetic risk. For those choosing testing, genetic counseling includes pretest counseling, testing, post-test counseling, and follow-up, so that clinical genetic laboratory tests are properly interpreted and patients are educated as to appropriate cancer prevention strategies given their level of risk (256,258,266). The counseling process also includes psychosocial assessment, support, and counseling appropriate to a family's culture and ethnicity. Because genetic risk affects biological relatives, contact with these relatives is often essential to collect an accurate family and medical history. Cancer genetic counseling may involve several family members, some of whom may have had cancer and others who have not, and it often involves multiple visits (256,267).

Informed consent is a crucial part of the testing process because of the risks of genetic testing (264). Risks include psychological harm and genetic discrimination (268–270). Positive test results may be accompanied by feelings of anger, anxiety, and depression. Even individuals that have already been diagnosed with cancer may be shocked and saddened to learn that this "trait" may be passed on to their children, or that they are at risk for further cancers. Individuals who test negative may experience relief and joy; they may also experience feelings of guilt and shame (survivor guilt) when dealing with the reality that others in the family carry the deleterious gene. Ambiguous results of tests may lead over time to anxiety and depression greater than a positive result (267,268).

The gravest negative consequence of genetic testing for hereditary CRC is the possibility of genetic discrimination (269). Discrimination may be purely social, such as with respect to dating and marriage. Genetic testing also may lead to the inability to obtain or keep a job or health, life, or disability insurance. Protections are in place to help prevent genetic discrimination against cancer susceptibility gene carriers, but they are imperfect and largely untested (270). The Federal Health Insurance Portability and Accountability Act (HIPAA) of 1996 prohibits employers or insurers from excluding individual employees from group health plans or charging them higher premiums based on genetic information. HIPAA does not bar insurers from excluding coverage, raising rates or capping benefits for all members of the group as long as individuals are not singled out, nor does this legislation protect individually insured persons. Further the HIPAA permits insurers to demand genetic testing as condition of coverage. Proposed legislation at the Federal level to provide further protections against genetic discrimination have broad bipartisan support but have not yet been passed into law at the date of this writing. A large number of states have passed laws to protect individuals against insurance and genetic discrimination, but these vary considerably. The impact of state laws can be limited by the Employee Retirement Income Security Act, which pre-empts self-insured employers from many of the state insurance provisions. Parties interested in genetic testing need to seek updated information about the laws in their state. The National Human Genome Research Institute website provides updated information about public policy and genetic testing (271). Documented insurance discrimination related to genetic testing for hereditary CRC is exceedingly rare (270). Furthermore, the hope is that as genetic predisposition testing becomes more common for a plethora of diseases, genetic discrimination will become increasingly untenable. Fear of genetic discrimination should not prevent patients from obtaining beneficial services, such as cancer predisposition testing, but they need to be made cognizant of these issues. However, vexing issues regarding professional disclosure of familial genetic information may confront health care professionals involved in genetic counseling and testing (272).

One of the biggest barriers to the full-scale implementation of genetic testing for hereditary CRC is cost. The genetic tests are expensive, ranging in price from $750 to $2000 for the germline FAP or HNPCC tests depending on the test and the vendor. Once a mutation has been identified, the cost of follow-up testing of other family members is far less expensive, being often in the range of $200 to $300 per test. Health insurance companies are increasingly willing to pay for these tests, though patients often remain reluctant to seek coverage because of fear of discrimination.

Indications and Strategy for Genetic Testing in Hereditary CRC

The American Society of Clinical Oncology (ASCO) recommends that cancer predisposition testing be offered only when: (i) the person has a strong family history of cancer or very

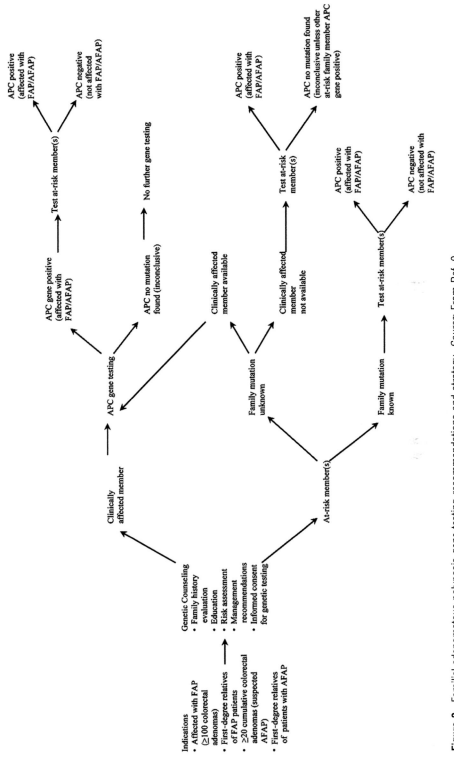

Figure 3 Familial adenomatous polyposis gene testing recommendations and strategy. *Source:* From Ref. 9.

Table 9 Appropriate Interpretation of Genetic Test Results

Proband result	Family member result	Interpretation
Positive	Positive	Positive
Positive	Negative	Negative
Negative	Do not test	Not informative[a]
Ambiguous	Do not test	Not informative[a]

[a]Must assume that family member carries the deleterious gene given the inability to prove otherwise because of the negative test in the proband. Proceed with cancer screening appropriate for a gene carrier in the family member.

early age of onset of disease; (ii) the test can be adequately interpreted; and (iii) the results will influence the medical management of the patient or family member (273). ASCO recognizes three general categories of indications for genetic testing. In the first category testing may already be considered part of the standard care; in the second category the value of testing is presumed, but not clearly established; and in the third category the benefit of testing is not yet established. There is no doubt that intensive cancer screening among individuals at risk for FAP and HNPCC will save lives and has been found to be cost effective (66,231–233). Detection of FAP and HNPCC gene carriers is beneficial because it will improve the efficiency of cancer prevention in families with these conditions by allowing those who do not carry the predisposition allele to avoid costly and burdensome screening tests, and has also been found to be cost effective (10,227,274). Therefore, genetic testing for FAP and HNPCC falls under the first ASCO category and is now the standard of care for families suspected of having these syndromes (9,10,256,258). Genetic testing for other rare polyposis syndromes and for the gene alterations that cause common familial CRC is becoming commercially available, but the benefits of such testing are not yet clearly established (65).

Familial Adenomatous Polyposis
Testing for FAP mutations is a standard part of the care of affected individuals and families (9,260). The indications and strategy for FAP testing are summarized in Figure 3. Genetic testing of an FAP family should start with an affected family member. If a mutation is found, then at-risk members of the family can proceed to testing. If the mutation is not found in an affected person, it does not mean that FAP is not present, but that the test is noninformative (Table 9) (266). Because up to one-third of individuals with FAP have a spontaneous germline *APC* mutation, testing should not be limited to members of classic FAP kindred. Individuals with the FAP phenotype, but without a family history, are also eligible for testing. As minors can develop polyposis and therefore require cancer screening, predisposition testing of minors is appropriate, though this is best deferred until early adolescence (258,275). Opthalmological exams of families with CHRPE can be used as a surrogate for genetic testing, but the validity of this approach to FAP screening has not been conclusively demonstrated. It may be difficult to determine whether an individual has the FAP phenotype and therefore merits testing, especially if the diagnosis of attenuated FAP is being considered. A finding of multiple polyps in an individual over age 45 to 50, especially in the absence of a family history, is far more

Table 10 Likelihood of Detecting a Germline *MSH2* or *MLH1* Mutation Depending on Family History and Tumor MSI Status

Clinical criteria met	Likelihood of detecting a mutation (%)
Amsterdam criteria met	40–70
Amsterdam criteria met and MSI-H tumor	80
Near Amsterdam criteria met	20–50
Near Amsterdam and MSI-H tumor	50–60
Bethesda guidelines met	30
Bethesda guidelines met and MSI-H tumor	50
Early onset CRC without family history	0–30
Early onset CRC and MSI-H tumor	30
Sporadic CRC	<1
Sporadic CRC with MSI-H tumor	10

Abbreviations: MSI, microsatellite instability; CRC, colorectal cancer.

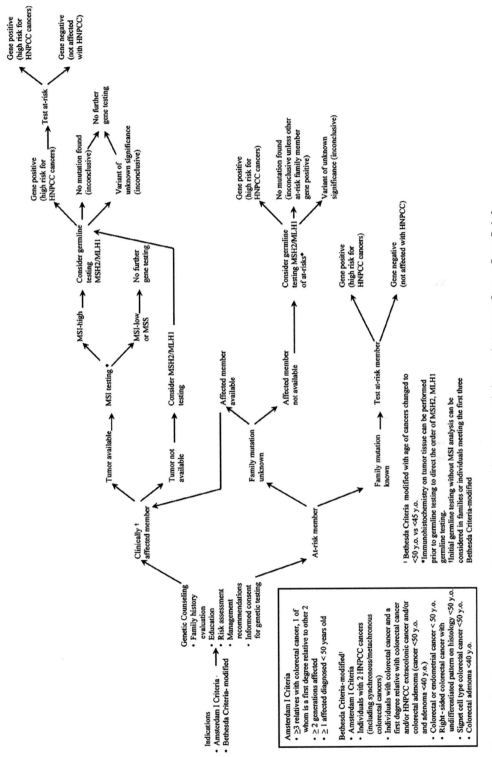
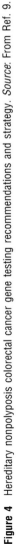

Figure 4 Hereditary nonpolyposis colorectal cancer gene testing recommendations and strategy. *Source:* From Ref. 9.

likely to be part of the spectrum of sporadic colonic neoplasms rather than FAP, but this remains an area of controversy. Some experts would test patients with 20 or more cumulative colorectal adenomas (3,10).

Hereditary Nonpolyposis Colorectal Cancer

Similar to FAP, genetic testing is a standard part of the care of individuals and families at risk for HNPCC (9,260). However, determining when genetic testing is indicated for HNPCC is a far more difficult problem than in FAP, because individuals with HNPCC do not have a unique phenotype to help establish the clinical diagnosis. Some investigators have suggested direct germline *MSH2* and *MLH1* testing of CRC patients that meet appropriate and fairly stringent clinical criteria, such as Amsterdam, Amsterdam II criteria, or the first three Bethesda guidelines (189,190). The likelihood of detecting a germline *MSH2* or *MLH1* mutation based on clinical criteria met is summarized in Table 10. Other investigators have suggested that tumor MSI testing or MSH2/MLH1 protein inmmunohistochemistry should be performed first, and that germline testing be reserved for those found to have MSI-H tumors or those with loss of MMR protein expression (192,194,224,276). The decision to perform tumor MSI or immunohistochemistry testing is again based on clinical criteria, though often less stringent criteria than used to decide for germline testing, such as modified Bethesda guidelines (10). The likelihood of detecting a germline mutation following a positive tumor MSI test also is summarized in Table 10.

Once a germline mutation is detected in the affected proband, germline testing can then be carried out in other family members. In this situation, if family members are found not to carry the family mutation, there result is considered a true negative, and their risk for cancer is that of the general population. As with FAP, if a mutation is not detected in a family suspected of having HNPCC, the test result is not informative. Failure to detect a mutation in a family without a known mutation does not mean that the family does not have HNPCC (Table 9). The indications and strategy for HNPCC gene testing are summarized in Figure 4 (9).

SUMMARY

Heredity plays an important causative role in a large percentage of CRCs. Clinical recognition of the hereditary polyposis syndromes, hereditary nonpolyposis CRC, and common familial CRC is essential because screening, surveillance, and treatment among affected individuals and their family members differs from that recommended to the general population. More intensive cancer screening and surveillance is required if premature death is to be avoided. Genetic testing is commercially available for most of the hereditary CRC syndromes and can greatly facilitate the management of patients if properly undertaken.

REFERENCES

1. Greenlee RT, Hill-Harmon MB, Murray T, Thun M. Cancer statistics, 2001. Calif Cancer J Clin 2001; 51:15–36.
2. Calvert PM, Frucht H. The genetics of colorectal cancer. Ann Intern Med 2002; 137:603–612.
3. Burt RW. Colon cancer screening. Gastroenterology 2000; 119:837–853.
4. Johns LE, Houlston RS. A systematic review and meta-analysis of familial colorectal cancer risk. Am J Gastroenterol 2001; 96:2992–3003.
5. Houlston RS, Tomlinson IP. Polymorphisms and colorectal tumor risk. Gastroenterology 2001; 121:282–301.
6. Terdiman JP, Conrad PG, Sleisenger MH. Genetic testing in hereditary colorectal cancer: indications and procedures. Am J Gastroenterol 1999; 94:2344–2356.
7. Samowitz WS, Curtin K, Lin H, et al. The colon cancer burden of genetically-defined hereditary nonpolyposis colon cancer. Gastroenterology 2001; 12:1005–1008.
8. Salovaara R, Loukola A, Kristo P, et al. Population-based molecular detection of hereditary non-polyposis colorectal cancer. J Clin Oncol 2000; 18:2193–2200.
9. American Gastroenterological Association Medical Position Statement: Hereditary colorectal cancer and genetic testing. Gastroenterology 2001; 121:195–197.
10. Giardiello FM, Brensinger JD, Petersen GM. AGA technical review on hereditary colorectal cancer and genetic testing. Gastroenterology 2001; 121:198–213.
11. Bisgaard ML, Fenger K, Bulow S, Niebuhr E, Mohr J. Familial adenomatous polyposis (FAP): frequency, penetrance and mutation rate. Hum Mutat 1994; 3:121–125.
12. Lindor NM, Greene MH. The concise handbook of family cancer syndromes. Mayo Familial Cancer Program. J Natl Cancer Inst 1998; 90:1039–1071.

13. Galle TS, Juel K, Bulow S. Causes of death in familial adenomatous polyposis. Scand J Gastroenterol 1999; 34:808–812.
14. Spirio L, Olschwang S, Groden J, et al. Alleles of the APC gene: an attenuated form of familial polyposis. Cell 1993; 75:951–957.
15. Lynch HT, Smyrk T, McGinn T, et al. Attenuated familial adenomatous polyposis (AFAP). A phenotypically and genotypically distinctive variant of FAP. Cancer 1995; 76:2427–2433.
16. Church JM, McGannon E, Hull-Boiner S, et al. Gastroduodenal polyps in patients with familial adenomatous polyposis. Diseases of the Colon and Rectum 1992; 35:1170–1173.
17. Campbell WJ, Spence RA, Parks TG. Familial adenomatous polyposis. Br J Surg 1994; 81:1722–1733.
18. Offerhaus GJ, Giardiello FM, Krush AJ, et al. The risk of upper gastrointestinal cancer in familial adenomatous polyposis. Gastroenterology 1992; 102:1980–1982.
19. Wallace MH, Phillips RK. Upper gastrointestinal disease in patients with familial adenomatous polyposis. Br J Surg 1998; 85:742–750.
20. Saurin JC, Chayvialle JA, Ponchon T. Management of duodenal adenomas in familial adenomatous polyposis. Endoscopy 1999; 31:472–478.
21. Spigelman AD. Screening modalities in familial adenomatous polyposis and hereditary nonpolyposis colorectal cancer. Gastrointest Endosc Clin North Am 1997; 7:81–86.
22. Belchetz LA, Berk T, Bapat BV, Cohen Z, Gallinger S. Changing causes of mortality om patients with familial adenomatous polyposis. Dis Colon Rectum 1996; 39:384–387.
23. Bjork J, Akerbrant H, Iselius L, et al. Periampullary adenomas and the adenocarcinomas in familial adenomatous polyposis: cumulative risks and APC gene mutations. Gastroenterology 2001; 121: 1127–1135.
24. Kadmon M, Tandara A, Herfath C. Duodenal adenomatosis in familial adenomatous polyposis coli. A review of the literature and results from the Heidelberg Polyposis Register. Int J Colorectal Dis 2001; 16:63–75.
25. Burke W, Daly M, Garber J, et al. Recommendations for follow-up care of individuals with an inherited predisposition to cancer. II. BRCA1 and BRCA2. Cancer Genetics Studies Consortium. JAMA 1997; 277:997–1003.
26. Hofgartner WTMT, Ramus MWGD, Chey WY, et al. Gastric adenocarcinoma associated with fundic gland polyps in a patient with attenuated familial adenomatous polyposis. Am J Gastroenterol 1999; 94:2275–2281.
27. Tiret A, Taiel-Sartral M, Tiret E, Laroche L. Diagnostic value of fundus examination in familial adenomatous polyposis. Br J Ophthalmol 1997; 81:755–758.
28. Ruhswurm I, Zehetmayer M, Dejaco C, Wolf B, Karner-Hanusch J. Ophthalmic and genetic screening in pedigrees with familial adenomatous polyposis. Am J Ophthalmol 1998; 125:680–686.
29. Clark SK, Smith TG, Katz DE, et al. Identification and progression of a desmoid precursor lesion in patients with familial adenomatous polyposis. Br J Surg 1998; 85:970–973.
30. Church JM, McGannon E. Prior pregnancy ameliorates the course of intra-abdominal desmoid tumors in patients with familial adenomatous polyposis. Dis Colon Rectum 2000; 43:445–450.
31. Soravia C, Berk T, McLeod RS, Cohen Z. Desmoid disease in patients with familial adenomatous polyposis. Dis Colon Rectum 2000; 43:363–369.
32. Rodriguez-Bigas MA, Mahoney MC, Karakousis CP, Petrelli NJ. Desmoid tumors in patients with familial adenomatous polyposis. Cancer 1994; 74:1270–1274.
33. Giardiello FM, Offerhaus GJA, Lee DH, et al. Increased risk of thyroid and pancreatic carcinoma in familial adenomatous polyposis. Gut 1993; 34:1394–1396.
34. Cetta F, Montalto G, Gori M, Curia MC, Cama A, Olschwang S. Germline mutations of the APC gene in patients with familial adenomatous polyposis–associated thyroid carcinoma: results for a European cooperative study. J Clin Endocrinol Metab 2000; 85:286–292.
35. Hamilton SR, Liu B, Parsons RE, et al. The molecular basis of Turcot's syndrome. N Engl J Med 1995; 332:839–847.
36. Paraf F, Jothy S, Van Meir EG. Brain tumor-polyposis syndrome: two genetic diseases? J Clin Oncol 1997; 15:2744–2758.
37. Kinzler KW, Nilbert MC, Su LK, et al. Identification of FAP locus genes from chromosome 5q21. Science 1991; 253:661–665.
38. Groden J, Thliveris A, Samowitz W, et al. Identification and characterization of the familial adenomatous polyposis coli gene. Cell 1991; 66:589–600.
39. Miyoshi Y, Ando H, Nagase H, et al. Germ-line mutations of the APC gene in 53 familial adenomatous polyposis patients. Proc Natl Acad Sci USA 1992; 89:4452–4456.
40. Polakis P. The adenomatous polyposis coli (APC) tumor suppressor. Biochim Biophys Acta 1997; 1332:F127–F147.
41. Dihlmann S, Gebert J, Siermann A, Herfath C, von Knebel Doeberitz M. Dominant negative effect of the APC 1309 mutation: a possible explanation for genotype-phenotype correlations in familial adenomatous polyposis. Cancer Res 1999; 59:1857–1860.
42. Bullions LC, Levine AJ. The role of beta-catenin in cell adhesion, signal transduction, and cancer. Curr Opin Oncol 1998; 10:81–87.
43. Behrens J, Jerchow BA, Wurtele M, et al. Functional interaction of an axin homolog, conductin, with beta-catenin, APC, and GSK3beta. Science 1998; 280:596–599.

44. Kishida S, Yamamoto H, Ikeda S, et al. Axin: a negative regulator of the wnt signaling pathway, directly interacts with adenomatous polyposis coli and regulates the stabilization of beta-catenin. J Biol Chem 1998; 273:10823–10826.

45. He TC, Sparks AB, Rago C, et al. Identification of c-MYC as a target of the APC pathway. Science 1998; 281:1509–1512.

46. Tetsu O, McCormick F. Beta-catenin regulates expression of cyclin D1 in colon carcinoma cells. Nature 1999; 398:422–426.

47. Wallis YL, Morton DGCMM, Macdonald F. Molecular analysis of the APC gene in 205 families: extended genotype-phenotype correlations in FAP and evidence for the role of APC amino acid changes in colorectal cancer predisposition. J Med Genet 1999; 36:14–20.

48. Hernegger GS, Moore HG, Guillem JG. Attenuated familial adenomatous polyposis: an evolving and poorly understood entity. Dis Colon Rectum 2002; 45:127–134; discussion 134–126.

49. Giardiello FM, Brensinger JD, Luce MC, et al. Phenotypic expression of disease in families that have mutations in the 5′ region of the adenomatous polyposis coli gene. Ann Intern Med 1997; 126: 514–519.

50. Gardner RJ, Kool D, Edkins E, et al. The clinical correlates of a 3′ truncating mutation (codons 1982–1983) in the adenomatous polyposis coli gene. Gastroenterology 1997; 113:326–331.

51. Brensinger JD, Laken SJ, Luce MC, et al. Variable phenotype of familial adenomatous polyposis in pedigrees with 3′ mutation in the APC gene. Gut 1998; 43:548–552.

52. Soravia C, Berk T, Madlensky L, et al. Genotype-phenotype correlations in attenuated adenomatous polyposis coli. Am J Hum Genet 1998; 62:1290–1301.

53. Rozen P, Samuel Z, Shomrat R, Legum C. Notable intrafamilial phenotypic variability in a kindred with familial adenomatous polyposis and APC mutation in exon 9. Gut 1999; 45:829–833.

54. O'Sullivan MJ, McCarthy TV, Doyle CT. Familial adenomatous polyposis: from bedside to benchside. Am J Clin Pathol 1998; 109:521–526.

55. Olschwang S, Tiret A, Laurent-Puig P, Muleris M, Parc R, Thomas G. Restriction of ocular fundus lesions to a specific subgroup of APC mutations in adenomatous polyposis coli patients. Cell 1993; 75:959–968.

56. Wallis YL, Macdonald F, Hultén M, et al. Genotype-phenotype correlation between position of constitutional APC gene mutation and CHRPE expression in familial adenomatous polyposis. Hum Genet 1994; 94:543–548.

57. Saurin JC, Ligneau B, Ponchon T, et al. The influence of mutation site and age on the severity of duodenal polyposis in patients with familial adenomatous polyposis. Gastrointest Endosc 2002; 55:342–347.

58. Caspari R, Olschwang SWF, Mandl M. Familial adenomatous polyposis: desmoid tumors and lack of opthalmic lesions (CHRPE) associated with APC mutations beyond codon 1995; 1444.

59. Betario L, Russo A, Sala P, et al. Genotype and phenotype factors as determinants of desmoid tumors in patients with familial adenomatous polyposis. Int J Cancer 2001; 95:102–107.

60. Vasen HFA, van der Luijt RB, Slors JFM, et al. Molecular genetic tests as a guide to surgical management of familial adenomatous polyposis. Lancet 1995; 348:433–435.

61. Wu JS, Paul P, McGannon EA, Church JM. APC genotype, polyp number, and surgical options in familial adenomatous polyposis. Ann Surg 1998; 227:57–62.

62. Friedl W, Caspari R, Sengteller M, et al. Can APC mutation analysis contribute to therapeutic decisions in familial adenomatous polyposis? Experience from 680 FAP families. Gut 2001; 48:515–521.

63. Jones S, Emmerson P, Maynard J, et al. Biallelic germline mutations in MYH predispose to multiple colorectal adenoma and somatic G:C to T:A mutations. Hum Mol Genet 2002; 11:2961–2967.

64. Sieber OM, Lipton L, Crabtree M, et al. Multiple colorectal adenomas, classic adenomatous polyposis, and germ-line mutations in MYH. N Engl J Med 2003; 348:791–799.

65. Dunlop MG. Guidance on gastrointestinal surveillance for hereditary nonpolyposis colorectal cancer, familial adenomatous polyposis, juvenile polyposis, and Peutz-Jeghers syndrome. Gut 2002; 51:v21–v27.

66. Heiskanen I, Luostarinen T, Jarvinen HJ. Impact of screening examinations on survival in familial adenomatous polyposis. Scand J Gastroenterol 2000; 35:1284–1287.

67. Alacorn FJ, Burke CA, Church JM, van Stolk RU. Familial adenomatous polyposis: efficacy of endoscopic and surgical treatment for advanced duodenal adenomas. Dis Colon Rectum 1999; 42: 1533–1536.

68. Heiskanen I, Kellokumpu I, Jarvinen H. Management of duodenal adenomas in 98 patients with familial adenomatous polyposis. Endoscopy 1999; 31:412–416.

69. Norton ID, Geller A, Petersen BT, Sorbi D, Gostout CJ. Endoscopic surveillance and ablative therapy for periampullary adenomas. Am J Gastroenterol 2001; 96:101–106.

70. de Vos tot Nederveen Cappel WH, Jarvinen HJ, Bjork J, Berk T, Griffioen G, Vasen HF. Worldwide survey among polyposis registries of surgical management of severe duodenal adenomatosis in familial adenomatous polyposis. Br J Surg 2003; 90:705–710.

71. Giardiello FM, Hamilton SR, Krush AJ, et al. Treatment of colonic and rectal adenomas with sulindac in familial adenomatous polyposis. N Engl J Med 1993; 328:1313–1316.

72. Steinbach G, Lynch PM, Phillips RK, et al. The effect of celecoxib, a cyclooxygenase-2 inhibitor, in familial adenomatous polyposis. N Engl J Med 2000; 342:1946–1952.

73. Madden MV, Neale KF, Nicholls RJ, et al. Comparison of morbidity and function after colectomy with ileorectal anastomosis or restorative proctocolectomy for familial adenomatous polyposis. Br J Surg 1991; 78:789–792.

74. Fazio VW, Ziv Y, Church JM, et al. Ileal pouch-anal anastomoses complications and function in 1005 patients. Ann Surg 1995; 222:120–127.

75. Kartheuser AH, Parc R, Penna CP, et al. Ileal pouch-anal anastomosis as the first choice operation in patients with familial adenomatous polyposis: a ten-year experience. Surgery 1996; 119:615–623.

76. Tonelli F, Valanzano R, Monaci I, Mazzoni P, Anastasi A, Ficari F. Restorative proctocolectomy or rectum-preserving surgery in patients with familial adenomatous polyposis: results of a prospective study. World J Surg 1997; 21:653–658; discussion 659.

77. Soravia C, Klein L, Berk T, O'Connor BI, Cohen Z, McLeod RS. Comparison of ileal pouch-anal anastomosis and ileorectal anastomosis in patients with familial adenomatous polyposis. Dis Colon Rectum 1999; 42:1028–1033; discussion 1033–1024.

78. Bjork J, Akerbrant H, Iselius L, et al. Outcome of primary and secondary ileal pouch-anal anastomosis and ileorectal anastomosis in patients with familial adenomatous polyposis. Dis Colon Rectum 2001; 44:984–992.

79. Tonelli F, Batignani G, Ficari F, Mazzoni P, Garcea A, Monaci I. Straight ileoanal anastomosis with multiple ileal myotomies as an alternative to pelvic pouch. Int J Colorectal Dis 1997; 12:261–266.

80. van Duijvendijk P, Slors JF, Taat CW, Oosterveld P, Vasen HF. Functional outcome after colectomy and ileorectal anastomosis compared with proctocolectomy and ileal pouch-anal anastomosis in familial adenomatous polyposis. Ann Surg 1999; 230:648–654.

81. Ko CY, Rusin LC, Schoetz DJ, et al. Does better functional results equate with better quality of life? Implications for surgical treatment in familial adenomatous polyposis. Dis Colon Rectum 2000; 43:829–837.

82. van Duijvendijk P, Slors JFM, Taat CW, et al. Quality of life after total colectomy with ileorectal anastomosis or proctocolectomy and ileo-anal anastomosis for familial adenomatous polyposis. Br J Surg 2000; 87:590–596.

83. Heiskanen I, Jarvinen HJ. Fate of the rectal stump after colectomy and ileorectal anastomosis for familial adenomatous polyposis. Int J Colorectal Dis 1997; 12:9–13.

84. Bulow C, Vasen H, Jarvinen H, Bjork J, Bisgaard ML, Bulow S. Ileorectal anastomosis is appropriate for a subset of patients with familial adenomatous polyposis. Gastroenterology 2000; 119:1454–1460.

85. Vasen HF, van Duijvendijk P, Buskens, E, et al. Decision analysis in the surgical treatment of patients with familial adenomatous polyposis: a Dutch-Scandinavian collaborative study including 659 patients. Gut 2001; 49:231–235.

86. Betario L, Russo A, Radice P, et al. Genotype and phenotype factors as determinants for rectal stump cancer in patients with familial adenomatous polyposis. Ann Surg 2000; 231:538–543.

87. Church J, Burke C, McGannon E, Pastean O, Clark B. Predicting polyposis severity by proctoscopy: how reliable is it? Dis Colon Rectum 2001; 44:1249–1254.

88. Church J, Burke C, McGannon E, Pastean O, Clark B. Risk of rectal cancer in patients after colectomy and ileorectal anastomosis for familial adenomatous polyposis: a function of available surgical options. Dis Colon Rectum 2003; 46:1175–1181.

89. Saigusa N, Kurahashi T, Nakamura T, et al. Functional outcome of stapled ileal pouch-anal canal anastomosis versus handsewn pouch-anal anastomosis. Surg Today 2000; 30:575–581.

90. Tuckson WB, McNamara MJ, Fazio VW, Lavery IC, Oakley JR. Impact of anal manipulation and pouch design on ileal pouch function. J Natl Med Assoc 1991; 83:1089–1092.

91. Remzi FH, Church JM, Bast J, et al. Mucosectomy vs. stapled ileal pouch-anal anastomosis in patients with familial adenomatous polyposis: functional outcome and neoplasia control. Dis Colon Rectum 2001; 44:1590–1596.

92. Hoehner JC, Metcalf AM. Development of invasive adenocarcinoma following colectomy with ileoanal anastomosis for familial polyposis coli. Report of a case. Dis Colon Rectum 1994; 37:824–828.

93. von Herbay A, Herfarth C, Otto HF. Cancer and dysplasia in ulcerative colitis: a histologic study of 301 surgical specimen. Z Gastroenterol 1994; 32:382–388.

94. Vuilleumier H, Halkic N, Ksontini R, Gillet M. Columnar cuff cancer after restorative proctocolectomy for familial adenomatous polyposis. Gut 2000; 47:732–734.

95. Wu JS, McGannon EA, Church JM. Incidence of neoplastic polyps in the ileal pouch of patients with familial adenomatous polyposis after restorative proctocolectomy. Dis Colon Rectum 1998; 41: 552–556; discussion 556–557.

96. Polese L, Keighley MR. Adenomas at resection margins do not influence the long-term development of pouch polyps after restorative proctocolectomy for familial adenomatous polyposis. Am J Surg 2003; 186:32–34.

97. van Duijvendijk P, Vasen HFA, Betario L, et al. Cumulative risk of developing polyps or malignancy at the ileal pouch-anal anastomosis in patients with familial adenomatous polyposis. J Gastrointest Surg 1999; 3:325–330.

98. Sugerman HJ, Sugerman EL, Meador JG, Newsome HH Jr., Kellum JM Jr., DeMaria EJ. Ileal pouch anal anastomosis without ileal diversion. Ann Surg 2000; 232:530–541.

99. Gullberg K, Liljeqvist L. Stapled ileoanal pouches without loop ileostomy: a prospective study in 86 patients. Int J Colorectal Dis 2001; 16:221–227.

100. Michelassi F, Hurst R. Restorative proctocolectomy with J-pouch ileoanal anastomosis. Arch Surg 2000; 135:347–353.

101. Giardiello FM, Yang VW, Hylind LM, et al. Primary chemoprevention of familial adenomatous polyposis with sulindac. N Engl J Med 2002; 346:1054–1059.

102. Cruz-Correa M, Hylind LM, Romans KE, Booker SV, Giardiello FM. Long-term treatment with sulindac in familial adenomatous polyposis: a prospective study. Gastroenterology 2002; 122:641–645.

103. Thorson AG, Lynch HT, Smryk TC. Rectal Cancer in FAP patient after sulindac. Lancet 1994; 343:180.

104. Utech M, Bruwer M, Buerger H, Tubergen D, Senninger N. Rectal carcinoma in a patient with familial adenomatous polyposis coli after colectomy with ileorectal anastomosis and consecutive chemoprevention with sulindac suppositories. Chirurg 2002; 73:855–858.

105. Jeghers H, McKusick VA, Katz KH. Generalized intestinal polyposis and melanin spots of the oral mucosa, lips and digits: a syndrome of diagnostic significance. N Engl J Med 1949; 241:993–1005.

106. McGarrity TJ, Kulin HE, Zaino RJ. Peutz–Jeghers Syndrome. Am J Gastroenterol 2000; 95: 596–604.

107. Bartholomew LG, Dahlin DC, Waugh JM. Intestinal polyposis associated with mucocutaneous melanin pigmentation (Peutz–Jeghers syndrome). Review of the literature and report of six cases with special reference to pathologic findings. Gastroenterology 1957; 32:434–451.

108. Foley TR, McGarrity TJ, Abt A. Peutz–Jeghers syndrome: a 38 year follow up of the "Harrisburg Family". Gastroenterology 1988; 95:1535–1540.

109. Utsunomiya J, Gocho H, Miyanaga T, Hamaguchi E, Kashimure A. Peutz–Jeghers syndrome: its natural course and management. Johns Hopkins Med J 1975; 136:71–82.

110. Boardman LA, Thibodeau SN, Schaid DJ, et al. Increased risk for cancer in patients with the Peutz–Jeghers syndrome. Ann Int Med 1998; 128:896–899.

111. Giardiello FM, Brensinger JD, Tersmette AC, et al. Very high risk of cancer in familial Peutz-Jeghers syndrome. Gastroenterology 2000; 119:1447–1453.

112. Perzin KH, Bridge MF. Adenomatous and carcinomatous changes in hamartomatous polyps of the small intestine (Peutz-Jeghers syndrome). Report of a case and review of the literature. Cancer 1982; 49:971–983.

113. Jenne DE, Reimann H, Nezu J, et al. Peutz-Jeghers syndrome is caused by mutations in a novel serine threonine kinase. Nat Genet 1998; 18:38–43.

114. Hemminki A, Markie D, Tomlinson I, et al. A serine/threonine kinase gene defective in Peutz-Jeghers syndrome. Nature 1998; 391:184–187.

115. Boardman LA, Couch FJ, Burgart LJ, et al. Genetic heterogeneity in Peutz-Jeghers syndrome. Hum Mutat 2000; 16:23–30.

116. Wirtzfeld DA, Petrelli NJ, Rodriguez-Bigas MA. Hamartomatous polyposis: molecular genetics, neoplastic risk, and surveillance recommendations. Ann Surg Oncol 2001; 8.

117. Amaro R, Diaz G, Schneider J, Hellinger MD, Stollman NH. Peutz-Jeghers syndrome managed with a complete intraoperative endoscopy and extensive polypectomy. Gastrointest Endosc 2000; 52: 552–554.

118. Rubio CA, Jaramillo E, Lindblom A, Fogt F. Classification of colorectal polyps: guidelines for the endoscopist. Endoscopy 2002; 34:226–236.

119. Woodford-Richens K, Bevan S, Churchman M, et al. Analysis of genetic and phenotypic heterogeneity in juvenile polyposis. Gut 2000; 46:656–660.

120. Giardiello FM, Offerhaus JG. Phenotype and cancer risk of the various polyposis syndromes. Eur J Cancer 1995; 31a:1085–1087.

121. Jarvinen H, Franssila KO. Familial juvenile polyposis coli: increased risk of colorectal cancer. Gut 1984; 25:792–800.

122. Howe JR, Mitros FA, Summers RW. The risk of gastrointestinal carcinoma in familial juvenile polyposis. Ann Surg Oncol 1998; 5:751–756.

123. Howe JR, Roth S, Ringold JC, et al. Mutations in the SMAD4/DPC4 gene in juvenile polyposis. Science 1998; 280:1086–1088.

124. Houlston R, Bevan S, Williams A, et al. Mutations in DPC4 (SMAD4) cause juvenile polyposis syndrome, but only account for a minority of cases. Hum Mol Genet 1998; 7:1907–1912.

125. Woodford-Richens KL, Rowan AJ, Poulsom R, et al. Comprehensive analysis of SMAD4 mutations and protein expression in juvenile polyposis: evidence for a distinct pathway and polyp morphology in SMAD4 mutation carriers. Am J Pathol 2001; 159:1293–1300.

126. Takagi Y, Kohmura H, Futamura M, et al. Somatic alterations of the DPC4 gene in human colorectal cancers in vivo. Gastroenterology 1996; 111:1369–1372.

127. Riggins GJ, Thiagalingam S, Rozenblum E, et al. Mad-related genes in the human. Nat Genet 1996; 13:347–349.

128. Olschwang S, Serova-Sinilnikova OM, Lenoir GM, Thomas G. PTEN germline mutations in juvenile polyposis. Nat Genet 1998; 18:12–13.

129. Zhou XP, Woodford-Richens K, Lehtonen R, et al. Germline mutations in BMPR1A/ALK3 cause a subset of cases of juvenile polyposis syndrome and of Bannayan-Riley-Ruvalcaba syndromes. Am J Hum Genet 2001; 69:704–711.

130. Doxey BW, Kuwada SK, Burt RW. Inherited polyposis syndromes; molecular mechanisms, clinicopathology, and genetic testing. Clin Gastroenterol Hepatol 2005; 3:633–641.

131. Liaw D, Marsh DJ, Li J, et al. Germline mutations of the PTEN gene in Cowden disease, an inherited breast and thyroid cancer syndrome. Nat Genet 1997; 16:64–67.
132. Zigman AF, Lavine JE, Jones MC, Boland CR, Carethers JM. Localization of the Bannayan-Riley-Ruvalcaba syndrome gene to chromosome 10q23. Gastroenterology 1997; 113:1433–1437.
133. Ward EM, Wolfsen HC. Review article: the non-inherited gastroinestinal polyposis syndromes. Aliment Pharmacol Ther 2002; 16:333–342.
134. Rashid A, Houlihan S, Booker S, Petersen GM, Giardiello FM, Hamilton SR. Phenotypic and molecular characteristics of hyperplastic polyposis. Gastroenterology 2000; 119:323–332.
135. Sumner HW, Wasserman NF, McClain CJ. Giant hyperplastic polyposis of the colon. Dig Dis Sci 1981; 26:85–89.
136. Warner AS, Glick ME, Fogt F. Multiple large hyperplastic polyps of the colon coincident with adenocarcinoma. Am J Gastroenterol 1994; 89:123–125.
137. Iino H, Jass JR, Simms LA, et al. DNA microsatellite instability in hyperplastic polyps, serrated adenomas, and mixed polyps: a mild mutator pathway for colorectal cancer? J Clin Pathol 1999; 52:5–9.
138. Jass JR, Iino H, Ruszkiewics A, et al. Neoplastic progression occurs through mutator pathways in hyperplastic polyposis of the colorectum. Gut 2000; 47:43–49.
139. Jass JR, Young J, Leggett BA. Hyperplastic polyps and DNA microsatellite unstable cancer of the colorectum. Histopathology 2000; 37:295–301.
140. Hawkins NJ, Ward RL. Sporadic colorectal cancers with microsatellite instability and their possible origin in hyperplastic polyps and serrated adenomas. J Natl Cancer Inst 2001; 93:1307–1313.
141. Jass JR, Biden KG, Cummings MC, et al. Characterisation of a subtype of colorectal cancer combining features of the suppressor and mild mutator pathways. J Clin Pathol 1999; 52:455–460.
142. Jass JR, Whitehall VLJ, Young J, Leggett BA. Emerging concepts in colorectal neoplasia. Gastroenterology 2002; 123:862–876.
143. Cronkhite LW, Canada WJ. Generalized gastrointestinal polyposis: an unusual syndrome of polyposis, pigmentation, alopecia and onychontrophia. N Engl J Med 1955; 252:1011–1015.
144. Burke AP, Sobin LH. The pathology of the Cronkhite-Canada polyps. A comparison to juvenile polyposis. Am J Surg Pathol 1989; 13:940–946.
145. Russell DM, Bhathal PS, St. John DJ. Complete remission in the Cronkhite-Canada syndrome. Gastroenterology 1983; 85:180–185.
146. Rappaport LB, Sperling HV, Stavrides A. Colon cancer in the Cronkhite-Canada syndrome. J Clin Gastroenterol 1986; 8:199–202.
147. Malhorta R, Sheffield A. Cronkhite-Canada syndrome associated wit colon carcinoma and adenomatous changes in C-C polyps. Am J Gastroenterol 1988; 83:772–776.
148. Ward E, Wolfsen HC, Ng CS. Medical management of the Cronkhite-Canada syndrome. South Med J 2002; 95:272–274.
149. Kelly JK, Gabos S. The pathogenesis of inflammatory polyps. Dis Colon Rectum 1987; 30:251–254.
150. Brozna JP, Fisher RL, Barwick KW. Filiform polyposis: an unusual complication of inflammatory bowel disease. J Clin Gastroenterol 1985; 7:451–458.
151. Taylor BA, Wolff BG. Colonic lipomas. Report of two cases and review of the literature. Dis Colon Rectum 1987; 30:888–893.
152. Swain VA, Young WF, Pringle EM. Hypertrophy of the appendices epiploicae and lipomatous polyposis of the colon. Gut 1969; 10:587–589.
153. Ramirez JM, Ortego J, Deus J, Bustamante E, Lozano R, Dominguez M. Lipomatous polyposis of the colon. Br J Surg 1993; 80:349–350.
154. Ranchord M, Lewin KJ, Dorfman RF. Lymphoid hyperplasia of the gastrointestinal tract. Am J Surg Pathol 1978; 2:383–400.
155. Levendoglu H, Rosen Y. Nodular lymphoid hyperplasia of the gut in HIV infection. Am J Gastroenterol 1992; 87:1200–1202.
156. Bastlein C, Burlefinger R, Hlozberg E, Voeth C, Garbrecht M, Ottenjann R. Common variable immunodeficiency syndrome and nodular lymphoid hyperplasia in the small intestine. Endoscopy 1988; 20:272–275.
157. Lynch HT, Smyrk TC, Watson P, et al. Genetics, natural history, tumor spectrum and pathology of hereditary nonpolyposis colorectal cancer: an updated review. Gastroenterology 1993; 104:1535–1549.
158. Ponz de Leon M, Sassatelli R, Benatti P, Roncucci L. Identification of hereditary nonpolyposis colorectal cancer in the general population. The 6-year experience of a population-based registry. Cancer 1993; 71:3493–3501.
159. Evans DG, Walsh S, Jeacock J, et al. Incidence of hereditary non-polyposis colorectal cancer in a population-based study of 1137 consecutive cases of colorectal cancer. Br J Surg 1997; 84:1281–1285.
160. Aaltonen LA, Salovaara R, Kristo P, et al. Incidence of hereditary nonpolyposis colorectal cancer and the feasibility of molecular screening for the disease. N Engl J Med 1998; 338:1481–1487.
161. Ravnik-Glavac M, Potocnik U, Glavac D. Incidence of germline hMLH1 and hMSH2 mutations (HNPCC patients) among newly diagnosed colorectal cancers in a Slovenian population. J Med Genet 2000; 37:533–536.
162. Lynch HT, Smyrk TC, Watson P, et al. Genetics, natural history, tumor spectrum, and pathology of hereditary nonpolyposis colorectal cancer: an updated review. Gastroenterology 1993; 104:1535–1549.

163. Lynch HT, Smyrk T, Lynch JF. Overview of natural history, pathology, molecular genetics and management of HNPCC Lynch Syndrome. Int J Cancer 1996; 69:38–43.
164. Kinzler KW, Vogelstein B. Lessons from hereditary colorectal cancer. Cell 1996; 87:159–170.
165. Watanabe T, Muto T, Sawada T, Miyaki M. Flat adenoma as a precursor of colorectal carcinoma in hereditary nonpolyposis colorectal carcinoma. Cancer 1996; 77:627–634.
166. Rijcken FEM, Hollema H, Kleibeuker JH. Proximal adenomas in hereditary nonpolyposis colorectal cancer are prone to rapid malignant transformation. Gut 2002; 50:382–386.
167. Lindgren G, Liljegren A, Jaramillo E, Rubio C, Lindblom A. Adenoma prevalence and cancer risk in familial nonpolyposis colorectal cancer. Gut 2002; 50:228–234.
168. Vasen HF, Wijnen JT, Menko FH, et al. Cancer risk in families with hereditary nonpolyposis colorectal cancer diagnosed by mutation analysis. Gastroenterology 1996; 110:1020–1027.
169. Dunlop MG, Farrington SM, Carothers AD, et al. Cancer risk associated with germline DNA mismatch repair gene mutations. Hum Mol Genet 1997; 6:105–110.
170. Aarnio M, Sankila R, Pukkala E, et al. Cancer risk in mutation carriers of DNA mismatch repair genes. Int J Cancer 1999; 81:214–218.
171. Vasen HFA, Stormorken A, Menko FH, et al. MSH2 mutation carriers are at a higher risk of cancer than MLH1 mutation carriers: a study of hereditary nonpolyposis colorectal cancer families. J Clin Oncol 2001; 19:4074–4080.
172. Mecklin JP, Järvinen H. Treatment and follow-up strategies in hereditary nonpolyposis colorectal carcinoma. Dis Colon Rectum 1993; 36:927–929.
173. Hemminki K, Li X, Dong C. Second primary cancers after sporadic and familial colorectal cancer. Cancer Epidemiol Biomarkers Prevention 2001; 10:793–798.
174. Jass JR, Smyrk TC, Stewart SM, Lane MR, Lanspa SJ, Lynch HT. Pathology of hereditary nonpolyposis colorectal cancer. Anticancer Res 1994; 14:1631–1634.
175. Michael-Robinson JM, Biemere-Huttmann A, Purdie DM, et al. Tumor infiltrating lymphocytes and apoptosis are independent features in colorectal cancer according to microsatellite instability status. Gut 2001; 48:360–366.
176. Young J, Simms LA, Biden KG, et al. Features of colorectal cancers with high-level microsatellite instability occurring in familial and sporadic settings: parallel pathways of tumorigenesis. Am J Pathol 2001; 159:2107–2116.
177. Lynch HT, Smyrk T. Colorectal cancer, survival advantage, and hereditary nonpolyposis colorectal carcinoma. Gastroenterology 1996; 110:943–947.
178. Sankila R, Aaltonen LA, Järvinen HJ, Mecklin JP. Better survival rates in patients with MLH1-associated hereditary colorectal cancer. Gastroenterology 1996; 110:682–687.
179. Myrhøj T, Bisgaard ML, Bernstein I, Svendsen LB, Søndergaard JO, Bülow S. Hereditary nonpolyposis colorectal cancer: clinical features and survival. Results from the Danish HNPCC register. Scand J Gastroenterol 1997; 32:572–576.
180. Watson P, Lin KM, Rodriguez-Bigas MA, et al. Colorectal carcinoma survival among hereditary nonpolyposis colorectal carcinoma family members. Cancer 1998; 83:259–266.
181. Bertario L, Russo A, Sala P, et al. Survival of patients with hereditary colorectal cancer: comparison of HNPCC and colorectal cancer in FAP patients with sporadic colorectal cancer. Int J Cancer 1999; 80:183–187.
182. Watson P, Lynch HT. Extracolonic cancer in hereditary nonpolyposis colorectal cancer. Cancer 1993; 71:677–685.
183. Lynch HT, Smyrk T. Hereditary nonpolyposis colorectal cancer (Lynch syndrome). An updated review. Cancer 1996; 78:1149–1167.
184. Park YJ, Shin KH, Park JG. Risk of gastric cancer in hereditary nonpolyposis colorectal cancer in Korea. Clin Cancer Res 2000; 6:2994–2998.
185. Kim JC, Kim HC, Roh SA, et al. hMLH1 and hMSH2 mutations in families with familial clustering of gastric cancer and hereditary nonpolyposis colorectal cancer. Cancer Detection Prevention 2001; 25:503–510.
186. Suspiro A, Fidalgo P, Cravo M, et al. The Muir–Torre syndrome: a rare variant of hereditary nonpolyposis colorectal cancer associated with hMSH2 mutation. Am J Gastroenterol 1998; 93:1572–1574.
187. Kruse R, Rütten A, Lamberti C, et al. Muir-Torre phenotype has a frequency of DNA mismatch-repair-gene mutations similar to that in hereditary nonpolyposis colorectal cancer families defined by the Amsterdam criteria. Am J Hum Genet 1998; 63:63–70.
188. Vasen HF, Mecklin JP, Khan PM, Lynch HT. The International Collaborative Group on Hereditary Non-Polyposis Colorectal Cancer (ICG-HNPCC). Dis Colon Rectum 1991; 34:424–425.
189. Wijnen JT, Vasen HF, Khan PM, et al. Clinical findings with implications for genetic testing in families with clustering of colorectal cancer. N Engl J Med 1998; 339:511–518.
190. Syngal S, Fox EA, Li C, et al. Interpretation of genetic test results for hereditary nonpolyposis colorectal cancer: implications for clinical predisposition testing. JAMA 1999; 282:247–253.
191. Syngal S, Fox EA, Eng C, Kolodner RD, Garber JE. Sensitivity and specificity of clinical criteria for hereditary non-polyposis colorectal cancer associated mutations in MSH2 and MLH1. J Med Genet 2000; 37:641–645.

192. Terdiman JP, Gum JR Jr., Conrad PG, et al. Efficient detection of hereditary nonpolyposis colorectal cancer gene carriers by screening for tumor microsatellite instability before germline genetic testing. Gastroenterology 2001; 120:21–30.

193. Vasen HF, Watson P, Mecklin JP, Lynch HT. New clinical criteria for hereditary nonpolyposis colorectal cancer (HNPCC, Lynch syndrome) proposed by the International Collaborative group on HNPCC. Gastroenterology 1999; 116:1453–1456.

194. Rodriguez-Bigas MA, Boland CR, Hamilton SR, et al. A National Cancer Institute Workshop on Hereditary Nonpolyposis Colorectal Cancer Syndrome: meeting highlights and Bethesda guidelines. J Natl Cancer Inst 1997; 89:1758–1762.

195. Cunningham JM, Kim CY, Christensen ER, et al. The frequency of hereditary defective mismatch repair in a prospective series of unselected colorectal carcinomas. Am J Hum Genet 2001; 69:780–790.

196. Leach FS, Nicolaides NC, Papadopoulos N, et al. Mutations of a mutS homolog in hereditary nonpolyposis colorectal cancer. Cell 1993; 75:1215–1225.

197. Papadopoulos N, Nicolaides NC, Wei YF, et al. Mutation of a mutL homolog in hereditary colon cancer. Science 1994; 263:1625–1629.

198. Bronner CE, Baker SM, Morrison PT, et al. Mutation in the DNA mismatch repair gene homologue hMLH1 is associated with hereditary non-polyposis colon cancer. Nature 1994; 368:258–261.

199. Nicolaides NC, Papadopoulos N, Liu B, et al. Mutations of two PMS homologues in hereditary nonpolyposis colon cancer. Nature 1994; 371:75–80.

200. Fishel R, Lescoe MK, Rao MR, et al. The human mutator gene homolog MSH2 and its association with hereditary nonpolyposis colon cancer. Cell 1994; 77:167.

201. Miyaki M, Konishi M, Tanaka K, et al. Germline mutation of MSH6 as the cause of hereditary nonpolyposis colorectal cancer [lett]. Nat Genet 1997; 17:271–272.

202. Peltomäki P, Vasen HF. Mutations predisposing to hereditary nonpolyposis colorectal cancer: database and results of a collaborative study. The International Collaborative Group on Hereditary Nonpolyposis Colorectal Cancer. Gastroenterology 1997; 113:1146–1158.

203. Kolodner RD, Tytell JD, Schmeits JL, et al. Germ-line msh6 mutations in colorectal cancer families. Cancer Res 1999; 59:5068–5074.

204. Wu Y, Berends MJ, Mensink RG, et al. Association of hereditary nonpolyposis colorectal cancer-related tumors displaying low microsatellite instability with MSH6 germline mutations. Am J Hum Genet 1999; 65:1291–1298.

205. Wang Q, Lasset C, Desseigne F, et al. Prevalence of germline mutations of hMLH1, hMSH2, hPMS1, hPMS2, and hMSH6 genes in 75 French kindreds with nonpolyposis colorectal cancer. Hum Genet 1999; 105:79–85.

206. Plaschke J, Kruppa C, Tischler R, et al. Sequence analysis of the mismatch repair gene hMSH6 in the germline of patients with familial and sporadic colorectal cancer. Int J Cancer 2000; 85:606–613.

207. Huang J, Kuismanen SA, Liu T, et al. MSH6 and MSH3 are rarely involved in genetic predisposition to nonpolypotic colon cancer. Cancer Res 2001; 61:1619–1623.

208. Wagner A, Hendriks Y, Meijers-Heijboer EJ, et al. Atypical HNPCC owing to MSH6 germline mutations: analysis of a large Dutch pedigree. J Med Genet 2001; 38:318–322.

209. Fishel R. The selection for mismatch repair defects in hereditary nonpolyposis colorectal cancer syndrome (HNPCC): revising the mutator hypothesis. Cancer Res 2001; 61:7369–7374.

210. Heinen CD, Schmutte C, Fishel R. DNA repair and tumorigenesis: lessons from hereditary cancer syndromes. Cancer Biol Ther 2002; 1:477–485.

211. Parsons R, Li LGM, Longley MJ, et al. Hypermutability and mismatch repair deficiency in RER+ tumor cells. Cell 1993; 75:1227–1236.

212. Peltomaki P, Lothe RA, Aaltonen LA, et al. Microsatellite instability is associated with tumors that characterize the hereditary non-polyposis colorectal carcinoma syndrome. Cancer Res 1993; 53:5853–5855.

213. Aaltonen LA, Peltomaki P, Mecklin JP, et al. Replication errors in benign and malignant tumors from hereditary nonpolyposis colorectal cancer patients. Cancer Res 1994; 54:1645–1648.

214. Dietmaier W, Wallinger S, Bocker T, Kullmann F, Fishel R, Rüschoff J. Diagnostic microsatellite instability: definition and correlation with mismatch repair protein expression. Cancer Res 1997; 57:4749–4756.

215. Boland CR, Thibodeau SN, Hamilton SR, et al. A National Cancer Institute Workshop on Microsatellite Instability for cancer detection and familial predisposition: development of international criteria for the determination of microsatellite instability in colorectal cancer. Cancer Res 1998; 58:5248–5257.

216. Markowitz S, Wang J, Myeroff L, et al. Inactivation of the type II TGF-beta receptor in colon cancer cells with microsatellite instability. Science 1995; 268:1336–1338.

217. Parsons R, Myeroff LL, Liu B, et al. Microsatellite instability and mutations of the transforming growth factor beta type II receptor gene in colorectal cancer. Cancer Res 1995; 55:5548–5550.

218. Rampino N, Yamamoto H, Ionov Y, et al. Somatic frameshift mutations in the BAX gene in colon cancers of the microsatellite mutator phenotype. Science 1997; 275:967–969.

219. Yamamoto H, Sawai H, Weber TK, Rodriguez–Bigas MA, Perucho M. Somatic frameshift mutations in DNA mismatch repair and proapoptosis genes in hereditary nonpolyposis colorectal cancer. Cancer Res 1998; 58:997–1003.

220. Yagi OK, Akiyama Y, Nomizu T, Iwama T, Endo M, Yuasa Y. Proapoptotic gene BAX is frequently mutated in hereditary nonpolyposis colorectal cancers but not in adenomas. Gastroenterology 1998; 114:268–274.

221. Cawkwell L, Gray S, Murgatroyd H, et al. Choice of management strategy for colorectal cancer based on a diagnostic immunohistochemical test for defective mismatch repair [comments]. Gut 1999; 45:409–415.

222. Salahshor S, Koelble K, Rubio C, Lindblom A. Microsatellite instability and hMLH1 and hMSH2 expression analysis in familial and sporadic colorectal cancer. Lab Invest 2001; 81:535–541.

223. Wahlberg SS, Schmeits J, Thomas G, et al. Evaluation of microsatellite instability and immunohistochemistry for the prediction of germline MSH2 and MLH1 mutations in hereditary nonpolyposis colon cancer families. Cancer Res 2002; 62:3485–3492.

224. Christensen M, Katballe N, Wikman F, et al. Antibody-based screening for hereditary nonpolyposis colorectal carcinoma compared with microsatellite analysis and sequencing. Cancer 2002; 95: 2422–2430.

225. Lin KM, Shashidharan M, Thorson AG, et al. Cumulative incidence of colorectal and extracolonic cancers in MLH1 and MSH2 mutation carriers of hereditary nonpolyposis colorectal cancer. J Gastrointest Surg 1988; 2:67–71.

226. Lin KM, Shashidharan M, Ternent CA, et al. Colorectal and extracolonic cancer variations in MLH1/MSH2 hereditary nonpolyposis colorectal cancer kindreds and the general population. Dis Colon Rectum 1998; 41:428–433.

227. Ramsey SD, Clarke L, Etzioni R, Higashi M, Berry K, Urban N. Cost-effectiveness of microsatellite instability screening as a method for detecting hereditary nonpolyposis colorectal cancer. Ann Intern Med 2001; 135:577–588.

228. Burke W, Petersen G, Lynch P, et al. Recommendations for follow-up care of individuals with an inherited predisposition to cancer. I. Hereditary nonpolyposis colon cancer. Cancer Genetics Studies Consortium. JAMA 1997; 277:915–919.

229. de Vos tot Nederveen Cappel WH, Nagengast FM, Griffioen G, et al. Surveillance for hereditary nonpolyposis colorectal cancer. A long-term study on 114 families. Dis Colon Rectum 2002; 45: 1588–1594.

230. Winawer SJ, Fletcher RH, Miller L, et al. Colorectal cancer screening: clinical guidelines and rationale [published erratum appears in Gastroenterology 1997; 112(3):1060]. Gastroenterology 1997; 112: 594–642.

231. Jarvinen HJ, Aarnio M, Mustonen H, et al. Controlled 15-year trial on screening for colorectal cancer in families with hereditary nonpolyposis colorectal cancer. Gastroenterology 2000; 118:829–834.

232. Vasen HF, van Ballegooijen M, Buskens E, et al. A cost-effectiveness analysis of colorectal screening of hereditary nonpolyposis colorectal carcinoma gene carriers. Cancer 1998; 82:1632–1637.

233. Syngal S, Weeks JC, Schrag D, Garber JE, Kuntz KM. Benefits of colonoscopic surveillance and prophylactic colectomy in patients with hereditary nonpolyposis colorectal cancer mutations. Ann Intern Med 1998; 129:787–796.

234. Dove-Edwin I, Boks D, Goff S, et al. The outcome of endometrial carcinoma surveillance by ultrasound scan in women at risk for hereditary nonpolyposis colorectal carcinoma and familial colorectal carcinoma. Cancer 2002; 94:1708–1712.

235. Renkonen-Sinisalo L, Sipponen P, Aarnio M, et al. No support for endoscopic surveillance for gastric cancer in hereditary nonpolyposis colorectal cancer. Scan J Gastroenterol 2002; 37:574–577.

236. Church JM. Prophylactic colectomy in patients with hereditary nonpolyposis colorectal cancer. Ann Med 1996; 28:479–482.

237. Rodríguez-Bigas MA, Vasen HF, Pekka-Mecklin J, et al. Rectal cancer risk in hereditary nonpolyposis colorectal cancer after abdominal colectomy. International Collaborative Group on HNPCC. Ann Surg 1997; 225:202–207.

238. Lichtenstein P, Holm NV, Verkasalo PK, et al. Environmental and heritable factors in the causation of cancer—analyses of cohorts of twins from Sweden, Denmark, and Finland [comments]. N Engl J Med 2000; 343:78–85.

239. Winawer SJ, Zauber AG, Gerdes H, et al. Risk of colorectal cancer in the families of patients with adenomatous polyps. National Polyp Study Workgroup. N Engl J Med 1996; 334:82–87.

240. Fuchs CS, Giovannucci EL, Colditz GA, Hunter DJ, Speizer FE, Willett WC. A prospective study of family history and the risk of colorectal cancer. N Engl J Med 1994; 331:1669–1674.

241. Sandler RS. Epidemiology and risk factors for colorectal cancer. Gastroenterol Clin North Am 1996; 25:717–735.

242. Laken SJ, Petersen GM, Gruber SB, et al. Familial colorectal cancer in Ashkenazim due to a hypermutable tract in APC. Nat Genet 1997; 17:79–83.

243. Gryfe R, Di Nicola N, Gallinger S, Redston M. Somatic instability of the APC I1307K allele in colorectal neoplasia [comments]. Cancer Res 1998; 58:4040–4043.

244. White RL. Excess risk of colon cancer associated with a polymorphism of the APC gene? [editorial; comment]. Cancer Res 1998; 58:4038–4039.

245. Woodage T, King SM, Wacholder S, et al. The APCI1307K allele and cancer risk in a community-based study of Ashkenazi Jews [comments]. Nat Genet 1998; 20:62–65.

246. Frayling IM, Beck NE, Ilyas M, et al. The APC variants I1307K and E1317Q are associated with colorectal tumors, but not always with a family history. Proc Natl Acad Sci USA 1998; 95: 10722–10727.
247. Rozen P, Shomrat R, Strul H, et al. Prevalence of the I1307K APC gene variant in Israeli Jews of differing ethnic origin and risk for colorectal cancer [comments]. Gastroenterology 1999; 116:54–57.
248. Gryfe R, Di Nicola N, Lal G, Gallinger S, Redston M. Inherited colorectal polyposis and cancer risk of the APC I1307K polymorphism. Am J Hum Genet 1999; 64:378–384.
249. Drucker L, Shpilberg O, Neumann A, et al. Adenomatous polyposis coli I1307K mutation in Jewish patients with different ethnicity: prevalence and phenotype. Cancer 2000; 88:755–760.
250. Syngal S, Schrag D, Falchuk M, et al. Phenotypic characteristics associated with the APC gene I1307K mutation in Ashkenazi Jewish patients with colorectal polyps. JAMA 2000; 284:857–860.
251. Stern HS, Viertelhausen S, Hunter AG, et al. APC I1307K increases risk of transition from polyp to colorectal carcinoma in Ashkenazi Jews. Gastroenterology 2001; 120:392–400.
252. Rozen P, Naiman T, Strul H, et al. Clinical and screening implications of the I1307K adenomatous polyposis coli gene variant in Israeli Ashkenazi Jews with familial colorectal neoplasia. Cancer 2002; 94:2561–2568.
253. Potter JD. Colorectal cancer: molecules and populations. J Natl Cancer Inst 1999; 91:916–932.
254. Rex DK, Johnson DA, Lieberman DA, Burt RW, Sonnenberg A. Colorectal cancer prevention 2000: screening recommendations of the American College of Gastroenterology. American College of Gastroenterology. Am J Gastroenterol 2000; 95:868–877.
255. Screening for colorectal cancer: recommendation and rationale. Ann Intern Med 2002; 137:129–131.
256. Petersen GM, Brensinger JD, Johnson KA, Giardiello FM. Genetic testing and counseling for hereditary forms of colorectal cancer. Cancer 1999; 86:2540–2550.
257. Eng C, Hampel H, de la Chapelle A. Genetic testing for cancer predisposition. Annu Rev Med 2001; 52:371–400.
258. Solomon CH, Burt RW. Current status of genetic testing for colorectal cancer susceptibility. Oncology 2002; 16:161–171.
259. www.geneclinics.org.
260. ACMG/ASHG statement. Genetic testing for colon cancer: Joint statement of the American College of Medical Genetics and the American Society of Human Genetics. Genet Med 2000; 2:362–366.
261. Wijnen J, van der Klift H, Vasen H, et al. MSH2 genomic deletions are a frequent cause of HNPCC [letter]. Nat Genet 1998; 20:326–328.
262. Yan H, Papadopoulos N, Marra G, et al. Conversion of diploidy to haploidy. Nature 2000; 403: 723–724.
263. Samowitz WS, Slattery ML, Kerber RA. Microsatellite instability in human colonic cancer is not a useful clinical indicator of familial colorectal cancer. Gastroenterology 1995; 109:1765–1771.
264. Thibodeau SN, French AJ, Roche PC, et al. Altered expression of hMSH2 and hMLH1 in tumors with microsatellite instability and genetic alterations in mismatch repair genes. Cancer Res 1996; 56: 4836–4840.
265. Geller G, Botkin JR, Green MJ, et al. Genetic testing for susceptibility to adult-onset cancer. The process and content of informed consent. JAMA 1997; 277:1467–1474.
266. Giardiello FM, Brensinger JD, Petersen GM, et al. The use and interpretation of commercial APC gene testing for familial adenomatous polyposis. N Engl J Med 1997; 336:823–827.
267. Lerman C, Marshall J, Audrain J, Gomez-Caminero A. Genetic testing for colon cancer susceptibility: anticipated reactions of patients and challenges to providers. Int J Cancer 1996; 69:58–61.
268. Aktan-Collan K, Haukkla A, Mecklin JP, Uutela A, Kaariainen H. Psychological consequences of predictive genetic testing for hereditary nonpolyposis colorectal cancer (HNPCC): a prospective follow-up study. Int J Cancer 2001; 93:608–611.
269. Coughlin SS, Miller DS. Public health perspectives on testing for colorectal cancer. Am J Prevent Med 1999; 16:99–104.
270. Hall MA, Rich SS. Laws restricting health insurers' use of genetic information: impact on genetic discrimination. Am J Hum Genet 2000; 66:293–307.
271. http://www.nhgri.nih.gov.
272. ASHG statement. Professional disclosure of familial genetic information. The American Society of Human Genetics Social Issues Subcommittee on Familial Disclosure. Am J Hum Genet 1998; 62:474–483.
273. Statement of the American Society of Clinical Oncology: genetic testing for cancer susceptibility, Adopted on February 20, 1996. J Clin Oncol 1996; 14:1730–1736; discussion 1737–1734.
274. Cromwell DM, Moore RD, Brensinger JD, Petersen GM, Bass EB, Giardiello FM. Cost analysis of alternative approaches to colorectal screening in familial adenomatous polyposis. Gastroenterology 1998; 114:893–901.
275. Giardiello FM. Genetic testing in hereditary colorectal cancer [clinical conference]. JAMA 1997; 278:1278–1281.
276. Lamberti C, Kruse R, Ruelfs C, et al. Microsatellite instability—a useful diagnostic tool to select patients at high risk for hereditary non-polyposis colorectal cancer: a study in different groups of patients with colorectal cancer. Gut 1999; 44:839–843.

26 | Ulcerative Colitis

Oded Zmora
Colon and Rectal Surgery, Department of Surgery and Transplantation, Sheba Medical Center, Tel Hashomer, and Sakler School of Medicine, Tel Aviv University, Tel Aviv, Israel

Rami Eliakim
Division of Gastroenterology, Department of Medicine, Rappaport School of Medicine, Rambam Medical Center and Technion–Israel Institute of Technology, Haifa, Israel

Hagit Tulchinsky
Colon and Rectal Surgery, Department of Surgery, Rabin Medical Center, Beilinson Campus, Petah Tikva, and Sakler School of Medicine, Tel Aviv University, Tel Aviv, Israel

DISEASE OVERVIEW

Ulcerative colitis (UC) is a chronic disease of inflammation confined to the mucosa and submucosa of the large bowel. The rectum is almost uniformly involved in the disease, and may occasionally be the only part of the bowel involved, termed ulcerative proctitis. In most patients, however, the inflamed mucosa extends proximal to the rectum and when encompassing the entire colon is termed pancolitis. Typically, the inflamed area is uniformly affected, in a continuous fashion, without the "skip lesions" typical to Crohn's colitis.

The large bowel is the principal target organ of ulcerative colitis, whereas other parts of the gastrointestinal tract are not involved in the disease. In patients with pancolitis, it is not unusual to find some inflammatory changes in the distal 20 to 30 cm of the terminal ileum, referred to as "backwash ileitis." However, when the terminal ileum is significantly diseased, differentiation between ulcerative pancolitis and Crohn's disease may be difficult.

Pathologically, the inflammatory response is confined to the mucosa, resulting in mucosal ulcerations and regeneration. Polymorphonuclear infiltration with the formation of crypt abscesses is typical, especially in the active phases of the disease. Features of chronic inflammation, such as lymphatic infiltration and eosinophils, are also the characteristics of this disease. Unlike Crohn's colitis, the inflammatory process of ulcerative colitis is confined to the mucosa, while deeper layers of the colonic wall are uninvolved.

Despite extensive research efforts in the past decades, the etiology of ulcerative colitis is still poorly understood. There is, however, accumulating evidence that the pathophysiology is autoimmune in part. It is presumed that some antigenic stress initiates an inflammatory cascade in individuals with a genetic and/or environmental predisposition. The imbalanced inflammatory response recruits inflammatory cells, releasing mediators that result in mucosal damage and dysfunction. However, the full spectrum of the etiology and pathophysiology of ulcerative colitis is still unclear; hopefully a better understanding of these features may assist in the development of more useful and specific treatment modalities.

The onset of ulcerative colitis in early childhood is uncommon, however, there is a significant peak in the second or third decades of life. Therefore, it is typical to diagnose patients in their active and productive phases of life, i.e., while growing a family and building a career. These patients may suffer from intestinal and extra-intestinal manifestations of the disease, which may severely alter their lifestyle. Care of these patients is aimed at providing a normal lifestyle and lifespan and can be rewarding to the physician. Ulcerative colitis may, however, become symptomatic only later in life, with the second peak of onset in the fifth to the sixth decades. Late onset of the disease may pose unique challenges to the treating physician, due to the patient's advanced age, general medical condition, and past medical history.

Typically, ulcerative colitis is a chronic disease, with relapses of acute colitis and periods of clinical remission between these two phases. The clinical course of the disease for any specific patient is difficult to predict. Although some may experience mild relapse being easily controlled with medical therapy and long periods of remission, other patients may suffer from severe exacerbations that may require urgent surgical therapy.

The majority of medical treatments for ulcerative colitis are aimed at modulating the immune process and reducing the inflammatory response of the colonic mucosa. Steroids remain the principal immunomodulatory agents affecting the disease, but their long-term use is associated with significant adverse effects and, therefore, not recommended for a prolonged period. Other immunomodulating systemic and topical drugs are often used for the induction and maintenance of remission and to wean these patients from steroids. 5-Aminosalicylic acid (5-ASA) compounds specifically affect the inflammatory response within the bowel, but cytotoxic agents such as 6-mercaptopurine (6-MP), imuran, and methotrexate have a significant systemic effect, and patients taking these agents need to be monitored to avoid severe adverse effects.

The chronic inflammatory process and continuous mucosal regeneration characteristic of ulceratives of ulcerative colitis renders these patients at increased risk for the development of colorectal cancer. It is estimated that patients with ulcerative pancolitis for 30 years have an almost 20% chance to develop cancer; this is a significantly higher rate compared to matched controls. The longer the patient is expected to live with ulcerative colitis, the higher the risk to develop cancer. The relation between a long-standing quiescence disease and a somewhat reduced risk to develop cancer is not clear yet, and patients with a long-standing remission may be at an increased risk to develop cancer as well.

Surgical treatment in the management of patients with ulcerative colitis may be divided into two main categories: urgent surgery for acute exacerbation and elective procedures. In the case of acute severe exacerbations unresponsive to medical therapy, surgery is mainly aimed at decreasing the local and systemic toxic effects of the disease in the safest fashion, while maintaining future treatment options. Urgent surgery will usually involve the minimal procedure required, as these patients are at increased risk of postoperative morbidity and mortality. This would usually consist of a subtotal colectomy (resection of the colon up to the mid-sigmoid colon) or a total abdominal colectomy (resection up to the upper rectum). Primary anastomosis is associated with higher risk of anastomotic complications, and most surgeons would elect to avoid anastomoses in such a setting. Once the patient has overcome the acute phase and is weaned off immunosuppressive drugs, a second-stage definitive surgery may be considered.

In the elective setting, surgery has the potential to cure ulcerative colitis by removing the entire colon and rectum. Total proctocolectomy essentially eliminates the inflammatory large bowel disease and practically eliminates the associated risk of colorectal cancer. Total proctocolectomy, however, carries a significant risk of early and late morbidity, and lifestyle alteration and thus the potential gain from surgery should always be weighed against the potential risks.

In the past few decades, reconstruction using various continent reservoirs after total proctocolectomy has been developed. First, an abdominal reservoir with a continent ileostomy was used, known as the Kock's pouch. In 1978, Park and Nichols first introduced the pelvic pouch, a reservoir consisting of the terminal ileum, attached to the anal canal, which allows defecation in the normal route. In the past two decades, the ileoanal pouch has become the restoration method of choice for patients requiring total proctocolectomy. With this method, most patients experience an average of 6 to 10 bowel movements a day, often with continence intact and report a good or excellent quality of life.

Despite the large experience with the ileoanal pouch in numerous centers around the globe, some controversies regarding the appropriate patient selection and best technique for this procedure still exist. Patients with severe dysplasia, or with a colonic mass associated with dysplasia, are best served with surgery. The role of prophylactic colectomy in patients with long-standing disease, or lower grades of dysplasia, is still controversial. Although it is widely agreed that failure of medical therapy is an indication for surgery, the definition of such a failure may vary. The use of routine mucosectomy of the anal transition zone is another controversy, as is the need for a routine temporary diversion proximal to the anastomosis.

This chapter aims to review the current concepts in the etiology, epidemiology, and pathophysiology of ulcerative colitis, its diagnosis and medical treatment, and surgery in the emergent, urgent, and elective settings. Controversies in medical and surgical treatment will be outlined and discussed, and the authors' personal bias, if expressed, will be mentioned as such.

MEDICAL ASPECTS OF ULCERATIVE COLITIS

Ulcerative colitis is a disease in which the chronic inflammatory response and subsequent morphologic changes are confined to the colon. Ulcerative colitis presents mainly with chronic bloody or mucoid diarrhea, tenesmus, urgency, and abdominal pain.

The disease "begins" in the distal rectum with variable degrees of extension proximally along the colon. Microscopically, the acute and chronic inflammatory process is confined to the mucosa accompanied by crypt abscesses, distorted mucosal glands, and goblet cell depletion.

Epidemiology

Ulcerative colitis is found worldwide, although with variable incidences in different regions of the world. As medical awareness and diagnostic modalities improve, the disease is being recognized more frequently in many countries. The incidence of ulcerative colitis follows distinct patterns. The highest rates have been reported in the northern countries, such as Britain, Sweden, and the United States, with ranges from 6 to 15 per 10^5 inhabitants (1,2). By contrast, southern countries in Europe and South Africa have lower annual incidence rates ranging between 2 and 7 per 10^5 inhabitants (3,4). In Asia, South America, and Japan, ulcerative colitis is quite rare with incidence rates as low as 0.5 per 10^5 (5,6).

When individuals from southern Asia migrate to Europe, the prevalence of ulcerative colitis becomes similar to Europeans within two decades (6). The same north-to-south pattern that has been seen on the global scale is also being recognized within individual countries (7), but at least in Europe, southern countries seem to be catching up to their northern neighbors (8,9), perhaps due to increasingly similar environmental exposures.

Trends Among Racial and Ethnic Groups

The incidence of ulcerative colitis is higher in Caucasian Americans compared to that of African-Americans or Asians (8,9). Incidence rates rise in populations that immigrate to high-risk geographic areas (Table 1). A higher incidence of ulcerative colitis is found among Jews compared to non-Jews (two to fourfold) and in Ashkenazi Jews compared with Sephardi Jews in many countries (10). The latter is true for the incidence in Israel as well, but is less pronounced than in other countries. The rate of disease in Jews varies from region to region parallel to the general population, suggesting an important role of environmental factors (11).

Age and Gender

Ulcerative colitis primarily affects young adults but may present at any age. Two peaks of the disease have been described—one between the ages of 15 to 30 years and the other, a smaller peak, between the ages of 60 and 80 years (1,8). Most studies reveal a male-to-female ratio that is close to 1 in all ages, with some studies suggesting a progressive decrease in the incidence of the disease in women older than 40 years (9,12).

Disease Course
Extent and Severity

The majority of patients with ulcerative colitis have a disease confined to the left colon at the time of diagnosis. Various studies found that up to 49% of patients have proctosigmoiditis and

Table 1 Epidemiology of Ulcerative Colitis

Incidence (per 10^5)	Northern countries 6–15; southern 2–7
Racial incidence	More frequent in Caucasians than non-Caucasians
Ethnic incidence	More frequent in Jews than non-Jews
	More frequent in Ashkenazi than Sephardi Jews
Genetics	Higher frequency within families, HLA system, twins
Urban-rural effect	More frequent in urban than rural communities
Socioeconomic class	More frequent in higher socioeconomic classes
Effect of smoking	Decreases the risk of disease
Effect of appendectomy	Decreases the risk of disease

Abbreviation: HLA, human leukocyte antigen.

Table 2 Local Complication of Ulcerative Colitis

Massive hemorrhage	3.5% of patients
Acute colonic dilatation	5% of severe attacks
Perforation	Very rare, 16% mortality
Strictures—benign malignant	Rare
Pseudopolyps inflammatory polyps	Not malignant
Colonic cancer	

14% to 37% have pancolitis (13–16). The clinical severity of disease at presentation usually correlates with the extent of the disease; patients with pancolitis having more severe symptoms and signs than patients with left-sided colitis. Most patients will present with moderate disease at time of first presentation (70%), whereas 20% will have mild disease and 10% will present with severe disease.

Most patients will experience a chronic intermittent course with remissions and execrations (80–90%); 16% will have a chronic continuous course, with a minority having a continuous unrelenting course requiring colectomy (0.1%) (7).

A course free of relapse was found in only 1% of patients after 18 years of follow-up. The clinical course over 25 years of follow-up is not influenced by the extent of disease at time of diagnosis, nor by the age at presentation, gender, presenting symptoms, or the length of time between onset of symptoms and diagnosis, but rather by the occurrence of systemic symptoms such as fever and weight loss (13). When patients who undergo colectomy are included in such analyses, investigators have found that the extent of disease at diagnosis influences later extent and severity (8).

Patients presenting with pancolitis have the highest probability of undergoing colectomy, which is close to 40%.

Local complications are relatively rare and generally related to the anatomic extent and severity of the disease. Massive hemorrhage occurs in up to 3.5% of ulcerative colitis patients; acute colonic dilatation in up to 5% of patients with severe colitis; and colonic perforation is even less, although this complication is associated with a mortality rate of 16% (17). Other local complications include benign or malignant strictures and colon cancer (Table 2).

Risk of Colon Cancer

The risk of colon cancer among ulcerative colitis patients is highest in patients with extensive involvement and duration of more than 10 years of disease. Although it is clear that patients with long-term ulcerative colitis have an increased risk of colorectal cancer, its exact magnitude has been difficult to estimate.

Early studies, conducted in referral tertiary care centers, tended to overestimate the risk, whereas later population-based studies describe more conservative risk estimates (16). Ekbom et al. (18) found a sixfold increase in incidence of colorectal cancer in ulcerative colitis patients followed up for 35 years compared to an age-matched cohort. The risk was proportional to the extent of disease: proctitis, risk not increased; left-sided colitis, intermediate risk ($\times$2-3); pancolitis, increased risk ($\times$15). A recent meta-analysis by Eaden et al. (19), based on 116 studies, found the overall prevalence of colorectal cancer in ulcerative colitis to be 3.7%. The incidence rates calculated corresponded to cumulative probabilities of 2% by 10 years, 8% by 20 years, and 18% by 30 years of disease. There was a slight worldwide geographical variation in cancer incidence, and a slight (although not significant) increase in overall incidence of cancer over the years studied. The overall annual incidence of colorectal cancer in ulcerative colitis of more than 10 years, duration is 0.5% to 1% (20). Several studies have indicated that a subset of patients with ulcerative colitis, those with primary sclerosing cholangitis, may be even at a higher risk for colorectal cancer and suggested annual colonoscopic surveillance from the time of diagnosis of primary sclerosing cholangitis in these patients (21). The influence of medical treatments on the risk of colon cancer in ulcerative colitis patients has not been thoroughly investigated, but it has been suggested that treatment with amino salicylates and folic acid supplementation may reduce this risk (Table 3).

Colorectal cancer in ulcerative colitis patients tends to differ from sporadic cancer. It tends to occur at younger age, often arises from flat mucosa, is more evenly distributed in the colon, and may present as synchronous tumors.

Table 3 Risk Factors and Manifestation of Colorectal Cancer in Ulcerative Colitis

Risk factor	Influence	Manifestations
Extent of disease	↑↑↑↑	Occurs at younger age
Longevity of disease	↑↑↑↑	Arises from flat mucosa
Young age at onset	↑↑	More evenly distributed
Sclerosing cholangitis	↑↑	Multiple tumors
Stricture (present)	↑↑	Increased at stricture sites
Drugs (5-ASA, folic acid)	↓	May be preceded by dysplasia, DALM

Abbreviations: 5-ASA, 5-aminosalicyclic acid; DALM, dysplasia-associated lesions or masses.

The present surveillance policy for colorectal cancer in ulcerative colitis advocates colononscopy after 8 to 10 years of disease followed by periodic colonoscopy during remission at intervals of 1 to 2 years beginning 8 to 10 years after disease onset for pancolitis and 15 years for left-sided colitis (16). During colononscopy the entire colon should be assessed with two to four random biopsies taken at 10-cm intervals throughout the entire colon. It is suggested that 33 biopsies are required to give a 95% chance of detecting dysplasia. Dysplasia is a precancerous marker that is defined as an unequivocal neoplastic transformation of the epithelium. The greater the degree of dysplasia the easier it is for the pathologist to make the diagnosis. If the diagnosis of dysplasia is confirmed, the patient should generally be referred for colectomy.

Assessing the impact of surveillance on cancer prevalence is difficult, as large numbers of patients and a long duration of follow-up are needed to determine the utility and cost effectiveness of this method. Definitive data supporting the efficacy of surveillance is lacking, but it is nonetheless considered standard management by most authorities.

Recently the approach to dysplasia-associated lesions or masses (DALM) has been re-evaluated. In the past, the presence of such a lesion led to surgery. Nowadays, if the lesion is a true dysplasia-associated lesion or mass, the patient should generally be referred for colectomy.

If a polypoid lesion has an adenoma-like appearance, many clinicians would take a different approach—polypectomy and multiple biopsies from the adjacent nonpolypoid mucosa. If the adjacent mucosa shows no dysplasia (suggesting an adenomatous polyp, rather than DALM) then the patient can probably be placed in a surveillance program and colonoscopy repeated in a year (22).

Molecular markers including P53, Ki-ras mutations CA-19–9, CA50, carcinoembryonic antigen (CEA), TAG-72, Sialosyl-Tn antigen, and the adenomatous polyposis coli gene are being investigated as markers to complement dysplasia in surveillance for pre-cancerous conditions in patients with ulcerative colitis (18).

Extra-Intestinal Manifestations

Ulcerative colitis is associated with a number of extra-intestinal manifestations, acute arthropathy being the most common of these, affecting up to 20% of patients (23). It may present as either large-joint pauciarticular arthritis or small-joint symmetric polyarthritis. The flares of large-joint arthritis generally parallel the state of the acute bowel disease. Sacroliitis and ankylosing spondylitis are less common than peripheral arthritis with frequencies up to 11% by plain radiography. Seventy percent of patients may have evidence of the disease, mostly asymptotic, by technetium bone scan (23). The majority of patients with sacroliitis are human leukocyte antigen (HLA)-B27 negative and do not progress to ankylosing spondylitis, whereas the majority of patients with ankylosing spondylitis are HLA-B27 positive (8). The course of spondylitis is independent of bowel activity and may not improve after successful medical therapy or colectomy. Ocular symptoms occur in up to 10% of ulcerative colitis patients and include episcleritis and anterior uveitis. Mild conjunctivitis is also common. These complications tend to parallel the activity of bowel disease.

The most common skin manifestations of ulcerative colitis include erythema nodosum, which occurs in up to 15% of patients, and less frequently pyoderma-gangrenosum and Sweet's syndrome (acute febrile neutrophilic dermatosis), all of which tend to parallel bowel activity (24).

Hepatobilliary complications are also common in patients with ulcerative colitis. Transient elevations of serum liver enzymes and fatty infiltration of liver cells may be found in up to 50% of the patients with acute colitis as a consequence of malnutrition, administration of parenteral nutrition, or sepsis (25). The most serious extra-intestinal manifestation of ulcerative colitis is primary sclerosing cholangitis, which occurs in up to 7% of patients with ulcerative colitis. This is a chronic, cholestatic hepatobilliary disorder characterized by inflammation and progressive obliterative fibrosis of the billiary tree, leading to cirrhosis, portal hypertension, and eventually hepatic failure (26). The disease usually affects men in their 30s, with a five-year survival of approximately 85%. There is an increased risk of cholangiocarcinoma in these patients which reaches 10% over six years. The diagnosis is made via endoscopic retrograde cholangiography, which shows beading, irregularity, and strictures of both the intra- and extrahepatic bile ducts. At present there is no effective medical treatment. Therapy with immunosuppressants, cupruretic agents, antifibrotic agents, and choleretic medications has been tried with no proven success (25). A variety of endoscopic and radiologic techniques are used to treat complications of mechanical obstruction, but orthotopic liver transplantation is the only effective treatment for localized disease, extending life expectancy of patients (27). Other disorders that have been described in association with ulcerative colitis and inflammatory bowel disease (IBD) include pericholangitis, chronic hepatitis, granulomatous hepatitis, primary billiary cirrhosis, and portal vein thrombosis (26). Extra-intestinal complications of ulcerative colitis are illustrated in Figure 1.

Etiology and Pathogenesis

The etiology of ulcerative colitis remains unknown. Clinical and laboratory studies indicate that both genetics and environmental factors are important (28). Other theories involve defects in the mucous gel barrier, which may be either primary or acquired by bacteria sulphatases, and a potential infectious etiology (29–31).

Genetic and Environmental Factors

The importance of genetic factors in the cause of ulcerative colitis has been strongly supported by genetic epidemiologic studies. Many lines of evidence indicate that genetic factors are involved in the pathogenesis of ulcerative colitis:

1. Jews appear to have a genetic predisposition to the disease.
2. The disease occurs with high frequency within families (10–20% of patients will have one other family member affected).
3. Familial cases are concordant for various characteristics of the disease, i.e., predominant ulcerative colitis or Crohn's disease.
4. Genetic anticipation occurs among children of ulcerative colitis patients, i.e., the disease develops at a younger age than the parents, similar to the age of others of their generation (32).

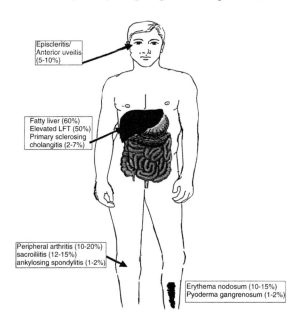

Episcleritis/Anterior uveitis (5-10%)

Fatty liver (60%)
Elevated LFT (50%)
Primary sclerosing cholangitis (2-7%)

Peripheral arthritis (10-20%)
sacroiliitis (12-15%)
ankylosing spondylitis (1-2%)

Erythema nodosum (10-15%)
Pyoderma gangrenosum (1-2%)

Figure 1 Extra-intestinal manifestations of ulcerative colitis.

5. There is highly concordant frequency of ulcerative colitis in monozygotic and dizygotic twin pairs.
6. Several studies found a significant association between the human leukocyte antigen (HLA) DR2 allele and ulcerative colitis, which is strongest in patients with pancolitis (33,34). In Japanese and Jewish patients there is an association between ulcerative colitis and the 1502 allele of HLA-DR2 (HLA-DRB1∗1502). In Northern Europe, an association with DRB1∗ 0103 and DRB1∗12 has been described (34,35). Specific HLA class II molecules may predict disease severity and extension, i.e., DRB1∗0301 DQB∗0201 (36–38).
7. Loci on chromosome 3, 7, and 12 have been linked to ulcerative colitis (34,36).
   Nevertheless, environmental factors are not less important as we can learn from the protective effect of smoking in these patients, as well as from the fact that the disease is more frequent in urban communities and in higher socioeconomic classes.

Human and animal studies suggest that ulcerative colitis can be initiated by environmental factors triggering a loss of tolerance to normal intestinal flora in genetically susceptible individuals (22).

Smoking has been the most consistent environmental association with ulcerative colitis (39–42). Ulcerative colitis is more common in nonsmokers than in smokers, with a relative risk of 2.6 of developing ulcerative colitis in nonsmokers as compared to smokers. The risk is particularly high for ex-smokers within the first years of cessation (43). The mechanisms underlying these effects are not clear but include effects on mucus production by colonic mucosa and on mucosal blood flow, intestinal trefoil factor (ITF), and somatostatin (40,41,44).

Oral contraceptive use was initially reported to be slightly increased in women with ulcerative colitis, but this weak association appears less significant if the data are corrected for other factors. Another consistent interesting finding is a low appendectomy rate in ulcerative colitis patients compared to controls (45,46).

Role of Intestinal Bacteria
Despite hopes and suggestions of an infectious etiology and extensive investigation, no organism has been consistently isolated from UC patients, and therefore ulcerative colitis is unlikely to be a simple infective disorder. Cooke and coworkers have found that strains of *Escherichia coli* isolated from patients with ulcerative colitis were more likely to produce hemolysins and necrotoxins, but this difference occurred after the disease relapsed (47). Later it was shown that *E. coli* from colitic patients expressed adhesins more frequently suggesting a greater potential for adherence to the epithelial cell and initiation of damage (48). This led to a trial in which Tobramycin was found to be significantly better than placebo in active ulcerative colitis (49,50). Other studies with antibiotics, such as rifaximin and ciprofloxacin, also proved to be beneficial, suggesting bacterial infections may play some role in the pathophysiology of ulcerative colitis (50). *Clostridium difficile* toxin and *Salmonella* infection have been associated with disease exacerbation. Moreover, an excess of sulfate-reducing bacteria have been found in fecal samples of patients with active ulcerative colitis. These bacteria result in overproduction of hydrogen sulfide, which is toxic to the mucosa by competing with short-chain fatty acids (50).

Abnormalities in mucosal permeability may also give rise to chronic inflammation induced by normal bacterial components in a genetically susceptible host (30,50).

Further evidence for the role of intestinal bacteria comes from studies in patients with pouchitis, which develops in patients with ulcerative colitis or familial polyposis who undergo an ileal pouch anal anastomosis. Ulcerative colitis patients are genetically susceptible to the development of pouchitis after colonization of the pouch by intestinal flora. Early treatment with antibiotics improves this condition.

Immunopathogenesis
Immunologic mechanisms involving both humoral and cellular responses are implicated in the pathogenesis of inflammation in ulcerative colitis.

Humoral Responses
The inflamed colon in ulcerative colitis shows an increase in cells that produce increased amounts of IgG1 and IgG3, a response that suggests that protein antigens may be the predominant trigger

in ulcerative colitis (57). A destructive inflammatory response directed toward self-antigens such as mucin, colonocytes, or other cells have been proposed as the underlying basis to ulcerative colitis (51,52). An increased association of ulcerative colitis with other autoimmune diseases such as thyroid, diabetes, and pernicious anemia has been described. Moreover, autoantibodies to colonic epithelium and lymphocytes as well as low titers of smooth muscle, parietal cell, and thyroid antibodies have been described (57). Antibodies against 40-kDa epithelial antigens and to epithelial cell–associated components have been described (53). An antibody to this 40-kDa molecule was eluted from the inflamed mucosa of patients with ulcerative colitis only and was found not only in the colon but also in the skin and billiary epithelium of these patients (53). These data may shed some light into the pathogenesis of some extra-intestinal manifestations of ulcerative colitis. High levels of antibodies to human intestinal tropomyosin isoform 5 have also been reported in patients with ulcerative colitis by the same group (54).

Finally another autoantibody, a perinuclear antineutrophil cytoplasmatic antibody (p-ANCA), has been found in up to 70% of patients with ulcerative colitis, almost all of whom developed pouchitis after ileal anal pouch anastomosis (55). The epitope recognized by p-ANCA in ulcerative colitis is located in the c-terminal basic random-coil domain of histone, H1 (30). The antibody titer is not affected by disease activity, but may decline after a prolonged remission or following colectomy. Thus, in summary, the endogenous antigens that drive the inflammatory events in ulcerative colitis remain ill defined.

Cellular Responses

The balance between Th1 and Th2 phenotypes of T lymphocytes determines the characteristics of a chronic inflammatory process. Th1 cells secrete proinflammatory cytokines like interleukin (IL) -2 and interferon γ (INFγ), whereas Th2 cells express regulatory or anti-inflammatory cytokines such as IL-4 and IL-10. Th2 responses have been shown to be important in conditions in which altered humoral immunity is present. Existing data suggest that ulcerative colitis more closely resembles a Th2 reaction (56). Many studies have found diminished suppressor activity during active ulcerative colitis.

Activation of the immune cells leads to the release of an extensive number of cytokines and inflammatory mediators. These include prostaglandin E_2 (PGE_2), leukotriene B_4 (LTB_4), thromboxane B_2, platelet activating factor (PAF), nitric oxide, IL-1β, IL-8, IL-6, INFγ, tumor necrosis factor (TNFα), MCP-1, and others (57,58). These mediators attract and activate leukocytes and other inflammatory cells, thus helping to intensify the inflammatory process (PGE_2, LTB_4, PAF, and TXB_2), alter epithelial cell permeability (LTB4, PAF, and INFγ), affect collagen synthesis (transforming growth factor β), and affect endothelial cells (IL-1, IL-6, TNFα, and INFγ).

Psychosomatic Effects

Both patients and doctors believe that psychological stress influences ulcerative colitis (59,60). Psychological stress was cited as a potential trigger by up to 40% of patients with ulcerative colitis (61). There is some evidence that links psychological stress with increased illness and possible increased susceptibility for infections (62). Psychological factors that possibly contribute to IBD include the patient's psychological status, life events that are particularly stressful, and history of physical or sexual abuse (59). Although the issue of stress and its role in the etiology and exacerbation of inflammatory bowel disease remains controversial, several studies noted a relationship between stressful life events and disease activity (63). A history of abuse of any sort has been shown to adversely affect the coping skills of the patient. Undoubtedly, the chronic disease itself has a major impact on the patient, and many of the psychological features described in ulcerative colitis may actually be secondary to the disease rather than its cause.

Clinical Features

Ulcerative colitis is associated with both intestinal and extra-intestinal manifestations. This section will concentrate on the intestinal manifestations of this disease. The most consistent feature of ulcerative colitis is the presence of blood and mucus in the stool, diarrhea, and lower abdominal pain that is most intense during bowel movements (Table 4). The symptoms tend to vary according to the extent and severity of the disease (31). Ulcerative colitis may have a slow,

Table 4 Symptoms and Signs in Ulcerative Colitis

Symptoms	Signs
Rectal bleeding	No signs
Diarrhea	Tachycardia±
Tenesmus	Abdominal tenderness± distention
Abdominal pain	Weight loss±
Fever	Pallor±
Weight loss	Leg edema±
Weakness	Extra-intestinal manifestations±

insidious onset but is generally diagnosed earlier than Crohn's disease after the onset of symptoms, as the gross blood often present in stool alerts the patient to consult with a physician.

Patients usually complain of passing fresh blood, either separate from the stool or streaked onto the surface of a loose, normal, or hard stool and thus may be mistakenly attributed to hemorrhoidal bleeding. When the disease extends beyond the rectum, there is usually diarrhea mixed with blood and mucus. Bloody diarrhea is the hallmark of ulcerative colitis but may not always be present, especially in patients in whom the disease is confined to the rectum/rectosigmoid. Diarrhea is often postprandial and nocturnal. Tenesmus, which is described as the urgency to defecate with a feeling of incomplete evacuation, is also common; patients with severe disease may report incontinence. The cause of diarrhea involves several mechanisms including the failure to absorb salt and water, inflammatory mediators, and increased colonic motility. Urgency and tenesmus are caused by poor compliance and loss of reservoir capacity of the inflamed rectum (64).

The location of the abdominal pain depends on the extent of colonic involvement and, although present in many patients, is not a predominant symptom. Pain is present in the left lower quadrant in distal disease, extending to the entire abdomen with pancolitis; severe cramps and pain may occur in severe attacks. Other symptoms include fever in up to 40% of patients at the time of presentation, usually accompanied by severe colitis. Weight loss may be a feature in both adults and children and is caused by nausea, hypercatabolism, and protein loss through the severely inflamed mucosa. Weakness and shortness of breath secondary to anemia due to blood loss and chronic inflammation are also occasionally present.

Signs

Most patients with ulcerative colitis exhibit no or minor physical signs. In some, the affected portion of the colon may be tender whereas in severe attacks, tachycardia, abdominal tenderness and distention, fever, and weight loss are often seen. Some extra-intestinal manifestations may also be present.

Disease Severity

The severity of ulcerative colitis can be determined by various criteria including clinical symptoms, sigmoidoscopic and histologic features, or a combination of these features.

The original criteria of Truelove and Witts using clinical symptoms are easy to use and are still applied, although they lack precision (Table 5). These take into account the number of bloody stools per day, body temperature, pulse rate, anemia, and sedimentation rate, and categorize the disease as mild, moderate, or severe (65). Another numeric index has been developed at St. Mark's in London, which takes into account general health, abdominal pain, bowel frequency, consistency, bloody stools, anorexia, nausea and vomiting, abdominal tenderness, extra-intestinal manifestations, temperature, and sigmoidoscopy with points ranging from 0

Table 5 Truelove and Witt's Activity Index

Mild	Moderate	Severe
Non-bloody diarrhea < 4/day	Anything between mild and severe	Diarrhea > 6/day bloody
No fever		Fever > 37°C
No tachycardia		Pulse > 90
Anemia "not severe"		Hemoglobin < 75% of expected
ESR < 30 mm/hr		ESR > 30 mm/hr

Abbreviation: ESR, erythrocyte sedimentation rate.

Table 6 Potential Markers of Activity

Serum	Stool	Tissue
ESR	α_1 antitrypsin	IL-8
CRP	Lactoferrin	IL-1/IL-1RA
Orsomucoid (α_1 acid glycoprotein)	IL-1β	Nitric oxide
TNFα	IL-8	
L-selectin	PGE$_2$, LTB$_4$, TXB$_2$	

Abbreviations: IL, interleukin; TNF, tumor necrosis factor; PGE$_2$, prostaglandin E$_2$; LTB$_4$, leukotriene B$_4$; ESR, erythrocyte sedimentation rate; CRP, C-reactive protein.

to 3 in most parameters. Unfortunately, this numeric index has not gained wide acceptance. An index that has gained recognition in recent years measures the effect of inflammatory bowel disease on the patient's quality of life, using the inflammatory bowel disease questionnaire (IBDQ) questionnaire developed by the MacMaster group (65). The scoring system covers four domains: bowel symptoms, systemic symptoms, emotional function, and social symptoms. The IBDQ has been extensively validated and found to be a reliable tool in assessing the impact of disease on patients (65).

The severity of macroscopic inflammation visualized on sigmoidoscopy can also be used to characterize disease severity. A convenient grading system from 0 to 4 has been suggested: 0, normal mucosa; 1, loss of vascular pattern; 2, granular, nonfriable mucosa; 3, friability on rubbing; and 4, spontaneous bleeding and ulceration (31).

Microscopic assessment on histologic analysis of biopsy specimens is less useful for decision making on medical therapy, as these changes occur more slowly than clinical symptoms or macroscopic appearance.

Active disease may be associated with a rise in acute-phase reactants, erythrocyte sedimentation rate, platelet count, and many other markers, both in serum and in stools (Table 6). Disease confined to the rectum or rectosigmoid rarely increases in any of these parameters (66). A combination of elevated orsomucoid, ESR, and α_2 globulin predicts relapse in 88% of patients, as does persistent elevation of C-reactive protein (CRP) or ESR.

Diagnosis

The diagnosis of ulcerative colitis relies mainly on the clinical history, stool examinations, endoscopic appearance, and histology of rectal or colonic biopsies.

Routine stool cultures should be performed in order to exclude *Salmonella, Shigella, Campylobacter, E. coli*, or *Yersinia* infections.

It is not uncommon to find a patient whose disease began with a documented infection that either revealed quiescent disease or initiated it. The presence of *C. difficile* toxin as well as amebiases must be excluded by examination of a fresh, warm stool sample. Viral infections of the colon (such as cytomegalovirus or herpes) should also be excluded.

Sigmoidoscopy and Colonoscopy

Sigmoidoscopy should be performed in an unprepared bowel with minimal air insufflation if severe inflammation is present. The earliest endoscopic signs of ulcerative colitis are blurring, or the loss of a vascular pattern of the mucosa (sigmoidoscopic score of 1) with blunted valves of Houston. Later the mucosa becomes granular (score of 2), friability and minute bleeding occurs upon rubbing (score of 3), followed by overt friability with spontaneous bleeding and the presence of fibrin and ulcerations (score of 4; Fig. 2). When the disease is long-standing, pseudopolyps may also be present (Fig. 3).

At remission, the mucosa may appear normal or become thin, pale, and atrophic.

Colonoscopy is not necessary for the diagnosis of ulcerative colitis, but is useful to determine disease extent. The best timing for endoscopy is when active disease is controlled and the procedure should be accompanied by multiple biopsies. The procedure is useful in patients in whom symptoms are out of proportion to other diagnostic modalities (X rays) and for cancer surveillance.

Radiology

Patients with a severe episode of ulcerative colitis should undergo a plain supine film of the abdomen in order to assess bowel and colonic dilatation (toxic megacolon) (Fig. 4). Plain

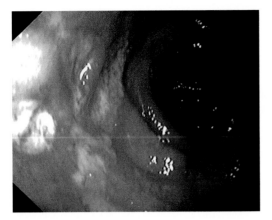

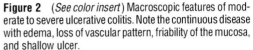

Figure 2 (*See color insert*) Macroscopic features of moderate to severe ulcerative colitis. Note the continuous disease with edema, loss of vascular pattern, friability of the mucosa, and shallow ulcer.

abdominal films are also useful in assessing the presence of fecal material, which is seldom present in inflamed mucosa and thus providing some information of disease extent (67). Barium enema should generally be avoided in severe disease and is contraindicated if the colon is dilated; this is considered safe in mild-to-moderate disease. The radiologic findings consist of mucosal granularity (the earliest change), followed by irregular mucosal lines that then become thickened and form superficial ulcers (collar-button ulcer). In severe colitis, deeper ulcerations follow. The folds may become edematous and thickened as the disease progresses, and loss of haustral folds is seen in patients with chronic disease (Fig. 5), along with shortening and narrowing of the colon; as well, the presacral space (between the sacrum and posterior wall of the rectum) is widened. Long-standing disease is radiologically characterized by pseudopolyps that may resemble a cobblestone appearance (68,69).

Computed tomography (CT) findings associated with ulcerative colitis include mural thickening (<1.5 cm), inhomogenous wall density, normal small bowel wall, increased perirectal and presacral fat, and adenopathy (69).

Pathologic Features
Macroscopic Findings
Approximately 15% to 20% of adults present with pancolitis, 30% to 40% will have left-sided colitis (disease extending beyond the sigmoid), and 40% to 55% will have proctitis or proctosigmoiditis (20). The typical changes are most severe in the rectum and extend proximally to a variable extent, except in patients receiving topical treatment (suppositories or enemas). In severe disease, the proximal colon may show a more severe pattern than the rectum, however, this is rare (70). Other rare situations include "skipped lesions"—areas of cecal or appendiceal inflammation in patients with left-sided colitis. In these cases, ileoscopy and multiple biopsies of the terminal ileum and entire colon are of importance to rule out Crohn's disease.

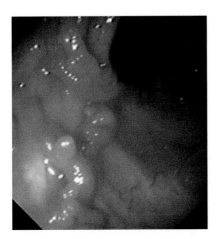

Figure 3 (*See color insert*) Macroscopic appearance of long-standing ulcerative colitis. Note the areas of quiescent disease and pseudopolyps.

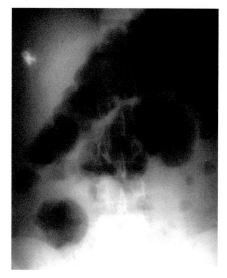

Figure 4 Toxic megacolon—plain radiograph. The transverse colon and sigmoid are dilated by gas. Note the course nodularity of the colonic wall and absence of haustra in the transverse colon. *Source*: Courtesy of Prof. Kleinhaus, Department of Radiology, Rambam Medical Center, Haifa, Israel.

Microscopic Findings

As mentioned earlier, the inflammatory process in ulcerative colitis is predominantly confined to the mucosa of the colon. Early signs include an edematous lamina propria with dilated capillaries. Acute and chronic inflammation with increased numbers of neutrophils, eosinophils, lymphocytes, plasma cells, mast cells, and macrophages are seen. There is a tendency for the neutrophils to invade the crypts epithelium creating what is known as a crypt abscess (Fig. 6). The migration of leukocytes and other inflammatory cells involves chemoattractant mediators from colonic bacteria, cytokines, as well as inflammatory mediators such as LTB_4, PAF, and others that are present in the inflamed mucosa and epithelial cells (58). Furthermore, mucus discharge from goblet cells and goblet cell depletion appears. Most of these changes are nonspecific and can occur in any infectious colitis. Distorted crypt architecture, crypt atrophy, increased intercrypt spacing, basal lymphoid aggregates, and chronic inflammatory cells are microscopic features that increase the likelihood of ulcerative colitis compared to self-limited colitis (71,72). With increased inflammation, the epithelial surface is flattened and shallow or deep ulcers appear. The submucosa may appear congested and inflamed, however, transmural inflammation is characteristic of Crohn's disease.

During remission, histologic features may return to normal, but usually some evidence of disease such as altered architecture or loss of glands can be seen (Fig. 7). Continuous

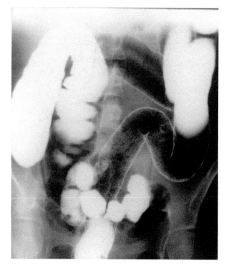

Figure 5 Radiologic features of long-standing (chronic) ulcerative colitis. Note absence of haustra in the presence of normal colonic width. Multiple pseudopolyps cause the diffuse nodularity seen along the wall of the sigmoid colon. *Source*: Courtesy of Prof. Kleinhaus, Department of Radiology, Rambam Medical Center, Haifa, Israel.

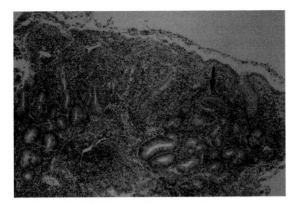

Figure 6 (*See color insert*) Microscopic findings showing active chronic ulcerative colitis including superficial ulcerations, crypt distortion, marked mononuclear inflammation within the lamina propria, and crypt abscess (*arrow*). *Source:* Courtesy of Prof. Groisman, Department of Pathology, Hillel-Yaffe Medical Center, Hadera, Israel.

microscopic inflammation in a patient with a clinical remission is a poor prognostic sign, indicating a high risk for relapse.

Laboratory Results

In mild or distal disease, laboratory findings may all be normal. Chronic bleeding may cause iron-deficiency anemia. Thrombocytosis, leukocytosis, and eosinophilia can also be seen during an acute attack. In severe or prolonged attacks, the sedimentation rate or C reactive protein may be elevated, hypoalbuminemia may develop, and minor reversible elevations of liver enzymes can be seen. If liver enzymes remain persistently elevated, further investigations should be undertaken to rule out or diagnose primary sclerosing cholangitis.

Differential Diagnosis

A differential diagnosis depends on the onset and type of predominant symptoms. When the patient presents with acute symptoms, infectious disease must be ruled out. *Shigella*, *Salmonella*, *Campylobacter*, or *E. coli:0157:H7* are the most common species that should be excluded. Sudden onset, the presence of disease in other family contacts, and abdominal pain with or without fever should suggest this possibility. As the endoscopic appearance cannot distinguish between ulcerative colitis and infectious colitis, one must rely on stool cultures or histology. The presence of chronic inflammatory infiltrate, distorted architecture, and basal lymphoid aggregates strongly suggest ulcerative colitis rather than an infectious process (71,72).

Biopsies with special stain will help diagnose some opportunistic infections that can mimic ulcerative colitis such as cytomegalovirus infection and herpes simplex virus. Sexually transmitted causes generally do not cause diarrhea, but rather watery pus. Diagnosis is made by clinical suspicion and appropriate cultures. Yersinia may cause chronic colitis that may continue for a few months and then resolve. Stool cultures or rising antibody titers are useful in the diagnosis of this condition.

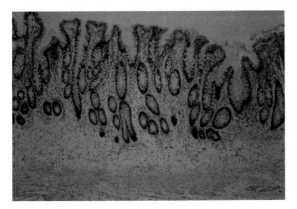

Figure 7 (*See color insert*) Microscopic findings showing inactive (quiescent) ulcerative colitis including crypt distortion and atrophy and paucity of inflammatory cells. *Source:* Courtesy of Prof. Groisman, Department of Pathology, Hillel-Yaffe Medical Center, Hadera, Israel.

Amebic dysentery may mimic ulcerative colitis in every aspect including chronicity. Microscopic examination of fresh, warm stool will usually help make a diagnosis. This is important as steroid therapy may cause dissemination of amebiasis.

A drug history must be obtained as several drugs may cause mild colitis including non-steroidal anti-inflammatory drugs, penicillamine, gold, methyldopa, and ticlopidine (73,74). Antibiotics may also induce colitis via *C. difficile* toxin–mediated or other pathways. Salicylates may rarely cause colitis and cause confusion, as patients who are diagnosed with ulcerative colitis may receive therapeutic salicylates and experience a relapse (75).

When patients present with long-standing complaints of many months, the major differential diagnosis is with Crohn's colitis. Patients with Crohn's colitis tend to have perianal lesions and, less frequently, bloody diarrhea. Rectal sparing is not uncommon and thus complaints of proctitis (tenesmus and bloody stools) may be absent. Crohn's colitis is relatively easy to diagnose using endoscopy, histology, and radiology. Rectal sparing, segmental disease, aphthous or linear ulcers within a normal mucosa, fistula, strictures, and small bowel involvement are all indicative of Crohn's disease. Transmural focal inflammation goblet cell preservation and granulomas on histology are also suggestive of Crohn's disease.

Indeterminate colitis refers to cases where there is diffuse colonic inflammation, in which macroscopic and microscopic features may make it difficult to determine whether it is ulcerative colitis or Crohn's disease. Serology may be helpful in some of these cases. Positive antineutrophil cytoplasmatic antibody (ANCA) and negative antisaachromyces cerevisiae antibody (ASCA) would suggest ulcerative colitis, whereas negative ANCA and positive ASCA would suggest Crohn's capsule endoscopy may be helpful in making the precise diagnosis in these patients. Patients with indeterminate colitis should generally be treated as if they have ulcerative colitis until there are more definite characteristics of Crohn's disease.

Radiation colitis, ischemic colitis and microscopic (MC) and collagenous colitis (CC), all covered elsewhere in this text, should also be considered in the differential diagnosis of patients with a long history of diarrhea. The clinical setting, disease history, and endoscopic and histologic findings are of great importance in the diagnosis of these conditions.

MC and CC are more frequently recognized. The clinical setting is typically one of chronic diarrhea, generally with normal laboratory studies and preserved well being. Macroscopically, the mucosa appears normal and the diagnosis is based only on the histology. CC appears as a thickened subepithelial collagen band and chronic inflammation, whereas MC shows increased intra-epithelial lymphocytes and chronic inflammatory infiltrate (Table 7).

Medical Treatment

Two major milestones during 1940s and 1950s made a dramatic impact on the treatment of ulcerative colitis; these were the introduction of sulfasalazine and corticosteroids. The medical treatment of ulcerative colitis is based on two major considerations—the extent and severity of the disease. Three major categories of drugs are routinely used in the treatment of ulcerative colitis: salicylates, corticosteroids, and immunosuppressive/immunomodulatory agents.

Table 7 Differential Diagnosis of Ulcerative Colitis

Infectious	Inflammatory	Others
Bacterial	Crohn's colitis	Segmental colitis assoociated
Shigella, Salmonella,	Indeterminate colitis.	with diverticulitis
Campylobacter, Escherichia coli	Microscopic colitis,	Drugs
0157:H7, Yersinia,	(lymphocytic, collagenous)	Lymphoma
Clostridium difficile	Ischemic colitis	Vasculitis
Viral	Radiation colitis	
Cytomegalovirus		
Herpes		
Parasites		
Amebiasis		

Table 8 New Salicylate Compounds

Enteric coated	Controlled release	AZO bond
Asacol (Eudragit S) pH $\geq$ 7.0 Salofalk (Eudragit L) pH $\geq$ 6.0 Claversal	Pentasa pH $\geq$ 6.0	Olsalazine

Salicylates

Aminosalicylates are the mainstay for induction and maintenance of remission in mild-to-moderate disease (76). Sulfasalazine, initially introduced for rheumatoid arthritis, was also found to be effective for the treatment of ulcerative colitis. This consists of 5-ASA linked by an azo bond to sulfapyridine. In the colon, bacterial azoreductases split the azo bond of the two compounds and the 5-ASA, the active moiety, is mainly excreted through the feces.

Sulfasalazine is effective in inducing and maintaining remission in mild-to-moderate disease. The mode of action involves a decreased synthesis of various inflammatory mediators (prostaglandins, leukotrienes, thromboxane, and PAF), suppression of IL-1 release, inhibition of nuclear factor-KB transcription, and protection from reactive oxygen metabolites (77). The incidence of adverse events associated with sulfasalazine is relatively high (78) and include those that are dose dependent (nausea, vomiting, anorexia, headache, and alopecia) and others that are not (hypersensitivity reaction, hepatitis, hemolytic anemia, agranulocytosis, alveolitis, and infertility). Most side effects are reversible with drug cessation due to the sulfapyridine moiety of the molecule. The fact that the active moiety of sulfasalazine is 5-ASA and most side effects are caused by the sulfapyridine moiety of the molecule has led to the development of new drugs that contain only 5-ASA (mesalamine and olsalazine). Two types of delivery systems have been applied: pH-sensitive–coating system or linkage of two 5-ASA molecules via an azo bond (Table 8). These new drugs were shown to be as effective as sulfasalazine for treating active ulcerative colitis and maintaining remission but with minimal side effects (headache, drug fever, rash, pancreatitis, hepatitis, pneumonitis, nephritis, and exacerbation of colitis) (78–80). 5-ASA compounds are available in various forms such as suppositories that extend to 15 to 20 cm, enemas that reach the level of the splenic flexure, or orally ingested pills; distal colitis is treated either per rectum or orally. The usual enema doses consist of 1 g once daily or 2 to 4 g pills daily. Topical treatment is more effective than oral in treating distal colitis and a combination of both is optimal (Table 9) (81,82). 5-ASA compounds are also effective in a dose-dependent manner as maintenance therapy for ulcerative colitis. In distal colitis, topical treatment seems more effective than oral (83,84).

Corticosteroids

Corticosteroids are the mainstay of treatment for moderate-to-severe ulcerative colitis. The mode of their anti-inflammatory action combines a decreased transcription of various inflammatory genes and an increased transcription of anti-inflammatory genes (77). When treatment with 5-ASA is inadequate or when a patient presents with moderate-to-severe colitis, oral corticosteroids are effective. There is no accepted optimal dose as a result of controlled trials, however, 40 mg daily prednisone has proven superior to 20 mg and nearly as effective as 60 mg, thus, this dose is often arbitrarily chosen (85,86). Parenteral steroids are the standard therapy for hospitalized patients with severe or fulminant ulcerative colitis (73,81). The most commonly used are hydrocortisone 100 mg q.i.d. or methylprednisone 16 mg q.i.d or a continuous infusion. Again, as with oral corticosteroids, an optimal dose has never been defined

Table 9 Therapeutic Options for Ulcerative Colitis

Distal colitis	Extensive colitis	Fulminant
Mild–moderate disease 5-ASA (suppositories, enema, oral) Corticosteroids (enema, foam)	5-ASA (oral)	Steroid (IV) cyclosporine (IV)
Severe disease 5-ASA/corticosteroids (rectal) corticosteroids (oral)	Corticosteroids (oral)	
Maintenance 5-ASA (rectal, oral) Azathioprine/6-MP (oral)	5-ASA (oral) azathioprine/6-MP (oral)	

through rigorous study (86). Topical steroids or 5-ASA compounds are often given as adjunctive therapy for severe colitis. Topical steroids are less effective than 5-ASA in the treatment of distal ulcerative colitis (87).

Several studies have compared hydrocortisone with adrenocorticotropic hormone in the treatment of ulcerative colitis. Intravenous corticotrophin was found to be more effective in patients not previously treated with steroids, whereas hydrocortisone was better in already treated patients who had already received steroid therapy (88). Steroids are ineffective in maintaining remission in ulcerative colitis patients (77,80).

Budesonide, a novel steroid with a high affinity to the glucocorticoid receptor and low systemic bioavailability, is available in enema form for distal ulcerative colitis (87) and, most recently, in oral form (89).

Immunomodulators

Cyclosporine A

Cyclosporine is increasingly used for the treatment of severe ulcerative colitis. It is very potent when administered intravenously to patients with acute severe refractory ulcerative colitis or to outpatients refractory to oral steroids who are unable to wait until the onset of action of azathioprine or 6-MP. As well, it is used as a bridge to other immunosuppressives or when surgery is not desirable. However, long-term maintenance is not advised due to toxicity (90). 60% to 80% of patients with severe ulcerative colitis failing to respond to intravenous steroids may avoid colectomy when given cyclosporine at a dose of 4 mg/kg/day, in a continuous infusion. The median response time is seven days (91). Subsequent studies have shown equal efficacy at 2 mg/kg (92). It is important to maintain cholesterol levels at >120 mg and serum magnesium at normal levels to reduce the risk of seizures. Furthermore, renal function should be closely monitored and cyclosporine dose adjusted to serum creatinine rise. Cyclosporine levels should also be monitored daily. Other side effects of cyclosporine include hypertension, hepatotoxicity, and electrolyte imbalance (90). With the onset of remission, cyclosporine should be given orally for six months at a dose of 6 to 8 mg/kg/day of Sandimmune or 5 mg/kg/day of Neoral (93). During this period azathioprine or 6-MP will generally be initiated.

Azathioprine and 6-Mercaptopurine

These drugs have been widely used for immunosuppression. Azathioprine is converted to 6-MP in the liver and then to thioinosinic acid, which impairs purine biosynthesis, thus inhibiting cellular proliferation. The major use of these compounds in ulcerative colitis is in the management of chronic active disease, which is either steroid dependent or resistant, and in maintenance of remission. It is also useful in left-sided colitis that fails to respond to steroids and 5-ASA compounds (94). The mode of action of both drugs includes antiproliferative effects on lymphocyte populations and inhibition of cytotoxic T-cell and natural killer (NK) cell function. The median time for these drugs to achieve clinical effects ranges between six weeks and three months. A prospective blinded study showed lack of effect of intravenous administration on time to respond to azathioprine (95). Despite the lack of dose-ranging trials of these drugs in ulcerative colitis, doses of 1.5 mg/kg/day for 6-MP and 2.5 mg/kg/day for azathioprine have proven effective. Some authors have suggested that lower doses may be effective for ulcerative colitis, whereas others advocate dosing to induce mild leukopenia and others recommend therapeutic monitoring of 6-MP metabolites (96–99). Prospective trials should define optimal dosing schedules and the utility and cost effectiveness of therapeutic monitoring of metabolites. Side effects of both drugs include nausea, arthralgia, rash, drug fever, leukopenia, thrombocytopenia, pancreatitis, hepatitis, and infections. Continuous monitoring of blood count and liver enzymes is required because of these potential side effects.

Infliximab (Remicaide)

Infliximab is a chimeric monoclonal antibody to tumor necrosis factor shown to be effective in Crohn's disease. Recent studies have shown it to be effective in moderate to severe ulcerative colitis.

Methotrexate

Methotrexate is an inhibitor of dihydrofolate reductase and is associated with anti-inflammatory properties related to decreased IL-1, ecosanoids production, and decreased chemotaxis (77,100).

The evidence of methotrexate benefits if ulcerative colitis remains unproven. The only controlled study to date comparing oral methotrexate, 12.5 mg/wk, to placebo demonstrated no benefit (101).

Nutrition

Inflammatory bowel disease is a condition in which there is an obvious link between the gastrointestinal tract and nutrition. In severe ulcerative colitis, there is high prevalence of protein-energy malnutrition, which is predominantly hypoalbuminemic. Insufficient amounts of short-chain fatty acids (butyrate) and defective oxidation of butyrate have been proposed as contributory to the pathogenesis of ulcerative colitis (102). The efficacy of butyrate enemas in patients with diversion colitis has led to trials in distal ulcerative colitis, some of which have shown no efficacy, whereas others showed some benefit (102). Fish oil supplements produced inconsistent effects when given to patients with ulcerative colitis, as some studies showed beneficial effects as an adjunct treatment whereas others found no benefit.

Investigational Therapies
Nicotine and Cigarettes

Clinical trials with nicotine related to ulcerative colitis were stimulated by observations that patients with ulcerative colitis who stopped smoking relapsed. Randomized trials with mild-to-moderate disease showed a modest benefit with patches or nicotine gum (103–105). However, nicotine was ineffective in maintaining remission (106). Although the application of nicotine enemas has been tried, they are not currently in clinical use (106). Nicotine treatment is associated with considerable side effects including contact dermatitis, lightheadedness, dizziness, nausea, vomiting, headaches, sleep disturbances, diaphoresis, sweating, tremor, tachycardia, and hypertension (107).

Heparin

Observation of a paradoxical improvement of patients with ulcerative colitis who were treated with heparin led to a blinded, randomized controlled trial. Several subsequent open-labeled studies demonstrated the benefits of unfractionated heparin in mild-to-moderate ulcerative colitis (108–110). Heparin affects the inflammatory and endothelial cells and its mode of action may include promotion of epithelial cell repair and interference with leukocyte recruitment (80).

Probiotics

Probiotics seem to be one of the most promising agents and have been tested in several controlled trials. Administration of nonpathogenic *E. coli* was shown to be equivalent to low-dose mesalamine in maintaining remission of ulcerative colitis (111). VSL 3, a preparation containing several strains of probiotic bacteria, was proven beneficial in the treatment and prevention of pouchitis after ileoanal anastomosis (112).

Interleukin-10

IL-10 is an anti-inflammatory cytokine produced by Th_2 cells, macrophages, and monocytes that suppresses cytokine production by Th_1 cells. Although recombinant IL-10 has proven to be safe and well tolerated by patients with ulcerative colitis, it was not found to be effective (113).

Mediator Antagonists/Inhibitors

Studies assessing inhibitors to LTB_4, thromboxane, and platelet-activating factor, all failed to show any effectiveness in the treatment of ulcerative colitis.

Fertility and Pregnancy in Ulcerative Colitis

Sexual health is an important aspect of quality of life, which may be impaired in patients with inflammatory bowel disease. However, there are no specific reports of sexual dysfunction in women with ulcerative colitis who have not had previous surgery (114). Furthermore, no data are available regarding thromboembolic complications of oral contraceptives in ulcerative colitis.

Women with ulcerative colitis generally appear to have normal fertility, although voluntary childlessness is probably greater in patients with inflammatory bowel disease (IBD) than in the general population (114). There is a large body of evidence showing that the frequency of spontaneous abortion, stillbirth, and congenital abnormalities are no different in ulcerative colitis than in the general population (115). The influence of pregnancy on ulcerative colitis depends on the disease activity at the time of conception. Quiescent disease at time of conception is no more likely to flare up than at any other time, whereas patients with active disease at conception are very likely to have continued active disease during pregnancy with potential worsening in 45% (114).

5-Aminosalicylates, sulphasalazine, and corticosteroids appear to be safe for use during pregnancy. Azathioprine and 6-MP have not been proven teratogenic in humans. Similarly, there was very little evidence of adverse events in renal transplant recipients who were unable to discontinue the drug during pregnancy; the same has proven true in a series of patients with IBD. In general, it is reasonably safe for pregnant patients with ulcerative colitis to continue receiving one of these drugs when cessation is not an option (114). However, it is not advisable to commence initial treatment during pregnancy.

Although it is not advisable to commence cyclosporine and methotrexate therapy during pregnancy, there is no medical indication to discontinue maintenance therapy.

SURGICAL MANAGEMENT
Indications for Surgery

Surgery for ulcerative colitis usually involves removal of the entire diseased colon and rectum (total proctocolectomy) or excision of a large part or most of the diseased organ (total abdominal colectomy). Surgical treatment may be categorized as urgent or emergent in which the indication is usually acute disease toxicity or as elective that is aimed to control chronic symptoms and eliminate the risk of cancer.

Indications for Urgent and Emergent Surgery

Acute fulminant ulcerative colitis is usually associated with a rapid development of severe symptoms such as abdominal pain, bloody diarrhea, urgency, tenesmus, and anorexia. The profound water and electrolytes loss may result in the rapid development of dehydration and shock, often with severe electrolyte imbalance, such as hyponatremia and hypokalemia. Frequent bloody diarrhea results in significant blood loss, which may not be adequately replenished by the suppressed bone marrow; anorexia combined with the severe catabolic state may lead to hypoalbuminemia and malnutrition. Fulminant colitis may progress to a toxic dilatation of the colon (toxic megacolon), which carries a high risk of colonic perforation. Mortality in these cases may exceed 16% to 44%. Thus, every effort should be made to anticipate and prevent toxic megacolon. Prompt surgical treatment should be undertaken before or with the first signs of the development of toxic megacolon (116,117).

Patients with acute fulminant colitis without signs of toxicity can be initially treated with intensive medical therapy and close monitoring. All patients with fulminant colitis should be admitted to the hospital; the joint assessment and collaboration of an experienced gastroenterologist and an experienced surgeon is essential in these cases. Prompt fluid and electrolyte resuscitation must be immediately initiated and stool cultured to exclude infectious colitis. Medical treatment should be initiated early and usually consists of high-dosage intravenous steroids (118). There are no comparative studies to determine the exact dosage of steroids in these cases, however, most clinicians use adult doses in the range of 300 mg of hydrocortisone, or its equivalent, per day.

The timeframe for which this conservative regiment should be continued is controversial. Clearly, patients who clinically deteriorate and develop signs of toxicity should emergently undergo surgery. Patients in whom symptoms fail to significantly improve within a few days are unlikely to respond to prolonged therapy. The optimal duration of a high-dose steroids course is not well determined and is based largely on clinical assessment. Long courses of high doses of steroids may, however, lead to worsened malnutrition and increased operative risk and an increased risk of toxic perforation. Traditional teaching suggests that failure to improve within five days is an indication for surgical intervention or cyclosporine A treatment; however, this "traditional" duration is not based on comparative studies and may serve more as a general guideline rather than a strict rule. The author's personal preference is to proceed with surgical treatment in most patients who fail to significantly improve within a timeframe of four to seven days.

Cyclosporine A is an immunosuppressant specifically inhibiting cytotoxic T-cell activation, attenuating cell-mediated immunity. The use of cyclosporine A in patients with acute fulminant colitis refractory to high doses of steroids was shown to induce remission in 60% to 80% of these patients, thus avoiding emergent colectomy; in some, however, the colitis flares up soon after cessation of the treatment. Hyde et al. (119) prospectively surveyed 50 patients who received cyclosporine A for steroid refractory acute colitis. Remission was achieved in 56% but almost one-third relapsed after discharge from the hospital, thus leaving only 40% of the patients in durable remission. Haslam et al. (120) found similar results, with an initial response rate of 63% but only a 30% maintained remission rate. Half of the patients in this study suffered from adverse effects of the cyclosporine A treatment, 12% of which were life-threatening. We believe that cyclosporine A is a valid option for patients who fail to respond to high-dose steroid therapy in an attempt to avoid emergent surgery and are cognizant of the moderate success rate and potential side effects. Surgery is clearly indicated at any point should deterioration of symptoms or any signs of toxicity develop, and for those patients who fail to improve with cyclosporine A treatment.

When urgent or emergent surgery is required in these seriously ill patients, the surgical procedure usually involves resection of enough diseased tissue to cease the acute exacerbation, while minimizing surgical trauma. Thus, pelvic dissection and excision of the rectum, as well as primary anastomosis, are frequently avoided and subtotal or total abdominal colectomy with an end ileostomy are most commonly used (121). A staged procedure, with an elective completion proctectomy, with or without restoration of the normal route of defecation, should be considered after remission has been achieved and systemic steroids are weaned. Some data suggest that a more extensive procedure such as a total proctocolectomy with ileal pouch anal anastomosis and a diverting ileostomy may be performed in well-selected patients with fulminant colitis. Ziv et al. (122) reviewed a limited series of 12 patients who had restorative proctocolectomy for fulminant colitis and did not find any early septic complications reported in this group.

Indications for Elective Surgery

Elective surgery for ulcerative colitis is usually indicated for one of two reasons: (i) failure of medical therapy or dependency on potentially toxic therapy with severe side effects, or (ii) prophylaxis of or treatment of colorectal cancer. Some controversies on the definitions of these categories still exist and the optimal timing of surgery is not always well defined. Thus, sound clinical and surgical judgment and the collaborative assessment of the gastroenterologist and the surgeon are often required to tailor the appropriate timing of surgery to each patient.

Failure of Medical Treatment

Patients with chronically active ulcerative colitis and those with frequently recurrent disease, despite appropriate medical therapy, are candidates for elective surgery. These patients usually suffer from frequent diarrhea and abdominal cramps, severely impacting on their quality of life. Although not in a fulminant state, these patients often suffer from mild-to-moderate chronic malnutrition and anemia. As well, they are in a chronically disabled state with diminished physical, emotional, and social quality of life and are usually best served by removal of the diseased organ (123,124). Infrequently, surgery is also indicated for intractable extraintestinal manifestations of ulcerative colitis such as arthritis or pyoderma gangrenosum. However, sclerosing cholangitis has not been shown to improve with proctocolectomy, nor, at times, does central arthritis.

Since these patients are chronically ill and frequently on systemic steroids, many surgeons elect to manage such cases in a staged fashion, performing a more limited initial procedure such as total abdominal colectomy. The patients are then weaned off steroids and an improvement in their nutritional status and general health is seen prior to performing the completion proctectomy and restoration. Penna et al. (125) have shown that the postoperative complication rate was decreased in 55 patients who had an initial subtotal colectomy compared to 78 patients who had a restorative proctocolectomy with a diverting ileostomy for active ulcerative colitis. This difference, however, did not translate to better long-term pouch function. Ziv et al. (126) reviewed the Cleveland Clinic experience of 361 patients who had a total proctocolectomy with ileal pouch anal anastomosis and a diverting ileostomy while on prolonged systemic steroids therapy and found no significant increase in the postoperative septic complication rate as compared to 310 patients who were not on steroids. These results are in line with several other published series (127,128). Our personal bias is that restorative proctocolectomy with a diverting ileostomy may be offered to active chronic ulcerative colitis patients, unless other risk factors coexist.

Steroid and Cytotoxic Agent Dependency

Although the etiology of ulcerative colitis is not yet completely understood, its pathophysiologic features suggest an autoimmune disease generally treated with immunomodulating drugs. The most effective, widely used, and time-honored immunomodulating therapy consists of steroidal medications. Although effective in the control of symptoms, prolonged use of steroids is associated with severe side effects, some of which are irreversible. Thus, prolonged treatment with systemic steroids for ulcerative colitis should be avoided (129). Although it is widely agreed that steroid-dependent disease is a clear indication for surgery, there is no strict definition of steroid dependency or an agreed time limit for this therapy. Whereas some practitioners tend to attempt to "save" patients from surgery by extending the time frame to declare dependency, sometimes resulting in steroid-related complications, others attempt to save the patients from steroids by offering early surgery, sometimes without an adequate duration of medical therapy. Thus, collaboration and mutual discussion between the gastroenterologist and the surgeon, combined with sound clinical judgment, are essential to determine the appropriate timing for surgery in these cases. Our personal bias is that any course of steroid treatment should have a defined end point, and if the patient cannot be placed on other remission maintaining drugs, they should be referred to surgery.

Cytotoxic agents, such as 6-MP and azathioprine, are widely used as steroid-sparing agents to control chronic symptoms and maintain remission (94,130), as discussed above. Although severe side effects of these drugs are less frequent, they are not risk free and may induce bone marrow depression and liver toxicity. Currently, there are no available data to determine whether long-term dependency on cytotoxic agents is indicative of surgery, and most practitioners would probably consider such a prolonged treatment acceptable.

Surgery for steroid-dependent disease usually consists of resection of the entire colon and rectum with restoration using an ileal pelvic pouch. The safety of performing this surgery in one procedure, with a diverting ileostomy, compared to a staged procedure with total abdominal colectomy first, is controversial, as discussed above.

Prophylaxis of Cancer

Long-standing ulcerative colitis is a predisposing factor for the development of colorectal cancer. Although the actual prevalence of colorectal cancer in patients with ulcerative colitis varies in different series, it is clear that cancer is more common in these patients compared with the age-matched general population. In a recent review of the literature, the cumulative probability of developing colorectal cancer was assessed at 18% for a patient who suffers from ulcerative colitis for a 30-year duration (26). The disease duration is proportionally correlated with an increased risk of cancer, as the cumulative probability to develop cancer in 10 years of disease was only 2%. The extent of disease also correlates with an increased risk of cancer, with the risk more prevalent in patients with pancolitis.

The ideal aim of cancer prophylaxis in patients with ulcerative colitis is to prevent any cancer from developing and to avoid unnecessary radical surgery in patients unlikely to develop cancer. Surveillance is aimed at identifying precancerous conditions, which should be considered as an indication for surgery. When adenocarcinoma is found, either by colonoscopy or in the surgical specimen, as cure rates are less than 100% some degree of cancer-related morbidity and mortality is expected.

The common practice is to start an annual or biannual surveillance colonoscopy program for a duration of approximately 10 years from the onset of disease and to refer patients with severe dysplasia found in endoscopic biopsy for surgery (131). Some controversies, however, do exist concerning this practice. The cost-effectiveness of intensive colonoscopic surveillance has not yet been determined, in light of the number of colonoscopic examinations and biopsies required to identify one potential precancerous lesion. Delco and Sonnenberg (132) in a hypothetical cohort calculated that a colorectal cancer cumulative probability of 27% is required for surveillance to become beneficial.

The ability of a surveillance colonoscopy program to reliably identify premalignant conditions before invasive cancer occurs, or to detect cancer at a very early stage, is also under debate. Biasco et al. (133) in a cohort study of 65 patients followed for a range of 6 to 12 years found that, although none of the patients without high-grade dysplasia developed cancer, all patients with high-grade dysplasia already had cancer at surgery.

Although there is a correlation between the grade of dysplasia and the incidence of cancer (134), the pathologic distinction between grades of dysplasia may be difficult and significant interobserver variation exists (135). Whereas confirmed high-grade dysplasia is considered as an indication for proctocolectomy, the approach to low-grade dysplasia is controversial. A conservative approach indicates a follow-up colonoscopy with repeat biopsies and surgical referral only if high-grade dysplasia develops. Gorfine et al. (136) have challenged this practice in a review of 160 patients who had a colonoscopy with multiple biopsies within a year prior to total proctocolectomy for chronic ulcerative colitis. Of the 51 endoscopic specimens interpreted as dysplasia, cancer was found in the surgical specimen of 26, and in 6 of the 103 cases who were considered negative in endoscopic biopsy, the colon also harbored a carcinoma. Although dysplasia was predictive for synchronous cancer, there was no correlation with the grade of dysplasia, and 7 of the 11 patients in whom dysplasia was interpreted as low-grade already harbored cancer.

Bernstein et al. (137) reviewed 10 prospective studies involving surveillance colonoscopy and concluded that when low-grade dysplasia was found endoscopically, 19% were already found to have cancer in immediate colectomy; this figure was increased to 42% with high-grade dysplasia. These studies suggest that confirmed dysplasia of any grade may be considered as an indication for surgery. Our personal view is that, although colonoscopy with biopsy is probably still the best surveillance tool, surgery should at least be discussed with any patient who is found to have any grade of dysplasia.

When dysplasia-associated lesion or mass (DALM) is found, the risk of already existing cancer is high and such a finding is widely accepted as a clear indication for surgery, unless the lesion has an adenoma-like appearance and the adjacent mucosa shows no dysplasia (138).

The diagnosis of an already existing colorectal carcinoma is an obvious indication for surgery and, if curable intent is possible, surgery should include removal of the entire colon and rectum, as the presence of one proven cancer puts the patient at a significant risk for a synchronous or developing metachronous carcinoma.

As surveillance colonoscopy with multiple biopsies has obvious limitations in accurately detecting precancerous conditions, additional surveillance methods are being evaluated. The use of cellular ploidity and molecular markers as adjuncts to colonoscopy is currently being assessed (139,140) in order to hopefully improve patient selection for surgery.

When elective surgery for ulcerative colitis is planned for prophylaxis of cancer, the extent of resection should encompass the entire tissue, namely the colon and rectum, which has the potential for neoplastic transformation. In cases where premalignant conditions are not found, several retrospective studies have advocated the use of total abdominal colectomy with ileorectal anastomosis, obviating the need for pelvic dissection (141). This may be a viable option for patients with a relatively low risk to develop cancer or those with a mildly diseased rectum who wish to avoid the potential risks and complications of a pelvic pouch. These patients must be aware of the need for routine rectal surveillance even if asymptomatic; this procedure should be avoided in cases of any evidence of dysplasia or long-standing pancolitis.

For most patients, total proctocolectomy is the most suitable procedure for cancer prophylaxis. Patients who are good at operative risks and with an adequate anal sphincter mechanism are generally suitable for reconstruction with the ileal pouch anal anastomosis. Two main techniques are used to anastomose the ileal pouch to the anus; one is anal mucosectomy with hand sewn anastomosis and the other is the double-stapled technique. The main difference between the two techniques is excision of the most distal 2 cm of rectal mucosa, or the anal transition zone, which is preserved with the stapled technique. Surgeons who routinely use mucosectomy feel that a complete eradication of all the potential cancer-bearing tissue is essential (142), whereas advocates of the stapled technique argue that the chance of cancer developing in the retained anal transition zone is very rare (143).

Subtotal and Total Abdominal Colectomy

Subtotal or total excision of the colon, leaving the rectum in place, is most commonly used in the urgent or emergent setting to minimize the extent of surgical trauma; this is accompanied

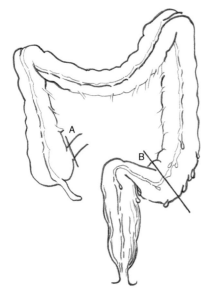

Figure 8 Extent of resection in subtotal colectomy.

by the construction of an end ileostomy (Fig. 8). In selected patients who require elective surgery for ulcerative colitis, total abdominal colectomy with an ileorectal anastomosis may also be considered (Tables 10 and 11).

Urgent and Emergent Setting

Urgent and emergent surgery for ulcerative colitis is usually indicated in acute fulminant colitis unresponsive to medical treatment or progressing to toxic megacolon. These patients are usually severely ill, malnourished, anemic, and often treated with high doses of steroids, which puts them at an increased surgical risk with concomitantly increased morbidity and mortality. In this setting, many surgeons opt for the least extensive procedure required to overcome the critical condition, leaving the definitive procedure for a later stage (121,152). In addition, acute fulminant colitis may frequently be the first presentation of the disease, making the distinction from Crohn's disease at that stage difficult. In these systemically ill patients, primary ileorectal anastomosis carries a considerable risk of anastomotic leak and disruption, and is thus usually avoided. A well-constructed Brooke end ileostomy is fashioned and care should

Table 10 Indications for Surgery in Ulcerative Colitis

Indication	Urgency	Consensus	Controversy
Fulminant colitis	Emergent/urgent	Surgery indicated in deterioration or failure to improve	Length of conservative treatment Type of procedure (STC and TAC vs. TPC)
Toxic megacolon	Emergent	Surgery indicated: STC or TAC	
Failure of medical therapy	Elective	Surgery indicated	Type of procedure: TAC vs. TPC + IPAA Staged vs. single-stage procedure
Steroid dependency	Elective	Surgery indicated	Type of procedure: TAC vs. TPC + IPAA Staged vs. single-stage procedure
High-grade dysplasia	Elective	Surgery indicated	
DALM	Elective	Surgery indicated	
Low-grade dysplasia	Elective		Indication is in controversy
Chronic ulcerative colitis without dysplasia	Elective		Indication controversial for long-standing pancolitis

Abbreviations: STC, subtotal colectomy; TAC, total abdominal colectomy; TPC, total proctocolectomy; IPAA, ileal pouch anal anastomosis.

Table 11 Subtotal and Total Abdominal Colectomy for Ulcerative Colitis (Series with More than 10 yr of Follow Up)

Authors	N	% Proctectomy	% Cancer
Baker et al. (144)	374	10	5.9
Gruner et al. (145)	57	50	6
Grundfast et al. (146)	84	21	4.8
Backer et al. (147)	59	22	5.1
Romano et al. (148)	86	8.1	4.6
Johnson et al. (149)	286	38	3.8
Oakley et al. (150)	288	55	1.8
Leijonmarck et al. (151)	51	57	0

be taken to preserve the length of the terminal ileum and its blood supply, to allow future pouch construction.

The blind rectal stump may also be at risk for leak in these ill patients, therefore its management is controversial. Many surgeons suture or staple the stump closed and leave it in the lower abdomen as a Hartmann's pouch, with or without an adjacent drain (153,154). If the stump is of adequate length, some prefer to bring it to the skin through a separate stoma site, or through the midline wound, to create a mucous fistula, whereas others bring the stump to above the abdominal fascia but below the skin, which can be opened should leak occur (155).

Elective Total Abdominal Colectomy with Ileorectal Anastomosis

Total proctocolectomy is associated with an altered lifestyle, even with adequate restoration, and the ileal pouch anal anastomosis carries a potential risk of short- and long-term complications. Thus, some surgeons advocate the use of total abdominal colectomy with ileorectal anastomosis for selected patients with ulcerative colitis (144–151,156–161). Appropriate candidates for this procedure are patients with mild rectal disease that appears distendable in lower endoscopy and those who are at low risk for developing rectal cancer. Elderly patients with a disease of short duration may be good candidates for this procedure. Younger patients wanting to avoid the potential risk of sexual dysfunction and infertility associated with the pelvic dissection or those who wish to return to their normal activity as soon as possible may also be considered for this procedure. These patients should be aware of the potential risk of rectal cancer and the need for adequate rectal surveillance, even if asymptomatic.

Technical Notes

When an urgent or emergent colectomy is performed for fulminant colitis, adequate fluid and electrolyte resuscitation prior to surgery is essential. A planned stoma site should be preoperatively marked by an enterostomal therapist. For patients on steroid therapy, an adequate stress dose should be considered. As well, perioperative broad-spectrum antibiotics should be administered prior to the skin incision.

The lithotomy position allows transanal access to the rectum for possible endoscopy and for the use of a stapling device and is a convenient location for the second assistant. The abdominal cavity is typically entered through a midline incision to allow adequate exposure of the pelvis and to protect potential stoma sites at the lateral abdominal wall. The peritoneal cavity is meticulously explored, paying specific attention to any stigmata of Crohn's disease.

Colectomy starts with complete mobilization of the right colon. A sharp incision is made over the lateral peritoneal line and the colon is mobilized to the base of its mesentery in precise anatomic planes. The hepatic flexure is then mobilized, followed by the transverse colon. If there is no evidence of cancer, the greater omentum may be left in place and the dissection is performed in the avascular plane between the transverse colon and the omentum. Alternatively, the gastrocolic ligament may be opened, allowing entrance to the lesser sac, with removal of the greater omentum attached to the transverse colon.

The left colon is then mobilized from the retroperitoneum in the same fashion, with careful attention paid to the splenic flexure. The extent of mobilization of the sigmoid colon and upper rectum depends on the extent of resection, and care should be taken at this point to identify and protect the left ureter.

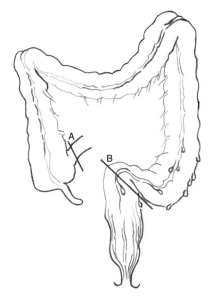

Figure 9   Extent of resection in total abdominal colectomy.

The terminal ileum is divided adjacent to the ileocecal valve (Fig. 9), and the mesentery of the cecum is divided close to the bowel wall, protecting the terminal branches and arcades of the ileocolic artery to allow future construction of an ileal pouch, if desired (Fig. 10). The large bowel mesentery is then serially divided and ligated. Division of the sigmoidal arteries depends on the level of resection; however, the superior hemorrhoidal vessels should remain intact. If a total abdominal colectomy is performed, the large bowel is divided in the rectosigmoid junction, at the level of the sacral promontory. In cases of subtotal colectomy, approximately half of the sigmoid colon is preserved. If a mucous fistula is planned, care should be taken to leave ample length of rectosigmoid stump that can easily reach the abdominal wall.

After specimen removal, an end Brooke's ileostomy at the right lower quadrant or an ileorectal anastomosis is performed.

In the postoperative period, attention must be paid to water and electrolyte loss with resumption of bowel function. Serum electrolytes should be monitored and adequate replacement given. In cases of high stomal output, antidiarrheal medication may be used to decrease gastrointestinal loss.

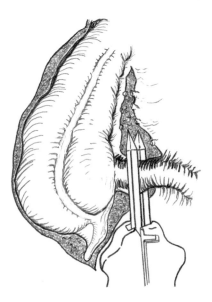

Figure 10   Division of the terminal ileum.

Total Proctocolectomy Without Restoration

Total proctocolectomy (removal of the entire colon and rectum) is the principal surgical treatment for most patients requiring elective surgery for ulcerative colitis. This procedure completely removes the diseased organ and eliminates the potential risk of colorectal cancer. Although most patients may be suitable for a restorative procedure such as an ileal pouch anal anastomosis, some may fare better without reconstruction. In this case, a permanent, well-constructed end ileostomy is fashioned at the completion of surgery and the perineal wound is primarily closed.

Patients Selection for Total Proctocolectomy Without Restoration

Restorative procedures obviate the need for an ileostomy continuously draining into a collection bag. However, reconstruction is associated with significantly increased early and late morbidity, compared with total proctocolectomy alone. Furthermore, patients who are likely to develop complications or are unlikely to enjoy the benefits of restoration should be offered total proctocolectomy with end ileostomy (156–158). Appropriate preoperative counseling and a mutual decision of the surgeon and patient are essential for maximizing patients' expectations and satisfaction.

Elderly patients with a significantly complex past medical history are at increased surgical risk and are less likely to survive complications and, thus, may benefit from the simplest, most effective procedure such as a nonrestorative proctocolectomy. A pelvic pouch is attached to the anal canal, challenging the anal sphincter mechanism with the need to control large amounts of liquid stool. Ileoanal surgery alone may temporarily or permanently affect the sphincter function, reducing anal sensation particularly when mucosectomy is performed (159–161). Patients with an attenuated sphincter mechanism may further suffer from a significant degree of anal incontinence following ileoanal pouch surgery and should therefore be considered for a nonreconstructive procedure.

Counseling patients as to the various options and their associated lifestyles will allow patients to select the option that best fits with their life. If well informed, the patient's preference should be respected, regardless of the surgeon's personal views.

Technical Notes

Nutritional status should be optimized as early as possible prior to surgery and any fluid and electrolyte imbalances should be promptly corrected. Preoperative stoma therapist counseling with careful stoma site marking is essential, as the permanent ileostomy will be an important determinant in the patients' future quality of life.

Preoperative prophylactic and perioperative broad-spectrum antibiotics should be administered, and patients who recently received systemic steroids should be given a steroidal stress dose.

The patient is placed in the lithotomy position with the perineum slightly over the edge of the table for an easy access to the perineal part of the proctectomy. A soft sand bag or folded sheet under the sacrum may assist in correctly positioning the buttocks. It is worthwhile to mention that a few surgeons find it easier to place the patient in the prone jack-knife position and perform the perineal part of the proctectomy first, then turn the patient onto the supine position to commence with the abdominal portion of the procedure.

A generous midline incision is used and the abdominal cavity is explored. In patients who have had previous abdominal surgery, adhesiolysis is performed with care to avoid small bowel injury. The abdominal colon is then mobilized free from the retroperitoneum and greater omentum (see Section on "Technical Notes" under "Subtotal and Total Abdominal Colectomy") and the mesentery is serially divided and ligated. The superior hemorrhoidal vessels are divided between clamps and securely ligated, allowing entrance to the postrectal space. Great care should be taken to identify and protect the hypogastric sympathetic nerves to avoid ejaculatory dysfunction in men (Fig. 11).

The posterior rectal mobilization then proceeds behind the mesorectum, in the presacral space, as far down as possible (Fig. 12). Many surgeons, trained to perform total mesorectal excision for rectal cancer, mobilize the posterior plane sharply under direct vision. Some may find it easier to bluntly separate this plane when operating for benign conditions.

Lateral and anterior mobilization is then carried out to the level of the pelvic floor, dividing the plane between the rectum and the prostate or vagina (Fig. 13). Care should be taken to protect the parasympathetic periprostatic nerve plexus, which innervates erectile function.

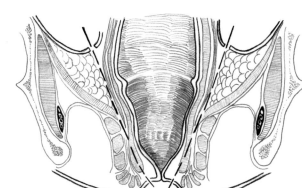

Figure 11 Pelvic dissection borders in proctectomy for ulcerative colitis.

Again, whereas some surgeons commonly mobilize the rectum external to the mesorectum, others feel that a dissection closer to the rectum, with ligation of the lateral stalks within the mesorectum, is safer to avoid nerve injury. The authors' preference, however, is that with appropriate training, the bloodless anatomic plane between the rectum and the prostate can be safely sharply dissected with identification of the periprostatic nerves.

Prior to commencing the perineal part of the proctectomy, the anus is sutured closed with a purse-string suture to prevent spillage of fecal content during the dissection. An incision is made internal to the intersphincteric groove and deepened in the plane between the internal and external sphincters into the perirectal fat. Dissection is initially carried out posteriorly, coring the rectum out of the levator ani muscle, to enter the already dissected postrectal space. The lateral and anterior planes are then dissected, dividing any puborectalis fibers attached to the rectum. The anterior dissection of the rectum near the prostate or vagina is more difficult, and the correct plane should be carefully maintained. Adequate assistance and exposure are essential for the precise dissection of this plane.

Following completion of the proctectomy, the pelvic floor and perineal wound are closed and a Brooke's ileostomy is fashioned at the previously marked site (Fig. 14). The ileal mucosa is everted using absorbable sutures passing through the edge of the ileum, the seromuscular layer proximal to that, and the dermis of the skin, in four quadrants.

Postoperatively, an enterostomal therapist should educate the patient and the patient's family regarding stoma care and early initiation of self–stoma care should be encouraged.

Continent Ileostomy

More than 30 years ago, patients undergoing total proctocolectomy were entitled to life with a conventional end ileostomy. During the 1970s, Kock gradually developed an ileal reservoir

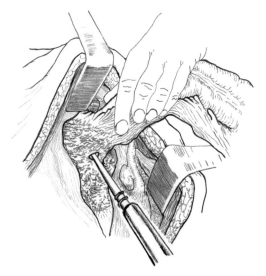

Figure 12 Posterior rectal dissection.

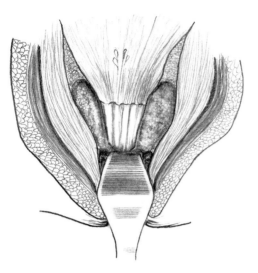

Figure 13 Anterior rectal dissection.

with a continent ileostomy that has become known as the Kock pouch (162–164). For some time, this was the only viable option for these patients to avoid a conventional ileostomy. However, with the development and popularization of the ileoanal pouch, the use of the Kock's pouch has become less frequent, and with few exceptions, even tertiary centers with a significant volume of ulcerative colitis patients currently have only limited experience with this procedure.

The main indication for the construction of a Kock's pouch in the era of the ileoanal pouch would be patients in whom the pelvic pouch has failed and needs to be excised or patients who had a total proctocolectomy with a conventional Brooke's ileostomy in the past, and wish to avoid wearing the conventional ileostomy bag (165). Patients should be aware that this type of surgery is associated with a significant rate of early and late complications, with the instability of the nipple valve being the most common reason for reoperation. In our experience, patients in whom the ileoanal pouch failed are usually reluctant to undergo another potentially morbid procedure, and prefer the end ileostomy. Most patients with a conventional ileostomy are satisfied with their quality of life, compared to their life before the operation. Highly motivated patients, however, who wish to avoid a conventional ileostomy for social or emotional reasons, are candidates for the continent ileostomy.

Technical Notes
Preoperatively, the stoma site should be marked just above the right pubic hairline, superior to the insertion of the rectus abdominus muscle. The abdomen is typically entered through a

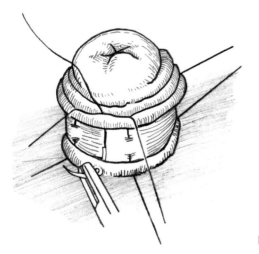

Figure 14 Brooke's ileostomy construction.

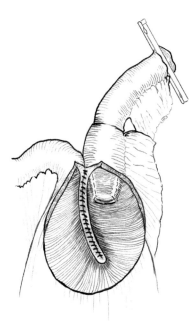

Figure 15 The pelvic ileal J pouch.

midline incision to protect possible stoma sites in the lateral abdominal wall. As most of these patients have had previous abdominal surgeries, careful adhesiolysis should be undertaken, avoiding injury to the small bowel. Any previous stoma is taken down and excised.

Approximately 45 to 50 cm of the terminal ileum is used for the construction of the Kock pouch (Figs. 15 and 16). The most distal end is used as the outlet and the length depends on the thickness of the abdominal wall. The segment of 10 to 12 cm bowel proximal to that site is used to construct a valve, and the proximal 30 cm is used for the reservoir. A wedge-shaped window is made at the mesentery of the segment used for the valve, preserving the main blood vessels. The purpose of this window is to reduce the mesenteric bulk between the intussuscepted small bowel loops and increase its stability.

To construct the reservoir, the 30-cm proximal loop is folded in a U shape and then secured with seromuscular stay sutures. The antimesenteric border is longitudinally incised and the posterior wall of the pouch is sutured together, leaving at least 2 cm toward the afferent and efferent limbs opened. The intussusception valve is then constructed. The bowel wall at the middle of the 10- to 12-cm segment planned for the valve is grasped through the lumen

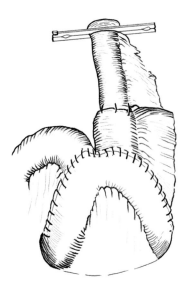

Figure 16 Construction of the Kock's pouch.

Table 12 Rate of Nipple Valve Dysfunction (Series of More than 50 Patients)

Author	N	% Dysfunction
Kock et al. (166)	220	42
Fazio and Church (167)	168	17
Dozios et al. (168)	299	33
Jarvinen et al. (169)	76	41
Palmu and Sivula (170)	51	29
Gerber (171)	100	4.1

of the pouch and pulled towards the pouch. The nipple valve is constructed by securing the intussuscepted bowel wall in this configuration. This may be achieved by placing sutures through both bowel walls, or by stapling them using a TA stapler without a pin or an S-GIA stapler without a knife, at three to four quadrants. Care should be taken to avoid compromising the mesentery of this loop and to prevent valve ischemia. The distal edge of the valve is transfixed to the outlet limb with sutures or with a stapler. The anterior wall of the pouch is then closed in a horizontal fashion and the pouch integrity tested by placing a catheter through the outlet and valve into the pouch followed by air installation. The catheter is then removed to test the valve function and reinserted to empty the pouch. The stoma site is prepared and the bowel end is fashioned at the skin level.

Postoperatively, the pouch is continuously intubated and drained for one or two weeks after which the catheter is removed. Patient education regarding frequent pouch emptying is important to prevent distention.

The most common long-term complication encountered in patients with Kock's pouch is nipple valve dessusception and malfunction (Table 12). A number of techniques have been suggested to reduce the rate of dessusception. Some surgeons believe that the use of the stapled technique for valve construction is associated with a lower failure rate. In addition, serosal incisions of the intussuscepted loop may facilitate adherence of the bowel walls to each other and to prevent slippage. Several authors have suggested the use of a peri-ileal collar (171), sutured to the junction of the valve with the outlet limb created from either a portion of the fascia, muscle, or a synthetic material. The use of these techniques, however, may be associated with an increased risk of valve fistula and are not routinely employed.

Restorative Proctocolectomy

Fifty-five years ago, Ravitch and Sabiston (172) described subtotal colectomy with mucosal proctectomy and straight ileoanal anastomosis in the treatment of patients with ulcerative colitis. The aim was to preserve the sphincter mechanism and fecal continence. However, this was often followed by high stool frequency and urgency (173–176).

In 1969, Kock (159) first described a small bowel reservoir fashioned from an ileal loop with which he formed a continent ileostomy. Parks and Nicholls in 1978 (177) combined the idea of an ileal reservoir with distal rectal mucosectomy for the restoration of bowel continuity in patients with ulcerative colitis requiring total proctocolectomy. The ileal reservoir is placed in the pelvis side and an ileoanal anastomosis is performed to maintain anal continence.

Over the last two decades, proctocolectomy with ileal pouch anal anastomosis has become the gold-standard elective surgical treatment for ulcerative colitis. It removes the diseased bowel while eliminating the necessity of a permanent ileostomy. The ability to eliminate the disease while preserving continence and relatively normal defecation has dramatically altered the concept of surgical management of ulcerative colitis.

Indications for Restorative Proctocolectomy

Patients with ulcerative colitis who require elective operative intervention because of intractability, complications of medical therapy, or cancer risk are potential candidates for restorative proctocolectomy. Patients with life-threatening complications, such as toxic megacolon, massive hemorrhage, or perforation, who need an emergent operation are usually not good candidates for an immediate ileoanal pouch procedure and may be best served with total colectomy, leaving a long rectal stump and end ileostomy. After a recovery period, a second-stage restorative proctocolectomy may be considered.

Patient Selection

While restoring the natural route of defecation and improved quality of life, restorative proctocolectomy may also be associated with a significant rate of early and late postoperative complications and failure, therefore, careful patient selection is essential for good outcome.

Anal Sphincter Incompetence

A well-functioning anal sphincter is mandatory for adequate outcome. Patients with a past history suggestive of sphincter injury should undergo preoperative sphincter assessment by anal physiology studies and endoanal ultrasonography, and a damaged sphincter may be considered for repair prior to the ileoanal procedure. The reported results of sphincter repair in preparation for ileoanal pouch surgery, however, are contradictory. Although Thompson and Quigley (178) reported two patients who underwent anal sphincter repair with satisfactory pouch function, Ogunbiyi et al. (179) reported the outcome in three patients who underwent pelvic floor repair and one treated by graciloplasty. Two of these patients had poor pouch function and two had their pouches eventually excised.

Concomitant Colorectal Carcinoma

Restorative proctocolectomy should not be carried out if a cancer is located at the lower rectum or the colorectal carcinoma is incurable.

Elderly Patients

Advanced age is a relative contraindication for pouch surgery because of increased operative risk and the greater probability of a weakened sphincter, which may result in postoperative fecal incontinence. Several studies have shown that a decrease in anal sphincteric strength is related to aging, especially in females (180). Thus, there must be a degree of caution when offering the operation to elderly patients, particularly females. Lewis et al. (181) compared the results of stapled ileoanal pouch operation in 18 patients, 50 to 60 (median 55) years of age, with those of 18 matched patients who were below 50 (median 34) years and showed slightly inferior clinical results in the older group. A few other authors have found no difference in the complication rate or functional results between patients older than 50 years and younger patients (182,183). Tan et al. (184) found some mild decrease in function only in patients older than 70 years at the time of surgery. These results suggest that restorative proctocolectomy may be offered to well-selected elderly patients requiring total proctocolectomy.

Psychological Unsuitability

Patients with severely disabling psychiatric disorders and emotional instability are not appropriate candidates for the ileoanal pouch procedure. Patients undergoing ileoanal pouch surgery must be cognizant of their disease, understand the necessity of surgery, able to endure the operative process, and continue with a strict follow-up regimen. Lastly and very important, these patients must be prepared to cope with the lifestyle alterations associated with this procedure.

Body Habitus

Massively obese patients tend to have a short and fatty mesentery, which may not allow the pouch to reach into the pelvis (185). Very tall individuals may pose the same problem, having inadequate mesentery length for the pouch to reach the anal canal. When offering surgery to these patients, they should be informed that it may be technically impossible to perform an ileal pouch anal anastomosis, and they might require a permanent ileostomy. Efron et al. (186) assessed the morbidity and functional outcome after restorative proctocolectomy in 31 obese patients, as compared to a matched cohort of 31 nonobese patients. Although the operative time was longer and the perioperative morbidity was higher in the obese group, the length of the hospital stay was similar. Overall pelvic sepsis was significantly higher in the obese group and in the long term, more stomal complications and incisional hernias occurred. However, at a mean follow-up of 51 months, the functional outcome of restorative proctocolectomy in obese patients was not significantly different compared to the nonobese patients. The authors' personal view is that, in most cases, obesity should not be a contraindication for the ileoanal pouch procedure provided that the patients are aware of the technical difficulty and increased risk.

Previous Abdominal and/or Anal Surgery

Previous abdominal and anal surgery was considered as a contraindication for restorative proctocolectomy. However, with increased experience, most surgeons are now willing to operate on these patients. Parker and Nicholls (187) reported the outcome of 13 patients with a past history of pelvic, abdominal, or perianal surgery, 12 of whom had an uncomplicated recovery, and only one patient required pouch removal. Currently, most patients who have had urgent or emergent total abdominal colectomy or other abdominal procedures are considered good candidates for ileal pouch anal anastomosis. Previous small bowel resections, however, may increase the technical difficulty of the operation and compromise mesenteric length. Pouch function may be altered in such cases because of watery output and high stool frequency.

Surgical Technique

Preparation for surgery, positioning of the patient, and the abdominal proctocolectomy procedure are described in section "Technical Notes" under "Subtotal and Total Abdominal Colectomy" and "Total Proctocolectomy without Restoration." Technically, the ileoanal anastomosis may be performed manually by suturing the ileal pouch to the dentate line or by using the stapled technique, attaching the pouch to the anal canal. Using the stapled anastomosis, the mucosa of the anal transition zone, the distal-most end of the rectum, is left below the anastomosis, whereas anal mucosectomy, excising the anal transition zone, requires a handsewn ileoanal anastomosis. When the rectum is completely mobilized, the next step depends on the type of anastomosis. For mucosectomy with a handsewn ileoanal anastomosis, the rectum is closed with a clamp and the distal part irrigated from below. The anorectal mucosa is dissected free of the muscular coat transanally, and the rectum is transected en-bloc with the excised mucosa at the upper border of the levator ani muscle. When applying the double stapling technique, the rectum is closed using a linear stapler, a clamp is placed proximal to the staple line, and the rectum divided along the edge of the staples.

Pouch Construction

The terminal ileum is transected flush at the ileocecal valve by a linear cutter. The small bowel mesentery should be mobilized from the retroperitoneum up to the third part of the duodenum and inferior border of the pancreas to allow the ileal reservoir to reach the anus without tension. If additional length is needed, the branches of the ileocolic vessels can be divided. It is wise to temporary block these branches using a noncrushing clamp to ensure viability of the pouch prior to transecting the vessels. The most common pouch configuration is the JQ-shaped pouch. The distal 30 to 40 cm of the terminal ileum is folded into two limbs of 15 to 20 cm each and is connected to form the reservoir. Seromuscular sutures may be placed to approximate the two limbs and a small enterotomy is made at the antimesenteric border of the pouch apex. A side-to-side anastomosis is created by two applications of a 100 mm linear cutter. After careful hemostasis, a purse-string suture is placed around the enterotomy, the anvil of the circular stapler is inserted into the pouch, and the purse-string suture is tied (Fig. 17C).

Ileal Pouch Anal Anastomosis

The most popular method of ileoanal anastomosis is the stapled technique (Fig. 18). Before construction of the anastomosis, the pelvis is thoroughly checked for hemostasis. The circular stapler is introduced through the anus and the center rod advanced through the center of the linear stapler line. The anvil is then engaged in the stapler shaft and the instrument slowly closed to avoid inadvertently catching the mesentery. The pouch position is reassessed to ensure a straight mesentery without rotation or tension. The stapler is then fired to form the circular anastomosis at the upper anal canal and the instrument is removed.

When the handsewn anastomosis is used, cooperation between the surgeon performing the anastomosis through the anus and the surgeon at the abdominal component is essential. The pouch must be brought into the pelvis without rotation or tension. The handsewn anastomosis between the anus at the dentate line and the enterotomy at the apex of the pouch is formed transanally using interrupted absorbable sutures. It is generally helpful to apply sutures at the four corners of the anastomosis first, to ensure correct orientation of the anastomosis. As the level of the anastomosis is lower using this technique, great care should be taken to avoid excess anastomotic tension due to the tethered mesentery.

(A)   **(B)**   **(C)**

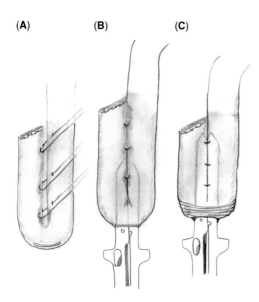
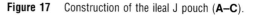

Figure 17   Construction of the ileal J pouch (**A–C**).

Drainage of the presacral space is usually performed using a suction drain. If a diverting ileostomy is used, a loop of ileum is brought out through the abdominal wall at the right lower quadrant and a rod is placed between the ileal loop and the skin. The bowel wall is then opened and the proximal portion is sutured to the skin, everted in Brooke's fashion.

Complications of Ileoanal Pouch Surgery

Restorative proctocolectomy is a complex procedure with a fairly high incidence of both major and minor complications even in experienced centers. The overall reported complication rate ranges between 13% and 63%. However, many of these complications are minor and most patients have a reasonable pouch function and a good quality of life. Fazio et al. (188) showed that despite an overall morbidity rate of 62.7% in a series of 1005 patients, 93% had a good or excellent quality of life. Meagher et al. (189) reported the complications and long-term outcome in 1310 ulcerative colitis patients and found that 91% had a functioning pouch at a 10-year follow-up. Poor functional result or pouch failure, however, are usually the end result of major unmanageable complications.

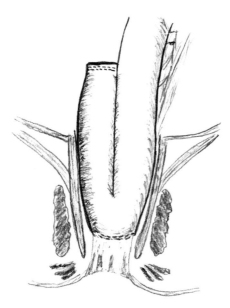

Figure 18   The pelvic ileal J pouch.

Pelvic Sepsis

Pelvic abscess is quite often the result of a leak or disruption of the ileoanal anastomosis, infected hematoma, or leak from the pouch suture line. The prevalence of postoperative pelvic sepsis varies between 5% and 25% (189–191) and this wide range is attributable in part to the lack of a standard definition. Signs and symptoms include fever, anal pain, tenesmus, purulent discharge, bleeding from the anus, and leukocytosis. The diagnosis may be established by examination under anesthesia alone or in combination with imaging studies such as contrast pouchography, CT, and magnetic resonance imaging (MRI) (useful for the detection of small occult collections). Severe pelvic sepsis may lead to poor pouch function, pouch excision, or permanent diversion (192,193).

Pelvic sepsis may be clinically evident in the immediate postoperative period, after ileostomy closure or after a long follow-up period (190). Late sepsis may present as pouch dysfunction with frequency, urgency, incontinence, or pouch-related fistula without systemic signs of sepsis.

Treatment depends on the severity of sepsis. Some patients can be successfully managed with antibiotics (193,194), whereas others may require operative or CT-guided percutaneous drainage. In most cases, the abscess can be transanally drained through the suture line and sometimes multiple local procedures are required to eradicate sepsis. A small proportion of patients require laparotomy for drainage of an abscess and diversion, if not already established (192). In this group, eventual pouch excision is more common and ileostomy closure is less frequent (194).

Pelvic abscess caused by anastomotic dehiscence must be drained and proximally diverted and the ileoanal anastomosis repaired at a later stage. There are two main surgical options for the delayed repair of an ileoanal anastomotic disruption. One is transanal repair of the anastomosis or endoanal pouch advancement and resuturing of the pouch to the anal canal (195), and the other is an abdomino-anal revision with complete pouch mobilization, extensive debridement, and a repeat handsewn ileoanal anastomosis (196). In some cases, complete excision of the existing pouch and reformation of a new pouch is required. A diverting ileostomy is required in these cases until complete healing of the anastomosis is ensured. It is clear, however, that severe pelvic sepsis with extensive anastomotic breakdown results in a high failure rate, despite salvage attempts (179,197).

Pouch Bleeding

Bleeding from the pouch in the early postoperative period is rare and usually from a pouch staple line. Other less common reasons are early pelvic sepsis, anastomotic breakdown, or a bleeding disorder. The treatment consists of hemodynamic stabilization, blood transfusions when needed, correction of coagulation disorders, and irrigation of the pouch through a large catheter. The bleeding is usually self-limited, persistent bleeding requires evaluation under anesthesia.

Bleeding from a suture line should be sutured or a tamponade should be attempted. If bleeding continues despite all measures, laparotomy with pouch mobilization, hemostasis, and diversion is mandatory. If bleeding is controlled, excision of the pouch can be avoided by bringing the apex of the pouch through the abdominal wall as a mucous fistula.

Small Bowel Obstruction

Small bowel obstruction is a common complication after major abdominal surgery. The reported risk of small bowel obstruction after restorative proctocolectomy ranges from 12% to 35% (188,189,198–200), and up to 17% of patients require laparotomy with adhesiolysis or small bowel resection (201–203). Although small bowel obstruction may occur before ileostomy closure, it is more common after closure. MacLean et al. (198) prospectively analyzed 1178 patients with a mean follow-up of 8.7 years. The overall risk of small bowel obstruction was 23% with 6.8% requiring surgical intervention. Forty-four percent of the obstructions occurred early in the postoperative course and 56% occurred later. In those patients who needed surgical intervention, obstruction was most commonly due to pelvic adhesions followed by adhesions at the ileostomy closure site. Fazio et al. (188) in their study of 1005 patients found a 25.3% overall risk of small bowel obstruction at a median follow-up of 2.3 years. Meagher et al. (189) reported that 202 out of 1310 patients (15%) developed at least one episode of small bowel obstruction following ileostomy closure. The cumulative probability of developing small bowel obstruction increases with longer duration of follow-up.

The risk varies between 14% and 26.7% at five years after ileostomy closure and increases to 31.4% at 10 years (189,198).

Pouch Dysfunction

Pouch function may vary among patients and even from day to day in the same individual. Therefore, "normal" or acceptable pouch function may be difficult to define. Most patients with pouch dysfunction have a stool frequency of 10 or more bowel movements per 24 hours, which is often associated with small amounts of stool. Urgency may be a feature and incontinence may be the predominant symptom or may occur in association with frequency and urgency.

The causes of pouch dysfunction can be divided into four categories, including mechanical or functional disorders, septic complications, and inflammation.

Diagnosis is based on an accurate history and physical examination, combined with one or more investigative methods such as evaluation under anesthesia, pouchoscopy, anorectal physiology tests, and various imaging techniques.

An important group to recognize is mechanical outlet obstruction as surgery can often relieve symptoms in these patients who may have ileoanal anastomotic stricture, a long efferent limb of an S pouch, and a retained rectal stump after a stapled ileoanal anastomosis. Patients most frequently present with symptoms of straining, increased number of movements per day, watery stool, urgency of defecation, a feeling of incomplete evacuation, and abdominal and anal pain.

Ileoanal Anastomotic Stricture

Stenosis of the ileoanal anastomosis is the most common perineal complication after ileoanal pouch surgery. The precise definition of an anastomotic stricture is unclear and contributes to the wide range of incidences reported in the literature. Narrowing which requires at least one dilatation under anesthesia has been reported in 4% to 40% of these cases (204–208). The main causative factors are pelvic sepsis with subsequent fibrosis and anastomotic tension leading to ischemia. Rectal examination confirms the diagnosis of anastomotic stricture and reveals its diameter and length. Imaging with contrast pouchography should be considered if a tight anastomosis is impassable with a finger or a pediatric proctoscope.

Anastomotic strictures can occur before or after ileostomy closure. Most strictures, especially those found during an outpatient clinic visit before ileostomy closure, are annular and web-like, due to lateral adhesions across the anastomosis and can be treated successfully with simple digital anal dilatation. Severe strictures resulting from anastomotic dehiscence and pelvic sepsis are often long and narrow and repeat dilatations using the finger or Hegar dilators are usually required for relief (206,208,209). Some patients may learn to intubate and drain the pouch in order to evacuate.

If a stricture persists in spite of repeated dilatations, operative therapy is required by either a transanal approach or a combined abdomino-anal approach. The transanal approach involves excision of the stricture, advancement of the pouch distally, and redo of the ileoanal anastomosis (210). The combined abdomino-anal procedure includes a laparotomy with complete pouch mobilization and excision of the anastomotic area, and the formation of a new transanal handsewn anastomosis of the pouch to the distal anal canal (209). Despite salvage attempts, up to 15% of patients with severe anastomotic stricture will eventually require pouch excision and permanent ileostomy (193,204–206).

Long Efferent Limb of an S Pouch

When the S pouch was first constructed, a 6 to 8 cm-long efferent limb was used to reduce the risk of fecal incontinence (177). In the long term, the long efferent limb was found to promote stasis and interfere with spontaneous defecation, thus causing straining during defecation and incomplete or delayed pouch emptying (209,211–213). A shorter limb of 2 to 3 cm or less leads to improved functional results with only 4% of the patients requiring catheterization (214,215).

When catheterization is difficult or accompanied by fecal incontinence, surgical correction should be considered. Nicholls and Gilbert (213) showed that 54% of 76 patients with an S pouch required catheterization in order to evacuate. In six patients, surgical correction of the efferent limb was required and all had significant improvement. Surgery consisted of shortening of the distal efferent limb and refashioning of the ileoanal anastomosis. This may be attempted transanaly, however, an abdominal approach seems to offer the greatest chance of success (211,213,216).

Retained Rectal Stump

Originally, restorative proctocolectomy included distal rectal mucosectomy and a manual endoanal anastomosis to the dentate line. Subsequently, the stapled ileoanal anastomosis was introduced placing the anastomosis at the level of the anorectal junction (217,218). In some patients it may be technically difficult to achieve a stapled anastomosis at the anorectal junction in which case the pouch is attached to the distal rectum. Choen et al. (219) in a prospectively randomized study of stapled versus handsewn ileoanal anastomosis showed that a few patients in the stapled group had an anastomosis significantly above the anorectal junction.

Several other authors have also reported a variable length of rectal mucosa left distal to the stapled anastomosis. Mucosal inflammation of some degree is a common finding in biopsies of the retained rectum (220–223). Approximately 2% to 9% of patients have symptomatic inflammation, which may be associated with persistent symptoms of proctitis such as bleeding, burning, urgency, and frequency (223–226).

Patients having symptoms due to residual rectal mucosa should be thoroughly investigated with a pouchography, rigid sigmoidoscopy, and biopsies. When the diagnosis is confirmed and pouch dysfunction is progressive, surgical correction is recommended (194,224,225). A combined abdomino-anal approach is usually used with complete mobilization of the pouch, detachment of the ileorectal anastomosis, and excision of the retained rectum. An endoanal mucosectomy of the anal stump is then performed followed by a handsewn anastomosis of the reservoir to the anal canal.

Tulchinsky et al. (227) reported 22 patients with pouch dysfunction resulting from a retained rectal stump who underwent abdomino-anal revision. Five patients had the pouch eventually excised and 17 had a functioning pouch at a median follow up of 22.5 (range 4–114) months; 15 patients reported marked improvement in pouch function and quality of life.

Pouch Fistulas

A fistula originating from the ileoanal anastomosis or the pouch itself is a serious complication. The incidence varies between 5% and 17% (228–230) and depends on the accuracy and duration of follow-up. It often requires further surgery and may alter ultimate functional outcome and lead to pouch excision. Fistulas may occur from the perineum, vagina, bladder, and abdominal wall skin. Etiologic factors include anastomotic dehiscence, pelvic sepsis, surgical experience, localized ischemia, entrapment of tissue (mainly the posterior vaginal wall) in the stapling device, and Crohn's disease. Pelvic sepsis is probably the major predisposing factor. Symptoms consist of purulent discharge and flatus or stool passing through the vagina, perineum, or abdominal wall. It may be associated with pelvic or abdominal pain, incontinence, and urgency. Diagnosis is based on history and physical examination and may be confirmed by examination under anesthesia. Other diagnostic modalities may be used to assess the tract including endoanal ultrasound, pouchography, fistulography, CT, and MRI. Initial management includes local procedures to drain the sepsis. Crohn's disease must be excluded as pouch fistulas associated with Crohn's disease tend to recur (231). Early postoperative fistulas may heal spontaneously if diverted and have a better prognosis than those occurring after ileostomy closure (229,232,233).

Pouch-Cutaneous Fistula.   Cutaneous fistulas from the pouch suture line or pouch appendage to the abdominal wall can usually be treated with fecal diversion, excision of the fistula tract, and closure of the pouch defect. Cutaneous fistulas related to Crohn's disease or chronic pelvic sepsis may not be amenable to surgical repair and may warrant pouch excision.

Pouch-Perineal Fistula.   Most pouch-perineal fistulas originate from the ileoanal anastomosis. When superficial, these fistulas can be managed by fistulotomy. If the fistula is trans-sphicteric, it can be managed by a staged fistulotomy using a seton or by a pouch advancement procedure.

Pouch-Vaginal Fistula.   Pouch-vaginal fistula following restorative proctocolectomy is disabling to the patient and is difficult to treat. The incidence varies between 3.6% and 12% (231–234) and postoperative pelvic sepsis is probably the major predisposing factor. Several various procedures have been described for pouch vaginal fistula repair, including transvagina and anal and abdominal procedures, with variable success rates. Initial management includes control of pelvic sepsis by drainage. Diversion may be considered to alleviate symptoms and control sepsis. In any case of fistula, Crohn's disease should be excluded. Definitive repair using an endoanal ileal advancement flap has a success rate of 20% to 80% (228,231,233,234). Lee et al. (234) reported 12 pouch vaginal fistulas repaired by transanal advancement flap with an over all success rate of 83.3% in the nine women without Crohn's disease. O'Kelly et al. (232) who described the endovaginal advancement flap, treated seven patients, and five (71%) had healed fistula and satisfactory pouch function at a mean follow up of 26 (range 4–72) months. Burke et al. (235) recently described a transvaginal approach for the treatment of pouch vaginal fistulas. In their series, 11 out of 14 patients (78.5%) had the fistula closed at a median follow up of 18 (6–60) months. Advanced procedures, including gracilis muscle repair and transposition of the rectus abdominus muscle may be used in cases of recurrent fistulas (236,237). High fistulas, entering the pouch above the ileoanal anastomosis, should be considered for repair using an abdominal approach.

Pouchitis

Symptomatic inflammation of the ileal pouch is a common complication following restorative proctocolectomy for ulcerative colitis. The etiology is poorly understood and several mechanisms have been suggested, including immune alterations, fecal stasis resulting in bacterial overgrowth (238), and lack of mucosal nutrients, and ischemia (239), but none of which have been definitively proven. Factors that may predispose to pouchitis include the presence of extra-intestinal manifestations (240,241), primary sclerosing cholangitis (242), and a previous course of extensive colonic disease and backwash ileitis (243). Smoking appears to protect the development of pouchitis (244). Pouchitis is considered by many to be a form of ulcerative colitis that recurs in the pouch and tends to occur in equal frequency irrespective of the pouch configuration. The reported prevalence of pouchitis in patients operated for ulcerative colitis varies between 5% and 59% (189,245–251). This variability may be partially explained by the lack of universally accepted diagnostic criteria that should be based on clinical, endoscopic, and histologic criteria (246–248). To address this issue, a Pouchitis Disease Activity Index (PDAI) was developed (252), taking into account the clinical symptoms, endoscopic findings, and histological changes. Shen et al. (253) used the PDAI score in 46 patients with ulcerative colitis and an ileoanal pouch and found that each of the three components in the score contributed with a similar magnitude to the overall PDAI score; symptoms alone did not reliably diagnose pouchitis. Furthermore, pouchitis may appear late in the postoperative course and its incidence increases with increases in length of follow-up (247).

Clinically, patients present with a marked increase of stool frequency, occasionally with bloody diarrhea (254), urgency, and incontinence. Abdominal and pelvic pain, fever, fatigue, anorexia, and malaise are often present and some patients may have extra-intestinal manifestations.

Pouchitis may appear as acute, acute relapsing, and chronic persistent phenomena. Pouchitis is usually well controlled with medical therapy and a variety of agents have been used. For the majority of patients a 10- to 14-day course of antibiotic treatment will rapidly control symptoms. Metronidazole is probably the most commonly used first-line agent and has been shown to be effective for active chronic pouchitis in a recent meta-analysis (255). However, the long-term use of metronidazole may cause peripheral neuropathy. Ciprofloxacin has been widely used as an alternative or in combination with metronidazole. In a randomized prospective trial, Shen et al. (253) compared ciprofloxacin and metronidazole and found that ciprofloxacin was associated with a greater reduction in the PDAI score and was better tolerated than metronidazole.

In patients with chronic pouchitis who respond to antibiotic treatment and are in remission, the use of probiotics seems to be effective in preventing further episodes. Gionchetti et al. (112) in a double-blind, placebo-controlled trial found that oral administration of a mixture of probiotic bacterial strains (VSL-3) was effective in secondary prevention of pouchitis.

When chronic pouchitis is refractory to antibiotic treatment, other medications such as anti-inflammatory agents, local or systemic steroids, or immunosuppressive agents may be used. Approximately 1% of patients develop chronic persistent pouchitis refractory to any medical treatment, therefore surgery may be necessary. Pouch excision is probably the only alternative in these cases as no other surgical approach has proven to alleviate symptoms and prevent recurrent pouchitis.

Controversies in Ileoanal Pouch Surgery

Despite the large experience gained with the ileoanal pouch procedure in the past decades, some controversies regarding the optimal surgical technique still exist. In some controversies, such as the pouch configuration, experience has led most surgeons to agree. Other controversies, however, such as the routine use of mucosectomy or a diverting ileostomy, are still in debate, and large series supporting each approach have been published.

Routine Mucosectomy with Handsewn Ileoanal Anastomosis vs. Stapled Anastomosis Without Mucosectomy

Since the introduction of restorative proctocolectomy in the late 1970s, there have been several modifications to the operative technique. The original approach of endoanal rectal mucosectomy down to the dentate line and a handsewn ileal pouch anal anastomosis has given way, in many centers, to a double-stapled technique with pouch anal anastomosis at the anorectal junction. Stapled ileoanal anastomosis was described at the mid-1980s with the claim of improved function (217,218). This procedure preserves the anal transitional zone, rich in sensory nerve supply, aiming to improve sensation and pouch function thereby resulting in decrease in stool frequency and fewer episodes of incontinence. However, none of the three prospective randomized controlled studies comparing stapled to handsewn anastomosis found a significant difference in the postoperative complication rate or function between these two techniques (219,256,257). The first study by Choen et al. from St. Mark's (219) Hospital, published in 1991, compared 32 consecutive patients matched by age and gender. There was no difference in the voluntary contraction pressure in the anal canal, the functional anal canal length, or anal sensation between the two groups. Clinical function, including continence and the ability to discriminate feces from flatus, was also similar. A later study by Luukkonen and Jarvinen (256) confirmed insignificant differences in operative aspects, postoperative complications, and functional outcome in 40 consecutive patients. The authors concluded that mucosectomy with handsewn anastomosis has the advantage of removing all disease-prone mucosa without functional compromise. In 1997, Reilly et al. from the Mayo Clinic (257) rechallenged this issue, randomizing 41 patients to either endoanal mucosectomy and hand sewn ileoanal anastomosis or a double-stapled anastomosis, sparing the anal transitional zone. Thirty-three percent of the handsewn group and 35% of the double-stapled anastomosis group had at least one postoperative complication. Resting anal pressures were higher in the stapled group, but other physiologic parameters were similar between the two groups. Nocturnal fecal incontinence occurred less frequently in the stapled group but this difference was not statistically significant.

More prospective randomized studies involving larger numbers of patients with longer follow-up are needed to determine the optimal surgical technique, taking into consideration the technical ease, postoperative complications, pouch function, and quality of life as well as the risk of dysplasia and cancer.

Using a stapled technique, a mucosal remnant of 1 to 2 cm is left behind. Even after mucosectomy, residual islands of rectal mucosa may be found in 20% of excised pouches (258,259). Therefore, there is the potential for neoplastic transformation in any retained mucosa. There have been reports of dysplasia in the residual anorectal cuff after stapled anastomosis associated with the presence of high-grade dysplasia or cancer in the proctocolectomy specimen (143). Nevertheless, only very few cases of adenocarcinoma have been reported (260), and cancer was rarely reported in the rectal stump after mucosectomy (261). At present, the risk of developing cancer seems to be very low in both groups, however, longer follow-up is required before this issue can be resolved.

The author's personal bias (OZ) is that the stapled anastomosis is technically easier, is potentially associated with improved postoperative function, and may be safely performed in patients without high grade dysplasia or cancer.

Type of Reservoir

Pouch configurations using two J, three S, or four W loops of small intestine have been performed throughout the years. The S pouch, introduced in 1978 by Parks and Nicholls (177), was the first to be used. Although it provides large volume, the early design was constructed with a long efferent limb, which led to pouch outlet obstruction. Today, the S pouch is constructed with almost no efferent limb and its function is comparable to other pouch configurations. The J pouch, first described by Utsunomiya in 1980 (262), is now the most commonly used reservoir as it is relatively easy to perform and can be rapidly constructed using a linear stapler. Furthermore, it is associated with adequate volume and function, while minimizing outlet obstruction complications. In 1985, Nicholls and Pezim (263) presented the W configuration, designed to provide a pouch with increased volume. A recent randomized, controlled trail comparing the functional results of the J and W configurations for ulcerative colitis showed a significantly lower frequency of defecation, nocturnal defecation, and the use of antidiarrheal medications with the W pouch during the first year after ileostomy closure (264). The long-term benefit of this pouch, however, remains to be proven.

Diverting Ileostomy

Continuous controversy exists regarding the necessity of a routine diverting loop ileostomy in restorative proctocolectomy. Advocates of the one-stage procedure, which avoids fecal diversion, argue that complication rates and functional results are comparable with those of the two-stage operation while avoiding the need for a second operation for ileostomy closure (265–268).

A recent matched-pair control study compared 57 patients with a one-stage procedure and 114 patients with a two-stage procedure. Early and late complication rates were significantly lower in the one-stage group, and anastomotic stricture was more common with the two-stage procedure. Likewise, Grobler et al. (269), in a randomized trial, showed no functional difference between the groups, and the use of a loop ileostomy was associated with a high complication rate. However, it should be emphasized that this study only included patients who were not on steroids and had an uneventful stapled anastomosis.

In contrast, many experienced surgeons believe that it is safer to perform a routine covering ileostomy to allow the ileal pouch anal anastomosis to heal completely prior to contact with the fecal stream. A temporary diverting loop ileostomy may potentially reduce septic consequences of anastomotic leakage, thereby minimizing the risk of pelvic sepsis and pouch failure.

We believe that the truth probably lies somewhere in between and careful patient selection should be undertaken for the use of a one-stage procedure. One can consider an ileoanal pouch operation without a diverting loop ileostomy if every aspect of the operative procedure was technically perfect and if the patient is not at risk for factors such as malnutrition, high-dose steroid administration, and immunomodulating therapy.

Laparoscopic Ileoanal Pouch Surgery

The introduction of laparoscopic techniques has been one of the most significant events in the evolution of general surgery in the 20th century. Advanced laparoscopic colon and rectal procedures were shown to be feasible and safe. The initial large series from the Cleveland Clinic Florida, published in 1994, suggested that morbidity may be higher using the laparoscopic technique (270). More recent series, however, revealed comparable complication rates using the laparoscopic and open techniques, with somewhat earlier return of the bowel function, shorter length of stay, and improved cosmesis with the laparoscopic approach (271,272).

Laparoscopic total proctocolectomy with ileal pouch anal anastomosis requires a high level of advanced laparoscopic skills and expertise, which are only partially translatable from traditional surgical training, and the utility of laparoscopy for this procedure is still limited to dedicated laparoscopic colon and rectal surgeons.

Sexual Function, Pregnancy, and Delivery

As a large proportion of the patients requiring restorative proctocolectomy are young, sexual function and fertility are very important factors in their postoperative quality of life. Data suggest that, in most patients, sexual activity increases and satisfaction improves after restorative proctocolectomy compared to the preoperative level, most likely due to improved general health. Dyspareunia, however, may be a frequent complication in females (273–275). Tiainen et al. (274) studied 95 patients who underwent restorative proctocolectomy. Among the 51 women, dyspareunia occurred in 13.7% before and 22% after surgery, although sexual satisfaction improved; the ability to achieve orgasm was unchanged in most patients. Among 44 men, 2.3% experienced retrograde ejaculation and 14.6% had erectile dysfunction, probably owing to damage to the sympathetic and parasympathetic nerves during surgery. The fear of leakage during coitus was significantly reduced after surgery in both genders.

Pregnancy and delivery have proven safe after restorative proctocolectomy, and problems associated with the pouch are relatively uncommon. Stool frequency and incontinence are increased during pregnancy, but seem to return to baseline after delivery (276,277).

There is debate as to whether female patients with an ileoanal pouch should be permitted to undergo a vaginal delivery for fear of damage to the anal sphincters. Several studies have shown, however, that the type of delivery, whether vaginal or cesarean section, did not influence pouch function and the choice should depend on obstetric indications. However, when the perineum is scarred and noncompliant, cesarean section is preferred. Farouk et al. (278) compared 85 pregnant women who had a vaginal delivery after surgery with 343 women who did not give birth. At a median follow-up of eight (range 5–17) years, stool frequency and continence were similar between the two groups.

Fertility of women with ulcerative colitis who have not undergone surgery correlates with the age-matched general population. However, for unknown reasons, fertility postileal pouch anal anastomosis is reduced. One possible explanation is the formation of adhesions obstructing the fallopian tubes. Olsen et al. (279) found that the birth rate was reduced to almost half of the expected in a group of 237 women postileal pouch procedure. In a more recent study by the same authors (280), 290 women postsurgery were included. A reference population of 1200 women from Denmark and Sweden was used as the control group. In the patient group, the fecundability (the probability of becoming pregnant per month with unprotected intercourse) ratio was decreased to 0.20. The cumulative incidence of pregnancy after surgery was 18% at 12 months, 27% at 24 months, and 36% at 60 months compared to 75%, 82% and 88%, respectively, in the reference population.

Women with ulcerative colitis in their reproductive years, who are candidates for restorative proctocolectomy, should be informed of the reduced probability of becoming pregnant after the operation.

Failure and Revision

Although most patients do well after restorative proctocolectomy, failure occurs in up to 17% of cases, and its rate increases with the length of follow-up. The main causes of failure include acute and chronic sepsis, poor function due to mechanical or functional complications, mucosal inflammation including pouchitis and retained rectal mucosa, and neoplastic transformation (189,191,281).

Salvage surgery is aimed at avoiding and correcting pouch failure, leading to pouch excision or indefinite diversion proximal to the pouch. Careful patient selection and counseling is essential and the patient must be given a realistic picture of the prospect of success, compared to the potential morbidity of removal of the reservoir with a permanent ileostomy.

Patients with outflow obstruction caused by a long efferent limb are probably the best candidates for pouch salvage surgery, with a success rate approaching 93% (211). Patients with peri-pouch fistulas and persistent anastomotic stenosis may have salvage rates of 50% to 85% (282–284), however, repeat procedures may be required to achieve this result. Patients must be aware that good functional results cannot be guaranteed. In motivated patients without Crohn's disease, however, surgical salvage attempts are worthwhile.

REFERENCES

1. Hiatt RA, Kaufman L. Epidemiology of inflammatory bowel disease in a defined northern California population. West J Med 1988; 149:541.
2. Lashner BA. Epidemiology of inflammatory bowel disease. Gastroenterol Clin North Am 1995; 24:467.
3. Martinez-Salemean JF, Rodrigo M, De Teresa J, et al. Epidemiology of inflammatory bowel disease in the province of Grenada Spain: a retrospective study from 1979–1988. Gut 1993; 34:1207.
4. Sandler RS. Epidemiology of inflammatory bowel disease. In: Taragan SR, Shanahan F, eds. Inflammatory Bowel Disease: From Bench to Bedside. Baltimore: Williams & Wilkins, 1994.
5. Yoshida Y, Murata Y. Inflammatory bowel disease in japan: studies in epidemiology and etiopathogenesis. Med Clin North Am 1990; 74:67.

6. Yang S-K, Loftus EV, Sandborn WJ. Epidemiology of inflammatory bowel disease in asia. Inflamm Bowel Dis 2001; 7:260–270.

7. Sonnenberg A, McCarty DJ, Jacobsen SJ. Geographic variations of inflammatory bowel disease within the united states. Gastroenterology 1991; 100:143.

8. Andreas PG, Friedman LS. Epidemiology and the natural course of inflammatory bowel disease. Gastroenterol Clin North Am 1999; 28:255–281.

9. Shivanada S, Lennard-Jones J, Logan R, et al. Incidence of inflammatory bowel disease across europe: is there a difference between the north and the south? Results of a European Collaborative Study in Inflammatory Bowel disease. Gut 1996; 39:690.

10. Roth MP, Petersen GM, McElree C, et al. Geographic origins of jewish patients with inflammatory bowel disease. Gastroenterology 1989; 97:900.

11. Gilat T, Grossman A, Fireman Z, et al. Inflammatory bowel disease in jews. In: McConnel R, Rozen P, Langman M, eds. The Genetics and Epidemiology of Inflammatory Bowel Disease in Frontiers of Gastrointestinal Research. New York: Karger, 1986.

12. Trallori G, Palli D, Saieva C, et al. A population based study of inflammatory bowel disease in florence over 15 years 1978–1992. Scand J Gastroenterol 1996; 31:892.

13. Langholz E, Munkholm P, Davidson M, et al. Causes of ulcerative colitis: analysis of changes in disease activity over years. Gastroenterology 1994; 107:3.

14. Farmer RG, Easley KA, Rankin GB. Clinical patterns natural history and progression of ulcerative colitis. Dig Res Sci 1993; 38:1137.

15. Langholz E, Munkholm P, Nielsen H, et al. Incidences and prevalence of ulcerative colitis in copenhagen county from 1962 to 1987. Scand J Gastroenterol 1991; 26:1247.

16. Eaden JA, Mayberry JF. Colorectal cancer complicating ulcerative colitis: a review. Am J Gastroenterol 2000; 95:2710–2718.

17. Greenstein AJ, Aufses AH Jr. Differences in pathogenesis incidence and outcome of perforation in inflammatory bowel disease. Surg Gynecol Obstet 1985; 160:63–69.

18. Ekbom A, Helmick C, Zack M, et al. Ulcerative colitis and colorectal cancer. N Eng J Med 1990; 323:1228–1233.

19. Eaden JA, Abrams KR, Mayberry JF. The risk of colorectal cancer in ulcerative colitis: a meta-analysis. Gut 2001; 48:526–535.

20. Ransohoff DF. Colon cancer in ulcerative colitis. Gastroenterology 1988; 29:206–217.

21. Jayaram H, Satsangi T, Chapman RWG. Increased colorectal neoplesia in chronic ulcerative colitis complicated by primary sclerosing cholangitis: fact or fiction? Gut 2001; 48:430–434.

22. Farrell RJ, Peppercorn MA. Ulerative colitis. Lancet 2002; 359:331–340.

23. Levine JB, Lukawski-Trubish D. Extra intestinal considerations in inflammatory bowel disease. Gastroenterol Clin N Am 1995; 24:633.

24. Jewell DP. Ulcerative colitis. In: Feldman M, Scharschmidt BF, Sleisenger MH, eds. Sleisenger and Fordtrans: Gastrointestinal and Liver Disease. Philadelphia: WB Saunders, 1998.

25. Loftus EV, Sandborn WJ, Linder KD, et al. Interactions between chronic liver disease and inflammatory bowel disease. Inflamm Bowel Dis 1997; 3:288.

26. Raj V, Lichtenstein DR. Hepatobilliary manifestations of inflammatory bowel disease. Gastroenterol Clinics N Am 1999; 28:491–513.

27. Narumi S, Roberts JP, Emond JC, Lake J, Ascher NL. Liver transplantation for sclerosing cholangitis. Hepatology 1995; 22:451–457.

28. Hendrickson BA, Gokhale R, Cho JH. Clinical aspects and pathophysiology of inflammatory bowel disease. Clin Mirobiol Rev 2002; 15:79–94.

29. Ghosh S, Shand A, Ferguson A. Ulcerative Colitis. BMJ 2000; 320:1119–1123.

30. Pullan RD, Thomas GA, Rhodes M, et al. Thickness of adherent mucus gel on colonic mucosa in humans and its relevance to colitis. Gut 1994; 35:353–359.

31. Tysk C, Riedesel H, Lindberg E, Panzini B, Podolsky D. Colonic glycoproteins in monozygotic twins with inflammatory bowel disease. Gastroenterology 1991; 100:419–423.

32. Lee JCW, Lennard-Jone JE. Inflammatory bowel disease in 67 families with three or more affected first degree relatives. Gastroenterology 1996; 3:587.

33. Toyoda H, Wang S-J, Yang H, et al. Distinct association of HLA class II genes with inflammatory bowel disease. Gastroenterology 1993; 104:741.

34. Karaban D, Eliakim R, Brant SR. Genetics of inflammatory bowel disease. IMAJ 2002; 4:798–802.

35. Satsangi J, Grootscholten C, Holt H, Jewell DP. Clinical patterns of familial inflammatory bowel disease. Gut 1996; 38:738.

36. Satsangi J, Welsh KI, Bunce M, et al. Contribution of genes of the major histocompatibility complex to susceptibility and disease phenotype in inflammatory bowel disease Lancet 1996; 347:1212–1217.

37. Satsangi J, Parkes M, Luis E, et al. Two stage geomic-wide search in inflammatory bowel disease provides evidence for susceptibility loci on chrosones 37 and 12. Nat Genet 1996; 14:199.

38. Papadakis KA, Targan SR. Current theories on the causes of inflammatory bowel disease. Gastroenterol Clin N Am 1999; 28:283–296.

39. Reif S, Lavy A, Keter D, et al. Lack of association between smoking and crohns disease but the usual association with ulcerative colitis in jewish patients in israel. A multicenter study. Am J Gastroenterol 2000; 95:471–475.

40. Eliakim R, Karmeli F, Rachmilewitz D, Cohen P, Fich A. Effect of chronic nicotine administration on trinitrobenzene sulfonic acid colitis. Eur J Gastroenterol Hepatol 1998; 10:1013–1019.
41. Eliakim R, Fam, Babyatsky MW. Chronic nicotine administration differentially alters jejunal and colonic inflammation in IL-10 deficient mice. Eur J Gastroenterol Hepatol 2002; 14:1–8.
42. Fiocchi C. Inflammatory bowel disease: ethiology and pathogenesis. Gastroenterology 1998; 115: 182–205.
43. Lindberg E, Tysk C, Andersson K, Jarnerot G. Smoking and inflammatory bowel disease: a case control study. Gut 1998; 29:352.
44. Eliakim R, Karmeli F, Cohen P, Heyman S, Rachmilewitz D. Dual effect of chronic nicotine administration: augmentation of jejunitis and amelioration of colitis induced by iodoacetamide. Int J Colorectal Dis 2001; 16:14–21.
45. Rutgeerts P, Dhaens G, Hiele M, et al. Appendectomy protects against ulcerative colitis. Gastroenterology 1994; 106:1251.
46. Reif S, Lavy A, Keer D, et al. Appendectomy in more frequent but not a risk factor for crohns disease while being protective in ulcerative colitis: a comparison of surgical procedures in IBD. Am J Gastroenterol 2001; 96:829–832.
47. Cooke EM, Ewins SP, Hywell-Jones J, Lennard-Jones JE. Properties of stains of E-coli carried in different phases of ulcerative colitis. Gut 1974; 15:143.
48. Burke DA, Axon ATR. Ulcerative colitis and escherichia coli with adhesive properties. J Clin Pathol 1987; 40:782.
49. Burke DA, Axon ATR, Clayden SA, et al. The efficacy of tobramycin in the treatment of ulcerative colitis. Aliment Pharm Ther 1990; 4:123.
50. Campieri MJ, Gionchetti P. Bacteria as the cause of ulcerative colitis. Gut 2001; 48:132–135.
51. Das KM. Relationship of extraintestinal involvement in inflammatory bowel disease: new insights into autoimmune pathogenesis. Dig Dis Sci 1999; 44:1–13.
52. Merger M, Croitoru K. Infections in the immunopathogenesis of chronic inflammatory bowel disease. Semin Immunol 1998; 10:69–78.
53. Das KM, Vecchi M, Sakemaki S. A shared and unique epitopes on human colon skin and biliary epithelium detected by a moncolonal antibody. Gastroenterology 1990; 98:464.
54. Onoma ER, Amenta PS, Ramaswany K, Lin JJ, Das KM. Autoimmunity in ulcerative colitis: a predominant colonic mucosal B-cell response against human tropomyosin isoform 5. Clin Exp Immunol 2000; 121:466–471.
55. Sandborn WJ, Landers CJ, Tremaine WJ, et al. Antineutrophil cytoplasmatic antibody correlates with chronic pouchitis after ileal pouch and anastomosis. Am J Gastroenterol 1999; 90:740–747.
56. Mosman R, Sod S. The expanding universe of t cell subsets – Th1, Th2 and more. Immunol Today 1996; 17:38–46.
57. MacDermott RP. Chemokines in inflammatory bowel disease. J Clin Immunol 1999; 19:266–272.
58. Eliakim R, Rachmilewitz D. Potential mediators and the pathogenesis of inflammatory bowel disease. Gastroenterol Int 1992; 5:48–56.
59. Drossman DA. Psychological factors in inflammatory bowel disease. In: Kirsner JB, Shorter RG, eds. Inflammatory Bowel Disease. Baltimore: Wiliams and Wilking, 1995:492.
60. Casati J, Toner BB. Psychological aspects of inflammatory bowel disease. Biomed Pharmacother 2000; 54:388–393.
61. Theis MK, Boyko EJ. Patients perceptions of causes of inflammatory bowel disease. Am J Gastroenterol 1994; 89:1920.
62. Herbert TB, Cohen S. Stress and immunity in humans – a meta-anaalysis. Psychosom Med 1993; 55:364–379.
63. Duffy LC, Zielezny MA, Marshall JR, et al. Relevance of major stress events as an indicator of disease activity prevalence in inflammatory bowel disease. Behav Med 1991; 17:101.
64. Rao SCC, Reed NW, Davison PA, et al. Anorectal sensitivity and responses to rectal distortion in patients with ulcerative colitis. Gastroenterology 1987; 93:1270.
65. Singleton JW. Measures of disease activity. In: Bayless TM, Hanauer SB, eds. Advanced Therapy of Inflammatory Bowel Disease. Hamilton, BC: Decker Inc., 2001:25–28.
66. Katz JA. Useful biologic markers as activity indices. In: Bayless TM, Hanauer SB, eds. Advanced Therapy of Inflammatory Bowel Disease. Hamilton, BC: Decker Inc., 2001:35–38.
67. Buckell NA, Williams GI, Bartram CI, Lennard-Jones JE. Depth of ulceration in acute colitis: correlation with outcome and clinical and radiologic features. Gastroenterology 1980; 79:19.
68. Caroline DF, Glick SN, O'Kane PL. Imaging of mucosal inflammation. In: Bayless TM, Hanauer SB, eds. Advanced Therapy of Inflammatory Bowel Disease. Hamilton, BC: Decker Inc., 2001:39–45.
69. Scotiniotis I, Rubesin S, Ginsberg GG. Imaging modalities in inflammatory bowel disease. Gastroenterol Clin N Am 1999; 28:391–421.
70. Ulcerative colitis. In: Whitehood R, ed. Gastrointestinal and Oesophageal Pathology. Edinburgh: Churchill Livingstone, 1989:522–531.
71. Surawicz CM, Belic L. Rectal biopsies helps to disinguish acute self-limited colitis from idiopathic inflammatory bowel disease. Gastroenterology 1984; 86:104.
72. Allison MC, Hamilton-Dutoit SJ, Dhillon AP, Pounder RE. The value of rectal biopsy in distinguishing self-limited colitis from early inflammatory bowel disease. Q J Med 1987; 65:985.

73. Robertson DJ, Grimm IS. Inflammatory bowel disease in the elderly. Gastroeneterol Clin N Am 2001; 300:409–425.

74. Berrebi D, Sautel, Flejou, et al. Ticlopidine induced colitis: a histopathological study including apoptosis. J Clin Pathol 1998; 51:280–283.

75. Austin CA, Cann PA, Jones TH, Holdsworth CD. Exacerbation of diarrhea and pain in patients treated with 5-amino salycilic acid for ulcerative colitis. Lancet 1984; 1:917.

76. Sutherland L, Roth D, Beck P, May G, Makiyama K. Oral 5-amino salicylic acid for inducing remission in ulcerative colitis cochrane review. The Cochrane Library, Issue 1. Oxford: Update Software, 2000.

77. Hanauer SB, Dossopoulos T. Evolving treatment strategies for inflammatory bowel disease. Annu Rev Med 2001; 52:299–318.

78. Ireland A, Jewell DP. Sulphasalazine and the new salicylates. Eur J Gastroenterol Hepatol 1989; 1:43.

79. Sutherland LR, May GR, Shaffer E. Sulphasalazine revisited: a meta-analysis of 5-aminosalicylic acid in the treatment of ulcerative colitis. Ann Int Med 1993; 118:540.

80. Sands BE. Therapy of inflammatory bowel disease. Gastroenterelogy 2000; 118:568–582.

81. Gionchetti P, Rizzello F, Venturi A, et al. Comparison of oral with rectal mesalazine in the treatment of ulcerative proctitis. Dis Colon Rectum 1998; 41:93–97.

82. Safdi M, DeMicco M, Sninsky C, et al. A double-blind comparison of oral versus rectal versus combination therapy in the treatment of distal ulcerative colitis. Am J Gastroenterol 1997; 92:1867–1871.

83. D'Albasio G, Pacini F, Camani E, et al. Combined therapy with 5-aminosalicylic acid tablets and enemas for maintaining remission in ulcerative colitis: a randomized double-blind study. Am J Gastroenterol 1997; 92:1143–1147.

84. D'Albasio G, Paoluzi P, Campieri M, et al. Maintenance treatment of ulcerative proctitis with mesalazine suppositories: a double blind placebo-controlled trial. The italian IBD study group. Am J Gastroenterol 1998; 93:799–803.

85. Baron JH, Connel AM, Kanaghinis TG, et al. Out patient treatment of ulcerative colitis: comparison between three doses of oral prednisolone. Br Med J 1962; 2:441–443.

86. Blomberg B, Jarnerot G. Clinical evaluation and management of acute severe colitis. Inflamm Bowel Dis 2000; 6:214–227.

87. Marshall JK, Irvine EJ. Rectal corticosteroids versus alternative treatments in ulcerative colitis: a meta-analysis. Gut 1997; 40:775–781.

88. Meyers S, Sacher DB, Goldberg TD, et al. Corticotropin versus hydrocortisone in the treatment of ulcerative colitis. A prospective randomized double-blind clinical trial. Gastroenterology 1985; 89: 1189–1191.

89. Lofberg R, Danielsson A, Suhr O, et al. Oral budesonide versus prednisolone in patients with active extensive and left-sided ulcerative colitis. Gastroenterology 1996; 110:1713–1718.

90. Shanahan F. Inflammatory bowel disease: immunodiagnostics immunotherapeutics and ecotherapeutics. Gastroenteroogy 2001; 120:622–635.

91. Lichtiger S, Present DH, Kornbluth A, et al. Cyclosporine in severe ulcerative colitis refractory to steroid therapy. N Engl J Med 1994; 330:1841–1845.

92. Atkinson KA, McDonald JW, Lamba B, Feagan BG. Intravenous cyclosporine for severe attacks of ulcerative colitis: a survey of canadian gastroenterologists. Can J Gastroenterol 1997; 11:583–587.

93. Actis GC, Aimo G, Priolo G, et al. Efficacy and efficiency of oral microemulsion cyclosporin versus intravenous and soft gelatin capsule cyclosporin in the treatment of severe steroid-refractory ulcerative colitis: an open-label retrospective trial. Inflamm Bowel Dis 1998; 4:276–279.

94. Nielsen OH, Vainer B, Rask-Madsen J. The treatment of inflammatory bowel disease with 6-mercaptopurine or azathioprine. Aliment Pharmacol Therapeut 2001; 15:1699–1708.

95. Sandborn WJ, Tremaine WJ, Wolf DC, et al. Lack of effect of intravenous administration on time to respond to azathioprine for steroid-treated Crohn's disease. North American Azathioprine Study Group. Gastroenterology 1999; 117(3):527–535.

96. Shanahan F, Bernstein CN. Safety of low-dose purine analogues in inflammatory bowel disease. Gastroenterology 1994; 107:1905–1906.

97. Colona T, Korelitz BI. The role of leukopenia in the 6-mercaptopurine – induced remission of refractory Crohn's disease. Am J Gastroenterol 1994; 89:362–366.

98. Cuffari C, Hunt S, Bayless T. Utilisation of erythrocyte 6-tioguanine metabolite levels to optimise azathioprine therapy in patients with inflammatory bowel disease. Gut 2001; 48:642–646.

99. Sandborn WJ. Rational dosing of azathioprine and 6-mercaptopurine. Gut 2001; 48:591–592.

100. Egan LJ, Sandborn WJ. Methotrexate for inflammatory bowel disease: pharmacology and preliminary results. Mayo Clin Proc 1996; 71:69–80.

101. Oren R, Arber N, Odes S, et al. Methotrexate in chronic active ulcerative colitis: a double-blind randomized israeli multicenter trial. Gastroenterology 1996; 38:1851–1856.

102. Cabre E, Gassull MA. Nurition in inflammatory bowel disease: impact on disease and therapy. Curr Opin Gastroenterol 2001; 17:342–349.

103. Lashner BA, Hanauer SB, Silverstein MD. Testing nicotine gum for ulcerative colitis patients. Dig Dis Sci 1990; 35:829–832.

104. Pullan RD, Rhodes J, Ganesh S, et al. Transdermal nicotine for active ulcerative colitis. N Engl J Med 1994; 330:811–815.

105. Sandborn WJ, Tremaine WJ, Offord KP, et al. Transdermal nicotine for mildly to moderately active ulcerative colitis. A randomized double-blind placebo-controlled trial. Ann Intern Med 1999; 126:364–371.

106. Thomas GA, Rhodes J, Mani V, et al. Transdermal nicotine as maintenance therapy for ulcerative colitis. N Engl J Med 1995; 332:988–992.

107. Ricart E, Sandborn WJ. Use of nicotine and tobacco in colitis. In: Bayless TM, Hanauer SB, eds. Advanced Therapy in Inflammatory Bowel Disease. Hamilton, BC: Decker Inc., 2001:99.

108. Gaffney PR, Doyle CT, Gaffney A, et al. Paradoxical response to heparin in 10 patients with ulcerative colitis. Am J Gastroenterol 1995; 90:220–223.

109. Torkvist L, Thorlacius H, Sjoqvist U, et al. Low molecular weight heparin as adjuvant therapy in active ulcerative colitis. Aliment Pharmacol Ther 1999; 13:1323–1328.

110. Korzenik JR, Robert ME, Bitton A, et al. A multicenter randomized controlled trial of heparin for the treatment of ulcerative colitis. Gastroenterology 1999; 116:A752.

111. Rembacken BJ, Snelling AM, Hawkey PM, et al. Non pathogenic escherichia coli versus mesalazine for the treatment of ulcerative colitis: a randomized trial. Lancet 1999; 354:635–639.

112. Gionchetti P, Rizzello F, Venturi A, et al. Oral bacteriotherapy as maintenance treatment in patients with chronic pouchitis: a double-blind placebo-controlled trial. Gastroenterology 2000; 119:305–309.

113. Schreiber S, Fedorak R, Wild G, et al. Safety and tolerance of rHuIL-10 treatment in patients with mild/moderate active ulcerative colitis. Gastroenterology 1998; 114:A1080.

114. Alstead E. Fertility and pregnancy in inflammatory bowel disease. World J Gastroenterol 2001; 7: 455–459.

115. Willoughby CP, Truelove SC. Ulcerative colitis and pregnancy. Gut 1980; 21:469–474.

116. Greenstein AJ, Sachar DB, Gibas A, et al. Outcome of toxic dilatation in ulcerative and crohns colitis. J Clin Gastroenterol 1985; 7(2):137–143.

117. Muscroft TJ, Warren PM, Asquith P, Montgomery RD, Sokhi GS. Toxic megacolon in ulcerative colitis: a continuing challenge. Postgrad Med J 1981; 57(666):223–227.

118. Danovitch SH. Fulminant colitis and toxic megacolon. Gastroenterol Clin North Am 1989; 18(1):73–82.

119. Hyde GM, Thillainayagam AV, Jewell DP. Intravenous cyclosporin as rescue therapy in severe ulcerative colitis: time for a reappraisal? Eur J Gastroenterol Hepatol 1998; 10(5):411–413.

120. Haslam N, Hearing SD, Probert CS. Audit of cyclosporin use in inflammatory bowel disease: limited benefits numerous side-effects. Eur J Gastroenterol Hepatol 2000; 12(6):657–660.

121. Binderow SR, Wexner SD. Current surgical therapy for mucosal ulcerative colitis. Dis Colon Rectum 1994; 37(6):610–624.

122. Ziv Y, Fazio VW, Church JM, Milsom JW, Schroeder TK. Safety of urgent restorative proctocolectomy with ileal pouch-anal anastomosis for fulminant colitis. Dis Colon Rectum 1995; 38(4):345–349.

123. Jowett SL, Seal CJ, Barton JR, Welfare MR. The short inflammatory bowel disease questionnaire is reliable and responsive to clinically important change in ulcerative colitis. Am J Gastroenterol 2001; 96(10):2921–2928.

124. Fazio VW, O'Riordain MG, Lavery IC, et al. Long-term functional outcome and quality of life after stapled restorative proctocolectomy. Ann Surg 1999; 230(4):575–584.

125. Penna C, Daude F, Parc R, et al. Previous subtotal colectomy with ileostomy and sigmoidostomy improves the morbidity and early functional results after ileal pouch-anal anastomosis in ulcerative colitis. Dis Colon Rectum 1993; 36(4):343–348.

126. Ziv Y, Church JM, Fazio VW, King TM, Lavery IC. Effect of systemic steroids on ileal pouch-anal anastomosis in patients with ulcerative colitis. Dis Colon Rectum 1996; 39(5):504–508.

127. Binder SC, Miller HH, Deterling RA Jr. Emergency and urgent operations for ulcerative colitis. The Procedure of Choice. Arch Surg 1975; 110(3):284–289.

128. Harms BA, Myers GA, Rosenfeld DJ, Starling JR. Management of fulminant ulcerative colitis by primary restorative proctocolectomy. Dis Colon Rectum 1994; 37(10):971–978.

129. Sher ME, Weiss EG, Nogueras JJ, Wexner SD. Morbidity of medical therapy for ulcerative colitis: what are we really saving? Int J Colorectal Dis 1996; 11(6):287–293.

130. Fraser AG, Orchard TR, Jewell DP. The efficacy of azathioprine for the treatment of inflammatory bowel disease: a 30 year review. Gut 2002; 50(4):485–489.

131. Levin B, Lennard-Jones J, Riddell RH, Sachar D, Winawer SJ. Surveillance of patients with chronic ulcerative colitis. Who collaborating centre for the prevention of colorectal cancer. Bull World Health Organ 1991; 69(1):121–126.

132. Delco F, Sonnenberg A. A decision analysis of surveillance for colorectal cancer in ulcerative colitis. Gut 2000; 46(4):500–506.

133. Biasco G, Brandi G, Paganelli GM, et al. Colorectal cancer in patients with ulcerative colitis. A prospective cohort study in Italy. Cancer 1995; 75(8):2045–2050.

134. Rozen P, Baratz M, Fefer F, Gilat T. Low incidence of significant dysplasia in a successful endoscopic surveillance program of patients with ulcerative colitis. Gastroenterology 1995; 108(5):1361–1370.

135. Odze RD, Goldblum J, Noffsinger A, Alsaigh N, Rybicki LA, Fogt F. Interobserver variability in the diagnosis of ulcerative colitis-associated dysplasia by telepathology. Mod Pathol 2002; 15(4):379–386.

136. Gorfine SR, Bauer JJ, Harris MT, Kreel I. Dysplasia complicating chronic ulcerative colitis: is immediate colectomy warranted? Dis Colon Rectum 2000; 43(11):1575–1581.

137. Bernstein CN, Shanahan F, Weinstein WM. Are we telling patients the truth about surveillance colonoscopy in ulcerative colitis? Lancet 1994; 343(8889):71–74.

138. Blackstone MO, Riddell RH, Rogers BH, Levin B. Dysplasia-associated lesion or mass dalm detected by colonoscopy in long-standing ulcerative colitis: an indication for colectomy. Gastroenterology 1981; 80(2):366–374.

139. Habermann J, Lenander C, Roblick UJ, et al. Ulcerative colitis and colorectal carcinoma: dna-profile laminin-5 gamma 2 chain and cyclin a expression as early markers for risk assessment. Scand J Gastroenterol 2001; 36(7):751–758.

140. Holzmann K, Weis-Klemm M, Klump B, et al. Comparison of flow cytometry and histology with mutational screening for 53 and Ki-ras mutations in surveillance of patients with long-standing ulcerative colitis. Scand J Gastroenterol 2001; 36(12):1320–1326.

141. Pastore RL, Wolff BG, Hodge D. Total abdominal colectomy and ileorectal anastomosis for inflammatory bowel disease. Dis Colon Rectum 1997; 40(12):1455–1464.

142. Horai T, Kusunoki M, Shoji Y, Yamamura T, Utsunomiya J. Clinicopathological study of anorectal mucosa in total colectomy with mucosal proctectomy and ileoanal anastomosis. Eur J Surg 1994; 160(4):233–238.

143. Ziv Y, Fazio VW, Sirimarco MT, Lavery IC, Goldblum JR, Petras RE. Incidence risk factors and treatment of dysplasia in the anal transitional zone after ileal pouch-anal anastomosis. Dis Colon Rectum 1994; 37(12):1281–1285.

144. Baker WN, Glass RE, Ritchie JK, Aylett SO. Cancer of the rectum following colectomy and ileorectal anastomosis for ulcerative colitis. Br J Surg 1978; 65(12):862–868.

145. Gruner OP, Flatmark A, Naas R, Fretheim B, Gjone E. Ileorectal anastomosis in ulcerative colitis. Results in 57 Patients. Scand J Gastroenterol 1975; 10(6):641–646.

146. Grundfest SF, Fazio V, Weiss RA, et al. The risk of cancer following colectomy and ileorectal anastomosis for extensive mucosal ulcerative colitis. Ann Surg 1981; 193(1):9–14.

147. Backer O, Hjortrup A, Kjaergaard J. Evaluation of ileorectal anastomosis for the treatment of ulcerative proctocolitis. J R Soc Med 1988; 81(4):210–211.

148. Romano G, Salzano De Luna F, Giamundo P, Santangelo ML. Role of ileorectal anastomosis in the treatment of ulcerative colitis and familial polyposis. Ital J Surg Sci 1987; 17(2):135–140.

149. Johnson WR, Hughes ES, McDermott FT, Pihl EA, Katrivessis H. The outcome of patients with ulcerative colitis managed by subtotal colectomy. Surg Gynecol Obstet 1986; 162(5):421–425.

150. Oakley JR, Lavery IC, Fazio VW, Jagelman DG, Weakley FL, Easley K. The fate of the rectal stump after subtotal colectomy for ulcerative colitis. Dis Colon Rectum 1985; 28(6):394–396.

151. Leijonmarck CE, Lofberg R, Ost A, Hellers G. Long-term results of ileorectal anastomosis in ulcerative colitis in stockholm county. Dis Colon Rectum 1990; 33(3):195–200.

152. Katz JA. Medical and surgical management of severe colitis. Semin Gastrointest Dis 2000; 11(1): 18–32.

153. McKee RF, Keenan RA, Munro A. Colectomy for acute colitis: is it safe to close the rectal stump? Int J Colorectal Dis 1995; 10(4):222–224.

154. Karch LA, Bauer JJ, Gorfine SR, Gelernt IM. Subtotal colectomy with hartmanns pouch for inflammatory bowel disease. Dis Colon Rectum 1995; 38(6):635–639.

155. Carter FM, McLeod RS, Cohen Z. Subtotal colectomy for ulcerative colitis: complications related to the rectal remnant. Dis Colon Rectum 1991; 34(11):1005–1009.

156. Hulten L. Proctocolectomy and ileostomy to pouch surgery for ulcerative colitis. World J Surg 1998; 22(4):335–341.

157. Hurst RD, Finco C, Rubin M, Michelassi F. Prospective analysis of perioperative morbidity in one hundred consecutive colectomies for ulcerative colitis. Surgery 1995; 118(4):748–754.

158. Mikkola K, Luukkonen P, Jarvinen HJ. Restorative compared with conventional proctocolectomy for the treatment of ulcerative colitis. Eur J Surg 1996; 162(4):315–319.

159. Goes R, Beart RW Jr. Physiology of ileal pouch-anal anastomosis. Current concepts. Dis Colon Rectum 1995; 38(9):996–1005.

160. Becker JM, LaMorte W, St Marie G, Ferzoco S. Extent of smooth muscle resection during mucosectomy and ileal pouch-anal anastomosis affects anorectal physiology and functional outcome. Dis Colon Rectum 1997; 40(6):653–660.

161. Cullen JJ, Kelly KA. Prospectively evaluating anal sphincter function after ileal pouch-anal canal anastomosis. Am J Surg 1994; 167(6):558–561.

162. Kock NG. Ileostomy without external appliances: a survey of 25 patients provided with intra-abdominal intestinal reservoir. Ann Surg 1971; 173(4):545–550.

163. Kock NG. Intra-abdominal reservoir in patients with permanent ileostomy. Preliminary observations on a procedure resulting in fecal continence in five ileostomy patients. Arch Surg 1969; 99(2): 223–231.

164. Kock NG, Myrvold HE, Nilsson LO, Philipson BM. Continent ileostomy. An account of 314 Patients. Acta Chir Scand 1981; 147(1):67–72.

165. Ojerskog B, Hallstrom T, Kock NG, Myrvold HE. Quality of life in ileostomy patients before and after conversion to the continent ileostomy. Int J Colorectal Dis 1988; 3(3):166–170.

166. Kock NG. Present status of the continent ileostomy: surgical revision of the malfunctioning ileostomy. Dis Colon Rectum 1976; 19(3):200–206.
167. Fazio VW, Church JM. Complications and function of the continent ileostomy at the Cleveland clinic. World J Surg 1988; 12(2):148–154.
168. Dozois RR, Kelly KA, Ilstrup D, Beart RW Jr, Beahrs OH. Factors affecting revision rate after continent ileostomy. Arch Surg 1981; 116(5):610–613.
169. Jarvinen HJ, Makitie A, Sivula A. Long-term results of continent ileostomy. Int J Colorectal Dis 1986; 1(1):40–43.
170. Palmu A, Sivula A. Kocks continent ileostomy: results of 51 operations and experiences with correction of nipple-valve insufficiency. Br J Surg 1978; 65(9):645–648.
171. Gerber A. The kock continent ileal reservoir for supravesical urinary diversion. An early experience. Am J Surg 1983; 146(1):15–20.
172. Ravitch MM, Sabiston DC Jr. Anal ileostomy with preservation of the sphincter a proposed operation in patients requiring total colectomy for benign lesions. Surg Gynecol Obstet 1947; 84:1095–1099.
173. Best RR. Evaluation of ileoproctostomy to avoid ileostomy in various colon lesions. JAMA 1952; 150:637–642.
174. Schneider S. Anal ileostomy; experience with new three-stage procedure. Arch Surg 1955; 70:539–544.
175. Martin LW, Le Coultre C, Schubert WK. Total colectomy and mucosal proctectomy with preservation of continence in ulcerative colitis. Ann Surg 1977; 186:477–480.
176. Taylor BM, Beart RW Jr, Dozois RR, Kelly KA, Phillips SF. Straight ileoanal anastomosis Vs ileal pouch-anal anastomosis after colectomy and mucosal proctectomy. Arch Surg 1983; 118:696–701.
177. Parks AG, Nicholls RJ. Proctocolectomy without ileostomy for ulcerative colitis. Br Med J 1978; 2:85–88.
178. Thompson JS, Quigley EMM. Anal sphincteroplasty for incontinence after ileal pouch anal anastomosis. Report of two cases. Dis Colon Rectum 1995; 38:215–218.
179. Ogunbiyi OA, Korsgen S, Keighley MRB. Pouch Salvage – long term outcome. Dis Colon Rectum 1997; 40:548–552.
180. McHugh SM, Diamant NE. Effect of age, gender, and parity on anal canal pressures. Contribution of impaired anal sphincter function to fecal incontinence. Dig Dis Sci 1987; 32:726–736.
181. Lewis WG, Sagar PM, Holdsworth PJ. Resrorative proctocolectomy with end to end pouch anal anastomosis in patients over the age of fifty. Gut 1993; 34:948–952.
182. Reissman P, Teoh TA, Weiss EG, Nogueras JJ, Wexner SD. Functional outcome of the double stapled ileoanal reservoir in patients more than 60 years of age. Am Surg 1996; 62(3):178–183.
183. Bauer JJ, Gorfine SR, Gelernt IM, Harris MT, Kreel I. Restorative proctocolectomy in patients older than fifty years. Dis Colon Rectum 1997; 40(5):562–565.
184. Tan HT, Connolly AB, Morton D, Keighley MR. Results of restorative proctocolectomy in the elderly. Int J Colorectal Dis 1997; 12(6):319–322.
185. Smith LE, Friend W, Medwell S. The superior mesenteric artery: The critical factor in pouch pull-through procedures. Dis Colon Rectum 1984; 27:741–744.
186. Efron JE et al. Restorative proctocolectomy with ileal pouch anal anastomosis in obese patients. Obes Surg 2001; 11:246–251.
187. Parker MC, Nicholls RJ. Restorative proctocolectomy in patients after previous intestinal or anal surgery. Dis Colon Rectum 1992; 35:681–684.
188. Fazio VW et al. Ileal pouch anal anastomoses complications and function in 1005 patients. Ann Surg 1995; 222:120–127.
189. Meagher AP, Farouk R, Dozois RR, Kelly KA, Pemberton JH. J ileal pouch anal anastomosis for chronic ulcerative colitis: complications and long-term outcome in 1310 patients. Br J Surg 1998; 85: 800–803.
190. Gemlo BT, Wong WD, Rothenberger DA, Goldberg SM. Ileal pouch anal anastomosis – patterns of failure. Arch Surg 1992; 127:784–787.
191. Setti Carraro P, Ritchie JK, Wilkinson KH, Nicholls RJ, Hawley PR. The first 10 years experience of restorative proctocolectomy for ulcerative colitis. Gut 1994; 35:1070–1075.
192. Farouk R, Dozois RR, Pemberton JH, Larson D. Incidence and subsequent impact of pelvic abscess after ileal pouch anal anastomosis for chronic ulcerative colitis. Dis Colon Rectum 1998; 41: 1239–1243.
193. Galandiuk S et al. Ileal pouch anal anastomosis: reoperation for pouch related complications. Ann Surg 1990; 212:446–454.
194. Scott NA, Dozois RR, Beart RW, Pemberton JH, Wolff BG, Ilstrup DM. Postoperative intra abdominal and pelvic sepsis complicating ileal pouch anal anastomosis. Int J Colorect Dis 1988; 3:149–152.
195. Fleshman JW, McLeod RS, Cohen Z, Stern H. Improved results following use of an advancement technique in the treatment of ileoanal anastomotic complications. Int J Colorect Dis 1988; 3:161–165.
196. Poggioli G, Marchetti F, Selleri S, Laureti S, Stocchi L, Gozzetti G. Redo pouches: salvaging of failed ileal pouch anal anastomosis. Dis Colon Rectum 1993; 36:492–496.
197. Sagar PM, Dozois RR, Wolff BG, Kelly KA. Disconnection, pouch revision and reconnection of the ileal pouch anal anastomosis. Br J Surg 1996; 83:1401–1405.
198. MacLean AR et al. Risk of small bowel obstruction after ileal pouch anal anastomosis. Ann Surg 2002; 235:200–206.

199. Francois Y, Dozois RR, Kelly KA, et al. Small intestinal obstruction complicating ileal pouch anal anastomosis. Ann Surg 1989; 209; 46–50.

200. Galandiuk S, Pemberton JH, Tsao J, et al. Delayed ileal pouch anal anastomosis. Complications and functional results. Dis Colon Rectum 1991; 34:755–758.

201. Marcello PW, Roberts PL, Schoetz DJ, et al. Long-term results of the ileoanal pouch procedure. Arch Surg 1993; 128:500–504.

202. Nicholls RJ. Restorative proctocolectomy with ileal pouch reservoir; indications and results. Schweiz Med Wochenschr 1990; 120:485–488.

203. McMullen K, Hicks TC, Ray JE, Gathright JB, Timmcke AE. Complications associated with ileal pouch and anastomosis. World J Surg 1991; 15:763–767.

204. Breen EM et al. Functional results after perineal complications of ileal pouch anal anastomosis. Dis Colon Rectum 1998; 41:691–695.

205. Schoetz DJ Jr., Coller JA, Veidenheimer MC. Can a pouch be saved? Dis Colon Rectum 1988; 31: 671–675.

206. Lewis WG, Kuzu A, Sagar PM, Holdsworth PJ, Johnston D. Stricture at the pouch anal anastomosis after restorative proctocolectomy. Dis Colon Rectum 1994; 37:120–125.

207. Beart RW. Proctocolectomy and ileoanal anastomosis. World J Surg 1988; 12:160–163.

208. Senapati A, Tibbs CJ, Ritchie JK, Nicholls RJ, Hawley PR. Stenosis of the pouch anal anastomosis following restorative proctocolectomy. Int J Colorectal Dis 1996; 11:57–59.

209. Herbst F, Sielezneff I, Nicholls RJ. Salvage surgery for ileal pouch outlet obstruction. Br J Surg 1996; 83:368–371.

210. Fazio VW, Tjandra JJ. Pouch advancement and neoileoanal anastomosis for anastomotic stricture and anovaginal fistula complicating restorative proctocolectomy. Br J Surg 1992; 79:694–696.

211. Fonkalsrud EW, Bustorff-Silva J. Reconstruction for chronic dysfunction of ileoanal pouches. Ann Surg 1999; 2:197–204.

212. de Silva HJ, de Angelis CP, Soper N, Kettlewell MG, Mortensen NJ, Jewell DP. Clinical and functional outcome after restorative proctocolectomy. Br J Surg 1991; 78:1039–1044.

213. Nicholls RJ, Gilbert M. Surgical correction of the efferent ileal limb for disordered defecation following restorative proctocolectomy with the s ileal reservoir. Br J Surg 1990; 77:152–154.

214. Vasilevsky CA, Rothenberger DA, Goldberg SM. The S ileal pouch-anal anastomosis. World J Surg 1987; (6):742–750.

215. Dozois RR et al. Restorative proctocolectomy with ileal reservoir. Int J Colorectal Dis 1986; 1:2–19.

216. Lilequist L, Linquist K. A reconstructive operation in malfunctioning S–shaped pelvic reservoir. Dis Colon Rectum 1985; 28:506–511.

217. Heald RJ, Allen DR. Stapled ileo anal anastomosis. A technique to avoid mucosal proctectomy in the ileal pouch operation. Br J Surg 1986; 73:571–572.

218. Johnston D, Holdsworth PJ, Nasmyth DG, et al. Preservation of the entire anal canal in conservative proctocolectomy for ulcerative colitis: a pilot study comparing end to end ileo-anal anastomosis without mucosal resection with mucosal proctectomy and endo-anal anastomosis. Br J Surg 1987; 74:940–944.

219. Choen S, Tsunoda A, Nicholls RJ. Prospective randomized trial comparing anal function after hand sewn ileoanal anastomosis with mucosectomy versus stapled ileoanal anastomosis without mucosectomy in restorative proctocolectomy. Br J Surg 1991; 78:430–434.

220. Thompson-Fawcett MW, Mortensen NJ. Anal Trasitional zone and columnar cuff in restorative proctocolectomy. Br J Surg 1996; 83:1047–1155.

221. Kmiot WA, Keighley MR. Totally stapled abdominal restorative proctocolectomy. Br J Surg 1989; 76:961–964.

222. Curran FT, Sutton TD, Jass JR, Hill GL. Ulcerative colitis in the anal canal of patients undergoing restorative proctocolectomy. Aust N Z J Surg 1991; 61:821–824.

223. Lavery JC, Sirimarco MT, Ziv Y, Fazio VW. Anal canal inflammation after ileal pouch and anstomosis. Dis Colon Rectum 1995; 38:803–806.

224. Thompson-Fawcett MW, Mortensen NJ, Warren BF. "Cuffitis" inflammatory changes in the columnar cuff anal transitional zone ileal reservoir after stapled pouch anal anastomosis. Dis Colon Rectum 1999; 42:348–355.

225. Curran FT, Hill GL. Symptomatic colitis in the anal canal after restorative proctocolectomy. Aust N Z J Surg 1992; 62:941–943.

226. Schmitt SL, Wexner SD, Lucas FU, James K, Nogueras JJ, Jagleman DG. Retained mucosa after double stapled ileal reservoir and ileoanal anastomosis. Dis Colon Rectum1992; 35:1051–1056.

227. Tulchinsky H et al. Salvage abdominal surgery in patients with a retained rectal stump after restorative proctocolectomy and stapled anastomosis. Br J Surg 2001; 88:1602–1606.

228. Ozuner G, Hull T, Lee P, Fazio VW. What happens to a pelvic pouch when a fistula develops? Dis Colon Rectum 1997; 40:543–547.

229. Keighley MRB, Grobler SP. Fistula complicating restorastive proctocolectomy. Br J Surg 1993; 80:1065–1067.

230. Paye F, Penna C, Chiche L, Tiret E, Frileux P, Parc R. Pouch related fistula following restorative proctocolectomy. Br J Surg 1996; 83:1574–1577.

231. Wexner SD, Rothenberger DA, Jensen L, et al. Ileal pouch vaginal fistula: incidence, etiology and management. Dis Colon Rectum 1989; 32:460–465.
232. O'Kelly TJ, Merrett M, Mortensen NJ, Dehn TCB, Kettlewell M. Pouch vaginal fistula after restorative proctocolectomy: aetiology and managment. Br J Surg 1994; 81:1374–1375.
233. Groom JS, Nicholls RJ, Hawley PR, Phillips RKS. Pouch vaginal fistula. Br J Surg 1993; 80:936–940.
234. Lee PY, Fazio VW, Church JM, Hull TL, Eu KW, Lavery IC. Vaginal fistula following restorative proctocolectomy. Dis Colon Rectum 1997; 40:752–759.
235. Burke D, VanLaarhoven CJHM, Herbst F, Nicholls RJ. Transvaginal repair of pouch vaginal fistula. Br J Surg 2001; 88:241–245.
236. Gorenstien L, Boyd JB, Ross TM. Gracilis muscle repair of rectovaginal fistula after restorative proctocolectomy. Report of two cases. Dis Colon Rectum 1988; 31:730–734.
237. Tran KT, Kuijpers HC, Van NieuwenhovenEJ, Van Goor H, Spauwen PH. Transposition of the rectus abdominus muscle for complicated pouch and rectal fistula. Dis Colon Rectum 1999; 42:486–489.
238. Fonkalsrud EW, Phillips JD. Reconstruction of malfunctioning ileoanal pouch procedures as an alternative to permanent ileostomy. Am J Surg 1990; 160:241–250.
239. Chaussade S, Denizot Y, Valleur P, et al. Presence of PAF-acether in stool of patients with pouch ileoanal anastomosis and pouchitis. Gastroenterology 1991; 100:1509–1514.
240. Lohmuller JL, Pemberton JH, Dozois RR, et al. Pouchitis and extraintestinal manifestations of inflammatory bowel disease after ileal pouch anal anastomosis. Ann Surg 1990; 211:622–627.
241. Oresland T, Fasth S, Nordgren S, Hulten L. The clinical and functional outcome after restorative procetocolectomy. A prospective study in 100 patients. Int J Colorectal Dis 1989; 4:50–56.
242. Penna C, Dozois R, Tremaine W, et al. Pouchitis after ileal pouch anal anastomosis for ulcerative colitis occurs with increased frequency in patients with associated primary sclerosing cholangitis. Gut 1996; 38:234–239.
243. Schmidt CM, Lazenby AJ, Hendrickson RJ, et al. Preoperative terminal ileal and colonic resection histopathology predicts risk of pouchitis in patients after ileoanal pull–through procedure. Ann Surg 1998; 227:654–662.
244. Merrett MN, Mortensen N, Kettlewell M, et al. Smoking may prevent pouchitis in patients with restorative proctocolectomy for ulcerative colitis. Gut 1996; 38:362–364.
245. Luukkonen P, Jarvinen H, Tanskanen M, Kahri M. Pouchitis-recurrence of the inflammatory bowel disease? Gut 1994; 35:243–246.
246. Svaninger G, Nordgren S, Oresland T, Hulten L. Incidence and characteristics of pouchitis in the kock continent ileostomy and the pelvic pouch. Scan J Gastroenterol 1993; 28:695–700.
247. Heuschen UA et al. Long-term follow up after ileoasnal pouch procedure. Dis Colon Rectum 2001; 44:487–499.
248. Simchuk EJ, Thirlby RC. Risk factors and true incidence of pouchitis in patients after ileal pouch anal anastomoses. World J Surg 2000; 24:851–856.
249. Moskowitz RL, Shepherd NA, Nicholls RJ. An assessment of inflammation in the reservoir after restorative proctocolectomy with ileoanal ileal reservoir. Int J Colorect Dis 1986; 1:167–174.
250. Madden MV, Farthing MJ, Nicholls RJ. Inflammation in ileal reservoirs: 'pouchitis'. Gut 1990; 31:247–249.
251. Sandborn WJ. Pouchitis following ileal pouch anal anastomosis: definition, pathogenesis and treatment. Gastroenterology 1994; 107:1856–1860.
252. Sandborn WJ, Tremaine WJ, Batts KP, Pemberton JH, Phillips S. Pouchitis after ileal pouch anal anastomosis: a pouchitic disease activity index. Mayo Clin Proc 1994; 69:409–415.
253. Shen B et al. Endoscopic and histologic evaluation together with symptom assessment are required to diagnose pouchitis. Gastroenterology 2001; 121:261–267.
254. Kelly DG, Phillips SF, Kelly KA, Wienstein WM, Gilchrist MJ. Dysfunction of the continent ileostomy: clinical features and bacteriology. Gut 1983; 24:193.
255. Sandborn WJ, McLeod R, Jewell DP. Medical therapy for induction and maintenance of remission in pouchitis: a systemic review. Inflamm Bowel Dis 1999; 5(1):33–39.
256. Luukkonen P, Jarvinen H. Stapled vs hand sutured ileoanal anastomosis in restorative proctocolectomy. A prospective, randomized study. Arch Surg 1993; 128:437–440.
257. Reilly WC, Pemberton JH, Wolff BG, et al. Randomized prospective trial comparing ileal pouch anal anastomosis performed by excising the anal mucosa to ileal pouch anal anastomosis performed by preserving the anal mucosa. Ann Surg 1997; 225:666–677.
258. O'Connel PR, Pemberton JH, Weiland LH, et al. Does rectal mucosa regenerate after ileoanal anastomosis? Dis Colon Rectum 1987; 30:1–5.
259. Heppell J, Weiland LH, Perrault J, Pemberton JH, Telander RL, Beart RW. The fate of rectal mucosa after rectal mucosectomy and ileoanal anostomosis. Dis Colon Rectum 1983; 26:768–771.
260. Sequens R. Cancer in the anal canal (tranzitional zone) after restorative proctocolectomy with stapled ileal pouch anal anostomosis. Int J Colorect Dis 1997; 12:254–255.
261. Stern H, Walfisch S, Mullen B, McLeod R, Cohen Z. Cancer in an ileoanal reservoir: a new late complication? Gut 1990; 31:473–475.
262. Utsunomiya J, Iwana T, Imajo M, et al. Total colectomy, mucosal proctectomy, and ileoanal anastomosis. Dis Colon Rectum 1980; 23:459–466.
263. Nicholls RJ, Pezim ME. Restorative proctocolectomy with ileal reservoir for ulcerative colitis and familial adenomatous polyposis: a comparison of 3 reservoir designs. Br J Surg 1985; 72:470–474.

264. Selvaggi F, Giuliani A, Gallo C, Signoriello G, Riegler G, Canonico S. Randomized, controlled trial to compare the J pouch and W pouch configurations for ulcerative colitis in the maturation period. Dis Colon Rectum 2000; 43:615–620.

265. Heuschen UA, Hinz U, Allemeyer EH, Lucas M, Heuschen G, Herfarth C. One or two stage procedure for restorative proctocolectomy. Rationale for a surgical strategy in ulcerative colitis. Ann Surg 2001; 234:788–794.

266. Mowschenson PM, Critchlow JH, Peppercorn MA. Ileoanal pouch operation. Long term outcome with or without diverting ileostomy. Arch Surg 2000; 135:463–466.

267. Sugerman HJ, Sugerman EL, Meador JG, Newsome HH, Kuller JM, DeMaria EJ. Ileal pouch anal anastomosis without ileal diversion. Ann Surg 2000; 232:530–541.

268. Gullberg K, Liljeqvist L. Stapled ileoanal pouches without loop ileostomy: a prospective study in 86 patients. Int J Colorectal Dis 2001; 16:221–227.

269. Grobler SP, Hosrie KB, Keighley MRB. Randomized trial of loop ileostomy in restorative proctocolectomy. Br J Surg 1992; 79:903–906.

270. Schmitt SL, Cohen SM, Wexner SD, Nogueras JJ, Jagelman DG. Does laparoscopic-assisted ileal pouch anal anastomosis reduce the length of hospitalization? Int J Colorectal Dis 1994; 9(3):134–137.

271. Marcello PW et al. Laparoscopic restorative proctocolectomy: case-matched comparative study with open restorative proctocolectomy. Dis Colon Rectum 2000; 43(5):604–608.

272. Dunker MS, Bemelman WA, Slors JF, van Duijvendijk P, Gouma DJ. Functional outcome, quality of life, body image, and cosmesis in patients after laparoscopic-assisted and conventional restorative proctocolectomy: a comparative study. Dis Colon Rectum 2001; 44(12):1800–1807.

273. Metcalf AM, Dozois RR, Kelly KA. Sexual function in women after proctocolectomy. Ann Surg 1986; 204:624–627.

274. Tiainen J, Matikainen M, Hiltunen KM. Ileal J pouch anal anastomosis, sexual dysfunction, and fertility. Scand J Gastroenterol 1999; 34:185–188.

275. Couniham TC, Robert PL, Schoetz DJ Jr, Coller JA, Murray JJ, Veidenheimer MC. Fertility and sexual and gynecologic function after ileal pouch anal anastomosis. Dis Colon Rectum 1994; 37:1126–1129.

276. Nelson H, Dozois RR, Kelly KA, Malkasian GD, et al. The effect of pregnancy and delivery on the ileal pouch anal anastomosis functions. Dis Colon Rectum 1989; 32:384–388.

277. Juhasz ES, Fozard B, Dozois RR, Ilstrup DM, Nelson H. Ileal pouch anal anastomosis function following childbirth. Dis Colon Rectum 1995; 38:159–165.

278. Farouk R, Pemberton JH, Wolff BC, Dozois RR, Browing S, Larson D. Functional outcomes after ileal pouch anal anastomosis for chronic ulcerative colitis. Ann Surg 2000; 231:919–926.

279. Olsen KØ, Joelsson M, Laurberg S, Oresland T. Fertility after ileal pouch anal anastomosis in women with ulcerative colitis. Br J Surg 1999; 86:493–495.

280. Olsen KØ, Juul S, Berndtsson I, Oresland T. Ulcerative colitis: female fecundity before diagnosis, during disease, and after surgery compared with a population sample. Gastroenterology 2002; 122:15–19.

281. Korsgen S, Keighley MRB. Causes of failure and life expectancy of the ileoanal pouch. Int J Colorect Dis 1997; 12:4–8.

282. Zmora O, Efron JE, Nogueras JJ, Weiss EG, Wexner SD. Reoperative abdominal and perineal surgery in ileoanal pouch patients. Dis Colon Rectum 2001; 44(9):1310–1314.

283. Fazio VW, Wu JS, Lavery IC. Repeat ileal pouch-anal anastomosis to salvage septic complications of pelvic pouches: clinical outcome and quality of life assessment. Ann Surg 1998; 228:588–597.

284. Cohen Z, Smith D, McLeod R. Reconstructive surgery for pelvic pouches. World J Surg 1998; 22: 342–346.

285. Heuschen UA et al. Risk factors for ileoanal j pouch-related septic complications in ulcerative colitis and familial adenomatous polyposis. Ann Surg 2002; 213:207–216.

286. Fazio VW, Tjandra JJ. Transanal mucosectomy – Ileal pouch advancement for anorectal dysplasia or inflammation after restorative prectocolectomy. Dis Colon Rectum 1994; 37:1008–1011.

27 | Crohn's Disease of the Colon

Uma Mahadevan
*Department of Gastroenterology, University of California–San Francisco,
San Francisco, California, U.S.A.*

Tonia Young-Fadok
Division of Colon and Rectal Surgery, Mayo Clinic Scottsdale, Scottsdale, Arizona, U.S.A.

INTRODUCTION

Crohn's disease (CD) is a chronic focal, transmural, and granulomatous inflammatory disorder that can affect any portion of the gastrointestinal tract. The condition was first described by Crohn, Ginzburg, and Oppenheimer in 1932 as an inflammatory condition limited to the terminal ileum (1). It was not until 1960 that it was recognized that the disease could affect the colon alone as an entity distinct from ulcerative colitis (UC) (2). This chapter reviews the etiology, clinical presentation, diagnosis, and medical and surgical management of CD of the colon.

EPIDEMIOLOGY

CD has an estimated incidence of 5 to 7 in 100,000 in Western populations, a number which is increasing worldwide (3). The incidence of CD limited to the colon is also increasing; one study in Stockholm found a rise in colonic CD from 14% to 32% in the period from 1955 to 1989 (4). However, it is unclear if this is due to increasing awareness of the disorder as an entity distinct from UC or a true increase in the disease subtype. The small bowel is usually involved in patients with CD, with 30% having small-bowel disease alone and 40% having ileocolonic disease. In a large population-based study, 26% of CD patients had disease limited to the colon (5). Of these patients, 31% had pancolitis, 40% had segmental involvement, 26% had left-sided colonic disease, and 3% had disease in the ascending colon only. Twenty-four percent of these patients subsequently developed disease in the small bowel as well. Disease location does not change dramatically over time. One large study found disease location (defined by the Vienna classification as terminal ileum, colon, ileocolonic, or upper gastrointestinal) changed in only 16% of patients over 10 years (6). However, disease within the colon does seem to progress. A study of 323 patients with Crohn's colitis reported 48.6% of patients having pancolitis at diagnosis, but 77% of patients having pancolitis after 15 years of disease (7). The risk of developing perianal fistulas in patients with colonic CD was 43% (7).

CD follows a chronic, relapsing course: 58% of all patients with CD relapse by two years from diagnosis and 88% relapse by 10 years (8). Anatomic location is not thought to affect clinical severity of disease. Patients with colonic CD, who achieve remission, have an estimated five-year cumulative relapse rate of 67% (5). Disease location does affect overall complication rates, with fibrostenosis and need for surgery being lower in those with colonic disease alone (9,10) and complications from bleeding and fistulizing disease being higher in this group (6). Approximately 50% of patients with Crohn's colitis will require surgery during their disease course (10). Among patients with perineal CD, those with rectal CD were more likely to receive permanent stomas than those without rectal involvement (67% vs. 11%, $p < 0.001$) (11). The cumulative risk for a permanent ileostomy in patients with colonic CD is estimated at 25% (5), though this may be changing with the increased use of biologic therapy and immunosuppressants.

Older patients, those diagnosed with CD after the age of 40, may be more likely to have colonic involvement than younger patients ($p < 0.05$) (9), although this association has not been confirmed in all studies (6). Gender does not appear to affect disease location (12). Overall mortality in CD patients is higher than in the general population, especially late in the course of the disease (13,14). Two English studies found a higher rate of standardized mortality ratios in patients with CD of the colon, which happened to be an older population (15,16). However, two large studies did not find a correlation between mortality and disease location (13,14). Quality of life also appears to be affected by disease location: Patients with CD of the colon have lower quality-of-life scores than patients with ileal CD (17).

ETIOLOGY

The etiology of CD is unknown, but is generally thought to result from the combination of an exaggerated inflammatory response in a genetically susceptible host exposed to an appropriate environmental trigger (18). Potential factors implicated in the development of CD include luminal flora, genetic factors, and smoking. The luminal flora may play a central role in the development of this disease. Support for this can be found in models of murine colitis where a germ-free environment or the use of antibiotics can prevent or attenuate colitis in susceptible populations; alternatively, bacterial load and concentration can determine the extent of inflammation (19,20). In humans, when the bacterial load and content of mucosal biopsy specimens were compared, patients with CD had a much higher bacterial concentration than healthy controls, self-limited colitis, and UC patients. However, there was no significant difference in the actual composition of mucosal flora in inflammatory bowel disease (IBD) patients versus controls (21).

A growing body of evidence supports the role of genetic susceptibility as a key factor determining this inflammatory response to normal luminal flora. Clinical observations such as the increased incidence and prevalence of CD in particular populations such as people belonging to Northern countries, Caucasians, and Jews (3), and in families support a genetic link. A study by Peeters et al. reported the age-corrected risk of developing CD among all first-degree relatives of an affected individual as 3.9% and 10.4% in the child of an individual with CD (22). Disease localization such as colonic disease versus small bowel disease also appears to have a high concordance (46%) among family members (23). Recently, the NOD2/CARD15 gene, on chromosome 16q12, has been linked to CD (24,25). The NOD2 gene appears to be associated with fibrostenosing and ileal disease (26) but is negatively associated with colonic disease (27,28).

Environmental factors may influence the development of CD and UC as well. A prime example is smoking, which has been clearly associated with the development of CD (29). An article by Bridger et al. found that in IBD families, 21/23 sibling pairs discordant for smoking and for disease type (UC vs. CD) developed CD in the smoker and UC in the nonsmoker (30). This supports the pivotal role of environmental factors such as smoking in the development and possibly in the differentiation of IBD in genetically predisposed individuals. Smoking can also affect the clinical course of CD, with active smokers having higher rates of clinical relapse (31), surgical intervention, postoperative recurrence (32), and need for immunosuppressive therapy (33). However, smoking has not been implicated in the anatomic distribution of CD.

Prior appendectomy is another factor that may be associated with the development of CD, although the evidence here is less consistent. While the rate of appendectomy prior to diagnosis appears to be higher in patients with CD compared to normal controls, it may (34,35) or may not (36) be statistically significant, and some authors argue that it is a marker for undiagnosed CD (37).

The appropriate combination of genetic and environmental factors, still to be defined, leads to a sustained activation of the mucosal immune response. In patients with CD, the dominant $CD4^+$ lymphocytes, type1 helper (Th1) cells, produce the proinflammatory cytokines—interferon-γ (IFN-γ) and interleukin-2 (IL-2). This leads to an inflammatory cascade that includes tumor necrosis factor (TNF) and other mediators of inflammation (18). It may be that these activated cells are no longer capable of apoptosis or preprogrammed cell death, resulting in ongoing, uninhibited mucosal inflammation. Attempts at medical therapy broadly (steroids) or specifically (infliximab) aim to inhibit this inflammatory cascade.

DIAGNOSIS AND EVALUATION

There is no gold standard for the diagnosis and assessment of disease activity in CD. The diagnosis is usually made based on the combination of clinical signs and symptoms, laboratory tests, endoscopy, pathology, and imaging studies.

Clinical Presentation

CD of the colon often presents with symptoms of inflammation such as fever, sweats, malaise, abdominal pain, diarrhea, weight loss, and hematochezia. The volume of diarrhea and hematochezia in Crohn's colitis is usually less than in UC (38). Clinical signs such as pallor, cachexia, right lower quadrant mass, tenderness, perianal "elephant" tags, fistulas, and abscesses can also be found, and the latter may help differentiate from UC (39). Disease limited to the colon is more likely to present with rectal bleeding than ileal disease, though major gastrointestinal hemorrhage is rare. Reports vary as to whether (40) or not (41) there is predilection for colonic sites in massive gastrointestinal bleeding due to CD.

Extraintestinal manifestations are common in CD, occurring in approximately 25% of patients (42). Complications such as uveitis, iritis, sacroilitis, and ankylosing spondylitis, and the skin manifestations erythema nodosum and pyoderma gangrenosum seem to occur without consistent propensity for disease location. However, peripheral arthritis (10) and primary sclerosing cholangitis (43) are more commonly associated with colonic CD.

Laboratory Findings

Patients with active CD will generally have elevated levels of acute phase reactants such as white blood cell count, platelet count, erythrocyte sedimentation rate (ESR), C-reactive protein, orosomucoid level, and ferritin. Patients with Crohn's colitis may also have significant anemia from gross or occult blood loss. In moderate-to-severe disease, evidence of malnutrition may present with hypoalbuminemia, hypocholesterolemia, and vitamin deficiencies. Serologic tests for the diagnosis of CD are discussed further below.

Stool studies should be sent on all patients during the initial workup of CD as well as during subsequent flares, especially when they do not respond to standard medical therapy. While parasitic and bacterial superinfection may be a relatively uncommon cause of flare in CD (44), *Clostridium dificile* toxin has been detected in immunosuppressed and steroid naïve patients with active CD, regardless of antibiotic use (45,46). Also, patients with severe steroid refractory Crohn's colitis may have underlying cytomegalovirus (47), which can be assessed by routine histopathology and shell vial culture of endoscopic biopsy specimens.

Radiology

The barium enema is comparable to colonoscopy in diagnosis and assessment of disease extent and activity in Crohn's colitis, save for very superficial or mild disease (48). However, the inability to take biopsies and the widespread availability and acceptance of endoscopy have limited this study's use mainly to the assessment of fistula tracts and segments of the colon proximal to narrow strictures. Transabdominal ultrasound may be useful in assessing strictures in small bowel CD (49), but its use in colonic CD is probably best applied with rectal endoscopic ultrasound for fistulizing disease. Endoscopic ultrasound is very effective in determining the extent and severity of perianal fistulas and in localizing abscesses. One study comparing magnetic resonance imaging (MRI), endoscopic ultrasound, and exam under anesthesia found all three modalities equivalent, with 100% accuracy rates when two modalities were combined (50).

Computer tomographic (CT) imaging is extremely useful in assessing intra-abdominal abscess formation in the patient with CD. Colonic CD may present with the "accordion sign" on CT, a marker of diffuse colonic edema (51). Disease extent and severity can be assessed, with one study finding that prominent pericolic or perienteric vasculature on CT scan correlated with increased disease activity and extent based on ESR, C-reactive protein, and barium enema results (52).

Magnetic resonance imaging (MRI) has also been found to be useful in assessing the activity of luminal CD and is more accurate than CT scan in assessing perianal CD (53). Bowel-wall thickening and increased mesenteric vascularity were markers of disease activity on MRI (54). Positron emission tomography (PET) is another noninvasive means of assessing activity in CD with high sensitivity and specificity as well as high cost (55). Finally, technetium-99 m-99mT$_c$-hexamethyl propleneamine oxime (HMPAO)-labeled leukocyte scintigraphy (white cell scan) is useful in detecting segmental inflammatory activity, but is not as accurate as CT scan in the detection of abdominal abscess formation (56).

Endoscopy

Colonoscopy is crucial in determining the extent and severity of disease activity in Crohn's colitis. It also provides the opportunity for mucosal sampling to confirm the diagnosis. Inter-observer agreement in colonic CD is good, regardless of the experience of the observer, when assessing ulcer size and stricture formation. More subtle findings in the ileum, such as mucosal thickening and erythema, are not as reproducible (57). Interestingly, the severity of the mucosal lesions on endoscopy has little to no correlation with the degree of clinical symptoms experienced by the patient with CD (58), making frequent, repeated colonoscopic assessment of disease unnecessary. Colonoscopic findings can, however, be predictive of disease course. Patients with deep and extensive ulcerations on colonoscopy are more likely to undergo colonic resection and suffer from penetrating complications including abscess and fistula formation (59). Colonoscopy 6 to 12 months after surgical resection is also useful in determining which patients are more likely to have postoperative recurrence and benefit from more aggressive medical therapy to maintain remission and avoid further surgical intervention (60).

Finally, colonoscopy is used for the assessment and treatment of gastrointestinal hemorrhage in Crohn's colitis (40), for colon cancer surveillance in longstanding disease (61), and for the treatment of colonic and anastomotic strictures (62). Patients with nonmalignant strictures that are short and moderate grade are more amenable to endoscopic balloon dilation than those with long, tight, and multiple strictures (63). A through-the-scope hydrostatic balloon catheter is most commonly used. Endoscopic balloon dilation is effective and can lead to long-term relief in over 50% of patients (62).

Pathology

CD is characterized by focal intestinal inflammation with crypt inflammation, aphthous ulcers, and intervening segments of normal mucosa. Transmural inflammation, fibrosis, and stricture are later manifestations. Granulomas may be found in 15% to 70% of patients with CD (64,65), but this finding is not pathognomonic. Transmural lymphoid aggregates are very characteristic of CD. However, the earliest lesion is the aphthous ulcer. As the disease progresses, architectural distortion occurs, suggesting healing and recurrence of the aphthous ulcers. The ulcers can extend to form longitudinal and transverse ulcers, giving the familiar cobblestone appearance of the disease. Edema can be reabsorbed or may undergo gradual fibrosis, possibly leading to stricture formation. Fissures arise from the bases of aphthoid ulcers, and fistula tracts are extensions of these lesions (66). Unfortunately, there is a significant interobserver variation in the histological diagnosis of colonic CD (67). In patients with indeterminate colitis (IC) being considered for surgery, an experienced gastrointestinal or IBD pathologist should review the histopathology for CD versus UC prior to making decisions on surgical intervention.

DIFFERENTIAL DIAGNOSIS

The majority of cases of inflammatory bowel disease are clear-cut, but it can be difficult to differentiate between UC and CD. Other colitides must also be ruled out (68), especially when the presentation is atypical, when the patient does not respond to standard therapy, or when there is suspected exposure to infectious or toxic agents capable of causing colitis. Table 1 lists a limited differential diagnosis.

Infection is a common cause of colonic inflammation. Hemorrhagic colitis can be seen in enterohemorrhagic *Escherichia coli* 0157:H7, *Shigella*, *Vibrio parahaemolyticus*, *Campylobacter* and *Salmonella* infections (69). *Yersinia enterocolitica* presents with enterocolitis and can mimic CD especially in the ileum (70). *C. difficile* and amebiasis are other infectious agents that can be mistaken for Crohn's colitis (71). Viral pathogens such as herpes simplex virus and cytomegalovirus can also cause colitis in an immunocompetent host, presenting with diarrhea, abdominal pain, subepithelial hemorrhage, and mucosal ulceration throughout the colon (72).

Mycobacterial species have long been suspected to play an etiologic role in CD. *Mycobacterium avium* subspecies *paratuberculosis* (MAP), found in pasteurized milk, causes chronic inflammation of the small bowel and colon in some hosts. MAP can be found in full-thickness samples of the gut wall in patients with CD and responds to antibiotic therapy (73). However, proof of MAP as a causative agent for CD has been elusive. *Mycobacterium tuberculosis* (MTB) can also involve the intestine, mimicking CD. Ulcerative lesions are seen in 60% of patients,

Table 1 Limited Differential Diagnosis for Crohn's Colitis

Bacterial/parasitic/viral infections	*Escherichia coli* 0157:H7
	Vibrio parahemolyticus
	Shigella
	Salmonella
	Campylobacter
	Yersinia enterocolitica
	Clostridium difficile
	Amebiasis
	Mycobacterium tuberculosis
	Mycobacterium avium paratuberculosis
	Cytomegalovirus
	Herpes simplex virus
Vascular infections	Ischemic colitis
	Radiation colitis
	Giant cell arteritis
	Systemic lupus erythematosus
Medication-induced colitis	Nonsteroidal anti-inflammatory agents
	Phosphosoda preparations
	Gold
	Penicillamine
	Oral contraceptives
	Estrogen/progesterone
	Mesalamine/sulfasalazine
Other colitides	Ulcerative colitis
	Indeterminate colitis
	Collagenous colitis
	Lymphocytic/microsopic colitis
	Diverticulosis
Malignancy	Lymphoma
	Adenocarcinoma

and granulomas can be found on biopsy (74). Colonoscopic findings include superficial ulceration and nodular friable mucosa affecting the ileocecal valve, colonic segments, or the entire colon (75). In patients from areas in which MTB is endemic, this diagnosis should be carefully excluded prior to making the diagnosis of CD and initiating immunosuppressive therapy.

Vascular complications including ischemic colitis, radiation colitis, and giant cell arteritis can mimic or exacerbate Crohn's colitis (76). Diverticular disease, common in western populations, can be associated with a surrounding localized inflammatory response that can be similar in appearance to CD. Although patients may grossly have "creeping" fat, ulceration, edematous mucosa, and evidence of transmural granulomatous inflammation on biopsy, most of them do not clinically fit the pattern for CD (77).

Various drugs can cause segmental ulcerations of the colon mimicking CD, most commonly nonsteroidal anti-inflammatory drugs, which can present with multiple colonic ulcers and perforation (78). Other drugs include phosphosoda bowel preparations, oral contraceptives (79), penicillamine, and gold (80).

There have been multiple cases of lymphoma of the colon mimicking CD (81). Colitides such as collagenous and lymphocytic colitis do not generally manifest gross endoscopic lesions; however, some histologic features normally associated with IBD such as crypt irregularity, neutrophilic cryptitis, and crypt abscesses may be seen, potentially confusing the diagnosis (82).

Distinguishing between UC and Crohn's colitis is often the most difficult. While the presence of perianal disease, skip lesions, concomitant small bowel disease, and granulomas support the diagnosis of CD, these markers are not universally present. The distinction is most obscure in patients with acute severe colitis where the histopathology demonstrates deep, extensive ulceration without definitive features of UC or CD, leading to the diagnosis of IC (83). The rates of IC have been estimated to be between 5% and 15% (84,85). Making the distinction between IC and either CD or UC is important when considering medical therapy such as infliximab or surgery. While patients with CD do much worse than those with UC with ileal pouch anal anastomosis (IPAA) for severe disease, IC patients fall in between with a 19% pouch failure rate versus 8% for UC (86).

Table 2 Medical Therapy in Crohn's Colitis: Induction and Maintenance of Remission

	Induction	Maintenance
Sulfasalazine	Yes (colonic disease)	No
Mesalamine	Maybe	No
Antibiotics	Maybe	No
Corticosteroids	Yes	No
Budesonide	Yes (right colon)	No
Azathioprine/6-mercaptopurine	Yes	Yes
Methotrexate	Yes	Yes
Cyclosporine/tacrolimus	Yes	No
Infliximab	Yes	Yes

Serological tests have been proposed to aid in the distinction between CD and UC. Perinuclear cytoplasmic antibody (pANCA) is found in 60% to 80% of patients with UC and 10% to 20% of patients with CD (87,88). Anti–*Saccharomyces cerevisiae* antibody (ASCA) is found in 50% to 60% of patients with CD (89–91). Unfortunately, patients with CD, who are pANCA positive, have colonic disease that is indistinguishable from UC (92). Combining ASCA and pANCA may increase the specificity (93). One study prospectively measured ASCA and pANCA levels in 97 patients with IC (94). About 31 of 97 patients had a definitive diagnosis on clinical grounds. In these patients, ASCA+/pANCA− was found in 8/17 CD patients, whereas ASCA-/pANCA+ was found in 7/14 UC patients. Of the 97 patients, 47 (48.5%) were negative for both ASCA and pANCA. Thus, while certain serological combinations may be suggestive of CD or UC, in the majority of IC patients, serology will not establish the diagnosis. Fortunately, 50% to 80% of patients with IC will be clinically diagnosed as CD or UC at some point in their disease course (85,95).

MEDICAL THERAPY

When choosing medical therapy for Crohn's colitis, decisions must be made based on disease severity, disease location, and whether the treatment is for induction or maintenance of remission (68). Table 2 lists commonly used medications.

Aminosalicylates

Sulfasalazine (SAS) and 5-aminosalicylate (5-ASA) preparations have a topical effect on the bowel mucosa and multiple anti-inflammatory effects including inhibition of IL-1, TNF, leukotriene production, and nuclear factor-κB (96–98). The varying formulations can be targeted to disease location with oral formulations effective for pancolonic disease and suppository or enema formation for proctitis and left-sided disease, respectively. While these agents are effective for induction and maintenance of remission in UC (99), their efficacy in CD is controversial.

Randomized controlled trials have found SAS to be effective for induction (100,101), but not maintenance of remission in CD. The subgroup of patients with colonic disease alone had a better response to SAS than the ileal group (101). Only one large double-blind study of mesalamine has found a benefit over placebo in induction of remission in CD (102); in this case, the benefit was more pronounced in ileal disease. By meta-analysis, mesalamine was not an effective maintenance therapy in medically (103) or surgically induced remission (104) of CD.

Both SAS and 5-ASA agents have a limited toxicity profile. SAS has lower tolerability rates than 5-ASA agents due to the sulfapyridine moiety (105), which can cause headache, nausea, and vomiting. However, overall, 5-ASA may have higher rates of serious adverse events such as interstitial nephritis and pancreatitis (106). Rarely, both SAS and 5-ASA can cause a paradoxical worsening of diarrhea that clinically and endoscopically mimics colitis (107). Overall, given the safety of the medications, in CD limited to the colon, which can have an "UC-like" phenotype, SAS and perhaps 5-ASA formulations may be useful as first-line therapy. However, based on current data, this benefit is limited.

Glucocorticoids

Glucocorticoids are effective for the treatment of CD, but chronic use is limited by side effects and loss of efficacy. The molecular mechanism of action of glucocorticoids results from modulation of gene expression and inhibition of the production of proinflammatory cytokines such as TNF and IL-1, leading to reduced leukocyte migration and function, and inhibition of numerous mediators of inflammation (108). Systemic steroid therapy by oral or intravenous administration is effective for the induction of remission in CD (101,109); however, most patients will relapse. A population-based study in Olmstead County, Minnesota found that 43% of patients with CD had received at least one course of steroids during their disease course. Of these patients, 58% had a complete response to therapy, 26% a partial response, and 16% no response in the short term. At one year, however, only 32% were disease-free without steroid dependence or need for surgery (110).

Toxicities observed with corticosteroid therapy include moon face (47%), acne (30%), infection (27%), ecchymoses (17%), hypertension (15%), hirsutism (7%), petechial subcutaneous bleeding (6%), and striae (6%) (109). Prolonged corticosteroid therapy can result in multiple serious adverse events including new onset diabetes mellitus, osteonecrosis, osteoporosis, myopathy, psychosis, cataracts, and glaucoma (111).

Formulations designed to administer topical glucocorticoids directly to the site of disease have been developed in an effort to reduce systemic glucocorticoid toxicity. Rectal enemas and suppositories can be used for left-sided disease with systemic bioavailability ranging from 15% to 30%, but with a continued potential for adrenal suppression (112,113). Budesonide, a synthetic analog of prednisolone, has proven efficacy as oral enteric release capsules in ileal and right-sided colonic CD (114). Budesonide has high topical potency with affinity to the glucocorticoid receptor 15 and 200 times greater than prednisolone and hydrocortisone (115), respectively. First-pass inactivation in the liver is 90%, resulting in only 10% systemic bioavailability (116). When selecting corticosteroid therapy for CD, one can minimize toxicity by using budesonide for mild-to-moderate disease limited to the right colon or enemas for limited proctosigmoiditis. However, if oral or intravenous steroids must be used, a steroid-sparing agent (below) should be added if the patients are unable to taper off the corticosteroids within a reasonable length of time.

Antibiotics

The first report of antibiotic therapy for luminal CD was from Moss in 1978 who described a case series of 44 patients with radiographic improvement in colonic disease after treatment with a variety of antibiotics (117). Trials of ciprofloxacin (118) and metronidazole (119) have found equivalent efficacy to mesalamine and SAS, respectively. In a randomized trial of 105 patients with active luminal CD (120), metronidazole resulted in reductions in Crohn's disease activity index (CDAI) scores, particularly in patients with colonic disease, but the proportion of patients in clinical remission at the end of the 16-week trial was low.

Antibiotic combination therapy has also been studied. Two uncontrolled case series reported that metronidazole 250 mg three times daily and ciprofloxacin 500 mg twice daily might result in synergistic benefit for inducing remission and steroid sparing in patients with active luminal CD (121,122). More recently, a controlled trial of 141 patients comparing controlled ileal release budesonide 9 mg/day with a combination of budesonide 9 mg/day, metronidazole 500 mg twice daily, and ciprofloxacin 500 mg twice daily in patients with active luminal CD showed no added benefit for antibiotic therapy. Significantly more adverse events occurred in the group who received antibiotics (123). Controlled trials of antimycobacterial agents have also not demonstrated efficacy (124). Based on these data, the role of antibiotic therapy for colonic CD is unclear, but may be of benefit in patients with mild-to-moderate disease.

Azathioprine/6-Mercaptopurine

6-mercaptopurine (6-MP) and its prodrug azathioprine are purine antimetabolite drugs demonstrated to be effective for the induction and maintenance of remission in CD. Controlled trials have shown that effective doses are azathioprine 2.0 to 3.0 mg/kg/day and 6-MP 1.0 to 1.5 mg/kg/day with an estimated time to onset of action of 17 weeks and a steroid-sparing effect (125). Azathioprine/6-MP is an effective induction agent in newly diagnosed CD and can be used in the adolescent and pediatric population (126). Finally, as a maintenance agent, azathioprine continues to be superior to placebo for the maintenance of remission in CD for at least five years (127).

Approximately 5% of patients will develop allergic-type reactions to azathioprine/6-MP including pancreatitis, fever, rash, malaise, diarrhea, and hepatitis (128). Nonallergic reactions to azathioprine/6-MP include bone marrow suppression leading to leukopenia, anemia or thrombocytopenia, opportunistic infection, some cases of hepatitis, and non-Hodgkin's lymphoma (129,130). The risk of malignancy, especially lymphoma, in patients receiving azathioprine/6-MP is controversial. Cumulatively, current data suggests that the risk of malignancy, if present, is very small, and the overall benefit of azathioprine/6-MP therapy outweighs these risks (131–133).

Methotrexate

Methotrexate (MTX) is a folate analogue and inhibitor of dihydrofolate reductase leading to decreased levels of tetrahydrofolate, a donor in several reactions of purine and pyrimidine synthesis (134). Randomized controlled trials have demonstrated that intramuscular MTX 25 mg/week is effective for inducing remission in patients with CD (135) and that intramuscular MTX 15 mg/week is effective for maintaining remission (104). Dose escalation from 15 mg/week to 25 mg/week may be effective in patients who relapse on lower doses, and subcutaneous administration is an alternative to intramuscular dosing (136).

Adverse events associated with MTX therapy include dose-dependent antiproliferative effects (bone marrow depression, gastrointestinal ulceration, stomatitis, and alopecia) and idiosyncratic allergic or hypersensitivity reactions (rash and pneumonitis) (137). Increased serum transaminases are observed in up to 30% of patients treated chronically with MTX (135,138). Risk factors for liver injury include greater cumulative doses, significant alcohol use, obesity, diabetes, and older age (139). Similar to rheumatoid arthritis, patients with CD appear to have a low risk of MTX liver toxicity making routine liver biopsies unnecessary (140,141).

Cyclosporine and Tacrolimus

Cyclosporine and tacrolimus are both calcineurin inhibitors that are powerful and specific inhibitors of T-lymphocyte activation, including IL-2 and IFN-γ (142). The use of intravenous cyclosporine and oral tacrolimus in CD is best described for the treatment of fistulizing disease (143,144); however, small series have documented benefit in refractory luminal CD (143,145). Both cyclosporine and tacrolimus have significant short-term and long-term side effect profiles including paresthesias, hypertension, hypertrichosis, renal insufficiency, infections, gingival hyperplasia, seizures, anaphylaxis, and death (146). Given the significant toxicity profile and need for close monitoring, cyclosporine and tacrolimus use is limited to patients with CD and fistulizing or luminal disease that is refractory to other therapy.

Infliximab

Infliximab is a chimeric mouse–human monoclonal antibody to TNF. Infliximab, administered as an intravenous infusion, binds free and membrane-bound TNF preventing the cytokine from binding to its cell-surface receptor and exerting biological activity (147). Initial studies demonstrated the efficacy of a single dose of 5 mg/kg of infliximab versus placebo in the treatment of moderate to severe CD (148) and of three doses at 0, 2, and 6 weeks in the treatment of perianal fistulas (149). Subsequent studies have documented the efficacy of infliximab in the induction and maintenance of remission in patients with luminal CD. In the ACCENT I trial, infliximab given at a dose of 5 mg/kg at 0,2 and 6 weeks followed by every 8 weeks was more effective than a single dose of infliximab followed by placebo at the same intervals (150).

Infliximab has been shown to be relatively safe when used as a long-term maintenance therapy. In the ACCENT I trial (150), the most common adverse events with infliximab were upper respiratory infection, abdominal pain, and headache. Serious adverse events were similar in the placebo and 5 and 10 mg/kg infliximab groups (7%, 8%, and 6%, respectively). Acute infusion reactions (anaphylactoid, non–IgE-mediated) were characterized by headache, dizziness, nausea, flushing, chest pain, dyspnea, and pruritus and occurred in approximately 22% of patients.

In postmarketing experience, severe infections have been reported, including reactivation of latent tuberculosis (>100 cases), pneumonia, sepsis, disseminated coccydiomycoses, histoplasmosis, listeriosis, *Pneumocystis carini* pneumonia, aspergillosis, and disseminated herpes zoster. All patients receiving infliximab should be screened for tuberculosis with a purified protein derivative (PPD) skin test and, if indicated, a chest radiograph. Patients with active tuberculosis should be treated accordingly and should not receive infliximab until the infection is cleared. Patients with evidence of latent tuberculosis should be treated according to the American Thoracic Society guidelines (151) and may initiate infliximab after completion of therapy. Patients in areas endemic for other opportunistic infections should be screened appropriately, and all patients should be watched closely for signs of infection.

Finally, all immunosuppressive agents carry the potential risk of malignancy. There have been 18 solid tumors and 6 lymphomas in 1372 patients treated with infliximab in clinical trials. The solid tumor rate was similar to that expected in the patient years of follow-up. Four of the lymphomas occurred prior to 1998, and the infrequent occurrence of lymphoma does not appear to be associated with dose or duration of therapy (152). In summary, infliximab is an effective therapy for induction and maintenance of remission in CD, including the colon. Care should be taken to avoid infectious complications during its use.

Medical Prophylaxis Against Postoperative Recurrence

The goals of medical therapy are to induce and maintain remission, avoid surgery, and, if surgery occurs, prevent recurrence. Disease location is an important factor in predicting recurrence. Patients with ileocolonic resection have the highest rates of recurrence, whereas patients with colonic resection have the lowest (153,154). Unfortunately, few drugs have been found to be effective for the prevention of postoperative recurrence in CD, and most of the studies have looked at ileal or ileocolonic resection as opposed to colonic resection alone.

As mentioned above, mesalamine has not consistently been found to be effective by meta-analysis (155) and by large individual trials (156) for the prevention of postoperative recurrence. Antibiotics, specifically metronidazole (157) and a related compound, ornidazol (158), are effective, but with significant side effects. Oral budesonide, at 6 mg/day, did not affect recurrence after resection for fibrostenotic disease, but did decrease recurrence in patients who underwent surgery for active disease (159). Finally, the immunosuppressive 6-MP has been found to be effective for preventing endoscopic relapse in 32% of patients versus 10% of placebo-treated patients (160). No published data exists on infliximab for the prevention of postoperative recurrence. Based on the above evidence and the low rates of recurrence in certain subgroups of patients (nonsmokers, first resection, and fibrostenotic disease), D'Haens and Rutgeerts recommend following such patients and performing colonoscopy 6 to 12 months after surgery. If there is evidence of recurrence, appropriate therapy can then be initiated. Patients at high risk for early recurrence (ileocolonic resection and multiple resections) can be started on 6-MP with or without a three-month course of metronidazole (60).

NEOPLASIA

It is now recognized that patients with extensive Crohn's colitis and UC have similarly increased risks of colonic adenocarcinoma. In one study, the risk of colon cancer in extensive Crohn's colitis was 18-fold that of the normal population with an absolute cumulative frequency of risk of 8% at 22 years from the onset of symptoms, nearly identical to the risk in UC in the same study (161). A study of screening and surveillance colonoscopy in chronic Crohn's colitis found that 16% of patients had dysplasia. Based on these findings, the authors' practice is to survey patients with extensive Crohn's colitis on an annual basis after eight years of disease. In patients at increased risk for colon cancer, such as those with primary sclerosing cholangitis (162) and a family history of colon cancer (163), surveillance is begun earlier.

Colonic strictures in the setting of IBD should always raise concern for malignancy. The percentage of malignant strictures in CD increases with disease duration. One study found that 3% of CD strictures were malignant with disease for less than 20 years compared to 11% of strictures in patients with disease greater than 20 years (164).

Finally, the increased risk of lymphoma in CD is controversial. Although some have suggested that immunosuppression increases the risk of lymphoma (131), large population-based studies have not found an increase risk of lymphoma in CD with or without immunosuppression (132), except, perhaps, in the subgroup of young men with CD (133).

SURGICAL MANAGEMENT
Operative Indications

Despite advances in medical therapy, the majority of patients diagnosed with CD ultimately require operative intervention. Data from the National Cooperative Crohn's Disease Study (153) reported the risk of undergoing an operation to be 78% and 90% at 20 and 30 years, respectively, from diagnosis. Although these figures may change with increasing use of newer therapies, it is clear that a substantial proportion of patients with CD will ultimately require an operation. It is helpful to consider the indications for operative intervention as either elective or emergent.

Elective Indications
Fistula

The commonest indication for operation in CD is fistula with or without abscess. This complication is more likely, however, to arise from the small bowel than the colon: Fistula was present in a series of patients undergoing operation in 32% of patients with small-bowel disease, 44% with ileocolitis, and only 23% with Crohn's colitis (165). In many cases of fistula involving the colon, the colon is a bystander involved by ileocolic disease. In general, only symptomatic fistulae that have not responded to medical therapy would be approached surgically.

Obstruction

Obstruction is an uncommon indication for operation in Crohn's colitis. Although obstruction is the indication in 55% of operations for small bowel disease, it accounts for only 12% of patients with colonic disease (165). The presence of a colonic stricture must raise suspicions regarding the presence of malignancy.

Failed Medical Therapy

In the absence of absolute indications for a surgical approach (perforation, massive bleeding, malignancy, and high-grade obstruction), initial therapy is medical. Such an approach is considered to have failed if the response to medical treatment does not produce resolution of symptoms, if medications cannot be discontinued within a planned time period, or if significant side effects develop. In prepubertal children, recognition of growth retardation is an additional reason for considering surgical intervention (166).

Carcinoma

Although there are some conflicting reports, the balance of information suggests that there is an increased incidence of colorectal cancer in Crohn's colitis. In England, the Cancer Epidemiology Research Project reported that the incidence of colorectal cancer was increased four times in extensive Crohn's colitis (167). In a series of 579 patients Greenstein concurred (168) and also noted that the carcinoma could arise in areas of the colon affected both macroscopically and microscopically by CD. A Swedish study of 1655 patients found a relative risk of 5.6 for colorectal cancer in patients with CD limited to the colon. Furthermore, patients in whom CD was diagnosed before the age of 30 years and had any element of disease in the colon had a relative risk of 21 (169).

Emergent Indications
Toxic Colitis and Megacolon

In order to minimize morbidity and mortality, it is imperative to rapidly recognize toxic colitis particularly in patients whose symptoms may be masked by steroids and immunosuppressives. The best definition incorporates both subjective and objective criteria (170), with toxic colitis defined as a "flare" of colitis plus two or more of the following: fever >38.6°C; albumin <3.0 g/dL; white cell count greater than 10.5×10^9 cells/L; or tachycardia >100 beats per minute. Megacolon is additionally present when colonic dilation is greater than 5 cm.

Medical therapy is initiated unless free perforation, peritonitis, and septic shock, or massive hemorrhage mandate emergent surgical intervention after fluid resuscitation. Serial abdominal examinations and radiographs monitor the development of peritonitis or colonic dilation. Clinical deterioration in the first 48 hours should prompt surgical intervention, as should lack of significant improvement after a week of intense medical therapy.

Perforation

Free perforation is rare, occurring in only 1% to 3% of patients with Crohn's colitis (171,172). Most often it occurs in the setting of an acute flare, associated with either toxic colitis or distal obstruction.

Hemorrhage

Massive hemorrhage is likewise rare, being reported in 1.4% of patients with CD (173). As with other forms of massive gastrointestinal bleeding, the principles of patient stabilization and localization of the bleeding apply, with emergent operation considered for inability to stabilize the patient after four to six units of blood transfused, significant recurrent bleeding, or a pre-existing reason to resect the diseased colon.

Principles of Operative Management
Goals

CD cannot be cured by surgical means. Thus the aim of surgical intervention, when indicated, is to achieve control of symptoms while minimizing morbidity, and attempting to maintain the function and integrity of the gastrointestinal tract.

Patient Preparation

In the absence of a colonic stricture associated with obstructive symptoms, patients undergo a bowel preparation the day before surgery, employing either polyethylene glycol or Fleets® (Fleets, Lynchburg, Virginia, U.S.A.) phosphosoda. Enemas are given on the day of operation for left-sided resections. Oral antibiotics may be given as part of the bowel preparation according to surgeon preference. Intravenous antibiotics are given within one hour before skin incision, and are continued for 24 hours postoperatively (174,175).

Stress dosages of corticosteroids are given perioperatively if the patient has used steroids within the previous six months. Our practice is to give 20 to 40 mg of methylprednisolone intravenously on induction of anesthesia, depending on the prior dose, a repeat dose 12 hours later, and then wean using daily or twice daily dosing as indicated (176). Although many surgeons will attempt to discontinue immunosuppressives such as azathioprine and 6-MP two weeks prior to operation (170), a recent study at the Mayo Clinic has indicated no increase in perioperative complications if these are continued until the time of operation (177).

Attempting to correct malnutrition preoperatively with total parenteral nutrition (TPN) is controversial. One study compared 49 patients receiving preoperative TPN with 64 patients proceeding directly to operation (178). In those with small bowel disease, the length of bowel resected was significantly shorter, but there was no such benefit in those with colonic disease.

Another important preoperative consideration is that of stoma marking. Preoperative consultation, preferably with an enterostomal therapist, ensures that a planned stoma is correctly positioned within the rectus abdominis muscle, away from scars and creases and is visible to the patient. This preparation and teaching may also help to allay patients' fears regarding living with a stoma.

Resection Margins

Resection margins are less of an issue in the large bowel than in the small intestine, as considerations to avoid the short gut syndrome do not apply to colonic resections. For this reason, studies have concentrated on evaluation of resection margins in the small bowel. Early studies suggested that a microscopically positive margin resulted in higher anastomotic recurrence rates (179). Hamilton (180), however, found no differences in recurrences rates between patients whose resection margins were based on gross inspection versus those evaluated by frozen section. Clinical recurrence rates were 66% and 60%, respectively at 10 years of follow-up. Fazio et al. (181) randomized 131 patients to grossly free margins of 2 cm and 12 cm and found no significant difference in recurrence rates. Microscopic evidence of disease at the resection margin did not increase recurrence. Thus current practice is to resect only visibly abnormal bowel, leaving in situ normal appearing bowel that is soft, pliable, and free of serosal injection and "fat creeping." The extent of disease in the colon is often more difficult to determine by these standard appearances, and intraoperative colonoscopy may be helpful to delineate the extent of disease.

Intraoperative Considerations
Anastomotic Configuration
The method employed for creating an anastomosis varies by surgeon. In general, however, the anastomosis used for resections limited to the right side of the colon is either side-to-side stapled or end-to-end sutured. There is some evidence from retrospective studies to suggest that the side-to-side–stapled method may result in lower recurrence rates (182). It is unclear whether this might be a result of the usually larger anastomosis afforded by this technique or whether the materials used (inert staples vs. suture material) have a bearing on the recurrence rate at the anastomosis. In addition, all the existing studies are confounded by different follow-up periods for their two comparison groups. To answer this question, a multicenter North American study is currently accruing patients, although no results are yet available. In the distal colon, the use of the endoanal circular stapler is frequently employed as an alternative to a hand-sewn anastomosis.

Use of a Stoma

The decision as to whether or not to use a temporary stoma is based on the standard surgical principle of creating a safe anastomosis.

Strictureplasty

Use of strictureplasty is limited to strictures of the small bowel, as the intent is to preserve length of small bowel in the face of diffuse disease. The technique may occasionally be used for fibrotic strictures at ileocolic or ileorectal anastomosis (IRA), but is contraindicated for colonic strictures, because there is no indication for length-preserving measures in the colon and because colonic stricturing raises the greater possibility of underlying malignancy.

SURGICAL OPTIONS—BY DISTRIBUTION

Approximately one-quarter of patients have CD limited to the colon. Of these, 25% will have relative rectal sparing (183). Only about 10% have limited segmental involvement of the colon (184). Although the colon is considered an "expendable" or "nonessential" organ, the decision-making process in deciding upon the most appropriate operation is often more complex than that for small bowel disease. Consideration must be given to extent of disease, prior operations, patient age, fecal continence, nutritional status, urgency of operative intervention, and underlying comorbidities.

Segmental Colitis

Use of segmental resection in Crohn's colitis is controversial given the relatively high risk of recurrent disease. It is worth, however, bearing in mind that most data describing recurrence rates are derived from periods prior to aggressive postoperative prophylactic therapy and that this therapeutic field is one of rapid change. Certainly, the patient with limited segmental disease should not undergo a proctocolectomy and Brooke ileostomy with excision of the sphincter complex without serious consideration of the alternatives. In one series of 53 patients undergoing segmental colon resection for limited Crohn's colitis, only 14% ultimately required completion proctectomy after a mean follow-up of 14 years (185). Even if a completion proctectomy is eventually required, the patient will have been spared the psychosocial issues related to a permanent stoma, particularly during the dating and childbearing years.

Resection of the ascending colon requires an awareness of the final positioning of the resultant anastomosis, as it may overlie the duodenum. Recurrence at the anastomosis may then result in a fistula to the duodenum. For this reason, the anastomosis may either be constructed slightly more distally in the transverse colon or may be wrapped with omentum.

When CD affects both the ascending and the transverse colon, resection of the disease alone will result in an anastomosis between the ileum and descending colon with an associated wide mesenteric defect. Thus extended resection with ileosigmoid anastomosis is preferred and does not seem to meaningfully compromise functional outcome.

If the area of colon involved includes the transverse, descending, and/or sigmoid colon, there are two main operative options. In younger patients and those without prior small bowel resection, the subsequent reoperative rate is thought to be reduced if both the diseased segment and the normal proximal bowel is resected with anastomosis of the ileum to the sigmoid or rectum. In those patients with prior small bowel resection of greater than 30 cm and in patients over 50 years of age, whose continence may be compromised, segmental left-sided resection may retain better function. Occasionally, the sigmoid colon may be involved in a phlegmon that derives primarily from ileocolic disease. In a comparison of patients found to have an ileosigmoid fistula, there were no differences in complication rates between repair of the sigmoid aspect of the fistula versus resection of the sigmoid. These results were achieved by reserving repair for those instances in which the sigmoid was a "bystander" only and resection was utilized in those patients in whom there was segmental CD in the sigmoid. Intraoperative colonoscopy was noted to be a useful intervention for intraoperative decision making (186).

Pancolitis

In the presence of extensive colonic involvement, proctocolectomy and Brooke ileostomy is commonly the most appropriate procedure. In a small subset of patients, however, the presence of rectal sparing allows for consideration of ileorectostomy, if continence is acceptable and there is no evidence of perianal disease. In a group of such patients, Keighley (187) found that a maximal tolerated rectal volume of less than 150 mL predicted poor functional outcome, whereas anal canal pressures were not a useful predictor of function.

In rare cases of pancolonic CD, there is an involvement of the upper rectum, with sparing of the lower rectum. A straight ileorectostomy results in poor function; so some authors have suggested creating an ileal J-pouch and anastomosing this to the midrectum (170). We do not support this approach, because the multiple staple/suture lines of the J-pouch are at equally high risk for recurrence as a J-pouch in the pouch-anal setting, which is contraindicated in the setting of CD. Instead, proctocolectomy and end ileostomy are recommended.

Proctitis

Infrequently, CD is limited to the rectum. Removal of the rectum alone with creation of an end colostomy may be an option for certain patients, particularly those with prior extensive small bowel resection and elderly patients considered at risk of dehydration, but only if there is no disease in the proximal colon. In most patients, however, proctocolectomy and end ileostomy are the preferred choice, because of the high risk of recurrence in the remaining colon.

SURGICAL OPTIONS—BY INDICATION
Malignancy and Dysplasia

Operative management of colorectal cancer in the face of Crohn's colitis requires the use of standard oncologic practices, but also consideration of the extent of resection. As with any colorectal carcinoma, high ligation of mesenteric vessels is indicated. In addition, more extensive resection should be considered, as synchronous carcinomas have been described in up to a third of patients (168). Indeed, in the patient with longstanding or extensive colitis, consideration should be given to total abdominal colectomy with IRA or proctocolectomy, depending on whether the carcinoma is in the colon or rectum, respectively, and whether the rectum is free of disease. The finding of dysplasia also warrants concern, because it may be closely associated with existing malignancy or even present in a portion of the colon distant from the primary tumor (188–190). The actual risk of a coexistent malignancy in the setting of dysplasia is less well established in Crohn's colitis than UC, but would also warrant resection as for malignancy (170).

Stricture

Colonic strictures are found in 5% to 17% of patients with Crohn's colitis. This finding should always raise concerns for malignancy, which may be present in 7% of colonic strictures (164), and merits endoscopic assessment. If the stricture is responsible for obstructive symptoms or if malignancy cannot be excluded, then resection is indicated. There is no role for strictureplasty in the primary management of colonic strictures. Stricturing secondary to recurrence of CD at a prior ileocolonic or IRA may, however, be amenable to strictureplasty. In a series of 22 patients with a mean of two-year follow-up, no patient demonstrated recurrent stricturing at the site of the anastomotic strictureplasty (191).

Toxic Colitis and Megacolon

Emergent laparotomy is indicated in the presence of colonic dilation, perforation, uncontrollable hemorrhage, peritonitis, and sepsis. Deterioration in the clinical presentation or minimal improvement after five to seven days of maximal therapy is also an indication for operative intervention.

The most commonly employed procedure for toxic colitis is total abdominal colectomy (subtotal colectomy), with end ileostomy and retention of the rectum. The rectum may be decompressed by employing a rectosigmoid mucous fistula or by closing the proximal rectum and decompressing with a rectal tube via the anus in order to avoid "blow-out" of the rectal stump. Despite retention of the diseased rectum, patients undergoing this procedure usually improve rapidly postoperatively. If the state of the rectum permits restoration of bowel continuity, this can be done at a later time. If the rectum produces bothersome symptoms, it can be excised, or if asymptomatic, it can be left in place providing the patient accepts continued surveillance for malignancy (192).

In the acute setting, proctocolectomy is usually avoided when possible. In these toxic patients, removal of the rectum is associated with a mortality of 9% to 30%, although these figures admittedly derive from older data (193–195). More recent data is not available, given that current practice is to avoid emergent proctectomy. There is increased risk of bleeding and damage to the autonomic nerves of the pelvis. In addition, in the setting of acute colitis, it may be impossible to distinguish between ulcerative and Crohn's colitis, and removal of the sphincter complex would preclude later ileal pouch-anal anastomosis if subsequent pathology were more consistent with UC.

Use of a loop ileostomy and decompression blowhole colostomy is now more of historical interest than of practical application. With significant advances in the management of these sick patients and the recognition of the need for early surgical intervention to avoid perioperative mortality, it has become rare indeed to encounter a patient too ill to undergo resection.

SURGICAL APPROACH

The vast majority of literature pertaining to surgical intervention in Crohn's colitis describes the use of standard laparotomy—an "open" procedure. With the success of laparoscopic techniques in small bowel CD, however, there is increasing interest in the application of minimally invasive techniques to Crohn's colitis, despite the fact that these operations require advanced laparoscopic skills in order to meet the attendant technical challenges. Resection of the colon and/or rectum mandates an ability to operate in multiple quadrants of the abdomen, divide major vascular pedicles, extract a bulky specimen, and then restore bowel continuity. CD presents additional, unique challenges. Even at laparotomy, dissection may be made difficult by the inflammatory manifestations of CD, such as abscess, fistula, and phlegmon. The mesentery is often thickened and foreshortened, requiring careful division. In addition, these patients may be malnourished and on steroids, rendering the tissues more fragile than usual. Not infrequently, patients have had prior resections. The patient with Crohn's colitis presents a further challenge, related to technical difficulty engendered by the extent of the procedure.

There are relatively few data specifically addressing laparoscopic colectomy and IRA or proctocolectomy for CD. Such cases are often included in overall series of laparoscopic resection for CD (196). Information may be drawn from series performed for other indications. Milsom has reported a series of 16 laparoscopic-assisted total colectomies with IRA performed for familial adenomatous polyposis (197). The experience gained from this was translated into performing the same procedure on a more challenging group of 13 patients with Crohn's colitis, reported as part of a larger experience of laparoscopic resection of CD (198). Both series reported benefits of the procedure.

The potential for benefits may also be extrapolated from series describing the more complex procedure of proctocolectomy and IPAA for UC. Early studies revealed excessively long operative times, often over seven hours (199,200), and no apparent benefits of the approach (201). These early techniques used four (199) or five (201) trocar sites as well as a Pfannenstiel incision to "complete the intra-abdominal portion of the operation" plus a separate site for the diverting ileostomy.

By simplifying the procedure, however, the laparoscopic approach has been shown to have patient benefits and reduced operative times. Early analysis of the initial cases performed using the simplified technique in a case-matched comparison with similar patients undergoing open IPAA demonstrated benefits (202). The laparoscopic patients had a median time to clear liquids of 2.0 versus 5.0 days ($p = 0.03$), time to regular diet of 3.0 versus 7.0 days ($p = 0.01$), and a reduced hospital stay of 4.0 versus 9.0 days ($p = 0.01$).

Given the success of laparoscopic approaches in ileocecal CD (202) and in the more complex IPAA performed for UC, it is reasonable to assume that this approach will become more widely utilized for patients with Crohn's colitis. For further discussion of laparoscopic approaches to colonic surgery, please see Chapter on "Laparoscopic Surgery."

SUMMARY

CD of the colon provides a therapeutic challenge to the gastroenterologist or surgeon caring for these complicated patients. Advances in medical therapy include the widespread use of immunosuppressants (azathioprine and MTX) and infliximab for the induction and maintenance of remission in moderate to severe and refractory disease. When medical therapy fails, multiple surgical techniques are available based on the indication for surgery and location of disease; increasing emphasis is being placed on bowel sparing and minimally invasive procedures when appropriate.

REFERENCES

1. Crohn BB, Ginzburg L, Oppenheimer GD. Regional ileitis. A pathological and clinical entity. JAMA 1932; 99:1323–1329.
2. Lockhart-Mummery HE, Morson BC. Crohn's disease (regional enteritis) of the large intestine and its distinction from ulcerative colitis. Gut 1960; 1:87–105.
3. Andres PG, Friedman LS. Epidemiology and the natural course of inflammatory bowel disease. Gastroenterol Clin North Am 1999; 28(2):255–281.
4. Lapidus A, Bernell O, Hellers G, Persson PG, Lofberg R. Incidence of Crohn's disease in Stockholm County 1955–1989. Gut 1997; 41(4):480–486.
5. Lapidus A, Bernell O, Hellers G, Lofberg R. Clinical course of colorectal Crohn's disease: a 35-year follow-up study of 507 patients. Gastroenterology 1998; 114(6):1151–1160.
6. Louis E, Collard A, Oger AF, Degroote E, Aboul Nasr El Yafi FA, Belaiche J. Behaviour of Crohn's disease according to the Vienna classification: changing pattern over the course of the disease. Gut 2001; 49(6):777–782.
7. Makowiec F, Schmidtke C, Paczulla D, Lamberts R, Becker HD, Starlinger M. Progression and prognosis of Crohn's colitis. Z Gastroenterol 1997; 35(1):7–14.
8. Munkholm P, Langholz E, Davidsen M, Binder V. Disease activity courses in a regional cohort of Crohn's disease patients. Scand J Gastroenterol 1995; 30(7):699–706.
9. Polito JM II, Childs B, Mellits ED, Tokayer AZ, Harris ML, Bayless TM. Crohn's disease: influence of age at diagnosis on site and clinical type of disease. Gastroenterology 1996; 111(3):580–586.
10. Farmer RG, Whelan G, Fazio VW. Long-term follow-up of patients with Crohn's disease. Relationship between the clinical pattern and prognosis. Gastroenterology 1985; 88(6):1818–1825.
11. Hurst RD, Molinari M, Chung TP, Rubin M, Michelassi F. Prospective study of the features, indications, and surgical treatment in 513 consecutive patients affected by Crohn's disease. Surgery 1997; 122(4):661–667; discussion 667–668.
12. Wagtmans MJ, Verspaget HW, Lamers CB, van Hogezand RA. Gender-related differences in the clinical course of Crohn's disease. Am J Gastroenterol 2001; 96(5):1541–1546.

13. Jess T, Winther KV, Munkholm P, Langholz E, Binder V. Mortality and causes of death in Crohn's disease: follow-up of a population-based cohort in Copenhagen County, Denmark. Gastroenterology 2002; 122(7):1808–1814.
14. Ekbom A, Helmick CG, Zack M, Holmberg L, Adami HO. Survival and causes of death in patients with inflammatory bowel disease: a population-based study. Gastroenterology 1992; 103(3):954–960.
15. Probert CS, Jayanthi V, Wicks AC, Mayberry JF. Mortality from Crohn's disease in Leicestershire, 1972–1989: an epidemiological community based study. Gut 1992; 33(9):1226–1228.
16. Farrokhyar F, Swarbrick ET, Grace RH, Hellier MD, Gent AE, Irvine EJ. Low mortality in ulcerative colitis and Crohn's disease in three regional centers in England. Am J Gastroenterol 2001; 96(2): 501–507.
17. Blondel-Kucharski F, Chircop C, Marquis P, et al. Health-related quality of life in Crohn's disease: a prospective longitudinal study in 231 patients. Am J Gastroenterol 2001; 96(10):2915–2920.
18. Podolsky DK. Inflammatory bowel disease. N Engl J Med 2002; 347(6):417–429.
19. Rath HC, Schultz M, Freitag R, et al. Different subsets of enteric bacteria induce and perpetuate experimental colitis in rats and mice. Infect Immun 2001; 69(4):2277–2285.
20. Rath HC, Ikeda JS, Linde HJ, Scholmerich J, Wilson KH, Sartor RB. Varying cecal bacterial loads influences colitis and gastritis in HLA-B27 transgenic rats. Gastroenterology 1999; 116(2):310–319.
21. Swidsinski A, Ladhoff A, Pernthaler A, et al. Mucosal flora in inflammatory bowel disease. Gastroenterology 2002; 122(1):44–54.
22. Peeters M, Nevens H, Baert F, et al. Familial aggregation in Crohn's disease: increased age-adjusted risk and concordance in clinical characteristics. Gastroenterology 1996; 111(3):597–603.
23. Annese V, Andreoli A, Astegiano M, et al. Clinical features in familial cases of Crohn's disease and ulcerative colitis in Italy: a GISC study. Italian Study Group for the disease of colon and rectum. Am J Gastroenterol 2001; 96(10):2939–2945.
24. Ogura Y, Bonen DK, Inohara N, et al. A frameshift mutation in NOD2 associated with susceptibility to Crohn's disease. Nature 2001; 411(6837):603–606.
25. Hugot JP, Chamaillard M, Zouali H, et al. Association of NOD2 leucine-rich repeat variants with susceptibility to Crohn's disease. Nature 2001; 411(6837):599–603.
26. Abreu MT, Taylor KD, Lin YC, et al. Mutations in NOD2 are associated with fibrostenosing disease in patients with Crohn's disease. Gastroenterology 2002; 123(3):679–688.
27. Cuthbert AP, Fisher SA, Mirza MM, et al. The contribution of NOD2 gene mutations to the risk and site of disease in inflammatory bowel disease. Gastroenterology 2002; 122(4):867–874.
28. Lesage S, Zouali H, Cezard JP, et al. CARD15/NOD2 mutational analysis and genotype-phenotype correlation in 612 patients with inflammatory bowel disease. Am J Hum Genet 2002; 70(4): 845–857.
29. Calkins BM. A meta-analysis of the role of smoking in inflammatory bowel disease. Dig Dis Sci 1989; 34(12):1841–1854.
30. Bridger S, Lee JC, Bjarnason I, Jones JE, Macpherson AJ. In siblings with similar genetic susceptibility for inflammatory bowel disease, smokers tend to develop Crohn's disease and non-smokers develop ulcerative colitis. Gut 2002; 51(1):21–25.
31. Duffy LC, Zielezny MA, Marshall JR, et al. Cigarette smoking and risk of clinical relapse in patients with Crohn's disease. Am J Prev Med 1990; 6(3):161–166.
32. Sutherland LR, Ramcharan S, Bryant H, Fick G. Effect of cigarette smoking on recurrence of Crohn's disease. Gastroenterology 1990; 98(5 Pt 1):1123–1128.
33. Cosnes J, Carbonnel F, Beaugerie L, Le Quintrec Y, Gendre JP. Effects of cigarette smoking on the long-term course of Crohn's disease. Gastroenterology 1996; 110(2):424–431.
34. Koutroubakis IE, Vlachonikolis IG, Kapsoritakis A, et al. Appendectomy, tonsillectomy, and risk of inflammatory bowel disease: case-controlled study in Crete. Dis Colon Rectum 1999; 42(2): 225–230.
35. Caserta L, de Filippo FR, Riegler G. Relationship between anamnestic evidence of appendectomy and onset and clinical course of Crohn's disease. Am J Gastroenterol 2002; 97(1):207–208.
36. Reif S, Lavy A, Keter D, et al. Appendectomy is more frequent but not a risk factor in Crohn's disease while being protective in ulcerative colitis: a comparison of surgical procedures in inflammatory bowel disease. Am J Gastroenterol 2001; 96(3):829–832.
37. Russel MG, Dorant E, Brummer RJ, et al. Appendectomy and the risk of developing ulcerative colitis or Crohn's disease: results of a large case-control study. South Limburg Inflammatory Bowel Disease Study Group. Gastroenterology 1997; 113(2):377–382.
38. Lashner B. Clinical features, laboratory findings, and course of Crohn's disease. In: Kirsner's Inflammatory Bowel Diseases. 5th ed. 2000:305–314.
39. Hanauer SB, Sandborn W. Management of Crohn's disease in adults. Am J Gastroenterol 2001; 96(3):635–643.
40. Driver CP, Anderson DN, Keenan RA. Massive intestinal bleeding in association with Crohn's disease. J R Coll Surg Edinb 1996; 41(3):152–154.
41. Pardi DS, Loftus EV Jr., Tremaine WJ, et al. Acute major gastrointestinal hemorrhage in inflammatory bowel disease. Gastrointest Endosc 1999; 49(2):153–157.
42. Veloso FT, Carvalho J, Magro F. Immune-related systemic manifestations of inflammatory bowel disease. A prospective study of 792 patients. J Clin Gastroenterol 1996; 23(1):29–34.

43. Rasmussen HH, Fallingborg JF, Mortensen PB, Vyberg M, Tage-Jensen U, Rasmussen SN. Hepato-biliary dysfunction and primary sclerosing cholangitis in patients with Crohn's disease. Scand J Gastroenterol 1997; 32(6):604–610.

44. Weber P, Koch M, Heizmann WR, Scheurlen M, Jenss H, Hartmann F. Microbic superinfection in relapse of inflammatory bowel disease. J Clin Gastroenterol 1992; 14(4):302–308.

45. Mathy CMU, Terdiman J. Clostridium dificile infection without antibiotic exposure in outpatients with inflammatory bowel disease. Gastroenterology 2002; 122:A606.

46. LaMont JT, Trnka YM. Therapeutic implications of clostridium difficile toxin during relapse of chronic inflammatory bowel disease. Lancet 1980; 1(8165):381–383.

47. Cottone M, Pietrosi G, Martorana G, et al. Prevalence of cytomegalovirus infection in severe refractory ulcerative and Crohn's colitis. Am J Gastroenterol 2001; 96(3):773–775.

48. Dijkstra J, Reeders JW, Tytgat GN. Idiopathic inflammatory bowel disease: endoscopic-radiologic correlation. Radiology 1995; 197(2):369–375.

49. Parente F, Maconi G, Bollani S, et al. Bowel ultrasound in assessment of Crohn's disease and detection of related small bowel strictures: a prospective comparative study versus x ray and intraoperative findings. Gut 2002; 50(4):490–495.

50. Schwartz DA, Wiersema MJ, Dudiak KM, et al. A comparison of endoscopic ultrasound, magnetic resonance imaging, and exam under anesthesia for evaluation of Crohn's perianal fistulas. Gastroenterology 2001; 121(5):1064–1072.

51. Mountanos GI, Manolakakis IS. The accordion sign at CT: report of a case of Crohn's disease with diffuse colonic involvement. Eur Radiol 2001; 11(8):1433–1434.

52. Lee SS, Ha HK, Yang SK, et al. CT of prominent pericolic or perienteric vasculature in patients with Crohn's disease: correlation with clinical disease activity and findings on barium studies. AJR Am J Roentgenol 2002; 179(4):1029–1036.

53. Solomon MJ. Fistulae and abscesses in symptomatic perianal Crohn's disease. Int J Colorectal Dis 1996; 11(5):222–226.

54. Koh DM, Miao Y, Chinn RJ, et al. MR imaging evaluation of the activity of Crohn's disease. AJR Am J Roentgenol 2001; 177(6):1325–1332.

55. Neurath MF, Vehling D, Schunk K, et al. Noninvasive assessment of Crohn's disease activity: a comparison of 18F-fluorodeoxyglucose positron emission tomography, hydromagnetic resonance imaging, and granulocyte scintigraphy with labeled antibodies. Am J Gastroenterol 2002; 97(8):1978–1985.

56. Molnar T, Papos M, Gyulai C, et al. Clinical value of technetium-99m-HMPAO-labeled leukocyte scintigraphy and spiral computed tomography in active Crohn's disease. Am J Gastroenterol 2001; 96(5):1517–1521.

57. Smedh K, Olaison G, Jonsson KA, Johansson KE, Skullman S, Hallbook O. Interobserver variation of colonoileoscopic findings in Crohn's disease. Scand J Gastroenterol 1995; 30(1):81–86.

58. Cellier C, Sahmoud T, Froguel E, et al. Correlations between clinical activity, endoscopic severity, and biological parameters in colonic or ileocolonic Crohn's disease. A prospective multicentre study of 121 cases. The Groupe d'Etudes Therapeutiques des Affections Inflammatoires Digestives. Gut 1994; 35(2):231–235.

59. Allez M, Lemann M, Bonnet J, Cattan P, Jian R, Modigliani R. Long term outcome of patients with active Crohn's disease exhibiting extensive and deep ulcerations at colonoscopy. Am J Gastroenterol 2002; 97(4):947–953.

60. D'Haens G, Rutgeerts P. Postoperative recurrence of Crohn's disease: pathophysiology and prevention. Inflamm Bowel Dis 1999; 5(4):295–303.

61. Friedman S, Rubin PH, Bodian C, Goldstein E, Harpaz N, Present DH. Screening and surveillance colonoscopy in chronic Crohn's colitis. Gastroenterology 2001; 120(4):820–826.

62. Breysem Y, Janssens JF, Coremans G, Vantrappen G, Hendrickx G, Rutgeerts P. Endoscopic balloon dilation of colonic and ileo-colonic Crohn's strictures: long-term results. Gastrointest Endosc 1992; 38(2):142–147.

63. Seidman EG. Role of endoscopy in inflammatory bowel disease. Gastrointest Endosc Clin N Am 2001; 11(4):641–657.

64. Chambers TJ, Morson BC. The granuloma in Crohn's disease. Gut 1979; 20(4):269–274.

65. Okada M, Maeda K, Yao T, Iwashita A, Nomiyama Y, Kitahara K. Minute lesions of the rectum and sigmoid colon in patients with Crohn's disease. Gastrointest Endosc 1991; 37(3):319–324.

66. Tanaka M, Riddell RH. The pathological diagnosis and differential diagnosis of Crohn's disease. Hepatogastroenterology 1990; 37(1):18–31.

67. Farmer M, Petras RE, Hunt LE, Janosky JE, Galandiuk S. The importance of diagnostic accuracy in colonic inflammatory bowel disease. Am J Gastroenterol 2000; 95(11):3184–3188.

68. The Mesalamine Study Group. An oral preparation of mesalamine as long-term maintenance therapy for ulcerative colitis. A randomized, placebo-controlled trial. Ann Intern Med 1996; 124(2):204–211.

69. Hamer DH GS. Infectious diarrhea and bacterial food poisoning. In: Feldman F, Sleisenger, eds. Sleisenger & Fordtran's Gastrointestinal and Liver Diseases. 7th ed. Saunders, 2022:1864–1906.

70. Simmonds SD, Noble MA, Freeman HJ. Gastrointestinal features of culture-positive Yersinia enterocolitica infection. Gastroenterology 1987; 92(1):112–117.

71. Kanani SR, Knight R. Relapsing amoebic colitis of 12 year's standing exacerbated by corticosteroids. Br Med J 1969; 2(657):613–614.

72. Sakamoto I, Shirai T, Kamide T, et al. Cytomegalovirus enterocolitis in an immunocompetent individual. J Clin Gastroenterol 2002; 34(3):243–246.

73. Hermon-Taylor J. Protagonist. Mycobacterium avium subspecies paratuberculosis is a cause of Crohn's disease. Gut 2001; 49(6):755–756.

74. Horvath KD, Whelan RL. Intestinal tuberculosis: return of an old disease. Am J Gastroenterol 1998; 93(5):692–696.

75. Shah S, Thomas V, Mathan M, et al. Colonoscopic study of 50 patients with colonic tuberculosis. Gut 1992; 33(3):347–351.

76. Colombat M, Imbert A, Bruneval P, Chatelain D, Gontier MF. Giant cell arteritis localized to the colon associated with Crohn's disease. Histopathology 2001; 38(1):21–24.

77. Gledhill A, Dixon MF. Crohn's-like reaction in diverticular disease. Gut 1998; 42(3):392–395.

78. Stamm C, Burkhalter CE, Pearce W, et al. Benign colonic ulcers associated with nonsteroidal antiinflammatory drug ingestion. Am J Gastroenterol 1994; 89(12):2230–2233.

79. Frossard JL, Spahr L, Queneau PE, Armenian B, Brundler MA, Hadengue A. Ischemic colitis during pregnancy and contraceptive medication. Digestion 2001; 64(2):125–127.

80. Ratnaike RN, Jones TE. Mechanisms of drug-induced diarrhoea in the elderly. Drugs Aging 1998; 13(3):245–253.

81. Son HJ, Rhee PL, Kim JJ, et al. Primary T-cell lymphoma of the colon. Korean J Intern Med 1997; 12(2):238–241.

82. Ayata G, Ithamukkala S, Sapp H, et al. Prevalence and significance of inflammatory bowel disease-like morphologic features in collagenous and lymphocytic colitis. Am J Surg Pathol 2002; 26(11): 1414–1423.

83. Price AB. Overlap in the spectrum of non-specific inflammatory bowel disease— 'colitis indeterminate'. J Clin Pathol 1978; 31(6):567–577.

84. Moum B, Vatn MH, Ekbom A, et al. Incidence of ulcerative colitis and indeterminate colitis in four counties of southeastern Norway, 1990–1993. A prospective population-based study. The Inflammatory Bowel South-Eastern Norway (IBSEN) Study Group of Gastroenterologists. Scand J Gastroenterol 1996; 31(4):362–366.

85. Meucci G, Bortoli A, Riccioli FA, et al. Frequency and clinical evolution of indeterminate colitis: a retrospective multi-centre study in northern Italy. GSMII (Gruppo di Studio per le Malattie Infiammatorie Intestinali). Eur J Gastroenterol Hepatol 1999; 11(8):909–913.

86. McIntyre PB, Pemberton JH, Wolff BG, Dozois RR, Beart RW Jr. Indeterminate colitis. Long-term outcome in patients after ileal pouch- anal anastomosis. Dis Colon Rectum 1995; 38(1):51–54.

87. Duerr RH, Targan SR, Landers CJ, Sutherland LR, Shanahan F. Anti-neutrophil cytoplasmic antibodies in ulcerative colitis. Comparison with other colitides/diarrheal illnesses. Gastroenterology 1991; 100(6):1590–1596.

88. Cambridge G, Rampton DS, Stevens TR, McCarthy DA, Kamm M, Leaker B. Anti-neutrophil antibodies in inflammatory bowel disease: prevalence and diagnostic role. Gut 1992; 33(5):668–674.

89. Ruemmele FM, Targan SR, Levy G, Dubinsky M, Braun J, Seidman EG. Diagnostic accuracy of serological assays in pediatric inflammatory bowel disease. Gastroenterology 1998; 115(4):822–829.

90. Peeters M, Joossens S, Vermeire S, Vlietinck R, Bossuyt X, Rutgeerts P. Diagnostic value of anti-Saccharomyces cerevisiae and antineutrophil cytoplasmic autoantibodies in inflammatory bowel disease. Am J Gastroenterol 2001; 96(3):730–734.

91. McKenzie H, Main J, Pennington CR, Parratt D. Antibody to selected strains of Saccharomyces cerevisiae (baker's and brewer's yeast) and Candida albicans in Crohn's disease. Gut 1990; 31(5): 536–538.

92. Vasiliauskas EA, Plevy SE, Landers CJ, et al. Perinuclear antineutrophil cytoplasmic antibodies in patients with Crohn's disease define a clinical subgroup. Gastroenterology 1996; 110(6):1810–1819.

93. Quinton JF, Sendid B, Reumaux D, et al. Anti-Saccharomyces cerevisiae mannan antibodies combined with antineutrophil cytoplasmic autoantibodies in inflammatory bowel disease: prevalence and diagnostic role. Gut 1998; 42(6):788–791.

94. Joossens S, Reinisch W, Vermeire S, et al. The value of serologic markers in indeterminate colitis: a prospective follow-up study. Gastroenterology 2002; 122(5):1242–1247.

95. Moum B, Ekbom A, Vatn MH, et al. Inflammatory bowel disease: re-evaluation of the diagnosis in a prospective population based study in south eastern Norway. Gut 1997; 40(3):328–332.

96. Cominelli F ZC, Dinarello CA. Sulfasalazine inhibits cytokine production in human mononuclear cells: a novel anti-inflammatory mechanism. Gastroenterology 1992; 96:A96.

97. Shanahan F, Niederlehner A, Carramanzana N, Anton P. Sulfasalazine inhibits the binding of TNF alpha to its receptor. Immunopharmacology 1990; 20(3):217–224.

98. Wahl C, Liptay S, Adler G, Schmid RM. Sulfasalazine: a potent and specific inhibitor of nuclear factor kappa B. J Clin Invest 1998; 101(5):1163–1174.

99. Gisbert JP, Gomollon F, Mate J, Pajares JM. Role of 5-aminosalicylic acid (5-ASA) in treatment of inflammatory bowel disease: a systematic review. Dig Dis Sci 2002; 47(3):471–488.

100. Summers RW, Switz DM, Sessions JT Jr., et al. National Cooperative Crohn's Disease Study: results of drug treatment. Gastroenterology 1979; 77(4 Pt 2):847–869.

101. Malchow H, Ewe K, Brandes JW, et al. European Cooperative Crohn's Disease Study (ECCDS): results of drug treatment. Gastroenterology 1984; 86(2):249–266.

102. Singleton JW, Hanauer SB, Gitnick GL, et al. Mesalamine capsules for the treatment of active Crohn's disease: results of a 16-week trial. Pentasa Crohn's Disease Study Group. Gastroenterology 1993; 104(5):1293–1301.
103. Camma C, Giunta M, Rosselli M, Cottone M. Mesalamine in the maintenance treatment of Crohn's disease: a meta- analysis adjusted for confounding variables. Gastroenterology 1997; 113(5):1465–1473.
104. Feagan BG, Fedorak RN, Irvine EJ, et al. A comparison of methotrexate with placebo for the maintenance of remission in Crohn's disease. North American Crohn's Study Group Investigators [see comments]. New England Journal of Medicine 2000; 342(22):1627–1632.
105. Sutherland LR, May GR, Shaffer EA. Sulfasalazine revisited: a meta-analysis of 5-aminosalicylic acid in the treatment of ulcerative colitis. Ann Intern Med 1993; 118(7):540–549.
106. Ransford RA, Langman MJ. Sulphasalazine and mesalazine: serious adverse reactions re-evaluated on the basis of suspected adverse reaction reports to the Committee on Safety of Medicines. Gut 2002; 51(4):536–539.
107. Iofel E, Chawla A, Daum F, Markowitz J. Mesalamine intolerance mimics symptoms of active inflammatory bowel disease. J Pediatr Gastroenterol Nutr 2002; 34(1):73–76.
108. Tillinger W, Gasche C, Reinisch W, et al. Influence of topically and systemically active steroids on circulating leukocytes in Crohn's disease. Am J Gastroenterol 1998; 93(10):1848–1853.
109. Singleton JW, Law DH, Kelley ML Jr., Mekhjian HS, Sturdevant RA. National Cooperative Crohn's Disease Study: adverse reactions to study drugs. Gastroenterology 1979; 77(4 Pt 2):870–882.
110. Faubion WA Jr., Loftus EV Jr., Harmsen WS, Zinsmeister AR, Sandborn WJ. The natural history of corticosteroid therapy for inflammatory bowel disease: a population-based study. Gastroenterology 2001; 121(2):255–260.
111. Talar-Williams C, Sneller MC. Complications of corticosteroid therapy. Eur Arch Otorhinolaryngol 1994; 251(3):131–136.
112. Cann PA, Holdsworth CD. Systemic absorption from hydrocortisone foam enema in ulcerative colitis. Lancet 1987; 1(8538):922–923.
113. Petitjean O, Wendling JL, Tod M, et al. Pharmacokinetics and absolute rectal bioavailability of hydrocortisone acetate in distal colitis. Aliment Pharmacol Ther 1992; 6(3):351–357.
114. Greenberg GR, Feagan BG, Martin F, et al. Oral budesonide for active Crohn's disease. Canadian Inflammatory Bowel Disease Study Group. N Engl J Med 1994; 331(13):836–841.
115. Spencer CM, McTavish D. Budesonide. A review of its pharmacological properties and therapeutic efficacy in inflammatory bowel disease. Drugs 1995; 50(5):854–872.
116. Edsbacker S. Budesonide capsules: scientific basis. Drugs of Today 2000; 38(suppl G):9–23.
117. Moss AA, Carbone JV, Kressel HY. Radiologic and clinical assessment of broad-spectrum antibiotic therapy in Crohn's disease. AJR Am J Roentgenol 1978; 131(5):787–790.
118. Colombel JF, Lemann M, Cassagnou M, et al. A controlled trial comparing ciprofloxacin with mesalazine for the treatment of active Crohn's disease. Am J Gastroenterol 1999; 94:674–678.
119. Ursing B, Alm T, Barany F, et al. A comparative study of metronidazole and sulfasalazine for active Crohn's disease: the cooperative Crohn's disease study in Sweden II. Result. Gastroenterology 1982; 83(3):550–562.
120. Sutherland L, Singleton J, Sessions J, et al. Double blind, placebo controlled trial of metronidazole in Crohn's disease. Gut 1991; 32(9):1071–1075.
121. Prantera C, Kohn A, Zannoni F, Spimpolo N, Bonfa M. Metronidazole plus ciprofloxacin in the treatment of active, refractory Crohn's disease: results of an open study. J Clin Gastroenterol 1994; 19(1):79–80.
122. Greenbloom SL, Steinhart AH, Greenberg GR. Combination ciprofloxacin and metronidazole for active Crohn's disease. Can J Gastroenterol 1998; 12(1):53–56.
123. Steinhart AH, Feagan BG, Wong CJ, et al. Combined budesonide and antibiotic therapy for active Crohn's disease: a randomized controlled trial. Gastroenterology 2002; 123(1):33–40.
124. Borgaonkar. Anti-tuberculous therapy for maintaining remission of Crohn's disease. The Cochrane Library. Oxford 1999.
125. Pearson DC, May GR, Fick GH, Sutherland LR. Azathioprine and 6-mercaptopurine in Crohn disease. A meta-analysis. Ann Intern Med 1995; 123(2):132–142.
126. Markowitz J, Grancher K, Kohn N, Lesser M, Daum F. A multicenter trial of 6-mercaptopurine and prednisone in children with newly diagnosed Crohn's disease. Gastroenterology 2000; 119(4):895–902.
127. Lemann MBY, Colombel JF, et al. Randomized, double-blind, placebo-controlled multicenter, azathioprine withdrawal trial in Crohn's Disease. Gastroenterology 2002; 122(suppl 4):A23.
128. Present DH, Meltzer SJ, Krumholz MP, Wolke A, Korelitz BI. 6-Mercaptopurine in the management of inflammatory bowel disease: short- and long-term toxicity. Ann Intern Med 1989; 111(8): 641–649.
129. Bouhnik Y, Lemann M, Mary JY, et al. Long-term follow-up of patients with Crohn's disease treated with azathioprine or 6-mercaptopurine. Lancet 1996; 347(8996):215–219.
130. Connell WR, Kamm MA, Ritchie JK, Lennard-Jones JE. Bone marrow toxicity caused by azathioprine in inflammatory bowel disease: 27 years of experience. Gut 1993; 34(8):1081–1085.
131. Dayharsh GA, Loftus EV Jr., Sandborn WJ, et al. Epstein-Barr virus-positive lymphoma in patients with inflammatory bowel disease treated with azathioprine or 6-mercaptopurine. Gastroenterology 2002; 122(1):72–77.

132. Lewis JD, Bilker WB, Brensinger C, Deren JJ, Vaughn DJ, Strom BL. Inflammatory bowel disease is not associated with an increased risk of lymphoma. Gastroenterology 2001; 121(5):1080–1087.

133. Bernstein CN, Blanchard JF, Kliewer E, Wajda A. Cancer risk in patients with inflammatory bowel disease: a population- based study. Cancer 2001; 91(4):854–862.

134. Cutolo M, Sulli A, Pizzorni C, Seriolo B, Straub RH. Anti-inflammatory mechanisms of methotrexate in rheumatoid arthritis. Ann Rheum Dis 2001; 60(8):729–735.

135. Feagan BG, Rochon J, Fedorak RN, et al. Methotrexate for the treatment of Crohn's disease. The North American Crohn's Study Group Investigators. N Engl J Med 1995; 332(5):292–297.

136. Egan LJ, Sandborn WJ, Tremaine WJ, et al. A randomized dose-response and pharmacokinetic study of methotrexate for refractory inflammatory Crohn's disease and ulcerative colitis. Aliment Pharmacol Ther 1999; 13(12):1597–1604.

137. Goodman TA, Polisson RP. Methotrexate: adverse reactions and major toxicities. Rheum Dis Clin North Am 1994; 20(2):513–528.

138. Kremer JM, Alarcon GS, Lightfoot RW Jr., et al. Methotrexate for rheumatoid arthritis. Suggested guidelines for monitoring liver toxicity. American College of Rheumatology. Arthritis Rheum 1994; 37(3):316–328.

139. Walker AM, Funch D, Dreyer NA, et al. Determinants of serious liver disease among patients receiving low-dose methotrexate for rheumatoid arthritis. Arthritis Rheum 1993; 36(3):329–335.

140. Te HS, Schiano TD, Kuan SF, Hanauer SB, Conjeevaram HS, Baker AL. Hepatic effects of long-term methotrexate use in the treatment of inflammatory bowel disease. Am J Gastroenterol 2000; 95(11):3150–3156.

141. Lemann M, Zenjari T, Bouhnik Y, et al. Methotrexate in Crohn's disease: long-term efficacy and toxicity [see comments]. Am J Gastroenterol 2000; 95(7):1730–1734.

142. Flanagan WM, Corthesy B, Bram RJ, Crabtree GR. Nuclear association of a T-cell transcription factor blocked by FK-506 and cyclosporin A. Nature 1991; 352(6338):803–807.

143. Egan LJ, Sandborn WJ, Tremaine WJ. Clinical outcome following treatment of refractory inflammatory and fistulizing Crohn's disease with intravenous cyclosporine. Am J Gastroenterol 1998; 93(3):442–448.

144. Sandborn WJ PD, Isaccs KL. Tacrolimus (FK506) for the treatment of perianal and enterocutaneous fistulas in patients with Crohn' disease: a randomized, double-blind, placebo-controlled trial. Gastronterology 2002; 122(4):A81.

145. Ierardi E, Principi M, Francavilla R, et al. Oral tacrolimus long-term therapy in patients with Crohn's disease and steroid resistance. Aliment Pharmacol Ther 2001; 15(3):371–377.

146. Sternthal M GJ, Kornbluth A. Toxicity associated with the use of cyclosporin in patients with inflammatory bowel disease. Gastroenterology 1996; 110:A1019.

147. Knight DM, Trinh H, Le J, et al. Construction and initial characterization of a mouse-human chimeric anti-TNF antibody. Mol Immunol 1993; 30(16):1443–1453.

148. Targan SR, Hanauer SB, van Deventer SJ, et al. A short-term study of chimeric monoclonal antibody cA2 to tumor necrosis factor alpha for Crohn's disease. Crohn's Disease cA2 Study Group. N Engl J Med 1997; 337(15):1029–1035.

149. Present DH, Rutgeerts P, Targan S, et al. Infliximab for the treatment of fistulas in patients with Crohn's disease. N Engl J Med 1999; 340(18):1398–1405.

150. Hanauer SB, Feagan BG, Lichtenstein GR, et al. Maintenance infliximab for Crohn's disease: the ACCENT I randomised trial. Lancet 2002; 359(9317):1541–1549.

151. American Thoracic Society. Targeted tuberculin testing and treatment of latent tuberculosis infection. MMWR Recomm Rep 2000; 49(RR-6):1–51.

152. Anon. Infliximab (Remicade). Physician's Desk Reference 2002.

153. Mekhjian HS, Switz DM, Watts HD, Deren JJ, Katon RM, Beman FM. National Cooperative Crohn's Disease Study: factors determining recurrence of Crohn's disease after surgery. Gastroenterology 1979; 77(4 Pt 2):907–913.

154. De Dombal FT, Burton I, Goligher JC. Recurrence of Crohn's disease after primary excisional surgery. Gut 1971; 12(7):519–527.

155. Sutherland LR. Mesalamine for the prevention of postoperative recurrence: is nearly there the same as being there? Gastroenterology 2000; 118(2):436–438.

156. Lochs H, Mayer M, Fleig WE, et al. Prophylaxis of postoperative relapse in Crohn's disease with mesalamine: European Cooperative Crohn's Disease Study VI [see comments] [published erratum appears in Gastroenterology 2000 Jul; 119(1):280]. Gastroenterology 2000; 118(2):264–273.

157. Rutgeerts P, Hiele M, Geboes K, et al. Controlled trial of metronidazole treatment for prevention of Crohn's recurrence after ileal resection [see comments]. Gastroenterology 1995; 108(6):1617–1621.

158. Rutgeerts PVAG, D'Haens G, et al. Ornidazol for prophylaxis of postoperative Crohn's Disease: final results of a double blind placebo controlled trial. Gastroenterology 2002; 122(4, suppl 1):A–80.

159. Hellers G, Cortot A, Jewell D, et al. Oral budesonide for prevention of postsurgical recurrence in Crohn's disease. The IOIBD Budesonide Study Group. Gastroenterology 1999; 116(2):294–300.

160. Korelitz B HS, Rutgeerts P. Postoperative prophylazxis with 6-MP, 5-ASA or placebo in Crohn's disease: a two year multicenter trial. Gastroenterology 1998; 114:A1011.

161. Gillen CD, Walmsley RS, Prior P, Andrews HA, Allan RN. Ulcerative colitis and Crohn's disease: a comparison of the colorectal cancer risk in extensive colitis. Gut 1994; 35(11):1590–1592.

162. Broome U, Lofberg R, Veress B, Eriksson LS. Primary sclerosing cholangitis and ulcerative colitis: evidence for increased neoplastic potential. Hepatology 1995; 22(5):1404–1408.

163. Askling J, Dickman PW, Karlen P, et al. Family history as a risk factor for colorectal cancer in inflammatory bowel disease. Gastroenterology 2001; 120(6):1356–1362.

164. Yamazaki Y, Ribeiro MB, Sachar DB, Aufses AH Jr., Greenstein AJ. Malignant colorectal strictures in Crohn's disease. Am J Gastroenterol 1991; 86(7):882–885.

165. Farmer RG, Hawk WA, Turnbull RB Jr. Indications for surgery in Crohn's disease: analysis of 500 cases. Gastroenterology 1976; 71(2):245–250.

166. Homer DR, Grand RJ, Colodny AH. Growth, course, and prognosis after surgery for Crohn's disease in children and adolescents. Pediatrics 1977; 59(5):717–725.

167. Gyde SN, Prior P, Macartney JC, Thompson H, Waterhouse JA, Allan RN. Malignancy in Crohn's disease. Gut 1980; 21(12):1024–1029.

168. Greenstein AJ, Sachar DB, Smith H, Janowitz HD, Aufses AH Jr. Patterns of neoplasia in Crohn's disease and ulcerative colitis. Cancer 1980; 46(2):403–407.

169. Ekbom A, Helmick C, Zack M, Adami HO. Increased risk of large-bowel cancer in Crohn's disease with colonic involvement. Lancet 1990; 336(8711):357–359.

170. Strong SA. Crohn's Disease. New York: Churchill Livingstone, 1997.

171. Softley A, Clamp SE, Bouchier IA, Myren J, Watkinson G, de Dombal FT. Perforation of the intestine in inflammatory bowel disease. An OMGE survey. Scand J Gastroenterol Suppl 1988; 144:24–26.

172. Bundred NJ, Dixon JM, Lumsden AB, Gilmour HM, Davies GC. Free perforation in Crohn's colitis. A ten-year review. Dis Colon Rectum 1985; 28(1):35–37.

173. Homan WP, Tang CK, Thorbjarnarson B. Acute massive hemorrhage from intestinal Crohn disease. Report of seven cases and review of the literature. Arch Surg 1976; 111(8):901–905.

174. de Lalla F. Surgical prophylaxis in practice. J Hosp Infect 2002; 50(suppl):AS9–AS12.

175. Song F, Glenny AM. Antimicrobial prophylaxis in colorectal surgery: a systematic review of randomized controlled trials. Br J Surg 1998; 85(9):1232–1241.

176. Coursin DB, Wood KE. Corticosteroid supplementation for adrenal insufficiency. JAMA 2002; 287(2):236–240.

177. Colombel JF LE, Tremaine WJ, et al. Perioperative infliximab and/or immunomodulator therapy is not associated with increased postoperative complications in Crohn's disease[abstr]. Gastroenterology 2003.

178. Lashner BA, Evans AA, Hanauer SB. Preoperative total parenteral nutrition for bowel resection in Crohn's disease. Dig Dis Sci 1989; 34(5):741–746.

179. Wolff BG, Beart RW Jr., Frydenberg HB, Weiland LH, Agrez MV, Ilstrup DM. The importance of disease-free margins in resections for Crohn's disease. Dis Colon Rectum 1983; 26(4):239–243.

180. Hamilton SR, Reese J, Pennington L, Boitnott JK, Bayless TM, Cameron JL. The role of resection margin frozen section in the surgical management of Crohn's disease. Surg Gynecol Obstet 1985; 160(1):57–62.

181. Fazio VW, Marchetti F, Church M, et al. Effect of resection margins on the recurrence of Crohn's disease in the small bowel. A randomized controlled trial. Ann Surg 1996; 224(4):563–571; discussion 571–573.

182. Munoz-Juarez M, Yamamoto T, Wolff BG, Keighley MR. Wide-lumen stapled anastomosis vs. conventional end-to-end anastomosis in the treatment of Crohn's disease. Dis Colon Rectum 2001; 44(1):20–25; discussion 25–26.

183. Block GE. Surgical management of Crohn's colitis. N Engl J Med 1980; 302(19):1068–1070.

184. Goligher JC. The long-term results of excisional surgery for primary and recurrent Crohn's disease of the large intestine. Dis Colon Rectum 1985; 28(1):51–55.

185. Prabhakar LP, Laramee C, Nelson H, Dozois RR. Avoiding a stoma: role for segmental or abdominal colectomy in Crohn's colitis. Dis Colon Rectum 1997; 40(1):71–78.

186. Young-Fadok TM, Wolff BG, Meagher A, Benn PL, Dozois RR. Surgical management of ileosigmoid fistulas in Crohn's disease. Dis Colon Rectum 1997; 40(5):558–561.

187. Keighley MR, Buchmann P, Lee JR. Assessment of anorectal function in selection of patients for ileorectal anastomosis in Crohn's colitis. Gut 1982; 23(2):102–107.

188. Simpson S, Traube J, Riddell RH. The histologic appearance of dysplasia (precarcinomatous change) in Crohn's disease of the small and large intestine. Gastroenterology 1981; 81(3):492–501.

189. Petras RE, Mir-Madjlessi SH, Farmer RG. Crohn's disease and intestinal carcinoma. A report of 11 cases with emphasis on associated epithelial dysplasia. Gastroenterology 1987; 93(6):1307–1314.

190. Hamilton SR. Colorectal carcinoma in patients with Crohn's disease. Gastroenterology 1985; 89(2):398–407.

191. Tjandra JJ, Fazio VW. Strictureplasty for ileocolic anastomotic strictures in Crohn's disease. Dis Colon Rectum 1993; 36(12):1099–1103; discussion 1103–1104.

192. Lavery IC, Jagelman DG. Cancer in the excluded rectum following surgery for inflammatory bowel disease. Dis Colon Rectum 1982; 25(6):522–524.

193. Scott HW Jr., Sawyers JL, Gobbel WG Jr., Graves HA, Shull HJ. Surgical management of toxic dilatation of the colon in ulcerative colitis. Ann Surg 1974; 179(5):647–656.

194. Binder SC, Miller HH, Deterling RA Jr. Emergency and urgent operations for ulcerative colitis. The procedure of choice. Arch Surg 1975; 110(3):284–289.

195. Koudahl G, Kristensen M. Toxic megacolon in ulcerative colitis. Scand J Gastroenterol 1975; 10(4):417–421.
196. Canin-Endres J, Salky B, Gattorno F, Edye M. Laparoscopically assisted intestinal resection in 88 patients with Crohn's disease. Surg Endosc 1999; 13(6):595–599.
197. Milsom JW, Ludwig KA, Church JM, Garcia-Ruiz A. Laparoscopic total abdominal colectomy with ileorectal anastomosis for familial adenomatous polyposis. Dis Colon Rectum 1997; 40(6):675–678.
198. Wong SK MP, Hammerhoffer KA, et al. Laparascopic surgery for Crohn's disease: an analysis of 92 cases. Surg Endosc 1999; 13 (suppl):4.
199. Liu CD, Rolandelli R, Ashley SW, Evans B, Shin M, McFadden DW. Laparoscopic surgery for inflammatory bowel disease. Am Surg 1995; 61(12):1054–1056.
200. Thibault C, Poulin EC. Total laparoscopic proctocolectomy and laparoscopy-assisted proctocolectomy for inflammatory bowel disease: operative technique and preliminary report. Surg Laparosc Endosc 1995; 5(6):472–476.
201. Schmitt SL, Cohen SM, Wexner SD, Nogueras JJ, Jagelman DG. Does laparoscopic-assisted ileal pouch anal anastomosis reduce the length of hospitalization? Int J Colorectal Dis 1994; 9(3):134–137.
202. Young-Fadok TM, HallLong K, McConnell EJ, Gomez Rey G, Cabanela RL. Advantages of laparoscopic resection for ileocolic Crohn's disease. Improved outcomes and reduced costs. Surg Endosc 2001; 15(5):450–454.

28 | Other Colitides: Microscopic Colitis, Eosinophilic Colitis, and Neutropenic Enterocolitis

Gregory D. Olds
Henry Ford Hospital, Detroit, Michigan, U.S.A.

Harry L. Reynolds and Jeffry A. Katz
Case Western Reserve University School of Medicine, University Hospitals of Cleveland, Cleveland, Ohio, U.S.A.

MICROSCOPIC COLITIS

In 1976, Linstrom introduced the term of collagenous colitis while describing a 48-year-old woman with watery diarrhea, normal rectal mucosa on proctoscopy, and a thickened subepithelial collagenous deposit on rectal biopsy (1). The term "microscopic colitis" was subsequently introduced by Read et al. in 1980 while reporting on eight patients with chronic diarrhea, normal endoscopic exam, and increased number of inflammatory cells on colonic biopsy (2). Lazenby et al. proposed replacing the term microscopic colitis with the less ambiguous term of lymphocytic colitis for patients with watery diarrhea and an increased number of intraepithelial lymphocytes on colonic biopsy, but without a thickened subepithelial collagen layer (3). Collagenous and lymphocytic colitis share many clinical and pathologic features. Whether they represent separate diseases or are just different pathologic manifestations of the same disease process is currently not known. For the purpose of this chapter, they will, when considered collectively, be referred to as microscopic colitis.

Epidemiology and Clinical Features

The incidence of collagenous colitis in Europe has been reported to be 1.1 to 1.8 cases per 100,000 inhabitants based upon two population based studies from Sweden and Spain (4,5). A recent study reported a higher incidence of 5.2 per 100,000 inhabitants in Iceland (6). Collagenous colitis, traditionally, has been considered a disease of middle age to elderly females with a male to female ratio of 1:5 to 1:9, and typically presenting in the sixth or seventh decade of life (5–7). However, there are several case reports of collagenous colitis in children and up to 25% of patients may present before the age of 45 (8–11). Lymphocytic colitis has an incidence of 3.1 to 4.0 cases per 100,000 inhabitants (5,6). It usually presents in the seventh decade with a mean age at diagnosis of 65 to 68 years and with a male to female ratio of 1:2.7 to 1:4.4 (5,6). Familial occurrences of both collagenous and lymphocytic colitis have been reported (12–15).

The signature symptom of microscopic colitis is watery, nonbloody diarrhea, with patients averaging five to nine bowel movements per day (11,16–20). When measured, daily stool output has ranged from 135 to 2000 cc, with one study reporting an average of 522 cc daily in 11 patients with collagenous colitis (16,18). Nocturnal diarrhea has been reported in 27% to 68% of patients (11,21). Fecal leukocytes and mild steatorrhea have also been noted (16,18,22).

Abdominal pain is usually mild, occurring in 20% to 80% of patients (11,17,20,21). Weight loss is seen in approximately 40% of patients, and in one study averaged 6 kg (11,20). Nearly one half of patients report a sudden onset of symptoms, while the remainder has an insidious onset (11). Laboratory studies are usually normal, although hypokalemia has been noted in patients with particularly severe diarrhea (11,20). The clinical features of lymphocytic as compared to collagenous colitis do not differ with respect to amount of stool, onset of symptoms, abdominal pain, and weight loss (20).

Many patients with microscopic colitis report rheumatologic and other autoimmune conditions, particularly arthralgias and arthritis (11,20,23). The most frequent associated conditions include celiac disease, rheumatoid arthritis, Sjoegren's syndrome, and autoimmune thyroid disorders (11,20,23). The coexistence of celiac disease with both collagenous and lymphocytic colitis has been demonstrated in multiple case reports (23–25). Large retrospective series on collagenous and lymphocytic colitis have also reported an increased prevalence of celiac disease compared to that seen in the general population, ranging from 3% to 9% (11,20). However, studies that have evaluated small bowel biopsies in patients with microscopic colitis have shown disparate results. In a study by Zins et al., 45 of 172 patients with collagenous colitis had a small bowel biopsy, but only one was noted to have celiac disease (26). In contrast, a smaller series found changes on small bowel biopsy consistent with celiac disease in 4 of 10 patients with collagenous colitis (27). Matteoni et al. reported that 4 of 27 with lymphocytic colitis and zero of 15 patients with collagenous colitis had small bowel biopsies consistent with celiac disease (28). Additionally, antiendomysium and antigliadin antibodies are no more prevalent in patients with collagenous colitis as compared to normal controls, arguing against an etiologic association between celiac disease and collagenous colitis (4).

It has long been known that the administration of rectal gluten enemas to patients with celiac disease elicits rectal inflammation, raising the question of whether gluten sensitivity may play a role in some cases of lymphocytic colitis (29). Two studies have carefully evaluated colonic biopsies in patients with known celiac disease. Wolber et al. reviewed colonic biopsies in 39 patients with documented celiac disease, noting a striking lymphocytic infiltration, histologically indistinguishable from lymphocytic colitis, in the superficial colonic epithelium of 12 patients (30). In contrast, Fine and Lee found colonic lymphocytosis in 19% of patients with untreated celiac disease, although this could be distinguished from lymphocytic colitis by a lack of surface epithelial damage and a lack of increased lamina propria cellularity (31). The same group evaluated patients with celiac disease and continued diarrhea despite a gluten-free diet, and found that 3 of the 11 had microscopic colitis (32).

Thus, although substantial portions of patients with celiac disease have changes on colon biopsy that are histologically consistent with or similar to lymphocytic colitis, the majority of patents with microscopic colitis do not have underlying celiac disease. It remains possible, however, that some cases of microscopic colitis may actually have undiagnosed celiac disease and some authors have recommended that all patients diagnosed with lymphocytic colitis should undergo small bowel biopsy (28). Additionally, colonoscopy should be considered in celiac patients whose diarrhea fails to respond to a gluten-free diet.

Approximately 10% of patients undergoing colonoscopy for the evaluation of diarrhea will be diagnosed with either lymphocytic or collagenous colitis (5,33,34). Although classically a normal colonoscopic exam is demonstrated in patients with microscopic colitis, nonspecific changes such as edema, erythema, and change in vascular pattern have been reported in approximately 30% of patients (11,21).

Microscopic colitis follows a variable clinical course, ranging from complete resolution, either spontaneously or after treatment to chronic intermittent symptoms, to intractable diarrhea unresponsive to medical therapy. The majority of patients in follow-up studies appear to have a benign natural history characterized by resolution of symptoms after a few years with many patients requiring no ongoing therapy. Goff et al. reported that 17 of 27 patients with collagenous colitis had either spontaneous or treatment-related resolution of symptoms at two years' follow-up (35). In another study of lymphocytic colitis, among 17 patients followed up four years after diagnosis, all 17 patients had improvement in symptoms, with 14 having complete resolution of symptoms and only 29% required continued medication (36). Unlike ulcerative colitis and Crohn's disease, patients with microscopic have no apparent increased risk of colon cancer (37).

Histology and Diagnosis

The histologic changes associated with collagenous colitis include both a thickened subepithelial collagen layer and associated mucosal inflammation (Fig. 1) (38,39). The subepithelial collagen layer in normal subjects is usually no greater than three to four μm (39–42). In collagenous colitis the collagen layer has been reported to be as thick as 230 micrometers, although most studies report a mean range of 10 to 20 μm (7,20,38,43,44). Qualitative in addition to quantitative changes

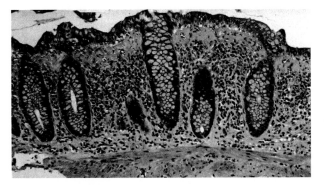

Figure 1 Collagenous colitis: colonic mucosa with prominent subepithelial collagen band. Moderate lamina propria mononuclear cell infiltrate is noted without any crypt distortion. (H&E stain—medium power). *Source*: Courtesy Dr. Joseph E. Willis, Case Western Reserve University School of Medicine, Cleveland, Ohio, U.S.A.

of the collagen layer have also been noted in collagenous colitis. These changes include entrapment of superficial capillaries within the thickened subepithelial collagen layer, along with an irregular border of the collagen layer adjacent to the lamina propria (3,38,39). The thickness of the collagen layer seen in collagenous colitis is usually not uniform throughout the colon, and up to 70% of patients with collagenous colitis may have rectal sparing.

A diagnosis of collagenous colitis also requires the demonstration of mucosal inflammation. An increased mixed inflammatory infiltrate in the lamina propria consisting predominantly of plasma cells and lymphocytes is always present. Additionally, an increase in intra-epithelial lymphocytes, similar to lymphocytic colitis, is often seen (3,38). Tangential section of biopsies may cause the collagen layer to appear artifactually thickened and the diagnosis of collagenous colitis should be questioned when a thickened collagen layer is reported in the absence of mucosal inflammation (39). Surface epithelial damage, manifested by cuboidal or thinned cellular appearance, presence of cytoplasmic vacuoles, decreased mucin and nuclear irregularity is also frequently present (38). With the exception of a thickened abnormal collagen layer, the same mucosal inflammatory features are seen in lymphocytic as in collagenous colitis (Fig. 2A) (3). However, in lymphocytic colitis there are always an increased number of intra-epithelial lymphocytes (Fig.2B). Sequential studies have shown both spontaneous and treatment-related resolution of the histologic changes found in both lymphocytic and collagenous colitis (45).

The histologic changes in both collagenous colitis and lymphocytic colitis can be patchy, with frequent rectal sparing (5,16,26,45,46), and the thickness of the collagen layer and extent of inflammation is usually not uniform throughout the colon (16,20,38,45). There have been reports that the changes of collagenous colitis are more prominent in the proximal colon, although in some studies this has not been the case (16,38,43). Rectal biopsy may be normal in some patients with collagenous colitis (5,26,43,45), however, when biopsies from both the rectum and sigmoid are obtained, a diagnosis can be made in 66% to 95% of cases (26,43). If the entire left colon is sampled, the yield increases to 82% to 97% (26,35,45). Therefore, in a large majority of cases the diagnosis can be made by flexible sigmoidoscopy as long as an

(A)   **(B)**

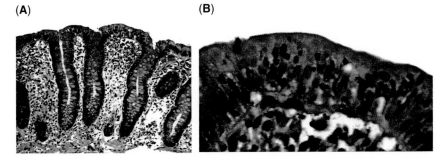

Figure 2 **(A)** Lymphocytic colitis: colonic mucosa with prominent intra-epithelial lymphocytosis. (H&E stain—medium power). **(B)** Lymphocytic colitis: multiple intra-epithelial lymphocytes on colonic surface epithelium. (H&E stain—high power). *Source*: Courtesy Dr. Joseph E. Willis, Case Western Reserve University School of Medicine, Cleveland, Ohio, U.S.A.

effort is made to obtain biopsies from the descending colon in addition to the rectum and sigmoid. If not done initially, colonoscopy should be considered when biopsies from the left colon are nondiagnostic and a clinical concern remains.

Etiology and Pathogenesis

Several theories regarding the etiology of the microscopic colitides and the underlying mechanism of diarrhea have been postulated. To date, no clear etiology has been determined, and the histologic pattern observed may represent nonspecific changes due to a variety of different etiologies.

Whether certain individuals are genetically prone to developing these diseases, is not clear, and studies of human leukocyte antigen (HLA) class I and II association have yielded conflicting results. Giardiello et al. reported an increased frequency of HLA-A1 and a decreased frequency of HLA-A3 in patients with lymphocytic colitis compared with normal controls. No HLA class II association was seen, and no difference in HLA class I or II frequency was noted in patients with collagenous colitis compared to controls (47). However, others have reported an increased frequency of HLA DQ2 (HLA class II antigen highly associated with celiac disease) in a mixed population of patients with either collagenous or lymphocytic colitis (48).

Diversion of the fecal stream has lead to a regression of the histologic abnormalities seen in collagenous colitis, suggesting that a noxious luminal factor may play a role in the etiology of the microscopic colitis (49). Potential noxious substances could include dietary factors, bacterial toxins, or unabsorbed bile salts. Bile salt malabsorption has been postulated to have a potential role in the pathogenesis of collagenous colitis (50,51). One study found that 44% of patients with collagenous colitis had bile salt malabsorption based upon 23-selena-25-homocholyltaurine testing, with nearly all patients improving with cholestyramine therapy (50). However, a follow-up study at a median of 4.2 years showed no histologic improvement in the patients who had continued cholestyramine therapy, calling into question the etiologic role of bile salts (52).

It is well established that Nonsteroidal anti-inflammatory drugs (NSAIDs) can cause inflammatory changes in the colonic mucosa (53). Previous reports have suggested a link between NSAIDs and collagenous colitis, including a case-control study that reported NSAIDs use was significantly more frequent in patients with collagenous colitis as compared to age matched controls (54,55). However, as already noted arthralgias and other rheumatologic conditions are also more common in patients with collagenous colitis, and whether NSAIDs are truly causative in some cases of collagenous colitis or just a surrogate for arthritic conditions remains unknown (11,20,23). Other medications implicated as potential causes of lymphocytic or collagenous colitis include lansoprazole, ticlopidine, ranitidine, simvastatin, and acarbose (11,56–61).

In collagenous colitis, the thickened collagen layer has been shown to be primarily type VI collagen and tenascin (62). The pericryptal subepithelial myofibroblast sheath is a population of mesenchymal cells in close association with the colonic epithelium. It has been suggested that a disorder of this pericryptal myofibroblast sheath may play a causative role in the accumulation of excessive collagen, perhaps via collagen overproduction (44,63). However, type VI collagen messenger ribonucleic acid expression is not increased in collagenous colitis compared to normal controls, suggesting that the thickened collagen layer is formed not by an increased production of collagen but by a decreased breakdown (62).

The mechanism of diarrhea in microscopic colitis is unknown. The thickened collagen layer may represent a barrier to water and electrolyte absorption thereby contributing at least in part to the diarrhea seen in collagenous colitis (1). However, most studies have shown that the degree of thickening does not correlate with the severity of diarrhea (16,40). Additionally, the presence of diarrhea despite the lack of thickened collagen layer in lymphocytic colitis argues against this being the primary cause. Colonic perfusion studies have shown decreased colonic fluid absorption in patients with microscopic colitis as a result of reduced passive and active transport of sodium and chloride and reduced bicarbonate and chloride exchange (64). This has been supported by a recent report citing reduced sodium and chloride absorption as the primary diarrheal mechanism in collagenous colitis, with some contribution of decreased absorption due to the thickened collagenous band (65). Active secretion of chloride ions and passive back leak of sodium and chloride into the intestinal lumen due to tight junction defects have also been implicated in the etiology of diarrhea in microscopic colitis (65).

Treatment

The first step in treating microscopic colitis is the withdrawal of any medication with a possible link to the illness, especially NSAIDs and ticlopidine. Caffeine avoidance may be prudent, although no data exist to support this recommendation (19). Antidiarrheal agents have traditionally been first-line therapy, which is appropriate, given the benign course of disease and the safety profile afforded by medications such as loperamide. In a retrospective study of 163 patients with collagenous colitis, loperamide 4 mg three times per day was effective in controlling diarrhea for 49/69 patients (11).

For those patients in whom antidiarrheals fail, bismuth subsalicylate (BSS) is often an effective therapy. A prospective open-label trial of BSS at a dose of eight 262 mg tablets per day for eight weeks reported resolution of diarrhea in all but one patient. Nine of the 12 patients remained free of diarrhea off treatment at follow-up intervals that ranged from 7 to 28 months (31). In a subsequent double blind, randomized, placebo controlled trial of 14 patients with microscopic colitis, all patients receiving BSS reported decreased stool frequency. About five of 7 patients who had not improved with placebo therapy were able to achieve remission when crossed over to active BSS (66).

Cholestyramine has also been used with success in patients with collagenous colitis. A prospective study reported, cholestyramine at a median dose of 10 g per day led to a marked or complete control of symptoms in 77% of patients, including 10 patients who had no evidence of bile acid malabsorption (50). However, cholestyramine is often poorly tolerated and many patients who initially respond, later discontinue therapy due to medication side effects (52).

5-aminosalicylates such as sulfasalazine and mesalamine are frequently used in the treatment of microscopic colitis; however, efficacy data comes only from retrospective studies. In the largest single series reporting treatment for collagenous colitis, sulfasalazine was effective in 37 of 108 (34%) patients and mesalamine in 8 of 16 (50%) (11). A review of all cases with collagenous colitis in the literature prior to 1995 reported a 66% clinical response to sulfasalazine and a 92% response to mesalamine (26). Therefore, despite the lack of prospective data, given the relative safety of these medications it is reasonable to attempt a trial of a 5-aminosalicylate, after conservative therapy has failed.

Although corticosteroids have been reported to be efficacious in the treatment of collagenous colitis, symptoms often return shortly after cessation of therapy, and side effects generally limit their long-term usage (67). Corticosteroid use is reserved for patients who have failed 5-aminosalicylic acid, bismuth, and antidiarrheal therapy. Some patients with chronic symptoms may become steroid dependent; azathioprine may allow for steroid withdrawal in this small group of patients (68). Budesonide, a topically acting corticosteroid with greatly decreased systemic bioavailability compared to traditional corticosteroids, has also been used in the treatment of microscopic colitis. A double-blind placebo controlled trial in patients with collagenous colitis reported that 8/14 patients had a clinical response to 9 mg of budesonide at eight weeks of therapy compared to only 3 of 14 patients receiving placebo. A subsequent larger trial of the same dose for only six weeks reported an 87% response with budesonide compared to 14% with placebo (69). Despite these encouraging results, when budesonide is tapered off over eight weeks, relapse is common (70). Therefore, budesonide should be considered in place of systemic corticosteroids in patients who have failed conservative therapy, although the optimal dose and duration of budesonide therapy has yet to be determined. Studies with longer follow-up and with prolonged therapy at lower maintenance doses may help clarify these questions.

Octreotide has been reported to control diarrhea in a single patient with refractory collagenous colitis (71). As a last resort, proctocolectomy or fecal diversion with an ileostomy has been used successfully in selective patients with severe disease refractory to medical therapy (49,68,72). In these cases, laparoscopic stoma creation may be the preferred approach.

EOSINOPHILIC COLITIS

Eosinophilic gastroenteritis is an infiltrative disease of unknown etiology that can involve the entire gastrointestinal tract. First described by Kaijser in 1937 (73), eosinophilic gastroenteritis is not likely a single disease entity, but rather a collection of disorders with similar clinico-pathologic features. Eosinophilic gastroenteritis most commonly involves the stomach and proximal small bowel, causing symptoms of postprandial nausea, vomiting, watery diarrhea, and weight loss (74). Peripheral eosinophilia occurs in approximately 25% of cases (75). Eosinophilic tissue infiltration localized to the colon, or eosinophilic colitis, appears to be a relatively rare disorder, with around 100 descriptions in the literature limited to case reports and small case series (76–88). Some have suggested that eosinophilic colitis may be underdiagnosed, with colonic involvement being overlooked in the face of prominent upper gastrointestinal symptoms and malabsorption (83).

Epidemiology and Clinical Features

Eosinophilic colitis affects men and women equally, with an age range from infants to the elderly. A careful review of 22 histologically proven cases of eosinophilic colitis reported a mean age of 41 years (85). Symptoms depend upon which part of the colon is involved with the illness. Mucosal and submucosal involvement causes typical colitic symptoms with diarrhea, cramps, and bleeding. Involvement of the muscle layer produces symptoms of bowel obstruction, particularly when the ileocolic region is involved, which may lead to an inaccurate diagnosis of Crohn's disease (77,86–88). Serosal involvement appears to be quite rare, but can cause eosinophilic ascites (79). As shown in Table 1, most patients present with relatively nonspecific symptoms. Over half of the reported patients with eosinophilic colitis have abdominal pain, diarrhea, nausea and vomiting, and weight loss, and between 20% and 25% will have blood in the stools and/or a palpable mass (85). The cecum and ascending colon are most commonly involved, followed by diffuse colonic involvement; isolated left colonic eosinophilic inflammation is rare (85,89). A predilection for involvement of the ileocecal region has been noted and may be confused with Crohn's disease (77,86–88). A single case report of eosinophilic colitis and perianal fistulous disease exists (78). Patients have also presented with colonic perforation and colonic intussusception (90,91).

Peripheral eosinophilia has been reported in between 25% and 50% of cases (75,85). The degree of peripheral eosinophilia has no relation to disease extent, severity, or prognosis. However, if elevated prior to the initiation of therapy, fluctuations in the peripheral eosinophil count can mirror improvement in clinical symptoms during treatment and can help guide medical therapy over time (92). Other laboratory findings are nonspecific. Mild to moderate anemia is often noted, along with decreases in serum albumin and total protein levels. Interestingly, the erythrocyte sedimentation rate often remains normal even in the presence of active disease (88). When ascites is present, eosinophilia in the ascitic fluid is often striking (77,79). Eosinophils and Charcot-Leyden crystals can be found on stool examination (82,92), but not in all cases (83). Immunoglobulin E (IgE) levels are generally normal, but are occasionally elevated (75,83,87,93).

The endoscopic findings in eosinophilic colitis are nonspecific, resembling the findings seen in other causes of chronic colitis. The mucosa may show focal areas of mucosal erythema, granularity, edema, and hemorrhage (83). The colon may also appear nodular and friable (83,94,95). Superficial shallow mucosal ulcers and erosions have been reported, but are not universal (83,87,89), and 1 to 2 mm hemorrhagic mucosal blebs have been described (96). The colon may also appear endoscopically normal, with eosinophilic tissue infiltration only evident on histologic examination (97).

A variety of colonic radiographic abnormalities have been reported with eosinophilic colitis, but none are diagnostic. Many barium enema findings have been reported in association with eosinophilic enterocolitis, with changes that can be indistinguishable from Crohn's disease (89). Strictures (86), rigid and fixed ileocecal valve with terminal ileal reflux (86,87),

Table 1 Presenting Symptoms in Patients with Eosinophilic Colitis

Symptom	Frequency
Abdominal pain	Common
Diarrhea	Common
Nausea/vomiting/weight loss	Common
Palpable mass	Occasional
Bleeding per rectum	Occasional

Source: From Ref. 85.

ulcerations (78), filling defects and polypoid lesions (80) have all been reported. It has been suggested that a stiff, rigid and fixed-open ileocecal valve can be used to differentiate eosinophilic enterocolitis from Crohn's disease (87). On rare occasions, eosinophilic colitis may present with an obstructing cecal mass (98) or an "applecore" lesion on barium enema suggesting colonic carcinoma (80). On computed tomography (CT), hyperenhancement of the outer bowel wall layers has been noted due to serosal and muscularis eosinophilic infiltration (99).

In the review of Naylor and Pollett, two-thirds of cases of eosinophilic colitis required laparotomy for diagnosis; five were performed to exclude carcinoma, four for presumed appendicitis, and three for unremitting symptoms despite medical treatment (85). With greater recognition of the syndrome and its clinical feature and more widespread use of colonoscopy, it is likely that eosinophilic colitis will be more frequently diagnosed preoperatively (89).

Histology and Diagnosis

Although the presence of peripheral eosinophilia or Charcot-Leyden crystals in the stool may serve as clues to the diagnosis of eosinophilic colitis, the clinical presentation is typically nonspecific and the diagnosis is often only made after histologic evaluation. Tissue infiltration with eosinophils and edema are the striking histologic features of eosinophilic colitis (Fig. 3) (75,76), and a chronic inflammatory cell infiltrate is typically also present (82,92). The degree of these findings varies significantly within and between cases of eosinophilic colitis, and tends to be less dense than that found with eosinophilic gastritis or eosinophilic enteritis. Instead of the normal distribution of eosinophils in the upper lamina propria, clusters or sheets of eosinophils are typically seen deeper in the epithelium (100). In eosinophilic colitis the colonic crypts are preserved. Although the whole thickness of the bowel may be involved, the mucosa often shows only a modest increase in eosinophils, compared to the more marked infiltration typically seen in the submucosa (75). In some cases of primarily muscle layer and serosal involvement by eosinophilic colitis, mucosal biopsies obtained at colonoscopy are entirely normal and laparotomy may be necessary for diagnosis (79). Associated lymph nodes may be engorged with eosinophils, but are otherwise structurally normal. Arteritis is not present, and perivascular eosinophilia is not typically prominent (76). The degree of tissue eosinophilia does not appear to be related to the number of eosinophils in the peripheral blood (75,88).

The differential diagnosis of eosinophilic colitis falls into two distinct categories: diseases associated with peripheral eosinophilia along with eosinophilic tissue infiltration, and diseases that mimic eosinophilic colitis clinically and radiologically and have a more mild to moderate increase in mucosal eosinophils (Table 2). Hypereosinophilic syndrome presents with very high peripheral eosinophilia and usually infiltration of multiple other organs besides the gastrointestinal tract. In the gut, involvement is usually diffuse, but isolated colonic involvement has been reported (101,102). Collagen vascular diseases, including polyarteritis nodosa, scleroderma, and eosinophilic fasciitis may be associated with peripheral eosinophilia, abdominal pain, diarrhea, and colonic eosinophilia (103–105). Clouse et al. described 10 patients with pericryptal eosinophilic colitis, chronic watery diarrhea, normal endoscopic evaluation, and collagen vascular disease (106). Biopsies revealed an eosinophilic

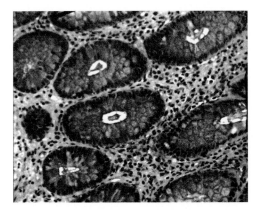

Figure 3 Eosinophilic colitis: eosinophilic infiltrate into colonic lamina propria. (H&E stain—medium power). *Source*: Courtesy Dr. Joseph E. Willis.

Table 2 Differential Diagnosis of Colonic Mucosal Eosinophilia

Crohn's disease
Ulcerative colitis
Infectious colitis with helminthes or ameba
Allergic colitis due to food or medications
Collagen vascular disease
Hypereosinophilic syndrome
Lymphoma
Colonic adenoma
Carcinoma

cellular infiltrate deep in the mucosa, separating crypt bases from the muscularis mucosae (105,106). Peripheral eosinophilia was present in four patients, and in seven patients, diarrhea improved with corticosteroid treatment. Symptom improvement correlated with histological changes, including resolution of the pericrypt eosinophilia, suggesting that chronic diarrhea was directly related to the presence of increased eosinophils.

Intestinal parasitism is another cause of peripheral eosinophilia and gastrointestinal symptoms, including pain and diarrhea. Eosinophilic colitis has been associated with the "herring worm" *Eustoma rotundatum* (107), the pinworm *Eustoma rotundatum* (108), the eggs of *Trichuris trichura* and an *Oxyuris* parasite (85), and the protozoa *Dientamoeba fragilis* (109).

Conditions presenting with nonspecific clinical or radiologic findings similar to those of eosinophilic colitis and also showing mild or moderate tissue eosinophilia include Crohn's disease, ulcerative colitis, allergic colitis, lymphoma, colonic adenomas and carcinoma. The differentiation of these conditions from eosinophilic colitis is usually made based on clinical characteristics specific to each diagnosis. As noted earlier, it may be quite difficult to distinguish ileocolic Crohn's disease from eosinophilic ileocolitis (77,86,88). Although there exists no definitive quantitative histologic measure relating tissue eosinophils to eosinophilic colitis, significantly fewer eosinophils are usually seen in inflammatory bowel disease. In eosinophilic colitis, eosinophils have been estimated at a density of 17 to 60 per high-power field; while in a small sample of Crohn's disease patients the density of colonic eosinophils has been estimated to average eight per high-power field (82,87,91). Thus, the marked increase in density of tissue eosinophils best distinguishes eosinophilic colitis from other colonic diseases with similar clinical presentations.

Etiology and Pathogenesis

The etiology of eosinophilic colitis is not well defined and the pathogenesis is poorly understood. Since its initial description (76), eosinophilic colitis has been assumed to be an allergic disorder in some patients, but not consistently so (75). Naylor and Pollet reported a history of allergic reactions in 7 of 22 (32%) (85). In two patients symptoms were clearly exacerbated by drugs or food ingestion. As mentioned earlier, elevated serum IgE, often associated with allergy, has been an inconsistent finding in eosinophilic colitis (75,83,87,93). Although specific correlation with food allergy has been described (110), sequential withdrawal of various food substances often fails to provide sustained symptom relief (111).

In the pediatric population, particularly infants between 2 to 16 weeks in age, eosinophilic colitis is more clearly an allergic inflammation of the gut. The offending allergen is typically cow's milk, although up to 35% of infants who are allergic to cow's mild develop an allergy to soy formula as well (112). Eosinophilic colitis has also been reported within one to two days of birth in exclusively breast-fed neonates; in these children transplacental sensitization of the colon to cow's milk antigens has been hypothesized (113–115). Compared to adults, infants more commonly present with hematochezia, with diarrhea being significantly less common, occurring in just 14% of cases in one series (116). These children typically improve with milk avoidance and substitution of soy or hydrolyzed formulas. The peripheral eosinophil count may remain elevated for weeks, despite clinical improvement (113).

Eosinophilic colitis has been associated with a number of different drugs and an offending medication should be considered in the differential diagnosis of all cases. In addition to their association with collagenous colitis (54), NSAIDs have also been reported in association with eosinophilic colitis (117). Other medications reported to cause eosinophilic colitis include carbamazepine (118), rifampicin (119), and gold sodium thiomalate (92). Most patients with medication induced eosinophilic colitis have peripheral eosinophilia. Stopping the offending medication generally results in prompt clinical improvement.

Whatever the underlying cause of eosinophilic infiltration of the bowel, it is the presence of eosinophils and the associated inflammation that leads to gastrointestinal symptoms (102,120). The major role of eosinophils in the gut is homeostasis and modulation of inflammation (74). Eosinophils can cause tissue damage through both cellular and antibody-dependent cytotoxicity. In addition, a large number of enzymes are found in eosinophilic granules, including major basic protein (MBP) and eosinophilic cationic protein (ECP), and are capable of tissue damage. Secretion and release of MBP into the surrounding tissue cause direct cytotoxicity; ECP has been reported to activate the coagulation system (102). Monoclonal antibody and immunohistochemical studies show that the eosinophils in eosinophilic gastroenteritis are activated and degranulated, and thus can directly contribute to tissue injury (102,120). Activated eosinophils and deposition of MBP have been identified in ulcerated colonic tissue in eosinophilic colitis (102), again supporting a direct role for eosinophils in tissue injury.

Recently, interleukin (IL) 5 has been reported to enhance activation, degranulation, differentiation, and proliferation of eosinophils, and has been implicated in the pathogenesis of hypereosinophilic syndrome (121,122). IL-5 may be derived from activated T-cells, mast cells, or eosinophils themselves (102). A case report has documented elevated serum IL-5 levels in a patient with hypereosinophilic syndrome and eosinophilic colitis, which fell to undetectable after steroid therapy (102). Serum-soluble IL 2 receptor levels may also be increased in eosinophilic syndromes (123).

Treatment

Treatment of eosinophilic colitis depends upon the underlying etiology. In cases of allergic eosinophilic colitis in infants, discontinuation of milk and substitution with noncasein formulas for feedings results in prompt improvement. Likewise, if an offending medication is suspected to have caused the eosinophilic colitis, discontinuation of the drug typically produces rapid benefit. Cases related to the hypereosinophilic syndrome will require systemic chemotherapy, with both hydroxyurea and cyclophosphamide being used successfully (101,124).

Most cases of eosinophilic colitis, however, are idiopathic and treatment is directed at suppression of immune-mediated colonic inflammation. Although most cases were treated surgically in earlier reports (75,76), the diagnosis of eosinophilic colitis is now typically made endoscopically and medical therapy is the mainstay of treatment. Most patients will respond rapidly to systemic corticosteroids, with doses of prednisone between 20 and 40 mg producing dramatic improvement within 48 hours (77,83,85,88,89,106). Seven to 10 days of therapy is often sufficient and most patients are able to taper off of steroids over several weeks. Although relapses are common, they typically respond to reinstitution of steroid therapy (85,89). Budesonide has been used to successfully treat eosinophilic gastroenteritis (125), but no reports of its use in eosinophilic colitis exist. Based on the pharmacokinetics of budesonide and its successful use in both Crohn's disease and microscopic colitis, one would expect it to be efficacious in eosinophilic ileocolitis. Sulfasalazine has also been effective (86,87). While no reports of mesalamine therapy for eosinophilic colitis exist, one would again expect it to be helpful in controlling disease symptoms (106). Immunomodulators, such as azathioprine, have been used as steroid sparing agents.

Therapies aimed at interrupting an allergic response within the gut have been tried as treatment for eosinophilic colitis. Several patients have responded to treatment with ketotifen, an H1 class of antihistamine that stabilizes mast cells and possibly impairs eosinophil migration to target organs (82,84,126). Oral cromolyn sodium, another mast cell stabilizer, has also been used (92). Some reports suggest that the selective leukotriene receptor antagonist montelukast can maintain prednisone remission in eosinophilic gastroenteritis (127); other reports show only an effect on peripheral eosinophilia without improvement in gastrointestinal symptoms (128).

Most cases of eosinophilic colitis improve with medical therapy and fatalities are extremely rare (129). For patients with persistent symptoms despite steroid therapy, steroid dependence, or severe steroid side effects, surgical resection of the involved bowel may be required, with resolved symptoms in most patients (85). Postoperative recurrence of eosinophilic ileocolitis requiring medical therapy has been reported (86).

NEUTROPENIC ENTEROCOLITIS

Neutropenic enterocolitis (NEC) is a syndrome of inflammatory changes of the intestine most frequently associated with cytotoxic chemotherapy and hematologic malignancies. A variety of terms have been used to describe NEC, including neutropenic colitis, ileocecal syndrome, necrotizing colitis, necrotizing enteropathy, and typhlitis (130). First reported in 1933 as appendiceal perforation, leukemic infiltration, and subserosal hemorrhage in association with leukemia (131), there have since been multiple reports of necrotizing lesions of the colon and small bowel in association with neutropenia occurring during treatment of hematologic malignancies and solid tumors. As the pathophysiology of NEC remains uncertain, the best treatment continues to be debated. A rational approach to the management of this life-threatening condition based upon a careful review of the available literature is presented here.

Epidemiology and Clinical Features

Occurring in both adults and children, NEC typically presents during or soon after intensive chemotherapy for hematologic malignancies; less frequently it occurs with chemotherapy for solid organ malignancies. Rarely NEC presents with primary marrow failure in patients with aplastic anemia, cyclic neutropenia, multiple myeloma, or HIV (132–137). It has also been described following solid organ transplantation (138). Vincristine, cytosine arabinoside and prednisone have been implicated as agents predisposing to NEC in a number of articles, however, multiple other agents and combination chemotherapy have also been associated with the development of NEC (139–141).

The precise incidence of NEC is uncertain, in part due to differing definitions of NEC used in the literature, and in part due to the lack of pathologic confirmation in many patients managed without surgical resection. Likewise, confusion with chemotherapy-induced diarrhea and pseudomembranous colitis can make diagnosis difficult. Mower estimated the incidence to be 2.6% (13 of 499) in a series of adults treated for acute leukemia (142), while Shamberger et al. reported a 32% (25/77) incidence in children with myelogenous leukemia (143). The universal initiating factor is neutropenia, with neutrophil counts typically less than $500/mm^3$, and NEC may recur with repeated cycles of chemotherapy (144,145).

The spectrum of disease presentation is wide, but typical presenting symptoms include fever, nausea, vomiting, diarrhea, and abdominal pain. Pain may be either diffuse or localized to the site of involvement. The diarrhea may be grossly bloody. Gomez reported fever, pain, and diarrhea in nearly all of their 29 patients with NEC (144). Stool was grossly bloody in about half of the patients, and two-thirds had nausea and/or vomiting.

Physical exam typically reveals an ill appearing, febrile patient, often with obvious sepsis and hypotension present. The abdomen may be distended, with diffuse or point tenderness, and signs of localized or diffuse peritonitis. However, in these immunocompromised patients, the abdominal examination can also be remarkably benign, despite significant intra-abdominal pathology. Fullness may be palpable in the right lower quadrant (130). The duration of neutropenia prior to development of symptoms is typically 7 to 10 days and a white blood cell count of $< 500/mm^3$ is expected (144). Patients are often pancytopenic as well, with low platelet counts contributing to the increased risk of gastrointestinal bleeding.

Plain films of the abdomen are frequently nonspecific, but may show bowel thickening or thumbprinting (Fig. 4). Free air or pneumatosis coli may also be present and are indications for surgical intervention. CT provides more useful information in securing a diagnosis and guiding therapy of NEC. Common findings include bowel wall thickening, inflammatory changes, intramural air, free air, or free intra-abdominal fluid (Fig. 5) (146). Ultrasound has also been described as useful in the evaluation of patients with NEC, particularly for identifying bowel wall thickening or free intra-abdominal fluid in children (147).

Endoscopic evaluation of the colon in patients with NEC has generally been avoided for fear of inducing hemorrhage or perforation. However, limited sigmoidoscopic evaluation may be useful for excluding other potentially confounding diagnoses, including Clostridia difficile colitis, ischemic colitis, or graft versus host disease (89,148,149). Peritoneal lavage may be

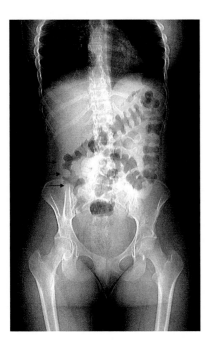

Figure 4 Plain radiograph of the abdomen in a patient with neutropenic enterocolitis demonstrating mucosal edema and "thumbprinting" (*arrows*) in the ascending colon. *Source*: Courtesy. Dr. Elmar Merkle, Duke University School of Medicine, Durham, North Carolina, U.S.A.

useful for demonstrating free perforation (150). Likewise, in equivocal cases, diagnostic laparoscopy may be useful in determining if an abdominal catastrophe has occurred (151).

Histology and Diagnosis

The pathologic spectrum of disease is wide, with findings ranging from mild edema to transmural necrosis. Histologic evaluation may show edema, ulceration, varying degrees of necrosis, focal hemorrhage, chronic inflammatory infiltrates, absent acute inflammatory cells, and rarely leukemic infiltrates (89,132,149,152). Secondary infection with host flora is thought to play a role in furthering tissue necrosis. Organisms reported in NEC associated sepsis include alpha-hemolytic *Streptococcus*, *Bacteroides*, *C. difficile*, *Clostridia perfringens*, *Clostridia septicum*, *Escherichia coli*, *Enterococcus faecium*, *Enterobacter*, *Klebsiella*, *Pseudomonas*, *Candida*, and Cytomegalovirus (89,132–134,138,144,149,152–156).

Etiology and Pathogenesis

NEC has a predisposition for involving the terminal ileum, appendix, and cecum. NEC is thought to originate from a mucosal injury, which predisposes the patient to secondary bacterial, viral or fungal infection with subsequent translocation, and the potential for systemic

(A)　　　　　　　　　　　　　**(B)**

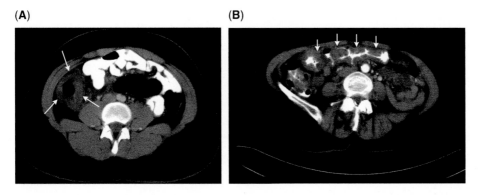

Figure 5 (**A** and **B**) Abdominal computed tomography in a patient with neutropenic enterocolitis demonstrating marked thickening of the colonic wall in the cecum (**A**) (*arrows*) and cecum, ascending, and transverse colon (**B**) (*arrows*). *Source*: Courtesy. Dr. Elmar Merkle, Duke Unversity School of Medicine, Durham, North Carolina, U.S.A.

sepsis. Mucosal injury may result from direct tissue damage due to chemotherapeutic agents, infiltration of the mucosa by lymphomatous or leukemic cells, necrosis of mural leukemic infiltrates, submucosal hemorrhage secondary to thrombocytopenia, fecal stasis with mucosal erosion, instrumentation-induced mucosal injury, or ischemia from sepsis-induced hypotension (89,132,157,158).

Treatment

Optimal management of NEC is controversial, with most treatment recommendations based on case reports or small case series. Some authors advocate initial medical therapy, while others have argued for early surgical intervention. Table 3 summarizes the available data

Table 3 Medical and Surgical Management of Neutropenic Enterocolitis

References	Year	Number	Medical management (N)	Medical management death	Surgical management (N)	Surgical management death
Sherman and Woolley (157)	1973	11	8	8	3	1
Rasmussen and Freeman (159)	1975	2	0	0	2	0
Matolo et al. (160)	1976	8	1	1	7	7
Kies et al. (161)	1979	2	0	0	2	0
Varki et al. (162)	1979	1	0	0	1	0
Lea et al. (163)	1980	2	0	0	2	0
Lehman and Armitage (164)	1980	2	0	0	2	0
Pokorney et al. (134)	1980	1	0	0	1	0
Dworkin et al. (148)	1981	1	1	0	0	0
Ikard (165)	1981	1	0	0	1	0
Abramson et al. (152)	1983	5	1	0	4	1
Gandy and Greenberg (166)	1983	2	2	0	0	0
Schaller and Schaller (167)	1983	3	0	0	3	1
Mulholland and Delaney (132)	1983	4	2	0	2	2
Shaked et al. (168)	1983	2	1	0	1	1
Alt et al. (133)	1985	2	0	0	2	0
Kunkel and Rosenthal (155)	1986	8	2	2	6	3
Moir et al. (169)	1986	16	10	5	6	2
Mower et al. (142)	1986	13	5	5	8	0
Shamberger et al. (143)	1986	25[a]	21	1	6	1
Starnes et al. (153)	1986	23	22	7	1	0
Villar et al. (170)	1987	19	15	14	4	1
Skibber et al. (171)	1987	16	3	3	13	1
O'Brien et al. (172)	1987	7	7	0	0	0
Baniel et al. (173)	1988	3	1	0	2	1
Koea and Shaw (174)	1989	3	0	0	3	0
Merine et al. (175)	1989	1	1	0	0	0
Sauter et al. (150)	1990	3	3	0	0	0
Frankel et al. (138)	1991	1	0	0	1	0
Cutrona et al. (176)	1991	2	2	0	0	0
Chakravarty et al. (177)	1992	1	0	0	1	1
Wade et al. (139)	1992	22	16	11	6	3
Vohra et al. (178)	1992	3	0	0	3	1
Or et al. (179)	1992	1	1	1	0	0
Winberger et al. (180)	1993	2	0	0	2	0
Chubachi et al. (181)	1993	1	1	0	0	0
Bajwa et al. (182)	1993	1	1	1	0	0
Dudiak (183)	1993	1	1	0	0	0
Coleman et al. (184)	1993	1	0	0	1	0
Anderson (185)	1993	1	0	0	1	0
Suarez et al. (186)	1995	1	1	0	0	0
Stein et al. (187)	1995	1	1	1	0	0
Gomez et al. (144)	1998	28[b]	29	8	0	0
Totals		253	159	68(43%)	97	27(28%)

[a]27 episodes in 25 patients.
[b]29 episodes in 28 patients.
Source: From Ref. 130.

comparing both medical and surgical management of NEC. No clear conclusion regarding the superiority of medical or surgical therapy can be made from this analysis. The tabulated data suggest a potentially better outcome in the surgically treated group (28% surgical mortality vs. 43% medical mortality), however, the groups are not comparable, and it is likely that many in the medical group were more debilitated and deemed unfit for surgery (130). Most recent series have suggested a selective approach tailored to the specific clinical situation of the individual patient and have emphasized a sequential management algorithm with medical management initially followed by prompt surgical intervention in those patients that fail or have obvious abdominal catastrophes (89,130,139,143,144,169,188).

Evaluation of these immunocompromised, extremely fragile patients can be difficult, and cooperative management with both the surgical and medical oncology teams is essential in ensuring optimal care. In patients who show no clear signs of free perforation, abscess, life-threatening hemorrhage, obstruction, or intestinal necrosis, initial management may be nonsurgical (169). Clinical decision making is complicated by the fact that a relatively benign abdomen may harbor an occult perforation (150). Likewise, an exam suggesting perforation and peritonitis may reveal negative findings at laparotomy (188). Medical therapy consists in keeping the patient nil per os and administering broad spectrum antibiotics and parenteral nutrition (139). Some reports have used granulocyte colony stimulating factor and white blood cell transfusion, though their efficacy is uncertain (144,169,172). Serial abdominal exams and follow-up abdominal CT are essential in guiding patient management and determining the need for surgical intervention. Patients developing obvious radiologic signs of perforation or necrosis, life-threatening hemorrhage, or obstruction should be considered for surgery. Some authors have suggested that NEC presenting during induction of chemotherapy should be handled more aggressively, with earlier surgical intervention, than those with end-stage malignancies not responding to chemotherapy, who would have a poor prognosis regardless of intervention (139).

Patients with an obvious intra-abdominal catastrophe, such as a perforated viscous clear peritonitis, or evidence of full-thickness necrosis should be surgically explored. Patients with a worsening abdominal exam or signs of progressive sepsis despite appropriate medical therapy should also be considered for laparotomy, or laparoscopy in equivocal cases. Likewise, patients in whom appendicitis cannot be ruled out should be considered for laparoscopy. Life-threatening hemorrhage localized to a specific colonic segment may also be an indication for surgical intervention, particularly if bleeding persists after correction of coagulopathy and platelet transfusion. Most authors recommend resection of all compromised intestine and creation of a diverting stoma. Typically this would involve a right colectomy with end ileostomy and mucous fistula or long Hartmann's pouch. Primary anastomosis should be avoided in these frequently malnourished, immunocompromised, critically ill patients (170,188). In neutropenic patients with apparent appendicitis, right hemicolectomy instead of appendectomy should be performed, as the extent of mucosal necrosis may not be apparent at initial laparotomy (155,171,173). In a small report, 2/8 neutropenic patients who died after appendectomy were found at autopsy to have cecal necrosis, which was not apparent at initial laparotomy (155). Certainly, in neutropenic patients with suspected appendicitis, careful attention must be paid to the cecum for subtle signs of necrosis, and a right hemicolectomy should be performed if there is any question of compromise. In patients with NEC who recover with medical therapy, some authors have recommended elective resection in those who need further chemotherapy (145).

REFERENCES

1. Lindstrom CG. "Collagenous colitis" with watery diarrhoea—a new entity? Path Europ 1976; 11: 87–89.
2. Read NW, Krejs GJ, Read MG, Santa Ana CA, Moraski SG, Fordtran JS. Chronic diarrhea of unknown origin. Gastroenterology 1980; 78:264–271.
3. Lazenby AJ, Yardley JH, Giardiello FM, Jessurun J, Bayless TM. Lymphocytic ("microscopic") colitis: a comparative histopathologic study with particular reference to collagenous colitis. Hum Pathol 1989; 20:18–28.
4. Bohr J, Tysk C, Eriksson S, Abrahamsson H, Jarnerot G. Collagenous colitis: a retrospective study of clinical presentation and treatment in 163 patients. Gut 1996; 39(96):846–851.

5. Fernandez-Banares F, Salas A, Forne M, Esteve M, Espinos J, Viver JM. Incidence of collagenous and lymphocytic colitis: a 5-year population-based study. Am J Gastroenterol 1999; 94:418–423.

6. Agnarsdottir M, Gunnlaugsson O, Orvar KB, et al. Collagenous and lymphocytic colitis in Iceland. Dig Dis Sci 2002; 47:1122–1128.

7. Bohr J, Tysk C, Eriksson S, Jarnerot G. Collagenous colitis in Oregro, Sweden, an epidemiological study 1984–1993. Gut 1995; 37:394–397.

8. Gremse DA, Boudreaux CW, Manci EA. Collagenous colitis in children. Gastroenterology 1993; 104:906–909.

9. Perisic VN, Kokai G. Diarrhoea caused by collagenous colitis. Arch Dis Child 1989; 64:867–869.

10. Busittil A. Collagenous colitis in a child. Am J Dis Child 1989; 143:998–1000.

11. Bohr J, Tysk C, Eriksson S, Abrahamsson H, Jarnerot G. Collagenous colitis: a retrospective study of clinical presentation and treatment in 163 patients. Gut 1999; 39:846–851.

12. Abdo AA, Zetler PJ, Halparin LS. Familial microscopic colitis. Can J Gastroenterol 2001; 15:341–343.

13. Freeman HJ. Familial occurrence of lymphocytic colitis. Can J Gastroenterol 2001; 15:757–760.

14. Jarnerot G, Hertervig E, Granno E, et al. Familial occurrence of microscopic colitis: a report on five families. Scand J Gastroenterol 2001; 36:959–962.

15. Van Tilburg AJ, Lam HG, Seldenrijk CA, et al. Familial occurrence of collagenous colitis: a report of two families. J Clin Gastroenterol 1990; 12:279–285.

16. Wang KK, Perrault J, Carpenter HA, Schroeder KW, Tremaine WJ. Collagenous colitis: a clinico-pathologic correlation. Mayo Clin Proc 1987; 62:665–671.

17. Mullhaupt B, Guller U, Anabitarte M, Guller R, Fried M. Lymphocytic colitis: clinical presentation and long term course. Gut 1998; 43:629–633.

18. Giardiello FM, Bayless TM, Jessurun J, Hamilton SR, Yardley JH. Collagenous colitis: physiologic and histopathologic studies in seven patients. Ann Intern Med 1987; 106:46–49.

19. Giardiello FM, Lazenby AJ, Bayless TM, et al. Lymphocytic (microscopic) colitis. Clinicopathologic study of 18 patients and comparison to collagenous colitis. Dig Dis Sci 1989; 34:1730–1738.

20. Baert F, Wouters K, D'Haens G, et al. Lymphocytic colitis: a distinct clinical entity? A clinical pathological confrontation of lymphocytic and collagenous colitis. Gut 1999; 45:375–381.

21. Pimentel RR, Achkar E, Bedford R. Collagenous colitis: a treatable disease with an elusive diagnosis. Dig Dis Sci 1995; 40:1400–1404.

22. Zins BJ, Tremaine WJ, Carpenter HA. Collagenous colitis: mucosal biopsies and association with fecal leukocytes. Mayo Clin Proc 1995; 70:430–433.

23. Hamilton I, Sander S, Hopwood D, Bouchier IA. Collagenous colitis associated with small intestinal villous atrophy. Gut 1986; 27:1394–1398.

24. Breen EG, Farren C, Connolly CE, Mccarthy CF. Collagenous colitis and coeliac disease. Gut 1987(28):364.

25. O'Mahony S, Nawroz IM, Ferguson A. Coeliac disease and collagenous colitis. Postgrad Med J 1990; 66:238–241.

26. Zins BJ, Sandborn WJ, Tremaine WJ. Collagenous and lymphocytic colitis: subject review and therapeutic alternatives. Am J Gastroenterol 1995; 90:1394–1400.

27. Armes J, Gee DC, Macrae FA, Schroeder W, Bhathol PS. Collagenous colitis: jejunal and colorectal pathology. J Clin Pathol 1992; 45:784–787.

28. Matteoni CA, Goldblum JR, Wang N, Brzezinski A, Achkar E, Soffer EE. Celiac diseases is highly prevalent in lymphocytic colitis. J Clin Gastroenterol 2001; 32:225–227.

29. Dobbins WO, Rubin CE. Studies of rectal mucosa in celiac sprue. Gastroenterology 1964; 47:471–479.

30. Wolber R, Owen D, Freeman H. Colonic lymphocytosis in patients with celiac sprue. Hum Pathol 1990; 21:1092–1096.

31. Fine KD, Lee EL. Efficacy of open-label bismuth subsalicylate for the treatment of microscopic colitis. Gastroenterology 1998; 114:29–36.

32. Fine KD, Meyer RL, Lee EL. The prevalence and causes of chronic diarrhea in patients with celiac sprue treated with a gluten-free. Gastroenterology 1997; 112:1830–1838.

33. Shah RJ, Fenoglio-Preiser C, Bleau BL, Giannella RA. Usefulness of colonoscopy with biopsy in the evaluation of patients with chronic diarrhea. Am J Gastroenterol 2001; 96:1091–1095.

34. Fine KD, Seidel RH, Do K. The prevalence, anatomic distribution, and diagnosis of colonic causes of chronic diarrhea. Gastrointest Endosc 2000; 51:318–326.

35. Goff JS, Barnett JL, Pelke T, Appelman HD. Collagenous colitis: histopathology and clinical course. Am J Gastroenterol 1997; 92:57–60.

36. Bonner GF, Petras RE, Cheong DM, Grewal ID, Breno S, Ruderman WB. Short- and long-term follow-up of treatment for lymphocytic and collagenous colitis. Inflamm Bowel Dis 2000; 6:85–91.

37. Chan JL, Tersmette AC, Offerhaus GJ, Gruber SB, Bayless TM, Giardiello FM. Cancer risk in collagenous colitis. Inflamm Bowel Dis 1999; 5:40–43.

38. Jessurun J, Yardley JH, Giardiello FM, Hamilton SR, Bayless TM. Chronic colitis with thickening of the subepithelial collagen layer (collagenous colitis): histopathologic findings in 15 patients. Hum Pathol 1987; 18:839–848.

39. Lazenby AJ, Yardley JH, Giardiello FM, Bayless TM. Pitfalls in the diagnosis of collagenous colitis: experience with 75 cases from a registry of collagenous colitis at the Johns Hopkins Hospital. Hum Pathol 1990; 21:905–910.

40. Lee E, Schiller LR, Vendrell D, Santa Ana CA, Fordtran JS. Subepithelial collagen table thickness in colon specimens from patients with microscopic colitis and collagenous colitis. Gastroenterology 1992; 103:1790–1796.
41. Gledhill A, Cole FM. Significance of basement membrane thickening in the human colon. Gut 1984; 25:1085–1088.
42. Van den Oord JJ, Geboes K, Desmet VJ. Collagenous colitis: an abnormal collagen table? Two new cases and review of the literature. Am J Gastroenterol 1982; 77:377–381.
43. Offner FA, Jao RV, Lewin KJ, Havelec L, Weinstein WM. Collagenous colitis: a study of the distribution of morphological abnormalities and their histological detection. Hum Pathol 1999; 30(451–457).
44. Widgren S, Jlid IR, Cox JN. Collagenous colitis: histologic, morphometric, immunohistochemical and ultrastructural studies. Report of 21 cases. Virchows Archiv A Pathol Anat 1988; 413:287–296.
45. Carpenter HA, Tremaine WJ, Batts KP, Czaja AJ. Sequential histologic evaluations in collagenous colitis: correlations with disease behavior and sampling strategy. Dig Dis Sci 1992; 37:1903–1909.
46. Tanaka M, Mazzoleni G, Riddell RH. Distribution of collagenous colitis: utility of flexible sigmoidoscopy. Gut 1992; 33:65–70.
47. Giardiello FM, Lazenby AJ, Yardley JH, et al. Increased HLA A1 and diminished HLA A3 in lymphocytic colitis compared to controls and patients with collagenous colitis. Dig Dis Sci 1992; 37:496–499.
48. Fine KD, Do K, Schulte K, et al. High prevalence of celiac sprue-like HLA-DQ genes and enteropathy in patient with microscopic colitis syndrome. Am J Gastroenterol 2000; 95:1974–1982.
49. Jarnerot G, Tysk C, Bohr J, Eriksson S. Collagenous colitis and fecal stream diversion. Gastroenterology 1995; 109:449–455.
50. Ung KA, Gillberg R, Kilander A, Abrahamsson H. Role of bile acids and bile acid binding agents in patients with collagenous colitis. Gut 2000; 46:170–175.
51. Rampton DS, Baithun SI. Is microscopic colitis due to bile-salt malabsorption? Dis Colon Rectum 1987; 30:950–952.
52. Ung KA, Kilander A, Nilsson O, Abrahamsson H. Long-term course in collagenous colitis and the impact of bile acid malabsorption and bile acid sequestrants on histopathology and clinical features. Scand J Gastroenterol 2001; 36:601–609.
53. Bjarnason I, Hayllar J, MacPherson AJ, Russell AS. Side effects of nonsteroidal anti-inflammatory drugs on the small an large intestine in humans. Gastroenterology 1993; 104:1832–1847.
54. Giardiello FM, Hansen FC, Lazenby AJ, et al. Collagenous colitis in the setting of nonsteroidal anti-inflammatory drugs and antibiotics. Dig Dis Sci 1990; 35:257–260.
55. Riddell RH, Tanaka M, Mazzoleni G. Non-steroidal anti-inflammatory drugs as a possible cause of collagenous colitis: a case-control study. Gut 1992; 33:683–686.
56. Feurle GE, Bartz KO, Schitt-Graff A. Lymphocytic colitis induced by ticlopidine. Z Gastroenterol 1999; 37:1105–1108.
57. Beaugerie L, Patey N, Brousse N. Ranitidine, diarrhoea, and lymphocytic colitis. Gut 1995; 37: 708–711.
58. Chagnon JP, Cerf M. Simvastatin-induced protein-losing enteropathy. Am J Gastroenterol 1992; 87:257.
59. Persoz CF, Cornella F, Kaeser P, Rochat T. Ticlopidine-induced interstitial pulmonary disease: a case report. Chest 2001; 119:1963–1965.
60. Piche T, Raimondi V, Schneider S, Hebuterne X, Rampal P. Acarbose and lymphocytic colitis. Lancet 2000; 356:1246.
61. Wilcox GM, Mattia A. Collagenous colitis associated with lansoprazole. J Clin Gastroenterol 2002; 34:164–166.
62. Aigner T, Neureiter D, Muller S, Kuspert G, Belke J, Kirchner T. Extracellular matrix composition and gene expression in collagenous colitis. Gastroenterology 1997; 113:136–143.
63. Hwang WS, Kelly JK, Shaffer EA, Hershfield NB. Collagenous colitis: a disease of pericryptal fibroblast sheath? J Pathol 1986; 149:33–40.
64. Bo-Linn GW, Vendrell DD, Lee E, Fordtran JS. An evaluation of the significance of microscopic colitis in patients with chronic diarrhea. J Clin Invest 1985; 75:1559–1569.
65. Burgel N, Bojarski C, Mankertz J, Zeitz M, Fromm M, Schulzke J. Mechanism of diarrhea in collagenous colitis. Gastroenterology 2002; 123:433–443.
66. Fine D, Ogunji F, Lee E, Lafon G, Tanzi M. Randomized, double-blind, placebo-controlled trial of bismuth subsalicylate for microscopic colitis. Gastroenterology 1999; 116:A880.
67. Sloth H, Bisgaard C, Grove A. Collagenous colitis: a prospective trial of prednisolone in six patients. J Intern Med 1991; 229:443–446.
68. Pardi DS, Loftus EV, Tremaine WJ, Sandborn WJ. Treatment of refractory microscopic colitis with azathioprine and 6-mercaptopurine. Gastroenterology 2001; 120:1483–1484.
69. Miehlke S, Heymer P, Bethke B, et al. Budesonide treatment for collagenous colitis: A randomized, double-blind, placebo-controlled, multicenter trial. Gastroenterology 2002; 123:978–984.
70. Bonderup OK, Hansen JB, Birket-Smith L, Vestergaard V, Teglbjaerg PS, Fallingorg J. Budesonide treatment of collagenous colitis: a randomised, double blind, placebo controlled trial with morphometric analysis. Gut 2003; 52:248–251.
71. Fisher NC, Tutt A, Sim E, Scarpello J, Green J. Collagenous colitis responsive to octreotide therapy. J Clin Gastroenterol 1996; 23:300–301.

72. Williams RA, Gelfand DV. Total proctocolectomy and ileal pouch anal anastomosis to successfully treat a patient with collagenous colitis. Am J Gastrenterol 2000; 95:2147.
73. Kaijser R. Zur kenntnis der llergischen affektionen des verdauungs-kanals vom standpunkt des chirurgan aus. Arch Klin Chir 1937; 188:36–64.
74. Cello JP. Eosinophilic gastroenteritis—a complex disease entitiy. Am J Med 1979; 67:1097–1104.
75. Johnstone JM, Morson BC. Eosinophilic gastroenteritis. Histopathology 1978; 2:335–348.
76. Dunstone GH. A case of eosinophilic colitis. Br j Surg 1959; 46:474–476.
77. Haberkern CM. Eosinophilic gastroenteritis presenting as ileocolitis. Gastroenterology 1978; 74:896–899.
78. Lee FI, Costello FT, Cowley DJ, Murray SM, Srimanker J. Eosinophilic colitis with perianal disease. Am J Gastroenterol 1983; 78:164–166.
79. Levinson JD, Rmanathan VR, Nozick JH. Eosinophilic gastroenteritis with ascites and colon involvement. Am J Gastroenterol 1977; 68:603–607.
80. Lim K, Black R. Eosinophilic colitis masquerading as colonic cancer. Aust NZ J Surg 2000; 70: 682–684.
81. Loffeld RJLF. Primary biliary cirrhosis associated with recurrent angiodysplastic lesions in the gastrointestinal tract, the lupus anticoagulant and eosinophilic gastroenteritis eosinophilic colitis. Netherlands J Med 1991; 39:101–104.
82. Moore D, Lichtman S, Lentz J, Stringer D, Sherman P. Eosinophilic gastroenteritis presenting in an adolescent with isolated colonic involvement. Gut 1986; 27:1219–1222.
83. Partyka EK, Sanowski RA, Kozarek RA. Colonoscopic features of eosinophilic gastroenteritis. Dis Colon Rectum 1980; 23:353–356.
84. Persic M, Stimac T, Stimac D, Kovac D. Eosinophilic colitis: a rare entity. J Ped Gastroenterol Nutr 2001; 32:325–326.
85. Naylor AR, Pollet JE. Eosinophilic colitis. Dis Colon Rectum 1985; 28:615–618.
86. Schulze K, Mitros FA. Eosinophilic gastroenteritis involving the ileocecal area. Dis Colon Rectum 1979; 22:47–50.
87. Tedesco FJ, Huckaby CB, Hamby-Allen M, Ewing GC. Eosinophilic enterocolitis. Expanding spectrum of eosinophilic gastroenteritis. Dig Dis Sci 1981; 26:943–948.
88. Zora JA, O'Connell EJ, Sachs MI, Hoffman AD. Eosinophilic gastroenteritis: a case report and review of the literature. Ann Allergy 1984; 53:45–47.
89. Ettinghausen SE. Collagenous colitis, eosinophilic colitis, and neutropenic colitis. Surg Clin NA 1993; 73:993–1016.
90. Steele RJC, Mok SD, Crofts TJ, Li AKC. Two cases of eosinophilic enteritis presenting as large bowel perforation and small bowl hemorrhage. Aust NZ J Surg 1987; 57:335–336.
91. Box JC, Tucker J, Watne AL, Lucas G. Eosinophilic colitis presenting as a left-sided colocolonic intussusception with secondary large bowel obstruction: an uncommon entity with a rare presentation. Am Surg 1997; 63:741–743.
92. Martin DM, Goldman JA, Gilliam J, Nasrallah SA. Gold-induced eosinophilic enterocolitis: response to oral cromolyn sodium. Gastroenterology 1981; 80:1567–1570.
93. Gilinsky NH, Kottler RE. Idiopathic obstructive eosinophilic enteritis with raised IgE: response to oral disodium cromoglycate. Postgrad Med J 1982; 58:239–243.
94. Ma TY, Hollander D, Freeman D, Nguyen T, Krugliak P. Oxygen free radical injury of IEC-18 small intestinal epithelial cell monolayers. Gastroenterology 1991; 100:1533–1543.
95. Moore KW, Vieira P, Fiorentino DF, Trounstine ML, Khan TA, Mosmann TR. Homology of cytokine synthesis inhibitory factor (IL-10) to the epstein-barr virus gene BCRFI. Sci 1990; 248:1230–1234.
96. Sullivan S, Troster M. Eosinophilic colitis (letter). Gut 1987; 28:506.
97. Anttila VJ, Valtonen M. Carbamazepine-induced eosinophilic colitis. Epilepsia 1992; 22:119–121.
98. Shweiki E, West JC, Klena JW, et al. Eosinophilic gastroenteritis presenting as an obstructing cecal mass—a case report and review of the literature. Am J Gastroenterol 1999; 94:3644–3645.
99. Wiesner W, Kocher T, Heim M, Bongartz G. CT findings in eosinophilic enterocolitis with predominantly serosal and muscular bowel wall infiltration. JBR-BTR 2002; 85:4–6.
100. Carpenter HA, Talley NJ. The importance of clinicopathological correlation in the diagnosis of inflammatory conditions of the colon: histological patterns with clinical implications. Am J Gastroenterol 2000; 95:878–896.
101. Shah AM, Joglekar M. Eosinophilic colitis as a complication of the hypereosinophilic syndrome. Postgrad med J 1987; 63:485–487.
102. Tajima K, Katagiri T. Deposits of eosinophil granule proteins in eosinophilic cholecystitis and eosinophilic colitis associated with hypereosinophilic syndrome. Dig Dis Sci 1996; 41:282–288.
103. Suen KC, Burton JF. The spectrum of eosinophilic infiltration of the gastrointestinal tract and its relationship to other disorders of angiitis and granulomatosis. Hum Pathol 1979; 10:31–43.
104. Naschitz JE, Yeshurun D, Miselevich I, Boss JH. Colitis and pericarditis in a patient with eosinophilic fasciitis. A contribution to the multisystem nature of eosinophilic fasciitis. J Rheumatol 1989; 16: 688–692.
105. DeSchryver-Kecskemeti K, Clouse RE. A previously unrecognized subgroup of "eosinophilic gastroenteritis": association with connective tissue diseases. Am J Surg Pathol 1984; 8:171–180.
106. Clouse RE, Alpers DH, Hockenberry DM, DeSchryver-Kecskemeti K. Pericrypt eosinophilic enterocolitis and chronic diarrhea. Gastroenterology 1992; 103:168–176.

107. Kuipers FC, Theil PHV, Rodenburg W, Wielinga WJ, Roskam RT. Eosinophilic phlegmon of the alimentary canal caused by a roundworm. Lancet 1960; 2:1171–1173.
108. Liu LX, Chi J, Upton MP, Ash LR. Eosinophilic colitis associated with larvae of the pinworm *Enterobius vermicularis*. Lancet 1995; 346:410–412.
109. Cuffari C, Oligny L, Seidman EG. *Dientamoeba fragilis* masquerading as allergic colitis. J Ped Gastroenterol Nutr 1998; 26:16–20.
110. Leinbach GE, Rubin CE. Is eosinophilic gastroenteritis caused by food allergy? (Abstract). Gastroenterology 1969; 56:1177.
111. Klein NC, Hargrove RL, Sleisinger MH, Jeffries GH. Eosinophilic gastroenteritis. Med (Baltimore) 1970; 59:299–319.
112. Moon A, Kleinman RE. Allergic gastroenteropathy in children. Ann Allergy Asthma Immunol 1995; 74:5–12.
113. Wilson NW, Self TW, Hamburger RN. Severe cow's milk induced colitis. Clin Pediatr 1990; 29:77–80.
114. Vetter V, Behrens R. Eosinophilic colitis: a differential diagnosis of allergic colitis (Letter). Eur J Pediatr 1997; 156:583.
115. Sherman MP, Cox KL. Neonatal eosinophilic colitis. J Pediatrics 1982; 100:587–589.
116. Berezin S, Schwarz SM, Glassman M, Davidian M, Newman LJ. Gastrointestinal milk intolerance of infancy. Am J Dis Child 1989; 143:361–362.
117. Bridges AJ, Marshall JB, Diaz-Arias AA. Acute eosinophilic colitis and hypersensitivity reaction associated with Naprosyn therapy. Am J Med 1990; 89:526–527.
118. Anttila VJ, Valtonen M. Carbamazepine-induced eosinophilic colitis. Epilepsia 1990; 33:119–121.
119. Lange P, Oun H, Fuller S, Turney JH. Eosinophilic colitis due to rifampicin (letter). Lancet 1994; 344:1296–1297.
120. Keshavarzian A, Saverymutu SH, Tai PC, et al. Activated eosinophils in familial eosinophilic gastroenteritis. Gastroenterology 1985; 88:1041–1049.
121. Metz J, McGrath KM, Savoia HF, Begley CG, Chetty R. T-cell lymphoid aggregates in bone marrow patients in idiopathic hypereosinophilic syndrome. J. Clin Pathol 1993; 46:955–958.
122. Lopez AF, Sanderson CJ, Gamble JR, Campbell HD, Young IG, Vadas MA. Recombinant human interleukin 5 is a selective activator of human eosinophil function. J Exp Med 1988; 167:219–224.
123. Plumas J, Gruart V, Capron M, Prin L. The interleukin 2 receptor in the hypereosinophilic syndrome. Leukemia 1992; 8:449–457.
124. Lee JH, Lee JW, Jang CS, et al. Successful cyclophosphamide therapy in recurrent eosinophilic colitis associated with hypereosinophilic syndrome. Yonsei Med J 2002; 43:267–270.
125. Tan AC, Kruimel JW, Naber TH. Eosinophilic gastroenteritis treated with non-enteric-coated budesonide tablets. Eur J Gastroenterol Hepatol 2001; 13:425–427.
126. Katsinelos P, Pilipilidis P, Xiarchos P, et al. Oral administration of ketotifen in a patient with eosinophilic colitis and severe osteoporosis. Am J Gastroenterol 2002; 97:1072–1074.
127. Schwartz DA, Pardi DS, Murray JA. Use of montelukast as steroid-sparing agent for recurrent eosinophilic gastroenteritis. Dig Dis Sci 2001; 46:1787–1790.
128. Daikh BE, Ryan CK, Schwartz RH. Montelukast reduces peripheral blood eosinophilia but not tissue eosinophilia or symptoms in a patient with eosinophilic gastroenteritis and esophageal stricture. Ann Allergy Asthma Immunol 2003; 90:23–27.
129. Tytgat GN, Grijm R, Dekker W, Hartog NAD. Fatal eosinophilic enteritis. Gastroenterology 1976; 71:479–483.
130. Williams N, Scott AD. Neutropenic colitis: a continuing surgical challenge. Br J Surg 1997; 84: 1200–1205.
131. Cooke JV. Acute leukemia in children. JAMA 1933; 101:432–435.
132. Mulholland MW, Delaney JP. Neutropenic colitis and aplastic anemia: a new association. Ann Surg 1983; 197:84–90.
133. Alt B, Glass NR, Sollinger H. Neutropenic enterocolitis in adults: review of the literature and assessment of surgical intervention. Am J Surg 1985; 149:405–408.
134. Pokorney BH, Jones JM, Shaikh BS, Aber RC. Typhlitis: a treatable cause of recurrent septicemia. JAMA 1980; 243:682–683.
135. Prolla JC, Kirsner JB. The gastrointestinal lesions and complications of leukemia. Ann Intern Med 1964; 61:1084–1103.
136. Till M, Lee N, Soper WD, Murphy RL. Typhlitis in patients with HIV-1 infection. Ann Intern Med 1992; 116:998–1000.
137. Wilson SE, Robinson G, Williams RA, et al. Acquired immune deficiency syndrome (AIDS). Indication for abdominal surgery, pathology, and outcome. An Surg 1989; 210:228–434.
138. Frankel AH, Barker F, Williams G, Benjamin IS, Lechler R, Rees AJ. Neutropenic enterocolitis in a renal transplant patient. Transplantation 1991; 52:913–914.
139. Wade DS, Nava HR, Douglas HO. Neutropenic enterocolitis: clinical diagnosis and treatment. Cancer 1992; 69:17–23.
140. Slavin RE, Dias MA, Saral R. Cytosine arabinoside induced gastrointestinal toxic alterations in sequential chemotherapeutic protocols. Cancer 1978; 42:1747–1759.
141. Kingry RL, Hobson RW, Muir RW. Cecal necrosis and perforation with systemic chemotherapy. Am Surg 1973; 39:129–133.

142. Mower WJ, Hawkins JA, Nelson EW. Neutropenic enterocolitis in adults with acute leukemia. Arch Surg 1986; 121:571–574.

143. Shamberger RC, Weinstein HJ, Delorey MJ, Levey RH. The medical and surgical management of typhlitis in children with acute nonlymphocytic (myelogenous) leukemia. Cancer 1986; 57:603–609.

144. Gomez L, Martino R, Rolston KV. Neutropenic enterocolitis: spectrum of the disease and comparison of definite and possible cases. Clin Infect Dis 1998; 27:695–699.

145. Keidan RD, Fanning J, Gatenby RA, Weese JL. Recurrent typhlitis. A disease resulting from aggressive chemotherapy. Dis Colon Rectum 1989; 32:206–209.

146. Vas WG, Seelig R, Mahanta B, et al. Neutropenic colitis: evaluation with computed tomography. J Comput Tomogr 1988; 12:211–215.

147. Alexander JE, Williamson SL, Seibert JJ, Golladay ES, Jimenez JF. The ultrasonographic diagnosis of typhlitis (netropenic colitis). Pediatr Radiol 1988; 18:200–204.

148. Dworkin B, Winawer SJ, Lightdale CJ. Typhlitis: report of a case with long term survival and reviews of the recent literature. Dig Dis Sci 1981; 26:1032–1037.

149. Dosik GM, Luna M, Valdivieso M, et al. Necrotizing enterocolitis in patients with cancer. Am J Med 1979; 67:646–656.

150. Sauter ER, Vauthey JN, Bolton JS, Sardi A. Selective management of patients with neutropenic enterocolitis using peritoneal lavage. J Surg Oncol 1990; 45:63–67.

151. Blair SL, Schwarz RE. Critical care of patients with cancer. Surgical considerations. Crit Care Clin 2001; 17:721–742.

152. Abramson SJ, Berdon WR, Baker DH. Childhood typhlitis: its increasing association with acute myelogenous leukemia. Radiology 1983; 146:61–64.

153. Starnes HF, Moore FD, Mentzer S, Osteen RT, Steele GD, Wilson RE. Abdominal pain in neutropenic cancer patients. Cancer 1986; 57:616–621.

154. McDonald GB, Shulman HM, Sullivan KM, Spencer GD. Intestinal and hepatic complications of human bone marrow transplantation II. Gastroenterology 1986; 90:770–784.

155. Kunkel JM, Rosenthal D. Management of the ileocecal syndrome: neutropenic enterocolitis. Dis Col Rectum 1986; 29:196–199.

156. Goodman MD, Porter DD. Cytomegalovirus vasculitis with fatal colonic hemorrhage. Arch Pathol 1973; 96:281–284.

157. Sherman NJ, Woolley MM. The ileocecal syndrome in acute childhood leukemia. Arch Surg 1973; 107:39–42.

158. Newbold KM. Neutropenic enterocolitis: clinical and pathological review. Dig Dis 1989; 7:281–287.

159. Rasmussen BL, Freeman JS. Major surgery in leukemia. Am J Surg 1975; 130:647–651.

160. Matolo NM, Garfinkle SE, Wolman EF. Intestinal necrosis and perforation in patients receiving immunosuppressive drugs. Am J Surg 1976; 132:753–754.

161. Kies MS, Luedke DW, Body JF, McCue MJ. Neutropenic enterocolitis: two case reports of long-term survival following surgery. Cancer 1979; 43:730–734.

162. Varki AP, Armitage JO, Feagler JR. Typhlitis in acute leukemia: successful treatment by early surgical intervention. Cancer 1979; 43:695–697.

163. Lea JW, Masys DR, Shackford SR. Typhlitis: a treatable complication of acute leukemic therapy. Cancer Clin Trials 1980; 3:355–362.

164. Lehman JA, Armitage JO. Surgical intervention in complications of acute leukemia. Postgrad Med 1980; 68:89–92.

165. Ikard RW. Neutropenic typhlitis in adults. Arch Surg 1981; 116:943–945.

166. Gandy W, Greenberg BR. Successful medical management of neutropenic enterocolitis. Cancer 1983; 51:1551–1555.

167. Schaller RT, Schaller JF. The acute abdomen in the immunologically compromised child. J Pediatr Surg 1983; 18:937–944.

168. Shaked A, Shinar E, Freund H. Neutropenic typhlitis. A plea for conservation. Dis Colon rectum 1983; 26:351–352.

169. Moir CR, Scudamore CH, Benny WB. Typhlitis: selective surgical management. Am J Surg 1986; 152:563–566.

170. Villar HV, Warneke JA, Peck MD, Durie B, Bjelland JC, Hunter TB. Role of surgical treatment in the management of complications of the gastrointestinal tract in patients with leukemia. Surg Gynecol Obstet 1987; 165:217–222.

171. Skibber JM, Matter GJ, Pizzo PA, Lotze MT. Right lower quadrant pain in young patients with leukemia > A surgical perspective. Ann Surg 1987; 206:711–716.

172. O'Brien S, Kantarjian HM, Anaissie E, Dodd G, Bodey GP. Successful medical management of neutropenic enterocolitis in adults with acute leukemia. South med J 1987; 80:1233–1235.

173. Baniel J, Lombrozo R, Ziv Y, Wolloch Y. Neutropaenic colitis. Case Report. Acta Chir Scand 1988; 154:71–73.

174. Koea JB, Shaw JHF. Surgical management of neutropenic enterocolitis. Br J Surg 1989; 76:821–824.

175. Merine D, Nussbaum AR, Fishman EK, Sanders RC. sonographic observations in a patient with typhlitis. Clin Pediatr (Phila) 1989; 28:377–379.

176. Cutrona AF, Blinkhorn RJ, Crass J, Spagnuolo PJ. Probable neutropenic enterocolitis in patients with AIDS. Rev Infect Dis 1991; 13:828–831.

177. Chakravarty K, Scott DGI, McCann BG. Fatal neutropenic enterocolitis associated with sulfasalazine therapy for rheumatoid arthritis. Br J Rheumatol 1992; 31:351–353.

178. Vohra R, Prescott RJ, Banerjee SS, Wilkinson PM, Schofield PF. Management of neutropenic colitis. Surg Oncol 1992; 1:11–15.

179. Or R, Mehta J, Nagler A, Craciun I. Neutropenic enterocolitis associated with autologous bone marrow transplantation. Bone Marrow Transplant 1992; 9:383–385.

180. Winberger M, Hollingsworth H, Feuerstein IM, Young NS, Pizzo PA. Successful surgical management of neutropenic enterocolitis in two patients with severe aplastic anemia. Case reports and review of the literature. Arch Intern Med 1993; 153:107–113.

181. Chubachi A, Hashimoto K, Miura AB. Successful treatment of methicillin-resistant Staphylococcus aureus (MRSA) enterocolitis in a neutropenic patient following cytotoxic chemotherapy [letter]. Am J Hematol 1993; 43:327.

182. Bajwa RP, Marwaha RK, Garewal G. Neutropenic enterocolitis and cecal perforation in acute lymphatic leukemia. Indian J Cancer 1993; 20:31–33.

183. Dudiak KM. Abdominal case of the day. Neutropenic enterocolitis associated with acute leukemia. Am J Roentgenol 1993; 160:1323–1324.

184. Coleman N, Speirs G, Khan J, Broadbent V, Wright DG, Warren RE. Neutropenic enterocolitis associated with Clostridium tertium. J Clin pathol 1993; 46:180–183.

185. Anderson PE. Neutropenic enterocolitis treated by primary resection with anastomosis in a leukaemic patient receiving chemotherapy. Aust NZ J Surg 1993; 63:74–76.

186. Suarez B, Kalifa G, Adamsbaum C, Saint-Martin C, Barbotin-Larrieu F. Sonographic diagnosis and follow-up of diffuse neutropenic colitis: case report of a child treated for osteogenic sarcoma. Pediatr Radiol 1995; 25:373–374.

187. Stein M, Zalik M, Drumea K, Lachter J, Militianu D, Haim N. Fatal neutropenic colitis complicating successful chemotherapy for small cell lung cancer: a case report. Isr J Med Sci 1995; 31:194–196.

188. Glenn J, Funkhouser WK, Schneider PS. Acute illness necessitating urgent abdominal surgery in neutropenic cancer patients: description of 14 cases and review of the literature. Surg 1989; 105: 778–779.

29 | Diversion Colitis and Pouchitis

Laurence R. Sands
Division of Colon and Rectal Surgery, University of Miami School of Medicine, Miami, Florida, U.S.A.

INTRODUCTION

Diversion colitis and pouchitis are two nonspecific inflammatory bowel conditions that affect a large number of patients. Although diversion colitis rarely presents as a significant clinical problem, pouchitis remains a challenging clinical entity for the patient, gastroenterologist, and colon and rectal surgeon. Although both of these conditions are often medically managed, surgical intervention may be necessary in medically refractory cases.

DIVERSION COLITIS

Diversion colitis occurs when the intestinal tract has been divided, thereby interrupting the normal route of fecal transit. Although there is no clear definition for this condition, it was initially recognized in 1981 when 10 patients without prior evidence of inflammatory bowel disease were noted to have bowel inflammation after undergoing either creation of a diverting ileostomy or colostomy for various medical indications. This initial report noted that those patients who underwent restoration of the fecal stream with stoma reversal had complete resolution of these inflammatory changes. Interestingly, only one of this small group of 10 patients was initially symptomatic whereas two others manifested mild symptoms after diagnosis (1).

The microscopic changes of diversion colitis are similar to those of mucosal ulcerative colitis (MUC) and include crypt abscesses, inflammation of the lamina propria, epithelial cell degeneration, and regenerative changes within the crypts. In extreme cases of diversion colitis, patients may present with significant nodularity secondary to lymphoid hyperplasia and inflammation of the mucosa and underlying submucosa (2). Today, it is recognized that the majority of patients who undergo fecal diversion have proctosigmoidoscopic findings of diversion colitis, although most patients remain completely asymptomatic (3).

The symptoms that are most commonly associated with this condition include anal passage of bloody mucus rarely associated with crampy lower abdominal pain. This occurs in the diverted segment of bowel and may involve either the entire diverted segment or only the distal aspect of the diverted rectum.

The etiology of diversion colitis is essentially unknown. It has been suggested that the colonic mucosa derives its nutrients from the mesenteric vasculature, in addition to the absorption of nutrients from the colonic lumen. When the intestinal tract is divided by fecal diversion, the distal bowel segment is no longer able to absorb nutrients from ingested food. Particularly, the lack of ingested short-chain fatty acids has been implicated as a causative agent in diversion colitis. Butyrate is a short-chain fatty acid that is generated by microbial fermentation of dietary substrates. This microbial fermentation occurs within the colonic lumen. The colonic cells then absorb the butyrate by passive diffusion within the colon along with sodium and water absorption and bicarbonate secretion. Although the exact role of butyrate remains elusive, this nutrient has been implicated in protecting against colorectal neoplasia, improving colonic motility, increasing colonic blood flow, and improving colonic anastomotic healing (4). Furthermore, butyrate may even reduce symptoms of MUC. In addition, short-chain fatty acids fuel the colonic epithelial cells and have trophic effects on the epithelium (5).

Diversion colitis is a common disorder among patients with a neuropathic large bowel requiring fecal diversion. Several studies have shown that patients with spinal cord injury who have undergone long-term fecal diversion have experienced complications due to diversion colitis (6,7). These patients complain of abdominal discomfort, rectal discharge, fever, and rectal bleeding. Colonoscopy of the diverted rectum in 94% of these patients has revealed mucosal friability and erythema, whereas mucosal biopsies have revealed severe inflammation in the majority of these patients (7). Radiographic studies of the diverted Hartman's stump have also been performed and have revealed abnormalities in 19% of patients studied (8). These abnormalities include leaks, fistulae, strictures, and recurrent cancers of the Hartman's stump.

The ideal therapy for symptomatic diversion colitis remains reversal of the stoma and restoration of the fecal stream. Prior to stoma reversal, patients should undergo a thorough evaluation of the Hartmann's stump and the proximal bowel. Radiographic evaluation of the diverted segment is best assessed by a water-soluble contrast agent in order to prevent barium contamination of the abdominal cavity in the event of a leak in this portion of bowel. A proctosigmoidoscopic evaluation may also be performed if there are significant abnormalities demonstrated on the radiographic study. Additionally, rigid proctoscopy will clearly define the length of the distal rectum. These studies are often complementary.

If the stoma cannot be closed, the diversion colitis may remain severe. If the patient remains symptomatic from the diversion colitis, the rectal stump may be treated with anti-inflammatory medications, such as Rowasa, or corticosteroid enemas administered twice daily. In addition, butyrate enemas have been used to aid in the healing of diversion colitis. Although there are no randomized controlled trials showing a benefit to any of these therapies, some patients have shown some improvement with local therapy to the distal bowel.

If there is no improvement after such medical therapy, surgical excision of the diverted bowel segment may be performed to relieve symptoms of diversion colitis. This resection may be performed as a perineal proctectomy if the diverted rectum is short enough. If this is not possible, then an abdominal procedure may be undertaken to remove the diverted bowel segment, thereby leaving the patient with a permanent stoma.

POUCHITIS

Ileal pouch inflammation has long been a recognized complication of restorative proctectomy. Although the etiology of this inflammatory condition remains unknown, the treatment is fairly well established. The entity, although quite common and affecting nearly 30% to 40% of all pouch patients, is generally short lived and transitory. There are, however, a small group of patients who will suffer from refractory and debilitating pouchitis, ultimately requiring pouch excision and a permanent ileostomy. These patients may have had indeterminate colitis and may ultimately prove to have Crohn's disease. Consequently, pouch failure may occur with recurrent episodes of pouchitis, pouch perineal fistulae, and possibly perianal sepsis.

Incidence

Pouchitis is the most common long-term complication of ileal pouch anal anastomosis affecting as many as 24% to 47% of patients with ulcerative colitis within 10 to 11 years after surgery (9–11). The probability of suffering a second episode after an initial attack may be as high as 64% (12). Interestingly, the incidence of pouchitis in patients with familial adenomatous polyposis (FAP) is considerably lower, ranging from 0% to 10%, thus implicating some aspect of the underlying inflammatory condition of ulcerative colitis that predisposes patients to this complication (13). The reason for such a wide range of reported incidences for pouchitis likely reflects the lack of consensus as to the definition and diagnostic criteria used to define this entity.

Etiology

Little is known about the pathogenesis of pouchitis. Several hypotheses have been proposed including immunologic mechanisms, bacterial etiologies, nutritional deficiencies, and ischemic phenomena.

An immunologic mechanism to explain pouchitis has been suggested particularly since pouchitis is considerably less common in patients undergoing total proctocolectomy with reconstruction for FAP. The Birmingham group has studied various cytokines in order to determine whether there is any correlation with pouchitis. Specifically, interleukin (IL)-1 beta (IL-1 beta), interleukin-6 (IL-6), interleukin-8 (IL-8), and tumor necrosis factor alpha (TNF alpha) in the mucosa of patients with pouchitis and controls were assessed. IL-1 beta, IL-6,

IL-8, and TNF alpha secretions were significantly greater in pouchitis and in patients with active ulcerative colitis than in the noninflamed ileoanal pouch and normal controls. In addition, there was a significant correlation between the levels of cytokines in pouchitis patients and those suffering from active ulcerative colitis (14). Another study has shown higher levels of CD4+ T cells as well as a higher number of interferon gamma–producing mononuclear cells in patients with ulcerative colitis and pouchitis compared with patients with ulcerative colitis without pouchitis. It has been suggested that these findings may lead to greater mucosal destruction as is commonly seen in pouchitis (15). In addition, matrix metalloproteinases, which have been suggested as a causative agent in tissue destruction in inflammatory disease states, have been shown to be present in higher concentrations in patients with ulcerative colitis with active pouchitis compared to patients with ulcerative colitis with uninflamed pouches and those with FAP (16).

Immunologic links to the development of pouchitis have also been suggested by the presence of preoperatively high levels of perinuclear antineutrophil cytoplasmic antibody (pANCA) in patients undergoing restorative ileoanal J-pouch surgery for ulcerative colitis. Patients with preoperatively high levels of pANCA were noted to be at significantly higher risk of developing pouchitis than those with lower levels (17).

A bacterial etiology has also been suggested since pouchitis responds positively to antibiotic therapy. An overgrowth of both aerobic and anaerobic bacteria has been noted even in healthy pouches. However, there have been several studies that failed to show that the bacterial flora in patients with pouchitis differs from the flora in healthy pouches (18). There have also been studies that have shown different bacterial flora in patients with pouchitis compared to controls; the patients with pouchitis had an increased number of aerobes, a decreased anaerobe-to-aerobe ratio, less bifidobacteria and anaerobic lactobacilli, and more *Clostridium perfringens*. In addition, patients with pouchitis also had several organisms, such as fungi, that were not found in control patients. Furthermore, the pH was significantly higher in patients with pouchitis than in control patients. A higher pH allows greater activity of glycosidases and proteases, thereby potentially causing greater mucosal destruction contributing to pouchitis (19). However, it is still unknown whether the alteration of bacterial flora changes the pH or the change in pH alters the bacterial flora of the pouch.

Some studies have confirmed the presence of increased numbers of *Bacteroides* species in patients with pouchitis, whereas other studies have refuted this claim (20). Currently, there remains no clear association between a specific bacteriologic pathogen and the development of pouchitis.

Nutritional considerations for the development of pouchitis have also been proposed. Ileoanal pouches often undergo colonic metaplasia over the course of time. This finding has led some to believe that the pouch mucosa behaves similarly to colonic mucosa. As previously mentioned, butyrate has long been shown to be the fuel of the colonocyte and has been used in the treatment of diversion colitis. Pouchitis has been associated with low luminal levels of short-chain fatty acids (21). This may be due to increased stool frequency, which may wash out luminal levels of short chain fatty acids. This theory is credible in that the treatment of pouchitis has been successful in some instances with short-chain fatty acid enemas (22).

Mucosal blood flow in patients with pouchitis has been shown via laser Doppler to be lower than in those patients without pouchitis, suggesting mucosal ischemia as a cause of this condition (23). Mucosal ischemia may produce oxygen free radicals, which may cause inflammation. Based on this theory, allopurinol, an oxygen free radical scavenger, has been suggested as a treatment regimen for pouchitis. Levin et al. demonstrated a 50% improvement in patients with allopurinol (24). However, a recent double-blind, prospective, randomized placebo-controlled trial with allopurinol failed to prove that prophylactic use of allopurinol reduces the risk of a first attack of pouchitis (25).

Diagnosis

Although the clinical picture of pouchitis may appear obvious based on symptomatology, patients are rarely appropriately diagnosed by pouchoscopy and biopsy. Patients are often treated based on the symptoms of increased stool frequency, fecal urgency, and pelvic discomfort. This practice may be responsible for the high incidence of pouchitis reported in the literature.

Patients may also experience low-grade fevers, bloody diarrhea, abdominal cramping, and other extra-intestinal manifestations of inflammatory bowel disease that may make the diagnosis more obvious. Patients with extra-intestinal manifestations of inflammatory bowel disease more often develop pouchitis while experiencing these manifestations (26). The extra-intestinal manifestations that may improve following colectomy are those that often reappear during episodes of pouchitis.

However, in order to properly diagnose pouchitis, the patient should undergo pouchoscopy after administering an enema to visually confirm active pouch inflammation. A biopsy will confirm this inflammation microscopically with neutrophilic inflammatory cell infiltration, while attempting to rule out the possibility of Crohn's disease. The biopsy findings, however, are often nonspecific. Scoring systems have been developed to grade the inflammation seen in biopsies of pouchitis. In one study, there were inflammatory changes in almost every patient biopsied regardless of symptoms of pouchitis. Acute inflammatory changes were seen in those patients with active pouchitis. There was no correlation between the degree of inflammation and the configuration of the pouch, the compliance of the pouch, or the degree of pouch emptying. In addition, and as seen in other studies, there was greater inflammation seen in pouches constructed for ulcerative colitis as opposed to those constructed for FAP (27).

The typical endoscopic appearance of pouchitis resembles that of any other inflammatory bowel condition, which is friable, hemorrhagic mucosa with edema and ulcerations. There has been a lack of definitive correlation between symptoms and endoscopic and microscopic findings of pouchitis most likely representing the wide spectrum of patients with this condition (28). As a result, a Pouch Disease Activity Index (PDAI) has been proposed to assist with the diagnosis and objectivity in defining pouchitis (29). This scoring system combines clinical, endoscopic, and histologic information in order to indicate active pouchitis. In addition to its research utility, such a system may help determine appropriate treatment for patients with pouchitis.

Treatment

There are numerous medical regimens that have been suggested for the treatment of pouchitis. These include antibiotics, probiotics, topical anti-inflammatory agents, and immunosuppressive medications. Surgical therapies for the treatment of pouchitis include fecal diversion and ultimately pouch excision. Fortunately, surgical therapy is rarely required to treat this condition and is reserved for severe medically refractory cases.

The most common therapy for pouchitis is oral antibiotics. Metronidazole is often the firstline agent, because it is extremely effective, inexpensive, and readily available. Approximately 80% to 90% of patients will have an excellent response to the use of metronidazole. This medication is usually dosed at either 250 or 500 mg two to three times daily for 14 days. It has both antianaerobic properties while inhibiting the production of superoxides (30). Long-term use of metronidazole may result in peripheral neuropathy as well as a metallic taste. Once these symptoms occur, this medication should be discontinued.

Ciprofloxacin, tetracycline, amoxicillin/clavulinic acid, doxycycline, and clarithromycin have all been used as alternative regimens for the treatment of pouchitis. A recent prospective randomized trial from the Cleveland Clinic Foundation comparing a two-week regimen of ciprofloxacin (1000 mg/day) to a two-week regimen of metronidazole (20 mg/kg/day) for the treatment of acute pouchitis showed greater efficacy with the former. Ciprofloxacin was more effective in reducing the overall PDAI and demonstrated a greater improvement in clinical symptoms and endoscopic scores. In addition there was less toxicity associated with the use of ciprofloxacin (31).

Most patients with acute pouchitis rapidly respond to antibiotics. However, up to 20% may develop refractory pouchitis or have relapsing symptoms (11). These patients should be placed on a more prolonged course of antimicrobial therapy in order to resolve their symptoms. There are some patients who will require frequent intermittent antibiotic use to keep the disease in a remissive state. Some reports, however, have found that long-term pouch function may be compromised even after only one bout of pouchitis, even in clinically inactive pouchitis (32).

Probiotics have been suggested as maintenance therapy when active pouchitis has been controlled (33). Probiotics probably maintain remission through several mechanisms. First, they likely suppress native pouch pathogens that cause pouchitis. Second, they promote glycoprotein production by the intestinal epithelial cells and prevent bacteria from adhering to these cells. Probiotics may also induce host immune responses (34). VSL #3 is an agent that has been studied in patients with refractory pouchitis. This contains $5 \times 10^{11}/g$ of viable bacteria consisting of four strains of lactobacilli, three strains of bifidobacteria, and one strain of *Streptococcus salivarius*. In a prospectively randomized, double-blinded, placebo-controlled trial studying VSL #3, only 15% of patients treated with VSL #3 had a relapse of pouchitis compared to 100% of the patients who were treated with placebo in a nine-month follow-up period. However, VSL #3 must be given in the inactive phase of pouchitis and continuously used in order to be effective (35).

Several topical agents have been suggested in the treatment of pouchitis including bismuth carbomer foam enemas, glutamine suppositories, butyrate enemas and suppositories, topical and oral mesalamine (Rowasa), Canasa suppositories, and corticosteroid enemas. Bismuth carbomer foam enemas have been compared to placebo in their effectiveness in the treatment of pouchitis. In a small study of 40 patients with active and chronic pouchitis who failed antibiotic and other medical therapies, the response rates between the treated and placebo groups were identical at 45%. Therefore, there appears to be no significant benefit in the use of bismuth carbomer foam enemas for the treatment of pouchitis (36).

Glutamine has been shown to be an essential nutrient for the enterocyte. Topical application of glutamine may be effective in reducing inflammation of the ileal pouch mucosa. However, ileoanal pouch cells undergo metaplasia and take on the appearance of colonic cells over time. Therefore, it has been proposed that the application of butyrate enemas to the inflamed mucosa of the ileoanal pouch will result in adequate treatment of pouchitis. In a small nonplacebo-controlled study assessing the effectiveness of glutamine and butyrate suppositories for the treatment of pouchitis, 40% of patients who received glutamine had relapses of pouchitis during treatment, whereas 67% who received butyrate had relapsing symptoms. This study also showed that total concentrations of short chain fatty acids were considerably lower in patients with pouchitis than in those without pouchitis (37).

Topical and oral use of mesalamine (Rowasa enemas, Canasa suppositories, and Asacol) may have some role in the treatment of pouchitis. These anti-inflammatory agents are effective in treating distal forms of ulcerative colitis. However, long-term use may be required in order to maintain states of remission (38). In addition, corticosteroid enemas, which may function through a systemic rather than a local mechanism of action, have been used. Patients have complained of systemic side effects of such steroid enema use. More recently, budesonide enemas have been used to treat chronic pouchitis without the systemic side effects of steroids.

In those individuals who ultimately prove to have Crohn's disease of the ileoanal pouch, infliximab as well as other immunosuppressive medications have been effective. In seven patients treated with anti TNF-alpha monoclonal antibody for active inflammatory disease of the pouch or fistulizing Crohn's disease, six patients had complete response. Other immunosuppressive medications were used to maintain remission (39).

Azathioprine and 6-mercaptopurine have been used anecdotally for the treatment of severe pouchitis and may also be effective (40). However, there are no prospective randomized trials looking at the efficacy of these drugs. The suggested starting dose for both drugs is generally 50 mg/day with dosing similar to that given for patients with ulcerative colitis and Crohn's disease (41). Careful monitoring with blood tests is essential for patients on immunosuppressive therapy. In addition, it may take several weeks for these medications to be effective.

Contrary to the deleterious effect of cigarette smoking on the status of Crohn's disease, a protective role of smoking against ulcerative colitis has been reported (42). Furthermore, there have been reports that smoking may have a positive effect in preventing pouchitis, although the exact mechanism for this is unknown. The first study to report this finding concluded that only 1 of 17 smokers had a single episode of pouchitis compared to 18 of 72 nonsmokers who had 46 episodes of pouchitis (43). This raises the question of whether there could be benefits using a nicotine patch in preventing pouchitis, although there is no current data addressing this issue.

Surgical therapy is generally limited to patients with severe medical refractory pouchitis. This will ultimately affect less than 2% of patients and should be reserved for those patients who have refractory disease with poor pouch function. In one series of 470 patients who had undergone total proctocolectomy with ileoanal pouch reconstruction, 1.4% of patients required pouch excision. One-half of these patients were ultimately shown to have Crohn's disease of the pouch and none of the patients had their pouches removed due to refractory pouchitis (44).

Pouch excision may be a technically challenging to perform with significant operative morbidity; therefore, proper patient counseling is imperative. Risks of this surgery include injury to the small bowel, ureters, or major vascular structures. In addition, pelvic fibrosis may result from the previous pelvic surgery as well as recurrent episodes of pouchitis and pelvic sepsis. This scarring may lead to a loss of the proper planes of pelvic dissection and may result in injury to pelvic nerves causing impotency or infertility in males, dyspareunia in females, and dangerous presacral bleeding.

Prior to pouch excision, consideration for proximal fecal diversion should be given since this procedure is easier to perform with less operative morbidity and is reversible. Fecal diversion will often eliminate the symptoms of medical refractory pouchitis. However, upon stoma reversal the patients may relapse and experience recurrent bouts of pouchitis. If the patient elects to undergo pouch excision consideration may be given to construction of a second pelvic pouch or a continent ileostomy. These operations are technically demanding and should only be undertaken by surgeons with significant expertise in reoperative pouch surgery.

CONCLUSIONS

Diversion colitis and pouchitis are both common inflammatory bowel conditions that require proper diagnosis prior to initiating treatment. Understanding the pathophysiology of these clinical entities helps the clinician in choosing the proper course of therapy. These treatments should be carried out with the patient, gastroenterologist, and the colon and rectal surgeon working together with open and clear lines of communication in order to provide the most effective therapy.

REFERENCES

1. Glotzer DJ, Glick ME, Goldman H. Proctitis and colitis following diversion of the fecal stream. Gastroenterology 1981; 80(3):438–441.
2. Murray FE, O'Brian M, Birkett DH, Kennedy SM, LaMont JT. Diversion colitis: pathologic findings in a resected sigmoid colon and rectum. Gastroenterology 1987; 93:1404–1408.
3. Fenton CM, Siegel RJ. A prospective evaluation of diversion colitis. Am Surg 1991; 57:46.
4. Velazquez OC, Lederer HM, Rombeau JL. Butyrate and the colonocyte. Production, absorption, metabolism, and therapeutic implications. Adv Exp Med Biol 1997; 427:123–134.
5. Cook SI, Sellin JH. Review article: short chain fatty acids in health and disease. Aliment Pharmacol Ther 1998; 12(6):499–507.
6. Lai JM, Chuang TY, Francisco GE, Strayer JR. Diversion colitis: a cause of abdominal discomfort in spinal cord injury patients with colostomy. Arch Phys Med Rehabil 1997; 78(6):670–671.
7. Frisbie JH, Ahmed N, Hirano I, Klein MA, Soybel DI. Diversion colitis in patients with myelopathy: clinical, endoscopic, and histopathologic findings. J Spinal Cord Med 2000; 23(2):142–149.
8. Cherukuri R, Levine MS, Maki DD, Rubesin SE, Laufer I, Rosato EF. Hartman's pouch: radiographic evaluation of postoperative findings. Am J Roentgenol 1998; 171(6):1577–1582.
9. Fazio VW, Ziv Y, Church JM, et al. Ileal pouch-anal anastomoses complications and function in 1005 patients. Ann Surg 1995; 222(2):120–127.
10. Penna C, Dozois R, Tremaine W, et al. Pouchitis after ileal pouch-anal anastomosis for ulcerative colitis occurs with increased frequency in patients with associated primary sclerosing cholangitis. Gut 1996; 38(2):234–239.
11. Madiba TE, Bartolo DC. Pouchitis following restorative proctocolectomy for ulcerative colitis: incidence and therapeutic outcome. J R Coll Surg Edinb 2001; 46(6):334–337.
12. Meagher AP, Farouk R, Dozois RR, Kelly KA, Pemberton JH. J ileal pouch-anal anastomosis for chronic ulcerative colitis: complications and long-term outcome in 1310 patients. Br J Surg 1998; 85(6):800–803.
13. Penna C, Tiret E, Kartheuser A, Hannoun L, Nordlinger B, Parc R. Function of ileal J pouch-anal anastomosis in patients with familial adenomatous polyposis. Br J Surg 1993; 80(6):765–767.
14. Patel RT, Bain I, Youngs D, Keighley MR. Cytokine production in pouchitis is similar to that in ulcerative colitis. Dis Colon Rectum 1995; 38(8):831–837.
15. Stallmach A, Schafer F, Hoffmann S, et al. Increased state of activation of CD4 positive T cells and elevated interferon gamma production in pouchitis. Gut 1998; 43(4):499–505.

16. Stallmach A, Chan CC, Ecker KW, et al. Comparable expression of matrix metalloproteinases 1 and 2 in pouchitis and ulcerative colitis. Gut 2000; 47(3):415–422.
17. Fleshner PR, Vasiliauskas EA, Kam LY, et al. High level perinuclear antineutrophil cytoplasmic antibody (pANCA) in ulcerative colitis patients before colectomy predicts the development of chronic pouchitis after ileal pouch-anal anastomosis. Gut 2001; 49(5):671–677.
18. O'Connell PR, Rankin DR, Weiland LH, Kelly KA. Enteric bacteriology, absorption, morphology and emptying after ileal pouch-anal anastomosis. Br J Surg 1986; 73(11):909–914.
19. Ruseler-van Embden JG, Schouten WR, van Lieshout LM. Pouchitis: result of microbial imbalance? Gut 1994; 35(5):658–664.
20. Nasmyth DG, Godwin PG, Dixon MF, Williams NS, Johnston D. Ileal ecology after pouch-anal anastomosis or ileostomy. A study of mucosal morphology, fecal bacteriology, fecal volatile fatty acids, and their interrelationship. Gastroenterology 1989; 96(3):817–824.
21. Clausen MR, Tvede M, Mortensen PB. Short-chain fatty acids in pouch contents from patients with and without pouchitis after ileal pouch-anal anastomosis. Gastroenterology 1992; 103(4):1144–1153.
22. de Silva HJ, Ireland A, Kettlewell M, Mortensen N, Jewell DP. Short-chain fatty acid irrigation in severe pouchitis. N Engl J Med 1989; 321(20):1416–1417.
23. Kienle P, Weitz J, Reinshagen S, et al. Association of decreased perfusion of the ileoanal pouch mucosa with early postoperative pouchitis and local septic complications. Arch Surg 2001; 136(10):1124–1130.
24. Levin KE, Pemberton JH, Phillips SF, Zinsmeister AR, Pezim ME. Role of oxygen free radicals in the etiology of pouchitis. Dis Colon Rectum 1992; 35(5):452–456.
25. Joelsson M, Andersson M, Bark T, et al. Allopurinol as prophylaxis against pouchitis following ileal pouch-anal anastomosis for ulcerative colitis. A randomized placebo-controlled double-blind study. Scand J Gastroenterol 2001; 36(11):1179–1184.
26. Lohmuller JL, Pemberton JH, Dozois RR, Ilstrup D, van Heerden J. Pouchitis and extraintestinal manifestations of inflammatory bowel disease after ileal pouch-anal anastomosis. Ann Surg 1990; 211(5):622–627.
27. Moskowitz RL, Shepherd NA, Nicholls RJ. An assessment of inflammation in the reservoir after restorative proctocolectomy with ileoanal ileal reservoir. Int J Colorectal Dis 1986; 1(3):167–174.
28. Shen B, Achkar JP, Lashner BA, et al. Endoscopic and histologic evaluation together with symptom assessment are required to diagnose pouchitis. Gastroenterology 2001; 121(2):261–267.
29. Sandborn WJ, Tremaine WJ, Batts KP, Pemberton JH, Phillips SF. Pouchitis after ileal pouch-anal anastomosis: a pouchitis disease activity index. Mayo Clin Proc 1994; 69(5):409–415.
30. Bjarnason I, Hayllar J, Smethurst P, Price A, Gumpel MJ. Metronidazole reduces intestinal inflammation and blood loss in non-steroidal anti-inflammatory drug induced enteropathy. Gut 1992; 33(9):1204–1208.
31. Shen B, Achkar JP, Lashner BA, et al. A randomized clinical trial of ciprofloxacin and metronidazole to treat acute pouchitis. Inflamm Bowel Dis 2001; 7(4):301–305.
32. Hurst RD, Chung TP, Rubin M, Michelassi F. The implications of acute pouchitis on the long-term functional results after restorative proctocolectomy. Inflamm Bowel Dis 1998; 4(4):280–284.
33. Gionchetti P, Amadini C, Rizzello F, et al. Probiotics—role in inflammatory bowel disease. Dig Liver Dis 2002; 34(suppl 2):S58–S62.
34. Sartor RB. Probiotics in chronic pouchitis: restoring luminal microbial balance. Gastroenterology 2000; 119(2):584–587.
35. Gionchetti P, Rizzello F, Venturi A, et al. Oral bacteriotherapy as maintenance treatment in patients with chronic pouchitis: a double-blind, placebo-controlled trial. Gastroenterology 2000; 119(2):305–309.
36. Tremaine WJ, Sandborn WJ, Wolff BG, Carpenter HA, Zinsmeister AR, Metzger PP. Bismuth carbomer foam enemas for active chronic pouchitis: a randomized, double-blind, placebo-controlled trial. Aliment Pharmacol Ther 1997; 11(6):1041–1046.
37. Wischmeyer P, Pemberton JH, Phillips SF. Chronic pouchitis after ileal pouch-anal anastomosis: responses to butyrate and glutamine suppositories in a pilot study. Mayo Clin Proc 1993; 68(10):978–981.
38. Miglioli M, Barbara L, Di Febo G, et al. Topical administration of 5-aminosalicylic acid: a therapeutic proposal for the treatment of pouchitis. N Engl J Med 1989; 320(4):257.
39. Ricart E, Panaccione R, Loftus EV, Tremaine WJ, Sandborn WJ. Successful management of Crohn's disease of the ileoanal pouch with infliximab. Gastroenterology 1999; 117(2):429–432.
40. Berrebi W, Chaussade S, Bruhl AL, et al. Treatment of Crohn's disease recurrence after ileoanal anastomosis by azathioprine. Dig Dis Sci 1993; 38(8):1558–1560.
41. Shen B. Diagnosis and treatment of patients with pouchitis. Drugs 2003; 63(5):453–461.
42. Abraham N, Selby W, Lazarus R, Solomon M. Is smoking an indirect risk factor for the development of ulcerative colitis? An age- and sex-matched case-control study. J Gastroenterol Hepatol 2003; 18(2):139–146.
43. Merrett MN, Mortensen N, Kettlewell M, Jewell DO. Smoking may prevent pouchitis in patients with restorative proctocolectomy for ulcerative colitis. Gut 1996; 38(3):362–364.
44. Becker JM, Stucchi AF, Bryant DE. How do you treat refractory pouchitis and when do you decide to remove the pouch? Inflamm Bowel Dis 1998; 4(2):167–169.

30 | Hemorrhoids

Martin Luchtefeld
Ferguson Clinic, MMPC, Grand Rapids, and Michigan State University, East Lansing, Michigan, U.S.A.

INTRODUCTION

Hemorrhoidal disease has plagued mankind since ancient times. It is one of the few diseases with a patron saint; St. Fiacre was accorded this honor in the time of Galen (1). Although a common disorder, this malady is still frequently misunderstood and inappropriately treated.

ANATOMY

Thomson (2) described hemorrhoids as vascular cushions in his master's thesis in 1975. The submucosa in each of the regions of the cushions is filled with blood vessels intertwined with muscular fibers (muscularis submucosa). These appear to be important in supporting the blood vessels and maintaining the position of the cushions in the anal canal by supporting the adherence to the internal anal sphincter.

Hemorrhoidal cushions are present at birth and, even at that stage of development, are present in the three classical locations: left lateral, right anterior, and right posterior (2). Secondary hemorrhoids are present between the three main cushions. The forces of aging, gravity, and any other pelvic pressure can lead to disruption or attenuation of the supportive fibers that help hold the cushions in place. Eventually, the cushions can engorge and/or start to prolapse out of the anal canal. It is this process that actually leads to the condition of "hemorrhoidal disease."

The blood supply of hemorrhoids is from the superior rectal (hemorrhoidal) artery, middle rectal artery, and inferior hemorrhoidal artery. There are corresponding superior, middle, and inferior hemorrhoidal veins that drain into the inferior mesenteric vein, and subsequently into the portal vein. The hemorrhoidal tissues themselves contain arteriovenous fistulas that do not contain muscle, therefore these structures should be considered sinusoids (3).

Hemorrhoids are not the result of portal hypertension (4). When portal hypertension is present, the portosystemic connections allow the superior and middle rectal veins to enlarge and form rectal varices; as many as 44% of patients with cirrhosis will have anorectal varices (5). While patients may have both anorectal varices and hemorrhoids, these two entities are not related.

The dentate line serves as the dividing line between the internal and external hemorrhoids. Internal hemorrhoids start at the dentate line and extend superiorly. The lining here is transitional epithelium initially and columnar epithelium at the most superior aspect. External hemorrhoids extend from the perianum up to the dentate line and are covered by the anoderm, which is a specialized squamous epithelium with no skin appendages (Fig. 1).

One of the clinically important anatomical differences between the internal and external hemorrhoids is their nerve supply. The richly innervated and highly sensitive anoderm that covers the external hemorrhoids has sensation provided by the inferior rectal branch of the pudendal nerve, a somatic nerve. Autonomic nerves (both sympathetic and parasympathetic fibers) from the pelvic plexus provide innervation to the mucosa overlying the internal hemorrhoids. This variance in the nerve supply is what allows for the interventions that treat internal hemorrhoids to be relatively pain free.

(A)　　　　　　　　　　　　　　　**(B)**

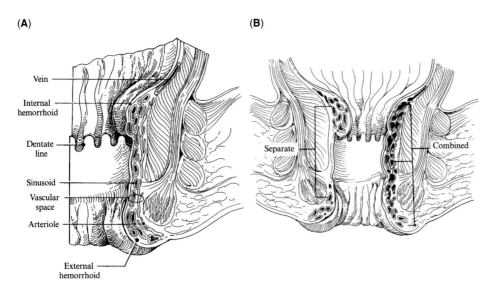

Vein

Internal
hemorrhoid

Dentate
line

Separate

Combined

Sinusoid

Vascular
space

Arteriole

External
hemorrhoid

Figure 1 Hemorrhoidal anatomy. (**A**) Arteriovenous anastomosis (AV shunts) forming hemorrhoidal plexus; (**B**) usual position of the hemorrhoids. Separate external and internal hemorrhoids are seen on the left and a combined internal–external hemorrhoidal complex is seen on the right.

CLASSIFICATION

The most commonly referenced classification system for hemorrhoidal disease uses the following definitions: *first degree*: bleeding hemorrhoids that visibly bulge on examination; *second degree*: hemorrhoids that prolapse with defecation, but spontaneously reduce; *third degree*: hemorrhoids that prolapse with defecation, but require manual reduction; *fourth degree*: permanently prolapsed hemorrhoids. This classification system is useful for comparing treatment groups but does not apply to those patients with primarily external hemorrhoidal disease such as with thrombosis or skin tags.

INCIDENCE

Although the true incidence and prevalence of symptomatic hemorrhoids is unknown, the prevalence was estimated to be approximately 4.4% in a 1990 study using data from the National Center for Health Statistics (6). The peak age group in this study was reportedly between 45 and 65 years of age. However, the incidence of hemorrhoids were self-reported, therefore it is difficult to determine the accuracy of this report. Another recent survey reported that 9% of adults were either surgically (4%) or medically (5%) treated for hemorrhoidal disease (7).

CLINICAL PRESENTATION

Pain, protrusion, and rectal bleeding are the hallmarks of hemorrhoidal disease. Burning and itching can sometimes be a component of the presentation. The exact nature of the patient's complaints can vary considerably among individuals. Severe pain from hemorrhoids is very unusual except in the setting of thrombosis or in the presence of a concomitant anal fissure; internal hemorrhoids are rarely painful. A call from the emergency room to see a patient with a "painful internal hemorrhoid" is almost guaranteed to be a condition other than a hemorrhoid.

The protrusion associated with hemorrhoids can be related to several variables. For those patients who complain of constant protrusion, large skin tags or fourth-degree prolapsed hemorrhoids are often the cause. The presence of these large hemorrhoids can be painless, although in some patients it can interfere with good hygiene. Other patients complain of transient protrusion that occurs after bowel movements, and then spontaneously reduces or requires manual reduction. Swelling that persists for several days to weeks but eventually resolves is often the result of thrombosis.

Bleeding associated with hemorrhoidal disease ranges from traces of blood on the toilet paper to accounts of blood spraying into the toilet bowl. The blood is usually bright red and generally not mixed into the stool. It is highly unusual for hemorrhoidal bleeding to be severe enough to lead to anemia (8). However, if anemia is present, a thorough investigation of the gastrointestinal tract before attributing the anemia to hemorrhoids should be undertaken.

Hemorrhoidal thrombosis can be a dramatic event. Some patients will have had few, if any, previous hemorrhoidal complaints, and usually describe a sudden swelling in the perianal region accompanied by significant pain. Depending on the severity and extent of the thrombosis as well as the patient's level of tolerance, these symptoms can lead to urgent trips to the office or emergency room. If left untreated, most of these episodes begin to resolve by the third or fourth day. The swelling typically takes considerably longer to reduce. Occasionally, the thrombosis can erode through the skin, leading to rather dramatic bleeding for a short period of time accompanied by a substantial decrease in pain.

EVALUATION

Before embarking upon a treatment course for hemorrhoids, a careful evaluation must be completed to insure that the condition is in fact hemorrhoids. A focused history will provide many clues as to whether or not the assumed diagnosis of hemorrhoids is correct. Most patients are not familiar with any perianal disorders other than hemorrhoids, therefore all symptoms emanating from the proximity of the anus are attributed to "hemorrhoids."

Physical examination starts with evaluation of the perianal skin. Any external hemorrhoids are noted as well as any other findings such as dermatoses or the superficial ulcerations and thickened skin consistent with pruritus ani. Slight eversion of the anal canal usually allow visualization of anal fissures. Digital rectal examination is undertaken to evaluate for masses and for any areas of induration or pain. Anoscopy with a side-viewing anoscope is the ideal method of evaluating hemorrhoids. Asking the patient to strain slightly during the examination can facilitate identification of the largest, most symptomatic hemorrhoids.

Bleeding should always be thoroughly evaluated; even a history that sounds convincingly like anorectal outlet in origin can be the sign of malignancy or inflammatory bowel disease. At a minimum, proctosigmoidoscopy and, if feasible, colonoscopy should be performed for every patient to exclude other sources of bleeding.

TREATMENT

There are a number of different options available for the treatment of hemorrhoidal symptoms. The ultimate decision as to which treatment to utilize will be based on the symptoms, the nature of the hemorrhoids (internal vs. external), and the patient's motivation. Some patients are content with the assurance that their symptoms are due to hemorrhoids and not other, more life-threatening disorders. The treatment of hemorrhoids is almost always elective, and many patients will defer treatment to a more convenient time.

Conservative Management of Hemorrhoids

The conservative management of hemorrhoids involves a careful examination and evaluation, as previously discussed, to insure that the symptoms are truly attributable to hemorrhoidal disease. For those patients who do require therapy, treatment generally consists of normalizing bowel movements and the use of topical ointments. Fiber supplements are also quite useful in the management of hemorrhoids. For those patients who tend to be constipated, the addition of a 3 to 6 g/day fiber supplement results in more frequent, softer bowel movements, thereby decreasing the amount of straining. However, it is also important to counsel the patient to avoid straining during evacuation.

Sitz baths using warm-to-hot tap water twice daily for 10 to 15 minutes can also be helpful, particularly during an acute flare-up of hemorrhoidal disease. It has been shown that for hemorrhoidal disease as well as other painful anorectal disorders, sitz baths actually decrease anal canal tone, providing a physiologic explanation for the associated pain relief (9).

Topical therapies can also be helpful; multiple various over-the-counter and prescription ointments are available. These salves contain a combination of skin protectants, astringents, and anti-inflammatory agents as well as topical anesthetics. The effectiveness of these various ointments varies among patients. Often, trial and error is the only way to isolate the most effective topical agent. It is important to avoid the use of a steroid-containing agent for prolonged periods of time, as this can lead to thinning of the perianal skin (10), and ultimately worsen the outcome. Regardless of any potential merits to these ointments, the results will most likely be less satisfactory when used for acute thrombosed hemorrhoids.

Procedures for Hemorrhoids

There are several options for the treatment of internal hemorrhoids because of the relatively insensitive nature of the mucosal lining in this area. These treatment options are associated with relatively minimal pain while effectively treating internal hemorrhoids. While external hemorrhoids may secondarily benefit from these therapies, treatment is intended primarily for internal hemorrhoids.

Nonexcisional Procedures

One of the numerous options available for the treatment of internal hemorrhoids is rubber band ligation. This appears to be the most effective and most widely used of the treatment modalities.

Rubber Band Ligation

The concept of ligating or tying off internal hemorrhoids has been in use for many years. Simple ligature of the internal hemorrhoids with silk suture was described in Dr. Joseph Mathew's textbook in 1899 (11). An instrument to allow rubber band ligation of hemorrhoids was first described in 1958 by Blaisdell (12). In 1963 (13), Barron reported on a series of patients treated by rubber band ligation with great success. This technique proved so popular that it replaced hemorrhoidectomy as the primary treatment of hemorrhoids among some surgeons (14). This method has proven particularly durable and useful for the treatment of stages II and III hemorrhoidal disease.

Rubber band ligation is generally undertaken in the office setting. The patient is asked to prepare for the procedure by using one or more disposable phosphate enemas; no anesthesia is necessary. The internal hemorrhoids are identified and exposed using an anoscope or retractor of choice. Once exposure has been accomplished, the hemorrhoids are treated by placing a band at the base of the internal hemorrhoid 1 to 1.5 cm above the dentate line (Fig. 2). Care

(A)

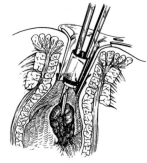

(B)

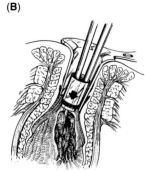

(C)

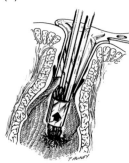

(D)

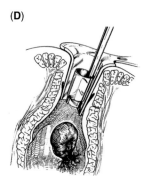

Figure 2 Rubber band ligation. (**A**) A suitable retractor exposes the hemorrhoid, which is firmly grasped. (**B**) The rubber band is carefully "eased" toward the hemorrhoid while traction is exerted on it. (**C**) One or two bands are placed at the base. (**D**) Satisfactory placement of the band causes no pain. *Source*: From Ref. 15.

must be taken to avoid hemorrhoidal banding too close to the dentate line as this distal place-ment may lead to significant patient discomfort; one to three bands can be placed at each encounter. While some studies have indicated that there is no difference in pain or complica-tions related to the number of bands placed (16,17), Lau et al. (18) reported severe pain in 29% of patients when three bands were used. Consequently, many clinicians limit the number of bands placed to one or two per session to avoid causing the patient undue pain.

Complications of hemorrhoidal banding are quite unusual; approximately 1% of patients will have significant delayed bleeding one to two weeks after the procedure when the band has fallen off (19). This bleeding can be profuse enough to require suture ligation while at other times it will resolve spontaneously. Postbanding sepsis is a rare but significant compli-cation. Although its exact incidence is unknown, it is a sentinel event that can lead to severe sepsis and even death. Postbanding sepsis was first definitively reported in 1980 (20), and can occur even after a single band is placed in young, otherwise healthy patients (20,21). The characteristic signs of postbanding sepsis are fever, inability to urinate, increasing pain, and bleeding. Patients undergoing banding should be made aware of the warning signs, and clin-icians need to promptly respond to any of these complaints following banding. Treatment includes broad-spectrum antibiotics and debridement of the banding site; a colostomy may be necessary in extreme cases.

Hemorrhoidal banding has been proven effective in 77% to 91% of patients who report good-to-excellent results, depending on how that is defined (7,22,23). However, banding is less effective for grade IV than for grades II and III hemorrhoids (22). For patients who are unresponsive to banding, have grade IV hemorrhoids, or large skin tags, excisional hemor-rhoidectomy should be considered.

Sclerotherapy

Injection of hemorrhoids with a caustic solution was first described in 1869 by Morgan (24), and has since been used as a nonsurgical means of treating hemorrhoids. Sodium morrhuate, 5% phenol in almond or vegetable oil, quinine, urea, and a number of other solutions have been used for this purpose; this method is inexpensive and easy to learn. Similar to other modalities of treating internal hemorrhoids, the principle of this treatment is to cause attenuation and scarring at the site of the internal hemorrhoid. Such treatment has not been deemed useful for patients with significant prolapse. However, the healing process that leads to fibrosis also helps reduce any partially prolapsed external hemorrhoid back into the anal canal.

An anoscope or anorectal retractor is used to expose the internal hemorrhoids. One to three internal hemorrhoids can then be injected using a small gauge needle with small amounts of 1 to 3 cc of sclerosing solution per hemorrhoid. It is important to inject 1 cm or more above the dentate line to minimize discomfort. A larger amount of sclerosant can seep toward the dentate line and cause pain. Although this method of treatment has been popular, particularly in the United Kingdom (25,26), randomized trials have shown that it is less effec-tive than rubber band ligation (27,28). However, it can be useful in the setting of bleeding hemorrhoids that are friable and/or not yet enlarged enough to place rubber bands.

Infrared Coagulation

Infrared coagulation, first described in 1979 by Neiger (29), is another option in the treatment of internal hemorrhoids. It shares many of the same characteristics as injection sclerotherapy, and is generally used for the same indications. The infrared radiation is generated by a tung-sten halogen lamp that is housed in a gold-plated box. The infrared light application has a width of 3 mm, and penetrates the tissue to a depth of 3 mm; the radiation causes protein coagulation. Infrared coagulation can be performed in an outpatient setting with minimal dis-comfort; one to three hemorrhoids can be treated per session. The manufacturer recommends three to five applications (or pulses) of infrared coagulation per hemorrhoid treated. Although the instrument can be calibrated for pulse lengths of 0.1 to 3 seconds, a pulse of 1 to 1.5 seconds is generally optimal.

Infrared coagulation is performed in the office or outpatient setting. An anoscope or retractor is used to gain exposure to the internal hemorrhoids. The tip of the instrument is a small flat circle that is directly applied to the mucosal surface of the intended treatment area. Each hemorrhoid is then treated with three to five applications at a level of 1 to 2 cm above the dentate line. It is important to treat at a level cephalad enough to minimize pain. A small white dot immediately appears after each application. Occasionally, an audible "pop" is heard as tissue is heated. Eventually, the treated area becomes ulcerated and edematous and produces a discharge before healing and scarring occurs.

The results of studies using infrared coagulation have indicated that this is an effective therapy for internal hemorrhoids. Prospective trials have found this modality to be equally efficacious compared to injection sclerotherapy, bipolar diathermy, and rubber band ligation (28,30–32). However, this method tends to preserve more tissue, which leads to less scarring than do some other methods described in this section. Consequently, infrared coagulation is less effective for prolapse than methods such as rubber band ligation.

Cryotherapy

Cryotherapy was initially described as a painless, effective method of treating hemorrhoids. Theoretically, cryotherapy could be used for both the internal and the external hemorrhoids. A probe of liquid nitrogen or liquid nitrous oxide leads to rapid freezing, followed by thawing and subsequent cellular destruction. Although initial reports were encouraging (33), subsequent literature has been less positive. Oh (34) found that many patients had prolonged drainage, which was also confirmed by Traynor and Carter (35). Other authors have reported that cryotherapy is effective only for internal hemorrhoids (36). One study compared cryotherapy versus standard hemorrhoidectomy and found that 65% of the patients preferred hemorrhoidectomy (37). Given the many options for the treatment of hemorrhoids and the relative lack of any supporting literature, there seems to be little role for cryotherapy at this time.

Direct Current Therapy

The direct current (Ultroid® device, Cabot Medical, Racine, Wisconsin, U.S.A.) device utilizes a special probe to deliver a 16 mA current to each of the hemorrhoids. A few reports have claimed good results (38–40). The primary drawback to this method is that the probe must be left in place for 10 minutes at each location. At the present time, there are too few data to endorse the routine use of this device.

Bipolar Diathermy

Another approach for the treatment of hemorrhoids with electrical current is bipolar diathermy. The Bipolar Circum Active Probe (BICAP®) device (Circon ACMI, Stamford, Massachusetts, U.S.A.) utilizes bipolar current through the tip of the device to produce coagulation, destruction of tissue and, ultimately, fibrosis at the treated area. A two-second pulse is applied to the internal hemorrhoids, which results in a 3-mm deep white coagulum. When compared to rubber band ligation (41), infrared coagulation (32), and direct current therapy (38), it was found to be equally efficacious.

Lord's Dilation

One type of nonexcisional therapy for hemorrhoids was reported by Lord in 1968 (42). He believed that increased anal canal pressure contributes to hemorrhoidal problems and symptoms and, for this reason, described dilation of the anus. Under appropriate sedation/ anesthesia, two fingers are initially inserted into the rectum, and the anus is then slowly dilated up until eight fingers can be inserted. Although some authors have reported good clinical results (42,43), this procedure does decrease anal canal pressures (44) and has been associated with the development of mild postoperative anal incontinence (45). A long-term follow-up study by Konsten and Baeten (46) revealed alarming rates of incontinence leading the authors to recommend that the procedure be abandoned. Given the multiple other treatment options for hemorrhoids, there would seem to be little role for this modality.

Hemorrhoidectomy

For patients who have failed conservative measures, have primary external hemorrhoidal disease, or for certain manifestations such as extensive thrombosis, excisional hemorrhoidectomy is the treatment of choice. Several variations on the technique of excisional hemorrhoidectomy have been reported and will be described in the following section. The choice of hemorrhoidectomy is based more on the surgeon's training and regional variations rather than scientific evidence.

Closed Ferguson Hemorrhoidectomy

Dr. Lynn Ferguson began closing all hemorrhoidectomy wounds in the 1950s and subsequently described his technique in 1959 (47). Prior to that time, the prevailing surgical wisdom was that closing the surgical wound would lead to extensive sepsis and prolonged healing times. Contrary to popular belief, Ferguson demonstrated that sepsis was rare and wound healing was rapid. Since his initial description and the subsequent publication of several large series of hemorrhoidectomies (48,49), most North American surgeons have adopted the technique of the Ferguson closed hemorrhoidectomy (Fig. 3A–H) (50).

Technique. Adequate anesthesia must first be established, which depends on surgeon and patient preference as well as body habitus and the anxiety level of the patient. General anesthesia, regional anesthesia, and heavy intravenous sedation with local anesthesia have all been successfully used. Ferguson described performing this procedure with the patient in the left lateral decubitus position as seen in Figure 4; other surgeons, however, prefer the lithotomy or prone jackknife positions. Once proper anesthesia and positioning have been achieved, the area is prepped and draped in a sterile fashion; local anesthesia is then infiltrated. A Hill-Ferguson retractor or similar instrument is used to gain optimal exposure of the anal canal. The hemorrhoids are incised in an elliptical fashion and dissected from the underlying sphincter muscle. The vascular pedicle is clamped, cut and then oversewn with an absorbable suture such as catgut or Vicryl (Ethicon Endosurgery Inc., Cincinnatti, Ohio, U.S.A.). The remaining mucosa and anoderm is then closed with a simple continuous stitch. The surgeon should take small portions of the underlying sphincter to close the potential dead space. The same sequence is repeated at each of the three classical hemorrhoidectomy sites: left lateral, right anterior, and right posterior. It is important to leave adequate tissue bridges between each excised site to minimize the incidence of stenosis. At the end of the procedure, each hemorrhoidectomy site should be reinspected for hemorrhage with a smaller retractor, as the larger retractors will sometimes tamponade bleeding (Figs. 3A–H).

Postoperative care consists of sitz baths, stool softeners, and pain control. Although this operation once required a five- to seven-day (or more!) hospitalization, it is now almost always performed on an outpatient basis or in a 23-hour observation unit.

Complications. Postoperative hemorrhage that is severe enough to require a return trip to the operating room occurs in approximately 1% of patients (51,52). The bleeding can be early (within 24 hours) or delayed (typically 10–14 days postoperatively). Delayed bleeding may be secondary to sepsis at the site of vascular ligation of the pedicle, whereas early bleeding is usually attributed to technical error or due to ineffectiveness of the epinephrine in the local anesthetic.

Surprisingly, the reported incidence of wound infection is quite low at less than 1% (51,52). However, it is quite possible that many patients develop small abscesses that drain and resolve spontaneously without medical intervention.

Urinary retention is a troublesome complication following hemorrhoidectomy. Catheterization rates as high as 14.9% to 52% (53,54) have been reported. Although multiple interventions have been tested to prevent this complication, perioperative fluid restriction and adequate perioperative pain control are the most efficacious. Both Scoma and the Ferguson Clinic group reported substantial decreases in catheterization rates by minimizing perioperative fluids (53,54). Narcotic pain medications are useful to maintain patient comfort. In addition, other authors have reported the use of ketorolac for dramatic improvement of pain control and decreased urinary retention (55,56).

Postoperative constipation is a constant threat; however, immediate preventative measures ensure that it rarely progresses to a significant problem. Less than 1% of patients go on to develop clinically significant fecal impaction. Skin tags, however, are a common long-term complication, and can generally be removed in the office under local anesthesia if they become bothersome. Anal stenosis is a rare but dreaded complication. The ideal treatment is prevention by leaving adequate skin bridges between the hemorrhoidal excision sites. However, if this complication does develop, several variations of anoplasty work quite well (57).

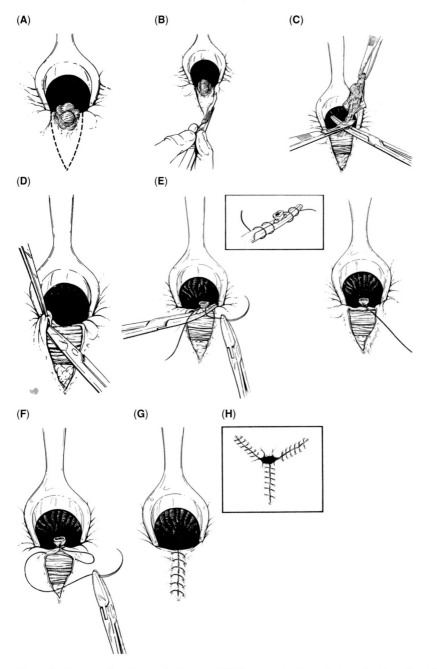

Figure 3 Ferguson closed hemorrhoidectomy. (**A**) The amount of tissue to be excised is outlined. (**B**) The hemorrhoidal complex is incised to the level of the subjacent muscle and superiorly to the anorectal ring. (**C**) Hemorrhoidal tissue is excised and the pedicle is secured. (**D**) Anoderm and perianal skin are sharply undermined and accessory hemorrhoidal tissue is excised. (**E**) The hemorrhoidal pedicle is secured with a suture if necessary. (**F**) A running suture closes the wounds. (**G**) The wound is secured without excessive tension. (**H**) The sutured wounds are properly separated. *Source*: From Ref. 15.

Results. Several large retrospective studies have reported excellent long-term results with hemorrhoidectomy. In a series from the Ferguson Clinic (52) of 1018 patients who responded to a survey, 95% had symptomatic relief. Most of the 28% of patients who had any rectal complaints suffered from pruritus ani. In another long-term study with follow-up of up to seven years, 7.7% of the 441 patients required further treatment of hemorrhoids, but only one actually required repeat hemorrhoidectomy (49). When prospectively evaluated, hemorrhoidectomy has been found effective, albeit more painful, than rubber band ligation (56–60).

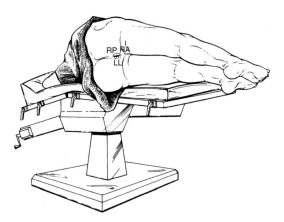

Figure 4 Patient in left lateral (Sims) decubitus position. The patient is tilted forward with the head down and shoulder below kidney rest. The table is canted away from the surgeon. The height of the table is variable. Orientation of hemorrhoids is shown as follows: RP, RA, and LL. *Abbreviations*: RP, right posterior; RA, right anterior; LL, left lateral. *Source*: From Ref. 15.

Open Hemorrhoidectomy

Outside the United States, many surgeons prefer the open hemorrhoidectomy technique, which is identical to the closed hemorrhoidectomy, except that after the vascular pedicle is oversewn, the anoderm and mucosa are not closed. Instead, they are allowed to heal by secondary intent. One variation of the open technique, which was popularized at St. Mark's Hospital in London, is referred to as the Milligan–Morgan hemorrhoidectomy (61). After gentle dilation of the anal canal, the hemorrhoids are everted by the use of a clamp placed at the mucocutaneous junction. After incising the anoderm and just slightly onto the mucosa, the vascular pedicle is tied off with a stout suture. The ligated hemorrhoid is then excised as is any skin tag or residual hemorrhoidal tissue. Three quadrants are usually excised in this fashion.

Several studies have compared the open versus closed techniques for hemorrhoidectomy (Table 1). Although proponents of each option feel very strongly that their choice is clearly superior, there is actually very little difference in these two methods in terms of healing or pain control that can be demonstrated on a consistent basis in the literature (62–65).

Alternative Energy Sources for Excisional Hemorrhoidectomy. In the recent past, there have been reports of alternative energy sources that have been used in lieu of the traditional scalpel or diathermy techniques for excisional hemorrhoidectomy. The promise of decreased pain, earlier return to work, and quicker wound healing has not been verified in randomized trials. Both Senagore et al. (66) and Nicholson et al. (67) compared Nd-YAG laser hemorrhoidectomy to excisional hemorrhoidectomy and found no difference in either pain control or wound healing. Ligasure (Tyco Healthcare, Massachusetts, U.S.A.), which is a type of bipolar electrocautery, was compared to conventional diathermy hemorrhoidectomy in 40 patients in a trial conducted by Jayne et al. (68); no statistically significant difference in pain control was noted in the Ligasure group. Similarly, no difference was seen when comparing scalpel excision to harmonic scalpel hemorrhoidectomy in other prospective randomized trials (69,70). Until a compelling reason and understandable pathophysiology can be presented, there appears to be little rationale for using alternative energy sources for hemorrhoidectomy.

Whitehead Hemorrhoidectomy

In 1882, Whitehead (71) described a type of hemorrhoidectomy that was designed to remove all hemorrhoidal tissue. In this technique, a circumferential incision is made at the dentate line and all the hemorrhoidal tissue excised through this incision. The redundant rectal

Table 1 Comparison of Open and Closed Hemorrhoidectomy Techniques

Authors, year	Number of patients	Findings
Arbman et al., 2000 (62)	77	Closed technique—wounds heal faster. Both methods "fairly efficient"
Carapati et al., 1999 (63)	35	No difference in outcome
Ho et al., 1997 (64)	67	No difference in pain. Open technique healed quicker
Gencosmanoglu et al., 2002 (65)	80	Open technique—longer healing, less pain

mucosa is excised and the proximal rectal mucosa is then sutured to the anoderm. Due to the technique of this operation, a circumferential ectropion known as a "whitehead deformity" may sometimes occur. This is a rather dreaded complication and is a large reason why most surgeons in North America have abandoned this procedure. However, there are still practitioners who argue that the Whitehead operation, when properly performed, is a good procedure (72,73).

Procedure for Prolapsed Hemorrhoid

In recent years there has been significant interest in a new procedure for hemorrhoidal disease that has been termed "procedure for prolapse and hemorrhoids," (PPH). Although a circular "stapled hemorrhoidectomy" was described in the mid-1980s (74), this procedure was used with increasing frequency after being popularized by Antonio Longo from Palermo, Italy, in the late 1990s (75). The term "stapled hemorrhoidectomy" is a misnomer. Sometimes referred to as a stapled anopexy, this technique does bring a new concept to the treatment of significant mixed hemorrhoidal disease. Instead of actually excising the internal and external hemorrhoids, the PPH technique partially excises some of the internal hemorrhoids but more importantly pulls the internal and external hemorrhoids up into their appropriate place in the anal canal. Conceptually, it is similar to a circumferential or "super banding" procedure. The primary allure of the PPH is the potential for less postoperative pain.

The procedure of PPH is illustrated in Figure 5A–F. Once the patient has been appropriately anesthetized and the field prepped and draped, the anus may require gentle dilatation to

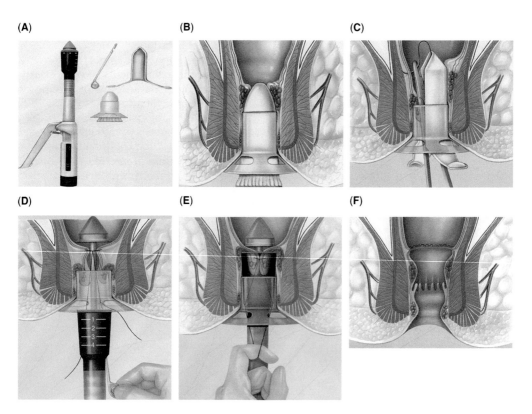

Figure 5 Procedure for prolapse and hemorrhoids. (**A**) Procedure for prolapsed hemorrhoid procedural set consisting of 33-mm hemorrhoidal circular stapler, suture threader, circular anal dilator, and purse-string suture anoscope. (**B**) After a gentle dilation of the anus, the circular anal dilator is inserted into the anus, and the obturator is removed. (**C**) The purse-string anoscope is introduced through the circular anal dilator. A purse-string suture is placed around the entire circumference of the rectum by rotating the anoscope. (**D**) The head of the hemorrhoidal circular stapler is introduced and placed proximal to the purse-string, which is then tied down. The suture threader is used to pull the ends of the suture, which are pulled through the lateral holes of the stapler. (**E**) With moderate traction on the purse string, the prolapse is drawn into the stapler. The stapler is closed and fired. The stapler is then opened slightly and removed. (**F**) When properly done, the staple line should lie at least 2 cm above the dentate line.

accept the flange. A prolene purse-string is then placed at the top of the internal hemorrhoids. The PPH instrument is then introduced into the anal canal and the previously placed purse-string is tied down in place. The instrument is fired and then removed. A large ring of tissue is usually excised. Any residual bleeding is controlled with electrocautery and/or suture ligature. Postoperative care consists mainly of stool softeners and analgesia, as needed. The most important claim associated with the PPH is less postoperative pain when compared to hemorrhoidectomy. There have now been a number of randomized prospective trials comparing PPH to various hemorrhoidectomy methods that support this notion (76–79). Boccasanta et al. (76) compared PPH to circular hemorrhoidectomy in 80 patients and found that, although both procedures were safe and effective, the PPH was less painful and associated with an earlier return to work. Similarly, Ho et al. (77) studied 119 patients undergoing either PPH or open diathermy hemorrhoidectomy and found that pain and time off work was decreased with the PPH. The complication rates were similar, but associated costs were significantly higher with the PPH. Other authors have compared PPH to diathermy hemorrhoidectomy and the Milligan–Morgan technique with similar results (78,79). One significant departure from this trend of positive results is a report from Cheetham et al. (80). A randomized, prospective trial comparing diathermy excisional hemorrhoidectomy to PPH was initiated but then terminated after accruing 22 patients, due to severe ongoing pain and fecal urgency in an excessively high number of patients. The authors summarized that incorporated muscle into the stapled anastomotic ring may have caused the excessive pain (80).

Complication rates seem to be similar to conventional excisional hemorrhoidectomy and consist primarily of bleeding, urinary retention, and stenosis. The dilation required to place the stapling instrument as well as the actual act of stapling has caused some concern for potential sphincter injury and incontinence. Ho et al. (77) used an intra-anal ultrasound and anorectal manometry to postoperatively evaluate both the diathermy hemorrhoidectomy and the PPH patients. Manometric changes were similar in both the groups. Intra-anal ultrasound revealed asymptomatic internal anal sphincter defects in one patient in each group, and in one incontinent patient in the diathermy hemorrhoidectomy group (77). In addition to the usual complications, there have been reports of rare but severe complications such as rectal perforation, retropneumoperitoneum, pneumomediastinum (81), and severe retroperitoneal sepsis (82,83).

The initial results support the view that there is less postoperative pain associated with the PPH procedure. As well, it does appear to provide good symptomatic relief of hemorrhoidal symptoms. Although to date, data collection has been primarily from European countries, preliminary results from a U.S. trial have also indicated less postoperative pain (84).

SELECTING THE APPROPRIATE PROCEDURE FOR INDIVIDUAL PATIENTS

Selection of the appropriate intervention for individual patients can sometimes be challenging because of the multiple options available. A meta-analysis of the literature of hemorrhoidal treatments was performed by MacRae and McLeod in 1995 (85) and subsequently updated in 2002 (86). The findings are summarized by the following guidelines: hemorrhoidectomy is the most effective treatment for grade III hemorrhoids. Although hemorrhoidectomy is more effective than rubber band ligation, the risk of complications is higher and pain is increased. Thus, rubber band ligation can be recommended as initial therapy of hemorrhoids. Rubber band ligation has proven more effective than both sclerotherapy and infrared coagulation. When comparing open to closed hemorrhoidectomy, no significant differences could be identified that supported the findings by Cheetham and Phillips (87). At the time of the meta-analysis, there were only three PPH trials published. In analyzing this small group, PPH was found to result in significantly less pain than other types of hemorrhoidectomy. However, follow-up has been short.

Based on this review, it would appear that rubber band ligation is an excellent first-line treatment for many patients with stage I, II, or III hemorrhoids. For those individuals who have stage IV hemorrhoids, recurrent or residual symptoms following banding, or simply prefer definitive therapy at the onset, hemorrhoidectomy is most effective. While the role of PPH has not been completely defined, this may very well expand if further long-term studies confirm its effectiveness.

SPECIAL CIRCUMSTANCES
Hemorrhoids and Crohn's Disease

One of the tenets of treatment for anorectal Crohn's disease is to minimize anorectal surgery. There has been significant concern that hemorrhoid surgery in patients with anorectal Crohn's disease can result in nonhealing wounds and even accelerate the timetable to requiring proctectomy. Jeffrey et al. (88) reported on a series of patients with inflammatory bowel disease and hemorrhoids. Of the 20 patients with Crohn's disease, six ultimately required proctectomy due to complications that seemed to date back to the time of the intervention for hemorrhoids (88). However, the Ferguson Clinic experience was quite different, as reported by Wolkomir and Luchtefeld in 1993 (89). At a mean follow-up of 11 years and five months, only one of the 17 patients required proctectomy. The authors emphasized that no patient had acutely active disease. It does appear, however, that with careful patient selection, hemorrhoid surgery can be safely and effectively performed in patients with Crohn's disease. The likely key to success is to ensure that the patient does indeed have symptomatic hemorrhoids rather than merely the skin tags that are the manifestation of severely active anorectal Crohn's disease.

Thrombosed External Hemorrhoids

The patient with a thrombosed external hemorrhoid usually recounts a history of perianal pain and swelling. The time course to presentation is variable with some patients enduring the condition for days, while others are in the doctor's office within 24 hours. Although many patients can relate the thrombosis to a specific event such as diarrhea or heavy lifting, others simply wake up one morning and discover the hemorrhoid.

Treatment varies and is based mainly on the time course of the thrombosed hemorrhoid. By three to five days, most patients start feeling better, and any surgical intervention will likely induce more pain rather than provide relief. For those early in their course or who remain in substantial pain, excision of the hemorrhoid can provide quick relief.

Excising a thrombosed external hemorrhoid is readily done in an office setting. The area of the thrombosis is infiltrated with local anesthetic, and a small wedge of skin is removed so that the underlying hemorrhoid and thrombosis can be excised; hemostasis is obtained using pressure and electrocautery, as needed. Postoperative care consists of twice daily sitz baths and appropriate analgesia.

Circumferential Thrombosed Gangrenous Hemorrhoids

The patient with circumferential thrombosed gangrenous hemorrhoids presents with a spectacular surgical problem. The patient usually recounts a short history of severe pain and swelling in the perianal region that may or may not have any precursor event. Physical examination confirms the diagnosis, usually at a single glance. At one point, there was significant concern regarding sepsis following hemorrhoidectomy in the setting of gangrenous hemorrhoids. For this reason, one treatment that evolved entailed extensive perianal block followed by manual reduction of the prolapsed hemorrhoids. Although this provided some pain relief, the hemorrhoidal problem still remained. Currently, a number of series have reported excellent results with excisional hemorrhoidectomy which is now the treatment of choice (90–92).

From a technical standpoint, there are some variations in technique that are worth mentioning. At the onset of the operation, the hemorrhoids are immensely edematous; therefore, the hemorrhoids and perianal region should be infiltrated with local anesthesia with 1:200,000 epinephrine. Manual pressure should then be applied for a minimum of several minutes to minimize the edema. This maneuver will dramatically shrink the hemorrhoids and simplify the operation. Intraoperatively, it is important to note that the entire thrombosis does not need to be removed to have a successful result. Adequate tissue bridges should be retained between the excision sites to minimize the incidence of anal stenosis. Significant hemorrhoidal tissue that remains between excision sites can be removed by mucosal undermining and excision.

Hemorrhoids in Pregnancy

Hemorrhoidal symptoms are common in pregnancy, but are rarely critical enough to require surgical intervention. Saleeby et al. (93) reported on 25 of 12,455 pregnant women (0.2%) who underwent hemorrhoidectomy. The procedures were performed under local anesthesia, and the majority of women were in the third trimester without any fetal or maternal complications. Although hemorrhoidectomy seems safe during pregnancy, prudence demands that surgical intervention be used only in unusual circumstances, and that appropriate maternal and fetal monitoring is instituted.

HIV and Hemorrhoidal Disease

Given the immunocompromised state of the human immunodeficiency virus (HIV) patients, there has been concern regarding hemorrhoidal surgery in this setting. Morandi et al. (94) studied a series of patients with either Centers for Disease Control (CDC) stage II asymptomatic disease ($N = 32$) or AIDS ($N = 16$). The healing rate was 66% at 14 weeks, and 100% at 32 weeks in patients with CDC stage II HIV infection; complications occurred in 22%. For those patients with AIDS, none had healed by 14 weeks, and only 50% at 32 weeks; complications occurred in 87.5%, including several wound infections with unusual organisms. In a retrospective study, Hewitt et al. (95) found that healing rates were similar in HIV+ and HIV− patients. Hemorrhoidectomy appears to be contraindicated in the patient with AIDS, but for patients with HIV infection, surgery should be approached with the knowledge that healing should occur but may possibly be delayed.

REFERENCES

1. Rachochot JE, Petourand CH, Riovoire JO. Saint Fiacre: the healer of hemorrhoids and patron saint of proctology. Am J Proctol 1971; 22:175–179.
2. Thomson WHF. The nature of haemorrhoids. Br J Surg 1975; 62:542–552.
3. Stelzner F, Staubesand J, Machleidt H. Das Cavernosum Recti-Die Grundlage der inneren Hamorrhoiden. Langenbecks Arch Klin Chir 1962; 299:302–312.
4. Thulsius O, Gjores JE. Arterio-venous anastomoses in the anal region with reference to the pathogenesis and treatment of hemorrhoids. Acto Chir Scand 1973; 139:476–478.
5. Hosking SW, Smart HL, Johnson AG, et al. Anorectal varices, haemorrhoids, and portal hypertension. Lancet 1989; 1:349–352.
6. Hohanson JF, Sonnenberg A. The prevalence of hemorrhoids and chronic constipation: an epidemiologic study. Gastroenterology 1990; 98:380–386.
7. Nelson RL, Abcarian H, Davis FG, et al. Prevalence of benign anorectal disease in a randomly selected population. Dis Colon Rectum 1995; 38:341–344.
8. Kluiber RM, Wolf BG. Evaluation of anemia caused by hemorrhoidal bleeding. Dis Colon Rectum 1994; 34:1006–1007.
9. Dodi G, Bogoni F, Infantino A, et al. Hot or cold in anal pain? A study of the changes in internal sphincter pressure profiles. Dis Colon Rectum 1986; 29:248–251.
10. Goldman L, Kitzmiller KW. Perianal atrophoderma from topical corticosteroids. Arch Dermatol 1973; 107:611–612.
11. Mathews JM. The ligature in the treatment of internal hemorrhoids. In: Mathews JM. A Treatise on the Diseases of the Rectum, Anus, and Sigmoid Flexure. New York, NY: D. Appleton and Co., 1899: 158–178.
12. Blaisdell PC. Prevention of massive hemorrhage secondary to hemorrhoidectomy. Surg Gynecol JM Mathews Obstet 1958; 106:485–488.
13. Barron J. Office ligation treatment of hemorrhoids. Dis Colon Rectum 1963; 6:109–113.
14. Corman ML, Veidenheimer MC. The new hemorrhoidectomy. Surg Clinic North Am 1973; 53: 417–422.
15. Mazier, WP. Hemorrhoids. In: Mazier WP, Levien DH, Luchtefeld MA, Senagore AJ, eds. Surgery of the Colon, Rectum, and Anus. Philadelphia: WB Saunders, 1995:229–254.
16. Khubchandani IT. A randomized comparison of single and multiple rubber band ligations. Dis Colon Rectum 1983; 26:705–708.
17. Poon GP, Chu KW, Lau WY, et al. Conventional vs. triple rubber band ligation for hemorrhoids–a prospective, randomized trial. Dis Colon Rectum 1986; 29:836–838.
18. Lau WY, Chow HP, Poon GP, et al. Rubber band ligation of three primary hemorrhoids in a single session. Dis Colon Rectum 1982; 25:336–339.
19. Bartizal J, Slosberg P. An alternative to hemorrhoidectomy. Arch Surg 1977; 112:534–536.
20. O'Hara VS. Fatal clostridial infection following hemorrhoidal banding. Dis Colon Rectum 1980; 23:570–571.
21. Russell TR, Donahue JH. Hemorrhoidal banding: a warning. Dis Colon Rectum 1985; 28:291–293.
22. Wrobleski DE, Corman ML, Veidenheimer MC, et al. Long-term evaluation of rubber ring ligation in hemorrhoidal disease. Dis Colon Rectum 1980; 23:478–482.

23. Gehamy RA, Weakley FL. Internal hemorrhoidectomy by elastic ligation. Dis Colon Rectum 1974; 17:347–353.
24. Morgan J. Varicose state of saphenous hemorrhoids treated successfully by the injection of tincture of persulphate of iron. Medical Press and Circular 1869:29–30.
25. Alexander-Williams J, Crapp AR. Conservative management of hemorrhoids. Clin Gastroenterol 1975; 4:595–601.
26. Senapati A, Nicholls RJ. Randomized trial to compare the results of injection sclerotherapy with a bulk laxative alone in the treatment of bleeding hemorrhoids. Int J Colorectal Dis 1988; 3:124–126.
27. Gartell PC, Sheridan RJ, McGinn FP. Outpatient treatment of haemorrhoids: a randomized clinical trial to compare rubber band ligation with phenol injection. Br J Surg 1985; 72:478–479.
28. Leicester RJ, Nicholls RJ, Mann CV. Comparison of infrared coagulation with conventional methods and the treatment of hemorrhoids. Coloproctology 1981; 5:313–315.
29. Neiger A. Hemorrhoids in everyday practice. Proctology 1979; 2:22–28.
30. Leicester RJ, Nichols RJ, Mann CV. Infrared coagulation: a new treatment for hemorrhoids. Dis Colon Rectum 1981; 24:602–605.
31. Ambrose NS, Hares MM, Alexander-Williams J, et al. A randomized trial of photocoagulation and rubber band ligation in treatment of haemorrhoids. Br Med J 1983; 286:1389–1391.
32. Dennison A, Whiston RJ, Rooney S, et al. A randomized comparison of infrared photocoagulation with bipolar diathermy for the outpatient treatment of hemorrhoids. Dis Colon Rectum 1990; 33:32–34.
33. Lewis MI. Cryosurgical hemorrhoidectomy: a follow-up report. Dis Colon Rectum 1972; 15:128–134.
34. Oh C. One thousand cryohemorrhoidectomies: an overview. Dis Colon Rectum 1981; 24:613–617.
35. Traynor OJ, Carter AE. Cryotherapy for advanced haemorrhoids: a prospective evaluation with 2-year follow-up. Br J Surg 1984; 71:287–289.
36. MacLeod JH. In defense of cryotherapy for hemorrhoids. Dis Colon Rectum 1982; 25:332–335.
37. Smith LE, Goodreau JJ, Fouty J. Management of hemorrhoids: operative hemorrhoidectomy versus cryosurgery. Dis Colon Rectum 1979; 22:10–16.
38. Hinton CP, Morris DL. A randomized trial comparing direct current therapy and bipolar diathermy in the outpatient treatment of third-degree hemorrhoids. Dis Colon Rectum 1990; 33:931–932.
39. Norman DA, Newton R, Nicholas GV. Direct current electrotherapy of internal hemorrhoids: an effective, safe, and painless outpatient approach. Am J Gastroenterol 1989; 84:482–487.
40. Zinberg SS, Stern DH, Furman DS, et al. A personal experience in comparing three nonoperative techniques for treating internal hemorrhoids. Am J Gastroenterol 1989; 84:488–492.
41. Griffith CDM, Morris DL, Wherry DC, et al. Outpatient treatment of haemorrhoids: a randomised trial comparing contact bipolar diathermy with rubber ring ligation. Coloproctology 1988; 6:332–334.
42. Lord PH. A new regime for the treatment of hemorrhoids. Proc R Soc Med 1968; 61:935–936.
43. Lord PH. Diverse methods of managing hemorrhoids: Dilatation. Dis Colon Rectum 1973; 16:180–183.
44. Creve U, Hubens A. The effect of Lord's procedure on anal pressure. Dis Colon Rectum 1979; 22:483–485.
45. McCaffrey J. Lord treatment of haemorrhoids: four-year follow-up of fifty patients. Lancet 1975; 1:133–134.
46. Konsten J, Baeten CG. Hemorrhoidectomy vs. Lord's method: 17-year follow-up of a prospective, randomized trial. Dis Colon Rectum 2000; 43:503–506.
47. Ferguson JA, Heaton JR. Closed hemorrhoidectomy. Dis Colon Rectum 1959; 2:176–179.
48. Ferguson JA, Mazier WP, Ganchrow MI, et al. The closed technique of hemorrhoidectomy. Surgery 1971; 70:480–484.
49. McConnell JC, Khubchandani IT. Long-term follow-up of closed hemorrhoidectomy. Dis Colon Rectum 1983; 26:797–799.
50. Wolf JS, Munoz JJ, Rosin JD. Survey of hemorrhoidectomy practices: open versus closed techniques. Dis Colon Rectum 1979; 22:536–538.
51. Buls JG, Goldberg SM. Modern management of hemorrhoids. Surg Clin North Am 1978; 58:469–478.
52. Ganchrow MI, Mazier WP, Friend WG, et al. Hemorrhoidectomy revisited-a computer analysis of 2038 patients. Dis Colon Rectum 1971; 14:128–133.
53. Bailey HR, Ferguson JA. Prevention of urinary retention by fluid restriction following anorectal operations. Dis Colon Rectum 1976; 19:250–252.
54. Scoma JA. Hemorrhoidectomy without urinary retention and catheterization. Conn Med 1976; 40:751–752.
55. ODonovan S, Ferrara A, Larach S, et al. Use of intraoperative Toradol facilitates outpatient hemorrhoidectomy. Dis Colon Rectum 1994; 37:793–799.
56. Place RJ, Coloma M, White PF, et al. Ketorolac improves recovery after outpatient anorectal surgery. Dis Colon Rectum 2000; 43:804–808.
57. Luchtefeld MA. Anal stenosis. In: Mazier WP, Levien DL, Luchtefeld MA, Senagore AJ, eds. Surgery of the Colon, Rectum and Anus. Philadelphia: WB Saunders, 1995:340–344.
58. Murie JA, Mackenzie I, Sim AJ. Rubber band ligation and hemorrhoidectomy for second and third degree hemorrhoids: a prospective clinical trial. Br J Surg 1980; 67:786–788.

59. Cheng FC, Shem DW, Ong GB. The treatment of second degree hemorrhoids by injection, rubber band ligation, maximal anal dilatation and hemorrhoidectomy, a prospective trial. Aust NZ J Surg 1981; 51:458–462.
60. Lewis AA, Rogers HS, Leighton M. Trial of maximal anal dilatation, cryotherapy and elastic band ligation as alternatives to hemorrhoidectomy in the treatment of large prolapsing hemorrhoids. Br J Surg 1983; 70:54–60.
61. Milligan ETC, Morgan CN, Nanto LE, et al. Surgical anatomy of the anal canal and the operative treatment of hemorrhoids. Lancet 1937; 2:1119–1124.
62. Arbman G, Krook H, Haapaniemi S. Closed vs. open hemorrhoidectomy–is there any difference? Dis Colon Rectum 2000; 43:31–34.
63. Carapati EA, Kamm MA, et al. Randomized trial of open versus closed day case haemorrhoidectomy. Br J Surg 1999; 86:612–613.
64. Ho YH, Seow-Choen F, Tan M, et al. Randomized trial of open and closed haemorrhoidectomy. Br J Surg 1997; 84:1729–1730.
65. Gencosmanoglu R, Sad O, Koc D, et al. Hemorrhoidectomy: open or closed technique? A prospective, randomized clinical trial. Dis Colon Rectum 2002; 45:70–75.
66. Senagore AJ, Mazier WP, Luchtefeld MA, et al. Treatment of advanced hemorrhoidal disease: a randomized, prospective trial of cold scalpel vs. contact Nd:YAG laser. Dis Colon Rectum 1993; 36: 1042–1049.
67. Nicholson JD, Halleran DR, Trivisonno DP, et al. The efficacy of the contact sapphire tip ND:YAG laser hemorrhoidectomy. St Louis: Poster presentation at the 89th Annual meeting of the American Society of Colon and Rectal Surgeons, April 29–May 4, 1990.
68. Jayne DG, Botterill I, Ambrose NS, et al. Randomized clinical trial of Ligasure versus conventional diathermy for day-case haemorrhoidectomy. Br J Surg 2002; 89:428–432.
69. Khan S, Pawlak SE, Eggenberger JC, et al. Surgical treatment of hemorrhoids: prospective, randomized trial comparing closed excisional hemorrhoidectomy and the Harmonic Scalpel technique of excisional hemorrhoidectomy. Dis Colon Rectum 2001; 44:845–849.
70. Tan JJ, Seow-Choen F. Prospective, randomized trial comparing diathermy and Harmonic Scalpel hemorrhoidectomy. Dis Colon Rectum 2001; 44:677–679.
71. Whitehead W. The surgical treatment of hemorrhoids. Br Med J 1882; 1:148–150.
72. Bonello JC. Who's afraid of the dentate line? The Whitehead hemorrhoidectomy. Am J Surg 1988; 156:182–186.
73. Wolff B, Culp CE. The Whitehead hemorrhoidectomy. An unjustly maligned procedure. Dis Colon Rectum 1988; 31:587–590.
74. O'Connor JJ. Staplers and hemorrhoids. Dis Colon Rectum 2000; 43:118–119 (letter).
75. Longo A. Treatment of hemorrhoids disease by reduction of mucosa and hemorrhoidal prolapse with a circular suturing device: a new procedure. Proceedings of the 6th World Congress of endoscopic surgery. Rome, June 1998:Italy 3–6.
76. Boccasanta P, Capretti PG, Venturi M, et al. Randomised controlled trial between stapled circumferential mucosectomy and conventional circular hemorrhoidectomy in advanced hemorrhoids with external mucosal prolapse. Am J Surg 2001; 182:64–68.
77. Ho YH, Cheong WK, Tsang C, et al. Stapled hemorrhoidectomy-cost and effectiveness. Randomized, controlled trial including incontinence scoring, anorectal manometry, and endoanal ultrasound assessments at up to three months. Dis Colon Rectum 2000; 43:1666–1675.
78. Roswell M, Bello M, Hemingway DM. Circumferential mucosectomy (stapled haemorrhoidectomy) versus conventional haemorrhoidectomy: randomised controlled trial. Lancet 2000; 355:779–781.
79. Mehigan BJ, Monson JR, Hartley JE. Stapling procedure for haemorrhoids versus Milligan–Morgan haemorrhoidectomy: randomised controlled trial. Lancet 2000; 355:782–785.
80. Cheetham MJ, Mortensen NJ, Nystrom PO, et al. Persistent pain and faecal urgency after stapled hemorrhoidectomy. Lancet 2000; 356:730–733.
81. Petti V, Caricato M, Arullami. Rectal perforation, retropneumoperitoneum, and pneumomediastinum after stapling procedure for prolapsed hemorrhoids: report of a case and subsequent considerations. Dis Colon Rectum 2002; 45:268–270.
82. Maw A, Eu KW, Seow-Choen F. Retroperitoneal sepsis complicating stapled hemorrhoidectomy: report of a case and review of the literature. Dis Colon Rectum 2002; 45:826–828.
83. Molloy RG, Kingsmore D. Life threatening pelvic sepsis after stapled hemorrhoidectomy. Lancet 2000; 355:810.
84. Singer MA, Cintron JR, Fleshman JW, et al. Early experience with stapled hemorrhoidectomy in the United States. Dis Colon Rectum 2002; 45:360–367.
85. MacRae HM, McLeod RS. Comparison of hemorrhoidal treatment modalities: a meta-analysis. Dis Colon Rectum 1995; 38:687–694.
86. MacRae HM, Temple LKF, McLeod RS. A meta-analysis of hemorrhoidal treatments. Seminars Colon Rectal Surg 2002; 13:77–83.
87. Cheetham MJ, Phillips RK. Evidence-based practice in haemorrhoidectomy. Colorectal Dis 2001; 3:126–134.
88. Jeffrey PJ, Ritchie JK, Parks AG. Treatment of hemorrhoids in patients with inflammatory bowel disease. Lancet 1977; 1:1084–1085.

89. Wolkomir AF, Luchtefeld MA. Surgery for symptomatic hemorrhoids and anal fissures in Crohn's disease. Dis Colon Rectum 1993; 36:545–547.
90. Ackland TH. The treatment of prolapsed gangrenous hemorrhoids. Aust NZ J Surg 1961; 30:201.
91. Heald RJ, Gudgeon AM. Limited haemorrhoidectomy in the treatment of acute strangulated haemorrhoids. Br J Surg 1986; 73:1002.
92. Mazier WP. Emergency hemorrhoidectomy: a worthwhile procedure. Dis Colon Rectum 1972; 15: 200–205.
93. Saleeby RG, Rosen L, Stasik JJ, et al. Hemorrhoidectomy during pregnancy: risk or relief? Dis Colon Rectum 1991; 34:260–261.
94. Morandi E, Merlini D, Salvaggio A, et al. Prospective study of healing time after hemorrhoidectomy: influence of HIV infection, acquired immunodeficiency syndrome, and anal wound infection. Dis Colon Rectum 1999; 42:1140–1144.
95. Hewitt WR, Sokol TP, Fleshner PR. Should HIV status alter indications for hemorrhoidectomy? Dis Colon Rectum 1996; 39:615–618.

31 | Anal Fissures, Ulcers, and Stenosis

Thomas E. Read
Division of Colon and Rectal Surgery, Department of Surgery, Western Pennsylvania Hospital, Clinical Campus of Temple University School of Medicine, Pittsburgh, Pennsylvania, U.S.A.

Peter J. Molloy and Owais Rahim
Division of Gastroenterology, Department of Medicine, Western Pennsylvania Hospital, Clinical Campus of Temple University School of Medicine, Pittsburgh, Pennsylvania, U.S.A.

ANAL FISSURE

Anal fissure is the most common cause of painful anal bleeding. The symptoms of anal fissure are often mistaken for those of hemorrhoidal disease, and patients may be reluctant to undergo detailed anal examination due to discomfort. However, when fissures are identified and promptly treated, patients may be extremely grateful for symptomatic relief.

Clinical Features

Fissures are most commonly diagnosed in the third decade of life, but may occur at any age. Fissures are the most common cause of anal bleeding in childhood and are associated with constipation. Men and women are affected equally (1). Fissures begin as acute linear tears in the anoderm, extending from the dentate line to the anal verge and develop after trauma to the anoderm, usually following a hard stool. Acute fissures can progress to chronic nonhealing ulcers, with exposed internal anal sphincter fibers, an overhanging sentinel skin tag, and/or a hypertrophied anal papilla at the base of the fissure (Fig. 1). Hypertonicity of the internal anal sphincter with poor arterial inflow to the area of the fissure, combined with repetitive trauma, results in nonhealing. There is no strict temporal definition to distinguish acute from chronic fissures. In general, a fissure that has been present for more than 8 to 12 weeks may be considered chronic. Many clinicians make the distinction based on the clinical appearance of the fissure. Patients typically recount a long history of chronic fissures that intermittently heal and recur.

Fissures are found in the posterior midline of the anal canal in approximately 90% of patients. The anterior midline is the second most common site; 10% of women and 1% of men have anal fissures located in the anterior midline. Fissures located in eccentric positions should raise the possibility of Crohn's disease, carcinoma, or syphilis. Pain with defecation and a small amount of anal bleeding, usually bright red, are the most common symptoms. Due to severe patient discomfort, a detailed examination of the anorectum may be difficult to perform on initial evaluation. However, gentle separation of the buttocks is usually adequate to expose the anal margin and the ulcer and/or overhanging sentinel skin tag (Figs. 2 and 3). This tag is usually mistaken for a hemorrhoid by inexperienced clinicians. Occasionally, it may be advisable to perform examination under anesthesia to determine the cause of severe anal pain in a patient who cannot be adequately examined in the office. However, neither a digital rectal examination nor anoscopy should be performed in the office setting in an awake patient with an acute painful anal fissure.

Patients with uncomplicated idiopathic anal fissure require no further diagnostic procedures prior to initiating treatment. However, atypical anal ulcers suspicious for Crohn's disease should prompt endoscopic examination of the colon and a more detailed assessment of the anal canal and rectum. If a malignant ulcer is suspected, biopsy should be performed. If an infectious etiology is suspected, culture and biopsy of the ulcer may be helpful.

Pathogenesis

Although most acute fissures develop secondary to local trauma from the passage of a large hard stool or forced evacuation, the pathogenesis of chronic anal fissures remains

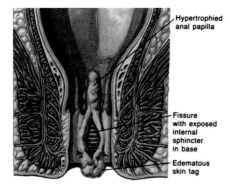

Hypertrophied
anal papilla

Fissure
with exposed
internal
sphincter
in base

Edematous
skin tag

Figure 1 Chronic anal fissure. *Source*: From Ref. 2.

incompletely understood. The progression of an acute tear in the anoderm to a chronic non-healing ulcer may be due to local ischemia that impairs healing. Spasm of the internal anal sphincter muscle and a paucity of blood vessels in the posterior midline may impede blood flow to the area of the fissure. Angiographic studies have shown that the blood vessels supplying the anal mucosa pass through the internal sphincter muscle, and that the vessels arise laterally, thus producing a relative area at risk for ischemia in the midline (3–5). Schouten et al. (6) have demonstrated an inverse relationship between anal sphincter tone and blood flow to the anal mucosa, suggesting that hypertonicity of the sphincter may lead to ischemia and a nonhealing ulcer. Manometric studies have shown that anal fissures occur in patients with high resting anal pressures (7). Although sphincter spasm due to the pain of the fissure may produce high pressures, other investigators have demonstrated that high pressures persist in the high anal canal after internal sphincterotomy in the low anal canal, suggesting that patients with anal fissures have intrinsic hypertonicity of the internal sphincter (8). Furthermore, division of a portion of the internal anal sphincter laterally (lateral internal sphincterotomy) can cause a reduction in anal resting pressures and lead to healing of midline fissures (9), supporting the hypothesis that sphincter spasm is a major contributor to the pathogenesis of chronic fissures. The other manometric findings of the overshoot phenomenon may correlate with the spasm and pain noted after bowel evacuation. Moreover, the overshoot phenomenon generally disappears after sphincterotomy.

Treatment

Initial therapeutic measures include oral fiber bulking agents and fluid, laxatives if necessary, and simple relaxation techniques such as soaking in warm water (10). The goal is to interrupt the cycle of constipation, hard stool, repetitive traumatic injury, pain, spasm, and nonhealing. Topical corticosteroids in the form of suppositories or ointments are sometimes effective. Anesthetic ointment applied immediately before bowel movements can be helpful by lessening the discomfort of defecation. Narcotic analgesics should be avoided as they can exacerbate constipation.

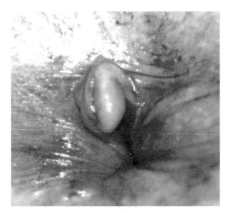

Figure 2 Sentinel tag overhanging anal fissure, often confused with a hemorrhoid.

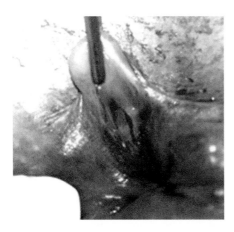

Figure 3 Anal fissure underlying sentinel skin tag.

These simple measures may produce healing in many patients with acute fissures and a proportion of patients with chronic fissures. In a randomized prospective trial, warm soaks in salt water and oral fiber therapy were more effective in healing fissures than topical lidocaine anesthetic gel or topical steroids (11). It could be argued that the conservative treatment of anal fissures simply allows time for the anus to heal as it would without any specific therapy. There are undoubtedly patients with anal fissures who never seek medical treatment, whose symptoms resolve spontaneously.

Glyceryl Trinitrate

In the past decade, alternative pharmacologic treatments have been developed that may be efficacious in the treatment of patients with acute and chronic fissures. The driving forces behind the development of these agents have been concern regarding fecal incontinence rates following surgical interventions for fissure (12,13), and a greater understanding of the physiology of the anal sphincter (14). Most of these therapies have been directed at the relaxation or temporary paralysis of the internal anal sphincter muscle in an attempt to transiently decrease resting tone, increase arterial blood flow to the area of the fissure, and promote healing. Relaxation of the internal anal sphincter is mediated by release of nitric oxide, and topical application of nitrates to the anal canal will decrease anal canal resting pressure by 20% to 25% (15). Topical glyceryl trinitrate (GTN) ointment, 0.2% to 0.4%, applied two to four times daily has been used to treat patients with both acute and chronic fissures.

Although early clinical trials of topical GTN in patients with anal fissure were promising (15), enthusiasm for its widespread use has been tempered by concerns over relapse and side effects. The majority of randomized controlled trials of GTN versus placebo for patients with chronic anal fissure have shown higher healing rates in patients treated with GTN (46–70% short term), although there is an overlap in rates of healing in the placebo and treatment groups between trials, and long-term follow-up has demonstrated symptomatic recurrences in 30% to 60% of patients initially thought to have healed (15–20). Trials comparing GTN with lateral internal sphincterotomy have shown that GTN is inferior to sphincterotomy in terms of healing (21–23). It is interesting to note that healing rates with GTN in these trials (39–45%) were lower than in trials of GTN versus placebo. The wide range of healing rates noted in GTN trials may be due to differences in patients recruited to the trial and to the difficulty in standardizing dosing. Most published series have used 0.2% to 0.3% GTN ointment, although frequency of application and duration of treatment have varied. In addition, patients are often given vague instructions as to the amount of ointment to apply.

One of the major limiting factors in the use of GTN has been side effects, primarily headaches, which reportedly occur in 30% to 70% of patients and may lead to the discontinuation of GTN therapy in up to 20% (15,16,19–23). Although tachyphylaxis is a concern in patients with cardiovascular disease managed with nitrates, there has not been clinical evidence that it occurs commonly. However, patients who have a history of hypotension or significant ischemic coronary disease have been excluded from most trials of GTN treatment and are probably optimally managed without utilization of vasoactive substances.

Calcium Channel Antagonists/Cholinergic Agonists

Investigators have demonstrated that the internal anal sphincter muscle can be inhibited by stimulation of parasympathetic muscarinic receptors or sympathetic beta-adrenoreceptors, and by inhibiting calcium entry into the muscle cells (24). Oral nifedipine causes a reduction in resting anal pressure in one-third of patients with anal fissure without decreasing maximum squeeze pressures (25); some patients have been treated with oral or topical nifedipine. Similarly, the application of topical calcium channel blockers or cholinergic agonists can lower resting anal pressure (26). Topical diltiazem and bethanechol have both been used in small numbers of patients with anal fissure with reasonable healing rates (26). However, the number of patients evaluated in all of these trials has been too small to allow for definitive conclusions as to the efficacy of any of these agents.

Botulinum Toxin Injection

Botulinum toxin A is a biologic toxin that binds irreversibly to presynaptic cholinergic nerve terminals, preventing the release of acetylcholine. Paralysis begins within hours, and resumption of neuromuscular impulse transmission occurs after the growth of new axon terminals. Reduction in muscle contraction strength is apparent for several months following injection. The use of botulinum toxin in patients with anal fissure is theoretically appealing as it offers the same advantage as topical agents in producing a reversible chemical sphincterotomy without the risk of permanent incontinence. Furthermore, it avoids the disadvantages of repeated dosing and the side effects associated with GTN therapy (27,28).

Investigators have utilized various dosing regimens and sites of injection. The majority of patients undergo injection of 10 to 40 units of botulinum toxin into the internal sphincter, although some investigators have injected into the external anal sphincter. Healing rates appear to be dose related (29,30). Some patients require more than one injection to effect healing. Side effects have been infrequent other than transient incontinence due to sphincter paralysis.

There has been increasing enthusiasm for the use of botulinum toxin due to the high healing rates reported in early trials (50–90%). However, because the anal sphincter paralysis is transient, it is intuitive that patients with an intrinsic tendency toward sphincter spasm may suffer a relapse. Longer-term follow-up suggests that up to 40% of patients may develop recurrent fissures (31). Comparison of botulinum toxin injection with lateral internal sphincterotomy at six months' follow-up demonstrated that healing rates were higher after sphincterotomy, although the risk of incontinence was also higher (32).

Lateral Internal Sphincterotomy

Division of the internal anal sphincter will produce healing of anal fissures in 90% to 95% of patients (23,33–35). Because of its proven efficacy, lateral internal sphincterotomy is the treatment against which new therapies should be measured.

Although some practitioners will perform lateral internal sphincterotomy in an office setting, the procedure is most frequently performed in the operating room on an outpatient basis. Patient discomfort due to anal manipulation in the setting of a fissure and sphincter spasm, as well as apprehension due to preexisting pain from the fissure, can make sphincterotomy under local anesthesia alone an uncomfortable procedure for both the patient and the surgeon. Deep intravenous sedation with a short-acting anesthetic just prior to injection of local anesthetic into the anal sphincter complex allows for excellent anesthesia with quick recovery (36). Alternatively, the procedure can be performed under regional or general anesthesia.

Lateral internal sphincterotomy can be accomplished with the patient in the prone jackknife, lithotomy, or left-lateral positions. Two techniques are most commonly utilized: open and closed. Open lateral internal sphincterotomy (Fig. 4) begins by insertion of an anoscope into the anal canal, palpation of the anal canal for a hypertrophied band of internal sphincter, and identification of the intersphincteric groove just outside the anal verge. A small incision of approximately 1 cm is made over the intersphincteric groove and the internal sphincter gently separated from the anoderm and external sphincter with a curved clamp. The internal sphincter fibers are brought into the wound and divided (usually with electrocautery), ensuring that the hypertrophied band of internal sphincter muscle has been included. The wound can then be

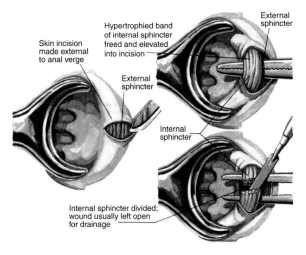

Figure 4 Lateral internal sphincterotomy, open technique. *Source*: From Ref. 37.

closed with fine absorbable sutures or left open. The primary advantages with the open technique include that the procedure is performed under direct vision, facilitating trainee instruction. Closed lateral internal sphincterotomy (Fig. 5) is performed by inserting a small scalpel into the intersphincteric groove with the blade parallel to the groove, rotating the scalpel 90°, and carefully dividing the internal sphincter fibers. Alternatively, the blade can be inserted in the submucosal space and then rotated to cut toward the intrasphincteric groove. Division of the muscle is usually accompanied by a gritty sensation noted by the hand manipulating the blade. The procedure is facilitated by insertion of an anoscope to make the intersphincteric groove more prominent, and by the insertion of the nondominant index finger into the anal canal to assess the exact position of the blade. The advantages of the closed technique are speed and small incision size. However, great care must be taken to avoid breaching the mucosa with the tip of the blade, which may result in an abscess and/or fistula formation. In addition, the risk of transmission of blood-borne pathogens makes the blind insertion of both scalpel and finger into close proximity hazardous to the inexperienced operator. A third option is to use a scissors after developing both the submucosal and the intrasphincteric space.

Prospective trials have demonstrated the effectiveness of lateral internal sphincterotomy, with a healing rate of 90% to 95% (21,23,34–36,38). Both nonhealing and recurrence after the procedure are unusual, occurring in fewer than 10% of patients. Anal endosonographic data suggest that nonhealing and recurrence may be due to inadequate division of the hypertrophied internal sphincter fibers, rather than an intrinsic failure of the technique (39). There is no appreciable difference in healing rates between the open and closed techniques of sphincterotomy (34,38).

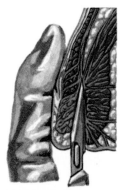

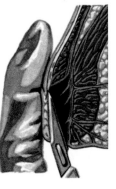

Figure 5 Lateral internal sphincterotomy, closed technique. *Source*: From Ref. 37.

Although lateral internal sphincterotomy is a rapidly performed, highly effective means of treating patients with anal fissures resistant to medical therapy, complications can occur following the procedure. In the immediate postoperative period, abscess or fistula may develop at the sphincterotomy site or if mucosal perforation occurs proximal to the sphincterotomy incision. Hematoma may also develop, which may become secondarily infected. Changes in continence have been difficult to interpret in the literature due to variability in reporting methods, lack of prospective data collection prior to and after the procedure, and lack of appropriate controls. Overall, it appears that worsening continence occurs in approximately 5% to 15% of patients after sphincterotomy, and the change in continence is usually minor (13,34,38,40–42). Occasionally patients will experience some fecal leakage after sphincterotomy due to change in contour of the anal canal. Although this deformity was thought to be most pronounced following sphincterotomy performed in the posterior midline, a recent meta-analysis of retrospective data failed to reveal a difference in continence following posterior midline versus lateral sphincterotomy (43).

Sphincterotomy should be cautiously approached in women due to the shorter sphincter length, lack of sphincter bulk anteriorly, and risk of past or future obstetrical injury to the anal sphincter. Similarly, patients who have chronic diarrhea or other conditions that reduce rectal compliance and/or continence (irritable bowel syndrome, diabetes, and advanced age) should consider all conservative treatment options to achieve healing of the fissure prior to considering sphincterotomy.

Anal Dilatation

Forceful anal dilatation under anesthesia has been utilized as an alternative to sphincterotomy. However, dilatation is associated with a higher fissure recurrence rate and an increased risk of fecal incontinence (up to 25%) when compared to sphincterotomy (43). These results are probably due to the uncontrolled nature of the procedure, with too gentle dilatation leading to inadequate reduction in internal sphincter tone and fissure recurrence, and over-vigorous tearing of the sphincter muscle causing incontinence. Although anal dilatation is still advocated by a few investigators (44), it is no longer commonly used as a treatment for fissure.

Fissurectomy

Excision of the fissure skin edges with or without closure of the defect (fissurectomy) has not been shown to add benefit to sphincterotomy. This would seem intuitive, as suture closure of the anoderm in a spastic anal canal will produce tension across the closure and ultimately cause wound breakdown. In addition, the cause of the fissure is most likely not an intrinsic problem with the skin edges (that could be extirpated), but rather lack of adequate anodermal blood flow.

Advancement Flap Anoplasty

In select patients with low sphincter pressures, dermal advancement flap procedures may allow reshaping of the anal canal and healing of chronic fissures. A diligent search for other causes of nonhealing anal ulcers should be sought in these patients prior to performing anoplasty, due to the rarity of idiopathic anal fissures in patients with poor sphincter tone.

ULCERS OF THE ANORECTUM
Anal Ulcers

Anal ulceration may occur in patients suffering from anal Crohn's disease. These lesions may be difficult to differentiate from idiopathic anal fissure if they occur in the absence of proctitis or other anal pathology. Anal ulcers secondary to Crohn's disease are often less painful than they appear and have a higher incidence of a lateral location and multiplicity when compared to idiopathic anal fissure occurring in the general population. Sphincterotomy should be performed only in carefully selected patients because of the risks of nonhealing and impaired continence if the patient develops other anorectal complications of the disease.

Ulcerated epidermoid carcinoma of the anal verge or anal canal may be confused with benign anal ulceration. If a fissure or ulcer is unresponsive to treatment, biopsy should be performed.

There are several infectious causes of anal ulceration, among them herpes simplex infection, syphilis, and lymphogranuloma venereum (Table 1). If an infectious etiology is suspected, bacterial and viral culture and biopsy of the ulcer may be helpful in guiding diagnosis and treatment. A few selected causes of rectal ulceration are considered in more detail below.

Stercoral Ulceration

Prolonged fecal impaction of hard fecal masses or scybalums can lead to ischemic pressure necrosis of the colorectal wall. The resultant ulcers are usually found in the rectum (70%) and sigmoid (20%), but have also been known to affect the transverse colon and cecum (45,46). The true incidence of these ulcers is unknown. The few available studies quote an incidence varying between 0.3% to as high as 4.6% with a slight female preponderance (47,48). Patients are generally elderly and debilitated, on constipating medications, residents of nursing homes and other chronic care facilities, and commonly have altered mental status (49). Younger patients are afflicted when there is neurological dysfunction, especially spinal cord injuries or diseases resulting in severe constipation and problems with painful defecation (50). Other risk factors include renal failure and transplantation, hypothyroidism and mechanical blockage of the colon due to strictures, foreign bodies, or extrinsic compression by noncolonic malignancies. Fecal impaction in the proximal colon should always raise the suspicion for an obstructing colon carcinoma. Stercoral ulcers are usually asymptomatic and only come to light after perforation or gross hematochezia (51). They should be considered in constipated patients with abdominal pain and leukocytosis.

Stercoral ulcers are large, irregular but well demarcated, and conforming to the faceted contours of the fecal masses. Histologically, there are acute and chronic inflammatory cells with a denuded and necrotic mucosa. On physical exam, fecal masses can sometimes be palpated in the left lower quadrant. Perforations can be localized or generalized, in which case patients may present with peritonitis (80–100%) (49,52). Plain abdominal X-ray series may reveal free air, marked fecal loading, or fecaliths in the colon. Water-soluble contrast enema or computed tomography may be helpful in making the diagnosis in patients with an unclear clinical presentation, and may show evidence of contained perforation or pericolonic inflammation (53,54). Perforations are round or ovoid, located at the base of the ulcer, and are usually found on the antimesenteric border of the colon. Stercoral perforations are distinct from the rare spontaneous colonic perforations that occur during a difficult bowel movement, which result in a transmural tear with edges devoid of inflammation (55).

Treatment options vary. Patients without signs of transmural inflammation or perforation usually benefit from manual disimpaction. Great care should be taken during the disimpaction, as the ulcer base is thin and easily perforated. An attempt should be made to

Table 1 Etiology of Ulcers of the Colorectum and Anus

Malignancy	Vasculitides
Crohn's disease	Systemic lupus erythematosus
Idiopathic anal fissure	Wegener's granulomatosis
Stercoral ulcer	Behcet's disease
Solitary rectal ulcer syndrome	Essential mixed granulomatosis
Dieulafoy type ulcer	Churg Strauss syndrome
Ischemia	Traumatic
Nonspecific ulcer of colon	Digital examination/manual disimpaction
Infectious	Insertion of rectal tubes or enema nozzles
Cytomegalovirus	Foreign body insertion
Lymphogranuloma venereum	Sodomy
Tuberculosis	Pharmacological agents
Syphilis	Levamisole
Actinomycosis	5-Fluorouracil
Histoplasmosis	Oral contraceptive agents
Amebiasis	Aminophylline suppositories
Herpes simplex	Ergotamine

soften up the stools prior to disimpaction with oral mineral oil or enemas. Occasionally colon-oscopic irrigation is required. Oral lavage solutions can be utilized with caution if there is no evidence of complete intestinal obstruction. Occasionally, the scybalums have been present for years and can only be evacuated surgically. Lactulose should be avoided until after disimpaction as bacterial fermentation gives rise to excessive gas and bloating.

Ulcers with free perforation usually require emergent surgery. Delay in operative intervention increases mortality, which is already high and increases with advanced age and comorbid conditions. Most mortality is due to sepsis, and broad-spectrum intravenous antibiotics should be started immediately on clinical presentation. The procedure associated with the least mortality is resection of the perforation with end colostomy and closure of the distal segment or mucous fistula (56). Decisions regarding primary anastomosis with or without intraoperative colonic lavage and proximal fecal diversion should be based on the overall condition of the patient and the condition of the remaining colorectum. As these patients are usually elderly and debilitated, the safest procedure is usually expeditious resection of the perforated segment with construction of proximal colostomy.

Patients with a contained perforation without peritonitis or fulminant sepsis can be considered for initial nonoperative treatment, which includes broad-spectrum antibiotics, fluid resuscitation, limitation of oral intake, and close observation. Unlike other microperforations of the colon and rectum, perforations due to stercoral ulceration are complicated by the continued presence of the inciting agent, namely, the hard stool ball. Manipulation of this mass of stool in attempted removal may acutely worsen the perforation; alternatively, leaving it in place may produce continued bowel wall erosion. This conundrum may prompt earlier surgical intervention than for patients presenting with a similar degree of pericolonic inflammation from a diverticular perforation.

In any patient treated for stercoral ulceration, a regular bowel regimen should be employed once the acute episode has resolved. Constipating medications should be avoided and fluid intake encouraged. Fiber bulking agents, laxatives, and exercise should be encouraged. Chronic care facility patients require particular attention to their bowel needs, and if needed, frequent enemas should be administered.

Solitary Rectal Ulcer

Solitary rectal ulcer is a chronic benign ulcer occurring typically in the anterior midrectum, which is thought to arise secondary to trauma from rectal prolapse or internal rectorectal intussusception. Initial descriptions by Cruveilheir date to 1829, but it was not until 1969 that a review by Madigan and Morson described the diagnostic criteria (57). "Solitary rectal ulcer" is a misnomer in that multiple ulcers, polypoidal tissue with ulceration, or a flat region of velvety erythematous mucosa with characteristic histologic findings may be present. Affected individuals are usually in their 30s and 40s, although patients in their 80s have been described. Patients often have a prior history of psychiatric illness including psychosis, anxiety, neurosis, or depression (58). Most patients present with symptoms of obstructed defecation and tenesmus. Rectal bleeding is present in 56% to 89% of patients, although rarely profuse, and mucorrhea is often present. Rectal pain usually is minimal, but can be severe and localized to the perineum, the sacral area, or left lower quadrant; it can be dull, intermittent, or continuous and unchanged by defecation. Up to 26% of patients are asymptomatic with incidental diagnosis occurring during endoscopy performed for unrelated indications (58). Asymptomatic ulcers are generally of the polypoidal variety and are more frequent in younger females and more amenable to treatment.

There is an association with rectal prolapse, which may be the main contributing factor in the pathogenesis of these lesions. Full-thickness rectal prolapse is noted in up to 30% of patients and mucosal prolapse or internal rectorectal intussusception in up to 45% of patients (57–60). One group of investigators found prolapse of at least rectal mucosa into the anal canal in 94% of patients suffering from solitary rectal ulcer. The differences in rates of prolapse reported in the literature may reflect differences in diagnostic evaluation, especially with regard to the use of defecography or pelvic dynamic magnetic resonance imaging.

Solitary rectal ulcers typically appear as single, small, oval, and shallow but well-demarcated ulcers 4 to 12 cm from the anal verge in the anterior midline. The exact pathogenesis remains somewhat controversial. Self-digitation, which is seen in 50% of patients in order to remove hard stools, is a suggested cause. However, quite often the ulcer is inaccessible to the patient's finger, and avoidance of the practice does not lead to healing. There is no convincing evidence that congenital anomalies of the anterior rectal wall, a localized form of inflammatory bowel disease, or infectious agents are etiologies. Localized ulceration due to suppository preparations containing ergotamine tartrate or a nonsteroidal inflammatory agent can usually be distinguished histologically from solitary rectal ulcer (61,62). The most plausible theory is that of local trauma and ischemia caused by the prolapsing rectal wall or mucosal rectal prolapse combined with high fecal voiding pressure, caused by overactivity of the external anal sphincter or failure of puborectalis relaxation during defecation (63–65).

A pathognomonic histologic feature of solitary rectal ulcer is replacement of the lamina propria by diffuse infiltration of collagen fibers (57,66). Combined with hypertrophy and disorganization of the muscularis mucosa, the picture is termed fibromuscular obliteration of the lamina propria. In addition, streaming of fibroblasts and muscle fibers up between crypts occurs. The mucosal glands are displaced into the submucosa, and erosion of the mucosal surface can be seen. Occasionally cystic glands can be seen in the submucosa, leading to speculation that colitis cystica profunda is a closely related syndrome (67). Histologic proof is necessary to differentiate solitary rectal ulcer from malignant conditions.

Barium enema examination may be normal in up to 20% of cases but can reveal ulceration, polypoidal lesion, stricture, granularity, and rectal fold thickening (68). Defecography demonstrates prolonged and incomplete evacuation in 75% of patients with solitary rectal ulcer syndrome and often demonstrates internal or external rectal prolapse. Transrectal ultrasound

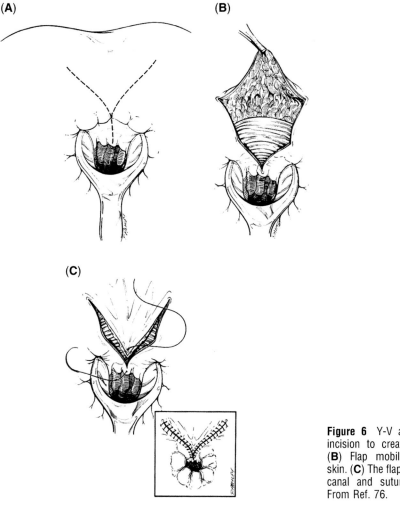

(A)

(B)

(C)

Figure 6 Y-V anoplasty. (**A**) Y-shaped incision to create a widely based flap. (**B**) Flap mobilization of full-thickness skin. (**C**) The flap is advanced into the anal canal and sutured into place. *Source*: From Ref. 76.

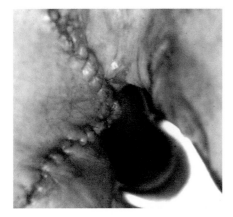

Figure 7 Completed Y-V anoplasty (intraoperative).

studies have marked thickening of the internal anal sphincter although thickening of the submucosa and external anal sphincter may be present (69,70).

Management depends on the severity of symptoms and whether rectal prolapse is identified. These ulcers are remarkably resistant to medical therapy; however, they do remain stable over a period of years, with minimal risk of perforation. Initially, conservative measures should be employed. Asymptomatic patients usually have polypoidal lesions that are somewhat more responsive to medical therapy. Medical management involves fiber bulking agents, high fluid intake, and bowel retraining to avoid straining and digital rectal manipulation. Steroids, 5-aminosalicylate (5-ASA) and sucralfate enemas can be tried, although no convincing evidence exists to support their effectiveness (71). Patients with suspected pelvic muscle dysfunction should also undergo anorectal physiologic evaluation and a trial of biofeedback, if indicated (72). Persistently troublesome symptoms warrant further evaluation with defecography.

If prolapse is present and medical management has failed, surgical intervention should be considered. However, the results of operative correction of prolapse will rarely translate into functional success. The number of patients reported in the literature undergoing surgical procedures for symptomatic solitary rectal ulcer is small; therefore it is difficult to draw definitive conclusions regarding the relative efficacy of any corrective procedure. Transabdominal rectopexy has been successful for some patients, presumably those in whom the rectal

(A)

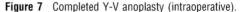

(B)

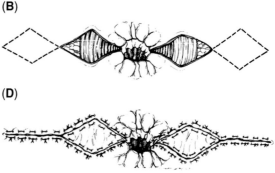

(D)

(C)

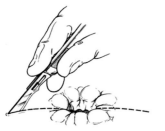
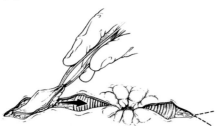

Figure 8 Diamond advancement flap anoplasty. (**A**) Release of cicatrix. (**B**) Diamond-shaped incisions. (**C**) Full-thickness skin flaps with underlying subcutaneous tissue attached. Undermining is minimized to protect against ischemia of the flap. (**D**) Flaps are rotated into the anal canal and sutured in place. *Source*: From Ref. 77.

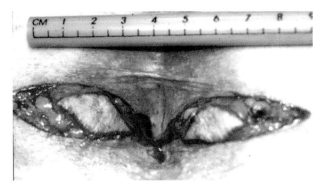

Figure 9 Diamond advancement flap ano-plasty, intraoperative photograph.

prolapse is mostly causative (58,73). Anterior resection of the rectosigmoid has occasionally been added to the rectopexy for constipated patients, but great care should be exercised as the rectum of these patients is often thick, scarred, and noncompliant. A few patients without overt prolapse have been managed successfully with local transanal excision of the ulcer. For patients who have failed all other methods of treatment, a diverting stoma is occasionally the best option.

Regardless of the surgical procedure, the patient should be extensively counseled in the preoperative period. They should not expect resolution or even improvement in any of their symptoms except the physical presence of the ulcer itself. In summary, surgery should be assiduously avoided and when performed should be in a patient with realistic expectations. Active pre- and postoperative psychiatric counseling is strongly recommended.

ANAL STENOSIS

Anal stenosis is a mechanical narrowing of the anal canal, which often results in difficult and painful defecation. The most common etiology is prior anal surgery in which excessive anoderm is removed, resulting in scarring and fixation of the anal canal (74). Excisional hemorrhoidectomy is the most common anorectal procedure associated with subsequent anal stenosis. Other common etiologies include congenital abnormalities, malignancy, laxative abuse, and fibrosis from anal Crohn's disease or external beam radiotherapy.

The diagnosis is relatively straightforward; symptoms include difficult defecation, anal pain, narrowed stools, and anal bleeding. Physical examination reveals the level and degree of stenosis. If a patient is too tender or anxious to be examined adequately in the office setting, examination under anesthesia should be performed. This technique is especially important if malignancy or Crohn's disease is entertained as a causative factor.

Nonsurgical management includes fiber bulking agents, fluids, and stool softeners or laxatives, as needed. Mild and moderate stenosis can often be managed with manual dilatations initially performed in the office by the physician and subsequently by the patient or family member at home. The simplest form of self-dilatation is to have the patient place a glycerin or hydrocortisone suppository per anus every night prior to retiring. Alternatively, the patient can use a well-lubricated finger or a tapered plastic dilator to gently dilate the anal canal on a regular basis. A short, tapered candle is also very effective, and has the added

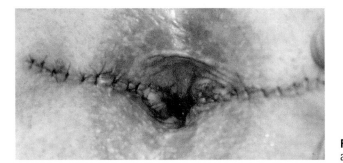

Figure 10 Diamond advancement flap anoplasty, completed (intraoperative).

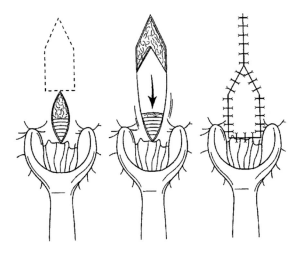

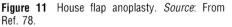

Figure 11 House flap anoplasty. *Source*: From Ref. 78.

benefit of the wax giving way if too much pressure is exerted. Most patients with anal stenosis will respond to these simple measures and never require surgical intervention.

For patients with severe stenosis, or for those who are unresponsive to nonoperative treatment, release of the cicatrix in the anal canal and augmentation of the anoderm with epithelialized tissue are indicated. Some patients will require only longitudinal division of the scarred anoderm to release the anal canal cicatrix, while others who have fibrosis of the internal anal sphincter will also require open internal sphincterotomy. A variety of flap ano-plasties have been devised to move epithelialized tissue into the anal canal in order to increase the circumference of the anal canal after the scar has been released (75). A Y-V anoplasty is rela-tively straightforward to perform (Fig. 6). A Y-shaped incision is made and a skin flap mobi-lized and advanced into the anal canal and sutured in place (Fig. 7). The tip of the flap should reach well up into the anal canal to ensure adequate coverage. One disadvantage of this tech-nique is that the tip of the flap is at risk for ischemia if under tension or lacks good perfusion at its narrow tip.

Alternative anoplasty techniques have been developed in order to provide greater mobility to the flap, so that it can be advanced further into the anal canal with less risk of ischemic necrosis. Diamond flap (Figs. 8–10), house flap (Fig. 11), and island flap techniques have all been successfully used to treat patients with anal stenosis (79–81). The operative prin-ciples are similar to those employed for any tissue transfer procedure. An S-anoplasty is a slightly more complicated procedure infrequently employed for patients with anal stenosis (75). The ultimate choice of anoplasty technique for a patient with severe anal stenosis is based on the experience and the anatomic configuration of the patient's anus and perineum.

REFERENCES

1. Lund JN, Scholefield JH. Aetiology and treatment of anal fissure. Br J Surg 1996; 83:1335–1344.
2. Fry RD, Kodner IJ. Benign anorectal conditions. Ciba-Geigy Clinical Symposia,1989; 37(6):12.
3. Klosterhalfen B, Vogel P, Rixen H, Mittermayer C. Topography of the inferior rectal artery: a possible cause of chronic, primary anal fissure. Dis Colon Rectum 1989; 32:43–52.
4. Lund JN, Binch C, McGrath J, Sparrow RA, Scholefield JH. Topographical distribution of blood sup-ply to the anal canal. Br J Surg 1999; 86:496–498.
5. Schouten WR, Briel JW, Auwerda JJ, De Graaf EJ. Ischaemic nature of anal fissure. Br J Surg 1996; 83:63–65.
6. Schouten WR, Briel JW, Auwerda JJ. Relationship between anal pressure and anodermal blood flow. The vascular pathogenesis of anal fissures. Dis Colon Rectum 1994; 37:664–669.
7. Gibbons CP, Read NW. Anal hypertonia in fissures: cause or effect? Br J Surg 1986; 73:443–445.
8. McNamara MJ, Percy JP, Fielding IR. A manometric study of anal fissure treated by subcutaneous lat-eral internal sphincterotomy. Ann Surg 1990; 211:235–238.
9. Chowcat NL, Araujo JG, Boulos PB. Internal sphincterotomy for chronic anal fissure: long term effects on anal pressure. Br J Surg 1986; 73:915–916.

10. Jiang JK, Chiu JH, Lin JK. Local thermal stimulation relaxes hypertonic anal sphincter: evidence of somatoanal reflex. Dis Colon Rectum 1999; 42:1152–1159.
11. Jensen SL. Treatment of first episodes of acute anal fissure: prospective randomised study of lignocaine ointment versus hydrocortisone ointment or warm sitz baths plus bran. Br Med J (Clin Res Ed) 1986; 292:1167–1169.
12. Speakman CT, Burnett SJ, Kamm MA, Bartram CI. Sphincter injury after anal dilatation demonstrated by anal endosonography. Br J Surg 1991; 78:1429–1430.
13. Khubchandani IT, Reed JF. Sequelae of internal sphincterotomy for chronic fissure in ano. Br J Surg 1989; 76:431–434.
14. O'Kelly TJ, Brading A, Mortensen NJ. In vitro response of the human anal canal longitudinal muscle layer to cholinergic and adrenergic stimulation: evidence of sphincter specialization. Br J Surg 1993; 80:1337–1341.
15. Lund JN, Scholefield JH. A randomised, prospective, double-blind, placebo-controlled trial of glyceryl trinitrate ointment in treatment of anal fissure. Lancet 1997; 349:11–14.
16. Kennedy ML, Sowter S, Nguyen H, Lubowski DZ. Glyceryl trinitrate ointment for the treatment of chronic anal fissure: results of a placebo-controlled trial and long-term follow-up. Dis Colon Rectum 1999; 42:1000–1006.
17. Altomare DF, Rinaldi M, Milito G, et al. Glyceryl trinitrate for chronic anal fissure-healing or headache? Results of a multicenter, randomized, placebo-controlled, double-blind trial. Dis Colon Rectum 2000; 43:174–179.
18. Bacher H, Mischinger HJ, Werkgartner G, et al. Local nitroglycerin for treatment of anal fissures: an alternative to lateral sphincterotomy? Dis Colon Rectum 1997; 40:840–845.
19. Carapeti EA, Kamm MA, McDonald PJ, Chadwick SJ, Melville D, Phillips RK. Randomised controlled trial shows that glyceryl trinitrate heals anal fissures, higher doses are not more effective, and there is a high recurrence rate. Gut 1999; 44:727–730.
20. Lund JN, Scholefield JH. Follow-up of patients with chronic anal fissure treated with topical glyceryl trinitrate. Lancet 1998; 352:1681.
21. Evans J, Luck A, Hewett P. Glyceryl trinitrate vs. lateral sphincterotomy for chronic anal fissure: prospective, randomized trial. Dis Colon Rectum 2001; 44:93–97.
22. Oettle GJ. Glyceryl trinitrate vs. sphincterotomy for treatment of chronic fissure-in-ano: a randomized, controlled trial. Dis Colon Rectum 1997; 40:1318–1320.
23. Richard CS, Gregoire R, Plewes EA, et al. Internal sphincterotomy is superior to topical nitroglycerin in the treatment of chronic anal fissure: results of a randomized, controlled trial by the Canadian Colorectal Surgical Trials Group. Dis Colon Rectum 2000; 43:1048–1057.
24. Bhardwaj R, Vaizey CJ, Boulos PB, Hoyle CH. Neuromyogenic properties of the internal anal sphincter: therapeutic rationale for anal fissures. Gut 2000; 46:861–868.
25. Cook TA, Humphreys MM, Mortensen NJM. Oral nifedipine reduces resting anal pressure and heals chronic anal fissure. Br J Surg 1999; 86:1269–1273.
26. Carapeti EA, Kamm MA, Evans BK, Phillips RK. Topical diltiazem and bethanechol decrease anal sphincter pressure without side effects. Gut 1999; 45:719–722.
27. Jost WH. One hundred cases of anal fissure treated with botulin toxin: early and long-term results. Dis Colon Rectum 1997; 40:1029–1032.
28. Brisinda G, Maria G, Bentivoglio AR, Cassetta E, Gui D, Albanese A. A comparison of injections of botulinum toxin and topical nitroglycerin ointment for the treatment of chronic anal fissure. N Engl J Med 1999; 341:65–69.
29. Brisinda G, Maria G, Sganga G, Bentivoglio AR, Albanese A, Castagneto M. Effectiveness of higher doses of botulinum toxin to induce healing in patients with chronic anal fissures. Surgery 2002; 131:179–184.
30. Minguez M, Melo F, Espi A, et al. Therapeutic effects of different doses of botulinum toxin in chronic anal fissure. Dis Colon Rectum 1999; 42:1016–1021.
31. Minguez M, Herreros B, Espi A, et al. Long-term follow-up (42 months) of chronic anal fissure after healing with botulinum toxin. Gastroenterology 2002; 123:112–117.
32. Mentes BB, Irkorucu O, Akin M, Leventoglu S, Tatlicioglu E. Comparison of botulinum toxin injection and lateral internal sphincterotomy for the treatment of chronic anal fissure. Dis Colon Rectum 2003; 46:232–237.
33. Weaver RM, Ambrose NS, Alexander-Williams J, Keighley MR. Manual dilatation of the anus vs. lateral subcutaneous sphincterotomy in the treatment of chronic fissure-in-ano. Results of a prospective, randomized, clinical trial. Dis Colon Rectum 1987; 30:420–423.
34. Kortbeek JB, Langevin JM, Khoo RE, Heine JA. Chronic fissure-in-ano: a randomized study comparing open and subcutaneous lateral internal sphincterotomy. Dis Colon Rectum 1992; 35:835–837.
35. Evans DA. Lateral subcutaneous sphincterotomy for treatment of anal fissure in children. Br J Surg 1996; 83:571.
36. Read TE, Henry SE, Hovis RM, et al. Prospective evaluation of anesthetic technique for anorectal surgery. Dis Colon Rectum 2002; 45:1553–1558.
37. Fry RD, Kodner IJ. Benign anorectal conditions. Ciba-Geigy Clinical Symposia, 1989; 37(6):14.
38. Boulos PB, Araujo JG. Adequate internal sphincterotomy for chronic anal fissure: subcutaneous or open technique? Br J Surg 1984; 71:360–362.

39. Garcia-Granero E, Sanahuja A, Garcia-Armengol J, et al. Anal endosonographic evaluation after closed lateral subcutaneous sphincterotomy. Dis Colon Rectum 1998; 41:598–601.

40. Nyam DC, Pemberton JH. Long-term results of lateral internal sphincterotomy for chronic anal fissure with particular reference to incidence of fecal incontinence. Dis Colon Rectum 1999; 42:1306–1310.

41. Lewis TH, Corman ML, Prager ED, Robertson WG. Long-term results of open and closed sphincterotomy for anal fissure. Dis Colon Rectum 1988; 31:368–371.

42. Garcia-Aguilar J, Belmonte C, Wong WD, Lowry AC, Madoff RD. Open vs. closed sphincterotomy for chronic anal fissure: long-term results. Dis Colon Rectum 1996; 39:440–443.

43. Nelson RL. Meta-analysis of operative techniques for fissure-in-ano. Dis Colon Rectum 1999; 42: 1424–1431.

44. Strugnell NA, Cooke SG, Lucarotti ME, Thomson WH. Controlled digital anal dilatation under total neuromuscular blockade for chronic anal fissure: a justifiable procedure. Br J Surg 1999; 86:651–655.

45. Lalla R, Enquist I, Oloumi M, Velez FJ. Stercoraceous perforation of the right colon. South Med J 1989; 82:80–82.

46. Russell WL. Stercoraceous ulcer. Am Surg 1976; 42:416–420.

47. Lal S, Brown GN. Some unusual complications of fecal impaction. Am J Proctol 1967; 18:226–231.

48. Grinvalsky HT, Bowerman CI. Stercoraceous ulcers of the colon: relatively neglected medical and surgical problem. JAMA 1959; 171:1941.

49. Serpell JW, Nicholls RJ. Stercoral perforation of the colon. Br J Surg 1990; 77:1325–1329.

50. Shatila AH, Ackerman NB. Stercoraceous ulcerations and perforations of the colon: report of cases and survey of the literature. Dis Colon Rectum 1977; 20:524–527.

51. Wang SY, Sutherland JC. Colonic perforation secondary to fecal impaction: report of a case. Dis Colon Rectum 1977; 20:355–356.

52. Gekas P, Schuster MM. Stercoral perforation of the colon: case report and review of the literature. Gastroenterology 1981; 80:1054–1058.

53. Rozenblit AM, Cohen-Schwartz D, Wolf EL, Foxx MJ, Brenner S. Case reports. Stercoral perforation of the sigmoid colon: computed tomography findings. Clin Radiol 2000; 55:727–729.

54. Berardi RS, Lee S. Stercoraceous perforation of the colon. Report of a case. Dis Colon Rectum 1983; 26:283–286.

55. Castleton K. Idiopathic perforation of the colon. Am Surgeon 1962; 27:329–331.

56. Guyton DP, Evans D, Schreiber H. Stercoral perforation of the colon. Concepts of operative management. Am Surg 1985; 51:520–522.

57. Madigan MR, Morson BC. Solitary ulcer of the rectum. Gut 1969; 10:871–881.

58. Tjandra JJ, Fazio VW, Church JM, Lavery IC, Oakley JR, Milsom JW. Clinical conundrum of solitary rectal ulcer. Dis Colon Rectum 1992; 35:227–234.

59. Halligan S, Nicholls RJ, Bartram CI. Evacuation proctography in patients with solitary rectal ulcer syndrome: anatomic abnormalities and frequency of impaired emptying and prolapse. AJR 1995; 164:91–95.

60. Martin JK Jr, Culp CE, Weiland LH. Colitis cystica profunda. Dis Colon Rectum 1980; 23:488–491.

61. Eckardt VF, Kanzler G, Remmele W. Anorectal ergotism: another cause of solitary rectal ulcers. Gastroenterology 1986; 91:1123–1127.

62. Gizzi G, Villani V, Brandi G, Paganelli GM, Di Febo G, Biasco G. Ano-rectal lesions in patients taking suppositories containing non-steroidal anti-inflammatory drugs (NSAID). Endoscopy 1990; 22:146–148.

63. Bogomoletz WV. Solitary rectal ulcer syndrome. Mucosal prolapse syndrome. Pathol Annu 1992; 27(Pt 1):75–86.

64. Mackle EJ, Parks TG. The pathogenesis and pathophysiology of rectal prolapse and solitary rectal ulcer syndrome. Clin Gastroenterol 1986; 15:985–1002.

65. Womack NR, Williams NS, Holmfield JH, Morrison JF. Pressure and prolapse—the cause of solitary rectal ulceration. Gut 1987; 28:1228–1233.

66. Levine DS, Surawicz CM, Ajer TN, Dean PJ, Rubin CE. Diffuse excess mucosal collagen in rectal biopsies facilitates differential diagnosis of solitary rectal ulcer syndrome from other inflammatory bowel diseases. Dig Dis Sci 1988; 33:1345–1352.

67. Levine DS. "Solitary" rectal ulcer syndrome. Are "solitary" rectal ulcer syndrome and "localized" colitis cystica profunda analogous syndromes caused by rectal prolapse? Gastroenterology 1987; 92:243–253.

68. Millward SF, Bayjoo P, Dixon MF, Williams NS, Simpkins KC. The barium enema appearances in solitary rectal ulcer syndrome. Clin Radiol 1985; 36:185–189.

69. Petritsch W, Hinterleitner TA, Aichbichler B, Denk H, Hammer HF, Krejs GJ. Endosonography in colitis cystica profunda and solitary rectal ulcer syndrome. Gastrointest Endosc 1996; 44:746–751.

70. Van Outryve MJ, Pelckmans PA, Fierens H, Van Maercke YM. Transrectal ultrasound study of the pathogenesis of solitary rectal ulcer syndrome. Gut 1993; 34:1422–1426.

71. Zargar SA, Khuroo MS, Mahajan R. Sucralfate retention enemas in solitary rectal ulcer. Dis Colon Rectum 1991; 34:455–457.

72. Binnie NR, Papachrysostomou M, Clare N, Smith AN. Solitary rectal ulcer: the place of biofeedback and surgery in the treatment of the syndrome. World J Surg 1992; 16:836–840.

73. Nicholls RJ, Simson JN. Anteroposterior rectopexy in the treatment of solitary rectal ulcer syndrome without overt rectal prolapse. Br J Surg 1986; 73:222–224.
74. Milsom JW, Mazier WP. Classification and management of postsurgical anal stenosis. Surg Gynecol Obstet 1986; 163:60–64.
75. Luchtefeld M. Anal stenosis. In: Read TE, ed. Problems in General Surgery: Benign Anorectal Problems. Soper NJ, series ed. Vol. 18. Philadelphia, PA: Lippincott, Williams and Wilkins, 1995:17–23.
76. Luchtefeld M. Anal stenosis. In: Mazier WP, Levien D, Luchtefeld MA, Senagore AJ, eds. Surgery of the Colon, Rectum and Anus. Philadelphia: WB Saunders, 1995:341.
77. Luchtefeld M. Anal stenosis. In: Mazier WP, Levien D, Luchtefeld MA, Senagore AJ, eds. Surgery of the Colon, Rectum and Anus. Philadelphia: WB Saunders, 1995:342.
78. Liberman H, Thorson AG. Anal stenosis. Am J Surg 2000; 179:325–329.
79. Caplin DA, Kodner IJ. Repair of anal stricture and mucosal ectropion by simple flap procedures. Dis Colon Rectum 1986; 29:92–94.
80. Sentovich SM, Falk PM, Christensen MA, Thorson AG, Blatchford GJ, Pitsch RM. Operative results of House advancement anoplasty. Br J Surg 1996; 83:1242–1244.
81. Pearl RK, Hooks VH III, Abcarian H, Orsay CP, Nelson RL. Island flap anoplasty for the treatment of anal stricture and mucosal ectropion. Dis Colon Rectum 1990; 33:581–583.

32 | Fistulas-in-Ano and Abscesses

Samir M. Yebara
Department of Colorectal Surgery, Cleveland Clinic Florida, Weston, Florida, U.S.A.

Mara R. Salum and Raúl Cutait
Department of Surgery, Syrian-Lebanese Hospital, São Paulo, Brazil

HISTORY AND EPIDEMIOLOGY

Discussions regarding fistula-in-ano date to ancient history. The oldest written testimony is the Hammurabi Code of the king of Babylonia, who in 2200 B.C. imposed the honoraries for the proctologist in that epoch. Hippocrates made reference to surgical therapy for fistulous disease in his book called *Peeri Siryggon* in 460 to 365 B.C. The English surgeon John Arderne (1307–1309) wrote *Treatises of Fistula in Ano and Haemmorhoids* in 1376, which illustrates fistulotomy and seton use. In the early 20th century, surgeons, namely, Goodsall and Miles, Milligan and Morgan, and Thompson and Lockhart-Mummery made important contributions to the treatment of anal fistula.

The mean incidence per 1,000,000 population studied among the inhabitants of the city of Helsinki (population 510,000) during a 10-year period, 1969 to 1978, was 8.6% (1). The mean age at the time of diagnosis of the idiopathic fistula was 38.3 years with a male:female ratio of 1.8:1; 35% of idiopathic anorectal abscess develop into a fistula (1). All published series report a male predominance, even in infants and children, implicating a possible role for gender hormones in fistulas (2,3).

ABSCESS
Perianal Anatomy

A thorough understanding of the pelvic floor and sphincter anatomy is a prerequisite for clearly understanding the classification system before choosing an appropriate surgical therapy. The anal canal is comprised of two muscular cylinders. The inner cylinder, the internal anal sphincter, is a 3-cm-long thickened continuation of the circular smooth muscle of the rectum. The outer cylinder, the external anal sphincter, is a 4-cm-long caudal extension of the skeletal muscle of the puborectalis. The levator ani muscle is above the puborectalis that divides the perineum from the abdominal cavity. The intersphincteric space lies between the internal and the external sphincters. The supralevator space is bounded superiorly by the peritoneum, laterally by the pelvic wall, medially by the rectal wall, and inferiorly by the levator ani muscle. The dentate or pectinate line separates the transitional and columnar epithelium of the rectum from the squamous epithelium of the anus. Anal crypts are present at the dentate line, and the anal glands are found at the base of the crypts (Fig. 1).

Pathophysiology

In more than 90% of cases, anorectal abscess may arise as a result of cryptoglandular infection. Fistulas may result from the extension of sepsis from an intramuscular anal gland, usually as a consequence of infection of one of the glands located within the anal canal. Bacteria that are normally present in the anal glands begin to multiply and form an abscess that burrows through the wall of the rectum into the skin surrounding the anus. There are between 4 and 10 anal glands with corresponding ducts entering the base of the anal crypts at the level of the dentate line. The duct becomes obstructed by debris, resulting in the stasis of glandular secretions. A fistula may develop when the tract that extends between the inside gland and the outside opening does not heal.

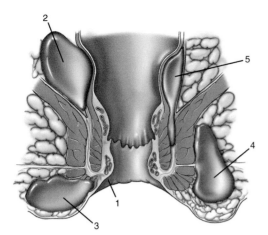

Figure 1 Anorectal abscesses: 1. submucosal abscess, 2. supralevator abscess, 3. perianal abscess, 4. ischioanal abscess, 5. intersphincteric abscess.

Clinical Presentation

Perianal pain, local swelling, and occasionally fever are the cardinal symptoms for perianal abscess (Fig. 2). On physical examination, there is erythema, tenderness, and swelling, while enlarged inguinal nodes may also be palpable. History and perianal inspection are usually sufficient, as digital examination may not be possible due to extreme tenderness. Palpation, if possible, will demonstrate tenderness, indurations, and possibly fluctuance.

Management of Abscess

Acute anorectal abscess is a common surgical emergency. The fundamental principle of treatment is adequate drainage, leaving the incision sufficiently open to help prevent rapid recurrence. A cruciate incision is made and/or the edges are excised to prevent coaptation of the edges. The patient is placed in the prone jackknife or left lateral position, and the area surrounding the abscess cavity is prepped with an antiseptic solution and then anesthetized with an injection of 1% lidocaine. Large ischiorectal, submucosal, and intramuscular abscesses may be better drained under regional or general anesthesia.

Technique

The drainage site for perineal and ischioanal abscesses is at or near the central zone of erythema, tenderness, and fluctuance. If an ischioanal abscess spreads over the buttocks, the site of the incision may be shifted toward the anal side of the abscess for postdrainage wound care. When an intersphincteric abscess is diagnosed, either by palpation or a protrusion into the anal canal or by needle aspiration, treatment consist of dividing the overlying internal sphincter from the anal verge to the cephalad extent of the cavity (4).

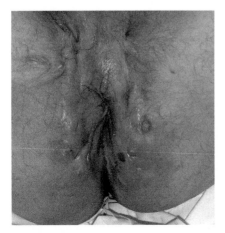

Figure 2 (*See color insert*) Chronic case of perianal abscess.

Supralevator abscesses are rare, but it is essential to determine their origin as they may arise in one of three ways. Upward extension of an intersphincteric abscess is drained into the rectum by dividing the overlying internal sphincter; upward extension of an ischioanal abscess is drained through the ischioanal space into the buttock; whereas a supralevator abscess arising from pelvic pathology may be drained into the rectum or through abdominal operation. In addition, although there are many imaging techniques that may reveal an abscess, such as computerized tomography, magnetic resonance imaging (MRI), ultrasonography, and radionucleotide white cell scanning, none of these are comparable in accuracy or therapeutic potential to an examination of the anal canal under anesthesia.

Most abscesses contain typical lower gastrointestinal tract bacteria such as *Bacteroides fragilis*, *Escherichia coli*, or *Enterococcus*. A culture of the abscess contents is generally superfluous and costly as the abscess resolves with proper drainage. However, unusual-appearing abscess cavities, extensive cellulites or soft tissue infection, diabetes, and immunosuppression are appropriately evaluated with Gram stain and culture. In general, postdrainage antibiotics are unnecessary.

Postoperative Care
If a mushroom-tipped catheter is placed within the abscess, it may be removed in 7 to 10 days. Packing is avoided as it is very painful and precludes free drainage. Sitz baths along with analgesics, stool softeners, and a dietary fiber supplement should be encouraged.

Primary Fistulotomy
There is debate whether fistulotomy should be performed at the time of the abscess drainage. Primary fistulotomy eliminates the source of infection and decreases the rate of recurrence, precluding the need for further surgery. However, the incidence of fistula after incision and drainage of acute cryptoglandular anorectal abscess is 37%, whereas another 10% of patients will develop recurrent abscess (5). Thus, in theory, drainage will avoid unnecessary fistulotomy in more than half of the patients (6). Cox et al. concluded that the optimal surgical management for ischiorectal abscess appears to be incision, drainage, and fistulotomy, resulting in a lower recurrence rate and decreased morbidity as compared to incision and drainage alone (7). A randomized clinical trial comparing simple drainage of anorectal abscess with and without fistula tract treatment of 200 consecutive patients showed that the internal opening of the fistula tract was found in 83% of the patients. The recurrence rate was related to the surgical technique employed; 29% in the group with drainage alone and 5% in the group for which treatment of the fistula tract was attempted (8). In cases of subcutaneous, intersphincteric, or low transphincteric fistulas, drainage with fistulotomy has a minimal morbidity and decreases the recurrence rate. Therefore, in these instances synchronous fistulotomy may be indicated. Conversely, high transphincteric or suprasphincteric fistulas may be treated with drainage alone with delayed treatment of the fistula tract (9–11).

Drainage with Primary Suture
Shorter healing time, shorter hospital stay, and less postoperative pain have been demonstrated following an incision, curettage, and primary suture under antibiotic cover when compared with simple incision and drainage (12,13). A prospective randomized trial showed shorter healing time with primary closure. Nevertheless, despite adequate treatment of any concomitant fistula, recurrence was common, occurring in 22% in the incision and drainage group and 39% in the primary suture group (13). This technique, although certainly intriguing, is not yet the standard therapeutic method.

Complications
Recurrence
Recurrence is more common in patients with a history of previous abscess, inadequate initial treatment, poor fistulotomy wound care, and underlying conditions such as Crohn's colitis. In addition to recurrence of the index abscess, missed infection occurrence may be secondary to persistent fistula. Other reasons of recurrence include missed infection or the presence of an undiagnosed fistula in adjacent anatomic spaces.

Morbidity

Anal incontinence may result if excessive division of the external sphincter is undertaken during drainage of an abscess. Thus, if a primary fistulotomy is undertaken, great care must be exercised to limit muscle division. There are many other reasons for ensuing incontinence, such as prolonged packing of the drained abscess preventing granulation tissue; conversely, failure by the patient to clean the wound may transcend to chronic infection with fibrosis.

The anorectal region may be the site of life-threatening necrotizing infections such as Fournier's gangrene; this condition results from unrecognized or inadequately treated suppurative disease, specifically in comorbid conditions such as diabetes or other immuno-compromised states. The portal of entry may be urethral, rectal, or cutaneous; the disease is rapidly progressive with a reported mortality of 3% to 38% (14,15). Death usually results from systemic illness such as sepsis, coagulopathy, acute renal failure, diabetic ketoacidosis, or multiple organ failure. The typical patient presents approximately two to four days after the onset of fever, appearing toxic and irritable with gangrenous genitalia and leukocytosis. Crepitus of the soft tissues is the physical hallmark of necrotizing fasciitis. Anorectal infection is the source of sepsis in 11% to 78.6% of cases (14–16). Current imaging techniques for the initial evaluation of Fournier's gangrene include radiography, sonography, and computed tomo-graphy (CT) scan. Treatment involves broad-spectrum antibiotic therapy for aerobic and anaerobic organisms and hemodynamic stabilization (17). Surgical treatment focuses on aggres-sive surgical debridement of all nonviable tissue (18). In some cases, fecal diversion and/or suprapubic catheterization may be necessary. The use of hyperbaric oxygen as an adjunctive therapy to surgical and medical treatment may promote wound healing and prevent the exten-sion of invading microorganisms (19). The interval from the onset of clinical symptoms to the initial surgical intervention may also cause an impact on outcome (20,21). Surgeons should be very aggressive with excisional debridement and should have a low threshold to return to the operating room on one or more occasions for additional debridement.

ANAL FISTULAS

Anal fistula is characteristic of the chronic phase of an unhealed perianal abscess. A fistula is a hollow tract lined with granulation tissue between the infected anal gland and a secondary opening in the perianal skin. It is unclear why some abscesses resolve after drainage and others persist, developing into a fistula. Fistulas are virtually always caused by a previous anorectal abscess; other fistulas develop secondary to trauma, Crohn's disease, anal fissures, carcinoma, radiation therapy, tuberculosis, and chlamydial infections. Some studies have shown that fistula persistence may be caused by epithelialization of the tract.

Classification

Successful surgical management of anal fistula depends upon accurate knowledge of anal sphincter topography and surgical anatomy. This classification should provide accurate infor-mation that permits simple, comprehensive, and comparable usage. The most comprehensive and practical classification that is the most widely used today is the Parks Classification (Fig. 3) (22). The classification is derived from the cryptoglandular hypothesis, which states that an infection begins in the anal gland and progresses into the muscular wall of the anal sphincter to cause an abscess; the majority of fistulas arise from an abscess in the inter-sphincteric plane that will terminate in a primary tract whose relation to the external sphincter will dictate the type of fistula and future management.

The classification is divided into four groups: intersphincteric, transsphincteric, supra-sphincteric, and extrasphincteric, as shown in Table 1.

Intersphincteric fistulas account for the vast majority of fistulas. They are typically simple, but occasionally deviate from this pattern and may have a high blind tract, a high opening into the rectum, no perineal opening, or a pelvic extension.

Transsphincteric fistulas may be uncomplicated, consisting simply of the primary tract or they may have associated secondary tracts terminating above or below the levator ani muscles. These tracts usually extend to the apex of the ischiorectal fossa and may undergo horseshoe formation at this level. Occasionally, the secondary tract may penetrate the levator plane to enter the supralevator space.

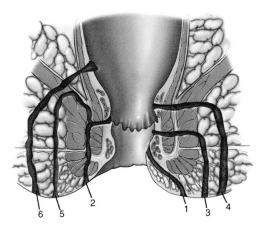

Figure 3 Classification of fistula-in-ano. 1. Superficial fistula, 2. intersphincteric fistula, 3. low transsphincteric fistula, 4. high transsphincteric fistula, 5. suprasphincteric fistula, 6. extrasphincteric fistula.

Suprasphincteric fistulas are rare. Although reported as common by Parks, this probably reflected his case selection through a tertiary referral pattern. It is very rare to encounter a suprasphincteric fistula that has not been previously operated upon. The inference is that most of these cases are likely to be iatrogenic. They are difficult to identify and some suprasphincteric fistulas are probably erroneously classified as suprasphincteric when in reality they are high trans-sphincteric in nature.

Extrasphincteric fistulas are rare, but should be suspected where an external opening is present in the perineum in the presence of a completely normal anal canal. These fistulas are not cryptoglandular in origin and are usually associated with pathology including trauma, Crohn's disease, infection, carcinoma, or its treatment.

Besides horizontal and vertical spread, sepsis may spread circumferentially in any of the three spaces—intersphincteric, ischiorectal, and pararectal. The posterior examples of these abscesses are superficial and deep postanal.

Preoperative Assessment

Surgical success depends upon accurate assessment including a full medical history and proctosigmoidoscopy. It is very important to exclude associated conditions.

Goodsall (23) described the five essentials of clinical assessment which include (i) identification of the internal opening, (ii) identification of the external opening, (iii) the course of the primary tract, (iv) any and all secondary extensions, and (v) any other diseases complicating the fistula.

The internal opening is the key to assessment. The relative positions of external and internal openings indicate the likely course of the primary tract. Palpable superficial indurations

Table 1 Classification of Fistula-in-Ano

Types of fistula	Primary tract	Frequency (%)	Other possible tracts
Intersphincteric	Via internal sphincter to the intersphincteric space and to the perineum	70	High blind tract, high opening into the rectum, no opening, or pelvic extension
Transsphincteric	Low via internal and external sphincters into the ischiorectal fossa	23	High tract with perineal opening; high blind tract
Suprasphincteric	Via intersphincteric space, superiorly above puborectalis muscle through ischiorectal fossa to the perianal skin	5	High blind tract
Extrasphincteric	From the rectum above the levators and through the levators to the perineal skin	2	

Source: From Ref. 22.

suggest a relatively superficial tract, whereas supralevator induration suggests a tract high in the ischiorectal fossa or more likely a secondary extension. The distance of the external opening from the anal verge may help differentiate an intersphincteric from a transsphincteric fistula; the greater the distance, the greater the likelihood of a complex cephalad extension. Goodsall's rule states that if the opening is anterior to a transverse anal line drawn across the tuberosities transecting the anal verge, the internal opening will be found on a straight radial tract into the anal canal. If the opening is posterior to the transverse line, the internal opening will show a curved tract to the posterior midline of the anal canal (Fig. 4). Exceptions include anterior openings more than 3 cm from the anal verge, which may be anterior extensions of posterior horseshoe fistulas, or fistulas associated with other diseases, especially Crohn's disease and cancer.

Primary Tract

Identify any external openings and assess the skin for the direction of the tract and palpate using a well-lubricated finger between the external opening and the anal orifice. An indurated tract suggests a fairly superficial course; its direction will give a hint to the circumferential location of the internal opening.

Feel for induration within the anal canal using the index finger applying counter pressure with the thumb to the perianal skin. The internal opening is likely to be located at the level of the dentate line. There is often an enlarged papilla in the region of the internal opening and, with experience, the opening itself can often be felt.

The level of the internal opening in relation to the puborectalis is then determined by asking the patient to contract the anal sphincter; it is possible to feel how much functioning muscle would remain were the primary tract to be laid open.

Secondary Tracts

Supralevator induration detects the presence of secondary tract formation. Although difficult to appreciate, there is often a difference between the two sides that will help to reveal its presence. A secondary tract usually arises from a transsphincteric primary tract, extending upwards to the apex of the ischiorectal fossa, or even through the levators. Alternatively, supralevator induration may arise from upward extension from an intersphincteric tract. Digital examination cannot distinguish between these two possibilities.

Radiographic Evaluation

Radiographic investigations have a limited role in the evaluation of fistula-in-ano. Most fistulas can be diagnosed and treated on the basis of clinical examination alone. Radiographic evaluation can be useful in atypical cases or after surgery has failed.

Fistulography

Fistulography may be useful when an extrasphincteric fistula is suspected. A sinogram using water-soluble contrast media may show a communication with the rectum, the sigmoid, or the small bowel. These fistulas are usually due to other pathology such as carcinoma, diverticular disease, or Crohn's disease.

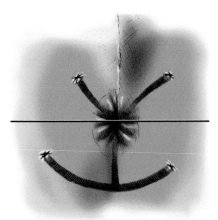

Figure 4   Goodsall rule.

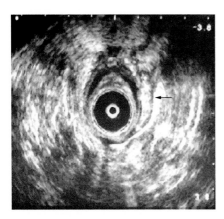

Figure 5 Horseshoe abscess (hydrogen peroxide–enhanced ultrasound) (*arrow*).

Computed Tomography Scanning

CT has also proven disappointing. The exact site of pathology in relation to the levators on axial CT scans can only be inferred indirectly through the relation of any abnormality to the piriformis and coccygeus muscles. The levators are not well identified, and internal and external sphincter resolutions are poor. Coronal imaging is rarely possible and there are many pitfalls in interpretation of the images.

Endoanal Ultrasound

Hydrogen peroxide can be used as a contrast medium for ultrasound to improve visualization of fistulas, particularly before treating recurrent fistulas. Endoanal ultrasonography may help detect supra- or extrasphincteric fistulas and horseshoe extensions, particularly in patients with Crohn's disease (Fig. 5) (24–27). Moreover, hydrogen peroxide–enhanced ultrasound yields location of internal opening of the anal fistula in approximately 60% to 93% of cases (28–31).

However, endoanal ultrasound can reveal sphincter defects in asymptomatic patients after anorectal surgeries including fistulotomy (32). Overall, the classification of fistulas was possible in 61% of patients with sonography, 89% with MRI, and 93% with surgery (33). Thus, MRI seems superior to endoanal ultrasound in the assessment of fistula-in-ano before major surgery (33,34). Anal ultrasound may be more useful than MRI merely because it is more widely available, can be performed in the office setting, and is less expensive. Therefore, although MRI is statistically superior, it may be inferior because of its limited availability and high cost. In addition, anal ultrasonography may be useful in patients in whom prior fistulotomy has been undertaken in order to quantify any muscle defects and help guide the extent of additional muscle division.

Magnetic Resonance Imaging

Patients with deep anorectal abscess may be better studied with magnetic resonance imaging (MRI). The accuracy of MRI is higher than is the accuracy of endoanal ultrasonography to determine the presence of ischiorectal or pelvirectal abscess, particularly when they occur simultaneously. The sensitivity and specificity for detecting fistula tracts have been reported at 100% and 86%, respectively; abscesses, 96% and 97%, respectively; horseshoe fistulas, 100% and 100%, respectively; and internal openings, 96% and 90%, respectively (33). MRI is accurate for detecting anal fistulas and provides important additional information in patients with Crohn's disease–related and recurrent anal fistulas (35). MRI and hydrogen peroxide–enhanced three-dimensional endoanal ultrasound have good agreement for classification of the primary fistula tract and the location of an internal opening and both are reliable methods for preoperative evaluation (36). Compared to endoanal ultrasound, endoanal MRI more accurately allows depiction and classification of fistulas (33). Nevertheless, phased array coil provides more valuable findings for supralevator/subcutaneous extension of fistula tracts than when an endoanal coil is used alone (37). Therefore, a combined approach reflects more accurate classification in complex cases (38).

Anal Manometry

Anal manometry has no role in patients with abscesses. Similarly, patients with de novo fistulas seldom require preoperative anorectal manometry. Patients with Crohn's disease, immunocompromised, advanced age, and in whom prior fistulotomies have been undertaken may benefit from preoperative manometry. Specifically, knowledge of preoperative resting and squeeze pressure may guide the extent and type of treatment rendered for the recurrent fistula.

Treatment

Treatment is surgical with the aim of abolishing the primary tract and draining any secondary tracts. The surgical anatomy should be known to the surgeon, if not preoperatively, then during the dissection. Most primary fistula operations are simple and can be performed without special preparation. Low fistulas can be operated upon under local anesthetic, but more complicated ones require regional or general anesthesia. Surgical approaches to preserve the sphincters (advancement flaps, "core-out" fistulectomy, and other approaches) require bowel preparation and perioperative antibiotics. Fistula procedures can be done with the patient in the lithotomy or the prone jackknife position. In general, anterior fistulas are more easily approached in the latter position and posterior fistulas in the former position. Lateral fistulas can be easily approached with either patient position.

Fistulotomy

Fistulotomy is the classic operation for anal fistula and is suitable for most uncomplicated fistulas. An appropriately shaped fistula probe is passed via the external opening along the length of the primary tract to emerge through the internal opening after which the tract is laid open (Fig. 6A–C). Granulation tissue is curetted and may be sent for histologic examination as adenocarcinoma has been detected in long-lasting fistulas (39–41). Any adherent granulation indicates a possible secondary extension and should be carefully analyzed. The wound is then trimmed and, in simple cases, marsupialized. Any secondary extensions need full and adequate drainage, either by direct widening of the wound or by the use of drains (42,43). Although laying open of an intersphincteric fistula is a simple and effective therapy, it can cause a significant decrease in postoperative resting anal pressure. In order to avoid poor continence, fistulotomy should be more conservative for patients with preoperative low-resting anal pressures (44) or any compromises in continence. Similarly, great care must be taken when prior fistulotomies have occurred. If careful gentle probing does not reveal the internal opening, the tract can be filled with hydrogen peroxide under pressure. Injection of hydrogen peroxide may reveal a bubbling of the peroxide through the internal opening. In these instances, as the location of the internal opening can be located, the surgeon can then gradually "cut down" both the internal and external openings or can simultaneously probe for both openings until the tract has been delineated.

Fistulotomy is generally not indicated in all high transsphincteric tracts; anterior transsphincteric fistulas in females, and most transsphincteric fistulas in patients with Crohn's disease. In these cases, there is a high chance of incontinence following a simple laying-open.

(A)   (B)   (C)

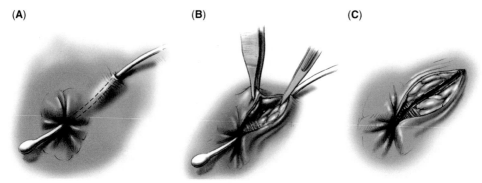

Figure 6   Tract laid open: (**A**) probe through the fistula; (**B**) tract being laid open; (**C**) final result.

It is more prudent to place a seton through the primary tract with drainage of secondary tracts and reassessment some weeks later.

Factors associated with recurrence include a complex fistula, horseshoe extension, lack of identification or lateral location of the internal fistulous opening, and previous fistula surgery. Incontinence has been associated with female gender, high anal fistula, type of surgery, and previous fistula surgery (45).

Fistulectomy

In fistulectomy, the tract is excised rather than laid open. Excision is best undertaken using diathermy to minimize bleeding and to optimize definition of the surgical anatomy of the fistula (46). False tracts caused by injudicious probing should be avoided and granulation tissue leading from the primary to any secondary tract is usually obvious. Healing after fistulectomy is slower than after fistulotomy (47).

When patients submitted to fistulectomy and fistulotomy were postoperatively assessed by endoanal ultrasound, Belmonte et al. noted that major injuries to the sphincter mechanism were much more likely to have been caused by the fistulectomy (48). Thus, fistulotomy rather than fistulectomy is our preferred technique.

Setons

The term seton is derived from the Latin word seta, meaning a bristle. It is used in fistula surgery in various ways. Setons may be classified as loose, tight, or chemical according to their different properties and modes of action.

The Loose Seton

A seton thread, loosely tied, may be used to mark a fistula tract when its exact position and level in relation to the external sphincter is unclear at the time of surgery. Scarring from previous surgery or the degree of relaxation of the external sphincter under anesthesia can make it impossible to determine the level of the tract. In such circumstances, it may be prudent to insert a seton to help determine the proportion of muscle above and below the tract at a later time when the patient is awake and with the tract palpably delineated by the seton. Similarly, a loosely tied seton can facilitate drainage of acute sepsis, allow acute inflammation to subside, and permit safer subsequent fistula surgery.

A seton may be part of a surgical strategy aimed to preserve the sphincter muscle by avoiding fistulotomy and is therefore chiefly applicable to a transsphincteric fistula (Fig. 7). A seton can be used in three ways: to preserve the entire external sphincter, to preserve the upper half of the voluntary muscle, or as part of a staged fistulotomy to reduce the degree of sphincter retraction following division of large amounts of muscle. The incidence of incontinence seen after division of the external sphincter following failure of the loose seton method demonstrates that any fibrosis that may result from the presence of the seton is insufficient to protect against incontinence (49).

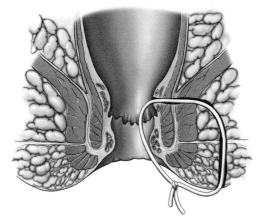

Figure 7 Seton.

A circumferential incision centered on the external opening is made outside the sphincter complex. The wound is deepened through the ischiorectal fossa, and any secondary tracts and chronic abscess cavities are laid open. The primary tract across the external anal sphincter is then identified and a seton is passed through and loosely tied. Various materials are suitable including a braided or monofilament nonabsorbable suture or silastic. A malleable fistula probe with an eye at its tip is useful to draw the seton through the tract. The seton can later be removed or converted to a cutting seton.

The Tight (Cutting) Seton

A tight or cutting seton achieves a staged fistulotomy by slow division of the muscle below the tract. The method was described by Hippocrates, who used a horse hair (50). This technique involves a slow transaction of the enclosed fistula tract and sphincter mechanism by a thread, leaving a trail of fibrosis thereby preventing muscle retraction.

Goldberg and co-workers recommended using a tight seton whenever more than 30% of the sphincter lies below the level of the primary tract, or where local sepsis or fibrosis preclude an advancement flap (51). The portion of the tract outside the sphincters is opened or drained with drains, and the anoderm and perianal skin covering the sphincter lying below the primary tract are incised. The intersphincteric space is drained by internal sphincterotomy, which is extended proximally as necessary to drain any cephalad intersphincteric extension after which the seton is placed. When suppuration has resolved, usually two to three weeks later, the seton is tightened at two-week intervals using a silk tie or baron band until it has cut through the muscle.

Although the cutting seton technique has shown low recurrence rates, gas incontinence may occur in up to 9.5% of the patients (52). Thus, cutting setons yield fairly good results relative to cure of the fistula but the risk of anal incontinence seems to be too high to justify its routine use for all high fistulas (6).

The Chemical Seton

In India, the Kshara sutra chemical seton technique has been used for centuries. It was probably first described by Sushruta, a surgeon who lived approximately 800 B.C.

A specially prepared thread is passed through the fistula and changed weekly. Slow division of the tract is achieved, about 1 cm of tract every six days, probably because of the caustic nature of the thread (pH 9.5) (53–55). The herbal-prepared thread also has antibacterial and anti-inflammatory properties.

A study by Ho et al. comparing pimary fistulotomy versus chemical seton for fistula reported that chemical seton was more painful than conventional fistulotomy in the first few days following surgery. However, ultimately there were no differences in time to wound healing, complications, or functional outcome (9).

Advancement Flaps

Advancement flaps were first proposed by Noble (56) to repair rectovaginal fistulas. Ten years later, Elting described their use in managing anal fistulas (57), stating two principles for their use: separation of the tract from the anal lumen and closure of the internal opening. The modern technique has added creation of a flap of adequate vascularity, and its anastomosis to the anoderm well distal to the internal opening (46,58–61). Modifications include the use of flaps of different thickness, different incisions such as curved or rhomboid, and the importance of closing the external defect. Detry et al. noted excellent functional results and high healing rates with a mucomuscular flap of the rectal wall (62).

Most surgeons would agree that an advancement flap should not be attempted in the presence of active sepsis. Furthermore, the tract should ideally be directed from the internal to the external opening. Adequate access to the anal canal is essential as a large amount of induration may preclude surgery. An Eisenhammer or Fansler retractor yields excellent exposure; this is then inserted and a flap of the lower rectum including mucosa and the underlying circular muscle is raised. The distal portion of the flap is advanced distally and sutured at a level below the internal opening. Fine PDS or Vicryl sutures are satisfactory. The external wound is then either left open or closed or a mushroom-tipped catheter may be left in the tract to facilitate drainage.

Initial reports suggest that patients with high transsphincteric or suprasphincteric anal fistulas achieved a 77% to 95% healing rate (63–65). In addition to high success rates, transanal rectal advancement flap repair also yields minimal or no disturbance of continence (66). Even in the Crohn's disease population, the advancement flap has reportedly reached a 71% success rate for healing. Unfortunately, more recent reports have failed to substantiate these earlier claims (67). Currently, success rates in the range of 50% are probably more realistic. Endorectal advancement flap is an effective surgical modality for the treatment of fistulas due to perianal Crohn's disease, but is less apt to succeed in patients with concomitant small bowel Crohn's disease (67). Moreover, cigarette smoking adversely affects the outcome of advancement flaps (68). Sonoda et al. had a 36.4% of recurrence rate (69), and Mizrahi et al. reported a 15.7% recurrence rate after advancement flap (70). Thus, success is mainly correlated with the presence of Crohn's disease.

Fibrin Glue

Two initial reports suggested success rates in excess of 65% to 75% (71,72). Both reports stressed the importance of thorough curettage to remove as much granulation tissue and debris as possible, as well as generous antibiotic administration, either parenterally or along the fistula tract itself. The success of the treatment of anal fistulas with fibrin glue–antibiotic mixture was independent of the vertical disposition of the fistula, but rather was dependent on the length of the fistulous tract (73). Park et al. have reported an overall success rate of 68% for closure of the fistula using fibrin sealant (74). Fibrin glue can be a simple and effective technique for anal fistulas. The advantage of this technique is that there is no risk of any compromise to continence. However, the disadvantage is that the realistic success rate is probably in the vicinity of 35%. Thus, patients should understand prior to fibrin glue procedures that the surgery will not alter continence but may not be efficacious. In this way, patients understand that fibrin glue will be a first, although innocuous attempt to heal the fistula; then failure should not result in undue disappointment.

Other Techniques
Direct Closure
An alternative to advancement flap is direct closure of the internal opening of a transsphincteric fistula. Functional results are excellent, although 22% of patients may present with suture line dehiscence, which may then lead to a recurrent or persistent fistula (75). Furthermore, this procedure puts little stress on the patient's continence.

Complex Fistulas

Fistulas may be complex, due to secondary tract formation recurrence despite adequate management, size, or underlying disease. Complexity due to secondary tracts can usually be reduced by drainage of these tracts after which the primary tract can be addressed. Preoperative physiologic assessment has a poor significance compared to a careful clinical assessment, but may help identify patients at risk of impaired continence after fistulotomy. If the primary tract is high, then an appropriate sphincter-preserving procedure should initially be undertaken; rarely, a temporary diverting stoma will be required.

Failure of sphincter-preserving methods and persistent symptoms will then make laying open or a long-term loose seton the only choices. After extensive fistulotomy, some patients are able to lead normal lives with the narrowest of (often fibrotic) anorectal rings (76). It is important to consider the possibility of an extrasphincteric fistula when a high "blind" tract is encountered, arising from pelvic or abdominal disease or from a presacral dermoid cyst. Failure to consider such a cause leads to delay in imaging by fistulography, barium studies, or MRI and is a major reason for delayed diagnosis. If a tract is truly high and blind, this may be due to an overlooked secondary extension. In such cases, the component of the tract outside the sphincters should be laid open and curetted; as the resulting wound may be large it is often wise to make a circular rather than a radial incision to avoid sphincter damage. Following granulation tissue with curettage, gentle probing should be carefully undertaken to avoid false tracts. If the tract cannot be traced to the intersphincteric space, it is safest to stop probing. If the tract enters the intersphincteric space but no internal opening can be identified, it is reasonable to assume that the opening has healed or is extremely small; internal sphincterotomy is then justified to obviate recurrence.

Special Considerations
Rectovaginal Fistula
The most common etiology of rectovaginal fistula is obstetric injury, followed by radiation injury, inflammatory bowel disease, operative trauma, infectious etiologies, and neoplasia. It is characterized by an epithelial-lined tract between the rectum and vagina.

Clinical Presentation
Most patients report passage of flatus or stool through the vagina, as well as vaginitis or cystitis. A proctosigmoidoscopic and vaginal speculum examination are essential and may confirm the size and location of the fistula.

The most important adjunctive measure is an examination under anesthesia; other procedures include instillation of methylene blue with assessment of a vaginal tampon for staining.

Treatment
Our preferred treatment is excision of the fistula, closure of the rectovaginal septum, and advancement of a transanal sliding rectal flap; fistulotomy is not recommended because it may result in incontinence.

Postoperative Care
The bladder catheter may be removed the following day; sitz baths, analgesics, and psyllium products can also be given. Bowel confinement and stoma are generally unnecessary (77). Sexual intercourse and the use of tampons should be avoided until complete healing. Success rates ranging from 85% to 100% have been reported (78–80).

Crohn's Disease
Fistulization is a common complication of Crohn's disease, with frequency varying from 17% to 43%. When a patient with Crohn's disease presents with perianal pain, the first complication that must be excluded is perianal abscess that may result from a cryptoglandular infection or obstructed fistula tract. The treatment of perineal abscess is adequate drainage. Successful management of fistula-in-ano in patients with Crohn's disease requires that initial therapy address any rectal inflammation. Such medical management includes corticosteroids, antibiotics, 6-mercaptopurine/azathioprine, methotrexate, cyclosporin, tacrolimus, infliximab, and other antitumor necrosis factors and agents. Due to the risk of failure of local treatment and recurrence, a fistula that causes minimal symptoms may be conservatively treated, perhaps with a draining seton. Surgical treatment of perianal fistulas in patients with Crohn's disease is based on the presence or absence of proctocolitis and the location and type of fistula. In the absence of active proctocolitis, most simple low trans-sphincteric, intersphincteric, and superficial fistulas can be treated with fistulotomy. In contrast, simple low fistulas in patients with active Crohn's proctocolitis should be treated with noncutting setons rather than fistulotomy, because of poor wound healing and the risk of incontinence. Complex fistulas and high fistulas involving a significant portion of the external sphincter such as high transsphincteric, suprasphincteric, or extrasphincteric fistulas necessitate a more conservative surgical approach to minimize the risk for incontinence. Noncutting setons (draining setons) are the treatment of choice in these situations. Some surgeons advocate the use of an endorectal advancement flap as an alternative to fistulotomy or noncutting setons in patients with a simple fistula who do not have active rectal inflammation. The success rate for flaps is lower in patients with Crohn's disease than in those without Crohn's disease.

Irradiation
Local repair, as described for traumatic fistulas, is associated with a high failure rate. Vascularized muscle flaps (gracilis, rectus abdominus, and bulbocavernosus) have been successfully interposed between the rectum and vagina to facilitate healing. Alternatively, successful abdominal approaches have been described and include the sleeve anastomosis technique and Bricker's on-lay patch anastomosis. The eventuality of treating a difficult fistula may be a permanent stoma.

Recurrent Fistula

Any of the previously proposed treatments are acceptable. However, consideration can also be given to a combined repair with muscle interposition (bulbocavernosus, gracilis, and rectus abdominus) or to diverting stoma.

High Fistulas

These fistulas, which are located between the mid rectum and posterior vaginal fornix, may be approached locally through a deep perineal incision with opening of the pouch of Douglas or a transsphincteric (York-Masson) approach.

Fistula-in-Ano in the HIV Positive Patient

Anorectal diseases in the HIV + patient are becoming increasingly more prominent. In a recent large series, Barrett et al. (81) reported 485 procedures performed on 178 patients (mean of 2.7 per patient). Current data have shown that wound healing and the outcome of surgery have been improved by better medical management of HIV infection. Regardless of the advanced immunomodulation therapy, delayed wound healing remains a serious complication after such procedures, and this can be correlated with preoperative CD4+ lymphocyte counts. In any case, the best treatment of anorectal disease in HIV-infected patients is still in question, but any patient with a CD4+ count of less than 50 cells/μL should generally not be offered an invasive procedure. If a procedure must be performed, aggressive preoperative identification of the specific pathogens allows more directed antibiotic therapy.

Asymptomatic fistulas do not require therapy. For the symptomatic patient, a thoughtful, risk–benefit analysis must be performed before performing any surgical procedure. In patients with an intersphincteric or low trans-sphincteric fistula who are good operative candidates, fistulotomy is appropriate. For high trans-sphincteric fistulas or candidates at high risk, placement of a draining (noncutting) seton appears to be the best option. Biopsy of the fistula tract is indicated because malignancy has been associated with perianal sepsis.

REFERENCES

1. Sainio P. Fistula-in-ano in a defined population. Incidence and epidemiological aspects. Ann Chir Gynaecol 1984; 73:219–224.
2. Duhamel J. Anal fistulae in childhood. Am J Proctol 1975; 6:40–43.
3. Longo WE, Touloukian RJ, Seashore JN. Fistula in ano in infants and children: implications and management. Pediatrics 1991; 87:737–739.
4. The American Society of Colon and Rectal Surgeons. Practice parameters for treatment of fistula-in-ano. The standards practice task force. Dis Colon Rectum 1996; 39:1361–1362.
5. Vasilevsky CA, Gordon PH. The incidence of recurrent abscesses or fistula-in-ano following anorectal suppuration. Dis Colon Rectum 1984; 27:126–130.
6. Hamalainen KP, Sainio AP. Incidence of fistulas after drainage of acute anorectal abscesses. Dis Colon Rectum 1998; 41:1357–1361; discussion 1361–1362.
7. Cox SW, Senagore AJ, Luchtefeld MA, Mazier WP. Outcome after incision and drainage with fistulotomy for ischiorectal abscess. Am Surg 1997; 63:686–689.
8. Inceoglu R, Gencosmanoglu R. Fistulotomy and drainage of deep postanal space abscess in the treatment of posterior horseshoe fistula. BMC Surg 2003; 3:10.
9. Ho YH, Tan M, Chui CH, Leong A, Eu KW, Seow-Choen F. Randomized controlled trial of primary fistulotomy with drainage alone for perianal abscesses. Dis Colon Rectum 1997; 40:1435–1438.
10. Knoefel WT, Hosch SB, Hoyer B, Izbicki JR. The initial approach to anorectal abscesses: fistulotomy is safe and reduces the chance of recurrences. Dig Surg 2000; 17:274–278.
11. Oliver I, Lacueva FJ, Perez Vicente F, et al. Randomized clinical trial comparing simple drainage of anorectal abscess with and without fistula track treatment. Int J Colorectal Dis 2003; 18:107–110.
12. Leaper DJ, Page RE, Rosenberg IL, Wilson DH, Goligher JC. A controlled study comparing the conventional treatment of idiopathic anorectal abscess with that of incision, curettage and primary suture under systemic antibiotic cover. Dis Colon Rectum 1976; 19:46–50.
13. Kronborg O, Olsen H. Incision and drainage vs. incision, curettage and suture under antibiotic cover in anorectal abscess. A randomized study with 3-year follow-up. Acta Chir Scand 1984; 150:689–692.
14. Yaghan RJ, Al-Jaberi TM, Bani-Hani I. Fournier's gangrene: changing face of the disease. Dis Colon Rectum 2000; 43:1300–1308.
15. Villanueva-Saenz E, Martinez Hernandez-Magro P, Valdes Ovalle M, Montes Vega J, Alvarez-Tostado FJF. Experience in management of Fournier's gangrene. Tech Coloproctol 2002; 6:5–10; discussion 11–13.

16. Gurdal M, Yucebas E, Tekin A, Beysel M, Aslan R, Sengor F. Predisposing factors and treatment outcome in Fournier's gangrene. Analysis of 28 cases. Urol Int 2003; 70:286–290.

17. Kovalcik PJ, Jones J. Necrotizing perineal infections. Am Surg 1983; 49:163–166.

18. Laucks SS II. Fournier's gangrene. Surg Clin North Am 1994; 74:1339–1352.

19. Korhonen K. Hyperbaric oxygen therapy in acute necrotizing infections. With a special reference to the effects on tissue gas tensions. Ann Chir Gynaecol 2000; 89(suppl 214):7–36.

20. Huber PJ, Kissack AS, Simonton CT. Necrotizing soft-tissue infection from rectal abscess. Dis Colon Rectum 1983; 26:507–511.

21. Korkut M, et al. Outcome analysis in patients with Fournier's gangrene: report of 45 cases. Dis Colon Rectum 2003; 46:649–652.

22. Parks AG, Gordon PH, Hardcastle JD. A classification of fistula-in-ano. Br J Surg 1976; 63:1–12.

23. Goodsall DH. Diseases of the Anus and Rectum. London: Longmans Green, 1900.

24. Cheong DM, Nogueras JJ, Wexner SD, Jagelman DG. Anal endosonography for recurrent anal fistulas: image enhancement with hydrogen peroxide. Dis Colon Rectum 1993; 36:1158–1160.

25. Felt-Bersma RJ, Sloots CE, Poen AC, Cuesta MA, Meuwissen SG. Hydrogen peroxide-enhanced trans-anal ultrasound in the assessment of fistula-in-ano. Dis Colon Rectum 1998; 41(9):1147–1152.

26. Ratto C, Gentile E, Merico M, et al. How can the assessment of fistula-inano be improved? Dis Colon Rectum 2000; 43:1375–1382.

27. Sloots CE, Felt-Bersma RJ, Poen AC, Cuesta MA. Assessment and classification of never operated and recurrent cryptoglandular fistulas-in-ano using hydrogen peroxide enhanced transanal ultrasound. Colorectal Dis 2001; 3:422–426.

28. Sudol-Szopinska I, Gesla J, Jakubowski W, Noszczyk W, Szczepkowsi M, Sarti D. Reliability of endosonography in evaluation of anal fistulae and abscesses. Acta Radiol 2002; 43:599–602.

29. Lengyel AJ, Hurst NG, Williams JG. Pre-operative assessment of anal fistulas using endoanal ultrasound. Colorectal Dis 2002; 4:436–440.

30. Ortiz H, Marzo J, Jimenez G, DeMiguel M. Accuracy of hydrogen peroxide-enhanced ultrasound in the identification of internal openings of anal fistulas. Colorectal Dis 2002; 4(4):280–283.

31. Moscowitz I, Baig MK, Nogueras JJ, et al. Accuracy of hydrogen peroxide enhanced endoanal ultrasonography in assessment of the internal opening of an anal fistula complex. Tech Coloproctol 2003; 7:133–137.

32. Felt-Bersma RJ, van Baren R, Koorevaar M, Strijers RL, Cuesta MA. Unsuspected sphincter defects shown by anal endosonography after anorectal surgery. A prospective study. Dis Colon Rectum 1995; 38:249–253.

33. Hussain SM, Stoker J, Schouten WR, Hop WC, Lameris JS. Fistula in ano: endoanal sonography versus endoanal MR imaging in classification. Radiology 1996; 200:475–481.

34. Maier AG, Funovics MA, Kreuzer SH, et al. Evaluation of perianal sepsis: comparison of anal endosonography and magnetic resonance imaging. J Magn Reson Imaging 2001; 14:254–260.

35. Beets-Tan RG, Beets GL, van der Hoop AG, et al. Preoperative MR imaging of anal fistulas: does it really help the surgeon? Radiology 2001; 218:75–84.

36. West RL, Zimmerman DD, Dwarkasing S, et al. Prospective comparison of hydrogen peroxide-enhanced three-dimensional endoanal ultrasonography and endoanal magnetic resonance imaging of perianal fistulas. Dis Colon Rectum 2003; 46:1407–1415.

37. Halligan S, Bartram CI. MR imaging of fistula in ano: are endoanal coils the gold standard? Am J Roentgenol 1998; 171:407–412.

38. deSouza NM, Gilderdale DJ, Coutts GA, Puni R, Steiner RE. MRI of fistula-in-ano: a comparison of endoanal coil with external phased array coil techniques. J Comput Assist Tomogr 1998; 22:357–363.

39. Ky A, Sohn N, Weinstein MA, Korelitz BI. Carcinoma arising in anorectal fistulas of Crohn's disease. Dis Colon Rectum 1998; 41:992–996.

40. Navarra G, Ascanelli S, Turini A, Lanza G, Gafa R, Tonini G. Mucinous adenocarcinoma in chronic anorectal fistula. Chir Ital 1999; 51:413–416.

41. Cirocchi R. Adenocarcinoma arising from a recurrent fistula-in-ano. Ann Ital Chir 1999; 70:771–774; discussion 774–775.

42. Friend WG. Anorectal problems: surgical incisions for complicated anal fistulas. Dis Colon Rectum 1975; 18:652–656.

43. Hanley PH. Rubber band seton in the management of abscess-anal fistula. Ann Surg 1978; 187:435–437.

44. Chang SC, Lin JK. Change in anal continence after surgery for intersphincteral anal fistula: a functional and manometric study. Int J Colorectal Dis 2003; 18:111–115.

45. Garcia-Aguilar J, Belmonte C, Wong WD, Goldberg SM, Madoff RD. Anal fistula surgery. Factors associated with recurrence and incontinence. Dis Colon Rectum 1996; 39:723–729.

46. Lewis P, Bartolo DC. Treatment of trans-sphincteric fistulae by full thickness anorectal advancement flaps. Br J Surg 1990; 77:1187–1189.

47. Kronborg O. To lay open or excise a fistula-in-ano: a randomized trial. Br J Surg 1985; 72:970.

48. Belmonte Montes C, Ruiz Galindo GH, Montes Villalobos JL, Decanini Teran C. Fistulotomy vs. fistulectomy Ultrasonographic evaluation of lesion of the anal sphincter function. Rev Gastroenterol Mex 1999; 64:167–170.

49. Lunniss PJ, Kamm MA, Phillips RK. Factors affecting continence after surgery for anal fistula. Br J Surg 1994; 81:1382–1385.
50. Adams F. In the genuine works of Hippocrates translated from the Greek and with a preliminary discourse and annotations. London: S Society, 1849.
51. Garcia-Aguilar J, Belmonte C, Wong DW, Goldberg SM, Madoff RD. Cutting seton versus two-stage seton fistulotomy in the surgical management of high anal fistula. Br J Surg 1998; 85:243–245.
52. Isbister WH, Al Sanea N. The cutting seton: an experience at King Faisal Specialist Hospital. Dis Colon Rectum 2001; 44:722–727.
53. Deshpande P, Sharma KR. Treatment of fistula-in-ano by a new technique. Review and follow-up of 200 cases. Am J Proctol 1973; 24:49–60.
54. Deshpande PJ, Sharma KR. Successful non-operative treatment of high rectal fistula. Am J Proctol 1976; 27:39–47.
55. Mohite JD, Gawai RS, Rohondia OS, Bapat RD. Ksharsootra (medicated seton) treatment for fistula-in-ano. Indian J Gastroenterol 1997; 16:96–97.
56. Noble G. A new operation for complete laceration of the perineum designed for the purpose of eliminating danger of infection from the rectum. Trans Am Gynecol Soc 1902:357–363.
57. Elting A. The treatment of fistula in ano. Ann Surg 1912; 56:744–752.
58. Jones IT, Jagelman DG. The use of transanal rectal advancement flaps in the management of fistula involving the anorectum. Dis Colon Rectum 1986; 30:919–923.
59. Wedell J, Meier zu Eissen P, Banzhaf G, Kleine L. Sliding flap advancement for the treatment of high level fistulae. Br J Surg 1987; 74:390–391.
60. Shemesh EI, Kodner IJ, Fry RD, Neufeld DM. Endorectal sliding flap repair of complicated anterior anoperineal fistulas. Dis Colon Rectum 1988; 31:22–24.
61. Stone JM, Goldberg SM. The endorectal advancement flap procedure. Int J Colorectal Dis 1990; 5: 232–235.
62. Detry R, Kartheuser A, Remacle G. Treatment of deep anal fistulas using a flap from the rectal wall. Ann Chir 1994; 48:178–182.
63. Miller GV, Finan PJ. Flap advancement and core fistulectomy for complex rectal fistula. Br J Surg 1998; 85:108–110.
64. Hyman N. Endoanal advancement flap repair for complex anorectal fistulas. Am J Surg 1999; 178: 337–340.
65. Cintron JR, Park JJ, Orsay CP, Pearl RK, Nelson RL, Abcarian H. Repair of fistulas-in-ano using autologous fibrin tissue adhesive. Dis Colon Rectum 1999; 42:607–613.
66. Kreis ME. Functional results after transanal rectal advancement flap repair of trans-sphincteric fistula. Br J Surg 1998; 85:240–242.
67. Joo JS, Weiss EG, Nogueras JJ, Wexner SD. Endorectal advancement flap in perianal Crohn's disease. Am J Surg 1998; 64:147–150.
68. Zimmerman DD, Delemarre JB, Gosselink MP, Hop WC, Briel JW, Schouten WR. Smoking affects the outcome of transanal mucosal advancement flap repair of trans-sphincteric fistulas. Br J Surg 2003; 90:351–354.
69. Sonoda T, Hull T, Piedmonte MR, Fazio VW. Outcomes of primary repair of anorectal and rectovaginal fistulas using the endorectal advancement flap. Dis Colon Rectum 2002; 45:1622–1628.
70. Mizrahi N, Wexner SD, Zmora O, et al. Endorectal advancement flap: are there predictors of failure? Dis Colon Rectum 2002; 45:1616–1621.
71. Hjortrup A, Moesgaard F, Kjaergard J. Fibrin adhesive in the treatment of perineal fistulas. Dis Colon Rectum 1991; 34:752–754.
72. Abel ME, Chiu YS, Russell TR, Volpe PA. Autologous fibrin glue in the treatment of rectovaginal and complex fistulas. Dis Colon Rectum 1993; 36:447–449.
73. Patrlj L, Kocman B, Martinac M, et al. Fibrin glue-antibiotic mixture in the treatment of anal fistulae: experience with 69 cases. Dig Surg 2000; 17:77–80.
74. Park JJ, Cintron JR, Orsay CP, et al. Repair of chronic anorectal fistulae using commercial fibrin sealant. Arch Surg 2000; 135:166–169.
75. Athanasiadis S, Helmes C, Yazigi R, Kohler A. The direct closure of the internal fistula opening without advancement flap for transsphincteric fistulas-in-ano. Dis Colon Rectum 2004; 47:1174–1180.
76. Milligan ETC. Surgical anatomy of the anal canal with special reference to anorectal fistulae. Lancet 1934:1150–1156.
77. Nessim A, Wexner SD, Agachan F, et al. Is bowel confinement necessary after anorectal reconstructive surgery? A prospective, randomized, surgeon-blinded trial. Dis Colon Rectum 1999; 42:16–23.
78. Mazier WP, Senagore AJ, Schiesel EC. Operative repair of anovaginal and rectovaginal fistulas. Dis Colon Rectum 1995; 38:4–6.
79. Pepe F, Panella M, Arikian S, Panella P, Pepe G. Low rectovaginal fistulas. Aust N Z J Obstet Gynaecol 1987; 27:61–63.
80. Tancer ML, Lasser D, Rosenblum N. Rectovaginal fistula or perineal and anal sphincter disruption, or both, after vaginal delivery. Surg Gynecol Obstet 1990; 171:43–46.
81. Barrett WL, Callahan TD, Orkin BA. Perianal manifestations of human immunodeficiency virus infection: experience with 260 patients. Dis Colon Rectum 1998; 41(5):606–611.

33 | Anorectal Neoplastic Disorders

David E. Beck
Department of Colon and Rectal Surgery, Ochsner Clinic Foundation, New Orleans, Louisiana, U.S.A.

Steven A. Guarisco
Department of Gastroenterology, Ochsner Clinic Foundation, New Orleans, Louisiana, U.S.A.

INTRODUCTION

This chapter reviews relevant anatomy and pathophysiology of anal lesions as well as some of the current limitations in terminology. Anal lesions have been divided into those occurring in the anal canal and margin and further subdivided into malignant and potentially malignant lesions (Table 1).

ANATOMY

Knowledge of the anatomy and physiology of the anus is essential to understanding the lesions in this area (1,2). Clinically the anus is divided into the anal canal and margin. The anal canal is defined by the American Joint Committee on Cancer as "running from the anorectal ring to the anal verge (intersphincteric groove)." Thus the anal canal, as depicted in Figure 1, is that portion of the anus that overlies the internal sphincter muscle. The lining of the anal canal is endodermal in origin and in adults contains several types of epithelium. At the superior or proximal edge, columnar mucosa is found whereas distally, toward the dentate line, a transitional epithelium is encountered. The area just above the dentate line contains elements of both columnar and squamous epithelium while squamous epithelium is seen distal to the dentate line. The proximity of the anal mucosa to the anal sphincters, the extensive blood supply, and lymphatic drainage in this area are important oncologic considerations (2). Lymphatic spread of anal canal lesions occurs in three different directions: superiorly to the pararectal and superior hemorrhoidal nodes, laterally to the internal iliac nodes, and inferiorly to the inguinal and external iliac nodes.

The anal margin runs from the intersphincteric groove (the distal portion of the internal sphincter) to approximately 5 cm caudal (cephalad) in a circumference on the perineum (Fig. 1) (2,3). This circular, doughnut-shaped area is covered by nonkeratinized squamous epithelium of ectodermal origin, which changes to keratinized squamous epithelium at its outer border at the perineal skin. The various epithelial types explain the differing symptoms and characteristics of lesions in this area. Metastatic anal margin lesions usually spread to the inguinal lymph nodes. However, if the primary lymphatic drainage is obstructed by tumor, metastatic spread may be redirected to the pelvic lymph nodes (4).

ANAL CANAL LESIONS

Anal cancers comprise approximately 1.5% of all digestive system cancers in the United States with an estimated 3500 new cases and 500 deaths in 2001 (5). Epidermoid or squamous cell carcinoma is the most common anal neoplasm. Additional names for these lesions include mucoepidermoid carcinoma, cloacogenic carcinoma, and basaloid carcinoma. Although these lesions have different histologic appearance, their evaluation, treatment, and prognosis are similar and will be discussed together.

EPIDERMOID CARCINOMA
Etiology

Studies have shown a high incidence of anal cancer in single males and in patients who practice anal intercourse (6). Other risk factors include sexually transmitted diseases and infection

Table 1 Anal Lesions

Anal canal	Anal margin
Epidermoid carcinoma	Malignant lesions
Melanoma	Squamous cell carcinoma
	Basal cell carcinoma
	Verrucous carcinoma
	Kaposi's sarcoma
	Potentially malignant lesions
	Intraepithelial neoplasias
	Adenomatous (Paget's disease)
	Squamous
	Bowen's disease
	Bowenoid papulosis
	AIN
	HSIN
	Leukoplakia

Abbreviations: AIN, anal intraepithelial neoplasia; HSIN, high-grade squamous intraepithelial neoplasia.

with human papillomavirus (HPV). The strongest evidence in support of this finding comes from a large case–control study in Denmark and Sweden (7). HPV DNA was present within tissue specimens in 88% of 388 patients with anal canal cancer. Recent experience suggests that perineal infection with HPV may be similar to cervical infections with development of intraepithelial neoplasms. HPV types 16 and 18 are integrated into host DNA and have been associated with a spectrum of perianal lesions ranging from subclinical infections to anal condylomata to anal intraepithelial neoplasia (AIN), and ultimately to invasive squamous cell carcinoma (8).

An increased risk of anal HPV infection has also been found in HIV-seropositive patients (9).There appears to be an inverse relationship between CD4 count and detection of HPV infection. The role of immunosuppression in the development of anal cancer is also seen in patients undergoing renal transplantations. These patients have a 100-fold increase in risk for the development of vulvar and anal cancer compared to the general population (10). Other risk factors include cigarette smoking, which has been shown to be associated with cervical cancer.

Diagnosis

Although there is a strong association between homosexuality and anal carcinoma, the majority of anal cancer patients have traditionally been females in their seventh decade of life (11). These patients generally present with bright red rectal bleeding and pain. Bleeding occurs in 27% to 74% of patients and is usually more constant than that associated with hemorrhoids, often preceding other symptoms (12). Twenty-one percent to 39% of patients have discomfort or pain,

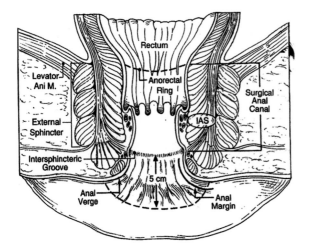

Figure 1 Anatomy of the anal canal and margin. *Source*: From Ref. 2.

which is less severe but more constant than is pain from an acute fissure (1). Patients may also occasionally complain of an ulcerated or mass lesion of the anus. The nonspecific nature of complaints may explain delays in diagnosis. However, appropriate questioning helps exclude other differential diagnoses.

The physical examination is helpful in the diagnosis and essential to determine the clinical stage of disease. Anal cancers are either visible or easily within reach of the examining finger. They tend to be hard, irregular, and ulcerated (Fig. 2). While most lesions remain undiagnosed until they have grown to between 1 and 5 cm in diameter, an occasional early lesion may be serendipitously diagnosed upon pathologic review of an operative specimen such as from a hemorrhoidectomy.

The exact location and size of any anal lesion must be documented prior to treatment and should include the vertical and horizontal diameter of the lesion, the location relative to the anal verge and dentate line, and position in the anus. An assessment of the lesion's fixity, relation to other structures, and status of the sphincteric muscles completes the perineal examination. Some series have reported that up to one-half of patients have sphincter invasion at presentation. In addition to evaluating the primary lesion, the patient should be examined for the presence of inguinal adenopathy as metastases to inguinal lymph nodes at the time of diagnosis have been found in 30% to 43% of patients (1).

Direct visualization of the anus and rectum is essential to exclude other lesions and to allow biopsy of the lesion to confirm the diagnosis. Anoscopy provides good exposure and is the least expensive method of examining and biopsying the anal canal. After identification, the lesion should be biopsied by taking several specimens from the edges of the lesion; a local anesthetic is not usually required. A rigid proctoscope or anoscope and biopsy forceps work well to accomplish an adequate biopsy. Histologically, approximately 70% are found to be squamous cell neoplasms, 25% are basaloid neoplasms, and 5% are mucoepidermoid. The majority of reports demonstrate that the different histologic types act in a similar clinical manner (2).

To assist in the clinical staging of these lesions, several modalities are currently available. These include, in order of decreasing sensitivity, intraluminal ultrasonography, computed tomography (CT) scanning, and magnetic resonance imaging (MRI) (11). Positron emission tomography (PET) scanning is also very sensitive but not anatomically specific. Intra-anal ultrasound is being used with ever-increasing frequency and is helpful in assessing the depth of anal tumors and in identifying the presence and characteristics of lymph nodes. Available intraluminal ultrasound probes have either a 7 MHz (2–5 cm focal length) or 10 MHz (1.5–4 cm focal length) transducer. More important than the type of transducer used, the quality of the examination depends greatly on the skill and experience of the operator. Further widespread experience and improved equipment are necessary before this technology can fulfill its potential (3). Until then, assessment with CT or MRI in addition to an intraluminal ultrasound is recommended.

Staging for anal cancer provides prognostic information and allows comparison of patient groups. Limitations of the current system as proposed by the American Joint Commission on Cancer include the inability to accurately stage patients by clinical means alone, alterations in specimens due to therapy, and the frequent absence of tissue for complete

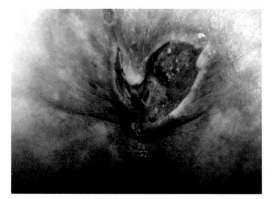

Figure 2 Epidermoid cancer of the anal canal. *Source:* From Ref. 2.

Table 2 Anal Cancer TNM Staging System[a]

Primary tumor (T)
TX: primary tumor cannot be assessed
Tis: no evidence of primary tumor
T0: carcinoma in situ
T1: tumor 2 cm or less in greatest dimension
T2: tumor more than 2 cm but no more than 5 cm in greatest dimension
T3: tumor more than 5 cm in greatest dimension
T4: tumor of any size invades adjacent organs except sphincter muscles
Lymph node (N)
NX: regional lymph nodes cannot be assessed
N0: no regional lymph node metastasis
N1: metastasis in perirectal lymph node(s)
N2: metastasis in unilateral internal iliac and/or inguinal lymph node(s)
N3: metastasis in perirectal and inguinal lymph nodes and/or bilateral internal iliac and/or inguinal lymph nodes
Distant metastasis (M)
MX: presence of distant metastasis cannot be assessed
M0: no distant metastasis
M1: distant metastasis

[a]American Joint Committee on Cancer, 1997.

evaluation if the therapy does not include surgery (Table 2). Additional deficiencies of this tumor node metastasis (TNM) system include difficulty in assessment of the external sphincter involvement, difficulty in estimating longitudinal tumor extension, ambiguity in the definition of neighboring structures, and the lack of consideration of mesenteric nodal involvement. Patients with late-stage disease fare worse than those with early disease, however, most reports lack comparable data from which to draw any meaningful conclusions. The available survival data are discussed below.

Treatment

Owing to the advances in the nonsurgical combined modality treatment of anal cancer, a discussion of the primary surgical management of this disease is generally of historical value (11). An abdominoperineal resection (APR) was the standard surgical therapy for anal cancer in the United States prior to 1974. An APR performed for anal cancer is similar to that utilized for rectal cancer with the exception that a slightly wider margin of perineal skin is removed and a posterior vaginectomy is added in patients with rectovaginal septal involvement. Results with APR included a five-year survival that ranges from 27% to 71% (averaging 50%) (11).

In 1974, Nigro and Vaitkenicius reported their initial results in three patients using 5-fluorouracil (5-FU), mitomycin-C, and radiotherapy (30 Gy) followed by an APR in two of the patients (13). The operative specimens had no residual tumor, and the third patient, who refused surgery, was clinically free of tumor at a 14-month follow-up.

Since this original report, many centers have published their results with multimodality treatment for anal canal carcinoma. A recent review of 26 published series totaled 1558 patients (11). The mean age was 62 years, and 71% were female. With variable follow-up, the mean local recurrence rate was 15%, the distal recurrence rate was 8%, and 75% of the patients remained continent. Three of the more recent randomized trials have convincingly demonstrated the additional benefit of concurrent chemotherapy in the treatment of invasive anal carcinoma (14–16). The United Kingdom Coordinating Committee on Cancer Research Anal Cancer Trial Working Party randomized 585 patients with anal cancer to receive either 45 Gy of radiotherapy alone or the same regimen with concurrent 5-FU and mitomycin (14). Patients with a good initial clinical response received a radiotherapy boost dose, whereas poor responders underwent salvage surgery. With a median follow-up of 42 months, the local failure rate was 36% in the combined treatment group versus 59% in patients receiving radiotherapy alone ($p < 0.0001$). Death owing to anal cancer was reduced ($p < 0.02$) for the combined modality group, although the improvement in overall survival was not statistically significant.

These results were supported by a study by the European Organization for Research and Treatment of Cancer of 110 patients with locally advanced (T3-4, node positive, or both) anal cancer (16). The addition of chemotherapy increased the complete remission rate from 54% to 80%. Patients receiving combined modality treatment had an 18% lower local recurrence rate ($p = 0.02$) and a 32% higher colostomy-free interval rate ($p = 0.0002$). Acute and late side effects were comparable between the arms, except for an increased incidence of anal ulcers in the combined treatment group. The rate of metastases was unchanged in the groups, resulting in similar overall survival rates (56% five-year overall survival).

An intergroup trial by the Radiation Therapy Oncology Group (RTOG) and Eartean Cooperative Oncology Group (ECOG) addressed the role of mitomycin in multimodality therapy (15). In this study of 291 patients, all received radiotherapy (45.0–50.4 Gy) and chemotherapy; randomization was between 5-FU alone and 5-FU with mitomycin C. At four years, patients in the mitomycin arm had lower colostomy rates (9% vs. 22%, $p = 0.002$), higher colostomy-free survival (71% vs. 59%, $p = 0.014$), and higher disease-free survival (73% vs. 51%, $p = 0.0003$); no differences were seen in overall survival. Grade 4 and 5 toxicities, mainly related to sepsis from neutropenia, were higher in the mitomycin group (23% vs. 7%, $p < 0.001$). These three trials clearly demonstrate that the current standard of care for invasive anal cancer is a combined modality approach consisting of radiotherapy, 5-FU, and mitomycin chemotherapy. The optimal timing, dose, and techniques when using this combined regimen await further investigation.

Due to the significant incidence of hematologic toxicity with the use of mitomycin C, new studies have focused on the use of platinum-based chemotherapy, which has been effective in the treatment of other squamous cell cancers (17–21). Initial studies have shown encouraging results. This has led to the initiation of a phase III randomized intergroup trial in which the current standard of care (5-FU, mitomycin, and radiotherapy) will be compared with a regimen of induction and concurrent 5-FU and cisplatin with radiotherapy. Pending adequate accrual, the results should clarify the possible benefits of cisplatin over mitomycin in terms of efficacy and treatment toxicity.

The management of HIV-positive patients with invasive anal cancer is expected to become a more common clinical scenario over the next several years. Currently, minimal data exist on the proper management of these patients. Generally, combination therapy seems effective if radiation and chemotherapy doses are kept relatively low. Tolerance to therapy is decreased when the pretreatment CD4 count is less than $200/mm^3$ (16,22).

In summary, the authors recommend combined therapy as initial treatment for patients with epidermoid anal canal cancer. Radiotherapy entails 30 Gy, administered over three to four weeks, using apposed fields with an additional boost of 15 to 20 Gy delivered to sites of macroscopic disease (11). Chemotherapy is given concomitantly with radiotherapy according to the following scheme: intravenous 5-FU ($1000 \, mg/m^2/day$) on day 1 to 5 and day 31 to 35 and mitomycin C ($15 \, mg/m^2$) on day 1. Patients undergo an evaluation that includes visual inspection of the lesion site one month after completion of radiotherapy; any suspicious finding warrants biopsy. Following chemoradiation, patients are examined every three months for the first two years, every six months for years 3 and 4, and annually thereafter. An APR, or in highly selected situations, additional chemoradiotherapy is offered to those patients with residual or recurrent disease following chemoradiation.

MELANOMA

Anorectal melanomas are rare; they account for 1% of all melanomas and 0.25% to 1% of anorectal tumors (23). The mean age of occurrence is in the fifth decade; females are affected more frequently than males. The most frequent presenting symptom is bleeding, followed by an anal mass or pain. The lesions are usually elevated, and 34% to 75% will be pigmented.

These tumors are locally invasive and have a high metastatic potential. Because many patients present late, the reported five-year survival rates range from 0% to 12%. The prognosis is related to tumor size, thickness, and clinical stage. Evaluation should include a biopsy and ruling out metastatic disease with CT of the abdomen, pelvis, and chest, liver function tests, chest X ray evaluation, and bone scans. Special stains or electron microscopy may be required to confirm the diagnostic biopsy.

Surgery provides the only potential for cure. However, the minimal chance for cure and limited experience have led to controversy regarding the appropriate procedure. Local excision has less associated morbidity. Compared to APR, recent reports have shown little difference in the mean survival rates following either procedure (11). Prophylactic lymphadenectomy is not indicated for clinically negative nodes but is helpful for clinically suspicious nodes. Radiotherapy and chemotherapy have demonstrated little benefit in this disease.

ANAL MARGIN LESIONS
Malignant Lesions

Malignant lesions of the anal margin include squamous cell carcinoma, basal cell carcinoma, verrucous carcinoma, and Kaposi's sarcoma (Table 1). These lesions, in general, tend to behave in a less invasive manner and have a better prognosis than malignant lesions of the anal canal.

Squamous Cell Cancer

Squamous cell cancer of the anal margin acts in a similar manner to lesions that occur in other cutaneous areas of the body. The lesions appear as raised hard flat masses that may ulcerate (Fig. 3). Any chronic unhealed cutaneous ulcer should be considered a potential squamous cell carcinoma (24). The lesions vary in size from small (<1 cm) to larger lesions that surround the anal orifice. Patients average in age between 62 and 70 years with an equal gender distribution (25). Symptoms usually include a mass, bleeding, pain, discharge, and itching (26). Despite what should be an obvious lesion, patients are often diagnosed late or misdiagnosed as having anal fissures, hemorrhoids, eczema, or abscesses (27). Pathologically, these lesions are usually well differentiated and keratinized. Local invasion can occur, but these lesions grow slowly. Lymphatic spread is mainly toward the inguinal lymph nodes.

The literature on managing these lesions is scant, and many series mix anal canal lesions with those of the anal margin. Appropriate therapy for most lesions is wide local excision with clear margins (2,28). With more advanced lesions, it may be difficult to obtain adequate margins and retain adequate anorectal function. Excision is inadequate if lymph nodes are involved. Chemoradiation provides an acceptable alternative for larger and advanced lesions (24,29–31). Dosages of radiotherapy have varied from 40 to 70 Gy (24). Residual or recurrent cancer following radiation has been treated with local excision or APR while residual or recurrent cancer after local excision has been managed with radiotherapy or APR. Early lesions have nearly a 100% cure rate, while five-year survival can drop to 60% for T2 lesions (27,32).

Basal Cell Cancers

Basal cell cancers of the anal margin are rare and appear as ulcerated masses. They are more frequent in men and usually occur in the sixth decade of life (4). Nonspecific complaints

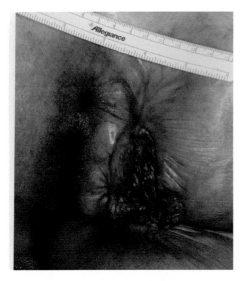

Figure 3 Squamous cell cancer of the anal margin.

include bleeding and pruritus (33,34). The lesions are similar to other basal cell cancers of the skin and usually have a central ulceration with a raised pearly border. Nielson and Jensen reported on 34 cases collected from the Danish Registry of Cancer (35). Nineteen (59%) patients had tumors less than 3 cm in diameter but 1% of the lesions were 5 to 10 cm in size. The larger lesions required an APR, and the smaller ones had wide excision. The importance of adequate margins is stressed by the 29% recurrence rate experienced by patients in this series. These lesions are slow growing and rarely metastasize, which explains why no patient in this series died of the disease. A wide local excision with clear margins is the treatment of choice. Incomplete excision results in a recurrence rate of up to 50% (36). The role of radiotherapy has not been determined. The five-year survival of reported patients exceeds 73% (35).

Verrucous Carcinoma

Verrucous carcinomas are rare low-grade, well-differentiated squamous cell cancers, which are locally aggressive but rarely metastasize (37). Originally described by Buschke in 1896 (38,39) and further elucidated by Buschke and Lowenstein in 1925 (40), these large cauliflower-like lesions resemble large anal condylomata and can affect the penis, vulva, scrotum, and perianal or anorectal region; hence the clinically synonymous terms "giant condylomata acuminata, malignant condylomata, or Buschke–Lowenstein tumor." These slowly but relentlessly enlarging warty tumors can only be distinguished histologically by local invasion and minimal dysplasia (2,37).

Since the first perianal case reported by Dawson et al. in 1965 (41), less than 50 cases of anorectal and perianal verrucous carcinoma have been reported in the literature, which documents the rarity of this condition (36,41–43). The average age of patients with this condition is 43 years, and the male to female ratio is approximately 2:1 (37). Common symptoms include pain, discharge, bleeding, defecatory disturbances, weight loss, anemia, and pruritus ani (43).

Surgical excision with an adequate margin is the treatment of choice. This allows histological evaluation and reduces the incidence of local recurrence. For large lesions an APR may be required to completely eradicate the tumor but appears to have little impact on survival (37). Inadequate information is available regarding multimodality therapy for this tumor; however, the high recurrence rate warrants further investigation of these adjuvant modalities.

Kaposi's Sarcoma

Kaposi's sarcoma is an uncommon malignancy that occurs in four forms. The lesion seen most commonly by the colorectal surgeon or gastroenterologist is associated with the acquired immunodeficiency syndrome. Previously, these lesions were seen in the preterminal stages of HIV infections. However, these patients were often too sick and debilitated to tolerate therapy; therefore, most patients died with or as a result of these tumors. However, newer and combination antiviral medications have helped in maintaining more of these patients in a healthy state and allowed them to tolerate therapy; Kaposi's sarcoma lesions are radioresponsive (44–46).

Potentially Malignant Lesions

Potentially malignant lesions of the anal margin are uncommon and include AINs such as Paget's disease, various squamous AINs (Bowen's disease, Bowenoid papulosis, and AIN), and leukoplakia (Table 1). An ongoing problem in this area has been a lack of standard and consistent terminology.

Paget's Disease

Paget's disease, a rare intraepithelial neoplasm or adenocarcinoma, was named for Sir James Paget who described 15 patients with a characteristic breast lesion in 1874 (47). The extramammary variety can be found wherever apocrine glands are located. The first case of perianal disease was reported in 1893 by Darier and Coulillaud (48). Since then, over 200 cases of perianal disease have been reported in the surgical literature (48–51).

Patients with perianal Paget's disease average 66 years of age (range, 37–90 years), and more than half have been females (48,49). In cases reported by Beck and Fazio (50), nine patients were symptomatic for an average of 21 months. They presented with nonspecific complaints of anal itching, burning, or bleeding. The perianal lesions were well-demarcated

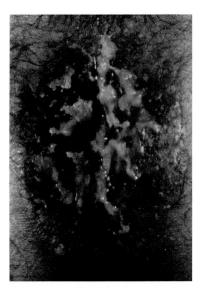

Figure 4 Perianal Paget's disease. *Source*: From Ref. 2.

eczematoid plaques that were either ulcerative and crusty or papillary (Fig. 4). Although less common, these lesions may have a gross appearance similar to other diseases as described in Bowen's disease (49).

A biopsy is performed in an office setting using the following technique: the lesion is cleansed with povidone-iodine solution, and analgesia is obtained with 0.5% xylocaine. Two to four full-thickness specimens (including subcutaneous tissue) are obtained from the central portion and edges of the lesion, using a 3 mm disposable punch biopsy (Baker Cummins Pharma-ceuticals, Inc., Miami, Florida, U.S.A.). After the punch biopsy is twisted in a circular manner to cut through the dermis, the biopsy specimen is elevated with small forceps, and the remaining attached subcutaneous tissue is cut with fine scissors. The specimen is immediately placed in 10% formalin or hollandaise solution. This technique allows the pathologist to compare lesion his-tology with adjacent normal skin. Any bleeding at the residual biopsy site is easily controlled with a silver nitrate stick; all biopsy specimens should be reviewed by an experienced pathologist.

On pathologic evaluation, perianal Paget's disease is characterized by large, faintly basophilic, or vacuolated cells located in the epidermis (Fig. 5). The nuclei are vesicular and demonstrate little mitotic activity. In contrast to Bowenoid cells, Paget's cells become highlighted with a periodic acid-Schiff (PAS) stain due to their high mucin content and also stain with a carcinoembryonic antigen (CEA) immunofluorescence stain (49).

The origin of Paget's cells has been debated for many years. Theories included primitive multipotential epidermal cells or elements of glandular cells (51). Recent work supports a glandular origin as these cells contain low–molecular weight cytokeratins and CEA. In addition they express the gross cystic disease fluid protein (51).

In Paget's disease, progression of the lesion into an invasive carcinoma has been report-edly as high as 40% in untreated lesions (50). However, the small number of reported patients

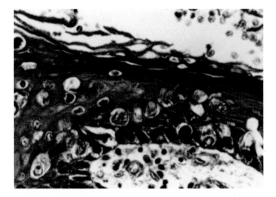

Figure 5 Perianal Paget's disease (photomicrograph, hematoxylin and eosin × 400). *Source*: From Ref. 2.

with these perianal lesions has limited our understanding regarding prognosis. The association of Paget's disease with other cancers has been much stronger than that for Bowen's disease. The incidence of associated malignancies with Paget's disease in reported series ranges from 38% to 86%, and the mortality has been high from this cancer despite aggressive therapy (51–55).

In the absence of invasive malignancy, wide local excision is adequate therapy (49). Curettage and radiotherapy have been associated with high recurrence rates. In the series reported by Jensen et al. (51), all seven patients managed with curettage or radiotherapy developed recurrent disease within six months.

If an associated malignancy is diagnosed, an aggressive approach is warranted to alter the historically poor prognosis (2,50). Long-term survival has been reported after APR in patients without metastatic disease at presentation (2). Long-term follow-up is essential as 61% of the patients in Jensen's series developed recurrent disease up to eight years after primary treatment. This high rate may be due to inadequate initial treatment.

Squamous Intraepithelial Neoplasias

Increasing experience has expanded our knowledge of these uncommon lesions. However, the lack of uniform and widely accepted terminology has led to some confusion. Lesions included in this group include Bowen's disease, Bowenoid papulosis, high-grade squamous intraepithelial neoplasia (HSIN) and AIN. These lesions have similar histologic and cytologic appearance and share some clinical characteristics. As described in the subsequent sections, there is substantial evidence that these lesions may have similar etiology.

Bowen's Disease

Bowen's disease is an uncommon intraepithelial squamous cell carcinoma named after John T. Bowen, who in 1912 described two patients with atypical epithelial proliferation of the skin (56). The first perianal case of Bowen's disease was reported by Vickers et al. (57) in 1939, and to date over 150 cases have been reported in the literature (58,59).

At the time of diagnosis, the age range of reported patients is 30 to 74 years (mean, 48 years) (60), and the majority of patients (64%) tend to be Caucasian females (58). A series reported by Beck et al. (59) showed that 40% of patients were diagnosed with perianal Bowen's disease after examination of hemorrhoidectomy specimen (incidental), whereas the remaining 60% presented with symptomatic perianal lesions that had been present for an average of 34 months (range, 1 month to 10 years).

Patients with perianal Bowen's disease commonly present with nonspecific complaints of anal itching, burning, or bleeding. Examination of the perineum in symptomatic patients usually reveals raised, irregular, scaly, brownish-red plaques with eczematoid features (Fig. 6). These lesions may have a gross appearance similar to other diseases such as leukoplakia, squamous cell cancer, condylomata acuminata, dermatitis, or eczema.

Any anal or perianal lesion that is unresponsive to appropriate therapy after two to four weeks should undergo biopsy (59). The microscopic appearance of these perianal lesions is characteristic and readily confirms the diagnosis. Bowen's disease demonstrates a disordered

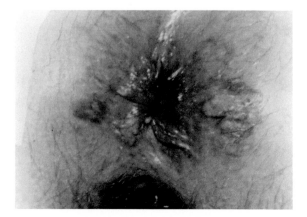

Figure 6 Perianal Bowen's disease. *Source:* From Ref. 2.

epidermal hyperplasia with parakeratosis and hyperkeratosis in the superficial surface layers. The Malpighian cells also reveal a disordered hyperplasia, with atypism and malignant dyskeratotic cells. Large atypical cells with haloed large hyperchromatic nuclei (Bowenoid cells) are present and are negative for a PAS stain; mitotic figures are present in all layers (Fig. 7).

An accurate diagnosis is important for both prognostic and therapeutic reasons. The clinical course of Bowen's disease has been relatively benign with progression toward invasive carcinoma in 2% to 6% of cases (61). In addition to concern about progression to an invasive cancer, a relationship of these epithelial lesions to nonepithelial malignancies has been proposed (62); although early reports have described such a relationship, a recent reexamination of the methods and analyses used in these published series demonstrated several flaws. The authors concluded that the evidence was insufficient to confirm a relationship between Bowen's disease and the subsequent development of internal malignancies (63). In addition, a recent collective survey of experience with perianal Bowen's disease found the incidence of subsequent nonsquamous malignancy to be only 4.7% (64).

Patients with perianal Bowen's disease should undergo proctoscopy and barium enema or colonoscopy to exclude an associated invasive cancer and to confirm the extent of the disease (2,59,61). If evaluation demonstrates an invasive carcinoma without metastases, an aggressive approach is warranted to improve the historically poor prognosis associated with these diseases. For adenocarcinoma of the lower rectum, the authors recommend an APR, and for epidermoid anal cancer the authors currently use combination chemoradiotherapy. In the absence of invasive cancer, the authors prefer local excision.

Adequate, microscopically normal margins are very important, as both Bowen's and Paget's cells may extend beyond the gross margins of the lesion (58). To insure a complete excision some authors utilize "lesion mapping." Biopsies are obtained 1 cm from the edge of the lesion and in all four quadrants of the perineum. As shown in Figure 8, 2 to 3 mm biopsies are taken at the dentate line, anal verge, and the perineum, approximately 2 to 3 cm from the anal verge. Utilizing this mapping as a guide, a wide local excision of the lesion is accomplished (58). The excision can either be done at the time of the anal mapping or after the final histopathologic assessment of the biopsies. The latter option saves countless hours of waiting in the operating room for additional frozen section diagnosis.

Following removal of the specimen, the margins of resection are examined by frozen section techniques to ensure complete excision. The wound defect is closed primarily in the wounds that encompass less than 30% of the anal circumference. Wounds greater than 30% are covered with a split thickness skin graft, either at the initial operation or three to four days later, or rotational or advancement flaps. Alternately, they may be left to heal by secondary intention. The low recurrence rate in patients treated by wide local excision supports this therapy as the appropriate method (65). For extensive lesions within the anal canal such as a circumferential distribution, a staged bilateral procedure possibly with temporary fecal diversion (such as a laparoscopically created loop stoma) may be considered.

Long-term follow-up is recommended to help limit recurrence of perianal Bowen's disease (65). However, the limited experience with this disease has hindered the development

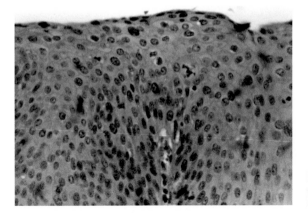

Figure 7   Perianal Bowen's disease (photomicrograph, hematoxylin and eosin × 400). *Source*: From Ref. 2.

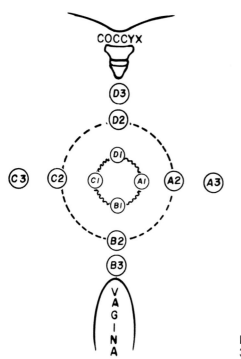

Figure 8 Anal mapping. 1—Dentate line, 2—anal verge, 3—perineum (2–3 cm from anal verge). *Source*: From Ref. 2.

of a standardized follow-up regimen. An annual complete physical examination, proctosigmoidoscopy, punch biopsy of any new lesion, and random biopsies at the edges of the split thickness skin graft or flaps are recommended (65). Colonoscopy is also generally performed at two to three year intervals. If a recurrence is found, it is excised with adequate clear margins using the methods described above.

Bowenoid Papulosis
Bowenoid papulosis is also a rare squamous premalignant lesion. While it is histologically similar to Bowen's disease, it has several significant clinical differences (54). The findings are usually multiple, 2- to 10-mm diameter lesions on the perineum. The lesions are flat, slightly elevated, and discrete. They are slightly pigmented, generally reddish to violaceous in color, and somewhat scaly. Occasionally the lesions will be continuous forming plaque-like lesions (55); ulcers are not present. Histologically they are indistinguishable from Bowen's disease.

These lesions occur in young patients (most are in their late 20s or early 30s) and have been reported more often in males (55). There has been a high incidence of prior viral infection (Herpes simplex virus or HPV). Hybridization studies have demonstrated HPV-16 DNA in 80% of examined lesions (66). HPV-16 and HPV-18 are associated with both anal malignancies and with condylomata acuminata. Therefore, condylomata may precede bowenoid papulosis or anal cancer especially in patients who practice anal receptive intercourse (60). Clinically these lesions have a benign course, and patients are usually treated for symptomatic relief. Eradication of these lesions has been accomplished by excision or destruction, as described for condylomata. A recent report of low-dose treatment with recombinant interferon-2c (5 million units subcutaneously daily) has proven to be promising (67).

AIN and HSIN
AIN and HSIN have recently received increased attention (68,69). While AIN is a histologic diagnosis, HSIN is a cytologic diagnosis. These lesions are well-described pathological precursors of invasive squamous cell carcinoma and can occur in several locations including the cervix, anal canal, and perineal skin. Lesions have been detected with increasing frequency in immunocompromised patients, particularly those with seropositivity for HIV (70). The epidemiology and natural history of these entities are unclear as the overall prevalence in

the HIV seronegative population is unknown. However, there is a clear etiological association between AIN and high-risk HPV subtype infection despite great variability in HPV DNA detection of cytological and histological materials. It appears that there is an antigen-specific hyporesponsiveness by cytotoxic lymphocytes against HPV peptide sequences or recombinant proteins encoded by oncogenic HPV subtypes in these patients, which is dependent upon the stage of their HIV-associated disease. Although the molecular biology of AIN and cervical or vulvar intraepithelial neoplasia are comparable, in AIN there is less significance of tumor suppressor gene mutations, proto-oncogenic growth factor activation, and genomic instability.

The need for surveillance and management of anal and perianal lesions is controversial. A recent prospective study of surgical treatment of HSIN by excision/cauterization of lesions visualized with high-resolution anoscopy was performed in 37 patients (70). Twenty nine of these patients were HIV positive, and the overall mean age was 45 years. With a mean follow-up of 32 months, there was no recurrence in the HIV negative patients, but 23 of the 29 HIV-positive patients had persistent or recurrent HSIN. No patient developed incontinence, stenosis, infection, or significant bleeding after surgical treatment. The authors concluded that surgical treatment was safe and capable of eliminating HSIN in HIV-negative patients, while in HIV-positive patients multiple staged procedures and continued surveillance may be necessary. Surveillance is performed with high-resolution anoscopy aided by the use of a topical solution of acetic acid.

Leukoplakia

Leukoplakia is a whitish thickening of the mucous membranes that may represent a precancerous dermatosis. Microscopically the lesions appear as hyperkeratosis and squamous metaplasia (71). Patients commonly present with itching, bleeding, and discharge and should be treated symptomatically with regular follow-up due to the questionable malignant potential. Any suspicious lesion should be biopsied to exclude a malignant lesion. If the leukoplakia is on a hemorrhoid, excisional biopsy is performed as a hemorrhoidectomy.

SUMMARY

Malignant and potentially malignant lesions of the anus are rare. Many physicians will only see one or two cases in their career. Knowledge of the anal anatomy aids in understanding pathology and management as well as avoiding excess morbidity.

REFERENCES

1. Billingham R. Neoplasms of the anus and the perianal skin. In: Mazier WP, Levien DH, Luchtefeld MA, Senagore AJ, eds. Surgery of the Colon, Rectum, and Anus. Philadelphia: WB, Saunders, 1995:205–228.
2. Beck DE, Wexner SD. Anal neoplasms. In: Beck DE, Wexner SD, eds. Fundamentals of Anorectal Surgery. 2nd ed. London: WB Saunders, 1998:261–277.
3. Beck DE. Malignancies of the colon, rectum and anus. In: Beck DE, ed. Handbook of Colon and Rectal Surgery. St Louis: Quality Medical Publishing, 1997:421–430.
4. Gordon PH. Current status-perianal and anal canal neoplasms. Dis Colon Rectum 1990; 33:799–808.
5. Greenlee RT, Hill-Harmon MD, Murray T, Thun M. Cancer statistics, 2001. CA Cancer J Clin 2001; 51:15–36.
6. Saclarides TJ, Klem D. Genetic alterations and virology of anal cancer. Semin Colon Rectal Surg 1995; 6:131–134.
7. Frisch M, Glimelius B, Van Den Brule AJC, et al. Sexually transmitted infection as a cause of anal cancer. N Engl J Med 1997; 337:1350.
8. Scholefield JH. The technique of anal colposcopy in the diagnosis of anal intraepithelial neoplasia. Semin Colon Rectal Surg 1995; 6:150–155.
9. Caussy D, Goedert JJ, Palefsky J, et al. Interaction of human immunodeficiency and papilloma viruses: association with anal epithelial abnormality in homosexual men. Int J Cancer 1990; 46:214.
10. Boman BM, Moertel CG, O'Connell MJ, et al. Carcinoma of the anal canal: a clinical and pathologic study of 188 cases. Cancer 1984; 54:114.
11. Wyn N, Beck DE. Epidermoid cancer of the anal canal. Clinics Colon Rectal Surg 2002; 15.
12. Montague ED. Squamous cell carcinoma of the anus. In: Flethcher GH, ed. Textbook of Radiotherapy. 3rd ed. Philadelphia: Lee & Febiger, 1980:717–718.
13. Nigro ND, Vaitkenicius VK. Combined therapy for cancer of the anal canal. Dis Colon Rectum 1974; 17:354–356.

14. UKCCR Anal Cancer Trial Working Party. Epidermoid anal cancer: results from the UKCCCR randomized trial of radiotherapy alone versus radiotherapy, 5-fluorouracil, and mitomycin. Lancet 1996; 348:1049–1054.
15. Flam M, John M, Pajak TF, et al. Role of mitomycin in combination with fluorouracil and radiotherapy, and of salvage chemoradiation in the definitive nonsurgical treatment of epidermoid carcinoma of the anal canal: results of a phase III randomized intergroup study. J Clin Oncol 1996; 14:2527.
16. Bartelink H, Roelofsen F, Eschwege F, et al. Concomitant radiotherapy and chemotherapy is superior to radiotherapy alone in the treatment of locally advanced anal cancer: results of a phase III randomized trial of the European Organization for Research and Treatment of Cancer Radiotherapy and Gastrointestinal Cooperative Groups. J Clin Oncol 1997; 15:2040.
17. Doci R, Zucali R, La Monica G, et al. Primary chemoradiation therapy with fluorouracil and cisplatin for cancer of the anus: results in 35 consecutive patients. J Clin Oncol 1996; 14:3121.
18. Martenson JA, Lipsitz SR, Wagner H Jr., et al. Initial results of a phase II trial of high dose radiation therapy, 5-fluorouracil, and cisplatin for patients with anal cancer (E4292): an Eastern Cooperative Oncology Group study. Int J Radiat Oncol Biol Phys 1996; 35:745.
19. Peiffert D, Seitz JF, Rougier P, et al. Preliminary results of a phase II study of high-dose radiation therapy and neoadjuvant plus concomitant 5-fluorouracil with CDDP chemotherapy for patients with anal canal cancer: a French cooperative study. Ann Oncol 1997; 8:575.
20. Rich TA, Ajani JA, Morrison WH, et al. Chemoradiation therapy for anal cancer. Radiation plus continuous infusion of 5-fluorouracil with or without cisplatin. Radiother Oncol 1993; 27:209.
21. Kuske RR Jr. Acute and late toxicity of radiation therapy in rectal cancer. In: Hicks TC, Beck DE, Opelka FG, Timmcke AE, eds. Complications of Colon and Rectal Surgery. Baltimore: Williams & Wilkins, 1996:382–404.
22. Hoffman R, Welton ML, Klencke B, et al. The significance of pretreatment CD4 count on the outcome and treatment tolerance of HIV-positive patients with anal cancer. Int J Radiat Oncol Biol Phys 1999; 44:127.
23. McNamara MJ. Melanoma and basal cell cancer. In: Fazio VW, ed. Current Therapy in Colon and Rectal Surgery. Philadelphia: BC Decker, 1990:62–63.
24. Nivatvongs S. Principles Practice of Surgery for the Colon Rectum Anus. In: Gordon PH, Nivatvongs S, eds. Principles and Practice of Surgery for the Colon, Rectum, and Anus. 2nd ed. St Louis: Quality Medical Publishing, 1999:447–471.
25. Papillon J, Chassard JL. Respective roles of radiotherapy and surgery in the management of epidermoid carcinoma of the anal margin. Dis Colon Rectum 1992; 35:422–429.
26. Beahrs OH, Wilson SM. Carcinoma of the anus. Ann Surg 1976; 184:422–428.
27. Jensen SL, Hagen K, Shokouh-Amiri MH, Nielsen OV. Does an erroneous diagnosis of squamous-cell carcinoma of the anal canal and margin at first physician visit influence prognosis? Dis Colon Rectum 1987; 30:345–351.
28. Localio SA, Eng K, Coppa GF. Anorectal presacral and sacral tumors. Philadelphia: WB Saunders, 1987:46–67.
29. Schraut WH, Wang C, Dawson PJ, Block GE. Depth of invasion, location, and size of cancer of the anus dictate operative treatment. Cancer 1983; 51:1291–1296.
30. Cummings BJ, Keane TJ, Hawkins NV, O'Sullivan B. Treatment of perianal carcinoma by radiation (RT) or radiation plus chemotherapy (RTCT). Int J Radiat Oncol Biol Phys 1986; 12:170–173.
31. Mendenhall WH, Zlotecki RA, Vauthey J, Copeland EM. Squamous cell carcinoma of the anal margin. Oncology 1996; 10:1843–1848.
32. Touboul E, Schlienger M, Buffat L, et al. Epidermoid carcinoma of the anal margin: 17 cases treated with curative intent radiation therapy. Radiother Oncol 1995; 34:195–202.
33. Corman ML. Less common tumors and tumor-like lesions of the colon, rectum, and anus. In: Corman ML, ed. Colon and Rectal Surgery. 2nd ed. Philadelphia: JB Lippincott, 1989:579–596.
34. Kuehn PG, Beckett R, Eisenberg H, Reed JF. Epidermoid carcinoma of the perianal skin and anal canal: a review of 157 cases. N Engl J Med 1964; 270:614–616.
35. Nielson OV, Jensen SL. Basal cell carcinoma of the anus: a clinical study of 34 cases. Br J Surg 1981; 68:856–857.
36. Armitage G, Smith I. Rodent ulcer of the anus. Br J Surg 1954; 42:395–398.
37. Cintrom JR. Buschke-Lowenstein tumor of the perianal and anorectal region. Semin Colon Rectal Surg 1995; 6:135–139.
38. Gold JA, Nurnberger FG. A tribute to Abraham Buschke. J Am Acad Dermatol 1992; 26:1019–1022.
39. Buschke A. Neisser's Sterokopischer Atlas. New York: Fisher, 1896.
40. Buschke A, Loewenstein L. Carcinomahnliche condylomata despenis. Klin Wochenschr 1925; 4: 1726–1728.
41. Dawson DF, Duckworth JK, Bernhardt H, Young JM. Giant condyloma and verrucous carcinoma of the genital area. Arch Pathol 1965; 79:2225–2231.
42. Chu QD, Vezeridis MP, Libbey NP, et al. Giant condylomata acuminatum (Buschke-Loewenstein Tumor) of the anorectal and perineal regions. Dis Colon Rectum 1994; 37:950–957.
43. Creasman C, Haas PA, Fox TA, et al. Malignant transformation of anorectal giant condylomata acuminatum (Buschke-Lowenstin tumor). Dis Colon Rectum 1989; 32:481–487.
44. Kaufman T, Nisce LZ, Coleman M. Case report: Kaposi's sarcoma of the rectum—treatment with radiation therapy. Br J Radiol 1996; 69:573–574.

45. Margolin DA, Beck DE, Wexner SD. Acquired immunodeficiency syndrome. In: Beck DE, Wexner SD, eds. Fundamentals of Anorectal Surgery. 2nd ed. London: WB Saunders, 1998:432–450.
46. Kirova YM, Belembaogo E, Frikha H, et al. Radiotherapy in the management of epidemic Kaposi's sarcoma: a retrospective study of 643 cases. Radiother Oncol 1998; 46(1):19–22.
47. Paget J. On disease of the mammary areola preceding cancer of the mammary gland. St Bartholomew's Hosp Rep 1874; 10:87–89.
48. Darier J, Coulillaud P. Sur un case maladie de Paget de la region perineo-anal et scrotale. Ann Dermatol Syphiligr 1893; 4:33.
49. Beck DE, Fazio VW. Premalignant lesions of the anal margin. South Med J 1989; 82:470–474.
50. Beck DE, Fazio VW. Perianal Paget's disease. Dis Colon Rectum 1987; 30:263–266.
51. Jensen SL, Sjolin KE, Shokouh-Amiri MH, Hagen K, Harling H. Paget's disease of the anal margin. Br J Surg 1988; 75:1089–1092.
52. Armitage NC, Jass JR, Richman PI, Thomson JPS, Phillips RKS. Paget's disease of the anus: a clinicopathologic study. Br J Surg 1989; 76:60–63.
53. Helwig EB, Graham JH. Anogenital (extramammary) Paget's disease: a clinopathological study. Cancer 1963; 16:387–403.
54. Gross G, Ikenberg H, Grosshans E, et al. Bowenoid papulosis. Presence of human papillomavirus (HPV) structural antigens and of HPV-16 related DNA sequences. Arch Dermatol 1985; 121:858–863.
55. Wade TR, Kopf AW, Ackerman B. Bowenoid papulosis of the genitalia. Arch Dermatol 1979; 115:306–308.
56. Bowen JT. Precancerous dermatoses: a study of 2 cases of chronic atypical epithelial proliferation. J Cutan Dis 1912; 30:241–255.
57. Vickers PM, Jackman RJ, McDonald JR. Anal carcinoma in situ: report of three cases. South Surgeon 1939; 8:503–507.
58. Beck DE. Paget's disease and Bowen's disease of the anus. Semin Colon Rectal Surg 1995; 6:143–149.
59. Beck DE, Fazio VW, Jagelman DG, Lavery IC. Perianal Bowen's disease. Dis Colon Rectum 1989; 32:252–255.
60. Wexner SD, Milson JW, Dailey TM. The demographics of anal cancers are changing: identification of a high-risk population. Dis Colon Rectum 1987; 30:942–946.
61. Graham JH, Helwig EB. Bowen's disease and its relationship to systemic cancer. Arch Dermatol 1961; 88:738–751.
62. Marfig TE, Abel ME, Galligher DM. Perianal Bowen's disease and associated malignancies: results of a survey. Dis Colon Rectum 1987; 30:782–785.
63. Arbesman H, Ransohoff DF. Is Bowen's disease a predictor for the development of internal malignancy? A methodological critique of the literature. JAMA 1987; 257:516–518.
64. Marchesea P, Fazio VW, Oliart S, et al. Perianal Bowen's disease: a clinicopathologic study of 47 patients. Dis Colon Rectum 1997; 40:1286–1293.
65. Beck DE, Timmcke AE. Anal margin neoplasms. Clinics Colon Rectal Surg 2002; 15:277–284.
66. Ikenberg H, Gissmann L, Gross G, et al. Human papillomavirus type-16-related DNA in genital Bowen's disease and in Bowenoid papulosis. Int J Cancer 1983; 32:563–565.
67. Gross G, Roussaki A, Schopf E, et al. Successful treatment of condylomata acuminata and Bowenoid papulosis with subcutaneous injections of low-dose recombinant Interferon-alpha. Arch Dermatol 1986; 122:749–750.
68. Kotlarewsky M, Freeman JB, Cameron W, Grimard LJ. Anal intraepithelial dysplasia and squamous carcinoma in immunosuppressed patients. Can J Surg 2001; 44:450–454.
69. Chang GJ, Berry JM, Palefsky JM, Welton ML. Surgical treatment of high-grade anal squamous intraepithelial lesions: a prospective study. Dis Colon Rectum 2002; 45:453–458.
70. Zbar AP, Fenger C, Efron J, Beer-Gabel M, Wexner SD. The pathology and molecular biology of anal intraepithelial neoplasia: comparisons with cervical and vulvar intraepithelial carcinoma. Int J Colorectal Dis 2002; 17(4):203–215.
71. Corman ML. Premalignant and malignant dermatoses. In: Colon and Rectal Surgery. Philadelphia: JB Lippincott, 1989:421–422.

34 ▌ Miscellaneous Colonic Disorders

Roanne R. E. Selinger and Kamran Ayub
*Division of Gastroenterology, Department of Internal Medicine,
University of Washington, Seattle, Washington, U.S.A.*

INTRODUCTION

In striving to make this text complete we found that there were several topics that did not fit neatly into other chapters, yet were important disorders worthy of inclusion. Accordingly, a separate chapter was created to include endometriosis, pneumatosis cystoides intestinalis (PCI), colitis cystica profunda (CCP), and malakoplakia.

ENDOMETRIOSIS

Endometriosis refers to the presence of endometrial tissue outside the uterus. It is estimated to be present in 5% to 20% of menstruating women (1,2), of whom 3% to 37% have intestinal involvement (3,4).

Clinical Features

Colonic endometriosis is usually asymptomatic, but when symptomatic, can have a varied presentation. In general, patients range in age from 20 to 60 years and are usually pre- or perimenopausal (2,5). Those who present postmenopausally usually have symptoms due to fibrosis or due to exogenous estrogen, most often in the form of hormone replacement therapy. Patients with colonic endometriosis can present with abdominal pain, bloating, cramps, abdominal mass, obstruction, rectal bleeding, which may or may not be catamenial, diarrhea, constipation, or an increase in urinary frequency (5–7). These symptoms most often occur in conjunction with dysmenorrhea, dyspareunia, pelvic pain, and/or infertility (8). The differential diagnosis includes diverticulitis, acute appendicitis, inflammatory bowel disease, ischemic colitis, tubo-ovarian abscess, ruptured ovarian cyst, irritable bowel syndrome, mucosal prolapse, and malignancy, including both carcinoma and lymphoma (5). The location of the implants is usually at a single site, but can be at multiple sites, and most commonly occurs on the serosal surface (primarily the muscularis propria, subserosa, or mesentery). However, submucosal and lamina propria implantation can also be seen, often with corresponding involvement of deeper layers of the colon. Any area of the colon can be involved, but the most common areas in decreasing order of frequency are the rectosigmoid, other areas of the colon, the appendix, and the cecum (5). Implants in the rectosigmoid area are more likely to present with changes in bowel habits, hematochezia, and diarrhea, which can occur either in relation to or independently of the menstrual cycle, and can mimic a colorectal carcinoma. On the other hand, implants in other areas of the colon can present with obstruction or perforation, the latter of which is more common during pregnancy (9). Additionally, both the glandular and stromal elements of these ectopic foci rarely can undergo neoplastic change, usually in the setting of unopposed estrogen therapy, and become endometrioid adenocarcinoma, endometrioid stromal sarcoma, or mullerian adenosarcoma (10).

Pathogenesis

The exact pathogenesis of endometriosis is not clear, but the prevailing theory is retrograde menstruation causing reflux of the endometrium into the fallopian tubes during the menstrual cycle (11). However, this is not likely to be the sole factor, as immunity and genetics also appear to play a role in the removal and proliferation of ectopic endometrial tissue (12,13). Other theories include (i) direct transplantation, evidenced by endometriosis developing in surgical scars, (ii) lymphatic and hematogenous dissemination, which explains endometrial implants distant to the pelvis, such as in the thorax, and (iii) the coelomic metaplasia theory, which states that because all of the pelvic organs are embryologically derived from cells lining the coelomic cavity, all cells in the peritoneal cavity have the potential to differentiate back into endometrial tissue (14).

Endometrial implants can cause a variety of changes within the colon. They can elicit an inflammatory response, causing subsequent fibrosis, and/or surrounding smooth muscle hypertrophy and hyperplasia. When the implants occur in the muscularis propria, fibrosis and hyperplasia occur, which can cause a consequent luminal stenosis. Alternatively, the implants can lead to the formation of mucosal, submucosal, or mural polyps and/or masses. These can then ulcerate or lead to serositis and intussusception (5).

Diagnosis

There are a variety of methods to diagnose colonic endometriosis. These include the physical examination including pelvic and rectal examinations, ultrasound, barium enema (BE), computerized tomography (CT), magnetic resonance imaging (MRI), flexible sigmoidoscopy, colonoscopy, endoscopic ultrasound (EUS), laparoscopy, and laparotomy. Physical examination can occasionally reveal the presence of an abdominal mass; the pelvic exam can demonstrate pain, tenderness, fixation, or a mass; and the rectal exam can reveal a mass or ulceration. However, the physical examination is most frequently normal. Radiologic studies can reveal luminal stenosis, obstruction, ulceration, polyp(s), or mass(es) (Figs. 1 and 2). The preferred method of diagnosis is direct visualization, such as with flexible sigmoidoscopy, colonoscopy, laparoscopy, or laparotomy. When suspicious areas are seen, such as patchy areas of gray-brown discoloration, also called "powder burns" (5), they can be biopsied for confirmation. However, biopsies, especially mucosal biopsies obtained by endoscopy, can be nondiagnostic because endometriosis more commonly involves the deeper layers of the wall (15). As there are no typical or pathognomonic radiologic or endoscopic features, diagnosis can be elusive.

Treatment

There are two approaches to medical treatment: (i) decreasing symptoms caused by the endometrial tissue and (ii) suppressing the endometrial tissue itself. Current medications to control symptoms include nonsteroidal anti-inflammatory drugs, progesterones, synthetic androgens (e.g., danazol and gestrinone), oral contraceptive pills, gonadotropin-releasing hormone (GnRH) agonists (e.g., nafarelin, goserelin, and leuprolide), or combinations of these agents (16,17).

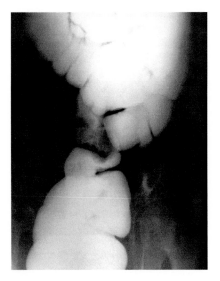

Figure 1 Endometriosis. Single-contrast barium enema demonstrating a high rectal obstructing lesion. *Source*: Courtesy of Dr. Charles Rohrmann, University of Washington Medical Center, Seattle, Washington, U.S.A.

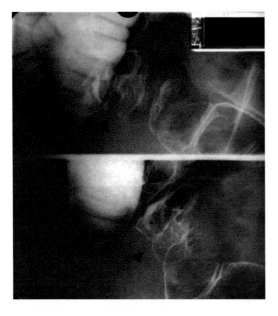

Figure 2 Endometriosis. Double-contrast barium enema of the same patient in Figure 1 demonstrating a focal area of luminal narrowing. *Source*: Courtesy of Dr. Charles Rohrmann, University of Washington Medical Center, Seattle, Washington, U.S.A.

Hormonal therapy is primarily used in two forms. The first form is combination therapy with estrogen and progesterone, such as in oral contraceptive pills, which induce a pregnancy-like state and cause decidualization and atrophy of endometrial tissue. The second form of hormonal therapy is the use of progestins alone; these have the same effects as combination oral contraceptive pills. Side effects of both of these therapies include bloating, weight gain, abnormal bleeding, hypertension, nausea, breast tenderness, and depression (16). Danazol is a steroid derivative, which causes anovulation by decreasing the midcycle surge of luteinizing hormone and follicle stimulating hormone, inhibiting enzymes in the steroid pathway, and increasing serum testosterone levels (18–20). Side effects include hirsutism, alterations in voice, hyperlipidemia, mood swings, and hepatotoxicity (21). Lastly, GnRH agonists also cause hypogonadal hypogonadism by inhibiting pituitary gonadotropin secretion. This leads to an estrogen deficient state and subsequent endometrial atrophy and anovulation (16). As this creates a menopausal-like state, the side effects include hot flashes, mood lability, abnormal bleeding, osteoporosis, vaginal dryness, and decreased libido. Many practitioners will combine GnRH agonists with combination hormonal therapy to reduce these side effects (22).

Surgery is often required both to establish the diagnosis of colonic endometriosis and to manage the symptoms, especially bleeding, obstruction, intussusception, and perforation. Conservative surgery is aimed at symptom control by removing all of the visible lesions while preserving the patient's reproductive potential (16). More extensive excisions can also be performed, depending on the severity of involvement or symptoms. Not infrequently definitive surgical therapy is required, which entails removal of the ovaries with or without the uterus and leads to the resolution of symptoms in the vast majority of patients (16,17). However, it also causes infertility, and is usually reserved for those patients who do not desire to preserve reproductive capacity.

In patients with symptomatic colonic involvement, suggested by complaints of constipation, diarrhea, rectal pain, obstructive symptoms, and/or cyclic rectal bleeding, surgical management originally entailed laparotomy. This is often still the case, especially when patients present in an urgent or a semiurgent manner, such as with an acute obstruction or with symptoms suggestive of appendicitis. In these situations, the actual pathophysiological process is often not elucidated until the resected specimen is analyzed. However, laparoscopic approaches, including superficial or partial-thickness excisions, full-thickness disc excision, segmental colectomy, proctectomy, proctocolectomy, appendectomy, and cecectomy, have been shown more recently to be safe, feasible, and effective alternative methods of treatment of colonic involvement, with the extent of resection dictated by the severity of the pelvic disease and the depth of implant invasion (23). In the hands of an experienced surgeon and otherwise equivalent procedures, the advantages of laparoscopy over laparotomy are shorter recovery times and lower costs. However, patients with extensive pelvic disease and adhesions may be more safely managed with laparotomy (16,23,24).

Several large series have demonstrated that surgical resection of areas of intestinal involvement is safe and effective for the treatment of colonic endometriosis, with rates of significant symptom improvement or complete resolution ranging from 80% to 100%. Contrary to original beliefs, both conventional and laparoscopic approaches have a low incidence of complications, which can include abscess, fistula, leak, and perforation, and both can be combined with gynecologic procedures if indicated (6,23,25,26).

Endometriosis is one of the most technically challenging surgical findings. Regardless of whether these procedures are done by laparotomy or laparoscopy, the intense fibrotic reaction makes tissue planes difficult to discern. Therefore laparoscopy, as mentioned, should only be contemplated by well-experienced laparoscopic surgeons. Moreover, if elective surgery is being performed for endometriosis, then additional precautions such as intraoperative placement of bilateral ureteric catheters may be of invaluable assistance. In order to fully resect the implants en bloc, resection may be required, and the patient should be appropriately prepared including a full mechanical and/or parenteral antibiotic bowel preparation as well as type and cross of blood and a full informed consent. Patients should even be preoperatively marked for the eventuality of a stoma if severe fibrosis prevents safe anastomosis. The informed consent presents a realistic view of the technical challenges of operating on pelvic endometriosis.

The bigger problem ensues when the general or colorectal surgeon unexpectedly encounters endometriosis. In these instances, ureteric catheters have not been employed, and a discussion with the patient may not have ensued. As always, meticulous dissection with maintenance of superb hemostasis and knowledge of tissue planes at all times is fundamental to help ensure a safe outcome. The unexpected finding of diverticulitis should be recognized and appropriately managed. If CCP coexists with solitary rectal ulcer and rectal endoanal intussusception realistic expectations should be offered to the patient. Specifically, although the ulcer itself will undoubtedly heal, the constipation and the associated symptoms such as pain and bleeding will undoubtedly linger. In fact, despite successful healing of the ulcer, it is not at all uncommon for patients to have exacerbation of both constipation and pain. Whether these procedures are performed by laparoscopy or laparotomy, the patient should understand that although the anatomic abnormality will be corrected, the functional disorder will remain. Therefore, one has to be exceptionally clear about the indication for surgery. While difficulty distinguishing between a solitary ulcer and a carcinoma is a reasonable surgical indication, attempting to relieve pelvic pain may be an unreasonable surgical indication.

PNEUMATOSIS CYSTOIDES INTESTINALIS

PCI is a rare disease, manifested by subserosal or submucosal gas-filled cysts in the intestine. It can be either a primary or a secondary condition due to a variety of causes, including other diseases and medications. The actual incidence is unknown, because most patients are asymptomatic (27).

Clinical Features

PCI can vary in presentation. The mean age of patients at presentation is 45 years old (28), with male-to-female ratios reported from 3.5:1 to equal (28–32). Some cases are incidental findings in an asymptomatic patient, while other patients are quite symptomatic with nausea, vomiting, abdominal distension, pain, flatulence, passage of mucus, hematochezia, weight loss, urgency, tenesmus, constipation and/or diarrhea (27,30,33). Roughly 15% of cases are primary or idiopathic, while the remainder are secondary and often due to a gastrointestinal disorder (29). Conditions associated with PCI are listed in Table 1.

The differential diagnosis of intramural bowel gas is extensive and includes ischemia, infarction, necrotizing enterocolitis, neutropenic colitis, volvulus, sepsis, trauma, obstruction, ulceration, and other mucosal disruptions (35). The most important distinction to make in a patient presenting with PCI is whether that individual has the benign or the life-threatening form, as this makes a significant difference in treatment and prognosis (27). The benign form is usually self-limited and has no significant complications. The life-threatening form, on the

Table 1 Gastrointestinal and Nongastrointestinal Conditions Associated with Pneumatosis Cystoides Intestinalis

Gastrointestinal	Nongastrointestinal
Mesenteric ischemia or ischemic colitis	Pulmonary disease—including bronchitis, asthma, chronic obstructive pulmonary disease, cystic fibrosis, pulmonary fibrosis
Intestinal obstruction	
Bowel infarction	
Inflammatory bowel disease—Crohn's disease, ulcerative colitis	HIV/AIDS
Diverticular disease	Collagen vascular disease—including progressive systemic sclerosis, systemic lupus erythematosus, polyarteritis nodosa, dermatomyositis, mixed connective tissue disease, overlap syndrome
Necrotizing enterocolitis	
Enteric infections—including *Clostridium perfringens*, cytomegalovirus, *Candida albicans*, cryptosporidiosis, coagulase-negative *Staphylococci*, *Lactobacillus*, *Klebsiella*, Varicella zoster, rotavirus, tuberculosis, adenovirus	Chemotherapy—including methotrexate, daunorubicin, cytosine arabinoside, 5-fluorouracil
	Immunosuppressive agents—steroids, cyclosporine, imuran
Endoscopy—including esophagogastroduodenoscopy, colonoscopy, flexible sigmoidoscopy, with or without biopsy, sclerotherapy, stent placement, or other therapy	Hemodialysis
	Other drugs—alkyl halides (trichloroethylene, chloral hydrate), lactulose, practolol, hydrogen peroxide, nitrous oxide
Pyloric stenosis	Organ transplantation—bone marrow, kidney, liver, heart
Gastric and duodenal ulcers	Graft vs. host disease
Chronic pseudo-obstruction	Leukemia
Jejunoileal bypass	Quadriplegia
Neutropenic typhlitis	Multiple sclerosis
Barium enema	Psychiatric diseases—including depression, anxiety
Esophageal stricture	Dementia
Cholelithiasis	Hypothyroidism
Appendicitis	Arthritis
Celiac sprue	Emphysematous pyelonephritis
Pseudomembranous colitis	Opportunistic infections—including toxoplasmosis of the central nervous system, *Mycobacterium avium* complex, *Candida krusei*
Hirschsprung's disease	
Idiopathic megacolon	Diabetes
Paralytic ileus	
Intestinal trauma	
Intestinal anastomoses	
Enteric tube placement	
Volvulus	
Adenomatous polyp	
Perineal descent	
Sphincter hypertrophy	
Meckel's diverticulum	
Rectal prolapse	
Intestinal malignancy—including carcinoma, lymphoma, sarcoma, cholangiocarcinoma, metastases	
Whipple's disease	
Toxin ingestion	

Abbreviations: HIV, human immunodeficiency virus; AIDS, acquired immunodeficiency syndrome.
Source: From Refs. 27, 30, 31, 33, 34.

other hand, is seen in those patients whose PCI is associated with intussusception (36), volvulus, infarction, obstruction, hemorrhage, perforation (31), and necrotizing enterocolitis (27)—in other words, due to significant bowel disease, and not an incidental finding. These patients are often very ill, presenting with an acute abdomen and/or shock, and should be rapidly assessed for further aggressive management.

Pathogenesis

The etiology of PCI is not clear, but there are currently three theories: mechanical, bacterial, and excessive intraluminal gas. The mechanical theory states that an increase in intraluminal pressure leads to the dissection of gas through the bowel wall. The bacterial theory states that PCI is caused by the entrance of gas-forming bacilli into the submucosa through a breach in the mucosa. The excessive intraluminal gas theory states that excessive hydrogen gas is produced by coliform bacteria, which subsequently diffuses across the mucosa (27,31,33).

The mechanical theory is supported by the observation of PCI in the setting of peptic ulcer disease and pyloric stenosis, where it is thought that obstruction of the upper intestinal tract causes pressurized gas to dissect through the mucosal lining (29,37), as well as by the observation that PCI can occur after endoscopy and BE (27,38). In this situation it is also theorized that the air can travel to other areas of the intestine along mesenteric blood vessels (27). The mechanical theory is further supported by the observation that patients with significant pulmonary disease and coughing can develop PCI, perhaps by the rupture of alveoli, leading to air dissection along blood vessels and bronchi to the mediastinum, and subsequently through the diaphragm to the mesenteric root and into the bowel (27,39). Alternatively, it is proposed that the pathogenic mechanism behind pulmonary disease and PCI may actually be due to the significant fluctuation in intraluminal pressure that occurs with coughing (33).

Conversely, the bacterial theory proposes that areas of loss of mucosal integrity allow gas-forming bacteria, such as *Clostridium perfringens*, to enter into the submucosa, where they subsequently produce gas-filled cysts (40–43). Evidence to support this theory is the observation that PCI caused by *Clostridia* in rats resolves with antibiotic treatment (44,45). Additionally, it has been noted that patients with PCI often have an elevated breath hydrogen level (46–48). However, there is a fair amount of evidence against this theory. This includes the observation that bacteria have not been cultured from the cysts, nor has electron microscopy revealed the presence of any bacteria in the cysts (49). Additionally, cyst rupture does not routinely lead to peritonitis, as would be expected if bacteria were present (27). Finally, even when PCI has been successfully treated, bacteria are still present on the mucosa and in the stool (44).

The excessive intraluminal gas theory proposes that PCI is caused by either excessive production or decreased utilization of hydrogen by bacteria. The subsequent high partial pressure of hydrogen causes the gas to dissect into the intestinal wall (27,31,33). This is supported by the abovementioned finding of elevated breath hydrogen levels (46–48), as well as by the finding that some patients with primary PCI lack methanogenic and sulfate-reducing bacteria, which normally use hydrogen (50). Additionally, patients with bacterial overgrowth, disaccharidase deficiency, and increased intestinal fermentation of carbohydrates have been observed to have PCI (27,51).

Analysis of the gas composition of the cysts has shown mixed findings. Some studies reveal a composition similar to air (52,53), which would support the mechanical theory, while others reveal high levels of hydrogen (54,55), supporting the latter two theories. It is likely that the gas contained in the cysts varies depending on the causative agent. For example, those patients with pulmonary disease or who have undergone endoscopy would have a cyst composition similar to air, while those with a gastrointestinal cause would have a composition similar to intestinal gas (27). However, once the cysts have been present for a period of time, intestinal gas may diffuse in, and even cysts that initially contained air may alter in composition and subsequently contain intestinal gas with a high hydrogen component (51).

PCI can be divided into three categories based on pathologic appearance: microvesicular, cystic, and diffuse (27). The microvesicular form has the gross appearance of a white plaque, and has also been referred to as "mucosal pseudolipomatosis" (56,57). Microscopically there are small (10–100 μm) spaces present within the lamina propria. This form of PCI is seen most often during endoscopy and likely is a result of the combination of air insufflation and small mucosal tears during the procedure. The cystic form can appear grossly as blebs, grape-like clusters, or sessile polypoid nodules, depending on whether the cysts are located within the submucosa or the subserosa (27). Microscopic examination reveals cystic spaces lined by multinucleated giant cells and macrophages, with an overlying mucosa that can exhibit granulomas or crypt architecture distortion (Fig. 3) (27,40,41,46). The diffuse form of PCI is recognized by its grossly spongy appearance. Microscopically it is similar to the cystic form with gas-filled spaces; however, these spaces have no epithelial lining (27).

Diagnosis

The physical examination is often normal in the benign form, but patients with either the benign or the life-threatening form can also present with a loss of liver dullness to percussion (58), diffuse abdominal tenderness, abdominal distention, decreased bowel sounds (30), apparent hepatomegaly, and/or an abdominal mass (28). Occasionally gas-filled cysts can be palpated on rectal examination (27). As mentioned above, fasting breath hydrogen levels can be elevated (46–48), but this is rarely used to establish the diagnosis. Rather, diagnosis is usually made by a radiologic study. Imaging methods include plain radiographs of the chest

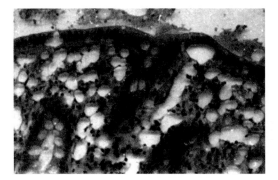

Figure 3 (*See color insert*) Microscopic picture of pneumatosis cystoides intestinalis. Hematoxylin and eosin stain. *Source*: Courtesy of Dr. Rodger Haggitt, University of Washington Medical Center, Seattle, Washington, U.S.A.

or abdomen, BE, CT, ultrasound, and MRI. Other methods of diagnosis include endoscopy, EUS, laparotomy, and laparoscopy. Two-thirds of patients will have air in the intestinal wall on plain radiograph (Fig. 4A) (28), and fewer will have free air under the diaphragm. The pattern of distribution of the air can be either circular or linear (27). BE can demonstrate circular or linear luminal filling defects (27,30) and can even mimic polyposis (Fig. 4B) (59). CT reveals the presence of low attenuation collections within the intestinal wall, consistent with gas (Fig. 5) (30), and is recommended as the subsequent method of evaluation following a suspicious X ray in order to define the extent of disease, to evaluate for causes, and to examine for complications (61). Endoscopy can reveal the presence of polyps (27) or of cystic, submucosal lesions, which collapse when punctured (Fig. 6) (27,34,62). Endoscopists must be aware of the risk of intestinal perforation and peritonitis if they accidentally attempt endoscopic polypectomy of polypoid-appearing cysts (34,63).

Treatment

Treatment depends on the etiology. Many patients who are asymptomatic can simply be monitored. Spontaneous cyst resolution is seen in up to 50% of cases (29,64–67). Patients who are symptomatic from the cysts have been managed in a variety of ways, including various combinations of hydration, elemental diets, parenteral nutrition, antibiotics, oxygen, antidiarrheals, sclerotherapy, and/or surgery. However, there have not been any randomized trials to assess the best method of management. There are many reports of success using inhaled oxygen with the goal of reducing the partial pressure of gases other than oxygen in the blood, causing a gradient of gases to form between the blood and the cysts, and leading to subsequent cyst deflation. This treatment has been performed using either high flow or hyperbaric oxygen for varying lengths of time and over varying periods of days, weeks, and even months (55,68–76). Many antibiotics have also been used with the goal of altering intestinal flora,

(A)   **(B)**

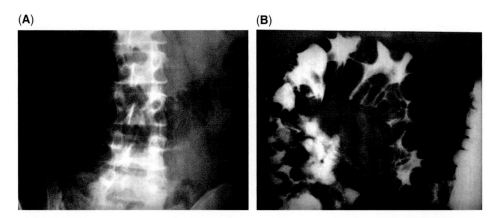

Figure 4 Primary pneumatosis cystoides intestinalis. (**A**) Plain abdominal X ray of an asymptomatic patient demonstrating multiple gas-filled pockets. This is more easily appreciated in (**B**), a single-contrast barium enema of the same patient. *Source*: Courtesy of Dr. Charles Rohrmann, University of Washington Medical Center, Seattle, Washington, U.S.A.

(A) **(B)** **(C)**

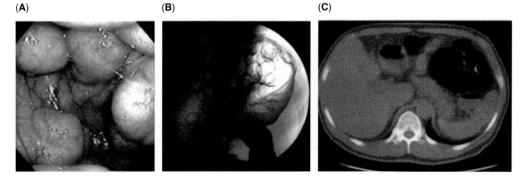

Figure 5 Pneumatosis cystoides intestinalis. (**A**) (*See color insert*) Endoscopic appearance of normal mucosa overlying gas-filled pockets. (**B**) Double-contrast barium enema illustrating the multiple pockets. (**C**) Abdominal computed
tomography scan demonstrating that the pockets are filled with gas. *Source*: From Ref. 60.

especially anaerobic bacteria. The antibiotics that have been used with success include metronidazole, tetracycline, ampicillin, and vancomycin (77). Again, the best dose and duration of
therapy have not been established (78,79). One article suggested using antibiotics in the setting
of hypomotility and bacterial overgrowth, as well as in the outpatient setting, where oxygen
therapy is not possible (27). The use of an elemental diet has also been reported to be successful (80). It is important to note that the cysts may take days, months, and even years to resolve.
Not infrequently the cysts will recur, and can often be retreated with success (33,74–76,78,80–83).
In one case series, symptom improvement was seen with therapy, but without the resolution
of the cysts (33).

In 2% of cases of colonic PCI the cysts can rupture and cause pneumoperitoneum (28).
However, the presence of pneumoperitoneum, in itself, does not warrant surgical exploration,
especially in the absence of other signs or symptoms of peritonitis, sepsis, or shock (84). Therefore, it is important to differentiate between benign pneumoperitoneum, which can be managed
conservatively, from the life-threatening form, which is associated with intestinal infarction
and/or perforation and which requires immediate surgery for management (27). In general,
the presence of portal venous gas (PVG) in a patient with PCI usually signifies an abdominal
catastrophe and often portends a poor prognosis (85). In one prospective study, the presence of
PCI and PVG had a mortality of 37% (32). Consequently, these patients should be rapidly
assessed for the need for immediate surgical management, although occasionally they can
be managed conservatively (86–89).

In terms of differentiating which approach to management to take—medical or surgical—
a recent review suggested using nonoperative therapy first while further evaluation is pursued
to determine whether there is a definitive indication for surgery. If an indication is found or if the
patient is not responding to medical management, such as in patients with signs of perforation,

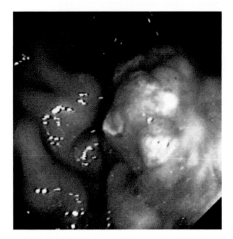

Figure 6 (*See color insert*) Colitis cystica profunda. Endoscopic
view of sigmoid involvement demonstrating edematous mucosa
overlying a mass. *Source*: From Ref. 62.

peritonitis, or abdominal sepsis, then surgery, usually entailing laparotomy with resection, should be performed (90). Additionally, patients with metabolic acidosis or hyperamylasemia are more likely to have infarcted bowel and should be strongly considered for surgery (28). In cases where it still remains unclear whether to operate or not, one report suggested using diagnostic laparoscopy as a tool to establish the diagnosis of PCI and to evaluate for perforation or infarction, reducing the possibility of a negative primary laparotomy (91), the latter of which has occurred in up to 27% of patients (28).

COLITIS CYSTICA PROFUNDA

CCP is a benign, uncommon disease of the colon and rectum. Fewer than 200 cases have been reported in the literature. It affects patients from ages 4 to 77 (92–94), but the peak incidence is seen in patients in their 20s and 30s (95). The actual prevalence and incidence are unknown. It is differentiated from colitis cystica superficialis (CCS), which is associated with pellagra and sprue, by the observation that in CCS the cystic lesions do not occur in the submucosa, but in the superficial mucosa (96–98).

Pathogenesis

CCP is characterized by the presence of mucus cysts in the submucosa (97). The exact etiology and pathogenesis are not clear, but the pathogenesis of disease localized to the rectum appears to be similar to that of solitary rectal ulcer syndrome (SRUS) and rectal prolapse (99). In fact, several authors have proposed that CCP, rectal prolapse, and SRUS may be simply different manifestations of the same pathologic entity (92,99–102). CCP is most common in patients in their 20s and 30s who have defecation disorders (103).

It is thought that CCP may be caused by chronic inflammation, such as from repetitive ulcerations followed by reepithelialization, as can occur with inflammatory bowel disease, prolapse, SRUS, and ischemia. This then leads to entrapment of colonic glands within the muscularis propria (92). An alternative mechanism of pathogenesis suggests that the muscularis mucosa may be abnormal due to this ulceration and inflammation, permitting the mucosa to herniate into the submucosa, subsequently forming glands (96). Another proposed contributing factor is chronic localized ischemia, perhaps due to this same trauma or inflammation, which may prevent complete healing (94,104).

Clinical Features

Patients with CCP most commonly present with the passage of blood and/or mucus per rectum (94,103). They can additionally complain of diarrhea, constipation, tenesmus, cramping/pain, distention, weakness, dizziness, fever, and weight loss (103,105–107). Rarely, they will present with obstructive signs and symptoms (97,107). In more than half of patients rectal examination will reveal the presence of one or more masses or cords (100,103,105).

There are three forms of CCP: diffuse (107–109), segmental, and localized (94,95,110–113). Localized disease is the most common and usually occurs in the rectum within 10 cm of the anal verge, but can occur more proximally (94,99,103,107). Endoscopic findings vary from mucosal irregularity and thickening (114), to broad-based polyps, which can have overlying normal, inflamed, or ulcerated mucosa (Fig. 6) (94,107). CCP has been reported in association with inflammatory bowel disease (108,115), SRUS (102), adenomatous polyps (116,117), infective dysentery (92), local trauma (118), previous colostomy site (119), and irradiation (104,106,120–123).

Diagnosis

Several studies have evaluated the efficacy of various imaging modalities and procedures to establish the diagnosis, including BE, CT, MRI (103), transrectal ultrasound (124), and EUS (62,114). BE can reveal mucosal irregularity, thickening of folds, and/or nodular or polypoid lesions (Fig. 7) (103). CT and MRI can reveal the presence of submucosal wall invasion without associated muscular invasion or lymphadenopathy, the loss of perirectal fat layers, and thickening of the levator ani on the affected side (103). Transrectal ultrasound can demonstrate multiple submucosal hypo- and/or hyperechoic cysts with posterior acoustic enhancement,

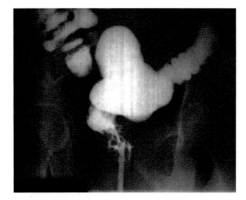

Figure 7 Colitis cystica profunda. Single-contrast barium enema demonstrating circumferential rectal involvement. *Source*: Courtesy of Dr. Charles Rohrmann, University of Washington Medical Center, Seattle, Washington, U.S.A.

ranging in size from 2 to 20 mm, which do not affect the muscularis propria and which have intervening areas of fibrosis seen as hyperechogenic bands (103,124). Similarly, EUS can demonstrate thickening of the mucosa and submucosa, a lack of tumor infiltration, and the presence of irregular, hyperechoic structures with an intact muscular layer and no lymphadenopathy (114). However, although these additional studies can be helpful, none of these have demonstrated a high diagnostic specificity (62,103,124).

The most sensitive method of diagnosis appears to be macrobiopsy with inclusion of the muscularis, either intraoperatively (125) or by deep endoscopic snare (114). When examined under the microscope there are colonic glands entrapped in the submucosa and muscularis propria, below the muscularis mucosae (Fig. 8) (92). These cysts are filled with mucus and are either unlined or lined with a single layer of columnar or squamous cells (126,127). The overlying mucosa can be edematous, hyperplastic, atrophic, or even ulcerated. The crypts reveal evidence of chronic inflammation with inflammatory cells and architecture distortion (94). There is a diffuse excess of collagen in the mucosa, which can mimic a desmoplastic reaction, and the use of saffron to stain this element has been shown to be useful in differentiating CCP and SRUS from inflammatory bowel disease, ischemic colitis, adenocarcinoma, and even collagenous colitis (128).

Not infrequently CCP is misdiagnosed as rectal carcinoma, especially mucosecretory rectal carcinoma, on clinical, gross, and histological grounds (126,129–131). However, it is important to be able to make a definitive diagnosis of one or the other in order to prevent unnecessary anguish and surgery, such as colonic or rectal resection. In contrast to invasive adenocarcinoma, there is no dysplasia present in the epithelium of the glands in CCP. Additionally, there is no cellular or

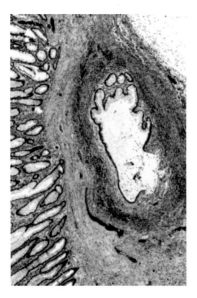

Figure 8 Colitis cystica profunda. Photomicrograph demonstrating a submucosal cyst lined by columnar epithelium and surrounding fibrosis. *Source*: From Ref. 62.

nuclear atypia, such as hyperchromasia, irregular contour, loss of polarity, or multiple cell layers. There is also no infiltrative growth pattern with abnormally shaped glands nor surrounding desmoplastic reaction as would be seen in neoplastic tissue (106).

Treatment

The vast majority of patients are treated with local excision, either transanally or transabdominally. This is considered to be the first-line therapy, especially for localized disease, and is curative in 79% of patients (95). There have also been reports of using repeated episodes of fulguration, but with less success, and of diverting colostomies (94,95). In a fair number of cases, lesions have been reported to recur, especially if rectal prolapse is present (94,95,107). In these situations, there are several procedures that have been successful. Pure repair of the prolapse, without associated bowel or mucosal resection, has been shown to be an effective management strategy (132). However, repair of the prolapse is most often performed in conjunction with local excision or segmental resection, depending on the extent of disease (94). Patients with more extensive disease, such as those with segmental or diffuse disease, have been treated with a variety of procedures with success, including segmental colectomy, subtotal colectomy, and total proctocolectomy, with or without colostomy, as well as abdominoperineal resection, depending on the extent and severity of disease (94). There is also a report of successful treatment of segmental rectal CCP using a mucosal sleeve resection and coloanal pull-through (133). Regardless of which procedure is performed, it is also important to keep in mind that CCP can coexist with adenocarcinoma (126); so excised specimens should be closely examined for any evidence of neoplasia, as described above.

Alternatively, resolution of CCP has been reported to be successful with conservative treatment, similar to that used for SRUS and rectal prolapse, as contributing factors to all three of these entities include constipation and prolapse (134). This includes establishing regular bowel habits, such as with lubricants, bulking agents, and a high fiber diet, and avoiding straining or other fecal removal maneuvers (103,132,134). However, improvement and resolution may take up to 6 to 18 months in some cases (103). Biofeedback has also been successful in some patients. Alternatively, some patients have been successfully treated with topical corticosteroids, such as in the form of enemas, to decrease the inflammation and facilitate healing (94). Finally, many authors have advocated the need to surgically correct rectal prolapse if it is present, in order for complete resolution to occur (94,132,135).

MALAKOPLAKIA

The word "malakoplakia" comes from the Greek "malakos" meaning soft and "plakos" meaning plaque, and was coined by Von Hansemann in 1903 after the disease was originally described the preceding year by Michaelis and Gutmann (136). It is a rare disease—less than 100 cases with intestinal involvement have been reported. Consequently, the actual incidence and prevalence are not known. Colorectal malakoplakia affects patients from ages 6 weeks to 88 years in a bimodal fashion with one peak for children under 13 years and a second peak for middle-aged adults (137), and males are affected more often than females, in a ratio of roughly 2:1 (138).

Clinical Features

Malakoplakia is a rare chronic inflammatory disease characterized by the presence of granulomas. It primarily affects the genitourinary tract—75% of reported cases—but affects the gastrointestinal tract in 11% of reported cases (137,139–141). It can also affect other organ systems, including the pulmonary system, central nervous system, eye, skin, adrenal glands, tonsils, bone, ear, breast, lymph nodes, pancreas, abdominal wall, and retroperitoneum (139,142). One review of the literature found that colonic malakoplakia most commonly affects the rectum (40% of cases), followed by the sigmoid colon (17%), cecum and ascending colon (12%), appendix (10%), descending colon (8%), entire colon (8%), transverse colon (4%), and anal canal and perianal region (1%) (138). When malakoplakia occurs in the setting of colonic adenocarcinoma or adenoma, the disease appears to occur primarily in the area surrounding the lesion, where it may be locally invasive, and not at sites distant to the lesion (143).

Patients most commonly present with rectal bleeding, diarrhea, abdominal pain, and/ or fever (138). Other complaints include weight loss, nausea, vomiting, malaise, constipation, and signs of obstruction (137). However, malakoplakia can also be an asymptomatic, incidental finding in association with neoplasia or inflammatory bowel disease (137,144,145).

Pathogenesis

The exact etiology and pathogenesis of malakoplakia are not known. In fact, the current thought is that there may be multiple causes, including infection, immunosuppression, malignancy, and systemic disease. Many patients with malakoplakia are chronically infected with *Escherichia coli*, *Klebsiella*, *Mycobacterium*, and *Staphylococcus* (141,146,147). Additional cases have been reported where *Pseudomonas aeruginosa* and *Aerobacter aerogenes* were recovered from tissue or stool (137). It is theorized that these patients may have defective killing and elimination of bacteria. This is supported by the findings of low levels of cyclic guanosine monophosphate (cGMP) and high ratios of adenosine monophosphate to cGMP in monocytes of patients with malakoplakia, leading to a subsequent defect in bactericidal activity (148–150). There are also a number of cases of malakoplakia, which have been reported in association with chemotherapy and immunosuppression (151,152). It has also been seen in patients with neoplasms, systemic lupus erythematosus, mycotic infections, liver disease, sarcoidosis, inflammatory bowel disease, cachexia, and drug addiction (138), and there has even been one report of a familial occurrence (153). The most common disease associated with malakoplakia is colorectal carcinoma, which is seen in 20% of reported cases (138).

Diagnosis

Endoscopy can demonstrate one of three patterns: a focal lesion (such as a nodule or polyp), multiple lesions, or a large mass (137,138,154). The mucosa has soft, yellowish, friable plaques or nodules, which can be ulcerated or umbilicated (Fig. 9) (138,155). Involved areas can also contain fistulae, mimicking Crohn's disease (145). Imaging studies such as BE, CT, MRI, and transrectal ultrasonography can provide adjunctive information regarding the extent of disease in other organs (156), but are less helpful in establishing a diagnosis of intestinal or colonic malakoplakia due to the often nonspecific and variable findings.

Definitive diagnosis is made upon review of tissue samples, which can be obtained by biopsy or by fine needle aspiration (157,158). Microscopic examination will reveal the presence of large macrophages, also known as Von Hansemann cells, which contain characteristic intracytoplasmic and extracellular calcified spheres with laminated concentric structures (Fig. 10) (141,144,159,160). These calculospherules, called Michaelis–Gutmann bodies, primarily consist of a glycolipid and calcium phosphate matrix and hence stain positively with periodic acid Schiff and calcium stains (141,144,159,160). Electron microscopy of these cells often reveals the presence of coliform bacteria in the cytoplasm (141,144,159,160). However, when malakoplakia occurs in the setting of colorectal adenoma or adenocarcinoma, Michaelis–Gutmann bodies are present, but microorganisms have not been identified (143,161).

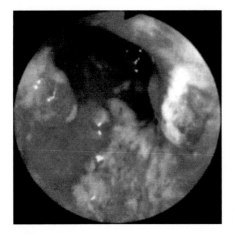

Figure 9 (*See color insert*) Malakoplakia. Endoscopic view of colonic involvement revealing yellowish mucosal discoloration with ulceration and irregularity. *Source*: From Ref. 138.

(A)   **(B)**

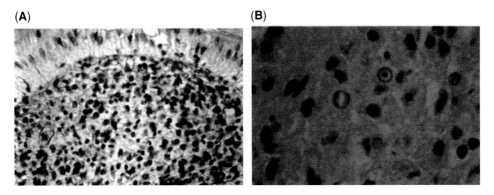

Figure 10 (*See color insert*) Malakoplakia. Photomicrograph at low (**A**) and high (**B**) power demonstrating characteristic Von Hansemann cells with Michaelis–Gutmann bodies. *Source*: From Ref. 138.

Treatment

As this disease is so rare, no studies have been done to determine the best modality of treatment. In fact, the current treatment regimens are based primarily on case reports or series (162,163). In general, treatment can be divided into either surgical or medical approaches. It is felt that the first line of therapy for symptomatic disease is surgical resection, particularly when it is associated with a malignancy. This is usually curative, especially in cases of localized malakoplakia. However, if surgery is not an option, then medical management can be tried as an alternative. This surgery is performed as the most common procedure with a segmental resection with anastomosis. However, under certain extenuating circumstances, either resection with a stoma or a subtotal colectomy could conceivably be necessary. Given the paucity of information on this condition no sweeping conclusions can be made. However, the important facet of the surgery is to resect the lesion with appropriate proximal and distal margins and to ensure the usual principles of a tension-free, well-vascularized circumferentially patent anastomosis.

Previous studies have demonstrated that intracellular levels of cGMP can be increased with the use of cholinergic agents, such as bethanechol, which improves monocyte bactericidal activity (148). However, this treatment has had mixed results in clinical practice (164–166). Alternatively, antibiotics, such as trimethoprim-sulfamethoxazole (162,166), rifampin, or fluoroquinolones (167), can be used, with the aim of interrupting the pathophysiological process through bacterial eradication. In immunosuppressed patients, withdrawal of the immunosuppressants has led to clinical improvement and return of normal leukocyte function (163,168). Consequently, this approach is often recommended if medically possible.

REFERENCES

1. Singh KK, Lessells AM, Adam DJ, et al. Presentation of endometriosis to general surgeons: a 10-year experience. Br J Surg 1995; 82(10):1349–1351.
2. Olive DL, Schwartz LB. Endometriosis. N Engl J Med 1993; 328(24):1759–1769.
3. Croom RD III, Donovan ML, Schwesinger WH. Intestinal endometriosis. Am J Surg 1984; 148(5): 660–667.
4. Prystowsky JB, Stryker SJ, Ujiki GT, Poticha SM. Gastrointestinal endometriosis. Incidence and indications for resection. Arch Surg 1988; 123(7):855–858.
5. Yantiss RK, Clement PB, Young RH. Endometriosis of the intestinal tract: a study of 44 cases of a disease that may cause diverse challenges in clinical and pathologic evaluation. Am J Surg Pathol 2001; 25(4):445–454.
6. Urbach DR, Reedijk M, Richard CS, Lie KI, Ross TM. Bowel resection for intestinal endometriosis. Dis Colon Rectum 1998; 41(9):1158–1164.
7. Collin GR, Russell JC. Endometriosis of the colon. Its diagnosis and management. Am Surg 1990; 56(5):275–279.
8. Roseau G, Dumontier I, Palazzo L, et al. Rectosigmoid endometriosis: endoscopic ultrasound features and clinical implications. Endoscopy 2000; 32(7):525–530.
9. Floberg J, Backdahl M, Silfersward C, Thomassen PA. Postpartum perforation of the colon due to endometriosis. Acta Obstet Gynecol Scand 1984; 63(2):183–184.

10. Yantiss RK, Clement PB, Young RH. Neoplastic and pre-neoplastic changes in gastrointestinal endometriosis: a study of 17 cases. Am J Surg Pathol 2000; 24(4):513–524.

11. Oral E, Arici A. Pathogenesis of endometriosis. Obstet Gynecol Clin North Am 1997; 24(2):219–233.

12. Lebovic DI, Mueller MD, Taylor RN. Immunobiology of endometriosis. Fertil Steril 2001; 75(1):1–10.

13. Simpson JL, Elias S, Malinak LR, Buttram VC Jr. Heritable aspects of endometriosis. I. Genetic studies. Am J Obstet Gynecol 1980; 137(3):327–331.

14. Schenken RS. Pathogenesis. In: Schenken RS, ed. Endometriosis: Contemporary Concepts in Clinical Management. Philadelphia: Lippincott, 1989:1.

15. Langlois NE, Park KG, Keenan RA. Mucosal changes in the large bowel with endometriosis: a possible cause of misdiagnosis of colitis? Hum Pathol; 25(10):1030–1034.

16. Olive DL, Pritts EA. Treatment of endometriosis. N Engl J Med 2001; 345(4):266–275.

17. Prentice A. Regular review: endometriosis. BMJ 2001; 323(7304):93–95.

18. Floyd WS. Danazol: endocrine and endometrial effects. Int J Fertil 1980; 25(1):75–80.

19. Barbieri RL, Canick JA, Makris A, Todd RB, Davies IJ, Ryan KJ. Danazol inhibits steroidogenesis. Fertil Steril 1977; 28(8):809–813.

20. McGinley R, Casey JH. Analysis of progesterone in unextracted serum: a method using danazol [17 alpha-pregn-4-en-20-yno (2, 3-d) isoxazol-17-ol] a blocker of steroid binding to proteins. Steroids 1979; 33(2):127–138.

21. Buttram VC Jr., Belue JB, Reiter R. Interim report a study of danazol for the treatment of endometriosis. Fertil Steril 1982; 37(4):478–483.

22. Moghissi KS. Medical treatment of endometriosis. Clin Obstet Gynecol 1999; 42(3):620–632.

23. Jerby BL, Kessler H, Falcone T, Milsom JW. Laparoscopic management of colorectal endometriosis. Surg Endosc 1999; 13(11):1125–1128.

24. Nezhat C, Nezhat F, Pennington E. Laparoscopic treatment of infiltrative rectosigmoid colon and rectovaginal septum endometriosis by the technique of videolaparoscopy and the CO_2 laser. Br J Obstet Gynaecol 1992; 99:664–667.

25. Bailey HR, Ott MT, Hartendorp P. Aggressive surgical management for advanced colorectal endometriosis. Dis Colon Rectum 1994; 37:747–753.

26. Bromberg SH, Waisberg J, Franco MI, Oliveira CV, Lopes RG, Godoy AC. Surgical treatment for colorectal endometriosis. Int Surg 1999; 84(3):234–238.

27. Heng Y, Schuffler MD, Haggitt RC, Rohrmann CA. Pneumatosis intestinalis: a review. Am J Gastroenterol 1995; 90(10):1747–1758.

28. Jamart J. Pneumatosis cystoides intestinalis. A statistical study of 919 cases. Acta Hepatogastroenterol Stuttg 1979; 26(5):419–422.

29. Koss LG. Abdominal gas cysts pneumatosis cystoides intestinorum hominis: an analysis with a report of a case and a critical review of the literature. Arch Pathol 1952; 53:523–549.

30. Diwakaran HH, Presti ME, Longo WE. Pneumatosis intestinalis. Am J Surg 2000; 179(2):110.

31. Boerner RM, Fried DB, Warshauer DM, Isaacs K. Pneumatosis intestinalis. Two case reports and a retrospective review of the literature from 1985 to 1995. Dig Dis Sci 1996; 41(11):2272–2285.

32. Knechtle SJ, Davidoff AM, Rice RP. Pneumatosis intestinalis. Surgical management and clinical outcome. Ann Surg 1990; 212(2):160–165.

33. Gagliardi G, Thompson IW, Hershman MJ, Forbes A, Hawley PR, Talbot IC. Pneumatosis coli: a proposed pathogenesis based on study of 25 cases and review of the literature. Int J Colorectal Dis 1996; 11(3):111–118.

34. Hoer J, Truong S, Virnich N, Fuzesi L, Schumpelick V. Pneumatosis cystoides intestinalis: confirmation of diagnosis by endoscopic puncture a review of pathogenesis associated disease and therapy and a new theory of cyst formation. Endoscopy 1998; 30(9):793–799.

35. Pear BL. Pneumatosis intestinalis: a review. Radiology 1998; 207(1):13–19.

36. Stern MA, Chey WD. Images in clinical medicine. Pneumatosis coli and colonic intussusception. N Engl J Med 2001; 345(13):964.

37. Dhall D, Mahaffy R, Matheson N. Intestinal pneumatosis treated by pyloroplasty. J R Coll Surg Edinb 1968; 13:226–229.

38. Marshak RH, Lindner AE, Maklansky D, Goldberg MD. Mesenteric fat necrosis simulating a carcinoma of the cecum. Am J Gastroenterol 1980; 74(5):459–463.

39. Elliot G, Elliott K. The roentgenologic pathology of so-called pneumatosis cystoides intestinalis. AJR 1963; 89:720–729.

40. Pieterse AS, Leong AS, Rowland R. The mucosal changes and pathogenesis of pneumatosis cystoides intestinalis. Hum Pathol 1985; 16(7):683–688.

41. Suarez V, Chesner IM, Price AB, Newman J. Pneumatosis cystoides intestinalis. Histological mucosal changes mimicking inflammatory bowel disease. Arch Pathol Lab Med 1989; 113(8):898–901.

42. Yale CE, Balish E. The natural course of *Clostridium perfringens*–induced pneumatosis cystoides intestinalis. J Med 1992; 23(3–4):279–288.

43. Ramer S, Bluestone R. Colitic arthropathies. Postgrad Med 1977; 61(1):141–147.

44. Holt S, Gilmour H, Buist T, et al. High flow oxygen for pneumatosis coli. Gut 1979; 20:493–498.

45. Wandtke J, Skucas J, Spataro R, et al. Pneumatosis intestinalis as a complication of jejunoileal bypass. AJR 1977; 129:601–604.

46. Shand AG, Penman ID, Ghosh S. Effects of a controlled challenge of chloral hydrate in pneumatosis cystoides coli—further evidence of a causal link? Am J Gastroenterol 2000; 95(12):3654–3655.
47. Read N, Al-Janabi M, Cann P. Is raised breath hydrogen related to the pathogenesis of pneumatosis coli? Gut 1984; 25:839–845.
48. Gillon J, Tadesse K, Logan R, et al. Breath hydrogen in pneumatosis cystoides intestinalis. Gut 1979; 20:1008–1011.
49. Haboubi N, Honan R, Hasleton P, et al. Pneumatosis coli: a case report with ultrastructural study. Histopathology 1984; 8:145–155.
50. Christl SU, Gibson GR, Murgatroyd PR, Scheppach W, Cummings JH. Impaired hydrogen metabolism in pneumatosis cystoides intestinalis. Gastroenterology 1993; 104(2):392–397.
51. Levitt MD, Olsson S. Pneumatosis cystoides intestinalis and high breath H2 excretion: insights into the role of H2 in this condition. Gastroenterology 1995; 108(5):1560–1565.
52. Kenney J. Pneumatosis intestinalis. Clin Radiol 1963; 14:70–76.
53. McGregor J, McKinnon D. Intestinal interstitial emphysema pneumatosis cystoides intestinalis. Gastroenterology 1958; 36:75–76.
54. Kennedy DK, Hughes ES, Masterton JP. The natural history of benign ulcer of the rectum. Surg Gynecol Obstet 1977; 144(5):718–720.
55. Forgacs P, Wright P, Wyatt A. Treatment of intestinal gas cysts by oxygen breathing. Lancet 1973; 1:579–581.
56. Snover DC, Sandstad J, Hutton S. Mucosal pseudolipomatosis of the colon. Am J Clin Pathol 1985; 84(5):575–580.
57. Waring JP, Manne RK, Wadas DD, Sanowski RA. Mucosal pseudolipomatosis: an air pressure-related colonoscopy complication. Gastrointest Endosc 1989; 35(2):93–94.
58. Maltz C. Benign pneumoperitoneum and pneumatosis intestinalis. Am J Emerg Med 2001; 19(3): 242–243.
59. Calne R. Gas cysts of the large bowel simulating multiple polyposis. Br J Surg 1959; 47:212–215.
60. Stollman NH, Lee KF. Primary pneumatosis cystoides intestinalis. Gastrointest Endosc 2000; 52:233.
61. Scheidler J, Stabler A, Kleber G, Neidhardt D. Computed tomography in pneumatosis intestinalis: differential diagnosis and therapeutic consequences. Abdom Imaging 1995; 20(6):523–528.
62. Petritsch W, Hinterleitner TA, Aichbichler B, Denk H, Hammer HF, Krejs GJ. Endosonography in colitis cystica profunda and solitary rectal ulcer syndrome. Gastrointest Endosc 1996; 44(6):746–751.
63. McCollister DL, Hammerman HJ. Air everywhere: pneumatosis cystoides coli after colonoscopy. Gastrointest Endosc 1990; 36(1):75–76.
64. Shallal JA, Van Heerden JA, Bartolomew RG, Chain JC. Pneumatosis cystoides intestinalis. Mayo Clin Proc 1974; 49:180–184.
65. Griffiths GJ. Pneumatosis cystoides intestinalis. Lancet 1955; II:905–906.
66. Mujahed Z, Evans JA. Gas cysts in the intestine pneumatosis intestinalis. Surg Gynecol Obstet 1958; 107:152.
67. Bloch C. The natural history of pneumatosis coli. Radiology 1977; 123:311–314.
68. Hoflin F, Van Der Linden W. Pneumatosis intestinalis treated by oxygen breathing. Scand J Gastroenterol 1974; 9:427–430.
69. Masterson J, Fratkin L, Osler T, et al. Treatment of pneumatosis cystoides intestinalis with hyperbaric oxygen. Ann Surg 1978; 187:245–247.
70. Mackinnon A, Frank J, Morris P. Treatment of pneumatosis cystoides coli by oxygen inhalation. Arch Dis Child 1977; 52:956–959.
71. Gruenberg J, Batra S, Priest R. Treatment of pneumatosis intestinalis with oxygen. Arch Surg 1977; 112(62):62–64.
72. Lee S. Oxygen therapy for pneumatosis coli: a report of two cases and a review. Aust N Z J Med 1977; 7:44–48.
73. Mirables M, Hinojasa J, Alonso J, et al. Oxygen therapy in pneumatosis coli. Dis Colon Rectum 1983; 26:458–460.
74. Wyatt A. Prolonged and symptomatic and radiological remission of colonic gas cysts after oxygen therapy. Br J Surg 1975; 62:837–839.
75. Case W, Hall R. Surgical treatment of pneumatosis coli. Ann R Coll Surg Engl 1985; 67:368–369.
76. Van Der Linden W. Reappearance of intestinal gas cysts after oxygen treatment. Lancet 1974; 2: 1388–1389.
77. Tak PP, Van Duinen CM, Bun P, et al. Pneumatosis cystoides intestinalis in intestinal pseudoobstruction. Resolution after therapy with Metronidazole. Dig Dis Sci 1992; 37(6):949–954.
78. Ellis B. Symptomatic treatment of primary pneumatosis coli with metronidazole. Br Med J 1980; 280:763–764.
79. Jauhonen P, Lehtola J, Karttunen T. Treatment of pneumatosis coli with metronidazole: endoscopic follow-up of one case. Dis Colon Rectum 1987; 30:800–801.
80. Van Der Linden W, Marsell R. Pneumatosis cystoides coli associated with high H2 excretion: treatment with an elemental diet. Scand J Gastroenterol 1979; 14:173–174.
81. Witkowski L, Pnotius G, Anderson R. Gas cysts of the intestine. Surgery 1955; 37:959–962.
82. Whitcomb DC, Martin SP, Trellis DR, Evans BA, Becich MJ. Diaphragm-like stricture and ulcer of the colon during diclofenac treatment. Arch Intern Med 1992; 152(11):2341–2343.

83. Hall MJ, Thomas WE, Cooper BT. Gastrocnemius myositis in a patient with inflammatory bowel disease. Digestion 1985; 32(4):296–300.
84. Rowe NM, Kahn FB, Acinapura AJ, Cunningham JN Jr. Nonsurgical pneumoperitoneum: a case report and a review. Am Surg 1998; 64(4):313–322.
85. Liebman PR, Patten MT, Manny J, Benfield JR, Hechtman HB. Hepatic-portal venous gas in adults: etiology pathophysiology and clinical significance. Ann Surg 1978; 187(3):281–287.
86. Ohtsubo K, Okai T, Yamaguchi Y, et al. Pneumatosis intestinalis and hepatic portal venous gas caused by mesenteric ischemia in an aged person. J Gastroenterol 2001; 36(5):338–340.
87. Faberman RS, Mayo-Smith WW. Outcome of 17 patients with portal venous gas detected by CT. AJR 1997; 169(6):1535–1538.
88. Hong JJ, Gadaleta D, Rossi P, Esquivel J, Davis JM. Portal vein gas a changing clinical entity. Report of 7 patients and review of the literature. Arch Surg 1997; 132(10):1071–1075.
89. Zhang D, Weltman D, Baykal A. Portal vein gas and colonic pneumatosis after enema with spontaneous resolution. AJR 1999; 173(4):1140–1141.
90. St Peter SD, Abbas MA, Kelly KA. The spectrum of pneumatosis intestinalis. Arch Surg 2003; 138: 68–75.
91. Terzic A, Holzinger F, Klaiber C. Pneumatosis cystoides intestinalis as a complication of celiac disease. Surg Endosc 2001; 15(11):1360–1361.
92. Wayte DM, Helwig EB. Colitis cystica profunda. Am J Clin Pathol 1967; 48:159–169.
93. Quzilbash AH, Meghji M, Castelli M. Pseudocarcinomatous invasion in adenomatous polyps of the colon and rectum. Dis Colon Rectum 1980; 23:529–535.
94. Guest CB, Reznik RK. Colitis cystica profunda: review of the literature. Dis Colon Rectum 1989; 32:983–986.
95. Martin JK Jr., Culp CE, Weiland LH. Colitis cystica profunda. Dis Colon Rectum 1980; 23(7):488–491.
96. Epstein SE, Ascari WQ, Ablow RC, Seaman WB, Lattes R. Colitis cystica profunda. Am J Clin Pathol 1966; 45:186–201.
97. Goodall HB, Sinclair IS. Colitis cystica profunda. J Pathol 1957; 73:33–42.
98. Denton J. The pathology of pellagra. Am J Trop Med 1925; 5:173–210.
99. Levine DS. Solitary rectal ulcer syndrome: are solitary rectal ulcer syndrome and localized colitis cystica profunda analogous syndromes caused by rectal prolapse? Gastroenterology 1987; 92: 243–253.
100. Madigan MR, Morson BC. Solitary ulcer of the rectum. Gut 1969; 10(11):871–881.
101. Talerman A. Enterogenous cysts of the rectum colitis cystica profunda. Br J Surg 1971; 58:643–647.
102. Rutter KR, Riddell RH. The solitary ulcer syndrome of the rectum. Clin Gastroenterol 1975; 4(3): 505–530.
103. Valenzuela M, Martin-Ruiz JL, Alvarez-Cienfuegos E, et al. Colitis cystica profunda: imaging diagnosis and conservative treatment: report of two cases. Dis Colon Rectum 1996; 39(5):587–590.
104. Gardiner GW, McAuliffe N, Murray D. Colitis cystica profunda occurring in a radiation-induced colonic stricture. Hum Pathol 1984; 15(3):295–298.
105. Walker JP, Wiener I, Rowe EB. Colitis cystica profunda: diagnosis and management. South Med J 1986; 79(9):1167–1170.
106. Ng WK, Chan KW. Postirradiation colitis cystica profunda. Case report and literature review. Arch Pathol Lab Med 1995; 119(12):1170–1173.
107. Bentley E, Chandrasoma P, Cohen H, Radin R, Ray M. Colitis cystica profunda: presenting with complete intestinal obstruction and recurrence. Gastroenterology 1985; 89(5):1157–1161.
108. Magidson JG, Lewin KJ. Diffuse colitis cystica profunda. Report of a case. Am J Surg Pathol 1981; 5(4):393–399.
109. Zidi SH, Marteau P, Piard F, Coffin B, Favre JP, Rambaud JC. Enterocolitis cystica profunda lesions in a patient with unclassified ulcerative enterocolitis. Dig Dis Sci 1994; 39(2):426–432.
110. Bernoulli RC, Spichtin HP, Meier AL. Localized colitis cystica profunda. Schweiz Med Wochenschr 1982; 112:1458–1462.
111. Nielsen OS, Sondergaard JO, Aru A. Colitis cystica profunda lokalisata. Acta Chir Scand 1984; 150(2):191–192.
112. Yashiro K, Murakami Y, Iizuka B, Hasegawa K, Nagasako K, Yamada A. Localized colitis cystica profunda of the sigmoid colon. Endoscopy 1985; 17(5):198–199.
113. Herman A, Nabseth D. Colitis cystica profunda. Arch Surg 1973; 106:337–341.
114. Doniec JM, Luttges J, Lohnert M, Henne-Bruns D, Grimm H. Rectal ultrasound in the diagnosis of localized colitis cystica profunda mucosal prolapse-related disease. Endoscopy 1999; 31(7):S55–S56.
115. Sakurai Y, Kobayashi H, Imazu H, et al. The development of an elevated lesion associated with colitis cystica profunda in the transverse colonic mucosa during the course of ulcerative colitis: report of a case. Surg Today 2000; 30(1):69–73.
116. Fechner RE. Polyp of the colon possessing features of colitis cystica profunda. Dis Colon Rectum 1967; 10:359–364.
117. Muto T, Bussey HJ, Morson BC. Pseudocarcinomatous invasion in adenomatous polyps of the colon and rectum. J Clin Pathol 1973; 26:25–31.
118. Lifshitz D, Cytron S, Yossiphov J, Lelcuk S, Rabau M. Colitis cystica profunda: self-inflicted by rectal trauma? Report of a case. Dig Dis 1994; 12(5):318–320.

119. Rosen Y, Vaillant JG, Yermakov V. Submucosal mucous cysts at a colostomy site: relationship to colitis cystica profunda and report of a case. Dis Colon Rectum 1976; 19(5):453–457.

120. Berthrong M, Fajardo LF. Radiation injury in surgical pathology. Part II: Alimentary tract. Am J Surg Pathol 1981; 5:153–178.

121. Black WCI, Ackerman LV. Carcinoma of the large intestine as a late complication of pelvic radiotherapy. Clin Radiol 1965; 16:278–281.

122. Valiulis AP, Gardiner GW, Mahoney LJ. Adenocarcinoma and colitis cystica profunda in a radiation-induced colonic stricture. Dis Colon Rectum 1985; 28(2):128–131.

123. Baratz M, Werbin N, Wiznitzer T, Rozen P. Irradiation-induced colonic stricture and colitis cystica profunda: report of a case. Dis Colon Rectum 1978; 21(1):75–79.

124. Hulsmans FJ, Tio TL, Reeders JW, Tytgat GN. Transrectal US in the diagnosis of localized colitis cystica profunda. Radiology 1991; 181(1):201–203.

125. Hrynyschyn K, Winkler R, Schaefer H. Colitis cystica profunda. Chirurg 1981; 52:93–95.

126. Silver H, Stolar J. Distinguishing features of well differentiated mucinous adenocarcinoma of the rectum and colitis cystica profunda. Am J Clin Pathol 1969; 51:493–500.

127. Stolar J, Silver H. Differentiation of pseudoinflammatory colloid carcinoma from colitis cystica profunda. Dis Colon Rectum 1969; 12:63–66.

128. Levine DS, Surawicz CM, Ajer TN, Dean PJ, Rubin CE. Diffuse excess mucosal collagen in rectal biopsies facilitates differential diagnosis of solitary rectal ulcer syndrome from other inflammatory bowel diseases. Dig Dis Sci 1988; 33(11):1345–1352.

129. Li SC, Hamilton SR. Malignant tumors in the rectum simulating solitary rectal ulcer syndrome in endoscopic biopsy specimens. Am J Surg Pathol 1998; 22(1):106–112.

130. Neumann H, Dietze W, Poll M, Willig F. Colitis cystica profunda—contribution to the differential diagnosis of rectum cancer. Leber Magen Darm 1985; 15:112–116.

131. Schein M, Veller M, Decker GA. Colitis cystica profunda simulating rectal carcinoma. A case report. S Afr Med J 1987; 72(4):289–290.

132. Stuart M. Proctitis cystica profunda: incidence etiology and treatment. Dis Colon Rectum 1984; 27:153–156.

133. Guy PJ, Hall M. Colitis cystica profunda of the rectum treated by mucosal sleeve resection and colo-anal pullthrough. Br J Surg 1988; 75:289.

134. Van Den Brandt-Gradel V, Huibregtse K, Tytgat GN. Treatment of solitary rectal ulcer syndrome with high-fiber diet and abstention of straining at defecation. Dig Dis Sci 1984; 29(11):1005–1008.

135. Beck DE. Surgical therapy for colitis cystica profunda and solitary rectal ulcer syndrome. Curr Treat Options Gastroenterol 2002; 5(3):231–237.

136. Michaelis L, Gutmann C. Ueber einschlusse in blasentumouren. Z Clin Med 1902; 47:208–215.

137. McClure J. Malakoplakia of the gastrointestinal tract. Postgrad Med J 1981; 57(664):95–103.

138. Cipolletta L, Bianco MA, Fumo F, Orabona P, Piccinino F. Malacoplakia of the colon. Gastrointest Endosc 1995; 41(3):255–258.

139. McClure J. Malakoplakia. J Pathol 1983; 140(4):275–330.

140. Long JP Jr., Althausen AF. Malacoplakia: a 25-year experience with a review of the literature. J Urol 1989; 141(6):1328–1331.

141. Stanton MJ, Maxted W. Malacoplakia: a study of the literature and current concepts of pathogenesis diagnosis and treatment. J Urol 1981; 125(2):139–146.

142. Zuk RJ, Neal JW, Baithun SI. Malakoplakia of the pancreas. Virchows Arch A Pathol Anat Histol 1990; 417:181–184.

143. Bates AW, Dev S, Baithun SI. Malakoplakia and colorectal adenocarcinoma. Postgrad Med J 1997; 73(857):171–173.

144. Lewin KJ, Harell GS, Lee AS, Crowley LG. An electron-microscopic study: demonstration of bacilliform organisms in malacoplakic macrophages. Gastroenterology 1974; 66:28–45.

145. Sanusi ID, Tio FO. Gastrointestinal malacoplakia: report of a case and review of the literature. Am J Gastroenterol 1974; 62:356–366.

146. Stevens S, McClure J. The histochemical features of the Michaelis-Gutmann body and a consideration of the pathophysiological mechanisms of its formation. J Pathol 1982; 137(2):119–127.

147. Miranda D, Vuletin JC, Kauffman SL. Disseminated histiocytosis and intestinal malacoplakia. Occurrence due to *Mycobacterium intracellulare* infection. Arch Pathol Lab Med 1979; 103:302–305.

148. Abdou NI, NaPombejara C, Sagawa A, et al. Malacoplakia: evidence for monocyte lysosomal abnormality correctible by cholinergic agonist in vitro and in vivo. N Engl J Med 1977; 297:1413–1419.

149. Lewin KS, Fair WR, Steigbigel R, Windberg CP, Droller MJ. Clinical and laboratory studies into the pathogenesis of malacoplakia. J Clin Pathol 1976; 29:354–363.

150. Thorning D, Vaco R. Malacoplakia: defect in digestion of phagocytosed material due to impaired vacuolar acidification? Arch Pathol 1975; 99:456–460.

151. Streem SB. Genitourinary malacoplakia in renal transplant recipients: pathogenic prognostic and therapeutic considerations. J Urol 1984; 132:10–13.

152. Biggar WD, Keating A, Bear RA. Malakoplakia: evidence for an acquired disease secondary to immunosuppression. Transplantation 1981; 31(2):109–112.

153. El Mouzan MI, Satti MB, Al Quorain AA, El Ageb A. Colonic malacoplakia—occurrence in a family. Report of cases. Dis Colon Rectum 1988; 31(5):390–393.

154. Moran CA, West B, Schwartz IS. Malacoplakia of the colon in association with colonic adenocarcinoma. Am J Gastroenterol 1989; 84(12):1580–1582.
155. Hayden AJ, Hardy DC, Jackson DE Jr. Malacoplakia of the colon. Mil Med 1986; 151(11):567–569.
156. Thrasher JB, Sutherland RS, Limoge JP, Donatucci CF. Transrectal ultrasound and biopsy in diagnosis of malacoplakia of prostate. Urology 1992; 13:70–73.
157. Kumar PV, Hambarsoomina B, Banani SA, Vaezzadeh K. Diagnosis of intestinal malacoplakia by fine needle aspiration cytology. Acta Cytol 1987; 31:53–56.
158. Perez-Barrios A, Rodriguez-Peralto JL, Martinez-Gonzalez MA, De Agustin P, Lozano F. Malacoplakia of the pelvis. Report of a case with cytologic and ultrastructural findings obtained by fine needle aspiration. Acta Cytol 1992; 36:377–380.
159. An T, Ferenczy A, Wilens SL, Melicow MM. Observation on the formation of Michaelis-Gutmann bodies. Hum Pathol 1974; 5(6):753–758.
160. Chaudhry AP, Saigal KP, Intengan M, Nickerson PA. Malakoplakia of the large intestine found incidentally at necropsy: light and electron microscopic features. Dis Colon Rectum 1979; 22(2):73–81.
161. Sandmeier D, Guillou L. Malakoplakia and adenocarcinoma of the caecum: a rare association. J Clin Pathol 1993; 46(10):959–960.
162. Maderazo EG, Berlin BB, Marhardt C. Treatment of malacoplakia with trimethoprim-sulfamethoxazole. Urology 1979; 13:70–73.
163. Van Der Voort HJ, Ten Velden JA, Wassenaar RP, Silberbusch J. Malacoplakia. Two case reports and a comparison of treatment modalities based on a literature review. Arch Intern Med 1996; 156(5):577–583.
164. Zornow DH, Landes RR, Morganstern SL, Fried FA. Malacoplakia of the bladder: efficacy of the bethanechol chloride therapy. J Urol 1979; 122:703–704.
165. Nieto-Zermeno J, Del Campo-Martinez M, Saenz-Urquidi E, Bulnes-Mendizabal D, Palet JA. Colonic malacoplakia: use of bethanechol. Bol Med Hosp Infant Mex 1984; 41:369–373.
166. Stanton MJ, Lynch JH, Maxted WC, Chun BK. Malacoplakia of the bladder: a case report of resolution with bethanechol trimethoprim-sulfamethoxazole and ascorbic acid. J Urol 1983; 130:1174–1176.
167. Van Furth R, Van't Wout JW, Wertheimer PA, Zwartendijk J. Ciprofloxacin for treatment of malakoplakia. Lancet 1992; 339(8786):148–149.
168. Biggar WD, Crawford L, Cardella C, Bear RA, Gladman D, Reynolds WJ. Malakoplakia and immunosuppressive therapy. Reversal of clinical and leukocyte abnormalities after withdrawal of prednisone and azathioprine. Am J Pathol 1985; 119(1):5–11.

35 | The Colon and Systemic Disease

Anton Emmanuel
Departments of Gastroenterology and Neurogastroenterology, University College Hospital, London, U.K.

INTRODUCTION

This content of this chapter will, by definition, be a wide-ranging description of the present state of knowledge pertaining to the colonic consequences of a wide variety of systemic disorders. The common thread that links the content is to focus on the symptoms of colonic disease that can occur in systemic disorders, to explain their pathophysiology and to consider the available treatments. The chapter is not intended to be a complete source of information about the impact of these conditions on the entire digestive tract; for some of the diseases the gastrointestinal burden may either primarily involve the hindgut (such as multiple sclerosis), mostly affect the upper gut (such as diabetes mellitus), or the entire digestive tract (such as systemic sclerosis). It can be seen that there is a wide range of diseases that potentially impact on colonic function, and these will be discussed sequentially, categorized in terms of the organ system that is primarily involved in the systemic disease. The emphasis is to dovetail with the content of the chapter on Miscellaneous Colonic Disorders in this textbook. This chapter will not address the corollary situation, namely the impact of colonic disease (specifically inflammatory bowel disease) on extra-intestinal organs. Greater detail of this aspect is available from recent comprehensive reviews (1).

INFILTRATIVE DISORDERS
Systemic Sclerosis

Progressive systemic sclerosis (frequently mistermed scleroderma) is a multisystem disease of unknown etiology which targets small arteries and connective tissue. The disease is approximately three times more common in women than men, with an annual incidence of 1/100,000 in the developed world (2). Characteristic systemic manifestations include Raynaud's phenomenon, dermatological involvement, polyarthritis, and progressive pulmonary and renal infiltration. Histologically, it is characterized by a vasculitis resulting in fibrous connective tissue proliferation, as well as smooth muscle atrophy (secondary to ischemia); in the gut this primarily involves the circular smooth muscle layer (3). The commonest site of gastrointestinal involvement is the esophagus, with over 90% of patients having dysphagia or atypical chest pain (4). However, more than half of all patients have anal or colonic involvement (5,6). Colonic disease seems to affect the distal bowel more than the right side (7,8). Pathophysiologically, involvement of the gastrointestinal tract seems to commence as a visceral neuropathy, becoming myopathic with advanced disease (9,10). The putative association between severity of disease and development of gastrointestinal symptoms remains unproven (11,12).

The most frequent clinical manifestation of colonic involvement with systemic sclerosis is episodic diarrhea, affecting over half of all patients (12). The symptom typically occurs at least monthly, and represents a major limitation of quality of life (12). Diarrhea may result from coexistent small bowel bacterial overgrowth (13), but there is often a mixture of neuropathic and myopathic attenuation of colonic motility (7,9). In approximately one-third of patients with systemic sclerosis (12), delayed colonic transit (7,14) in tandem with reduced rectal compliance (6) may result in constipation or evacuatory difficulty.

Fecal incontinence affects a minority of patients but causes major limitations in quality of life (15,16). Typically patients passively leak stool or flatus rather than reporting urge incontinence (6). Passive fecal incontinence has a number of possible etiologies, including altered rectal compliance, impaired rectal sensitivity, impairment of the recto-anal inhibitory reflex, and atrophy of the internal anal sphincter (15,17). Magnetic resonance imaging of the anal sphincters does not provide additional helpful diagnostic information beyond that provided by endoanal ultrasonography (17,18). An important potential cofactor causing fecal incontinence, and a not infrequent comorbidity of systemic sclerosis, is rectal prolapse (15), which results from chronic straining at stool and connective tissue infiltration.

Gastrointestinal bleeding may occur from a variety of causes in patients with progressive systemic sclerosis. Classically, there may be telangiectasia (19), but bleeding may also arise from diverticulosis and stercoral ulcerations, both of which are known to occur with increased frequency in patients with systemic sclerosis (3). The diverticula occurring in the context of systemic sclerosis are often described as being "fish-mouthed" in view of their macroscopic appearance and result from focal muscle fibrosis adjacent to uninvolved smooth muscle. Rarely, these wide-mouthed diverticula may trap stool, resulting in local fecal impaction and stercoral ulceration, or even more rarely, colonic perforation (20). Another rare acute colonic presentation of progressive systemic sclerosis includes colonic obstruction secondary to either benign stricture or volvulus (21).

In evaluating a patient with progressive systemic sclerosis who presents with new gastrointestinal symptoms, consideration of infectious, inflammatory, and neoplastic conditions is the initial priority. If such investigations are normal, the symptoms can be considered as secondary to the underlying systemic disorder. Colonic motility studies are unnecessary, but a plain abdominal radiograph may show colonic dilatation (see above); presence of a dilated upper gut in such a patient suggests the diagnosis of chronic intestinal pseudo-obstruction secondary to systemic sclerosis. Anorectal physiology testing and endoanal ultrasonography are helpful in patients with fecal incontinence, both to exclude coexisting sphincter defects (obstetric or postsurgical) and to determine if there is internal sphincter atrophy and weakness (16,18). Endosonographic appearances of thickening of the anal subepithelium and internal sphincter raise the possibility of rectal prolapse, which needs to be actively sought by examining the patient during feigned or attempted evacuation. If diarrhea is present, bacterial overgrowth should be excluded by a hydrogen breath test or ^{14}C-xylose breath test (22).

If bacterial overgrowth is present, broad-spectrum antibiotics (tetracycline or ciprofloxacin) or anaerobic agents (metronidazole) should be prescribed for courses of between one to three weeks (22). There is an invariably good initial result that may last for months. In patients with frequent relapse, cyclical courses of antibiotics for one week in every four have been advocated (23). In cases of persistent diarrhea, use of a low-residue diet is preferred to antidiarrheal which may cause profound constipation due to the potential for exacerbating the underlying tendency to delayed transit.

In patients with constipation, secondary to systemic sclerosis, a low-residue diet is again preferred, because excess fiber may exacerbate abdominal bloating and flatulence. Laxatives should be judiciously used, as in patients with functional constipation. Particular care should be taken with the use of magnesium salts in patients with comorbid renal involvement, due to the risk of hypermagnesemia. The symptomatic effect of existing enterokinetic drugs, such as erythromycin and cisapride, is almost invariably poor despite improvement of measured transit (13,24). Subtotal colectomy is not indicated in systemic sclerosis, because the underlying dysmotility is panenteric.

Conventional dietary (low-residue) and pharmacological (antidiarrheal) treatment of fecal incontinence in systemic sclerosis is frequently unsuccessful (16). Direct sacral nerve stimulation is a recently developed technique that has been shown to be effective in patients with idiopathic fecal incontinence (18,25). The technique has been safely and successfully applied to a small number of patients with fecal incontinence associated with systemic sclerosis, and this beneficial effect is maintained in to the medium term at least (18).

Systemic Amyloidosis

Systemic amyloidosis results from the widespread extracellular deposition of insoluble amyloid fibrils. Amyloidosis is subclassified according to the underlying clinical cause of the production of amyloid and the biochemical properties of the deposited fibrils (26,27). Five main subtypes are recognized, all of which may involve the digestive tract. Histologically, the primary gastrointestinal sites of amyloid protein deposition are perivascular (resulting in ischemia), the muscularis mucosa (predisposing to malabsorption), and the smooth muscle myocytes (resulting in dysmotility). Mucosal infiltration is seen only when the disease burden is massive (28). The five main subtypes of systemic amyloidosis recognized are:

1. AL amyloidosis: secondary to clonal expansion of myelomatous cells in the bone marrow, which in turn produce amyloidogenic immunoglobulins;
2. AA amyloidosis: secondary to overproduction of serum amyloid protein in chronic inflammatory or infectious conditions such as rheumatoid arthritis, inflammatory bowel disease, tuberculosis, and bronchiectasis;
3. AH amyloidosis: dialysis-associated production of β_2-microglobulin;
4. AF amyloidosis: autosomally inherited conditions (familial amyloid polyneuropathy) resulting in expression of abnormal liver proteins and hence overproduction of amyloid;
5. Senile amyloidosis.

Gastrointestinal symptoms can occur in any of the subtypes of systemic amyloidosis, and are present approximately 50% of the time (27,29). Colonic symptoms of amyloid are much less frequent than are gastric and small intestinal manifestations of gastroparesis and malabsorption. Colonic amyloid most frequently manifests as constipation or diarrhea (30). Colonic dilatation (with predisposition to volvulus) may be present as part of an amyloid-associated chronic intestinal pseudo-obstruction (30). Other more rarely recognized manifestations include colonic obstruction (mimicking carcinoma) secondary to an amyloid colonic stricture (32,33), colonic perforation (33), rectal bleeding (34), inflammatory colitis (30), and fecal incontinence (especially if secondary to an inherited familial amyloid polyneuropathy). Almost invariably, patients with colonic symptoms of amyloid will have generalized disease; there are, however, a minority of patients who have been described as having localized colonic amyloidosis complicating AL amyloid disease (35). A patient with amyloidosis presenting with abdominal pain, constipation, and a colonic stricture should raise the possibility of ischemic colitis.

Diagnosis of amyloid depends on obtaining and staining a biopsy specimen with Congo red dye, the material then being viewed under polarizing microscopy to reveal the characteristic apple-green birefringence. Liver biopsy is regarded as the gold standard (100% sensitivity), but is invasive. Although not frequently involved in disease, the colon is important in amyloidosis as the rectum is a readily accessible source of histological material. The sensitivity of rectal biopsy is 94% and just 73% for colonic biopsy (29). Rectal biopsy does not, however, give information about burden of amyloidosis or response to treatment, for which radioisotope serum amyloid P protein (SAP) testing is required (36).

Colonic involvement can be defined by contrast radiology, characteristically showing multiple filling defects, ischemic ulceration, or narrowing and rigidity most manifest in the rectum and sigmoid (27). Endoscopically, appearances are not as impressive in the lower gut as in the duodenum (37). The commonest colonoscopic abnormality is granularity of the mucosa (present in 34% of patients); more rarely there may be erosions (11%) or ulcers (9%), abnormalities being distributed throughout the colon (37).

If untreated, systemic amyloidosis is almost always rapidly fatal. However, an evolving range of therapeutic options now exists in the treatment of amyloidosis. Chemotherapy (with melphalan and prednisolone) has been used for AL amyloidosis, with a prolongation of median survival from 6 to 12 months (35). Chemotherapy as an adjuvant to autologous hematopoietic stem cell transplant has been successfully employed for the particular high-risk group of AL amyloidosis patients with cardiac involvement (38). Such treatment has been shown to effectively reduce the burden of gastrointestinal disease (38).

Treatment of AA amyloidosis centers on optimally suppressing the source of inflammation or chronic suppuration. Colchicine has been shown to be effective in reducing disease burden in this setting (39). Familial amyloidotic polyneuropathy is successfully treated by liver transplantation, which halts production of the aberrant transthyretin protein that results in systemic AF amyloidosis. The critical factor for this definitive therapy is timing—it should be delayed until peripheral neuropathic symptoms begin, but not be delayed to the point that there is significant cardiac or autonomic nerve dysfunction (39,40). In particular, if liver transplantation is delayed until after the development of anorectal denervation and sphincter compromise, the outcome in terms of improving fecal continence and evacuation difficulty is significantly worse compared to when the procedure is performed while anorectal physiology tests are still normal (Emmanuel and Kamm, unpublished observations).

Gastrointestinal complications, such as obstruction or perforation, can be successfully surgically treated (32,34). A beneficial response to cisapride, a 5HT[4] agonist with enterokinetic properties, has been reported in one patient (41). There is, however, no evidence that amyloidosis involves the enteric nerves (42), so it would be surprising if such serotonergic agents were of use in the majority of patients.

Familial Mediterranean Fever-Associated Amyloidosis

Familial Mediterranean fever is an autosomally recessive inherited condition characterized by episodic bouts of fever, arthritis, and pleuroperitonitis (39,43). The disease is rare, affecting mostly—but not exclusively—people of Mediterranean descent. The amyloidosis that complicates familial Mediterranean fever primarily affects the heart and kidney. Gastrointestinal involvement, although usually occurring early, is very rarely symptomatic (39). Once these patients have undergone renal transplantation, however, their gastrointestinal symptoms tend to become more prominent (43), with diarrhea and malabsorption. Parenteral nutrition is a helpful, albeit usually only short-term solution for such patients. Colchicine treatment is the cornerstone of management, although this therapy can exacerbate the diarrhea.

Amyloidosis Secondary to Inflammatory Bowel Disease

Amyloidosis secondary to inflammatory bowel disease is a rare, but potentially severe complication of chronic Crohn's disease or ulcerative colitis (44,45). The incidence of amyloidosis secondary to Crohn's disease is 0.9% (more common in ileocolitis than isolated ileal disease), and secondary to ulcerative colitis the incidence is 0.07% (45). The incidence rates from autopsy studies are considerably higher, suggesting that the disease is mostly asymptomatic (46). The mean time from onset of inflammatory bowel symptoms to diagnosis of amyloidosis was 15 years, but there were some cases in which this "lag-period" was as short as a year. There is a male preponderance to the development of amyloidosis in Crohn's disease, and patients tend to have had a history of suppurating complications (fistulae, abscess); an association with the presence of extra-intestinal manifestations of disease has not been described (45).

Amyloidosis secondary to inflammatory bowel disease can affect any organ, but the commonest presentation is with proteinuria or renal impairment (45). Colchicine can provide effective primary (47) and secondary (48) prevention of renal dysfunction in patients with Crohn's disease and proven amyloidosis. Effective renal replacement is also mandatory if renal function deteriorates, or if the amyloidosis is diagnosed only after there is significant renal impairment. In patients with Crohn's disease whose renal dysfunction results in kidney transplantation, the antirejection therapy seems to induce regression of the amyloid (49).

What is certain is that regular monitoring of renal function is important in at-risk patients (male gender, ileocolitis, septic complications, long history of disease) with Crohn's disease. A more controversial area of the literature relates to the role of intestinal resection in inducing amyloid regression. While some early reports suggested that resecting the inflamed colon was beneficial (50), the consensus of the majority of series is that there is no evidence of amyloid regression after resectional surgery (45,46).

Other Infiltrative Disorders
Sarcoidosis
Sarcoidosis is a multisystem disorder, characterized by granulomatous infiltration, primarily affecting the lymph nodes, lungs, skin, and eye. The digestive tract is relatively rarely involved, and when it is, the stomach is the most commonly involved organ. Colonic sarcoid is uncommon and may present as either a granulomatous colitis similar to Crohn's disease (51), a colonic obstruction similar to carcinoma (52), or a rectal mass (53). Endoscopic appearances are nonspecific and generally minor (54). The key differential is with Crohn's colitis where noncaseating granulomata are also the histological hallmarks. An elevated serum angiotensin converting enzyme level would indicate sarcoidosis, because the enzyme is not elevated in Crohn's disease (51,55).

Systemic Mastocytosis

Systemic mastocytosis is characterized by proliferation of mast cells in skin, lymph nodes, bone, and visceral organs. Symptoms relate to the release of histamine and prostaglandins secondary to mast cell degranulation. The disease may involve the digestive tract, the primary manifestation being diarrhea and malabsorption related to small intestinal disease. Colonic involvement is reported, presenting as diarrhea with mucosal edema and inflammatory mucosal infiltrate (56).

THE VASCULITIDES AND RHEUMATOLOGICAL DISEASES

The vasculitides are a family of multisystem diseases which may produce a wide range of gastrointestinal symptoms, of a severity ranging from minor dysmotility to severe ischemia. The classification of vasculitides revolves around the size of vessel that is primarily affected for each given disease. This pathological classification has important clinical sequelae. Diseases involving large or medium arteries tend to cause extensive full-thickness ischemia leading to intestinal infarction and perforation; diseases affecting small vessels tend to cause more localized ischemia resulting in mucosal ulceration (57,58).

Large- and Medium-Vessel Vasculitides

The two chief types of large vessel vasculitis are Takayasu's arteritis and giant cell arteritis. There is an association between Takayasu's arteritis and inflammatory bowel disease (59). It is possible to hypothesize that the basis of the link is that the gut inflammation is primary, with increased mucosal permeability allowing absorption of antigen and immune complexes in to the circulation, which may then provoke vasculitis (58). Alternatively, gut inflammation may be secondary to mucosal ischemia predisposed to by the vasculitic condition. The medium-sized-vessel vasculitides do not generally involve the digestive tract with the exception of polyarteritis nodosa.

Polyarteritis Nodosa

Polyarteritis nodosa is a necrotizing focal segmental vasculitis which results from deposition of immune complexes in the walls of medium-sized arteries (60). Unusually for the vasculitides, there is a relative male predisposition. Clinical features in the early stages are typically nonspecific with fever, malaise, and weight loss. Later in the course of the illness renal, peripheral nerve, and joint involvement are prominent. Visceral angiography may show the classical appearance of tapered arteries and microaneurysms at vessel branching points, but formal diagnosis requires histology. Gut involvement is seen in about half of all patients (60), the commonest complaint being abdominal pain (as the presenting symptom of intestinal ischemia). Typically, the superior mesenteric artery is involved and small intestinal ulcerations occur, although lesions can also be seen in the colon. Extensive involvement can result in intestinal or colonic necrosis (61,62). The presentation can also be with a severe diarrhea mimicking fulminant inflammatory bowel disease (62) and pseudomembranous colitis (63). If the involved vessel becomes aneurysmal, it may rupture resulting in major gastrointestinal or intra-abdominal bleeding. Colonic perforation may result from such aneurysmal rupture, but may also arise secondary to deep penetrating ulcers (64,65). Survival after such abdominal catastrophes is rare, the prognosis unfortunately not being significantly improved by surgery (64,66).

Treatment of polyarteritis nodosa depends on use of cyclophosphamide (or azathioprine) and steroids (57). Patients presenting with abdominal pain should be reviewed by a surgeon at an early stage, with a view to early surgery so as to avoid the above-described intra-abdominal catastrophes.

Small-Vessel Vasculitides
Antineutrophil Cytoplasmic Autoantibody-Associated Vasculitides

This family of conditions includes Wegner's granulomatosis and Churg-Strauss syndrome. Gastrointestinal involvement occurs in about 50% of patients, but usually involves the stomach and small intestine. Ischemic colitis is the most frequent of the colonic presentations, although it occurs in only a small minority of patients (67).

Immune Complex–Mediated Vasculitides

Systemic Lupus Erythematosus

Systemic lupus erythematosus (SLE) is the best described of the small-vessel immune complex vasculitides, in terms of involvement of the digestive tract. SLE is a multisystem vasculitis characterized by the presence of serum antinuclear antibodies. The disease affects 0.1% of the population, affecting primarily women and being much more common in black than white populations. The disease most commonly involves the joints, skin, lungs, nervous system, and kidneys. Gastrointestinal symptoms occur in over half of all SLE patients, but they are not commonly present at initial diagnosis (68).

Gastrointestinal vasculitis usually presents as abdominal pain, nausea, and vomiting, and in severe cases may present to the emergency room as an acute abdomen (69). The range of presentation reflects the degree of vasculitic mucosal involvement, in terms of surface area and depth of the bowel wall ischemia. Milder SLE gut vasculitis may mimic inflammatory bowel disease presenting as diarrhea or gastrointestinal bleeding from mucosal ulceration (70) or ischemic colitis (71). Rarely there may be colonic perforation (72), pneumatosis cystoides intestinalis (73,74), or intussusception (75) as manifestations of the vasculitis. At its most life threatening, SLE enteric vasculitis affects only about 2% of patients, but is fatal in over 50% of patients who develop the problem (74). A major problem with the clinical recognition of these problems is that most patients are taking corticosteroids, which may mask abdominal signs.

A minority of patients with SLE will have high titers of anticardiolipin antibody and are predisposed to recurrent arterial and venous thromboses (the antiphospholipid syndrome). This condition may also occur in the context of other autoimmune diseases (76). Patients may present with features similar to the above, depending on the degree of ischemia or mucosal congestion resulting from the thromboses (76). SLE-related conditions such as mixed connective tissue disease, Sjogren's syndrome, and polymyositis-dermatomyositis have a predilection for involvement of the esophagus and stomach, but do not usually have any colonic complications. There is, however, an interesting association between Crohn's disease and the myositides, and it has been suggested that there is subclinical bowel inflammation in patients with polymyositis-dermatomyositis (77).

Because SLE vasculitis is a disease of the small vessels of the bowel wall, mesenteric angiography is frequently normal despite the presence of marked disease (74). Bowel ischemia may manifest as bowel wall edema, "thumbprinting," and ileus (68). The diagnosis of SLE vasculitis primarily depends on clinical suspicion and the presence of elevated serum markers of disease activity.

Corticosteroid treatment of gastrointestinal SLE vasculitis is usually of only minimal benefit. Pulsed intravenous cyclophosphamide has been successfully employed (74) for this otherwise frequently fatal condition. Patients not infrequently end up having laparotomies as part of the workup of a presentation with an acute abdomen.

Henoch-Schonlein Purpura

Henoch-schonlein purpura is caused by immunoglobulin A (IgA)-immune complex deposition in small vessels. It primarily affects children around five years of age. Characteristically, following an upper respiratory tract infection, patients develop a purpuric rash on the buttocks and legs in association with abdominal pain and arthralgia. The central abdominal pain is usually due to extravasation of blood and fluid into the bowel wall (78). This phenomenon can also result in gastrointestinal bleeding, usually from the upper gastrointestinal tract. Petechial lesions may, however, be visible on colonoscopy. Worsening abdominal pain occurring with the passage of "redcurrant jelly" stool in the presence of an abdominal mass is the textbook presentation of an ileal or ileocolonic intussusception. Intussusceptions occur as the bowel telescopes over a localized submucosal hematoma (78). Previous teaching that a barium meal could help both diagnose and reduce such intussusceptions has been modified as the risks of gut perforation with contrast medium have been described (79). The diagnostic method of choice is an abdominal ultrasound, and treatment is surgical. Traditionally, laparotomy was required in approximately 10% of patients with Henoch-Schonlein purpura (80), usually for complications such as intussusception, infarction, hemorrhage, or perforation. However, a laparoscopic resection may now be preferable. In uncomplicated disease, the basis of therapy is immunosuppression with steroids, and rarely azathioprine (78).

Behcet's Disease

Behcet's disease is a clinically diagnosed disorder characterized by the triad of uveitis, aphthous mucosal ulceration, and genital ulceration (81). It is, however, a multisystem disease, and recurrent phlebitis and synovitis are common manifestations. In the colon, there may be a large-vessel arteritis or venulitis as part of a panintestinal vasculitis (81). Classically, there are ileocecal ulcers mimicking Crohn's disease on contrast radiology (63,82). Cytotoxic agents (such as cyclophosphamide) are indicated for the significant minority of patients who have a large-vessel arteritis, but the majority of patients are managed with glucocorticoids. There is ongoing controversy as to the effect of steroids in treating the mucosal manifestations of Behcet's disease (81).

Rheumatoid Arthritis

Rheumatoid arthritis (RA) affects about 2% of the adult population. Approximately 10% of patients have gastrointestinal complaints, and gut vasculitis affects only 1% of patients (83). Vasculitis occurs in patients at the more severe end of the disease spectrum, often in association with rheumatoid skin nodules and high titers of rheumatoid factor (83). The clinical presentation of RA vasculitis depends, as with SLE, on the degree of mucosal involvement. At its mildest there may be diarrhea and edema, but with more severe disease there may be frank gastrointestinal hemorrhage and mucosal ulceration, pain and visceral ischemia, or perforation (84). Histologically, colonic mucosa may show signs of an inflammatory infiltrate, but symptoms are relatively unusual (85). In RA cases where there is a marked colonic inflammation, there may be an accompanying subepithelial collagen band indicative of a collagenous colitis (86). Such patients present with the characteristic symptoms of watery diarrhea and abdominal distension.

There are some additional special situations that can cause colonic symptoms in the RA patient. There may be colonic manifestations of the drugs used to treat RA. In particular, there is the nonsteroidal-associated coloenteropathy (resulting in colonic strictures, or more rarely perforation) and gold-induced enterocolitis. Another possibility is development of the complication of secondary amyloidosis (see above), which occurs in between 5% and 20% of patients (87).

The Arthritides

Gastrointestinal manifestations of RA are either related to an RA vasculitis (rare) or are nonspecific, as part of the systemic features of a chronic illness (more common). The seronegative spondyloarthropathies are a family of rheumatological disorders in which rheumatoid factor is not present in the blood. There is a strong association with clinical or subclinical gut inflammation and HLA-B27 positivity (77).

Reactive Arthritis

Reactive arthritis (Reiter's syndrome) is characterized by joint inflammation (primarily lower limb), urethritis, and uveitis occurring after an infection elsewhere in the body (most frequently the gut). The most frequent enteric bacterial culprits are *Salmonella, Shigella, Clostridium difficile, Campylobacter, Yersinia, Cryptosporidia,* and *Giardia.* Up to two-thirds of patients who have a reactive arthritis will have ileocolonoscopic abnormalities (88), many of which may be asymptomatic. The presence of these gut lesions seems to predispose to progression of reactive arthritis to ankylosing spondylitis (AS) (89). The inflammatory gut lesions may mimic inflammatory bowel disease or collagenous colitis (90).

It has been suggested that gut (or other) infection results in increased absorption of antigen from the lumen, predisposing to formation of immune complexes that migrate to the joints. The strong relationship with HLA-B27 suggests a degree of cross-reactivity between the gut antigens and the protein produced by that region of the histocompatibility gene complex. Alternatively, there may be cross-reaction between the antigen-derived immune response in the gut and the joints.

The treatment of reactive arthritis is with nonsteroidal anti-inflammatory drugs (NSAIDs). There is no evidence that these drugs predispose to worsening of gut inflammation (88), although the typical gastrointestinal complications of NSAIDs may occur.

Ankylosing Spondylitis

AS is a systemic disorder with a primarily rheumatological and gastrointestinal symptom focus. There is a strong association with HLA-B27, and the condition is more frequent and more severe in men. The typical joint symptoms are axial, beginning classically with pain and stiffness in the lower back, most marked after rest or immobility.

Almost two-thirds of patients with AS have endoscopic abnormalities resembling features of Crohn's disease, although less than 10% of patients with AS develop inflammatory bowel disease (91). HLA-B27 negativity and elevated serum markers of disease activity predict the development of chronic inflammatory bowel disease in these patients (91). There is no temporal association between the exacerbation of gut and joint symptoms. In particular, surgical treatment of the inflammatory bowel disease does not improve joint stiffness. This is in stark contrast to the arthropathy that complicates inflammatory bowel disease in which joint symptoms improve with optimal gut disease management.

Psoriatic Arthritis

About one-third of patients with psoriasis get joint involvement, typically an asymmetric arthritis (although some may manifest as a symmetrical arthritis or spondylitic-type presentation). Endoscopic inflammation is present in about 10% of patients with psoriasis, particularly in those who are HLA-B27 positive (92). These gut lesions, as with AS, are frequently asymptomatic.

Endocrine Disorders

The hormonal environment acting in concert with local and central neural innervation critically influences colonic and anorectal function. Thus, it is unsurprising that a number of endocrine diseases may result in perturbation of colonic function.

Diabetes Mellitus

In the developing world, approximately one person in every 300 is treated with insulin. The incidence is increasing, with an approximate doubling in the last 30 years. Noninsulin-dependent diabetes affects about 7% of people in the United States (93). Autonomic neuropathy occurs in approximately one-quarter of diabetic patients (94). While subclinical autonomic neuropathy occurs within one to two years of the diagnosis of diabetes (95), clinical symptoms of neuropathy do not typically occur within the first 10 years (93). The neuropathy may involve both extrinsic autonomic and enteric nervous systems, and the potential range of gastrointestinal symptoms is panenteric. Approximately 75% of diabetics develop gastrointestinal symptoms (dysphagia, vomiting, constipation, diarrhea, and fecal incontinence) at some point in the course of their disease, and typically these are recurrent and unpredictable (96). Not all of these symptoms are related to diabetic autonomic neuropathy (DAN), however. For example, mean colonic transit time is similar for both patients with and without DAN (97), and furthermore there is a high prevalence of psychological dysfunction in diabetic patients (98). It is also clear that the development of chronic gastrointestinal symptoms has a profound negative effect on the already impaired quality of life of patients with diabetes (99).

Constipation is the commonest colonic manifestation of diabetes, affecting 60% of diabetics (100). The constipation is usually related to both a slowing of whole gut transit (101) and attenuation of the gastro–colic reflex (102), and only very rarely may be part of a chronic intestinal pseudo-obstruction picture (103). Diarrhea occurs in approximately 20% of diabetic patients (94). There are a number of possible noncolonic causes for diarrhea, which need to be considered (and treated). These etiologies include small bowel bacterial overgrowth treated by broad-spectrum antibiotics, exocrine pancreatic insufficiency managed with pancreatic enzyme supplementation, DAN addressed with clonidine, an a_2-adrenoceptor agonist, increased intestinal secretion treated with octreotide, somatostatin analogue, or comorbidity with an associated condition such as celiac disease or thyrotoxicosis.

It was previously thought that fecal incontinence in diabetes occurred secondary to diarrhea; however, the majority of fecal incontinent diabetic patients do not have stool weights compatible with true diarrhea. Rather, there is almost invariably evidence of DAN and impaired hindgut sensitivity (104), which attenuates resting anal tone and the rectoanal reflexes (104), thus leading to impaired continence.

Abdominal pain occurs in a significant minority of patients with diabetes. Once diabetic gastroparesis has been excluded as a cause, and especially if the nature of the pain is suggestive, diabetic radiculopathy of thoracic or lumbar nerve roots should be considered as a cause of pain (105). An alternative cause of abdominal pain in diabetic patients, especially if there is coexistent rectal bleeding, is mesenteric arterial ischemia and ischemic colitis.

Investigating the diabetic patient with gut symptoms focuses on two distinct, but related aspects: firstly, investigation for the presence of DAN, and secondly, investigation specifically of gastrointestinal function. Diabetic autonomic neuropathy is traditionally documented by testing of cardiovascular autonomic function with tests such as measurement of the heart rate response to deep breathing or standing, and the blood pressure and heart rate responses to the Valsalva maneuver. Recent refinements have encompassed measurement of heart rate variation by power spectral analysis, a technique that is independent of patient participation and bias. Assessment of gut function depends on the symptom. Whole gut transit time assessment in diabetes does not reflect degree of dysfunction and as such is of little value (102). Investigation of diarrhea centers on excluding extracolonic causes (see above). Fecal incontinence needs assessment with anorectal physiology and endoanal ultrasound as in nondiabetic subjects. If diabetic radiculopathy is suspected as a cause of pain, abdominal wall electromyography (EMG) studies may be performed (105). It must be remembered that whatever the gastrointestinal presentation, organic disease needs to be considered, and endoscopy and cross-sectional imaging should be applied as appropriate.

The primary aspect of the treatment of gut symptoms in diabetic patients is to ensure that the symptoms are not related to hyperglycemia and poor diabetic control (106). This assessment may occasionally require hospitalization of the patient to maintain euglycemia through intravenous therapy. If symptoms persist despite this therapy, they will need specific therapy. Treatment of constipation complicating diabetes mellitus is no different to that of patients with functional constipation. Although theoretically attractive, the efficacy of enterokinetic drugs in diabetes-associated constipation is disappointing (107). In treating diarrhea, assuming comorbidity has been excluded (bacterial overgrowth, pancreatic exocrine insufficiency, etc.), restriction of dietary fiber intake is beneficial (94). Some authors have recommended that idiopathic diabetic diarrhea be best treated with a prokinetic in order to avoid the vicious cycle of constipation and diarrhea that may occur with the use of drugs such as loperamide (94). The evidence base for this recommendation is not present. By contrast, other workers have advocated use of drugs such as loperamide or diphenoxylate with atropine (108), although again there is no evidence base. The experience of this author has been that judicious use of loperamide, particularly in syrup formulation for ease of dose adjustment, allows safe titration to reduce diarrhea and incontinence. Behavioral therapy (biofeedback) has also been shown to be effective in treating fecal incontinence associated with diabetes (109). Although not formally studied, agents for neuropathic pain (such as the tricyclic antidepressants and antiepileptics such as gabapentin) may be effective in patients with intractable diabetic radiculopathy causing abdominal pain.

Thyroid Disease

Hyperthyroidism is classically recognized as causing diarrhea, and this problem is likely to be related to acceleration of small bowel transit due to mucosal round cell infiltration (110). Successful treatment of the endocrine dysfunction results in normalization in mucosal histology, cessation of diarrhea and hence weight gain (110). With regard to the colon, there is a 4% prevalence of Grave's disease in association with ulcerative colitis (compared to less than 1% in the general population), and the thyrotoxicosis usually precedes colonic disease. The symptoms of the thyroid disease may exacerbate colitis, and the reverse is also true.

Hypothyroidism is most commonly caused by Hashimoto's thyroiditis. The association of this autoimmune thyroiditis with colitis provided early evidence of an immune component to the etiopathogenesis of ulcerative colitis. Hypothyroidism per se classically results in reduced whole gut motility, and the colonic manifestation of this can range from mild constipation to fecal impaction and megacolon (111).

Other Endocrine Diseases

Approximately 10% of patients with hyperparathyroidism report constipation as their initial presenting symptom (112). This problem is held to be secondary to hypercalcemia resulting

from increased serum levels of parathyroid hormone, and it is, therefore, unclear why constipation is also commonly reported in patients with hypoparathyroidism. Another symptom of
unknown causation is the diarrhea observed in patients with Addison's disease. Finally, the
colon may be involved in the multiple endocrine neoplasia syndromes, specifically Type 2b
where colonic mucosal neuromas and formation of diverticula may result in constipation
and abdominal pain (113).

Neurological Disorders

A complex interplay at three levels of the nervous system (the central nervous system, the
autonomic nerves, and enteric nervous system "mini-brain") maintains the integrity of colonic
and anorectal function. Accordingly, dysfunction of the nervous system at cortical, spinal, or
enteric levels may result in gastrointestinal symptoms. As described in the previous section,
diabetes mellitus may involve the nervous system at all three sites, and the major part of the
pathogenesis of gut symptoms in diabetes relates to neuropathy. The interconnections of these
nervous systems mean that nervous disorders usually result in dysfunction at a variety
of levels.

Central Nervous System Disorders

After a stroke, fecal incontinence occurs in up to 40% of patients within a month, especially in
diabetics, falling to less than 10% by six months (114). The impression of clinicians is that
prevalence of constipation after a stroke is high, although this has not formally been studied.

Up to two-thirds of patients with multiple sclerosis have colorectal dysfunction on transit and anorectal physiological assessment (115), with approximately one-third complaining of
constipation and one-quarter of fecal incontinence (115,116). The distribution of demyelinating
lesions through the nervous system results in a combination of upper and lower motor neu-
rone lesions in the gut, resulting in reduced colonic compliance and reduced internal and
external sphincter function. In addition to this range of motor dysfunction, the majority of
patients demonstrate reduced anorectal sensitivity (117). Treatment tends to be empiric, with
laxatives representing the most frequently depended upon intervention. Biofeedback has been
found to improve constipation and incontinence in some patients with multiple sclerosis, particularly those running a nonprogressive milder course (118).

Parkinson's disease causes report of the symptom of constipation in 30% of sufferers
(119), but prolongation of whole gut transit is seen in 80% of patients (95). Megacolon may also
occur, but only very rarely. In addition to slowing of transit, the symptom of constipation is
exacerbated by pelvic floor dyssynergia (present in over 50% of patients) (120). Anorectal
reflexes are impaired and there is dystonia and loss of function in external and internal anal
sphincters (121). The etiology of gut dysfunction in Parkinson's disease is loss of dopaminergic
neurons in both the brain stem and enteric nervous systems (122). Therapeutic trials of
available prokinetics to date have been of little value (95); therefore, treatment relies on use
of laxatives. Defecatory difficulty has been successfully treated in some patients with injection of botulinum toxin into the puborectalis, although the development of fecal incontinence
is a significant potential complication of such therapy (123).

Spinal Cord Disorders

Patients with paraplegia following spinal cord injury have a normal life expectancy, and those
with tetraplegia have a life expectancy only 10 years less than average (124). Because the
majority of patients suffer their injury below the age of 30, this means that spinally injured
patients suffer their gut symptoms for more than half their life. The estimated prevalence of
gut symptoms varies enormously in the literature according to referral practice. Constipation
is reported in over 50% and up to 90% of chronically injured patients (125,126). Monthly
episodes of fecal incontinence are reported in about one-third of patients, and a majority is
dependent on a caregiver for bowel management, spending as much as 2 hr/day (126,127).
Patients rate gut dysfunction as second only to the loss of mobility in terms of being their most
limiting problem.

Pathophysiologically, lesions can be classified as upper motor neuron type (supraconal
lesions) or lower motor neuron (cauda equina lesions). Whereas, the former typically have
delayed whole gut transit, the bowel slowing in the latter is usually confined to the distal
colon. The rectum in patients with supraconal lesions is typically noncompliant, whereas in

cauda equina the characteristic change is of a dilated and flaccid rectum. The rectoanal reflex tends to be pronounced in supraconal lesions and attenuated in cauda equina lesions (127,128). The approach to treatment between these two groups, therefore, tends to be rather different. In patients with a supraconal "reflexic" bowel, the aim is to use mild osmotic agents and softening laxatives to obtain a soft stool with as little rectal stimulation as possible. By contrast, the intention in patients with a cauda equina "flaccid" bowel is to pass a firm, formed stool that can be removed manually or with an enema. This is similar in approach to the treatment of gut dysfunction complicating myelomeningocele (129).

On balance, however, the management of bowel symptoms in spinally injured patients tends to be unsatisfactory for the majority of afflicted individuals. A number of more interventional approaches have received some attention. Irrigating the bowel in a retrograde fashion with an enema continence catheter (comprising a rectal tube with a balloon cuff that is inflated in the anal canal during irrigation in order to preserve continence) has been mostly employed in children. Improvements are seen mostly in terms of reducing episodes of fecal leakage in between bowel openings (130,131). Antegrade irrigation via an appendicostomy that can be intubated by the patient or caregiver allows delivery of laxative or irrigation directly to the right colon. Success rates similar to that with retrograde irrigation are reported, but it remains unknown how long these beneficial effects persist (132). Finally, electrical stimulation of sacral anterior roots (133) and formation of a colostomy (134) have been studied in isolated reports in carefully selected patients with refractory symptoms.

REFERENCES

1. Su CG, Judge TA, Lichtenstein GR. Extraintestinal manifestations of inflammatory bowel disease. Gastroenterol Clin North Am 2002; 31:307–327.
2. Silman A, Jannini S, Symmons D, et al. An epidemiological study of scleroderma in the West Midlands. Br J Rheumatol 1988; 27:286–290.
3. Rohrmann CA, Ricci MT, Krishnamurthy S, et al. Radiologic and histologic differentiation of neuromuscular disorders of the gastrointestinal tract: visceral myopathies, visceral neuropathies and progress systemic sclerosis. Am J Radiol 1981; 143:933–941.
4. Kahan A, Menkes C. Gastrointestinal involvement in systemic sclerosis. Clin Dermatol 1994; 12: 259–265.
5. Hamel-Roy J, Devroede G, Arhan P, et al. Comparative esophageal and anorectal motility in scleroderma. Gastroenterology 1985; 88:1–8.
6. Engel A, Kamm MA, Talbot IC. Progressive systemic sclerosis of the internal anal sphincter leading to passive fecal incontinence. Gut 1994; 35:857–859.
7. Battle WM, Snape WJ, Wright S, et al. Abnormal colonic motility in progressive systemic sclerosis. Ann Intern Med 1981; 94:749–752.
8. Whitehead WE, Taitelbaum G, Wigley FM, et al. Rectosigmoid motility and myoelectric activity in progressive systemic sclerosis. Gastroenterology 1989; 96:428–432.
9. Rees WDW, Leight RJ, Christofides ND, et al. Interdigestive motor activity in patients with systemic sclerosis. Gastroenterology 1982; 83:575–580.
10. Goldblatt F, Gordon TP, Waterman SA. Antibody-mediated gastrointestinal dysmotility in scleroderma. Gastroenterology 2002; 123:1144–1150.
11. Govoni M, Muccinelli M, Panicali P, et al. Colonic involvement in systemic sclerosis: clinical-radiological correlations. Clin Rheumatol 1996; 15:271–276.
12. Trezza M, Krogh H, Egekvist P, et al. Bowel problems in patients with systemic sclerosis. Scand J Gastroenterol 1999; 34:409–413.
13. Sjogren RW. Gastrointestinal motility disorders in scleroderma. Arthritis Rheum 1994; 9:1265–1272.
14. Wang SJ, Lan JL, Chen YH, et al. Colonic transit disorders in systemic sclerosis. Clin Rheumatol 2001; 20:251–254.
15. Leighton JA, Vladivinos MA, Pemberton JH, et al. Anorectal dysfunction and rectal prolapse in progressive systemic sclerosis. Dis Colon Rectum 1993; 6:182–185.
16. Jaffin BW, Chang P, Spiera H. Fecal incontinence in scleroderma: clinical features, anorectal manometric findings, and their therapeutic implications. J Clin Gastroenterol 1997; 25:513–517.
17. De Souza NM, Williams AD, Wilson HJ, et al. Fecal incontinence in scleroderma: assessment of the anal sphincter with thin-section endoanal MR imaging. Radiology 1998; 208:529–535.
18. Kenefick NJ, Vaizey CJ, Nicholls RJ, et al. Sacral nerve stimulation for fecal incontinence due to systemic sclerosis. Gut 2002; 51:881–883.
19. Marshall JB, Moore GF, Settles RH. Colonic telangiectasias. Arch Intern Med 1980; 140:1211–1216.
20. Regan PT, Weiland LH, Geall MGL. Scleroderma and intestinal perforation. Am J Gastroenterol 1977; 68:566–571.

21. Haque U, Yardley J, Talamini M, et al. Colon stricture and volvulus in a patient with scleroderma. J Rheumatol 1999; 26:2268–2272.
22. Rose S, Young MA, Reynolds JC. Gastrointestinal manifestations of scleroderma. Gastroenterol Clin N Am 1998; 27:563–594.
23. Kahn IJ, Geffries GH, Sleisinger MH. Malabsorption in scleroderma: correction by antibiotics. N Engl J Med 1966; 274:1339–1342.
24. Wang SJ, Lan JL, Chen DY, et al. Effects of cisapride on colonic transit in patients with progressive systemic sclerosis. Clin Rheumatol 2002; 21:271–274.
25. Malouf AJ, Vaizey CJ, Nicholls RJ, et al. Permanent sacral nerve stimulation for fecal incontinence. Ann Surg 2000; 232:143–148.
26. Cohen AS. History of amyloidosis. J Intern Med 1992; 232:509–516.
27. Buxbaum J. The amyloidosis. Mt Sinai J Med 1996; 63:16–27.
28. Rocken C, Saegar W, Linke RP. Gastrointestinal deposits in old age: report on 110 consecutive autopsical patients and 98 retrospective biopsy specimens. Pathol Res Pract 1994; 190:641–649.
29. Lee JG, Wilson JAP, Gottfried MR, et al. Gastrointestinal manifestations of amyloidosis. South Med J 1994; 87:243–253.
30. Kumar SS, Appavu SS, Abcarian H, et al. Amyloidosis of the colon: report of a case and review of the literature. Dis Colon Rectum 1983; 26:541–548.
31. Chen JH, Lai SJ, Tsai PP, et al. Localised amyloidosis mimicking carcinoma of the colon. Am J Roentgenol 2002; 179:536–537.
32. Rives S, Pera M, Rosinol L, et al. Primary systemic amyloidosis presenting as a colonic stricture: successful treatment with left hemi-colectomy followed by autologous haematopoietic stem-cell transplantation: report of a case. Dis Colon Rectum 2002; 45:1263–1266.
33. Gonzalez Sanchez JA, Molinero M, Sayans D, et al. Colonic perforation by amyloidosis: report of a case. Dis Colon Rectum 1989; 32:437–442.
34. Thaler W, Schwartzer G, Eder P, et al. Amyloidosis—an unusual cause of recurrent intestinal bleeding and sigmoid perforation: case report with review of the literature. Int J Colorectal Dis 1999; 14:297–299.
35. Kyle RA, Gertz MA, Lacy MQ, et al. Localised AL amyloidosis of the colon: an unrecognised entity. Amyloid 2003; 10:36–41.
36. Hawkins PN, Pepys MB. Imaging amyloidosis with radio labelled SAP. Eur J Nucl Md 1995; 22:595–598.
37. Tada S, Iida M, Iwashita A, et al. Endoscopic and biopsy findings of the upper digestive tract in patients with amyloidosis. Gastrointest Endosc 990; 36:10–15.
38. Moreau P, Milpied N, Defaucal P. High dose melphalan and autologous bone marrow transplantation for systemic AL amyloidosis with cardiac involvement. Blood 1996; 87:3063–3068.
39. Zemer D, Pras M, Sohar E, et al. Colchicine in the prevention and treatment of the amyloidosis of familial Mediterranean fever. N Engl J Med 1986; 314:1003–1005.
40. Coelho T. Familial amyloid polyneuropathy: new developments in genetics and treatment. Curr Opin Neurol 1996; 9:355–339.
41. Fraser AG, Arthur JF, Hamilton I. Intestinal pseudo-obstruction secondary to amyloidosis responsive to cisapride. Dig Dis Sci 1991; 36:532–535.
42. Anan I, el-Salhy M, Ando Y, et al. Comparison of amyloid deposits and infiltration of enteric nervous system in the upper with those in the lower gastrointestinal tract in patients with familial amyloidotic polyneuropathy. Acta Neuropathol 2001; 102:227–232.
43. Friedman S, Janowitz HD. Systemic amyloidosis and the gastrointestinal tract. Gastroenterol Clin N Am 1998; 27:595–614.
44. Gitking MJ, Wright SC. Amyloidosis complicating inflammatory bowel disease. Dig Dis Sci 1990; 35:906–912.
45. Greenstein AJ, Sachar DB, Panday AK, et al. Amyloidosis and inflammatory bowel disease: a 50 year experience with 25 patients. Medicine 1992; 71:261–269.
46. Werther JL, Schapira A, Rubenstein O, et al. Amyloidosis in regional enteritis. Am J Med 1960; 40:416–422.
47. Becker SA, Bass D, Nissim F. Crohn's ileitis complicated by amyloidosis: observations and therapeutic considerations. J Clin Gastroenterol 1985; 7:296–300.
48. Meyers S, Janowitz HD, Gumaste V, et al. Colchicine therapy of the renal amyloidosis of ulcerative colitis. Gastroenterol 1988; 94:1503–1507.
49. Lovat LB, Madhoo S, Pepys MB, et al. Long term survival in systemic amyloid A amyloidosis complicating Crohn's disease. Gastroenterol 1997; 112:1362–1367.
50. Fitchen JH. Amyloidsis and granulomatous ileocolitis: regression after trmoval of the involved bowel. N Engl J Med 1975; 292:352–354.
51. Dumot JA, Adal K, Petras RE, et al. Sarcoidosis presenting as granulomatous colitis. Am J Gastroenterol 1998; 93:1949–1951.
52. Hilzenrat N, Spanier A, Lamoureux E, et al. Colonic obstruction secondary to Sarcoidosis: nonsurgical diagnosis and management. Gastroenterol 1995; 108:1556–1559.
53. Zech JR, Kroger E, Bonnin AJ, et al. Sarcoidosis: unusual cause of a rectal mass. South Med J 1993; 86:1054–1055.

54. Ell SR, Frank PH. Spectrum of lymphoid hyperplasia: colonic manifestations of Sarcoidosis, infectious mononucleosis and Crohn's disease. Gastrointestin Radiol 1981; 6:329–334.
55. Silverstein E, Fierst SM, Simon MR, et al. Angiotensin converting enzyme in Crohn's disease: case report and review of the literature. Gastroenterol 1984; 87:421–425.
56. Legman P, Sterin P, Vallee C, et al. Colonic involvement and systemic mastocytosis. Sem Hop Paris 1981; 58:1460–1462.
57. Jennette JC, Falk RJ. Small-vessel vasculitis. N Engl J Med 1997; 337:1512–1523.
58. Bailey M, Caplin W, Licht H, et al. The effects of vasculitis on the gastrointestinal tract and liver. Gastroenterol Clin N Am 1998; 27:747–782.
59. Yasinger S, Adelman R, Cantor D, et al. Association of inflammatory bowel disease and large vascular lesions. Gastroenterology 1996; 101:844–846.
60. Krupski W, Selzman C, Whitehall T. Unusual cases of mesenteric ischemia. Surg Clin N Am 1997; 77:471–502.
61. Wood MK, Read DR, Kraft AR, et al. A rare cause of ischemic colitis: polyarteritis nodosa. Dis Colon Rectum 1979; 22:428–433.
62. Gullichsen R, Ovaska J, Ekfors T. Polyarteritis nodosa of the descending colon: case report. Eur J Surg 1991; 157:421–422.
63. Lee RG. The colitis of Behcet's syndrome. AM J Surg Path 1986; 10:888–893.
64. Roikjaer O. Perforation and necrosis of the colon complicating polyarteritis nodosa: case report. Acta Chir Scand 1987; 153:385–386.
65. Tanakaya K, Konaga E, Takeuchi H, et al Penetrating colon ulcer of polyarteritis nodosa: report of a case. Dis Colon Rectum 2001; 44:1037–1039.
66. Edwards WH Jr., Martin RS, Edwards WH Sr., et al. Surviving gastrointestinal infarction due to polyarteritis nodosa: a rare event. Am Surg 1992; 58:167–172.
67. Guillevin L, Lhote F, Amouroux J, et al. Antineutrophil cytoplasmic antibodies, abnormal angiograms and pathological findings in polyarteritis nodosa and Churg-Strauss syndrome: indications for the classification of vasculitides of the polyarteritis nodosa group. Br J Rheumatol 1996; 35:958–964.
68. Hoffman B, Katz WA. The gastrointestinal manifestations of systemic lupus erythematosus: a review of the literature. Semin Arthritis Rheum 1980; 9:23–27.
69. Zizic TM, Classen JN, Stevens MB, et al. Acute abdominal complications of systemic lupus erythematosus and polyarteritis nodosa. Am J Med 1982; 73:525–531.
70. Helliwell TR, Flook D, Whitworth J, et al. Arteritis and venulitis in systemic lupus erythematosus resulting in massive gastrointestinal haemorrhage. Histopathology 1985; 9:1103–1107.
71. Gore RM, Narn CS, Ujiki GT, et al. Ischaemic colitis associated with systemic lupus erythematosus. Dis Colon Rectum 1983; 26:449–453.
72. Zizic TM, Shulman LE, Stevens MB, et al. Colonic perforations in systemic lupus erythematosus. Medicine 1975; 54:411–416.
73. Derksen OS. Pneumatosis intestinalis in a female patient with systemic lupus erythematosus. Radiologia Clin 1978; 47:334–337.
74. Laing TJ. Gastrointestinal vasculitis and pneumatosis intestinalis due to systemic lupus erythematosus: successful treatment with pulsed intravenous cyclophosphamide. Am J Med 1988; 85:555–560.
75. Mekori YA, Sheider M, Yaretsky A, et al. Pancreatitis in systemic lupus erythematosus—a case report and review of the literature. Postgrad Med J 1980; 56:145–148.
76. Cappell MS, Mikhail N, Gujral N, et al. Gastrointestinal haemorrhage and intestinal ischemia associated with anticardiolipin antibodies. Dig Dis Sci 1994; 39:1359–1364.
77. Mielants H, Veys EM, Cuvelier C, et al. The evolution of spondyloarthropathies in relation to gut histology: III Relationship between gut and joint. J Rheumatol 1995; 22:2279–2284.
78. Robson WL, Leung AK. Henoch-Schonlein purpura. Adv Pediatr 1994; 41:163–194.
79. Jeong YK, Hu HK, Yoon CH, et al. Gastrointestinal involvement in Henoch-Schonlein syndrome: CT findings. Am J Roentgenol 1997; 168:965–968.
80. Martinez-Frontanilla LA, Hasse GM, Ernster JA, et al. Surgical complications in Henoch-Schonlein purpura. J Paediatr Surg 1984; 19:434–443.
81. O'Duffy JD. Behcet's disease. Curr Opin Rheumatol 1994:639–643.
82. Tolia V, Abdullah A, Thiraimoorthy MC, et al. A case of Behcet's disease with intestinal involvement due to Crohn's disease. Am J Gastroenterol 1989; 84:322–326.
83. Scot DGI, Baco PA, Tribe CR. Systemic rheumatoid vasculitis: a clinical laboratory study of 50 cases. Medicine 1981; 60:288–297.
84. Finkbiner RB, Decker JP. Ulceration and perforation of the intestine due to necrotising arteriolitis. N Engl J Med 1963; 268:14–18.
85. Marcolongo R, Bayeli PF, Montagnani M. Gastrointestinal involvement in rheumatoid arthritis: a biopsy study. J Rheumatol 1979; 6:163–173.
86. Wengrower D, Pollak A, Okon E, et al. Collagenous colitis and rheumatoid arthritis with response to sulphasalazine: a case report and review of the literature. J Clin Gastroenterol 1987; 9:456–460.
87. Dhillon V, Woo P, Isenberg D. Amyloidosis in the rheumatic diseases. Ann Rheumatol Dis 1989; 48:696–701.
88. De Vos M, Uvelier C, Mielants H, et al. Ileocolonoscopy in seronegative spondyloarthropathy. Gastroenterology 1989; 96:339–344.

89. Mielants H, Veys EM, Cuvelier C, et al. The evolution of spondyloarthropathies in relation to gut histology: I Clinical aspects. J Rheumatol 1995; 22:2266–2272.
90. Khan MA. Seronegative spondyloarthropathies: ankylosing spondylitis. Primer Rheum Dis 1993; 10:154–158.
91. Mielants H, Veys EM, Cuvelier C, et al. The evolution of spondyloarthropathies in relation to gut histology: II Histologic aspects. J Rheumatol 1995; 22:2273–2278.
92. Schatteman L, Mielants H, Veys EM, et al. Gut inflammation in psoriatic arthritis: a prospective ileo-colonoscopic study. J Rheumatol 1995; 22:680–683.
93. World Health Organisation. Diabetes mellitus: report of a WHO study group. WHO Technical report series 1985, Geneva; 727.
94. Vinik AI, Maser RE, Mitchell BD, et al. Diabetic autonomic neuropathy. Diabetes Care 2003; 26: 1553–1579.
95. Pfeiffer RE. Gastrointestinal dysfunction in Parkinson's disease. Lancet Neurol 2003; 2:107–116.
96. Bytzer P, Talley NJ, Leemon M, et al. Prevalence of gastrointestinal symptoms associated with diabetes mellitus: a population-based survey of 15,000 adults. Arch Intern Med 2001; 161:1989–1996.
97. Jung HK, Kim DY, Moon IH, et al. Colonic transit time in diabetic patients–comparison with healthy subjects and the effect of autonomic neuropathy. Yonsei Med J 2003; 44:265–272.
98. Clouse RE, Lustman PJ. Gastrointestinal symptoms in diabetic patients: lack of association with neuropathy. Am J Gastroenterol 1989; 84:868–874.
99. Talley NJ, Young L, Bytzer P, et al. Impact of chronic gastrointestinal symptoms in diabetes mellitus on health-related quality of life. Am J Gastroenterol 2001; 96:71–76.
100. Battle WM, Snape WJ, Alavi A, et al. Colonic dysfunction in diabetes mellitus. Gastroenterology 1980; 79:1217–1222.
101. Iber FL, Parveen S, Vandrunen M, et al. Relation of symptoms to impaired stomach, small bowel and colonic motility in long-standing diabetes. Dig Dis Sci 1993; 38:45–50.
102. Deen KI, Premaratna R, Fonseka MM, et al. The recto-anal inhibitory reflex: abnormal response in diabetics suggests an intrinsic neuroenteropathy. J Gastroenterol Hepatol 1998; 13:1107–1110.
103. Anuras S, Shirazi SS. Colonic pseudo-obstruction. Am J Gastroenterol 1984; 79:1217–1227.
104. Sun WM, Read NW, Miner PB. Relation between rectal sensation and anal function in normal subjects and patients with fecal incontinence. Gut 1990; 31:1056–1061.
105. Streib EW, Sun SF, Paustian FF, et al. Diabetic thoracic radiculopathy: electrodiagnostic study. Muscle Nerve 1986; 9:548–556.
106. Maleki D, Camilleri M, Zinsmeister, et al. Effect of acute hyperglycaemia on colorectal motor and sensory function in humans. Am J Physiol 1997; 273:G859-G864.
107. Camilleri M. Gastrointestinal problems in diabetes. Endocrinol Metab Clin North Am 1996; 25: 361–378.
108. Ryan JC, Sleisenger MH. Effects of systemic and extraintestinal disease on the gut. In: Sleisenger MH, Fordtran JS, eds. Gastrointestinal Disease. 5th ed. Philadelphia: Saunders Co, 1993:193–239.
109. Marzuk PM. Biofeedback for gastrointestinal disorders: a review of the literature. Ann Intern Med 1985; 103:240–245.
110. Shafer RB, Prentiss RA, Bond JH. Gastrointestinal transit in thyroid disease. Gastroenterology 1984; 86:852–857.
111. Chapoy P, Balzing P. Left micro-colon syndrome and hypothyroidism. Gastroenterol Clin Biol 1985; 9:365–368.
112. Gardener EC Jr., Hersh T. Primary hyperparathyroidism and the gastrointestinal tract. South Med J 1981; 74:197–204.
113. Griffiths AM, Mack DR, Byard RW, et al. Multiple endocrine neoplasia IIb: an unusual cause of chronic constipation. J Pediatr 1990; 116:285–287.
114. Nakayama H, Jorgensen HS, Pedersen PM, et al. Prevalence and risk factors of incontinence after stroke. Stroke 1997; 28:58–62.
115. Chia YM, Fowler CJ, Kamm MA, et al. Prevalence of bowel dysfunction in patients with multiple sclerosis and bladder dysfunction. J Neurol 1995; 242:105–108.
116. Hinds JP, Eidelmann BH, Wald A. Prevalence of bowel dysfunction in multiple sclerosis: a population study. Gastroenterology 1990; 98:1538–1542.
117. Waldron DJ, Horgan PG, Patel FR, et al. Multiple sclerosis: assessment of colonic and anorectal function in the presence of fecal incontinence. Int J Colorectal Dis 1993; 8:220–224.
118. Wiesel PH, Norton C, Roy AJ, et al. Gut focussed behavioural therapy (biofeedback) for constipation and fecal incontinence in multiple sclerosis. J Neurol Neu Osurg Psychiatr 2000; 67:240–243.
119. Edwards LL, Pfeiffer RE, Quigley EMM, et al. Gastrointestinal symptoms in Parkinson's disease. Mov Disord 1991; 6:151–156.
120. Stocchi F, Badiali D, Vacca L, et al. Anorectal function in multiple system atrophy and Parkinson's disease. Mov Disord 2000; 15:71–76.
121. Ashraf W, Pfeiffer RF, Quigley EMM, et al. Anorectal manometry in the assessment of anorectal function in Parkinson's disease: a comparison with chronic idiopathic constipation. Mov Disord 1994; 9:655–663.
122. Singaram C, Ashraf W, Gaumintz EA, et al. Dopaminergic defect of enteric nervous system in Parkinson's disease patients with chronic constipation. Lancet 1995; 346:861–864.

123. Albanese A, Maria G, Bentivoglio A, et al. Severe constipation in parkinson's disease relieved by Botulinum toxin. Mov Disord 1997; 12:764–766.

124. Biering-Sorensen F, Pedersen V, Clausen S. Epidemiology of spinal cord lesions in Denmark. Paraplegia 1990; 28:105–111.

125. Kannisto M, Rintala R. Bowel function in adults who have sustained spinal cord injury in childhood. Paraplegia 1995; 33:701–703.

126. Glickmann S, Kamm MA. Bowel dysfunction in spinal cord injury patients. Lancet 1996; 347: 1651–1653.

127. Krogh K, Nielsen J, Djurhuus JC, et al. Colorectal function in patients with spinal cord lesions. Dis Colon Rectum 1997; 40:1233–1239.

128. Stiens SA, Bergman SB, Goetz LL. Neurogenic bowel dysfunction after spinal cord injury: clinical evaluation and rehabilitative management. Arch Phys Med Rehabil 1997; 78:S86-S102.

129. Lie HR, Lagergren J, Rasmussen F, et al. Bowel and bladder control of children with myelomeningocele: a Nordic study. Dev Med Child Neurol 1991; 35:1053–1061.

130. Shandling B, Gilmour RF. The enema continence catheter in spina bifida: successful bowel management. J Pediatr Surg 1987; 22:271–273.

131. Christensen P, Kvitzau B, Krogh K, et al. Neurogenic colorectal dysfunction-use of new antegrade and retrograde wash-out methods. Spinal Cord 2000; 38:255–261.

132. Malone PS, Ransley PG, Kieley EM. Preliminary report: the antegrade continence enema. Lancet 1990; 336:1217–1218.

133. Binnie NR, Smith AN, Creasey GH, et al. Constipation associated with chronic spinal cord injury: the effect of pelvic parasympathetic stimulation by the Brindley stimulator. Paraplegia 1991; 29:436–439.

134. Stone JM, Wolfe VA, Nino-Murcia M, et al. Colostomy as treatment for complications of spinal cord injury. Arch Phys Med Rehabil 1990; 71:514–518.

36 | Medications, Toxins, and the Colon

Chad J. Long
Department of Medicine, University of Chicago Hospitals, University of Chicago Medical Center, Chicago, Illinois, U.S.A.

Eli D. Ehrenpreis
Section of Gastroenterology, Department of Medicine, University of Chicago Hospitals, University of Chicago Medical Center, Chicago, Illinois, U.S.A.

INTRODUCTION

The effects of medications and toxins on the colon range from the developmen t of mild symptoms of diarrhea and constipation to the very serious complications of perforation and toxic megacolon. Although some medications, such as laxatives, are designed to produce specific effects on the colon, the majority of medication-induced alterations of colonic function are unintended. Manifestations of medication and toxin-induced colonic damage predominantly fall into four main categories: histological changes (colitis), ischemic injury, diarrhea, and constipation. This chapter will discuss all major medications and toxins that affect the colon in these ways. Other, less common, forms of medication-induced colonic injury will also be briefly discussed.

COLITIS

Colitis is an inflammatory condition of the large intestine, which is often characterized by severe diarrhea, bleeding, and ulceration of the intestinal mucosa. Many agents cause histological changes suggestive of inflammation in the colon. Antibiotics and occasionally chemotherapeutic agents may produce pseudomembranous enterocolitis, comprehensively presented in the respective chapter(s). Medications have also been linked to lymphocytic and collagenous colitis (Table 1) as well as eosinophilic colitis (Table 2). Comprehensive evaluation of these entities can be found in Chapter on other colitides Chapter 28. Neutropenic enterocolitis, also comprehensively described in Chapter on other colitides Chapter 28, has a well-known relationship with antineoplastic agents but has also been linked to other less familiar medications (Table 3). Even though the classic histological changes of pseudomembranous, microscopic, and neutropenic enterocolitis can result from several medications and toxins, a nonspecific colitis characterized by generalized mucosal inflammation or ulceration is the most commonly elicited drug-induced histological change in the colon. Nonsteroidal anti-inflammatory drugs (NSAIDs) are the most prevalent drug class associated with this form of nonspecific colitis. NSAID-induced colitis as well as nonspecific colitides caused by antineoplastics, gold compounds, penicillin derivatives, and corrosive agents will be reviewed in this section. These and other less common agents associated with the development of nonspecific histological changes in the colon are listed in Table 4.

Nonsteroidal Anti-inflammatory Drugs

NSAIDs are used worldwide among the most commonly prescribed group of medications. The role of these agents in causing gastroduodenal mucosal lesions is well described; however, NSAIDs also produce pathologic changes in the colon. NSAIDs administered via oral and parenteral routes may cause nonspecific bleeding, colitis, colonic ulceration, perforation, and diaphragm-like strictures. Rectal administration of NSAID suppositories is frequently associated with inflammation, ulcers, and strictures of the anus and rectum.

Table 1 Agents Associated with Microscopic Colitis

Agent	Histological colitis
Ranitidine	Lymphocytic
Levodopa/benserazide	
Ticlopidine	
Flavonoid veinotonic agents	
Carbamazepine	
Iron sulfate preparation	
NSAIDs	Collagenous
Cimetidine	
Simvastatin	

Abbreviation: NSAIDs, nonsteroidal anti-inflammatory drugs.

Epidemiology

The prevalence of NSAID-induced colitis is difficult to ascertain. The requirement of endoscopy in examining the gastrointestinal tract, often employed only after the most significant complications of disease becomes clinically apparent, limits much of the literature to case-reports. Idiopathic colonic ulceration not associated with NSAIDs also occurs, so attribution of colonic ulceration to NSAID use, even in its presence, is often presumptive. The few studies designed to investigate the prevalence of NSAID-induced colonic damage have revealed conflicting data. Some studies demonstrate very little increased risk for histological change in the colon (1–3), whereas others document a significant correlation between NSAID use and newly documented colonic inflammation (4,5). An increased risk of colonic perforation has also been linked to NSAID use (6). All classes of NSAIDs have been associated with colitis, but fenemates, indomethacin, and slow-release formulations appear to have the strongest relationship with colonic pathology. NSAIDs with high biliary excretion have been associated with an increased rate of damage to the small intestine in clinical and experimental studies, but this association has not yet been adequately documented in the colon (7–9). The time period from initiation of NSAID use to the development of colitis or ulceration is variable, but review of the literature indicates that 75% of patients with NSAID-induced colonic lesions used NSAIDs for less than one year and 15% took the drugs for less than four weeks (10). NSAID-induced colonic ulceration is thought to be a precursor to stricture formation, and more than one year of drug exposure is usually reported in patients with NSAID-induced diaphragm-like strictures.

Pathogenesis

NSAIDs are believed to exert damage to the colon through both local and systemic effects. Many observations suggest that a local effect of NSAIDs on colonic mucosa plays the predominant role. For example, NSAID pill fragments have been found at the site of colonic strictures, ulcers, and within the peritoneal cavity following perforation (11,12). The majority of ulcerations and strictures associated with NSAIDs appear to occur in the ascending colon. This finding is compatible with a local effect due to topical damage, because the right side of the colon functions as a reservoir. NSAID suppository–induced rectal damage also suggests direct mucosal toxicity of these drugs.

Table 2 Agents Associated with Eosinophilic Colitis

NSAIDs
Carbamazepine
Auranofin
Elemental gold
Gemfibrozil
Trimethoprim–sulphamethoxazole
Methylprednisolone
Cyclosporine
Tacrolimus
Clofazimine
Perazine

Abbreviation: NSAIDs, nonsteroidal anti-inflammatory drugs.

Table 3 Non-antineoplastic Agents Associated
with Neutropenic Enterocolitis

Sulphasalazine
Clozapine
Methimazole
Mianserin

Other evidence supports a systemic mechanism of damage. Right-sided colonic lesions have occurred with intramuscular and rectal routes of NSAID administration (13–15). An NSAID-induced stricture arising in a bypassed ileal segment has also been described (16).

Whichever mechanism predominates, NSAIDs, by local or systemic effects, decrease the integrity of the colonic mucosa and increase its susceptibility to inflammation and injury. The exact mechanisms for these effects are multifactorial and incompletely understood, but appear to result primarily from inhibition of prostaglandin formation. NSAIDs inhibit cyclooxygenase, diverting arachidonic acid metabolism to the lipoxygenase pathway and thereby inhibiting the formation of prostaglandins (Fig. 1). Prostaglandins have been suggested to act in an anti-inflammatory capacity in the large bowel (18). NSAIDs also appear to uncouple mitochondrial oxidative phosphorylation, which reduces enterocyte adenosinetriphosphate (ATP) levels and results in the loss of control of the intercellular junctions and an increase in bowel permeability (19). NSAID-induced disruption of the microcirculation, as observed in gastric mucosa, may also be involved (20). Leukocyte adhesion in the setting of decreased prostaglandins may play a role in colonic injury, as well. NSAID use can result in elevated catecholamine levels, normally suppressed by prostaglandins, which may lead to granulocyte activation, free radical and superoxide production, and resultant colonic injury (21). Aspirin has been shown to promote leukocyte–endothelial cell adhesion in the microvasculature of rat mesenteric venules, and administration of a monoclonal antibody against leukocyte–adhesion glycoprotein has been shown to be protective against indomethacin-induced mucosal injury in rabbits (22,23). Another animal study has shown a direct correlation between the number of circulating neutrophils and the severity of NSAID-induced mucosal damage (24).

Clinical Symptoms

Clinical manifestations of NSAID-induced colitis are variable. With nonspecific colitis or ulceration, patients may be asymptomatic but can present with bloody or nonbloody diarrhea, weight loss, fatigue, abdominal pain, or anorexia. Obstructive symptoms can be associated with NSAID-induced diaphragm-like strictures. NSAID suppositories may cause proctalgia, tenesmus, watery or bloody diarrhea, or fecal incontinence.

Diagnosis

Diagnosis of NSAID-induced colitis is based on a history of NSAID use, clinical symptoms, laboratory studies, endoscopic visualization, and histological findings. Laboratory findings can be unremarkable or reflect low-grade blood or protein loss. Lesions are frequently not appreciated on barium enema, as radiological findings are often subtle or undetectable. Single or multiple frank ulcerations are the most common finding on colonoscopy (Fig. 2) (25), but generalized inflammation, diffuse ulcerations that may mimic inflammatory bowel disease,

Table 4 Agents Associated with Nonspecific Colitis

NSAIDs
Antineoplastics
Elemental gold
Auranofin
Penicillin derivatives
Cyclosporine
Methyldopa
Isotretinoin
Penicillamine
Flucytosine

Abbreviation: NSAIDs, nonsteroidal anti-inflammatory drugs.

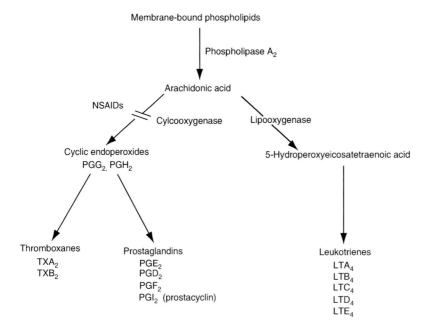

Figure 1 Effect of nonsteroidal anti-inflammatory drugs on arachidonic acid metabolism. *Source*: From Ref. 17.

or diaphragm-like strictures may also be seen (9). The right side of the colon is the most common site of ulceration and stricture. Pathological examination of NSAID-induced ulcerations reveals well-demarcated superficial ulcerations with overlying fibrosis and normal mucosa surrounding the lesion (26). An increase in lymphocytes in the lamina propria and epithelium, with an associated elevation in apoptic cells, may have some value for the histological diagnosis of lesions caused by NSAIDs (27). Diaphragm-like strictures are pathognomonic for NSAID-induced pathology. These are generally multiple (3–70), thin (2–4 mm), concentric, septate-like mucosal projections that can narrow the colonic lumen to 0.1–2 cm (Fig. 3) (28).

Treatment and Prognosis

Discontinuation of NSAIDs is the treatment of choice in those with NSAID-induced colonic injury. For individuals who require NSAID therapy, finding the minimum acceptable dose and avoiding fenemates, indomethacin, and sustained-release formulations is recommended. Treatment with prostaglandins, sulphasalazine, and metronidazole has not shown utility in reliable clinical trials. Prodrugs, such as sulindac, have also failed to show benefit and have been implicated in NSAID-induced colitis (29,30). To date, there have been only limited

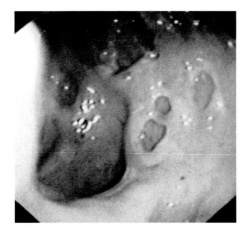

Figure 2 Nonsteroidal anti-inflammatory drug–induced colonic ulcerations. *Source*: From Ref. 25.

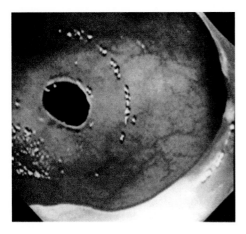

Figure 3 Endoscopic appearance of diaphragm-like stricture with pinhole lumen. *Source:* From Ref. 28.

studies to address colonic safety profiles of cyclooxygenase (COX)-2 selective agents. Experimental studies indicate that COX-2 plays a dominant role in the healing of preexisting colitis, and its inhibition may result in colitis exacerbation (Section "NSAIDs and Inflammatory Bowel Disease" for complete discussion). Some animal studies testing COX-2 selective agents, however, do not seem to find an increased risk of colitis with this medication class (31,32). A small retrospective clinical study has demonstrated some promise for the tolerability of COX-2 inhibitors in inflammatory bowel disease (IBD) patients (33), but episodes of acute colitis in non-IBD patients have been associated with these drugs (34,35). Further studies will be required to define the safety of COX-2 inhibitors on the normal and inflammatory bowel-diseased colon.

Upon discontinuation of NSAIDs, symptoms usually cease within days to weeks with accompanying restoration of normal histology. If symptoms and histology do not normalize, other etiologies, especially inflammatory bowel disease or ischemic colitis, should be considered. Discontinuation of NSAIDs is not believed to reverse diaphragm-like stricture formation. Reduction of diaphragm-like strictures is not always necessary in the absence of obstructive symptoms, but endoscopic dilation with a balloon dilator has been used to alleviate symptomatic strictures (30). Surgical management of NSAID-induced colonic strictures requires segmental colonic resection. The resection may be followed by primary anastomosis with or without a proximal diverting stoma or a Hartmann's procedure. Anorectal stenoses occurring from NSAID suppositories may warrant dilations, whereas perforation or severe hemorrhage secondary to ulceration obviously warrants surgical intervention, usually primary repair.

NSAIDs and Preexisting Disease
NSAIDs and IBD

Initially, NSAIDs were believed to hold a therapeutic role in patients with ulcerative colitis because the diseased mucosa produces increased amounts of prostaglandins. Subsequent cases, however, have linked the use of NSAIDs with inflammatory bowel disease exacerbations and an increased risk of emergency hospital admissions for IBD-associated colitis (36). Reactivation of IBD following NSAID intake ranges from hours to weeks (37). NSAID-induced injury in IBD is multifactorial and related to the general mechanisms of injury discussed above. COX-2, however, seems to play the dominant role in the repair of preexisting colitis, and its inhibition may be paramount in NSAID-induced IBD exacerbation.

NSAIDs are known to inhibit COX-1 and COX-2 isoforms of cyclooxygenase (Fig. 1). Prostaglandins derived from COX-1 were initially believed to be solely responsible for maintenance of gastrointestinal mucosal integrity, and prostaglandins produced in the context of inflammation were thought to be derived exclusively from COX-2. It is now apparent that this hypothesis is an oversimplification and considerable evidence suggests that prostaglandins from COX-2 contribute to gastrointestinal mucosal defense and prostaglandins from COX-1 play a role in inflammatory response and pain. In patients with a preexisting colitis, however,

COX-2 seems to be the more important isoform for natural repair and damage control. In humans and animal models, COX-2 expression in the normal colon is at low levels (7,38). In the presence of human IBD exacerbation or experimental colitis, there is a marked up-regulation of COX-2 expression with little change in the expression of COX-1 (7,38). Prostaglandins produced by the inflamed colon are also derived predominantly from COX-2 (7). COX-2 function has been shown to be essential for the healing of experimental colitis (7,38), and animal models that lack a functional gene for COX-2 exhibit significantly worse colitis than normal animals (39). Therefore, the mechanisms by which NSAIDs exacerbate colitis in IBD appear to be predominantly by compromise of COX-2–mediated repair.

NSAIDs and Diverticular Disease

The relationship between NSAID use and the development of bleeding, perforation, and fistula formation from diverticular disease is well established. Patients admitted with complications of diverticular disease have a significantly higher incidence of NSAID use. In one controlled prospective study, individuals presenting with complications of diverticular disease were more than twice as likely to be consuming NSAIDS than age- and gender-matched controls (40). Diverticular perforations have been reported to be three times more common in individuals taking NSAIDs (41).

It is unclear whether the predisposition toward diverticular complications with NSAID use is identical to the mechanisms of de novo damage or whether there is a more specific pathophysiology. It is possible that inhibition of cyclooxygenase by NSAIDs reduces the concentration of mucosal prostaglandins in diverticula, predisposing them to inflammation and perforation. COX-2–related inflammatory response might also have an important role. In one animal study, COX-2 inhibition led to inflammation-associated colonic injury and perforation (7). The possible link between NSAIDs and decreased inflammatory response with diverticular perforation is supported by evidence that immunosuppression also contributes to perforation. Patients receiving steroids, immunosuppressives after organ transplantation, and patients with acquired immune deficiency syndromes have an increased risk of perforated diverticular disease (42–45). Perforation in these immunocompromised patients is generally best treated by resection and fecal diversion. Laparoscopic colectomy may be the best option to limit further compromise to the immune system. Platelet dysfunction secondary to NSAID use also likely plays a role in the increased diverticular bleeding seen in patients consuming these medications.

Antineoplastics

The rapidly dividing cells of the gastrointestinal epithelium are especially susceptible to the toxic effects of cancer chemotherapeutic agents. Almost all classes of antineoplastics may contribute to gastrointestinal mucosal damage. Antimetabolites, such as cytosine arabinoside and methotrexate, have a particularly strong association with colonic damage, as does 5-fluorouracil, which is a fluorinated pyrimidine. Colonic ulceration has been demonstrated in up to 70% of patients receiving combination cytosine arabinoside therapy (46). The pathogenesis of damage is multifactorial and includes direct epithelial injury by chemotherapeutic agents, invasion of the mucosa by intestinal pathogens, and ischemic injury (46–48). Clinical symptoms may include abdominal pain, fever, and bloody or nonbloody diarrhea. Mucosal damage ranges from mild segmental colitis to fulminant ulcerative colitis and toxic megacolon. Antineoplastics also alter normal bowel flora and may predispose to *Clostridium difficile* infection (analyzed in Chapter 13 "Pseudomembranous Colitis"). Chemotherapy-induced agranulocytosis is a risk factor for the development of neutropenic enterocolitis (presented in Chapter 28 "Other Colitides").

Gold

For many years, elemental gold has been used for the treatment of rheumatoid arthritis. Colitis associated with gold therapy is a rare but well-described and dangerous complication that may progress to fulminant enterocolitis and toxic megacolon. Gold-induced enterocolitis has been associated with several different preparations of gold salts in both parenteral and oral formulation. At least five different gold salts have been incriminated (49). For this reason, elemental gold is believed to be the toxigenic agent responsible for the reaction rather than any other moiety. Gold toxicity is likely to be a hypersensitivity reaction, as it occurs relatively early in therapy and is seen after low-dose administration. Most described cases have occurred within 10 weeks of starting gold therapy, usually with less than a total dose of 500 mg of the chosen preparation. Temporary development of circulating immune complexes has also been observed in relationship to the onset of enterocolitis during gold therapy (50). Gold-induced eosinophilic colitis has reportedly responded to cromolyn therapy, further suggesting an allergic etiology of the process (51). Severe watery diarrhea, which is frequently bloody, heralds the onset of this reaction. Fever, skin rash, vomiting, and abdominal pain are often part of the presentation. The reaction typically occurs within three months of instituting gold therapy.

Diagnosis is based on the temporal association with gold therapy, clinical symptoms, laboratory studies, and colonoscopic findings. Gold-associated enterocolitis should be suspected in a patient with acute diarrhea, negative stool cultures, and gold administration in the past three months. Serum eosinophilia is often, but not universally, present (52). Differentiating between the mild and self-limited diarrhea due to Na^+-K^+ ATPase inhibition that commonly occurs in patients on oral therapy is important, as this mild diarrhea can be treated with reduction of dose or temporary discontinuation. Diffuse injury involving the entire gastrointestinal tract is common, and histological examination reveals nonspecific inflammatory changes. An early transient eosinophilic infiltration has also been described on histological examination (49).

The clinical course of gold-induced enterocolitis is generally prolonged and frequently complicated by hypoproteinemia and bacterial sepsis. Therapy is directed toward nutritional, antibiotic, and fluid support. Systemic corticosteroids have been used but their efficacy is unproven. The initially reported mortality for gold-induced enterocolitis was about 25%, but this percentage has decreased in recent years (49).

Antibiotic-Associated Hemorrhagic Colitis

Antibiotic-associated hemorrhagic colitis is a rare, self-limited process that may be experienced by patients receiving oral penicillin derivatives; no report of this entity has been described in any patient receiving intravenous or intramuscular drugs. The etiology of antibiotic-associated hemorrhagic colitis is unknown as *C. difficile* toxins and pseudomembranes are absent. Some clinicians postulate that a hypersensitivity reaction may be responsible. The colitis occurs independently of dosage and is most commonly described in those being treated for upper respiratory tract infections, with approximately 70% of patients reported in the literature receiving treatment for upper respiratory tract infections (53). An unidentified pathogen from the respiratory tract may interact with a penicillin derivative, or perhaps a specific toxic reaction to a structural component of penicillin occurs. Though originally thought to be associated exclusively with penicillin derivatives, a recent report has linked quinolones to a late-onset form of this colitis (54).

Penicillin-related hemorrhagic colitis presents with bloody diarrhea and a predominantly right-sided colitis. Symptoms usually begin within two to seven days of antibiotic use. Lower abdominal pain with loose stools is subsequently followed within hours by hematochezia. Laboratory and stool studies are usually normal. Barium enema features include spasm, "thumbprinting," luminal narrowing, loss of haustral markings, and punctuate ulceration (55). Colonoscopic findings include mucosal hemorrhage, aphthous ulcers, friability, edema, and spasm (55). Histological findings include an increase in subepithelial erythrocytes, edema, desquamation of surface epithelium, and inflammatory changes (55).

Bloody diarrhea with negative stool studies and negative *C. difficile* testing in a patient receiving oral penicillin derivatives is consistent with antibiotic-associated hemorrhagic colitis. Neither barium enema nor colonoscopy is indicated for diagnosis if a close correlation exists under stable patient conditions. The condition is self-limited and resolves spontaneously within a few days of discontinuation of the offending antibiotic. Symptoms persisting more than a few days after antibiotic discontinuation warrant a more thorough and invasive evaluation.

Corrosive Colitis

The oral administration of corrosives is a well-recognized source of damage in the esophagus and upper gastrointestinal tract and while colonic toxicity may occur less commonly, multiple case-reports of corrosive colitis have been described in the literature. Colitis has reportedly occurred due to intrarectally administered medications, contrast materials, detergents, illicit drugs, acids, bases, and other substances. Detergent enemas, water-soluble contrast media,

Table 5 Agents Associated with Corrosive Colitis

Detergent enemas
Hydrogen peroxide enemas and cleansing solutions
Hyperosmolar water-soluble contrast media
Acetic acid
Ethyl alcohol
Ergotamine
Herbal enemas
Sodium hydroxide
Hydrofluoric acid
Chloro-*m*-xylenol
Potassium permanganate

and hydrogen peroxide enemas and cleansing solutions have been the agents most often associated with corrosive colitis. These agents and others documented to cause corrosive colitis are listed in Table 5.

The clinical presentation is most dependent upon the toxin, concentration, exposure duration, and presence of preexisting colonic disease. Symptoms often include fever, abdominal pain, nonbloody or bloody diarrhea, tenesmus, and rectal tenderness. Leukocytosis is common and endoscopic findings of mucosal edema, erythema, friability, ulceration, and stenosis are often present. Pathology may show inflammation, neutrophilic infiltration, edema, submucosal fibrosis, ulceration, necrosis, or infarction. Treatment is primarily supportive with bowel rest, intravenous fluids, and antibiotics, if indicated. Emergent laparotomy is indicated for obstructing strictures, necrotic bowel, and perforation. Resection with fecal diversion may be the most prudent option in these patients.

ISCHEMIC COLITIS

Ischemic colitis is one of the most serious side effects that can result from medications and toxins. Though associated mainly with agents having vasoconstrictive or vasospastic properties, drugs that decrease splanchnic blood flow via systemic hypotension, vasculitis, induced thrombosis, and increased intracolic pressures (through constipation or an enema) have also been linked to colonic ischemia. Other medications have been associated with ischemic colitis, though their mechanism of action has yet to be determined. Table 6 lists medications that have been associated with ischemic colitis and their proposed mechanism of ischemia.

The clinical symptoms, laboratory findings, and imaging of medication and toxin-related ischemic colitis parallel cases of ischemic colitis not associated with these agents. Clinical evaluation may be difficult in overdose situations in which a patient may be comatose and reporting no abdominal symptoms. Other findings may be specific to nongastrointestinal side effects of the offending agent including cocaine, ergotamine derivatives, and amphetamines. Diagnosis depends on history, symptoms, examination, and relationship with an offending agent. Discontinuation of the inciting agent and medical management is generally warranted. Surgical resection is required in patients with fulminant ischemic colitis or subsequent colonic strictures. Elective resection with primary anastomosis is usually preferred for surgical treatment of strictures. Ischemic colitis generally requires a subtotal colectomy with an end Brooke ileostomy and either a rectosigmoid mucus fistula or a rectal Hartmann's pouch. Patients with lesser degrees of ischemia respond to conservative medical management including intravenous fluid therapy and bowel rest (see full discussion in Chapter 14 "Colon Ischemia").

DRUG-INDUCED DIARRHEA

Agents that induce diarrhea by affecting the colon do so via augmentation of fluid and electrolyte secretion, alteration of normal intestinal flora and/or bile acid metabolism, and by enhancement of colonic motility.

Secretory Diarrhea

Agents that induce secretory diarrhea generally have dual effects on the small intestine and colon. In many cases, the primary site of excess fluid and electrolyte secretion is the small

Table 6 Agents Associated with Ischemic Colitis

Agent	Mechanism
Vasopressin analogues	Vasoconstriction/vasospasm
Cardiac glycosides	
Pseudoephedrine	
Ergot derivatives	
Cocaine	
Amphetamines	
NSAIDs	
Alosetron	
Sumatriptan	
Cyclosporine	
ACE inhibitors	Systemic hypotension
Beta blockers	
Interleukin-2	
Phenobarbitol	
Antipsychotics	
Tricyclic antidepressants	
Amphetamines	Vasculitis
Gold compounds	
Oral contraceptives	Thrombotic lesion induction
Progestational agents	
Danazol	Increased intracolic pressure
Alosetron	
Glycerin enemas	
Flutamide	Undetermined
Mycophenolate mofetil	
Interferon-alpha	
Paclitaxel	
Hyperosmotic saline laxatives	

Abbreviations: NSAIDs, nonsteroidal anti-inflammatory drugs;
ACE, angiotensin-converting enzyme.

intestine; the absorptive function of the colon is then subsequently overwhelmed. Direct pharmacological effects of drugs on the colon may also become clinically relevant when incomplete absorption occurs in the small intestine. With these considerations, all medications included in this section have been documented to exert a specific direct effect on the colon. Agents that can cause colonic secretory diarrhea include those substances that activate adenylate cyclase and those compounds which inhibit the Na^+–K^+ exchange pump.

Activation of Adenylate Cyclase

Certain drugs bind specific receptors on the mucosal cells of the small and large intestine and impair fluid absorption by activating adenylate cyclase, which increases cyclic AMP levels. This results in active secretion of Cl^- and HCO_3^-, passive efflux of Na^+, K^+, and water, and inhibition of Na^+ and Cl^- entry into the enterocyte. Prostaglandins of the E series are known to stimulate intestinal water and electrolyte secretion chiefly through this mechanism. Ricinoleic acid also causes cyclic AMP–mediated intestinal fluid secretion (56). Many stimulant laxatives have been reported to increase the colonic formation of prostaglandins and could directly and indirectly work through this mechanism. Adenylate cyclase–mediated diarrhea is dose dependent and can usually be treated with dosage reduction.

Inhibition of the Na^+–K^+ Exchange Pump

Drugs can cause diarrhea by inhibiting the ileal and colonic Na^+–K^+ exchange pump that regulates intraluminal transport of water and electrolytes, leading to decreased fluid absorption and net secretion. The concentration-dependent inhibition of colonic Na^+–K^+ ATPase usually occurs in the setting of high doses that escape ileal absorption. Agents known to affect the colon in this manner are listed in Table 7.

Alteration of Normal Intestinal Flora and/or Bile Acid Metabolism

Diarrhea can result from alterations of normal intestinal flora and/or bile acid deconjugation, absorption, transport, and binding. In animal models, olsalazine inhibits ileal bile acid

Table 7 Agents that Inhibit the Na$^+$–K$^+$ Exchange Pump

Digoxin
Auranofin
Colchicine
Olsalazine
Sulfasalazine
Mesalazine
Chenodeoxylic acid

transport, resulting in excess bile acids reaching the colon and a bile acid–induced diarrhea (57). Although the primary cause of antineoplastic-associated diarrhea involves changes in the absorptive and secretory function of the small intestine, antineoplastics also alter the normal microflora of the colon that may augment diarrhea caused by other mechanisms. Antibiotics represent the most common agent associated with diarrhea resulting from alteration of the normal microflora and/or bile acid metabolism.

Antibiotics

Antibiotics are responsible for the greatest percentage of drug-induced diarrhea, and antibiotic-associated diarrhea may occur in 5% to 25% of those receiving antibiotics (58). Although pseudomembranous enterocolitis is its most serious form, only 10% to 20% of cases of antibiotic-associated diarrhea are caused by infection with *C. difficile* (58–60). Most cases of antibiotic-associated diarrhea are due to functional disturbances of intestinal carbohydrate or bile acid metabolism. Nearly all antibiotics can cause diarrhea, but antibiotics with broad-spectrum coverage, poor intestinal absorption, and high biliary excretion pose the greatest risk. In general, antibiotic-associated diarrhea is more common with oral drugs than with parenteral agents, with the exception of drugs excreted in the bile. The antibiotics reported to produce the highest incidence of diarrhea are the aminopenicillins, combinations of amoxicillin and clavulanic acid, cephalosporins, and clindamycin (58).

Antibiotic-associated alteration of the normal intestinal flora can result in impaired fermentation of poorly absorbed carbohydrates, leading to osmotic diarrhea and the reduced production of short-chain fatty acids (SCFAs) that normally enhance the colonic absorption of fluid (61,62). Decreased bacterial carbohydrate metabolism due to antibiotics may also result in functional disturbances of the colonic mucosa. In the distal colon, the SCFA *n*-butyrate is an important source of energy for the mucosa through cellular oxidation (63,64). Reduction in SCFA production via diminished digestion of carbohydrates normally metabolized by colonic bacteria may deprive the colonic mucosa of an energy source, as demonstrated by the clinical model of "diversion colitis" (65).

Primary bile acids that escape absorption in the small bowel are deconjugated and then dehydroxylated to secondary bile acids by bacteria in the colon (66). Dihydroxy bile acids, such as the primary bile acid chenodeoxycholic acid and the secondary bile acid deoxycholic acid, are potent colonic secretory agents and their presence in the colon results in secretory diarrhea (67,68). The effects of antibiotics in decreasing carbohydrate metabolism and dehydroxylation of bile acids may be synergistic because a decrease in carbohydrate metabolism results in higher fecal pH, which increases the solubility of dihydroxy bile acids (66,68).

Discontinuation of the offending antibiotic usually leads to rapid resolution of antibiotic-associated diarrhea. *C. difficile*-associated diarrhea might not respond in this manner. Although, conceptually, the use of probiotics to replenish the colonic microflora for prevention of symptoms caused by antibiotic disruption of the normal flora seems promising, there are only limited clinical data to support probiotic use in clinical practice.

Enhancement of Neuromuscular Motility

Agents may cause diarrhea by enhancement of gastrointestinal motility through direct action on either the smooth muscle or the myenteric nervous system. Agents may also increase motility by antagonizing the effects of inhibitory agents. Medications and toxins that exert these effects on the colon are listed in Table 8.

Table 8 Agents Associated with Neuromuscular-Induced Diarrhea

Agent	Mechanism
Erythromycin	Motilin-receptor agonist
Cisapride	5-HT4 receptor agonist
Metoclopramide	Dopamine D2 receptor antagonist
	5-HT4 receptor agonist
Opiate antagonists	Mu-receptor antagonist
Somatostatin analogs	Blocked release of VIP and substance P
Irinotecan	Cholinesterase inhibition
Tacrine	
Carbamates	
Huperzine A	

Abbreviations: HT, hydroxytryptamine; VIP, vasoactive intestinal peptide.

LAXATIVES

Laxatives are an important group of medications and, unlike other agents mentioned in this chapter, are intended for action on the colon. Nevertheless, unintentional effects of these agents on the colon are numerous. Stimulant laxatives, osmotic laxatives, lubricants, and bulk laxatives will be addressed in this section.

Stimulant Laxatives

Stimulant laxatives, more than any other class of laxative, have been associated with pathological effects on the colon. Stimulant laxatives have been demonstrated to induce histological, neuronal, anatomical, and radiographic changes in the colon. Electrolyte abnormalities may be associated with stimulant laxative use. A relationship between stimulant laxative use and colonic neoplasia has also been proposed.

Stimulant laxatives include diphenylmethane derivatives (phenolphthalein, bisacodyl, and sodium picosulfate), anthraquinones (senna and cascara), ricinoleic acid (castor oil), and surface-acting agents (docusates). These compounds facilitate evacuation through acceleration of bowel transit and an augmentation of epithelial transport of water and electrolytes, though the precise mechanisms of actions are incompletely known (69). Several mechanisms of action appear to occur simultaneously. Stimulant laxatives increase the colonic formation of histamine, serotonin, and prostaglandins, potential mediators of increased colonic secretions associated with these drugs. Like other drugs that produce diarrhea, stimulant laxatives also activate adenylate cyclase and inhibit Na^+–K^+ ATPase. Furthermore, colonic motility is augmented by every class of stimulant laxative.

Histological Alterations Associated with Stimulant Laxatives

Long-term use of stimulant laxatives has been linked to changes in both the myenteric plexus and the colonic smooth muscle. Electron microscopic studies have shown ballooning of axons, reduction of whole nerve-specific cell structures, and degeneration of nerve fibers (70–72). In the colonocytes of individuals taking stimulant laxatives, a change in microvilli, mitochondrial damage, and increased lysosomes have been reported (72–74). Intracellular space widening and colonocytic granular inclusions have also been observed (72,75). Similar findings have been reported in patients with diabetic autonomic neuropathy and chronic inflammatory bowel disease and may not be specific to stimulant laxative use (71). Other studies have not supported the deleterious effect that stimulant laxatives might have on the ultrastructure of colonic nerves (76). Some reports propose that these ultrastructural findings might be the changes associated with the condition of constipation, rather than a direct effect of stimulant laxatives (77). The clinical significance of the nervous system and cellular changes associated with stimulant laxative use are unknown.

Pseudomelanosis coli

Pseudomelanosis coli (or melanosis coli) is a discoloration of the colonic mucosa due to pigment-laden macrophages within the submucosa of colonocytes (Fig. 4) (78). It is commonly associated with chronic use of stimulant laxatives, especially anthraquinones, and was first

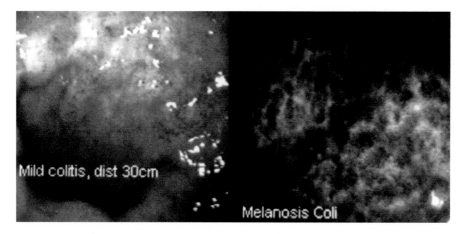

Figure 4 Colonoscopic view of melanosis coli associated with the chronic use of stimulant laxatives. There is little or no pseudomelanin pigment in the distal 30 cm of colon in the presence of active mild colitis (*left*), in contrast to the heavy pigmentation in the remaining colon (*right*). *Source*: From Ref. 78.

described in 1830 (79). Anthraquinones exert direct toxic effects on colonic mucosa, which can facilitate the infiltration of inflammatory cells and the formation of apoptic bodies in the tissue. Increased numbers of apoptotic bodies have been found in the surface epithelium and lamina propria in pseudomelanosis coli (80). It is thought that the precursors of the melenic substance are derived from anthranoid free radicals (81,82). Pigment formation is caused by the degradation of apoptotic bodies of colonic epithelial cells within macrophages. Though the nature and composition of pigments may vary with location in the gastrointestinal tract, the pigment granules seem to have similarities with lipofuscin, ceroids, and melanin (82). A majority of patients with long-term anthraquinone laxative use will exhibit melanosis coli. Pigment changes can occur in any part of the gastrointestinal tract, but it is more common in the proximal colon (83). One study showed that "melanosis" seems to appear within an average time of nine months following laxative initiation. Resolution of pigment changes after withdrawal of anthraquinones occurs in approximately nine months, as well (84). The clinical significance of pseudomelanosis coli is uncertain, but it appears to be a benign finding. Though concern for a relationship between pseudomelanosis coli and colorectal neoplasm has been proposed based on the findings of a retrospective/prospective study (85), subsequent prospective case–control studies fail to document this association (86).

Cathartic Colon

Cathartic colon is a historic radiological term, based on barium enema features such as loss of haustration, colonic dilatation, colonic redundancy, and gaping of the ileocecal valve (Fig. 5) (87). These findings have been related exclusively to long-term stimulant laxative abuse, especially anthraquinones, historically in female laxative abusers. The precise mechanism is unknown and reversal of these features can occur after discontinuation of stimulant laxative use (88). Pathologic changes in resected specimens of cathartic colon include mucosal atrophy, inflammation, thickening of the muscularis mucosa, and fibrosis. Although the existence of cathartic colon as a true entity has been questioned secondarily to an absence of recent description in the medical literature (89), subsequent publications have documented an association with stimulant laxatives and radiographic changes consistent with the cathartic colon (87).

Stimulant Laxatives and Neoplasm

The relationship between stimulant laxatives, especially anthraquinones, and neoplasm is controversial. In vitro studies indicate that stimulant laxatives have genotoxic and mutagenic effects (90–95). Anthraquinones have been shown to be mutagenic in malignant mammalian cell lines; however, they do not appear to affect normal colorectal epithelial cells in vitro (96,97). Stimulant laxatives have been shown to be carcinogenic in animal studies and may

(A)   **(B)**

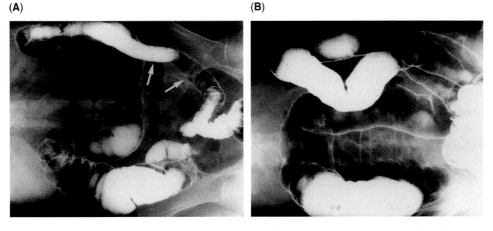

Figure 5 Loss of haustra seen on barium enema in two patients who were chronic stimulant laxative users. Haustral loss is seen in the left colon (**A**) in one patient and throughout the colon (**B**) in the other. *Source*: From Ref. 87.

act as tumor promoters (98,99). Senna and its extracts do not appear to be carcinogenic alone at concentrations that produce mild laxative effects, but are associated with premalignant lesions when given at high doses in combination with other mutagens (100,101).

Human studies have demonstrated that anthranoid exposure causes mucosal cell loss by apoptosis, increased cell proliferation, and inhibition of restoration of normal cellularity (102,103). However, the results of large epidemiologic studies evaluating the possible carcinogenic effects of stimulant laxative use in humans have been inconclusive (86,104–108). Further research will be necessary to conclusively demonstrate whether a link between stimulant laxative use and colorectal neoplasia exists.

Osmotic Laxatives

Osmotic laxatives include salts of poorly absorbable cations (magnesium); anions (phosphate, sulfate); molecules that are not absorbed in the small bowel but metabolized in the colon, such as sorbitol and lactulose; and metabolically inert compounds such as polyethylene glycol. The presence of these molecules in the lumen results in water retention. Sorbitol-containing elixirs, alpha glucosidase inhibitors, magnesium-containing antacids, and tube feeding can also result in diarrhea via osmotic effects. Side effects of these agents are predominantly related to metabolic disturbances resulting from excessive ion absorption. Hypermagnesemia, hyperphosphatemia, and hypernatremia have all been reported with the use of osmotic laxatives. Hypokalemia may be caused by these agents as loss of potassium in watery feces is aggravated by secretion of aldosterone following laxative-induced volume depletion (109). These agents should be used very cautiously in patients with renal impairment. A few reports have also linked the use of osmotic laxatives with hypoalbuminemia (110,111). Additional risk factors for complications from osmotic laxatives include ileus and bowel obstruction.

Lubricants

Liquid paraffin, or mineral oil, is the major lubricant laxative. Seed oils of arachis and croton are also included in this class. Lubricants can be given orally or rectally and decrease water absorption leading to softer stools and easier defecation. Lubricants are not chemically active and rarely have systemic side effects, though aspiration can result in lipoid pneumonia. The unpleasant side effect of oily rectal discharge is also frequently reported by patients on these agents.

Bulking Agents

Bulk laxatives include dietary or processed natural fibers such as bran and psyllium, synthetic polymers such as calcium polycarbophil, and chemically modified cellulose (methycellulose).

These organic polymers increase intraluminal volume via water retention and decrease stool transit time through the colon. Once subjected to bacterial fermentation in the colon, some of these agents produce SCFAs that may also increase luminal osmolarity and water retention, potentiating their laxative effect. Complications rarely occur from this class of laxative, but colonic obstruction and perforation have been reported after bulk laxative use (112,113). Life-threatening anaphylaxis has been reported after ingestion of psyllium-containing laxatives (114).

DRUG-INDUCED CONSTIPATION

Drug-induced constipation is most commonly due to changes in neuromuscular function. Thus, drugs that induce constipation predominantly affect the autonomic nervous system or smooth muscle function.

Anticholinergics

Cholinergic muscarinic receptors mediate smooth-muscle tone, amplitude of contractions, and peristaltic activity of the bowel. The colonic hypomotility that results from atropine-like effects of drugs makes constipation a common effect of anticholinergic drugs. Anticholinergic drugs elicit their effects by directly altering cholinergic function in the gut. Many medications, including antispasmodics, neuroleptics, anti-Parkinsonian medications, antidepressants, antipsychotics, and antihistamines, have anticholinergic properties.

Opioids

Opioids act centrally and peripherally on Mu, Kappa, and Delta receptors. Opioid agonism of the Mu receptor in the myenteric plexus is most responsible for the decreased gastrointestinal motility seen with opioid use. Opioids act to cause an increase in colonic tone while decreasing the frequency of propulsive peristaltic waves. Overall, opioids cause a disorganized pattern of contractions in the small and large bowel. Decreased colonic peristalsis subsequently causes an increase in the amount of time that intestinal contents are exposed to the mucosal lining, thus allowing for more absorption of water and sodium. Opioid-induced constipation is dose dependent and coadministration of laxatives is currently the mainstay of treatment. Methylnaltrexone, a peripheral opioid antagonist, has been investigated for reversal of opioid-induced constipation. This modified agent does not cross the blood–brain barrier so that analgesia is maintained, whereas inhibition of opioid effects in the myenteric plexus occurs (115,116). Naloxone, which undergoes extensive first-pass metabolism, also has minimal central effects and has been reported to be efficacious in the reversal of opioid-induced constipation (117).

Calcium Channel Antagonists

Calcium channel antagonists are potent inhibitors of intestinal smooth muscle contractility. Extracellular calcium is required for the contraction of colonic smooth muscle and for the generation of colonic slow waves (118,119). Impairment of peristaltic activity results from blockade of both neuronal and muscular calcium channels (120). Drug-sensitive calcium channels are likely to be present on neurons of the enteric plexuses and are involved in the modulation of both acetylcholine release and nonadrenergic, noncholinergic-mediated neuronal inhibition (120). Calcium channel antagonists also bind to high-affinity calcium channel sites on smooth muscle membranes and reduce contractile activity by blocking the influx of calcium (121–123). Individual calcium channel antagonists show different nervous-muscular activity properties.

Vinca Alkaloids

Although antineoplastic agents cause diarrhea predominantly by effects on the small intestine, they may also damage large intestinal smooth muscle cells and inhibit neuromuscular transmission to such an extent that constipation can result. Vinca alkaloids associated with constipation include vincristine, vindesine, vinblastine, bleomycin, and cytosine-arabinoside.

Clonidine

Constipation is a commonly described side effect of clonidine. Clonidine impairs the release of noradrenaline by stimulating presynaptic noradrenergic receptors. This results in the inhibition of propulsive peristalsis by decreasing acetylcholine release.

Stercoral Ulceration

Stercoral ulceration, a defect in the colonic wall caused by pressure necrosis and an inflammatory response to impacted feces, is a rare cause of rectal bleeding, obstruction, and, rarely, spontaneous perforation of the colon. A variety of potentially constipating medications have been associated with stercoral ulceration including tricyclic antidepressants (124), aluminum-based antacids (125), opioids (126,127), and NSAIDs (128). NSAIDs are thought to contribute to stercoral ulceration, secondarily to decreased prostaglandin cytoprotection and resultant compromise of intestinal integrity. Peritonitis and need for emergent laparotomy secondary to perforation is the most serious consequence of stercoral ulceration. Resection with either stoma construction or primary anastomosis with or without proximal fecal diversion is generally the selected surgical management.

OTHER DRUG EFFECTS ON THE COLON
Colonic Bezoar

Bezoars are most commonly associated with ingestion of foods that contain large amounts of nondigestible dietary fiber. Bezoars composed of concretions of medications have also been described. Although bezoars are most common in the stomach, they have occasionally been implicated as causes of colonic obstruction. Patients taking resin-coated extended-release medications designed to resist digestion in the stomach appear to be particularly at risk (129). Colonic bezoar formation has been associated with the use of calcium channel antagonists (129,130), vitamins (131), cholestyramine (132), and psyllium seed husks (133). The majority of patients have predisposing factors that contribute to bezoar formation including altered gastrointestinal anatomy from prior surgery, altered intestinal motility secondary to diabetes or Parkinson's disease, or the concurrent use of medications which diminish intestinal motility. Colonic bezoars may be asymptomatic. Symptoms develop if progression to obstruction occurs. Occasionally, toxic concentrations of medications, such as NSAIDS, can be locally released at the bezoar site potentially causing inflammation, ulceration, or perforation. Diagnosis of bezoars of the lower gastrointestinal tract may be clinically challenging. Radiologic studies may be useful but are often inconclusive. Colonic bezoars often require colectomy for removal, but the administration of clear fluids, colonic lavage, enemas, or colonoscopy may be useful in select cases. If surgery is required, then laparoscopic procedures such as colectomy or resection with primary repair or anastomosis, respectively, may be indicated.

Colonic Pseudo-Obstruction

Colonic pseudo-obstruction is a clinical syndrome in which a patient experiences signs and symptoms of colonic obstruction without an actual anatomical obstructing lesion (see Chapter 21 "Pseudo-obstruction"). Acute colonic pseudo-obstruction has been described with multiple medications that inhibit colonic motility including opioids, clonidine, and calcium channel antagonists. However, colonic pseudo-obstruction is especially associated with phenothiazines, tricyclic antidepressants, and laxative abuse. Anticholinergic properties of the phenothiazines and tricyclics are felt to predispose to this condition. Phenothiazines also act as calmodulin antagonists (134). The calcium–calmodulin complex is important in smooth muscle contraction, and phenothiazines have been shown to decrease colonic slow wave frequency and amplitude (135). The mechanism of laxative-abuse–related colonic pseudo-obstruction is incompletely understood.

Pancreatic Enzymes and Fibrosing Colonopathy

Approximately 90% of patients with cystic fibrosis depend on pancreatic enzyme supplements to relieve the symptoms of exocrine pancreatic insufficiency (136). Several cases of submucosal fibrosis and stricturing affecting primarily the proximal colon have been described in cystic fibrosis patients taking high-strength pancreatic enzyme supplements. It is possible that the decreased absorptive surface area of the intestines and the high unit dose per kilogram of body weight explains why this complication has only occurred in pediatric patients. Additionally, patients with rapid delivery of enzyme to the cecum combined with colonic stasis may be especially susceptible to damage, as there appears to be an increased incidence of fibrosing colonopathy in patients that are also using laxatives and prokinetic medications. In fact, the only report that has documented fibrosing colonopathy after low-strength pancreatic enzyme use was one that involved a patient ingesting high doses of the enzymes in combination with cisapride (137).

Patients with fibrosing colonopathy present with obstructive symptoms ranging from severe constipation to the development of a meconium ileus equivalent. Surgical intervention is usually required. Proposed mechanisms of fibrosing colonopathy include direct toxicity with digestion of the mucosal surface (138), activation of fibrogenic cytokines and fibrocyte stimulation (139,140), pressure-induced ischemia from excessive intraluminal accumulation of dehydrated lipid-free fecal material (141), enzymes other than lipase in the supplements (140), and damage caused by the enteric coating of these preparations (140,142).

Toxic Epidermal Necrolysis

Toxic epidermal necrolysis (TEN) is the most severe manifestation of the cutaneous condition erythema multiforme. Although the etiology of TEN is unknown, certain drugs play a role in triggering the mechanism. Sulfonamide and penicillin antibiotics, NSAIDs, anticonvulsants, and barbiturates are the most frequently associated inciting agents. TEN affects mucosal surfaces, most commonly the lips, buccal mucosa, tongue, conjunctivae, urethral meatus, vagina, and anus. Colonic involvement is rare, but has been reported (143–145). Patients with colonic TEN present with abdominal pain and bloody diarrhea. Colonoscopy demonstrates diffuse superficial mucosal lesions, friability, and erosions with a predilection for the rectum and sigmoid colon. A lymphocytic inflammatory infiltrate is seen on histological examination of affected tissue. Treatment is supportive and requires discontinuation of the offending agent, fluid replacement, nutritional support, and antibiotics. The role of surgical intervention is not well studied, but in cases of full-thickness involvement or perforation, resection with creation of a proximal stoma has been performed. Patients with TEN and colonic involvement generally have a poor prognosis.

REFERENCES

1. Mielants H, Veys EM, Cuvelier C, De Vos M. Ileocolonoscopic findings in seronegative spondyloarthropathies. Br J Rheumatol 1988; 27(suppl 2):95–105.
2. Mielants H, Veys EM, Cuvelier C, De Vos M, Botelberghe L. HLA-B27 related arthritis and bowel inflammation. Part 2. Ileocolonoscopy and bowel histology in patients with HLA-B27 related arthritis. J Rheumatol 1985; 12:294–298.
3. Cuvelier C, Barbatis C, Mielants H, De Vos M, Roels H, Veys E. Histopathology of intestinal inflammation related to reactive arthritis. Gut 1987; 28:394–401.
4. Holt S, Rigoglioso V, Sidhu M, Irshad M, Howden CW, Mainero M. Nonsteroidal anti-inflammatory drugs and lower gastrointestinal bleeding. Dig Dis Sci 1993; 38:1619–1623.
5. Tanner AR, Raghunath AS. Colonic inflammation and nonsteroidal anti-inflammatory drug administration: an assessment of the frequency of the problem. Digestion 1988; 41:116–120.
6. Langman MJS, Morgan L, Worrall A. Use of anti-inflammatory drugs by patients admitted with small or large bowel perforations and hemorrhage. BMJ 1985; 290:347–349.
7. Reuter BK, Asfaha S, Buret A, Sharkey KA, Wallace JL. Exacerbation of inflammation-associated colonic injury in rat through inhibition of cyclooxygenase-2. J Clin Invest 1996; 98:2076–2085.
8. Wallace JL. Nonsteroidal anti-inflammatory drugs and gastroenteropathy: the second hundred years. Gastroenterology 1997; 112:1000–1016.
9. Kurahara K, Matsumoto T, Iida M, Honda K, Yao Y, Fujishima M. Clinical and endoscopic features of nonsteroidal anti-inflammatory drug-induced colonic ulcerations. Am J Gastroenterol 2001; 96:473–480.
10. Davies NM. Toxicity of nonsteroidal anti-inflammatory drugs in the large intestine. Dis Colon Rectum 1995; 38:1311–1321.
11. Day TK. Intestinal perforation associated with osmotic slow release indomethacin capsules. BMJ 1983; 287:1671–1672.
12. Whitcomb DC, Martin SP, Trellis DR, Evans BA, Becich MJ. Diaphragm-like stricture and ulcer of the colon during diclofenac treatment. Arch Intern Med 1992; 152:2341–2343.

13. Gleeson M, Ramsay D, Hutchinson S, Spencer D, Monteith G. Colitis associated with non-steroidal anti-inflammatory drugs [Lett]. Lancet 1994; 344:1028.
14. Buchman AL, Schwartz MR. Colonic ulceration associated with the systemic use of nonsteroidal anti-inflammatory medication. J Clin Gastroenterol 1996; 22:224–226.
15. Hooker GD, Gregor JC, Ponich TP, McLarty TD. Diaphragm-like strictures of the right colon induced by indomethacin suppositories: evidence of a systemic effect. Gastrointest Endosc 1996; 44:199–202.
16. Monihan JM, Hensley SD, Sobin LH. Nonsteroidal anti-inflammatory drug-induced diaphragm disease arising in a bypassed ileal segment. Am J Gastroenterol 1994; 89:610–612.
17. Bernsdorff KR, Agrawal RM, Brodmerkel GJ Jr. Nonsteroidal anti-inflammatory drugs: gastroduodenal injury and beyond. Dig Dis 1995; 13(4):251–266.
18. Wallace JL, Tigley AW. New insights into prostaglandins and mucosal defence. Aliment Pharmacol Ther 1995; 9:227–235.
19. Madara JL, Moore R, Carlson S. Alteration of intestinal tight junction structure and permeability by cytoskeletal contraction. Am J Physiol 1987; 253:C854–C861.
20. Kauffman G. Aspirin-induced gastric mucosal injury: lessons learned from animal models. Gastroenterology 1989; 96:606–614.
21. Yamagiwa S. Yoshida Y, Halder RC, et al. Mechanisms involved in enteropathy induced by administration of nonsteroidal anti-inflammatory drugs (NSAIDs). Digestive Diseases and Sciences 2001; 46:192–199.
22. Asako H, Kubes P, Wallace J, Wolf RE, Granger DN. Modulation of leukocyte adhesion in rat mesenteric venules by aspirin and salicylate. Gastroenterology 1992; 103:146–152.
23. Wallace JL, Arfors KE, McKnight GW. A monoclonal antibody against the CD18 leukocyte adhesion molecule prevents indomethacin-induced gastric damage in the rabbit. Gastroenterology 1991; 100:878–883.
24. Wallace JL, Keenan CM, Granger DN. Gastric ulceration induced by nonsteroidal anti-inflammatory drugs is a neutrophil-dependent process. Am J Physiol 1990; 259:G462–G467.
25. Puspok A, Kiener HP, Oberhuber G. Clinical, endoscopic, and histologic spectrum of nonsteroidal anti-inflammatory drug-induced lesions in the colon. Dis Colon Rectum 2000; 43(5):685–691.
26. Kaufman HL, Fischer AH, Carroll M, Becker JM. Colonic ulceration associated with nonsteroidal anti-inflammatory drugs. Dis Colon Rectum 1996; 39:705–710.
27. Lee FD. Importance of apoptosis in the histopathology of drug related lesions in the large intestine. J Clin Pathol 1993; 46:118–122.
28. Gargot D, Chaussade S, d'Alteroche L, et al. Nonsteroidal anti-inflammatory drug-induced colonic strictures: two cases and literature review. Am J Gastroenterol 1995; 90(11):2035–2038.
29. Haque S, Haswell JE, Dreznick JT, West AB. A cecal diaphragm associated with the use of nonsteroidal anti-inflammatory drugs. J Clin Gastroenterol 1992; 15:332–335.
30. Monahan DW, Starnes EC, Parker AL. Colonic strictures in a patient on long-term non-steroidal anti-inflammatory drugs. Gastrointest Endosc 1992; 38:385–388.
31. Karmeli F, Cohen P, Rachmilewitz D. Cyclo-oxygenase-2 inhibitors ameliorate the severity of experimental colitis in rats. Eur J Gastroenterol Hepatol 2000; 12:223–231.
32. Lesch CA, Kraus ER, Sanchez B, Gilbertsen R, Guglietta A. Lack of beneficial effect of COX-2 inhibitors in an experimental model of colitis. Meth Findings Exp Clin Pharmacol 1999; 21:99–104.
33. Mahadevan U, Loftus EV, Tremaine WJ, Sandborn WJ. Safety of selective cyclooxygenase-2 inhibitors in inflammatory bowel disease. Am J Gastroenterol 2002; 97:910–914.
34. Garcia B, Ramaholimihaso F, Diebold MD, Cadiot G, Thiefin G. Ischaemic colitis in a patient taking meloxicam. Lancet 2001; 357:690.
35. Freitas J, Farricha V, Nascimento I, Borralho P, Parames A. Rofecoxib: a possible cause of acute colitis. J Clin Gastroenterol 2002; 34:451–453.
36. Evans JMM, McMahon AD, Murray FE, McDevitt DG, MacDonald TM. Nonsteroidal anti-inflammatory drugs are associated with emergency admission to hospital for colitis due to inflammatory bowel disease. Gut 1997; 40:619–622.
37. Gibson GR, Whitacre EB, Ricotti CA. Colitis induced by nonsteroidal anti-inflammatory drugs: report of four cases and review of the literature. Arch Intern Med 1992; 152:625–632.
38. Singer II, Kawka DW, Schloemann S, Tessner T, Riehl T, Stenson WF. Cyclooxygenase 2 is induced in colonic epithelial cells in inflammatory bowel disease. Gastroenterology 1998; 115:297–306.
39. Morteau O, Morham SG, Sellon R, et al. Impaired mucosal defense to acute colonic injury in mice lacking cyclooxygenase-1 or cyclooxygenase-2. J Clin Invest 2000; 105:469–478.
40. Campbell K, Steele RJC. Non-steroidal anti-inflammatory drugs and complicated diverticular disease: a case-control study. Br J Surg 1991; 78:190–191.
41. Goh H, Bourne R. Non-steroidal anti-inflammatory drugs and perforated diverticular disease: a case-control study. Ann R Coll Surg Engl 2002; 84:93–96.
42. Fenton JJ, Cicale MJ. Sigmoid diverticular perforation complicating lung transplantation. J Heart Lung Transplant 1997; 16:681–685.
43. Weiner HL, Rezai AR, Cooper PR. Sigmoid diverticular perforation in neurosurgical patients receiving high-dose corticosteroids. Neurosurgery 1993; 33:40–43.
44. Tyau ES, Prystowsky JB, Joehl RJ, Nahrwold DL. Acute diverticulitis: a complicated problem in the immunocompromised patient. Arch Surg 1991; 126:855–859.

45. Corder A. Steroids, nonsteroidal anti-inflammatory drugs, and serious septic complications of diverticular disease. BMJ 1987; 295:1238.

46. Slavin RE, Dias MA, Saral R. Cytosine arabinoside induced gastrointestinal toxic alterations in sequential chemotherapeutic protocols. Cancer 1978; 42:1747–1759.

47. Milles SS, Muggia AL, Spiro HM. Colonic histologic changes induced by 5-fluorouracil. Gastroenterology 1962; 43:391–399.

48. Mitchell EP, Schein PS. Gastrointestinal toxicity of chemotherapeutic agents. Semin Oncol 1982; 9:52–64.

49. Jackson CW, Haboubi NY, Whorwell PJ, Schofield PF. Gold induced enterocolitis. Gut 1986; 27:452–456.

50. Wright A, Benfield GFA, Felix-Davies D. Ischaemic colitis and immune complexes during gold therapy for rheumatoid arthritis. Ann Rheumatic Dis 1984; 43:495–497.

51. Martin DM, Goldman JA, Gilliam J, Nasrallah SM. Gold-induced eosinophilic enterocolitis: response to oral cromolyn sodium. Gastroenterology 1981; 80:1567–1570.

52. Edelman J, Davies P, Owen ET. Prevalence of eosinophilia during gold therapy for rheumatoid arthritis. J Rheumatol 1983; 10:121–123.

53. Moulis H, Vender RJ. Antibiotic-associated hemorrhagic colitis. J Clin Gastroenterol 1994; 18:227–231.

54. Koga H, Aoyagi K, Yoshimura R, Kimura Y, Iida M, Fujishima M. Can quinolones cause hemorrhagic colitis of late onset? Dis Colon Rectum 1999; 42:1502–1504.

55. Iida M, Matsui T, Fuchigami T, Iwashita A, Omae T. Radiographic and endoscopic findings in penicillin-related non-pseudomembranous colitis. Endoscopy 1985; 17:64–68.

56. Binder HJ, Dobbins JW, Whiting DS. Evidence against importance of altered mucosal permeability in ricinoleic acid induced fluid secretion [Abstr]. Gastroenterology 1977; 72:1029A–6.

57. Chawla A, Karl PI, Reich RN, et al. Effect of olsalazine on sodium-dependent bile acid transport in rat ileum. Dig Dis Sci 1995; 40:943–948..

58. Bergogne-Berezin E. Treatment and prevention of antibiotic associated diarrhea. Int J Antimicrobial Agents 2000; 16:521–526.

59. Bartlett JG. Antibiotic-associated diarrhea. Clin Infect Dis 1992; 15:573–581.

60. Kelly CP, Pothoulakis C, LaMont JT. *Clostridium difficile* colitis. N Engl J Med 1994; 330:257–262.

61. Clausen MR, Bonnen H, Tvede M, Mortensen PB. Colonic fermentation to short-chain fatty acids is decreased in antibiotic-associated diarrhea. Gastroenterology 1991; 101:1497–1504.

62. Ruppin H, Bar-Meir S, Soergel KH, Wood CM, Schmitt MG. Absorption of short-chain fatty acids by the colon. Gastroenterology 1980; 78:1500–1507.

63. Roediger WEW. Role of anaerobic bacteria in the metabolic welfare of the colonic mucosa in man. Gut 1980; 21:793–798.

64. Roediger WEW. The colonic epithelium in ulcerative colitis: an energy-deficiency disease? Lancet 1980; 2:712–715.

65. Harig JM, Soergel KH, Komorowski RA, Wood CM. Treatment of diversion colitis with short-chain fatty acid irrigation. N Engl J Med 1989; 320:23–28.

66. Hogenauer C, Hammer HF, Krejs GJ, Reisinger EC. Mechanisms and management of antibiotic-associated diarrhea. Clin Infect Dis 1998; 27:702–710.

67. Hofmann AF. Bile acids, diarrhea, and antibiotics: data, speculation, and a unifying hypothesis. J Infect Dis 1977; 135(suppl):S126–S132.

68. McJunkin B, Fromm H, Sarva RP, Amin P. Factors in the mechanism of diarrhea in bile acid malabsorption: fecal pH—a key determinant. Gastroenterology 1981; 80:1454–1464.

69. Schiller LR. Cathartics, laxatives, and lavage solutions. In: Friedman et al., eds. Gastrointestinal Pharmacology and Therapeutics. Philadelphia: Lipincott-Raven Publishers, 1997:159–174.

70. Smith B. Effect of irritant purgatives on the myenteric plexus in man and the mouse. Gut 1968; 9:139–143.

71. Riemann JF, Schmidt H. Ultrastructural changes in the gut autonomic nervous system following laxative abuse and in other conditions. Scand J Gastroenterol 1982; 71(suppl):111–124.

72. Balazs M. Melanosis coli: ultrastructural study of 45 patients. Dis Colon Rectum 1986; 29:839–844.

73. Riemann JF, Schenk J, Ehler R, Schmidt H, Koch H. Ultrastructural changes of colonic mucosa in patients with chronic laxative misuse. Acta Hepato-Gastroenterol 1978; 25:213–218.

74. Dufour P, Gendre P. Ultrastructure of mouse intestinal mucosa and changes observed after long term anthraquinone administration. Gut 1984; 25:1358–1363.

75. Ghadially FN, Parry EW. An electron-microscope and histochemical study of melanosis coli. J Path Bact 1966; 92:313–317.

76. Riecken EO, Zeitz M, Emde C, et al. The effect of an anthraquinone laxative on colonic nerve tissue: a controlled trial in constipated women. Z Gastroenterol 1990; 28:660–664.

77. Krishnamurthy S, Schuffler MD, Rohrmann CA, Pope CE. Severe idiopathic constipation is associated with a distinctive abnormality of the colonic myenteric plexus. Gastroenterology 1985; 88:26–34.

78. Blumberg D, Wald A. Other diseases of the colon and rectum. In: Feldman M, Friedman LS, Sleisenger MH, eds. 7th ed. Gastrointestinal and Liver Disease. SAUNDERS, Philadelphia, Pennsylvania USA 2002.

79. Bockus HL, Williard JH, Bank J. Melanosis coli. The etiologic significance of the anthracene laxatives: a report of forty-one cases. JAMA 1933; 101:1–6.

80. Walker NI, Bennett RE, Axelsen RA. Melanosis coli: a consequence of anthraquinone-induced apoptosis of colonic epithelial cells. Am J Pathol 1988; 131:465–476.

81. Krbavcic A, Pecar S, Schara M, Muller K, Wiegrebe W. Anthranoid free radicals found in *Pseudomelanosis coli*. Pharmazie 1998; 53:336–338.
82. Benavides SH, Morgante PE, Monserrat AJ, Zarate J, Porta EA. The pigment of melanosis coli: a lectin histochemical study. Gastrointest Endosc 1997; 46:131–138.
83. Koskela E, Kulju T, Collan Y. Melanosis coli: prevalence, distribution, and histologic features in 200 consecutive autopsies at Kuopio University Central Hospital. Dis Colon Rectum 1989; 32:235–239.
84. Speare GS. Melanosis coli: experimental observations on its production and elimination in twenty-three cases. Am J Surg 1951; 82:631–637.
85. Siegers CP, von Hertzberg-Lottin E, Otte M, Schneider B. Anthranoid laxative abuse—a risk for colorectal cancer?. Gut 1993; 34:1099–1101.
86. Nusko G, Schneider B, Schneider I, Wittekind C, Hahn EG. Anthranoid laxative use is not a risk factor for colorectal neoplasia: results of a prospective case control study. Gut 2000; 46:651–655.
87. Joo JS, Ehrenpreis ED, Gonzalez L, et al. Alterations in colonic anatomy induced by chronic stimulant laxatives: the cathartic colon revisited. J Clin Gastroenterol 1998; 26(4):283–286.
88. Campbell WL. Cathartic colon: reversibility of roentgen changes. Dis Colon Rectum 1983; 26:445–448.
89. Muller-Lissner S. What has happened to the cathartic colon? Gut 1996; 39:486–488.
90. Tikkanen L, Matsushima T, Natori S. Mutagenicity of anthraquinones in the Salmonella preincubation test. Mutat Res 1983; 116:297–304.
91. Brown JP, Brown RJ. Mutagenesis by 9,10 anthraquinone derivatives and related compounds in *Salmonella typhimurium*. Mutat Res 1976; 40:203–224.
92. Venturini S, Tamaro M. Mutagenicity of anthraquinone and azo dyes in Ames' *Salmonella typhimurium* test. Mutat Res 1979; 68:307–312.
93. Krivobok S, Seigle-Murandi F, Steiman R, Marzin DR, Betina V. Mutagenicity of substituted anthraquinones in the Ames/Salmonella microsome system. Mutat Res 1992; 279:1–8.
94. Heidemann A, Volkner W, Mengs U. Genotoxity of aloeemodin in vitro and in vivo. Mutat Res 1996; 367:123–133.
95. Sandnes D, Johansen T, Teien G, Ulsaker G. Mutagenicity of crude senna and senna glycosides in *Salmonella typhimurium*. Pharmacol Toxicol 1992; 71:165–172.
96. Muller SO, Eckert I, Lutz WK, Stopper H. Genotoxicity of the laxative drug components emodin, aloe-emodin and danthron in mammalian cells: topoisomerase II mediated? Mutat Res 1996; 371:165–173.
97. Schorkhuber M, Richter M, Dutter A, Sontag G, Marian B. Effect of anthraquinone-laxatives on the proliferation and urokinase secretion of normal, premalignant and malignant colonic epithelial cells. Eur J Cancer 1998; 34:1091–1098.
98. Dunnick JK, Hailey JR. Phenolphthalein exposure causes multiple carcinogenic effects in experimental model systems. Cancer Res 1996; 56:4922–4926.
99. Dunnick JK, Hardisty JF, Herbert RA, et al. Phenolphthalein induces thymic lymphomas accompanied by loss of the p53 wild type allele in heterozygous p53 deficient ($+/-$) mice. Toxicol Pathol 1997; 25:533–540.
100. Mereto E, Ghia M, Brambilla G. Evaluation of the potential carcinogenic activity of Senna and Cascara glycosides for the rat colon. Cancer Lett 1996; 101:79–83.
101. Mascolo N, Mereto E, Borrelli F, et al. Does senna extract promote growth of aberrant crypt foci and malignant tumors in rat colon? Dig Dis Sci 1999; 44:2226–2230.
102. Kleibeuker JH, Cats A, Zwart N, Mulder NH, Hardonk MJ, de Vries EGE. Excessively high cell proliferation in sigmoid colon after an oral purge with anthraquinone glycosides. J Natl Cancer Inst 1995; 87:452–453.
103. Van Gorkom BAP, Karrenbeld A, van Der Sluis T, Koudstaal J, de Vries EGE, Kleibeuker JH. Influence of a highly purified senna extract on colonic epithelium. Digestion 2000; 61:113–120.
104. Jacobs EJ, White E. Constipation, laxative use, and colon cancer among middle-aged adults. Epidemiology 1998; 9:385–391.
105. Sonnenberg A, Muller AD. Constipation and cathartics as risk factors of colorectal cancer: a meta-analysis. Pharmacology 1993; 47(suppl 1):224–233.
106. Kune GA. Laxative use not a risk for colorectal cancer: data from the Melbourne colorectal cancer study. Z Gastroenterol 1993; 31:140–143.
107. Longnecker MP, Sandler DP, Haile RW, Sandler RS. Phenolphthalein-containing laxative use in relation to adenomatous colorectal polyps in three studies. Environ Health Perspect 1997; 105:1210–1212.
108. Dukas L, Willet WC, Colditz GA, Fuchs CS, Rosner B, Giovannucci EL. Prospective study of bowel movement, laxative use, and risk of colorectal cancer among women. Am J Epidemiol 2000; 151:958–964.
109. Fleischer N, Brown H, Graham DY, Delena S. Chronic laxative-induced hyperaldosteronism and hypokalemia simulating Bartter's syndrome. Ann Intern Med 1969; 70:791–798.
110. Nataf C, Desmazures C, Giraudeaux V, Bernier JJ. Laxative-induced intestinal protein loss in normal subjects. Gastroenterol Clin Biol 1981; 5:187–192.
111. Pahor M, Guralnik JM, Chrischilles EA, Wallace RB. Use of laxative medication in older persons and associations with low serum albumin. J Am Geriatr Soc 1994; 42:50–56.

112. Elliot D, Glover GR. Large bowel perforation due to excessive bran ingestion. Br J Clin Pract 1983; 37:32–33.
113. Souter WA. Bolus obstruction of gut after use of hydrophilic colloid laxatives. BMJ 1965; 1:166–168.
114. Suhonen R, Kantola I, Bjorksten F. Anaphylactic shock due to ingestion of psyllium laxative. Allergy 1983; 38:363–365.
115. Yuan CS, Foss JF, O'connor M, Osinski J, Roizen MF, Moss J. Effects of intravenous methylnaltrexone on opioid-induced gut motility and transit time changes in subjects receiving chronic methadone therapy: a pilot study. Pain 1999; 83:631–635.
116. Yuan CS, Foss JF, Osinski J, Toledano A, Roizen MF, Moss J. The safety and efficacy of oral methyl-naltrexone in preventing morphine-induced delay in oral-cecal transit time. Clin Pharmacol Ther 1997; 61:467–475.
117. Meissner W, Schmidt U, Hartmann M, Kath R, Reinhart K. Oral naloxone reverses opioid-associated constipation. Pain 2000; 84:105–109.
118. Snape WJ. Effect of calcium on neurohumoral stimulation of feline colonic smooth muscle. Am J Physiol 1982; 243:G134–G140.
119. Anuras S. cAMP and calcium in generation of slow waves in cat colon. Am J Physiol 1982; 5:G124–G127.
120. Lecchini S, Marcoli M, De Ponti F, Castelletti CA, Frigo GM. Selectivity of Ca^{2+} channel blockers in inhibiting muscular and nerve activities in isolated colon. Br J Pharmacol 1991; 102:735–741.
121. Janis RA, Triggle DJ. New developments in Ca^{2+} channel antagonists. J Med Chem 1983; 26:775–785.
122. Janis RA, Triggle DJ. 1,4-Dihydropyridine Ca^{2+} channel antagonists and activators: a comparison of binding characteristics with pharmacology. Drug Dev Res 1984; 4:257–274.
123. Schwartz A, Triggle DJ. Cellular action of calcium channel blocking drugs. Ann Rev Med 1984; 35: 325–339.
124. Cass AJ. Stercoral perforation: case of drug-induced impaction. Br Med J 1978; ii:932–933.
125. Aguilo JJ, Zincke H, Woods JE, Buckingham JM. Intestinal perforation due to fecal impaction after renal transplantation. J Urol 1977; 116:153–155.
126. Haley TD, Long C, Mann BD. Stercoral perforation of the colon: a complication of methadone main-tenance. J Substance Abuse Treatment 1998; 15:443–444.
127. Stringer MD, Greenfield S, McIrvine AJ. Stercoral perforation of the colon following postoperative analgesia. J Roy Soc Med 1987; 80:115–116.
128. Hollingworth J, Alexander-Williams J. Non-steroidal anti-inflammatory drugs and stercoral perfor-ation of the colon. Ann Roy Coll Surg Engl 1991; 73:337–340.
129. Taylor JR, Streetman DS, Castle SS. Medication bezoars: a literature review and report of a case. Ann Pharmacother 1998; 32:940–946.
130. Reid T, Rubins JB, Levine J, DeCelles J, Silvis S. Colonic medication bezoar from extended-release nifedipine and procainamide. Arch Fam Med 1995; 4:715–717.
131. Hunt-Fugate AK, Schmidt HJ. Cecal vitamin bezoar formation inducing abdominal discomfort. Ann Pharmacother 1992; 26:485–487.
132. Cohen MI, Winslow PR, Boley SJ. Intestinal obstruction associated with cholestyramine therapy. N Engl J Med 1969; 280:1285–1286.
133. Agha FP, Nostrant TT, Fiddian-Green RG. "Giant colonic bezoar": a medication bezoar due to psyllium seed husks. Am J Gastroenterol 1984; 79:319–321.
134. Cheung WY. Calmodulin plays a pivotal role in cellular regulation. Science 1980; 207:19–27.
135. Anuras S. Role of calmodulin in slow wave generation of cat colon. Clin Res 1981; 29:758A.
136. FitzSimmons SC. The changing epidemiology of cystic fibrosis. J Pediatr 1993; 122:1–9.
137. Jones R, Franklin K, Spicer R, Berry J. Colonic strictures in children with cystic fibrosis on low-strength pancreatic enzymes. Lancet 1995; 346:499.
138. Oades PJ, Bush A, Ong PS, Brereton RJ. High-strength pancreatic enzyme supplements and large-bowel stricture in cystic fibrosis. Lancet 1994; 343:109.
139. Knabe N, Zak M, Hansen A, et al. Extensive pathological changes of the colon in cystic fibrosis and high-strength pancreatic enzymes. Lancet 1994; 343:1230.
140. Lloyd-Still JD. Cystic fibrosis and colonic strictures: a new "iatrogenic" disease. J Clin Gastroenterol 1995; 21:2–5.
141. Smyth RL, van Velzen D, Smyth AR, Lloyd DA, Heaf DP. Strictures of ascending colon in cystic fibrosis and high-strength pancreatic enzymes. Lancet 1994; 343:85–86.
142. van Velzen D. Colonic strictures in children with cystic fibrosis on low-strength pancreatic enzymes. Lancet 1995; 346:499–500.
143. Carter FM, Mitchell CK. Toxic epidermal necrolysis—an unusual cause of colonic perforation. Dis Colon Rectum 1993; 36:773–777.
144. Zweiban B, Cohen H, Chandrasoma P. Gastrointestinal involvement complicating Stevens-Johnson syndrome. Gastroenterology 1986; 91:469–474.
145. Chosidow O, Delchier JC, Chaumette MT, et al. Intestinal involvement in drug-induced toxic epidermal necrolysis. Lancet 1991; 337:928.

Index